INTEGRATIVE MEDICINE
for CHILDREN

INTEGRATIVE MEDICINE
for CHILDREN

May Loo, MD

Assistant Clinical Professor, Department of Pediatrics and
Department of Pediatric Anesthesiology, Stanford Medical
Center, Palo Alto, California

Director, Neurodevelopmental Program, Department
of Pediatrics, Santa Clara County Valley Medical Center,
San Jose, California

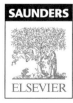

SAUNDERS

ELSEVIER

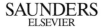

SAUNDERS
ELSEVIER

11830 Westline Industrial Drive
St. Louis, Missouri 63146

INTEGRATIVE MEDICINE FOR CHILDREN   ISBN: 978-1-4160-2299-2
Copyright © 2009 by Saunders, an imprint of Elsevier Inc.

Notice

Knowledge and best practice in this field are constantly changing. As new research and experience broaden our knowledge, changes in practice, treatment and drug therapy may become necessary or appropriate. Readers are advised to check the most current information provided (i) on procedures featured or (ii) by the manufacturer of each product to be administered, to verify the recommended dose or formula, the method and duration of administration, and contraindications. It is the responsibility of the practitioner, relying on their own experience and knowledge of the patient, to make diagnoses, to determine dosages and the best treatment for each individual patient, and to take all appropriate safety precautions. To the fullest extent of the law, neither the Publisher nor the Editors assume any liability for any injury and/or damage to persons or property arising out of or related to any use of the material contained in this book.

The Publisher

Library of Congress Cataloging-in-Publication Data
Integrative medicine for children / [edited by] May Loo.
     p. ; cm.
  Includes bibliographical references and index.
  ISBN 978-1-4160-2299-2 (hardcover : alk. paper) 1.
Children--Diseases--Alternative treatment. 2. Integrative medicine.
I. Loo, May, 1946-
  [DNLM: 1. Complementary Therapies--methods. 2. Adolescent. 3.
Child. 4. Infant. WB 890 I6084 2009]
  RJ53.A48I58 2009
  618.92--dc22
                       2008020998

Vice President and Publisher: Linda Duncan
Senior Editor: Kellie White
Senior Developmental Editor: Jennifer Watrous
Editorial Assistant: April Falast
Publishing Services Manager: Patricia Tannian
Project Manager: Jonathan M. Taylor
Designer: Amy Buxton

Printed in the United States of America

Last digit is the print number: 9 8 7 6 5 4 3 2 1

This book is dedicated to all the healthcare professionals who wish to broaden their knowledge for the well-being of children, to all the loving parents who seek safe and comprehensive care for their children, and especially to all children throughout the world who deserve to live healthy and happy lives.

✳ Contributors

Matthew I. Baral, ND
Naturopathic Physician
Assistant Professor, Pediatrics
Southwest College of Naturopathic Medicine
Tempe, Arizona

Jane Carreiro, DO
Associate Professor and Chair
Department of Osteopathic Manipulative Medicine
College of Osteopathic Medicine
University of New England
Biddeford, Maine

Maria Choy, MD, FAAN
Attending Physician, Neurology
CentraState Medical Center,
    Affiliate of Rutgers University
Freehold, New Jersey
Attending Physician, Neurology
Bayshore Community Hospital
Holmdel, New Jersey
Vice President
New Jersey Chapter of the American Academy
    of Medical Acupuncture
Morganville, New Jersey

Effie Poy Yew Chow, PhD, RN, LicAc(CA),
DiplAc(NCCAOM), Qigong Grandmaster
Founder and President
East West Academy of Healing Arts
San Francisco, California

Agatha P. Colbert, MD
Senior Investigator
Helfgott Research Institute
National College of Natural Medicine
Clinical Research Assistant Professor
Family Medicine
Oregon Health and Science University
Portland, Oregon

Stephen Cowan MD, FAAP
Clinical Instructor
Department of Pediatrics
New York Medical College
Valhalla, New York
Founder
The Holistic Developmental Center for Children
Mt. Kisco, New York
Cofounder
Riverside Pediatrics
Croton, New York

Timothy Culbert, MD
Medical Director, Integrative Medicine Program
Children's Hospitals and Clinics of Minnesota
Minneapolis, Minnesota

Lana Dvorkin-Camiel, PharmD
Associate Professor of Pharmacy Practice Director
Applied Natural Products Programs Natural
    Products Division
Coordinator
Center for Drug Information and Natural Products
    Massachusetts College of Pharmacy and Health Sciences
Boston, Massachusetts

Lynda Richtsmeier Cyr, PhD, LP
Program Lead, Pediatric Psychologist
Integrative Medicine
Children's Hospitals and Clinics of Minnesota
Clinical Instructor
Behavioral Pediatrics Program
Department of Pediatrics
University of Minnesota
Minneapolis, Minnesota

Maura A. Fitzgerald, RN, MS, MA, PCNS-BC
Clinical Nurse Specialist
Integrative Medicine Program
Children's Hospitals and Clinics
Minneapolis, Minnesota

Paula M. Gardiner, MD, MPH
Assistant Professor
Department of Family Medicine
Boston University Medical Center
Boston, Massachusetts

Russell H. Greenfield, MD
Director
Greenfield Integrative Healthcare
Charlotte, North Carolina
Clinical Assistant Professor
University of North Carolina–Chapel Hill School of Medicine
Chapel Hill, North Carolina
Visiting Assistant Professor
The University of Arizona College of Medicine
Tucson, Arizona

Tobin Hart, PhD
Professor
Department of Psychology
University of West Georgia
Carrollton, Georgia

Janet L. Levatin, MD
Clinical Instructor
Department of Pediatrics
Harvard Medical School
Boston, Massachusetts
Private Practice
Brookline, Massachusetts

Gerhard Litscher, MSc, PhD, MDsc
Professor
Research Unit of Biomedical Engineering in Anesthesia and
    Intensive Care Medicine and TCM Research Center Graz
Medical University of Graz
Graz, Austria

Jack Maypole, MD
Director of Pediatrics
South End Community Health Center
Boston, Massachusetts
Assistant Professor of Pediatrics
Boston Medical Center
Boston University School of Medicine
Boston, Massachusetts

Mary C. McLellan, BSN, RN, CMT, CPN
Massage Therapy Director
Integrative Therapies Team
Staff Nurse III, Education Coordinator
Inpatient Cardiology
Cardiovascular Program
Children's Hospital
Boston, Massachusetts

Randall Neustaedter, OMD, LAc, CCH
Classical Medicine Center
Redwood City, California

Karen Olness, MD, FAAP
Professor of Pediatrics
Family Medicine and Global Health
Case Western Reserve University
Cleveland, Ohio

David Rindge, DOM, LAc, RN
Center for Cooperative Medicine, PA
Healing Light Seminars, Inc.
Melbourne, Florida

Deborah Risotti, RN
Private Consultation
Pediatric Medical Education and Advocacy
North Reading, Massachusetts

Detlef Schikora, DR.sc.nat.
Faculty of Science
Institut for Biophotonics
University of Paderborn
Paderborn, Germany

Anne Spicer, DC, DACCP
Associate Professor, Clinical Mentor
Bloomington Natural Care Center
Northwestern Health Sciences University
Bloomington, Minnesota

Anna Tobia, PhD
Psychologist
Jefferson Myrna-Brind Center for Integrative Medicine
Thomas Jefferson University Hospital
Philadelphia, Pennsylvania

Catherine Ulbricht, PharmD
Founder
Natural Standard Research Collaboration
Cambridge, Massachusetts
Senior Attending Pharmacist
Massachusetts General Hospital
Boston, Massachusetts

Jennifer Woods, BS
Editorial Assistant
Natural Standard Research Collaboration
Cambridge, Massachusetts

Alan D. Woolf, MD, MPH
Associate Professor
Pediatrics
Harvard Medical School
Boston, Massachusetts
Director, Pediatric Environmental Health Center
General Pediatrics
Children's Hospital
Boston, Massachusetts

Joy A. Weydert, MD, FAAP
Integrative Medicine and Pain Management
Department of Pediatrics
Children's Mercy Hospital
Assistant Professor
University of Missouri–Kansas City School of Medicine
Kansas City, Missouri

Mark Wright
Contributing Author
Natural Standard Research Collaboration
Cambridge, Massachusetts

Chinese Herb Consultants

Harriet Beinfield, LAc
San Francisco, California

Jake Paul Fratkin, OMD, LAc
Boulder, Colorado

Efrem Korngold, OMD, LAc
San Francisco, California

✳ Preface

A powerful reference tool for pediatricians and complementary and alternative medicine (CAM) practitioners, *Integrative Medicine for Children* accumulates the best practices of experts in the field, offering conventional medical treatment blended with appropriate CAM therapies. Parents can also use this versatile guide for practical recommendations on using CAM therapies for specific childhood conditions.

Conceptual Approach

Following the success of *Pediatric Acupuncture* (Churchill Livingstone, 2002), a reference integrating Western medicine with acupuncture, *Integrative Medicine for Children* answers the call for a manual that addresses the broader scope of CAM therapies in relation to conventional treatments. As more practitioners and parents look to CAM to treat pediatric conditions, the need for an authoritative reference encompassing both conventional Western medicine and major CAM therapies is evident.

Organization

The first section of *Integrative Medicine for Children* presents the history, theory, current evidence-based information, applications, and contraindications on various CAM therapies.

The second section serves as a focused reference for 55 chronic and acute pediatric conditions, featuring:

- Conventional medical diagnosis and treatment
- Appropriate CAM therapies, including condition-specific, evidence-based information
- Treatment recommendations based on clinical experience
- Contraindications and potential adverse effects

As CAM therapies become more acceptable in mainstream medicine, *Integrative Medicine for Children* can be used as a textbook to provide a wider breadth of training for future practitioners.

Why Is This Book Important to Healthcare Professionals?

Current trends favor enhanced cooperation among various healthcare professionals and the integration of CAM therapies into conventional medical treatments. However, the reality is that it is difficult for any one conventional or CAM practitioner to comprehensively learn the nuances of other disciplines. Providers now can turn to this book for a single, concise volume covering the basics of major CAM fields and applicable modalities.

The significance of this unique, encyclopedic, and integrative reference book is evident as pediatricians and parents seek more collaborative treatment plans for children, especially difficult conditions that are not responsive to one particular type of treatment. *Integrative Medicine for Children* will hopefully lead to increased communication among practitioners.

Integrative Medicine for Children is based on the cooperative and diligent efforts of more than 30 expert contributors, who provide erudite information and share their personal, clinical experiences for the enhancement of healthcare for children.

May Loo, MD

June 2008

✳ Acknowledgments

With thanks to all the contributors and their assistants whose expertise, hard work, and thoughtfulness have made this book possible. Thanks to the Elsevier staff: Kellie White, Jennifer Watrous, and Jonathan Taylor, whose patience, persistence, and encouragement were invaluable for carrying this task to completion.

Thanks also to my family, Bill, Alyssa, and Alexandra, for their love and support through the innumerable, long, and arduous hours.

✳ Contents

CHAPTER 1

Introduction

Book Organization | May Loo

Integrative Medicine for Children is intended as a reference book that provides pediatricians with evidence-based information on complementary and alternative medicines (CAM) and practical CAM treatment recommendations from prominent CAM practitioners. At the same time, it provides CAM practitioners with information on conventional pediatric diagnoses and management. It is hoped that this book will promote communication among pediatric disciplines so that various modalities can be integrated to provide comprehensive, safe, and effective treatments for children.

The National Center for Complementary and Alternative Medicine (NCCAM) at the National Institutes of Health defines CAM as "those treatments and health care practices not taught widely in medical schools, not generally used in hospitals, and not usually reimbursed by medical insurance companies" and further indicates that "some approaches are consistent with physiologic principles of Western medicine, while others constitute healing systems with a different origin... [some] are becoming established in mainstream medicine."[1]

In recent years the use of CAM has exploded,[2,3] with adult usage as high as 62%[4,5] and pediatric usage ranging from estimates of 10% to 15% to as high as 40%.[6-16]

The escalation in pediatric CAM is global and is most prevalent in the Western world, especially in the United States, Canada, Australia, and Western Europe.[6,17-23] Usually children who see CAM practitioners have educated parents who also use CAM.[8,14,16,21,24-26]

Pediatric CAM is being used to treat a wide variety of acute and chronic physical and emotional conditions. The acute conditions can be common, routine outpatient problems,[14,16,24,27-29] such as gastrointestinal complaints,[22,30] skin disorders,[20,22] and musculoskeletal complaints.[8] As many as 50% to 70% of the parents of children with chronic, recurrent, or incurable conditions seek CAM.[11,15,31-34] The most common chronic conditions are asthma, arthritis, cystic fibrosis, cancer, inflammatory bowel disease (IBD), and cerebral palsy.[17,19,26,28,36-40] Parents may seek CAM even when their children are in tertiary children's hospitals.[29,41] CAM therapy is also increasingly used for psychoemotional and behavioral pediatric disorders.[22] For example, studies indicate that as many as 50% of children with autism in the United States may be using CAM therapies.[42,43]

Although some families incorporate CAM into their biomedical regimen, other families completely substitute CAM for conventional care of their children.[44] Five of the most common CAM modalities for children are homeopathy, naturopathy, acupuncture, chiropractic, and massage.[45] The motivation to seek CAM is so strong that patients are willing to pay billions of dollars out of pocket.[2-4,8,18,46]

Parents give numerous reasons for seeking CAM for their children: dissatisfaction with allopathic medicine*; concern about side effects[18,40]; desire for a more holistic, more natural, and safer form of healing[6,25,28,40]; parental satisfaction with self-use of CAM[8,26]; and a belief that CAM works[25,28] and is more compatible with their personal beliefs about health.[25] In addition, parents of children with chronic conditions often express the frustration that their children are unresponsive to conventional therapy[6]; that biomedicine has little or nothing to offer[28,43]; that the conventional treatments are complex, uncomfortable, too technological, and unnatural[43]; or that they are not sufficiently involved in the planning and management of their child's care.[17] Some parents even view hospitals as dangerous places.[47]

CAM offers these parents a sense of control and autonomy over their child's chronic illness or disability and in improving quality of life.[6,40,43] Children also appear to readily accept CAM therapies and report positively on their experiences.[13,21,49-51]

The abundance of resources—the media, the Internet, condition-specific publications, parent groups, health food stores, and even family members and friends who have used CAM—has contributed to the swaying of parents toward CAM.[6,19,25,43] Even the American Academy of Pediatrics (AAP) recognizes failure of biomedicine as the reason for parents to turn to CAM.[43]

Although the majority of pediatric CAM is used in conjunction with conventional therapies,[5,19] parents have been reluctant to discuss CAM treatments with pediatricians.† Reasons for this hesitancy include fear of ridicule and the belief that the pediatrician has little information about CAM practices. A U.S. survey of 348 pediatricians revealed a marked discrepancy between the pediatricians' perceptions of use and actual CAM use by children.[53] As pediatric CAM treatments become more accepted and as pediatricians become less judgmental and more knowledgeable about CAM, parents will be

---

*References 18, 25, 28, 40, 43, 47, 48.

†References 2, 3, 5, 14, 16, 29, 45, 52.

more comfortable discussing CAM therapy with their child's physician.[24,27,28,43,53]

Pediatricians, like most of the conventional medical community, have traditionally regarded CAM as being unscientific and supported mainly by anecdotal evidence. The AAP criticizes CAM because of the paucity of randomized, controlled, double-blinded clinical trials to prove its safety and efficacy in children.[43,45] However, it is important to realize that the lack of data does not signify a lack of CAM efficacy, but rather is a reflection of multiple difficulties in applying strict scientific research standards and evidence-based practice guidelines to CAM disciplines. Recognizing this problem in funding research, NCCAM issued a statement that "CAM has divergent belief systems and theories about health and illness, focuses on individualized care, and has varied measures of effectiveness."[54] The placebo response in CAM is strong and ever present, as it is generated simply by the close, more "hands-on" relationship between the practitioner and the patient.[55] Gradually, scientifically acceptable data in children are emerging, such as the use of acupuncture to treat pain,[13] massage therapy to lower anxiety and stress hormones,[57] herbs to treat colic,[58] and homeopathic remedies to reduce the duration of acute childhood diarrhea.[32] Currently, the NCCAM has a budget of more than $122 million to promote sound research in CAM. The AAP predicts that, in time, proven CAM therapies may come into wider use and lose their "alternative" status.[43]

Parental demand for CAM, their willingness to pay out of pocket, and the increasing scientific data are all factors that are changing the role of the pediatrician and are fueling physicians' interest in and positive attitudes toward CAM.[7,58] The pediatrician now must ask about CAM use in their patients,[7,16,29,37] be better informed about and provide parents with information on available CAM treatments,[37,43,59] consider nontraditional therapies when treating patients,[43] and be aware of the potential adverse effects of CAM or possible interactions with conventional management.[29,37,45] All of these are now incorporated into the AAP policy recommendations for pediatricians.[43,45] Because biomedicine expertise does not adequately prepare pediatricians to discuss CAM, the dire need to educate the physicians coincides with rising physician interest in learning about CAM.[7,43,58-62] Physicians themselves have turned to CAM use personally and are making referrals for CAM treatments.[4,53,58]

The increasing physician interest in CAM is counterbalanced by concern about CAM therapy: the ability of CAM practitioners to identify serious or complex medical conditions that require medical treatment,[63] the lack of uniform CAM standards for pediatric care, the appropriateness of treatment, legal liabilities[9] (especially in the absence of evidence-based studies[45,64]), and ethical issues.[31] When advising patients concerning CAM therapies, pediatricians face two major legal risks: medical malpractice and professional discipline.[9] The ethical issues revolve around the possibility of causing harm,[31,45,65] abuse and neglect in withholding proven medical treatments, and parental freedom of choice of therapy.[9,31] Although in general CAM is beneficial in pediatrics,[66] specific adverse events have been reported in the literature, varying from chemical burns to exacerbation of illness to quadriplegia

to fatal hypermagnesemia.[67-78] The Federation of Medical Boards specifies that the selected CAM therapies should provide "a favorable risk/benefit ratio compared with other treatments for the same condition."[65]

The current trend is in favor of integration of mainstream medicine with CAM therapies, with a majority of medical centers offering educational programs in CAM.[72-86] In March 2002, the White House Commission on Complementary and Alternative Medicine Policy (WHCCAMP) issued a lengthy report recommending across-the-board "integration" of CAM into government health agencies and the nation's medical, medical education, and insurance systems, which suggests that CAM is close to the mainstream.[87] In 1998, Children's Hospital Boston successfully established the first integrated CAM medical education and clinical services into an urban pediatric teaching hospital, where 2100 CAM consultations were provided over 5.5 years, and acupuncture and massage therapies were eventually incorporated into a Clinical Practice Guideline.[7] By tapping into the wealth of knowledge and experience of biomedicine and CAM modalities, this book hopes to contribute in some way to the integration of various modalities for treating children.

Book Organization

The first part of the book provides historical background of each CAM therapy, especially with respect to usage by children; theory behind each CAM practice; up-to-date, evidence-based information; current pediatric use; and any contraindications. The second part of the book discusses 55 pediatric conditions, beginning with conventional medical diagnosis and treatment and followed by pertinent CAM therapies. Each discussion includes available evidence-based information specific to that condition; practical treatment recommendations from the literature (when available), from the expert's clinical experience, or both; and contraindications and potential adverse effects for use.

This book is a cooperative effort by more than 30 qualified and dedicated practitioners and took more than 4 years to be produced. It is the hope of this editor that the book will serve as a helpful reference for pediatric health practitioners of different disciplines.

References

1. National Center for Complementary and Alternative Medicine: *What is CAM?* Available at http://nccam.nih.gov/heath/whatiscam. Accessed April 2004.
2. Eisenberg DM, Kessler RC, Foster C et al: Unconventional medicine in the United States. Prevalence, costs, and patterns of use, *N Engl J Med* 328:246-252, 1983.
3. Eisenberg DM, Davis RB, Ettner SL et al: Trends in alternative medicine use in the United States, 1990-1997: results of a follow-up national survey, *J Am Med Assoc* 280:1569-1575, 1998.
4. Barnes P, Powell-Griner E, McFann K et al: *CDC advance data report #343. Complementary and alternative medicine use among adults: United States, 2002. May 27, 2004.* Available at http://nccam.nih.gov/news/camstats.htm. Accessed July 2004.
5. Spigelblatt LS: Alternative medicine: should it be used by children? *Curr Probl Pediatr* 25:180-188, 1995.

6. Gardiner P, Wornham W: Recent review of complementary and alternative medicine used by adolescents, *Curr Probl Pediatr* 12:298-302, 2000.

7. Highfield ES, McLellan MC, Kemper KJ et al: Integration of complementary and alternative medicine in a major pediatric teaching hospital: an initial overview, *J Altern Complement Med* 11:373-380, 2005.

8. Bellas A, Lafferty WE, Lind B et al: Frequency, predictors, and expenditures for pediatric insurance claims for complementary and alternative medical professionals in Washington State, *Arch Pediatr Adolesc Med* 159:367-372, 2005.

9. Cohen MH, Kemper KJ: Complementary therapies in pediatrics: a legal perspective, *Pediatrics* 115:774-780, 2005.

10. Davis MP, Darden PM: Use of complementary and alternative medicine by children in the United States, *Arch Pediatr Adolesc Med* 157:393-396, 2003.

11. Chan E, Rappaport LA, Kemper KJ: Complementary and alternative therapies in childhood attention and hyperactivity problems, *J Dev Behav Pediatr* 24:4-8, 2003.

12. Kemper KJ, Wornham WL: Consultations for holistic pediatric services for inpatients and outpatient oncology patients at a children's hospital, *Arch Pediatr Adolesc Med* 155:449-454, 2001.

13. Kemper KJ, Sarah R, Silver-Highfield E et al: On pins and needles? Pediatric pain patients' experience with acupuncture, *Pediatrics* 105:941-947, 2000.

14. Ottolini MC, Hamburger EK, Loprieato JO et al: Complementary and alternative medicine use among children in the Washington, DC area, *Ambul Pediatr* 1:122-125, 2001.

15. Sanders H, Davis MF, Duncan B et al: Use of complementary and alternative medical therapies among children with special health care needs in southern Arizona, *Pediatrics* 111:584-587, 2003.

16. Sawni-Sikand A, Schubiner H, Thomas RL: Use of complementary/alternative therapies among children in primary care pediatrics, *Ambul Pediatr* 2:99-103, 2002.

17. Day AS, Whitten KE, Bohane TD: Use of complementary and alternative medicines by children and adolescents with inflammatory bowel disease, *J Paediatr Child Health* 40:681-684, 2004.

18. Shenfield G, Lim E, Allen H: Survey of the use of complementary medicines and therapies in children with asthma, *J Paediatr Child Health* 38:252-257, 2002.

19. Quattropani C, Ausfeld B, Straumann A et al: Complementary alternative medicine in patients with inflammatory bowel disease: use and attitudes, *Scand J Gastroenterol* 38:277-282, 2003.

20. Johnston GA, Bilbao RM, Graham-Brown RA: The use of complementary medicine in children with atopic dermatitis in secondary care in Leicester, *Br J Dermatol* 149:566-571, 2003.

21. Fong DP, Fong LK: Usage of complementary medicine among children, *Aust Fam Physician* 31:388-391, 2002.

22. Wilson K, Busse JW, Gilchrist A et al: Characteristics of pediatric and adolescent patients attending a naturopathic college clinic in Canada, *Pediatrics* 115:e338-e343, 2005.

23. Complementary medicine is booming worldwide, *Br Med J* 313:131-133, 1996.

24. Spigelblatt L, Laine-Ammara G, Pless IB et al: The use of alternative medicine by children, *Pediatrics* 94:811-814, 1994.

25. Losier A, Taylor B, Fernandez CV: Use of alternative therapies by patients presenting to a pediatric emergency department, *J Emerg Med* 28:267-271, 2005.

26. Hurvitz EA, Leonard C, Ayyangar R et al: Complementary and alternative medicine use in families of children with cerebral palsy, *Dev Med Child Neurol* 45:364-370, 2003.

27. Pitetti R, Singh S, Hornyak D et al: Complementary and alternative medicine use in children, *Pediatr Emerg Care* 17:165-169, 2001.

28. Friedman T, Slayton WB, Allen LS et al: Use of alternative therapies for children with cancer, *Pediatrics* 100:1-6, 1997.

29. Lim A, Cranswick N, Skull S et al: Survey of complementary and alternative medicine use at a tertiary children's hospital, *J Paediatr Child Health* 41:424-427, 2005.

30. Day AS: Use of complementary and alternative therapies and probiotic agents by children attending gastroenterology outpatient clinics, *J Paediatr Child Health* 38:343-346, 2002.

31. Cohen MH, Kemper KJ, Stevens L et al: Pediatric use of complementary therapies: ethical and policy choices, *Pediatrics* 116:e568-e575, 2005.

32. Jacobs J, Jiminez LM, Gloyd SS et al: Treatment of acute childhood diarrhea with homeopathic medicine: a randomized clinical trial in Nicaragua, *Pediatrics* 93:719-725, 1994.

33. Breuner CC, Barry PJ Kemper KJ: Alternative medicine use by homeless youth, *Arch Pediatr Adolesc Med* 152:1071-1075, 1998.

34. Hagen LE, Schneider R, Stephens D et al: Use of complementary and alternative medicine by pediatric rheumatology patients, *Arthritis Rheum* 49:3-6, 2003.

35. Southwood TR, Malleson PN, Roberts-Thomson PJ et al: Unconventional remedies used for patients with juvenile arthritis, *Pediatrics* 85:150-154, 1990.

36. Stern RC, Canda ER, Doershuk CF: Use of nonmedical treatment by cystic fibrosis patients, *J Adolesc Health* 13:612-615, 1992.

37. Sawyer MG, Gannoni AF, Toogood IR et al: The use of alternative therapies by children with cancer, *Med J Aust* 160:320-322, 1994.

38. Fernandez CV, Stutzer CA, MacWilliam L et al: Alternative and complementary therapy use in pediatric oncology patients in British Columbia: prevalence and reasons for use and nonuse, *J Clin Oncol* 16:1279-1286, 1998.

39. Grootenhuis MA, DeCraaf-Nijkerk JH, Wel MVD: Use of alternative treatment in pediatric oncology, *Cancer Nurs* 21:282-288, 1998.

40. Quattropani C, Ausfeld B, Straumann A et al: Complementary alternative medicine in patients with inflammatory bowel disease: use and attitudes, *Scand J Gastroenterol* 38:277-282, 2003.

41. Cincotta DR, Crawford NW, Lim A et al: Comparison of complementary and alternative medicine use: reasons and motivations between two tertiary children's hospitals, *Arch Dis Child* 91:153-158, 2006.

42. Nickel RE: Controversial therapies for young children with developmental disabilities, *Infants Young Child* 8:29-40, 1996.

43. AAP Policy Statement: Counseling families who choose complementary and alternative medicine for their child with chronic illness or disability, *Pediatrics* 107:598-601, 2001.

44. Coppes MJ, Anderson RA, Egeler RM et al: Alternative therapies for the treatment of childhood cancer [letter], *N Engl J Med* 339:846-847, 1998.

45. AAP Policy: Scope of practice issues in the delivery of pediatric health care—Committee on Pediatric Workforce, *Pediatrics* 111:426-435, 2003.

46. Bridevaux IP: A survey of patients' out-of-pocket payments for complementary and alternative medicine therapies, *Complement Ther Med* 12:48-50, 2004.

47. Rawsthorne P, Shanahan F, Cronin NC et al: An international survey of the use and attitudes regarding alternative medicine by patients with inflammatory bowel disease, *Am J Gastroenterol* 94:1298-1303, 1999.

48. Eisenberg L: Complementary and alternative medicine: what is its role? *Harvard Rev Psychiatr* 10:221-230, 2002.

49. Loman DG: The use of complementary and alternative health care practices among children, *J Pediatr Health Care* 17:58-63, 2003.

50. Zeltzer LK, Tsao JC, Stelling C et al: A phase I study on the feasibility and acceptability of an acupuncture/hypnosis intervention for chronic pediatric pain, *J Pain Symptom Manage* 24:437-446, 2002.

51. Simpson N, Roman K: Complementary medicine use in children: extent and reasons: a population-based study, *Br J Gen Pract* 51:914-916, 2001.

52. Sibinga EM, Ottolini MC, Duggan AK et al: Parent-pediatrician communication about complementary and alternative medicine use for children, *Clin Pediatr (Phila)* 43:367-373, 2004.

53. Sikand A, Laken M: Pediatricians' experience with and attitudes toward complementary/alternative medicine, *Arch Pediatr Adolesc Med* 152:1059-1064, 1998.

54. National Center for Complementary and Alternative Medicine: *Clinical practice guidelines in CAM,* 1997.

55. Harrington A editor: *The placebo effect: an interdisciplinary exploration*, Cambridge, Mass, 1997, Harvard University Press.

56. Hernandez-Reif M, Field T, Krasnego J et al: Children with cystic fibrosis benefit from massage therapy, *J Pediatr Psychol* 24:175-181, 1999.

57. Weizman Z, Alkrinawi S, Goldfarb D et al: Efficacy of herbal tea preparation in infant colic, *J Pediatr* 122:650-652, 1993.

58. van Haselen RA, Reiber U, Nickel I et al: Providing complementary and alternative medicine in primary care: the primary care workers' perspective, *Complement Ther Med* 12:6-16, 2004.

59. Kemper KJ, O'Connor KG: Pediatricians' recommendations for complementary and alternative medical (CAM) therapies, *Ambul Pediatr* 4:482-487, 2004.

60. Wetzel MS, Kaptchuk TJ, Haramati A et al: Complementary and alternative medical therapies: implications for medical education, *Ann Intern Med* 138:191-196, 2003.

61. Wetzel MS, Eisenberg DM, Kaptchuk TJ: Courses involving complementary and alternative medicine at US medical schools, *J Am Med Assoc* 280:784-787, 1998.

62. Graham-Pole J: "Physician, heal thyself": how teaching holistic medicine differs from teaching CAM, *Acad Med* 76:662-664, 2001.

63. Lee AC, Kemper KJ: Homeopathy and naturopathy: practice characteristics and pediatric care, *Arch Pediatr Adolesc Med* 154:75-80, 2000.

64. Kemper KJ, Cassileth B, Ferris T: Holistic pediatrics: a research agenda, *Pediatrics* 103:902-909, 1999.

65. Federation of State Medical Boards. Available at www.fsmb.org. Accessed August 2005.

66. Perrin JM, Kemper KJ: Holistic pediatrics—good medicine, *Pediatrics* 105(suppl):214-218, 2000.

67. Ernst E: Second thoughts about safety of St John's wort, *Lancet* 354:2014-2016, 1999.

68. Boyer E, Kearney S, Kemper KJ et al: Poisoning from a dietary supplement administered during hospitalization, *Pediatrics* 109: e49, 2002. Available at: www.pediatrics.org/cgi/content/full/109/3/e49. Accessed November 16, 2007.

69. Fugh-Berman A: Herb-drug interactions, *Lancet* 355:134-138, 2000.

70. Adams KE, Cohen MH, Jonsen AR et al: Ethical considerations of complementary and alternative medical therapies in conventional medical settings, *Ann Intern Med* 137:660-664, 2002.

71. Korkmaz A, Sahiner U, Yurdakok M: Chemical burn caused by topical vinegar application in a newborn infant, *Pediatr Dermatol* 17:34-36, 2000.

72. Bakerink JA, Gospe SM, Dimand RJ et al: Multiple organ failure after ingestion of pennyroyal oil from herbal tea in two infants, *Pediatrics* 98:944-947, 1996.

73. Yu EC, Yeung CY: Lead encephalopathy due to herbal medicine, *Chinese Med J* 100:915-917, 1987.

74. Shafrir Y, Kaufman BA: Quadriplegia after chiropractic manipulation in an infant with congenital torticollis, *J Pediatr* 120:266-269, 1992.

75. Bose A, Vashista K, O'Loughlin BJ: Azarcon por Empacho—another cause of lead toxicity, *Pediatrics* 72:106-108, 1983.

76. Aberer W, Strohal R: Homeopathic preparations—severe adverse effects, unproven benefits, *Dermatologica* 182:253, 1991.

77. Goodyear HM, Harper JI: Atopic eczema, hyponatraemia, and hypoalbuminaemia, *Arch Dis Child* 65:231-232, 1990.

78. Montoya-Cabrera MA, Rubio-Rodriguez S, Velazquez-Gonzalez E et al: Mercury poisoning caused by a homeopathic drug [in Spanish], *Gac Med Mex* 127:267-270, 1991.

79. Brinkhaus B, Joos S, Lindner M et al: Integration of complementary and alternative medicine into German medical school curricula—contradictions between the opinions of decision makers and the status quo, *Forsch Komplementarmed Klass Naturheilkd* 12:139-143, 2005.

80. Burke A, Peper E, Burrows K et al: Developing the complementary and alternative medicine education infrastructure: baccalaureate programs in the United States, *J Altern Complement Med* 10:1115-1121, 2004.

81. Owen D, Lewith GT: Teaching integrated care: CAM familiarisation courses, *Med J Aust* 181:276-278, 2004.

82. Kligler B, Maizes V, Schachter S et al: Education Working Group, Consortium of Academic Health Centers for Integrative Medicine: core competencies in integrative medicine for medical school curricula—a proposal, *Acad Med* 79:521-531, 2004.

83. Barnes L, Risko W, Nethersole S et al: Integrating complementary and alternative medicine into pediatric training, *Pediatr Ann* 33:256-263, 2004.

84. Saxon DW, Tunnicliff G, Brokaw JJ, et al: Status of complementary and alternative medicine in the osteopathic medical school curriculum, *J Am Osteopath Assoc* 104:121-126, 2004.

85. Levine SM, Weber-Levine ML, Mayberry RM: Complementary and alternative medical practices: training, experience, and attitudes of a primary care medical school faculty, *J Am Board Fam Pract* 16:318-326, 2003.

86. Forjuoh SN, Rascoe TG, Symm B, et al: Teaching medical students complementary and alternative medicine using evidence-based principles, *J Altern Complement Med* 9:429-439, 2003.

87. White House Commission on Complementary and Alternative Medicine Policy: *Final report, March 2002*. Available at: www.whccamp.hhs.gov. Accessed November 16, 2007.

CHAPTER 2

Mind/Body Approaches: Biofeedback, Hypnosis, Spirituality

General Mind/Body | Timothy Culbert, Lynda Richtsmeier Cyr

Hypnosis | Karen Olness

Spirituality in Pediatric Care | Tobin Hart

General Mind/Body

History and Theory

Emerging paradigms of "holism" and "integrative medicine" agree that, as a core principle, the unity of mind-body-spirit in all manifestations of health and wellness must be recognized. Underscoring this assertion, the World Health Organization (WHO) defines *health* as "a state of complete physical, mental and social well-being and not simply the absence of disease or infirmity." Historically, across most systems of healthcare around the world, mind and body have always been recognized as an integrated whole. It is only in the recent history of Western, allopathic biomedicine that a more reductionist model has briefly predominated (and, although recognized for its contributions, is now being reconsidered). In 1977, Kenneth Pelletier[1] wrote about the mind as both "healer" and "slayer" to denote that what we think, feel, and believe can have profound implications for the quality of our health and the length of our lives. With 30 years of solid research (and hundreds of years of experience), mind/body medicine is a concept that has now achieved wide acceptance and credibility in the twenty-first-century healthcare landscape.

Mind/body medicine (M/BM) refers to the understanding that mind and body (and spirit) represent a unitary entity, that mind and body influence each other bidirectionally and frequently, and that the nature of many health challenges, symptoms, and disorders is fundamentally psychophysiological. In other words, the etiology of the symptoms or disease and the experience of illness for each patient include biological as well as emotional, behavioral, and cognitive components. It would follow that appropriate assessment and treatment activities consider and address these components. Of all the complementary and alternative interventions, M/BM is supported by the largest body of scientific evidence for a surprisingly broad variety of conditions. Evidence is also mounting to support the complex interplay of the nervous, immune, and endocrine systems and the links to positive and negative emotional states as well as the impact of acute and chronic stress on these axes. The mind and body communicate messages to each other that result in biochemical and physiological changes that can in turn either promote or detract from health, wellness, and recovery from illness.

It is arguable that for much of the world, morbidity from medical conditions linked to psychosocial issues such as poverty, lifestyle choices, dietary habits, stress, lack of exercise, violence, and family dysfunction are as important and prevalent as traditional medical problems such as infectious disease, trauma, and genetic disorders. Additionally, many children and adolescents who suffer from various chronic illnesses (e.g., cancer, pain syndromes, diabetes, cystic fibrosis, inflammatory bowel disease, juvenile rheumatoid arthritis) experience concurrent emotional/behavioral challenges that can exacerbate and complicate their underlying illness and cause further functional impairment. As many as 25% of visits to pediatric offices are for symptoms related to psychosocial factors.[2] More than 50% of visits to primary care clinics in general are secondary to psychophysiological concerns.[3] Haggerty[2] has coined the term "the New Morbidity" to reflect this identified shift in the nature of illness and recognize the need for a corresponding shift in the healthcare service structure and delivery that mirrors this reality. It is difficult to understand ourselves and our experience of disease when we separate our body from our mind and spirit. In a holistic view, body-mind-spirit is seen as interconnected and interactive. Mental and emotional well-being alters our physical health in many ways.

Even though M/BM is widely accepted with an excellent database to support its relevance and the efficacy of mind/body treatment approaches, change in healthcare delivery systems is slow to come. Words such as *psychophysiological*, *biobehavioral*, *functional*, and *psychosomatic* have all been used in the past to denote this area. Some have a rather negative connotation that suggests, "It's all in your head." The abbreviation *M/BM* is used in this text for *mind/body medicine* to reflect a unified concept of mind/body.

Complementary and alternative medicine (CAM) pioneer Ken Pelletier has described six principles of M/BM[5]:

1. Mind, body, and spirit are interrelated, not only with one another but also with the external environment. Mind/body interventions help physically as well as mentally, and physical interventions help mentally as well as physically.

2. Stress and depression contribute powerfully to chronic disease. Stress responses usually compromise immunity, as does depression. Stress and depression can double the mortality rate of certain chronic illness conditions.

3. The mind affects the body through psycho-neuro-endocrine-immune pathways. These physical effcets of the mind are mediated by central nervous system biochemicals including peptides, neuropeptides, and hormones.

4. Mental outlook has an impact on physical health. Health is improved by optimism and acceptance, and it is diminished by anger, pessimism, and chronic, unrelenting stress.

5. Placebo effects can induce healing. They can have a profound influence on many physical characteristics and are an important element in many mind/body interactions.

6. Social support enhances and sustains health. Friends, family, and supportive clinicians bolster both effective conventional and CAM therapies.

Current Practice in M/BM: Assessment

Biopsychosocial factors should always be examined in the etiology and maintenance of illness/disease. It is therefore recommended that a "holistic lens" be used when assessing a patient; family's perception of medical symptoms and history; psychological symptoms and history; perceptions of the role of spirituality and religious beliefs; and the experience of the current illness or disease to the patients and their family members.

Lifestyle factors (e.g., diet, exercise, sleep), stressors and stress management strategies, psychosocial context (e.g., family constellation, family medical history, family psychological history, impact of illness on the family), recent major life events, perceived strengths, job and academic activities, hobbies, peer supports, meaning of illness, functional impairment (what the patient can or cannot do), and cultural factors (e.g., meaning of illness, preferred treatment approaches, involvement of elders and religious leaders) are also important factors to review.

Current Practice in M/BM: Treatment

One aspect of many (if not all) M/BM techniques is support of self-management and self-care. Closely related to the mind/body paradigm is the concept of self-regulation. Author Donald Bakal[6] in *Minding the Body* describes a key aspect of "humanness": our ability to examine and regulate our own inner life and experience. He states that "there is considerable evidence that individuals who are actively engaged in some form of self-regulation have an improved quality of life." Enough evidence has been accumulated to support the efficacy of M/BM approaches that many authors have agreed these techniques should be a standard part of primary ambulatory care settings and be included in healthcare training.[3,7,8]

Common themes in M/BM are self-awareness, self-regulation, and self-care. Training children and adolescents in self-regulation skills means assisting them in identifying and cultivating strategies that develop their innate abilities to control and contribute to their own health and wellness. Self-regulation skills training taps into the individual's natural drives for mastery and self-control. Children and adolescents can learn to modulate thoughts, emotions, and physiological functions in desired directions that support the recovery and maintenance of health,

wellness, and optimal performance. Studies in pediatric populations support the fact that children and adolescents as a group are very good at self-regulation techniques such as self-hypnosis and biofeedback and in many ways learn these techniques more quickly than adults. In 1985 Attansio et al. offered additional support for this assertion and described the following[9]:

- Children are more enthusiastic.
- Children learn more quickly.
- Children have more psychophysiological ability.
- Children are less skeptical.
- Children have more confidence in special abilities.
- Children can be reliable at symptom monitoring.
- Children enjoy practicing self-regulation skills.

The therapist-patient relationship, positive expectation, true collaboration and shared decision-making, and related factors can also be mediating factors in health outcomes that affect mind/body pathways.

M/BM often evokes images of specific techniques, such as relaxation training, imagery (self-hypnosis), meditation, or biofeedback, that fall within its overall domain. In an effort to be inclusive, the authors would hold that M/BM includes a broad variety of techniques and strategies, all of which embrace and reflect to some extent the reciprocal influence of mind and body and acknowledge the power of the mind to have quite remarkable influence over physical symptoms and the experience of illness and wellness. Historically, the list of techniques broadly considered M/BM has included the following:

- Yoga
- Tai Chi
- Qigong
- Hypnosis, guided imagery, and visualization techniques
- Biofeedback and applied psychophysiology
- Eye movement desensitization and reprocessing (EMDR)
- Meditation
- Cognitive/behavioral therapy and psychological therapies
- Stress management
- Relaxation training (progressive muscle relaxation, deep breathing, autogenics)
- Social support
- Music and expressive arts therapies
- Spiritual beliefs and practices, religious rituals, and prayer

Common goals of many M/BM approaches include the following:

- Enhanced access to subconscious material
- Cultivation of lowered state of autonomic nervous system (ANS) arousal
- Facilitation of sense of mastery and internal health locus of control
- Increased awareness of internal events and sensations
- Narrowed focus of attention
- Facilitation of imagery abilities
- Heightened suggestibility
- Altered state of awareness

This text will focus on two mind/body therapies in particular, biofeedback and hypnosis, for which there is solid evidence in children and adolescents. Reference will be made to other therapies in the mind/body realm as appropriate for specific conditions (e.g., yoga for asthma, meditation for chronic pain).

In this introductory section, specific additional comments will be provided about hypnosis and hypnotherapy with children.

A few key definitions follow:

Biofeedback is the use of electronic or electromechanical instruments to measure feedback information about physiological processes such as muscle activity, heart rate variability, breathing, finger temperature, sweat gland activity, and electroencephalogram activity.

Hypnosis is an altered state of awareness usually but not always involving relaxation, within which individuals experience heightened suggestibility. Within this altered state of awareness, individuals also experience increased concentration on a particular word or idea for the purpose of altering a chosen phenomenon (symptom/physiologic function/emotional reaction pattern) in a desirable (therapeutic) direction.

Meditation is an inner art and science practiced in various forms, with most types usually involving quiet contemplation, sometimes with a focus on breathing or a specific word or phrase.

Yoga is an ancient philosophy of life developed over the course of thousands of years, which includes ethical principles, dietary restrictions, and physical exercises to bring mind, body, and spirit into equilibrium.

Clinical conditions in pediatrics for which mind/body approaches have been studied and are particularly useful include the following:

- Chronic acute and recurrent pain, including headaches, recurrent abdominal pain, and pain associated with chronic illness, sickle cell anemia, burns, and medical procedures
- Asthma
- Diabetes
- Sleep disorders
- Enuresis
- Encopresis
- Habits such as thumbsucking, nail biting, and habitual cough
- Anxiety and stress-related disorders
- ANS dysregulation
- Tics and Tourette's syndrome
- Warts
- Neuromuscular rehabilitation
- Learning disorders, attention-deficit hyperactivity disorder, and autism
- Support for chronic illness such as cancer, autoimmune disorders, fibromyalgia, chronic fatigue syndrome, irritable bowel disease, and irritable bowel syndrome

Hypnosis

Children learn self-hypnosis easily and are able to apply it to solve many problems. These include acute and chronic pain, habit problems, anxiety associated with chronic illnesses, performance anxiety, and enuresis. The teaching and application of self-hypnosis is often enhanced by the addition of biofeedback. This provides proof to the child that changes in thinking result in changes in body responses.

The choice of strategies for teaching self-hypnosis to children depends on the age and developmental stage, preferred type of mental imagery (i.e., visual, auditory, kinesthetic, olfactory), likes, dislikes, fears, and learning style of the child. It is essential that the coach or teacher emphasize that the child is in control and can decide when and where to use self-hypnosis. The variability in preferences, learning styles, and developmental stages among children complicates the design of research protocols that study hypnosis with children. These protocols are often written to describe identical hypnotic inductions, often tape recorded, to be used at prescribed times. Measured variables do not include whether a child likes the induction, listens to it, or focuses on entirely different mental imagery of his or her own choosing. Furthermore, learning disabilities are often subtle and may not be recognized without detailed testing, which is not usually done prior to research studies involving child hypnosis. Each of these variables complicates efforts to perform metaanalyses on hypnosis and related interventions. Additionally, some investigators who have no training in hypnosis will study interventions called "relaxation imagery," "imagery," "visual imagery," or "progressive relaxation," each of which leads to a hypnotic state. The proper analyses of studies on efficacy of hypnosis in children should be to combine all strategies that induce hypnosis in children.

Some studies are defined as controlled but mix therapeutic interventions. For example, Scharff et al. reported "a controlled study of minimal contact thermal biofeedback treatment in children with migraine."[1] Children were randomly assigned to thermal biofeedback, attention, or wait-list control groups. The hand-warming biofeedback group received four sessions of cognitive behavioral stress management training, thermal biofeedback, progressive muscle relaxation, imagery training of warm places, and deep breathing techniques. Thus these children were also taught self-hypnosis. Results from this study found that children assigned to the hand-warming biofeedback group were more likely to achieve clinical improvement than the attention group.

Child patients referred for alternative treatments may not have had adequate diagnostic evaluations. In a study that reviewed 200 cases of children referred for treatment with hypnosis and/or biofeedback, we found that 25% had unrecognized biological bases for symptoms such as enuresis, headache, anxiety, and recurrent abdominal pain.[2] For example, some children with headache were diagnosed as having sinusitis, food allergies, brain tumor, and carbon monoxide poisoning. Interpretations of randomized clinical trials often assume that subjects have had equivalent diagnostic evaluations. This may not be true, and results of the trials are confounded when diagnoses are in error.

Safety Issues and Contraindications

In general, there are few situations or disorders for which mind/body skills are contraindicated. It is not ethical or appropriate to treat a minor or incompetent client without informed consent. Learning specific mind/body skills techniques or therapies does confer the right to use these therapies for populations or conditions that a practitioner would not normally treat.

Persons with acute, severe, or unstable medical illness should first receive appropriate medial care and stabilization. Mind/body therapies are not an alternative to key treatments such as medication, chemotherapy, or surgery. Individuals suffering from significant psychiatric disorders (schizophrenia, mania, major depression, paranoia, severe obsessive compulsive disorder, posttraumatic stress disorder) may not be suitable candidates for mind/body therapies or at least must be handled with special care and expertise. Caution is also recommended when using mind/body techniques in clients with severe impairments of memory or attention or in neurological conditions such as seizure. Children with disorders that involve severe, unstable ANS or metabolic functions should be under the care of an appropriate medical professional, and although mind/body therapies may play a supporting role, they do not generally represent first-line therapies in acute illness.

During self-regulation training and any form of deep relaxation, patients commonly enter altered states of awareness in which they may process information differently. In addition, as they become relaxed, some persons are prone to experience dissociative states. People with a history of abuse, severe stress, schizophrenia, or other psychoses are at risk for experiencing distress and/or dissociative phenoemena called *abreactions*. Although these reactions are uncommon, pediatric healthcare professionals who are using and teaching mind/body skills to children or adolescents must be prepared to deal effectively with these reactions should they manifest during a clinical session.

Patients taking medications for conditions such as diabetes, hypertension, anxiety, hypothyroidism, asthma, and headache should be made aware of the possible need for medication adjustments as they learn and practice mind/body skills. Medication status and adjustments should be reviewed and coordinated with the prescribing physician. Other ongoing treatments (e.g., physical therapy, massage, psychotherapy) are not a contraindication to concurrent mind/body skills training. Practical issues such as time, affordability, and absence from school to attend appointments should also be openly and honestly examined and discussed as possible impediments to successful treatment.

Spirituality in Pediatric Care

The nature of spirituality is vast and mysterious. It neither lends itself to complete definitions or verification, nor does it necessarily serve as a tool to treat symptoms in the same fashion that, say, medication or acupuncture might. Yet spirituality is of rising significance in contemporary society and may have something potent to offer both children and medicine. Both The Joint Commission (TJC) and the Commission on Accreditation of Rehabilitation Facilities (CARF) have new standards that call for the inclusion of spirituality in the assessment and treatments of all patients. The standards, however, perhaps to their credit, offer no real concept of what spirituality might entail or how it might be applied in clinical settings.

Instead of a primary emphasis on symptom reduction, spirituality may touch deep taproots of conditions. This is especially important because similar symptoms may emerge from different origins—the concept of equifinality. Spirituality represents a more subtle and encompassing dimension of human existence that can affect other levels (e.g., biophysical, behavioral, subtle energy) in the chain of being and can serve as a complement to other interventions. In some instances a spiritual change may not affect a symptom at all, but instead change one's relationship with that symptom and, in turn, with life and even death.

Background and History

The spiritual child

There is a growing body of evidence that children have innate spiritual capacities and experiences—particular moments and ways of knowing, both little and large, that shape their lives in enduring ways.[1-8] From moments of wonder to finding inner wisdom, from metaphysical musings, to expressing compassion, and even to seeing beneath the surface of the material world, these experiences may be powerfully formative for a child's worldview and life course, perhaps providing among the most fundamental source of motivation and healing and, at times, a source of difficulties. These experiences and capacities reveal a rich and significant spiritual life that has gone largely unrecognized in the annals of child development and medicine. Traditionally, developmental theory has been largely dismissive of the idea that children have genuine spiritual experiences and capacities.[9,10] Consequently, there is very little literature on the role of spirituality in pediatric care.[11-13] Until recently, most researchers have concluded that children, especially preadolescents, do not and cannot have a genuine spiritual life and therefore its consideration in everything from pediatrics to education and parenting would be simply irrelevant.[14] However, children's spirituality may exist apart from adult rational and linguistic conceptions and beyond religious knowledge. Children's personal experience of divinity—what William James understood as *personal religion* as opposed to *institutional religion*—may emerge as a sense of interconnection with the cosmos, a revelatory insight, a sense of a life force, and so forth.[15] These phenomena emerge as ways of being in the world, intuitive epistemic styles, and types of immediate, ontologically shifting awareness or perception that may take place within or outside the context of religion.[16] A child's openness and directness of perception allow for such intimate awareness and direct questioning of the world. Although they may not be able to articulate a moment of wonder or conceptualize a religious concept, their *presence*—their mode of being in the world—may be distinctly spiritual. As Gordon Allport suggested, "the religion of childhood may be of a very special order." [17]

Spiritual healing

Although not specific in any way to pediatric care, the history of spiritual healing in general has a great many threads and provides some context for understanding the application of spiritual principles to children. Only a few threads are mentioned here to give a hint of the range of approaches that might be considered spiritual: biopsychomedical, shamanism, dreams, prayer, and influences of past lives.

Biopsychomedical. The rise of anatomical understanding of the human body followed by comprehension of physiological processes and later biochemical mechanisms has largely defined the basis for modern Western medicine. By definition, this biomechanistic view of illness has largely excluded any consideration of the spiritual. The further development of psychosomatic medicine beginning in the early part of the twentieth century and followed by psychoneuroimmunology extended the understanding of what makes people well or ill. For example, a feeling of hope may have an effect on immune response and, in turn, on health or recovery. Levin suggests that the experience of meaning of illness or wellness plays a powerful role in health.[18] The contemporary health provider can lead the young person to consider what meaning an illness or injury may have or heighten bodily awareness for more precise and subtle recognition of physical and mental sensations. Working with chronic pain patients is a good example.[19]

Shamanism. Shamanism is generally considered the world's oldest form of religion, one that continues to exist among indigenous populations and has had a renewed interest among contemporary Westerners. The shaman serves as priest and healer, typically offering both guidance and medical intervention. The process of healing generally involves a shift in states of consciousness for the shaman and often for the individual seeking assistance. The underlying principle is that health or disorder is in some way influenced by a spiritual realm. Therefore to gain insight or healing it is necessary to shift consciousness (often through ritual dance or chanting, intoxicants, or fasting) and travel closer to that nonphysical realm. Through contemporary mind/body understanding, one can see how the power of belief and ceremony may play a role in the efficacy of such practices. In addition, the shamanic presupposition is that the world of spirit and intention (of self or by others) influence health and well-being. The use of dreams and prayers for insight and intervention relate to the same understanding.

Dreams. Hippocrates, regarded as the father of Greek medicine, sought advice on healing in dreams and invited his patients to do the same. Aristotle suggested that dreams may be sensitive indicators of bodily conditions.[20] The influential Persian physician Avicenna (980-1037 CE) not only looked to dreams for insight, but also suggested that in "dreamtime" one could also influence a condition: "The imagination of man can act not only on his own body but even on others and very distant bodies. It can fascinate and modify them; make them ill, or restore them to health."[21] More recently, particularly since the beginning of the twentieth century, the use of dreams in therapeutic intervention has been employed in some psychological models.

Prayer. Prayer is a common practice across culture and history. For example, the ancient Greeks invoked the Muses for inspiration, prayed to one or more gods for healing, or to their genius—their guardian spirit—for assistance. Although modern Western medicine has no place for such otherworldly interventions, contemporary practices are showing a resurging interest in prayer.[22,23]

Influence of past lives. Approaching health from a different tack, Hindu tradition, among others, recognizes that karma may play a role in current well-being. The concept is that past life experiences may carry over into consciousness in some way, including physical or psychological symptoms, such as phobias. In the West, Ian Stevenson has documented some compelling evidence for apparent past life influence.[24,25] Bowman provides an approach in working with children to overcome the current difficulty through a recollection, clarification, and release of alleged past-life memories.[26]

These concepts represent only a few diverse threads of spiritual-related interventions that can address spiritually rooted concerns or enhance efficacy of other approaches (e.g., increasing immune response or patient compliance by improving one's attitude or sense of hope). A wide range of other methods that can be applied to pediatrics include meditation, creative visualization, practicing energetic boundaries, making sense of and integrating near-death or out-of-body experiences, facing fears, creative expression, beholding beauty, finding inspiration, identifying sources of hope and guidance, tuning into inner guidance, sharing in community, practicing acts of compassion and service, finding meaning and life lesson in a situation, uncovering limiting beliefs, taking responsibility, practicing constructive surrender, practicing discernment, and so forth. These can take place both within and outside of a particular faith tradition.[12,27]

Theory: Dimensions of Spirituality

Although spirituality may be difficult to grasp precisely, its *movement* in our patients and in healers can be perceived. The following four general dimensions of spirituality—meaning, boundaries and connections, wisdom, and multidimensionality—are briefly elaborated and brought "down to earth" to treat pediatric patients. These cut across religious differences, tend to emphasize an expansion of awareness, and may represent deep structures of spiritual consciousness. They may provide trailheads for diagnosis and intervention.

Meaning

Meaning and purpose in life shape one's actions and attitudes. The search for truth and meaning is part of what defines humanity. Without a sense of meaning, a task becomes just something to do. And when life as a whole has little meaning, it becomes a plod through a vast flatland: draining, hopeless, without much contour or color. Meaning is fundamental to well-being. Just as the body needs food and water, the psyche needs meaning. When a child is able to find meaning, he or she finds self-sustaining energy. Victor Frankl, physician and Nazi concentration camp survivor, had first-hand experience with Nietzsche's famous maxim, "He who has a *why* to live can bear with almost any *how*."[28]

Children have everyday questions and crises of meaning such as, "Why should I bother doing my math homework?" They also ask the big questions: "Who am I?" "What is life about?" "What am I here to do?" Theologian Paul Tillich called this search for meaning, purpose, and truth *ultimate concerns*.[29] Children's openness, vulnerability, and tolerance for mystery enable them to entertain these big, perplexing, and paradoxical questions and wonder about the meanings and assumptions that are so central to life. They are natural philosophers searching for and creating their own worldview.

Practitioners can look for both little meaning that motivates and big meaning that inspires. One of the author's teenage patients shows how central these questions are to well being:

> I'm not sure that I really belong here. I know there is more to it [life], but no one is talking about it. I can't be the only one who sees it. Everything seems like a game. Don't they [adults] see the phoniness?... the adults don't seem to get it.... Doesn't anyone understand?

This is a child hungry for meaning and truth. Unless the big questions are addressed genuinely, children may find little point in getting up in the morning or getting well. Confusion may lead to anxiety or hopelessness.

The meaning ascribed to an illness or injury may help or hinder healing. As Levin suggests, meaning is central to postmodern medicine.[18] What is the meaning of the illness? Is this considered punishment for some moral bankruptcy or an opportunity to learn, or is it just bad luck? Although pain in life is inevitable, suffering (and healing) may be modulated by attitude and beliefs toward the difficulty.

Illness or injury may offer lessons of humility, patience, trust, prudence, responsibility, or all sorts of other considerations. When meaning is brought to a central position, individual consciousness can join with the healing process without resistance. This may reduce stress, improve immune responses, or increase compliance and personal responsibility with treatment.

Even after an acute healing crisis is over, a crisis of meaning may ensue. For example, children who experience near-death experiences often feel split between worlds; without validation or acknowledgement, serious complications may result. Unity of life and death, awe or wonder can be overwhelming and difficult to integrate. St. John of the Cross described this mystical knowing that is beyond the intellect's ability to understand as "infinite incomprehension."[30] For example, in one study on children's near-death experiences, one third of children studied turned to alcohol within 5 to 10 years after their experience. More than half experienced serious bouts of depression. A staggering 21% actually attempted suicide (this number compares with 4% among adult near-death experiencers).[31] Confusion, guilt, shame, lack of understanding, and family members who felt threatened contributed to the difficulty in balancing the worlds.

Considerations of meaning may range from understanding the patient's view of the difficulty to offering explanations to simply pondering big questions together. The task as healthcare providers is not to *give* children meaning or truth, but to legitimize their natural search for it by taking their considerations seriously and recognizing their need for meaning. Practitioners need to discover how their inner life and outer symptoms are organized around their emerging worldview.

Boundaries and connections

Every religion has considered the paradox of humans as both self-separate individuals and as interconnected, as part of the all, the One. Each person confronts a metaphysical dilemma of setting personal boundaries while being connected with the world.

Personal boundaries may be thought of as being more or less permeable or, one could say, thick or thin. At the thin or more permeable end is increased sensitivity that enables empathy, the quality described as the base of moral development and compassion.[32] But such openness can also leave one vulnerable and confused and can actually be a root source of a wide range of symptoms. When children understand and regulate the way they connect or close out the world, they can confront life without being overwhelmed by it.

A great many children and adults are sensitive to such a degree that they are confused or tugged by feelings or thoughts of others. Others may feel swamped by the deluge of feelings that wash over them or become overwhelmed by influences from multidimensional realms. Sixteen-year-old Sarah feels like a psychic sponge: "I'm an empath, and I hate school... I [feel other people's] anger, frustration, even happiness or joy. But it's no fun."

Along with moodiness, withdrawal, and feeling overwhelmed, some children try to manage their sensitivity by creating a kind of barbed perimeter around them with a hostile personality or even aggressive behavior. The tough, hostile, or impulsively violent child may be responding to all sorts of unintended boundary violations.

This is not only an issue of emotional sensitivity but also one of general sensory difficulty. Recently problems such as sensory integration dysfunction, although not necessarily or directly a spiritual concern, have reflected increased awareness of the role of hypersensitivity in young people.[33] Such sensitivity may be interpreted as a marker of various forms of giftedness.[34]

The general systems theory recognizes that families operate as systems.[35] If something is happening in one part of a system, the other parts will be affected. Children are often the emotional barometers of their parent's relationships. How might the child be manifesting the energy of the family, even present sympathetically with symptoms of a parent's illness? Is the child taking on a parent's depression or acting out the unspoken conflict between parents? Does the child's illness or difficulty symbolically reflect the anger or hopelessness of the family? Is the child working hard to be the "good child" in order to fulfill parents' unfulfilled hope, or are they serving as a scapegoat to release tension in the system? Empathically sensitive children are particularly adept at filling the needs of the system, sometimes at the cost of their own health and growth. Those unhealthy roles begin to unwind when family members attend to their conflicts and difficulties directly and teach the child to develop effective boundaries.

The other side of the coin of boundaries is connection. How does a child connect with the world? To whom or to what are they connected? Paradoxically, having some control of boundaries may enable intimacy. Children may be willing to risk allowing someone in if they know they have the power to keep them out. This opens up questions about the art of meeting the world: How do children open to the world? How do they protect themselves? What do they perceive that others might not? How do they process what they perceive? What are the sources of love and connection in their life? These are not simply social considerations but potentially deeply spiritual ones, as they express the fundamental nature of connection, compassion, and community.

Wisdom

The spiritual traditions are also referred to as the *wisdom traditions*. Wisdom may not be a body of knowledge so much as a way of knowing and being in the world. Surprisingly, even children have access to wisdom.[2,5] Where does a child draw comfort and guidance? What are the sources both within and without that provide wisdom? What happens when a child is cut off from the contemplative mind? This dimension is about awareness, silence, and finding sources of comfort and counsel.

Outside wisdom. Resilient children—children who have grown up in very difficult, abusive, or neglectful situations but have thrived nonetheless—often have had a *leg-up person*, someone who made a difference in their life, who saw a spark in them, who noticed them, who offered a kind word, or took genuine interest. These are spiritual friends who validate, comfort, and provide wisdom for life.

Sometimes comfort emerges from a special place. A practitioner might ask a child, "Do you have a special spot where you go in person or in your imagination?" Children sometimes find a special place of spiritual sustenance in their own backyard or bookshelf—a *bliss station*, as Joseph Campbell called it.[36] This can be a physical place, such as the steps outside the house to avoid parental conflict, or a stable to be with a beloved horse, or even a mental place such as dreaming.

Inner wisdom. The bliss station can also be a place within the child—a gateway in the consciousness that opens into the depths of mystery and to the still small voice within, which mystics and sages have recognized throughout history as a source of spiritual guidance. The thirteenth century Persian poet Rumi captured it this way[37]:

> There is another kind of tablet, one
> already completed and preserved inside you.
> A spring overflowing its springbox. A freshness
> in the center of the chest. This other intelligence
> does not turn yellow or stagnate. It's fluid,
> and it doesn't move from outside to inside
> through the conduits of plumbing-learning.
> The second knowing is a fountainhead
> from within you, moving out.

Throughout the world's spiritual traditions, various modalities such as contemplative practice (e.g., prayer, meditation) can lead to that still place. Through silence, daydreaming, and even sports, children may open to the contemplative mind and find their own inner fountainhead that reminds them what is most important and most just and may offer unexpected wisdom and comfort. It may emerge as an inner feeling, thought, or image pertaining to a deceased animal or relative that can offer counsel and comfort; for example, remembering a deceased pet can teach a child about grief and letting go.

Healthcare providers do not need to attach concrete reality of the inner wisdom, but they do need to be sensitive to its impact on the child's life. Listening to the messages from the wise self may provide information for healing. A simple relaxation, turning inward, and then a request to see what would be helpful for this situation can tap the intuitive wisdom of both child and healthcare provider: "What would be of service to this person right now?" "What would assist his or her healing?" Intuition invites the spiritual realm to respond. An experienced practitioner can regularly tap into the child's intuition and thereby connect with the child's spirituality to help with healing. A simple method is just asking children to relax, close their eyes, and imagine themselves in a very special and comfortable spot. Children can then be guided to sense

what their pain needs or has to offer. They will often be able to describe an image that entered the consciousness, such as an animal or an imaginary friend, make a drawing, or in some other way provide information that may help direct healing. The practitioner may also be able to enter into a dialogue with the symptom, such as pain, by asking yes or no questions about treatment (e.g., "Would such and such help?"). This kind of inquiry not only provides immediate direction, but also reinforces awareness of one's own sense of well-being and inner ability for healing.

A *multidimensional world*

Children sometimes have a remarkable capacity for "seeing the invisible"—that is, for perceiving the multidimensional nature of consciousness.[2] Spiritual traditions recognize the multidimensional nature of the universe. It is not uncommon to hear children describe deceased souls, angelic beings, guides, and energy. It is actually an ancient notion that some disorders may be influenced, for better or worse, by the multidimensional realms.

It is common knowledge that the world is more than what meets the eye. Science continues to disclose previously invisible dimensions to us, while mystics reveal a world that is multidimensional, interconnected, alive, and evolving—and perhaps one that is increasingly transparent. Both ancient and contemporary traditions offer maps of a multidimensional universe. These maps often share commonalities. For example, ancient writings in the Kabbalah contend that everything existing in the physical world originates in the nonphysical realm of the Sephirot: both the individual and the universe as a whole are composed of 10 dimensions, the 10 Sephirot, meaning "ten emanations" of light; that is, waves of light emanating out from a concentrated center—"a never-to-be-exhausted fountain of light."[38] Each of these waves represents a different dimension or level of consciousness or reality. Remarkably, more than 2000 years later, the superstring theory from theoretical physics also suggests 10 dimensions of existence that are likewise emanated from a kind of supernal luminescence—the Big Bang. Physicists retrieve the familiar four-dimensional universe by assuming that during the Big Bang, 6 of the 10 dimensions curled up, or "compactified," whereas the remaining 4 dimensions expanded explosively, engendering the visible universe we recognize.[39] The compactified dimensions exist not only in the here and now, but also in other dimensions or frequencies not ordinarily recognized in human reality.

Human awareness sometimes makes its way between dimensions through a kind of wormhole of consciousness that may be entered spontaneously, in altered states such as sleep, or more intentionally through such practices as meditation. For example, during out-of-body and near-death experiences, as well as *dreamtime*, as Australian aboriginal peoples call it, consciousness leaves the dominant magnetic pull of the physical body and awareness opens in another dimension. Some children (and adults) have a naturally open perceptual style that allows them to recognize a multidimensional universe firsthand. This can provide both a source of information or wonder and a source of pain and confusion in a society that may not accept the reality of such perception.

The phase "seeing the invisible" implies that in some way many children are able to perceive the more subtle levels and nonconcrete aspects of the multidimensional universe. These perceptions can be comforting or disturbing, such as seeing "colors and shapes around" other people, "sensing" the deceased, seeing angels that may make them feel safe, or "seeing" their own death in past lives.

Objective measure is obviously not possible. Contemporary culture often dismisses or assigns a pathology to these perceptions, not realizing that a multidimensional universe can open up the door to all sorts of possibilities. The ancients might have understood an angel's visit as manifestation of *genius*, a guardian spirit. In the Middle Ages, the genius became known as a guardian angel.[35] The significance of the child's encounter with the vision depends on its impact on the child's life.

Ian Stevenson, formerly head of psychiatry at the University of Virginia Medical School, researched historical documents such as municipal records and news reports (e.g., birth, marriage, death, hospital records, accidents, property deeds) for evidence of alleged past-life events.[24,25] He was able to confirm that children's recollection of and emotional responses to images from the multidimensional world do correspond to events that happened before their current lives. In addition, these events apparently still exert influence in the children's lives. He even found that physical symptoms—a chronic sore throat, a rash on the arm, or even a birthmark—correlated with the location of an injury that occurred to a person in this alleged past life. Symptoms often disappeared with some form of reconciliation with that past experience.[26]

In a survey of recalled childhood spiritual experiences, 90% responded affirmatively to at least one of several questions that addressed "non-ordinary perception" (e.g., telepathy, clairvoyance, pre/post-cognitions, near-death experience, out-of-body experience). Sixty-five percent of those who experienced non-ordinary perceptions claimed that they occurred frequently, and more than 85% said they occurred before the age of 18, with 52% indicating first occurrence between the ages of 12 and 17 years and 31% between ages 6 and 12 years.[5,40]

Current Pediatric Use

If the absence of literature is an accurate indicator, there is very little use of explicit spiritual approaches in pediatric care. However, increasingly families, healthcare providers, and educators are looking for alternatives for their children, and a few areas do appear in the literature.[11-13,23] For example, the use of meditation or other contemplative practices derived from spiritual traditions demonstrates the potential for behavioral change and even enhanced school performance.[42] Likewise, contemplative practices such as mindfulness have been applied in chronic pain situations and specifically with children.[19] Pediatric oncology, because of the imminent existential considerations raised by the presence of a dying child, has sometimes explored questions of meaning or "ultimate concern" explicitly.[43]

In response to TJC requirements, there is also some initiative to bring a spiritually oriented assessment and treatment to behavioral health.[44]

Some families and providers regularly use religious support and/or prayer, dream work, distant healing, spiritual guides, and many other methods in a variety of situations. It is difficult to assess prevalence, as most of them are anecdotal accounts and do not make their way into clinical reports or academic journals.

Contraindications

Most spiritual approaches present little chance for harm. However, two considerations must be taken into account for optimal spiritual healing: the conflict between the practitioner's methodology and the family's worldview, and the practitioner's intent versus conventional goal for healing. Parents may not accept some spiritual methodology, such as the notion of past life regression, or they may be suspicious of meditative practice. The conventional practitioner's goal of treatment is usually clearly delineated, such as remission of tumor or improving concentration. The spiritual intent of treatment may be larger than physical healing, such as prescribing healing guided by the benevolence of the universe. This is a bit tricky in a culture that emphasizes individual will and a science built on achieving control and predictability.

Spirituality alone is contraindicated in acute and dangerous conditions, such as an asthma attack or a serious infection. In these situations, spirituality may complement other modalities. In chronic situations, when a physical problem has emerged over a period of time and has physical symptoms as well as manifestations in other levels (e.g., subtle energy, social/family, spiritual), a multimodal approach can include spirituality.

It is important not to reduce spirituality to the level of a technique. Doing so uses the shell and leaves the nut behind. Spirituality is better understood as a way of being, rather than a tool. A spiritual healthcare provider may want to first consider his or her own spiritual life and its intersection with the patient. How does spirituality reorient healing? One common spiritual principle is that of interconnection. From revelatory moments of unity to compassionate concern for others, there is a common recognition that all life is interconnected. Recognition of interdependence is also increasingly being confirmed in spheres outside of spirituality, from ecology to quantum physics to global economics. This principle plays out in a variety of ways in the healing professions. For example, an attitude of caring versus simply technical curing may be an important shift in bringing spirituality to medicine. In an interdependent and multidimensional world, the intention and attitude of the healthcare provider may influence the well-being and ultimate cure of the patient. This shifts from a more Newtonian principle of "doing to" (curing) to a more interactive partnership, one that looks more like "being with." Through a lens of interdependence, one may even see that a particular patient has something to offer us. For example, caregivers of dying children are sometimes stunned by the lessons of courage, compassion, or wisdom offered by their young charges. One might even speculate that in some mysterious fashion a child's illness provides some healing lesson for those who care for him or her. A spiritual perspective opens all sorts of possibilities.

References

General Mind/Body

1. Pelletier K: *Mind as healer, mind as slayer,* St Lawrence, 1977, Delacorte Press.
2. Haggerty R, Roughman K, Pless I: *Child health in the community,* ed 2, New Brunswick, NJ, Transaction, 1993.
3. Sobel DS: The cost effectiveness of mind-body medicine interventions, *Prog Brain Res* 122:393-412, 2000.
4. Shannon S, editor: *Handbook of complementary and alternative therapies in mental health,* San Diego, 2002, Academic Press.
5. Pelletier K: *The best alternative medicine,* New York, 2000, Simon & Schuster.
6. Bakal D: *Minding the body: clinical applications of somatic awareness,* New York, 1999, Guilford Press.
7. Davies TA: Comprehensive approach to primary care medicine: mind and body in the clinic. In Moss D, McGrady V, Davies T et al, editors: *Handbook of mind-body medicine for primary care.* Thousand Oaks, Calif, 2003, Sage.
8. Pelletier K: Mind-body medicine in ambulatory care: an evidence-based assessment, *J Ambul Care Manage* 278:25-42, 2004.
9. Attanasio V et al: Clinical issues in utilizing biofeedback with children, *Clin Biofeed Health* 8:134-141, 1985.

Hypnosis

1. Scharff L, Marcus D, Masek B: A controlled study of minimal-contact thermal biofeedback treatment in children with migraine, *J Pediatr Psychol* 27:109-119, 2002.
2. Olness K, Libbey P: Unrecognized biologic bases of behavioral symptoms in patients referred for hypnotherapy, *Am J Clin Hypnos* 30:1-8, 1987.

General Mind/Body and Hypnosis Suggested Readings

Culbert T, Banez G. Pediatric applications other than headache. In Schwartz M, Andrasik F: *Biofeedback: a practitioner's guide,* New York, 2003, Guilford Press.

Olness K, Kohen D: *Hypnosis and hypnotherapy with children,* ed3, New York, 1996, Guilford Press.

Schwartz M, Andrasik F: *Biofeedback: a practitioner's guide,* ed3, New York, 2003, Guilford Press.

Spirituality in Pediatric Care

1. Armstrong T: *The radiant child,* Wheaton, Ill, 1985, Theosophical.
2. Hart T: *The secret spiritual world of children,* Makawao, Hawaii, 2003, Inner Ocean.
3. Hay D, Nye R: *The spirit of the child, London,* 1998, Fount/Harper Collins.
4. Hoffman E: *Visions of innocence: spiritual and inspirational experiences of childhood,* Boston, 1992, Shambhala.
5. Nelson PL, Hart T: A survey of recalled childhood spiritual and non-ordinary experiences, *Int J Child Spiritual* (in press).
6. Piechowski M: Childhood spirituality, *J Transpersonal Psychol* 33:1-15, 2001.
7. Robinson E: *Living the questions: studies in the childhood of religious experience,* Oxford, 1978, The Religious Experience Research Unit, Manchester College.
8. Robinson E: *The original vision: a study of the religious experience of childhood,* New York, 1983, Seabury Press.
9. Goldman R: *Religious thinking from childhood to adolescence,* London, 1964, Routledge Kegan & Paul.
10. Wilber K: *The Atman project: a transpersonal view of human development,* Wheaton, Ill, 1996, Quest.
11. Houskamp BM, Fisher LA, Stuber ML: Spirituality in children and adolescents: research findings and implications for clinicians and researchers, *Child Adolesc Psychiatr Clin N Am* 13:221-230, 2004.
12. Barnes LL, Plotnikoff GA, Fox K, et al: Spirituality, religion, and pediatrics: intersecting worlds of healing, *Pediatrics* 106 (4 suppl):899-908, 2000.
13. Hiatt JF: Spirituality, medicine, and healing, *South Med J* 79:736-743, 1986.
14. Dillon JJ: The spiritual child: appreciating children's transformative effects on adults, *Encounter Edu Meaning Social Justice* 13:4-18, 2000.
15. James W: *The varieties of religious experience,* New York, 1936, The Modern Library.
16. Hart T, Nelson P, Puhakka K, editors: *Transpersonal knowing: exploring the horizon of consciousness,* Albany, NY, 2000, State University of New York Press.
17. Allport G: *The individual and his religion,* New York, 1955, MacMillan.
18. Levin DM. Meaning and history of the body: toward a postmodern medicine, *Noetic Sci Rev* 33:5-11, 1995.
19. Kabat-Zinn J: *Full catastrophe living: using the wisdom of your body and mind to face stress, pain, and illness,* New York, 1990, Dell.
20. Dossey L. *Reinventing medicine: beyond mind-body to a new era of healing,* San Francisco, 1999, Harper.
21. Regardie I: *The philosopher's stone,* St Paul, Minn, 1970, Llewellyn.
22. Dossey L: *Living words: the power of prayer and the practice of medicine,* San Francisco, 1995, Harper.
23. O'Hara DP: Is there a role for prayer and spirituality in health care? *Med Clin North Am* 86:33-46, vi, 2002 [review].
24. Stevenson I: *Twenty cases suggestive of reincarnation,* Charlottesville, Va, 1974, University Press of Virginia.
25. Stevenson I: *Children who remember previous lives,* Charlottesville, Va, 1987, University Press of Virginia.
26. Bowman C: *Children's past lives: how past life memories affect your child,* New York, 1997, Bantam Books.
27. Dunn CM: *Religion that harms, religion that heals,* Wilmington, Del, 2002, Crimson Light Books.
28. Frankl VE: *Man's search for meaning,* New York, 1971, Washington Square Press.
29. Tillich P: *Dynamics of faith,* New York, 1957, Harper & Row.
30. Underhill E: *Mysticism,* New York, 1961, EP Dutton.
31. Atwater PMH: *Children of the new millennium: children's near-death experiences and the evolution of humankind,* New York, 1999, Three Rivers Press.
32. Hoffman ML: Empathy and justice motivation, *Motivation Emotion* 14:151-172, 1990.
33. Ayers JA: *Sensory integration and the child,* Los Angeles, 1994, Western Psychological Services.
34. Dabrowski K: On the philosophy of development through positive disintegration and secondary integration, *Dialectics Humanism* 3-4:131-144, 1976.
35. von Bertalanffy L: *General systems theory: foundations, development, applications,* New York, 1968, George Braziller.
36. Campbell J, Moyers B: *The power of myth,* Garden City, NY, 1991, Anchor.
37. Rumi: *The essential Rumi,* San Francisco, 1995, Harper (Translated by C Barks, J Moyne, AJ Arberry et al).
38. Scholem GG, editor: *Zohar: the book of splendor,* New York, 1995, Schocken.
39. Michio K: *Hyperspace,* New York, 1994, Oxford University Press.
40. Liester MB: Inner voices: distinguishing transcendent and pathological characteristics, *J Transpersonal Psychol* 28:1, 1996.

41. Nelson PL, Hart T: *A survey of recalled childhood spiritual and non-ordinary experiences: age, rate and psychological factors associated with their occurrence.* Available at: www.socialscienceservices.com/papers/Nelson-Hart.pdf. Accessed August 26, 2004.

42. Hart T: Opening the contemplative mind in the classroom, *J Transform Edu* 2:28-46, 2004.

43. Kuttner L: *No fears, no tears,* Harriman, NY, 1985, Fanlight Productions.

44. Hart T, Waddell A: *Spiritual issues in counseling and psychotherapy: toward assessment and treatment.* Available at www.childspirit.net/hart%20and%20waddell.pdf. Accessed August 26, 2004.

CHAPTER 3

Manual Therapies

Chiropractic | Anne Spicer
Massage Therapy | Mary C. McLellan

Osteopathy | Jane Carreiro
Psychology | Anna Tobia

Chiropractic

History

According to David D. Palmer in his text *Three Generations: A Brief History of Chiropractic*, chiropractic was founded in 1895 by his grandfather Daniel David Palmer, intimately known as "D.D."[1] When his wife died, leaving him with three small children, D.D. set out to find the cause of disease. He felt certain that disease came from within the body and that this must also be where the cure lies. D.D. surmised that if the nerves from the brain, through the spine, controlled organ function, then it would be possible that irritation to the nerve at the vertebral level could interrupt and alter normal organ function. He then reasoned that it was possible for these spinal vertebrae to have abnormal positioning that may cause this irritation. Furthermore, if this were true, then realigning the vertebra could enhance normal organ function, thereby reducing disease.

D.D. called this misalignment the chiropractic *subluxation*. This differed from the medical *luxation*, which referred to a dislocated joint. The subluxation was somewhat less than a partial dislocation. The root meaning of the term *sub-* derives from "less" or "low" and *lux* from "light," equating to "a state of having less light." D.D. stated that "every act and thought is controlled by nerves; they furnish the life of the body."[2] Also, he said that "we are well when the... nerves are free to act."[2] Disease, he reasoned, occurred when impingement from the subluxation interfered with the ability of the nerve to transmit impulses from brain to body and body to brain. The body then could only do its best with incomplete or erroneous information, creating a situation of disease or less than optimum health.

As much as D.D. was the discoverer of chiropractic, Bartlett Joshua (B.J.) was its developer. Together they established the Palmer School of Chiropractic (PSC). B.J. also spread the word of the science behind chiropractic to multitudes through print and radio. Through his own print media, B.J.'s clear writing engendered chiropractic treatment of infants and children with typhoid, diphtheria, polio, and the like.[2] (Reportedly, very ill children recovered after the neurologically restorative spinal adjustment.) Largely due to the lifetime efforts of B.J. Palmer, the PSC, now Palmer College of Chiropractic, continues to flourish at the original building site today as well as at campuses in Florida and California, with approximately 30,000 graduates to date.[4]

Although the early chiropractic education taught only the science and application of the adjustment, nutritional considerations and other musculoskeletal techniques are now commonly used supportively to the adjustment and toward the better health of the patient. Some chiropractors also incorporate other natural care procedures such as craniosacral therapy, homeopathic remedies, herbal remedies, and acupuncture as well as electrical therapies such as ultrasound, electromuscle stimulation, and cold laser.

Legalization

In order to define and regulate the practice of chiropractic, each state establishes rules and licensure through a state board or other state licensing body.

Proliferation

To date, there are 17 accredited chiropractic colleges in the United States, five of which are incorporated into universities, although all but the University of Bridgeport were first established with a chiropractic college as its central focus.[5]

There are six colleges of chiropractic in the United Kingdom and two colleges each in Australia, Canada, and South Africa. Brazil, Denmark, France, Japan, Korea, and New Zealand each have one college of chiropractic. Most of these international colleges function within already established universities.

The agency that accredits U.S. chiropractic colleges is the Council on Chiropractic Education (CCE), an accrediting body recognized by the U.S. Department of Education.

Education

A chiropractor must meet stringent criteria in academics, competency examinations, and ongoing professional requirements. The requirements for admission to an accredited college of chiropractic include a minimum of 2 years or 90 hours of undergraduate science-focused courses, with some states requiring a 4-year degree to be considered for licensure.

The chiropractic degree program consists of a minimum of 4200 hours of classroom, laboratory, and clinical experience. These courses are focused on basic and clinical sciences as well as other health-related subjects. This program includes approximately 550 hours of specific instruction devoted to spinal analysis and adjustment techniques.

Chiropractors in practice take a history including presenting symptoms, previous and other medical history, trauma history, family history, review of systems, lifestyle, diet, and exercise habits. The chiropractic examination includes inspection, auscultation, and palpation of joints, muscles, and indicated organ; orthopedic examination; and primary neurological examination. Where indicated, chiropractors will take or order radiographs or advanced imaging as well as laboratory studies. Chiropractors are trained to refer to a variety of health-care providers.

Chiropractic Licensure

In preparation for licensure, students and doctors must pass the nationally standardized examinations set by the National Board of Chiropractic Examiners, along with any additional examinations required by the state in which they wish to practice. Individual states may also have other requirements for licensure. The National Board of Chiropractic Examiners (NBCE) has developed and delivered four levels of nationally standardized examinations. Part I covers basic science subjects. Part II is a clinical science examination. Parts I and II are available to chiropractors or students in a chiropractic degree program who have completed the requisite coursework. Parts I and II are required by all states. Part III of the NBCE examination is a written clinical competency exam. Since 1993 the NBCE has offered Part IV (a practical clinical competency evaluation) of the nationalized examinations. Passage of Part IV is accepted by 47 states and the District of Columbia as adequate assurance of competency.[6] Individual states may require additional proof of competency, primarily in state legal issues pertaining to chiropractic, but typically reciprocity is garnered between states that accept Part IV as a licensing requirement.

Theory

A multitude of articles and entire textbooks have been written to describe the theories of chiropractic. To understand chiropractic care of children, one must first understand the view of health that doctors of chiropractic hold true: health is a dynamic continuum in every body at all times, not merely a lack of illness or disease. The body is in a continual attempt to balance its internal and external environments to maintain the best possible health status under the given circumstance. The body is responsive to both great and subtle changes in these environments and responds appropriately in time and fashion when optimal health exists. This attempt at homeostasis is the health of the organism: the more able the body is to maintain homeostasis, the healthier it is. The less able the body is to balance itself, the unhealthier it is. When less than optimal health is the state of affairs with the body, the response may be too much or too little to create the necessary change, or it may be too rapid or too slow. Asthma, for instance, is an overreaction of mucous production in the bronchioles. If asthma is a child's only challenge, he or she may be commonly considered a healthy individual. The chiropractor would place the child's health at least a notch down on the health continuum.

The person's position on the health continuum may not be readily noticeable. For instance, by the time a person has symptoms of pancreatic cancer, they are often at the brink of death. On the other hand, an ingrown toenail can be red, swollen, quite painful, and perhaps even debilitating, but rarely is life threatening. Therefore the chiropractor does not rely solely on symptoms to determine the vital health of the individual.

It is understood by the chiropractor that every encounter has influence over the body and its neurobiochemical fluctuations.

A cool breeze will cause the body to regulate temperature. Approach by a hostile person will cause the hormonal levels to shift. Eating spoiled food will trigger an immune reaction. With this understanding, a chiropractor does not view fever, vomiting, and anxiety as abnormal signs, but signs of a healthy body doing the work only it knows how to do for itself. Support of this body regulation is the rule, as chiropractors consider any attempt to suppress or counter the body's own self-regulation to be a direct interference to healthy body function. (Of course, this is a simplification of the balance between health and disease, as extreme situations do occur that require measures to maintain life while addressing underlying causes.) Now, having said this, what about the child who has daily episodes of vomiting without evidence of immune attack? Chiropractors see this as the body having lost its ability to self-regulate within physiologic parameters—a state of less than optimal health. Many causal factors can be surmised, although the chiropractic approach is to say that the body must require this vomiting based on internal feedback and regulation. A doctor of chiropractic will attempt to rule out organic causes of this condition and then will look to the nervous system for interference to optimal self-regulation.

Chiropractors understand that the health continuum can be influenced long before symptoms, degeneration, and disease are apparent. To the chiropractor, maintaining health is a higher goal than managing symptoms. This focus on prevention is a large portion of the chiropractic management.

At the hub of chiropractic management is identification of the subluxation complex (SC). The existence of the SC has been established by science.[7] The SC is described as an abnormal functional, structural, or pathological relationship between adjacent joints, which has a neurological effect to some degree and may influence organ systems or general health.[8] Perhaps the most prevalent of current theories espouses that the SC has several foundational components, including the following:

- Kinesiopathology
- Neuropathology
- Myopathology
- Histopathology
- Biochemical abnormalities

Although not all components need be identified to classify the condition as an SC,[9] these abnormalities generally exist and may also include local vascular changes. It is impossible to separate the individual components of the SC owing to the nature of body physiology. Any component can be the primary initiating factor of an SC and its consequences. For instance, inflammatory states at the spinal level or within organ systems alter the body's responses at a biochemical and cellular level, affecting a degenerative cascade and disrupting the normal joint physiology. This then can lead to muscle contracture; affect other local tissues such as tendons, cartilage, ligaments, articular capsule, or bone; and necessarily afferently stimulate the nervous system.[9]

Causes of the pediatric SC are varied. Evidence suggests that in utero constraint due to an abnormal fetal position can result in biomechanical stressors on the cartilagenous framework of the baby and, left unaddressed, can have lasting impact such as torticollis and scoliosis.[10] Even the normal birth process has been demonstrated to cause considerable disruption to the musculoskeletal system.[11–14] Accidental injury can occur any time after birth and result in an enduring SC. Chemical exposure (including food allergens) can result in a viscerosomatic SC. Emotional stressors have also been known to underlie the SC.

Evidence-Based Support

The science supporting the chiropractic theories grows annually. This literature helps to shed light on the importance of the SC in the management and prevention of disease as well as the enhancement of health. Understanding the neurology of the joint is an important starting point.

The two main types of sensory receptors in the joints are mechanoreceptors (pacinian Ruffini and Meissner's corpuscles, Merkel's receptors, muscle spindles, and Golgi tendon organs) and nociceptors. The mechanoreceptors are abundant in the joint but may also be found in surrounding tissue such as the intervertebral disc,[15,16] local blood vessels, and spinal ligaments.[17-19] The mechanoreceptors fire based on physiological movement and touch. Joint mechanoreceptors directly synapse to the thalamus, cerebellum, and brainstem, establishing a coordinated reflexive feedback to striated musculature in various parts of the body.[20] Mechanoreceptors also serve to inhibit nociception at the spinal cord. The nociceptors fire based on noxious mechanical stimulation or presence of chemical mediators as a result of local tissue injury. Mechanoreceptors and nociceptors have no direct influence over joint movement, but instead provide afferent information to the higher centers as to the physiological state of the joint.

The nociceptors synapse from the cord directly to the thalamus, which then relays nociceptive information to the hypothalamus, amygdala, and cortex.[21] The hypothalamus reads the internal well-being of the body and, under nociceptive stress, stimulates the pituitary hormones.[22] Facilitation of the amygdala releases corticosteroids and catecholamines,[22] initiating a fear/anxiety/stress response in the organ systems as well as cognitively and emotionally.[23] It is only when (and if) the nociception reaches the cortex that the individual feels pain. Pain is the conscious perception of nociceptive input to the cortex. Abnormal afferentation can and does occur in the absence of pain. Compromised afferent input may in turn compromise efferent response.[7] It is imperative that accurate afferent information remain constant to the central nervous system in order for the body to accurately perceive and respond to the internal and external environments.

Nociceptive facilitation has the capacity to become habitual[24] and self-perpetuating for as long as 4 years after removal of the original insult, depending on severity and duration.[25,26] Muscle control at the injured joint is also disordered (myopathology), creating instability.[27] This may be due to a significantly diminished position sense postinjury.[28] Pertinence in early detection and removal of dysafferentation due to SC is suggested. Slosberg states, "It is important to respond to repetitive noxious stimuli because it may cause progressive tissue damage."[29] Chiropractic adjustments to restore joint movement and enhance mechanoreception may be vital in rehabilitation of an injured joint.[30,31]

One cause of this nociceptive facilitation may be immobilization of a joint. Continual stimulation of the mechanoreceptors by restricted joint motion (kinesiopathology) causes an increase in the firing of nociceptors and a decrease in the firing of the mechanoreceptors.[29,32,33] This dysafferentation from an SC reflexively activates a response in the sympathetic nervous system.[34-36] This somatoautonomic response may cause seemingly unrelated symptoms such as sweating, pallor, nausea, vomiting, abdominal pain, sinus congestion, dyspnea, cardiac palpitations, and chest pain.[37,38] In infants, this immobilization-induced dysafferentation may present as irritability and sleeplessness[39] and may predispose to bradycardic apnea.[40] It is also important to note that infants and children require movement for proper brain development.[41] Lack of movement generally in children is associated with such changes as intellectual inefficiency, bizarre thoughts, exaggerated emotional reactions, and unusual bodily sensations due to decreased afferent stimulation of the cerebellum.[41]

In addition to the systemic effects of joint immobilization on the autonomic nervous system, local tissues also affected include the articular cartilage[42] and capsule, synovium, periarticular ligaments, subchondral bone, intervertebral discs, and meninges.[43] Afferent stimulation also results in reflexive contraction of the local musculature (myopathology).[44,45] Long-term effects of joint immobilization include degeneration (histopathology) of intervertebral discs, decreased bone density, deficient ligamentous collagen density, muscular atrophy, irreversible joint changes within 8 weeks, and even cardiopulmonary sequelae.[46-49] Although immobilization kinesiopathology leads directly to degeneration of the joint, hypomobility has been known to lead to a compensatory hypermobility in contiguous joints.[50] These effects make the SC a concern for the longevity of the joints and the health of the individual. The degree and permanence of the degeneration from an SC is greatly dependent upon the degree and duration of kinesiopathology. In some cases, complete reversal of degenerative change is possible.[51-53]

Chiropractors have also long discussed the "pinched nerve" hypothesis of neuropathology. Although pinching clearly does not occur in an average subluxation, an SC in the spine has the ability to cause nerve root compression.[54] Pressure on the root of as little as 10 mm Hg causes a nerve conduction block,[55] whereas as little as 5 mm Hg decreases blood flow to spinal roots.[56] This nerve conduction block and venous congestion, with subsequent diminished nutrient exchange, lead to local inflammatory changes and sympathetic stimulation.[57] Histological evidence associating the SC with pathologies of the gastrointestinal tract, heart, lung, uterus, and other organ systems[58-62] may be sequelae of this cascade of events. Removal of this pressure results in some level of recovery, although with diminishing levels of recovery at higher levels of pressure or when applied for longer durations.[55,63,64] Because it is clear that spinal root compression can occur without the presence of pain,[57] evaluation for SC prior to irreversible root damage is appropriate.

Science makes clear that the SC is a correctable condition. Stimulation of mechanoreceptors through the chiropractic adjustment reduces abnormal nociceptive afferents and their impact on the autonomic system. The chiropractic adjustment also restores normal joint motion, which reduces autonomic response and minimizes or reverses degenerative change. Therefore management of the SC by the chiropractor is the highest priority. The chiropractor uses a high-velocity, low-amplitude thrust to the affected joint to reestablish normal joint motion. The smaller the child, the lower the amplitude and velocity necessary to make the desired correction.

The importance of the SC in the health of the child can be understood through the concepts of neuropathology called *dysafferentation*, through the effects of kinesiopathology with its subsequent myopathology and degeneration, and through the physiological mechanisms of the inflammatory response.

Current Pediatric Use

Chiropractors have been evaluating and treating children since the origin of the profession more than 100 years ago.[2] Specific courses in pediatrics have been taught at the chiropractic colleges nearly since their inception.[65]

Of those children who use alternative healthcare, the modality most commonly sought is that of chiropractic at 36%. Although approximately 80% of adult visits to the chiropractor are for musculoskeletal conditions, Spigelblatt et al. found that 60% of childhood visits to chiropractors are for respiratory or ear, nose, and throat conditions. Twenty-two percent of visits are for musculoskeletal conditions, and approximately 4% to 9% each are for skin, gastrointestinal, and allergy-related conditions.[66]

An interesting statistic exposed in this study was that a child was more likely to require hospital services when that child did not participate in alternative healthcare modalities.

The NBCE has published a job analysis of chiropractic in which 18% of the patient population of U.S. chiropractors were children ages newborn to 17 years.[67] According to statistics derived in part from the job analysis of chiropractic, an estimated 23 million visits per year have been made to chiropractors by pediatric patients in the United States alone.[68] A summary estimate of the total number of visits between 1966 and 1998 was calculated by Richard Pistolese to be 502,184,156.[69]

Because the average spine doubles in length in the first 5 years of life,[70] the chiropractic effort to evaluate children in infancy and early childhood is motivated by an interest in prevention of long-term challenges to the neuromuscular system, chronic degeneration, and subsequent health consequences due to the uncorrected SC. The spine requires periodic maintenance by the chiropractor to ensure normal motion and minimize fibrosis, contracture, adhesions, deformity, structural derangements,[71] and their neurological sequelae.

Safety

In any care modality, the benefits must always outweigh the risks to the patient. Chiropractic care for the pediatric patient is exceedingly safe. The most commonly reported and arguably the most serious injury allegedly associated with the chiropractic adjustment is that of neurological and/or vertebrobasilar incidence/stroke after an adjustment to the cervical spine. The incidence of stroke in children from all possible causes reaches 2.7 per 100,000,[72] but it is rare that pediatric stroke would result from a vertebral artery dissection.[73]

During the past nearly 40 years, only two cases have been reported in the literature inferring injury to a child from a chiropractic adjustment to the cervical spine. The first case was that of a 7 year old with reports of headaches and intermittent cranial nerve abnormalities.[74] The child was being seen regularly by a chiropractor, who provided adjustments to the cervical spine, while the child was also simultaneously participating in a rigorous gymnastics program. It was determined that the child was suffering from vertebral artery thrombosis, and the physicians suggested that the stretching of the cervical soft tissues by the chiropractor was causal. It is interesting to note that the literature supports incidence of vertebral obstruction in athletes who perform hyperextensions of the neck.[75] This makes the link between the chiropractic adjustment and the child's condition tenuous at best.

The second case was a child who was examined by a chiropractor as an infant with a chief complaint of torticollis.[76] It was later discovered that the child had a spinal cord tumor in the cervical spine. The child subsequently became quadriplegic. The question still remains as to whether the adjustments or the tumor itself was responsible for the paralysis.

Assessment of the risks is especially prudent in light of the continually growing interest in complimentary care modalities for pediatric patients. Assessment of risk, however, requires that certain data be available for review. In the field of chiropractic, few data exist to quantify the number of adjustments given annually to pediatric patients. With the millions of chiropractic visits by children, it is reassuring to find only two cases on record of suspected injury. According to Pistolese, this puts the risk of neurological and/or vertebrobasilar injury at 1 in every 250 million visits.[69]

This author recommends that all infants and children be evaluated by a chiropractor to rule out the presence of the SC. There may in fact be a protective benefit to having an infant evaluated for the need of an adjustment. Even a mild mechanical irritation at the upper cervical spine can lead to severe bradycardia, possibly followed by apnea, which are common cofactors in the development of sudden infant death syndrome. The younger the infant, the more severe the effect. "Chiropractic treatment seems to be the most successful therapy which helps to treat such disorders,"[40] said Kocha, who reported 20,000 children safely treated with chiropractic. The mechanical irritation can be corrected with the chiropractic adjustment to prevent devastating permanent consequences.

Massage Therapy

History

The medical use of therapeutic massage has been documented in historical texts as early as 2000 BCE by the ancient Egyptians, Chinese, Japanese, Persians, Greeks, Romans, Incas, and Mayans.[1,2] During the Middle Ages, European knowledge of massage therapy remained only within folk traditions until the seventeenth century when French doctors began incorporating massage into postoperative care.[2] In the eighteenth century, Per Henrik Ling of Sweden expanded upon the French techniques.[1,2] Under his direction, the Royal Gymnastic Central Institute of Stockholm established the professional practice of what is now referred to as *Swedish massage*.[1] Swedish massage is defined as "the systematic and scientific manipulation of the soft tissues of the body"[1] that integrates movement with anatomy and physiology into a systematic approach of therapy. By the turn of the 20th century, medical texts, animal studies, and clinical trials on the effects of massage had been published.[1-4]

Unfortunately, the recreational use of nontherapeutic massage in brothels became prevalent in the late 1800s, discrediting the legitimacy of the therapy. Inconsistencies in massage training as well as the unsubstantiated and unethical claims touted by lay massage practitioners resulted in such scandals that massage therapy fell out of favor in the medical community.[2] Even today the massage profession battles the stigma inflicted upon it. A renewed interest in massage as a therapy occurred in response to the physical disabilities that occurred from the polio epidemic of 1918.[2] Over the next 30 years, other modalities within the Swedish massage framework were developed and investigated: connective tissue massage, manual lymphatic drainage, friction massage, and proprioceptive neuromuscular facilitation (Table 3-1).[2]

The focus on physical fitness and preventive medicine during the 1960s demonstrated benefits of exercise and massage for conditioning and stress reduction, resulting in incorporation of massage techniques into sports medicine practice.[2]

Exposure of Western medicine to acupuncture in the 1970s led to controlled clinical trials of acupressure during the 1970s and 1980s.[2] Nursing and rehabilitation medicine also began examining the therapeutic uses of massage for decubitus ulcer prevention[2] and as an adjunct to physical therapy. In the 1980s, the gate control theory of pain and its application to massage and cryotherapy (application of ice) for pain management[2] made its debut and substantiated the efficacy and application of massage. Medical advances in unraveling the mechanism of endorphin release through sensory hyperstimulation of the tissues also added evidence-based application of massage techniques.[2]

In the 1980s and 1990s, infant massage gained popularity. Many community hospitals offered and continue to offer prenatal and postnatal classes in infant massage for parents. Extensive randomized controlled clinical trials on the effects of massage therapy for a variety of pediatric and adult conditions were initiated under the direction of Tiffany Field, director of the Touch Therapy Institute in Miami. Some of these trials revolutionized standards of touch therapy and the introduction of touch to neonates and premature infants during hospitalization.

Licensure of massage therapists remains inconsistent in the United States; only 39 states have statewide licensure programs. The remainder of states rely on municipal regulations, which vary considerably even within a region.[5] Beginning in 1992, a national certification for massage therapists was implemented by the National Certification Board for Therapeutic Massage and Bodywork (NCBTMB) in the United States. A therapist with a minimum of 500 hours of massage education must pass a standardized exam to be certified. Recertification requires a minimum of 50 hours of continuing education credits and 200 hours of massage treatments every 4 years.[6] The American Massage Therapy Association maintains a Code of Ethics for Massage to be observed by members and grants membership

to massage therapists with at least 500 hours of massage education.[5] Additionally, the American Organization for Bodywork Therapies of Asia (AOBTA) offers membership for therapists with more than 500 hours of massage education from an AOBTA-approved school.[6]

Theory and Effects

The effects of therapeutic massage are psychological, mechanical, physiological, and reflexive.[1] Although many schools of thought exist as to the approach and application of massage techniques, modalities follow the basic principles of Swedish massage:

- *Effleurage*: Long, broad strokes to warm up the body's broad muscles to facilitate stretching; provides a passive stretch to the muscles or muscle groups to which it is applied; stimulates parasympathetic responses of the body.[1]
- *Petrissage*: Kneading or compression action to relax and stretch the muscles; softens the connective tissue (i.e., fascia, tendons) around the muscles by creating more space within the tissues.[1,2]
- *Tapotement*: Percussion to activate the tendon reflexes that assist with relaxation of spastic and/or tense muscle groups. Superficial tapotement initially causes cutaneous blood vessel contraction followed by dilatation from histamine, which may enhance the effects of cryotherapy.[2]
- *Friction*: Deep pressure applied in a cross-fiber direction to loosen subcutaneous and restrictive connective tissue.[2]
- *Vibration*: Gentle and rhythmic vibration applied to large muscle groups to promote relaxation.[1]

Basic scientific laws of anatomy and physiology are used to assess and determine the proper application of these techniques (Table 3-2).[2] Based on these laws and controlled clinical trials, the effects of massage therapy are as follows:

1. *Assists circulation to the soft tissues.* Active, healthy muscles provide a pumping action that assists venous return.[1] In the setting of weak or inactive muscles, this action may be less efficient, resulting in vasostasis. Massage may be an effective therapy to reduce vasostasis in individuals with impaired mobility by mechanically providing the pumping action in the direction of venous return. It is also theorized that massage techniques have a direct action on the vessel walls through a reflex action of the vasomotor nerves causing relaxation and constriction of the vessels that improves venous return.[1] A study on the effects of massage on arterial blood flow and diameter demonstrated no change measured by Doppler.[8] However, studies on effects on venous flow are lacking.

    Muscle cells maintain a metabolic homeostasis through the arrival of arterial flow of nutrients and the venous removal of muscle byproducts.[1] During episodes of overactivity, there is insufficient time for adequate inflow of nutrients while simultaneously producing excessive waste products,[1] resulting in delayed-onset muscle soreness. Although massage following exercise-induced muscle injury has demonstrated no effect on blood lactate levels, range of motion (ROM), muscle torque, or electomyographic activity, it did significantly lower fatigue indexes and soreness intensity.[8-12]

2. *Assists lymphatic flow.* Lymphatic vessels are noncontractile, relying partly on muscular contraction for lymphatic

✳ **TABLE 3-1**

Types of Massage Therapy

TYPE	DEFINITION	OTHER COMMON NAMES
Connective tissue massage	Mechanically softening the connective tissue through pressure, pulling, movement, and stretch on the tissues to rebalance the body by releasing tension in the fascia	Myofascial release* Mechanical link Myofascial mobilization Soft tissue mobilization
Deep tissue massage	Releases chronic patterns of tension in the body through slow strokes and deep pressure on the contracted areas, either following or going across the grain of muscles, tendons and fascia; focuses on the deeper layers of muscle tissue; applies concentrated pressure to "trigger points" to break cycles of spasm and pain	Trigger point therapy*
Lymphatic drainage	Applies light, short pumping strokes toward lymphatic drainage points to stimulate lymphatic flow	Lymphatic drainage therapy Manual lymphatic drainage
Neuromuscular therapy	Applies principles of reciprocal innervation, tonus receptor activation, reflex arc and positional receptor stimulation, and the application of stretching and lengthening to treat specific muscle groups	Myotherapy Neuromuscular facilitation* Muscle energy techniques Strain/counterstrain
Oriental bodywork	Oriental-based systems of finger pressure and massage to treat special points along acupuncture meridians; composed of compressive manipulations and stretches	Shiatsu Acupressure Tui-na* AMMA Thai massage Jin Shin Do Watsu
Energy approaches	Light touch to initiate reflexive responses and restore energy balance; based on ancient concepts of body energy	Reflexology* Therapeutic touch* Reiki* Rosen Method Zero balancing
Sports massage*	Focuses on muscle systems relevant to a particular sport to improve or restore function; can be used to stimulate the body for performance or as an adjunct to sports injury rehabilitation	
Structural integration	Balances the body within gravity through techniques involving manual soft tissue manipulation, joint mobilization, stretching, and exercises	Rolfing Trager psychophysical integration Bindegewebs massage Hellerwork Soma
Swedish massage*	Systematic and scientific manipulation of the body's tissue (NOTE: Technically, most massage types may be encompassed within Swedish massage)	Relaxation massage Therapeutic massage

*These therapies are readily adapted to infant and pediatric massage treatments.

flow.[1] Muscle immobilization from injury or denervation may interfere with lymphatic drainage, resulting in edema.[1] Although muscle activity is the most beneficial for lymphatic flow, slow, rhythmic massage may be a mechanical substitute when active exercise in not feasible.[1]

3. *Reduces edema* (see earlier discussion of stasis-induced edemas). In the case of injury, massage applied proximal to the injury site may help decrease swelling after the acute injury phase. Of note, pitting edema potentially compromises the integrity of the affected tissues, and massage can damage this fragile tissue. Massage therapy is contraindicated over areas of pitting edema.

4. *Prevents adhesions.* Fibrosis can occur in immobilized, injured or denervated muscles, resulting in contractures through the formation of subcutaneous scar tissue. This restrictive connective tissue leads to decreased ROM and sometimes pain. Stretching, ROM exercises, and massage application of friction may help to reform the connective tissue matrix to decrease restriction and improve mobility.

✳ **TABLE 3-2**

Scientific Laws Incorporated into Massage Theory

All-or-none law	Once sufficient stimuli are applied, a predicted response will occur. Even the weakest of stimuli will produce the maximum response.
Law of specificity of nervous energy	Excitation of a receptor always gives rise to the same sensation regardless of the nature of the stimuli.
Hilton's law	A nerve trunk that supplies a joint also supplies the muscles of the joint and the skin over the muscle insertions.
Law of symmetry	If stimulation is sufficiently increased, motor reaction is manifested not only in the side stimulated, but also in a similar manner on the opposite side of the body.
Gate control theory	Pain impulses may be overridden by other stimuli through activation of the large-diameter nerve fibers to the area. Counterirritation can produce an analgesic effect.
Reciprocal innervation	When one muscle group contracts, the antagonist muscle must relax.

From Fritz S: *Mosby's fundamentals of therapeutic massage,* St Louis, 1995, Mosby.

5. *Assists with muscle rehabilitation.* Although massage therapy may not prevent muscle mass loss or strength due to injury, it may accelerate voluntary and reflexive actions of the muscle once reinervation is present.[1] In controlled studies comparing massage therapy with physical therapy, education, or exercise to treat neck and back pain, massage did not show increased benefit but did decrease pain cycles and increase tolerance to other approaches,[13] which suggests that massage would be a helpful adjunct to a rehabilitation plan. Controlled studies have found massage to be more effective than relaxation techniques for musculoskeletal pain reduction.[14-16] Studies comparing effectiveness of massage therapy versus traditional therapies (e.g., traditional Chinese acupuncture, self-care measures, progressive muscle relaxation, soft tissue manipulation, exercise, placebo) for chronic low back pain demonstrated massage to be more effective for reducing symptoms and improving function.[16-19] In addition, massage therapy had beneficial effects for almost a year after active treatment when used in conjuction with exercise and education.[18] A recent systematic Cochrane review of massage for low back pain concluded from the eight studies reviewed that massage therapy may be beneficial for patients with subacute and chronic low back pain, especially when combined with exercise and education.[20] A randomized controlled trial demonstrated massage therapy to be effective in improving range of motion and reducing pain in patients with chronic shoulder pain.[21] Another systematic review of 23 articles suggested there is evidence for massage therapy to be a useful approach for pain relief in numerous chronic, nonmalignant pain conditions, specifically musculoskeletal pain complaints.[22] Just as an athlete stretches before activity to prevent injury and warm the muscle groups, massage can be used to warm the tissues prior to active and passive ROM in physical therapy for maximum benefits. Massage therapy was more effective at increasing ROM and decreasing pain in patients with shoulder or back pain compared with placebo, soft tissue manipulation, posture education, or remedial exercises.[19,21]

6. *Improves skin nutrition.* Massage stimulation to the peripheral nerve endings increases vasodilatation of the cutaneous circulation and may increase sebaceous and sweat gland activity.[1] The use of massage oils or lotions during treatment may help to hydrate dry skin. (Of note, mineral oil–based massage products should be avoided, as they may clog the pores. Individuals with nut allergies should avoid nut-based oils.)

7. *Improves respiration.* Massage applied to the accessory muscles of breathing (scalenes, intercostals, serratus, diaphragm, and abdominal and leg muscles) can relax these muscles and decrease chest wall restriction. Individuals with rounded shoulders may benefit from anterior chest massage to decrease pectoral contractures that restrict lung capacity. These pectoral contractures may develop at a young age and become restrictive by school age in children with chronic pulmonary disease or abnormal neuromuscular tone. Individuals with restrictions from prolonged mechanical ventilation (see discussion of adhesion prevention) may especially benefit from these treatments. Although research has not been done on this topic, the author and her colleagues, who are experienced pediatric massage therapists working with critically and chronically ill children, have reported infants and children with chronic pulmonary disease or abnormal neuromuscular tone who have benefited from anterior chest massage. Massage improved thoracic gas volumes, peak flows, forced vital capacity, oxygen saturations, and breath-holding times in a pilot study of adults with chronic obstructive lung disease.[23] Children with reactive airway disease (asthma) or cystic fibrosis showed improved pulmonary function tests following regular massage treatments from their parents.[24,25]

8. *Reduces pain.* Pain reduction through massage therapy has several mechanisms of action. The gate control theory suggests that painful stimuli transmitted by the large- and small-diameter nerve fibers may be overridden when pressure stimulation is applied to the large-diameter fibers, inhibiting the small-diameter fibers from transmitting the painful stimuli.[2] Massage pressure applied to trigger points—areas of hypersensitive tissue—can be effective in achieving this effect.[26] Levels of plasma beta-endorphins, biochemicals produced by the body to decrease pain, have been elevated following massage treatment.[27] Improved ROM and decrease in musculoskeletal restrictions can

be beneficial in pain reduction (see earlier discussion of muscle rehabilitation). Studies have shown massage therapy to be effective in reducing pain scores[14-22, 28-40] and more effective than relaxation techniques for musculoskeletal pain reduction.[14-17,35,37] Use of massage in postoperative pain trials reduced pain scores[36,41] and, in some studies, also decreased postoperative analgesic usage.[21,42-44]

9. *Promotes relaxation and reduces stress.* Physiological indicators suggestive of relaxation and increased parasympathetic nervous system (PNS) activity have been well documented following massage therapy: decreased heart rate, systolic and diastolic blood pressures, and respiratory rates[45-49]; decreased alpha and beta wave activity on electroencephalogram readings[50,51]; and decreased saliva and blood cortisol levels.[24,38,40,51-55] In addition to promoting opportunities for relaxation, receiving massage therapy on a regular basis decreased anxiety* and depression scores† in a large number of randomized controlled trials.

10. *Stimulates the autonomic nervous system.* Physical and psychological relaxation occurs from massage stimulation of the PNS. Sports massage is one of the few massage treatments that stimulates the sympathetic nervous system (SNS), which increases musculoskeletal blood flow, catecholamines, blood sugar, and cardiac output and decreases visceral and cutaneous circulation to prepare an athlete for performance. Pressure, speed, frequency, temperature, and duration of the massage treatment are factors that influence which part of the autonomic nervous system is activated. Deep and/or maintained pressure stimulates the PNS and decreases sensitivity to touch, whereas light touch can stimulate a sympathetic response. Strokes directed toward the torso have a more relaxing effect than strokes away from the torso. Slow, rhythmic strokes increase relaxation and inhibit tone in contrast to brisk or arrhythmic strokes of sports massage, which stimulate the muscles.

11. *Improves digestion.* Stimulation of the PNS increases stomach gastrin levels, intestinal peristalsis, and circulation to the gastrointestinal tract. Direct application of massage to the abdomen assists with the mechanical action of peristalsis. In a randomized controlled trial of preterm neonates, patients had increased vagal activity during a 15-minute massage and increased gastric motility after massage, compared to controls.[61] Before the use of current medical therapies, parents of children with cystic fibrosis massaged their child's abdomen to prevent blockage. A "colic routine" is taught to parents during infant massage classes to provide comfort to their infants.

Pediatric Massage Therapy

Many cultures worldwide incorporate infant massage into their parental practices. Western use of infant massage became popular in the 1990s with many community hospitals providing parents with infant massage classes as part of their postpartum experience. Infant massage certification courses became available to massage therapists and are included in some massage

school curriculums.[62] Despite these developments, instruction or information about pediatric massage may be difficult to obtain. The topic is frequently not covered in massage school curricula owing to the complexity of pediatric massage: musculoskeletal developmental changes, behavioral considerations, and acceptance of nonparental touch are all factors in its exclusion. As a result, many massage therapists are reluctant to work on pediatric patients unless they have sought continuing education in pediatrics and the parent is present during treatment. Despite the limitation of availability, research has demonstrated massage therapy to be highly beneficial to the pediatric population. The same effects previously described for adults occur in the pediatric population, with a few additional considerations, as follows:

1. *Improves parent-child interaction.* Parents who provide massage to their chronically ill child have reported decreased parental anxiety.* Providing a beneficial therapy to their child provides parents with a sense of purpose and an opportunity to participate in their child's comfort. Communication can improve through touch interaction.[65,66]

2. *Facilitates growth and development.* Childhood development may be enhanced through PNS activation and stress reduction. Infant learning occurs best while the infant is in a quiet alert state. Studies have shown that massage increased the quiet alert states in premature infants.[67,69] Infants receiving massage increase the quantity and quality of their vocalizations during the treatment.[67] In addition, preschoolers have shown improved cognitive performance following massage treatment,[70] perhaps due to a more relaxed state that facilitates concentration.

3. *Facilitates physical therapy in children with neuromotor dysfunction.* Tactile and visual stimulation in combination with proprioceptive input can help nervous system development and enhance body awareness. Children with hypotonic abdominal muscles may develop elevated rib cages and contracted anterior chest muscles, resulting in ineffective breathing patterns. Chest massage to elongate the pectorals and intercostal muscles can increase chest wall expansion. Children with truncal hypotonia may benefit from massage to the abdominal area to facilitate excretion. Using treatment techniques that incorporate slight traction while preventing subluxation to facilitate postural control is also beneficial for hypotonia. Providing massage to the extremities in midline position can promote visual contact with the extremities. Massage used with the intent to stimulate the SNS through quick, asymmetrical strokes may help to arouse the lethargic infant or child to a quiet alert state in preparation for physical therapy, ROM exercises, or feeding. Massage in conjunction with antigravity positioning may improve venous and lymphatic stasis in children with neuromotor impairments.[63]

Children with hypertonicity will develop contractures and joint deformities through constant spasticity of the muscles. Massage may help to decrease excessive tone prior to physical therapy or ROM to maximize stretching and elongation of the large muscle groups (e.g., the obliques, hamstrings, heel tendons).[63] Parents of children with developmental delay

---

*References 16, 28, 34-39, 48, 51, 52, 54-61.
†References 35, 37, 51, 54, 55, 57, 58, 60.

---

*References 24, 25, 39, 40, 56, 57, 63, 64.

have reported increased muscle tone and joint mobility, improved sleep patterns, and improved response to other therapies in their children in addition to self-reported decreased parental stress after participating in massage therapy classes.[71]

4. *Improves growth and development in premature infants.* Use of gentle human touch (GHT), a gentle placement of the hands on the head and abdomen or back with pressure but without stokes, has been used to positively touch premature infants.[72] Dr. Field developed a massage routine for premature neonates composed of 5 minutes of slow massage and 5 minutes of kinesthetic stimulation of the extremities followed by 5 minutes of slow massage. GHT or Field's approaches did not increase episodes of bradycardia, cyanosis, seizure activity, apnea, or temperature changes often associated with touching premature neonates.[72] GHT decreased stress response behaviors and improved sleep patterns in premature neonates.[69,72] Use of Field's approach improved daily and overall weight gain in premature infants by as much as 47%,[61,68,73,74] decreased startle responses and stress behaviors,[68] improved Neonatal Brazelton Assessment Scale scores, decreased oxygen requirements, and decreased length of hospital stay in massaged neonates compared with the nonmassaged neonates.[68,72]

5. *Improves sleep patterns.* Studies have demonstrated improved sleep patterns[68,69,75] and improved circadian rhythms in infants who receive massage therapy.[75]

6. *Decreases symptoms of psychiatric disorders.* Several controlled trials have studied massage therapy for pediatric psychiatric disorders. Autistic children[77] and children with attention-deficit disorder[77] had improved behavior scores after receiving massage therapy compared with controls. Bulimic or depressed adolescents had decreased anxiety and depression as well as lower salivary cortisol levels, increased dopamine levels, and improved behavioral ratings after regular massage was added to their treatment regimen.[78,79]

Safety and Precautions

Contraindications, dependent upon massage modalities used, do exist for massage therapy. Massage should not be done over areas of skin or tissue integrity loss, acute injury or inflammation, pitting edema, local tumor, or location of indwelling devices such as shunts, catheters, or central lines.[1] Massage is contraindicated in circulation disorders with increased risk of thrombus (i.e., bruit, varicose veins, phlebitis, thrombophlebitis, aneurysm).[1] Infectious pathological conditions that could be spread along the skin, through the circulation, or via the lymphatic system (i.e., varicella, sepsis, lymphangitis) are also contraindications.

Caution should be observed in areas of abnormal skin sensation, as sensory feedback to the massage pressure may be lacking.[1] Caution should also be observed in patients with prolonged bleeding times (i.e., anticoagulation therapy, platelet counts <50,000, hemophilia), because bruising could occur.[1]

Parents and massage therapists should always be attentive to the child's disposition during a massage treatment. Fidgeting, crying, or pulling away indicates the child has reached their touch quotient. This should be respected at all times, and the treatment should be terminated. Touch therapy should never be provided against a child's will. Often the length of treatment provided varies with a child's developmental level or disposition; for example, it is not uncommon for a toddler to reach the touch quotient after just 5 minutes, whereas a school-age child may reach it at 20 minutes. Some parents may use an "on-the-go" approach, massaging different body parts throughout the day as the opportunities arise. Infant and pediatric massage typically is provided with enough pressure to visualize some skin blanching during application of the strokes. Pressure that is too light can have an irritating or tickling effect, whereas pressure that is too deep can cause pain or discomfort. It is always important for parents to be observant of their child's response to the massage treatment as a gauge of how much pressure their child prefers.

Before teaching infant or pediatric massage to parents, it is important to consider the parent's goals so that the teaching session may be individualized to meet the family's needs. Some parents of chronically ill children may be feeling overwhelmed or exhausted and find massage therapy yet another burden, whereas some parents find massage an excellent opportunity to relax with their child. It should be reiterated with parents that they should provide massage therapy only if they enjoy the mutual experience as well.

Danger points caused by unprotected nerves or blood vessels are to be avoided during massage to prevent injury (Figure 3-1).[1]

Osteopathy*

History

Osteopathic medicine is a complete system of heathcare with a philosophy that combines the needs of the patient with the current practice of medicine, surgery, and obstetrics. The osteopathic philosophy emphasizes the interrelationship between structure and function and has an appreciation of the body's ability to heal itself.[1] Osteopathic medicine was developed during the American Civil War by Andrew Taylor Still, a medical doctor practicing on the midwestern frontier. Many of the pharmaceuticals and practices of the time were quite dangerous and mortality rates remained high. Osteopathic medicine and the osteopathic manipulative approach were developed as a mechanism of facilitating the normal self-regulating/self-healing mechanisms of the body. Today's pharmaceuticals and medical practices are much more advanced than during Still's time; nevertheless, osteopathic manipulative techniques can act as a complementary or alternative therapy in the management and treatment of many conditions.

Osteopaths and osteopathic physicians practice throughout the world, incorporating manual therapies into the healthcare of their patients. Two forms of osteopathic practice are primarily recognized internationally: fully licensed, medically trained osteopathic physicians and limited licensed osteopaths. In the United States, osteopathy is exclusively practiced by osteopathic physicians who have graduated from an accredited osteopathic

*This section is adapted in part from Carreiro JE: *An osteopathic approach to children*, London, 2003, Churchill Livingstone.

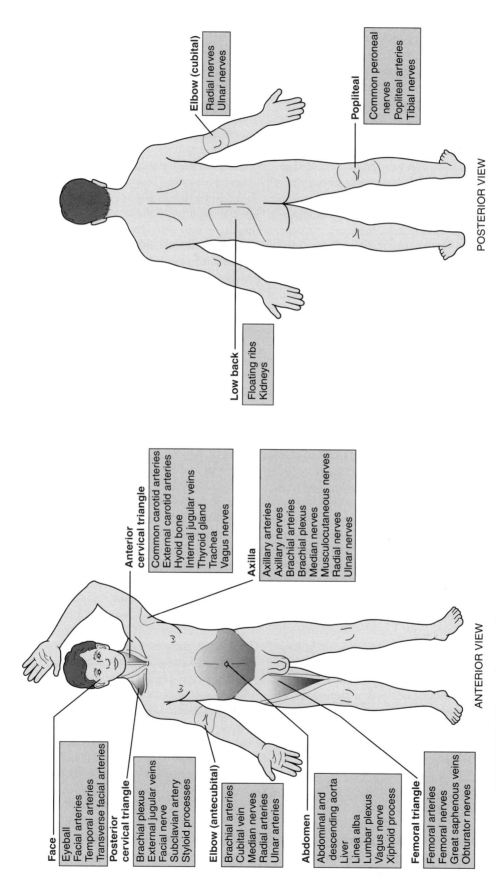

FIGURE 3-1 Massage therapy endangerment site map. *From Salvo S: Massage therapy: principles and practice, ed 3, St Louis, 2008, Saunders.*

POSTERIOR VIEW

ANTERIOR VIEW

Elbow (cubital)
Radial nerves
Ulnar nerves

Popliteal
Common peroneal nerves
Popliteal arteries
Tibial nerves

Low back
Floating ribs
Kidneys

Anterior cervical triangle
Common carotid arteries
External carotid arteries
Hyoid bone
Internal jugular veins
Thyroid gland
Trachea
Vagus nerves

Axilla
Axillary arteries
Axillary nerves
Brachial arteries
Brachial plexus
Median nerves
Musculocutaneous nerves
Radial nerves
Ulnar nerves

Face
Eyeball
Facial arteries
Temporal arteries
Transverse facial arteries

Posterior cervical triangle
Brachial plexus
External jugular veins
Facial nerve
Subclavian artery
Styloid processes

Elbow (antecubital)
Brachial arteries
Cubital vein
Median nerves
Radial arteries
Ulnar arteries

Abdomen
Abdominal and descending aorta
Liver
Linea alba
Lumbar plexus
Vagus nerve
Xiphoid process

Femoral triangle
Femoral arteries
Femoral nerves
Great saphenous veins
Obturator nerves

medical school and completed an appropriate postgraduate residency training program.

Training and Practice

In the United States, osteopathic physicians follow a training sequence similar to that of allopathic physicians: university degree, medical degree, post-doctoral residency, and specialty certification. The curriculums of allopathic and osteopathic medical schools are similar in terms of medical science; however, the osteopathic medical education includes osteopathic philosophy, practice, and manipulative medicine, and all the scientific and practical content needed to support that training. Upon graduation, U.S. osteopathic physicians enter post-doctoral residency training programs at osteopathic or combined (osteopathic/allopathic) hospitals, where they are educated to practice as primary care providers or specialists. In some European countries, postgraduate osteopathic training programs are available for medical doctors who wish to practice osteopathy. Outside the United States, individuals who are not physicians may train at osteopathic colleges or in osteopathic programs to practice as osteopaths. These practitioners do not receive full medical or osteopathic medical training, nor do they include pharmacology, obstetrics, or surgery in their practices. However, these osteopaths have 4 or more years of training in osteopathic principles, clinical diagnosis, and manual skills. Nonphysician osteopaths graduate from accredited osteopathic programs and are usually registered or licensed within their country. All osteopathic physicians and osteopaths are trained in many forms of manual therapies, including gentle myofascial, ligamentous, visceral, and cranial techniques suitable for children. Most practitioners who treat children employ the approaches described by William Sutherland, D.O. These are very gentle techniques that use the inherent forces within the patient's body, such as respiration, to achieve a change in tissue balance. Craniosacral therapy, as described by John Upledger, has some similarities to Sutherland's approach, but these therapists are not trained osteopathically.

Osteopathy and Children

The osteopathic profession has a long history of treating children. Andrew Taylor Still, the originator of osteopathy, discussed approaches to pediatric problems in his earliest writings.[2] In part, he founded osteopathic medicine in response to his experiences treating his own children when they had meningitis. During the first half of the twentieth century, William Sutherland[3-5] focused aspects of his teachings on newborns and infants and the anatomical relationships unique to that population. Between 1944 and 1967, Beryl Arbuckle, D.O., spent an entire career researching and working with children, especially those with cerebral palsy.[6] Recent publications have explored specific pediatric neurological problems[7] and general pediatric healthcare from an osteopathic perspective.[7-9] Outcomes research into the efficacy of osteopathic treatment in managing childhood diseases is beginning to emerge.[9-11] However, like much of the pediatric medical and CAM literature available, this data does not always meet the double-blinded, controlled, placebo group criteria of pharmaceutical studies performed

with adults. Nevertheless, osteopathy has a strong tradition of pediatric healthcare.

Philosophy and Theory

The basic tenets of osteopathy stress the interrelatedness of the neuromusculoskeletal system with the endocrine/immune system and the respiratory-circulatory system. The musculoskeletal system is the largest system in the body and is often overlooked in disease processes. For more than 100 years, osteopathic practitioners have used finely developed palpatory skills to evaluate and treat changes in tissue structure that might impede or compromise tissue function. During the great influenza epidemic of the early 1900s, osteopathic practitioners used their skills to aid thousands with an impressive decrease in morbidity and mortality in their patients. There was a 1% mortality rate among those patients treated osteopathically compared with 12% to 15% percent among those treated by medical doctors.[12] Contemporary research suggests that osteopathic treatment influences immune function and may have a role in the treatment of various disease processes.[13-17] Furthermore, research into the neuroendocrine immune network demonstrates that pain pathways and somatic nociception strongly influence endocrine and immune function through the hypothalamic-pituitary-adrenal axis.[18-24]

Within the osteopathic concept, the structural relationships among the various tissues of the body play a significant role in normal homeostatic processes. Osteopathic palpatory diagnosis is employed to evaluate impaired or altered function of the skeletal, arthrodial, and myofascial structures, as well as their related vascular, lymphatic, and neural elements. Impaired or altered function of these elements is termed *somatic dysfunction* and is treatable using osteopathic manipulative treatment.[25,26] However, osteopathic care is not limited to manual techniques. Medical, surgical, nutritional, pharmaceutical, and other aspects may be incorporated into the treatment plan as appropriate. Furthermore, unlike some other manual approaches, osteopathy does not emphasize alignment or radiographic evidence of biomechanical relationships. Rather, osteopathy acknowledges that although all human bodies have the same basic components and functions, individuals develop their own series of biomechanical adaptations to the physical events affecting them. Consequently, osteopaths and osteopathic physicians place less emphasis on whether or not bones "line up" and more emphasis on the integration of functional biomechanical relationships into the entire body framework.

The osteopathic approach can be described by five models of body function that are employed in thinking about patient care and the most appropriate means of supporting health within the patient.[27,28] The five models are the respiratory circulatory model, the bioenergetic model, the nociception/spinal facilitation model, the postural/biomechanical model, and the psychosocial model. Understanding these models allows the osteopathic physician to think about how the patient is responding to the disease, injury, or condition and consider the best means of supporting that response.

A schematic representation of the osteopathic approach is illustrated in Figure 3-2. The large box represents the child. Each child is a unique combination of genetic, environmental,

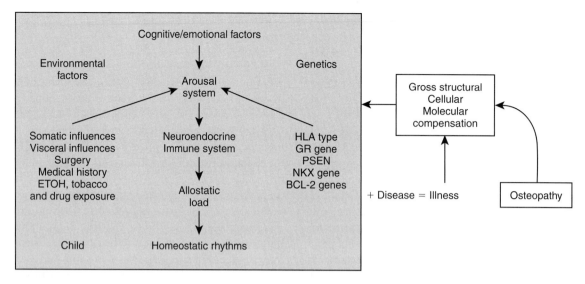

FIGURE 3-2 Schematic representation of the "host + disease = illness" model. *Used with permission of Frank H. Willard.*

cognitive, and emotional factors that influence his or her homeostatic rhythms. The symptoms of any illness or condition are a manifestation of the child's homeostatic processes and rhythms trying to function in the presence of disease or injury. The molecular, cellular, and structural physiology of the child adapts to or compensates for the influence of the disease or injury. This in turn affects the homeostatic state of the child. In addition to addressing the disease process or condition directly, osteopathy also attempts to intervene at the level of the individual's compensatory responses to facilitate the child's ability to function optimally. Different disease process and conditions affect a child in different ways. The osteopathic approach uses the aforementioned models of body function to understand the compensatory responses and to develop an effective therapeutic management plan for the child.

Models for the osteopathic approach to patient care

Respiratory/circulatory model. The respiratory/circulatory model concerns itself with the maintenance of extracellular and intracellular environments through the unimpeded delivery of oxygen and nutrients and the removal of waste products via the arterial, venous, and lymphatic systems. A.T. Still often stated that the "rule of the artery was supreme." Ultimately, proper cellular function is dependent upon the effective biomechanical function of gross anatomical structures of the body. Within the osteopathic concept, the respiratory/circulatory model includes the function of central and peripheral structures involved with the delivery of nutrients and removal of waste products. For example, limb movements affect drainage in deep lymphatic and venous structures[29-32] through altered tensions in the fascias and muscles. In addition to pulmonary ventilation, the biomechanical functions of the diaphragm, ribs, and other muscles of respiration play a role in venous and lymphatic drainage of the abdomen and pelvis and hence the removal of cellular waste products.[29,33-42] The integrity of the respiratory/circulatory system is influenced on a microscopic level through the tissue stress created by postural changes and macroscopically through respiratory mechanics. Most of the

muscles of the back, thorax, neck, and upper extremities play a role in respiratory mechanics. Altered respiratory mechanics can contribute to tissue congestion and decreased clearance, altered ventilation and increased energy expenditure, and altered lymphatic and venous return pressures. Factors that can affect respiratory mechanics include but are not limited to respiratory illnesses, scoliosis, thoracic or abdominal surgery, obesity, and postural changes. The osteopath or osteopathic physician will take into consideration the various factors influencing tissue respiration and their effect on the patient's ability to recover from an acute illness or function with a chronic condition.

Bioenergetic model. The human body requires a balance between energy expenditure and energy supply to maintain homeostasis. This fact forms the basis for the bioenergetic model. Efficient operation of internal body systems conserves energy that can be used to adapt to external stressors such as nutritional deficiencies, trauma, infection, nociceptive stimulation, and others. When several stressors occur simultaneously, their influence may become cumulative or synergistic, further compromising the body's ability to maintain homeostasis. Changes in the musculoskeletal system may increase the body's energy requirement.[43-45] For example, restriction in joint motion because of somatic dysfunction will alter biomechanics and reduce efficiency of motion. More work will be required to use the joint, which increases the metabolic demands placed upon the patient. Now imagine that there are many restricted joints, all in the thorax, and the patient is a 4-month-old infant with respiratory syncytial virus. The restricted joint mechanics will increase the work of breathing and increase the metabolic demands on the child. Within the osteopathic concept, any process that interferes with local or systemic homeostasis has the potential to increase the body's energy requirements.

Nociception/spinal facilitation model. The nociception/spinal facilitation model concerns the direct and indirect influences of nociception on normal body function. Spinal facilitation is one of the primary diagnostic clues garnered from an osteopathic examination. It manifests as a localized area of change in the muscles and fascia adjacent to the spine. Depending upon the acuity, these changes may manifest as tissue swelling or edema, increased or decreased temperature, and stiffness or loss of tone. Although these tissue texture changes may represent localized areas of inflammation that occur in response to direct local insult, they may also arise in response to damage or irritation to distal tissues through viscerosomatic reflexes. Viscerosomatic reflexes may be mediated by spinal facilitation. Recent scientific investigation into the mechanism and effects of viscerosomatic interactions has shed new light on the intimate relationship between the musculoskeletal system and the viscera through the SNS.[46-52] Viscerosomatic reflexes were first described by osteopaths in the early part of the 20th century.[53,54] The short restrictor paraspinal muscles are usually involved. The tissue texture characteristics and precise spinal level of the reflex are specific to the organ of involvement.[54-56]

Osteopathic clinicians use viscerosomatic reflexes to aid in their diagnosis and treatment of patients.[57-60] Chapman's points or Chapman's reflexes are another form of viscerosomatic integration[61,62] and may also be mediated by spinal facilitation. These superficial areas of tissue texture change have a high correlation with visceral pathology. They are pea-sized areas of edema usually found on the anterior and posterior aspects of torso. The site of location and presence of both anterior and posterior findings suggests a visceral problem.[61] They are very easily integrated into the general physical examination and provide another tool in developing a differential diagnosis. A general understanding of the viscerosomatic map and Chapman's reflexes can give the clinician clues about what may be causing the patient's symptoms and can provide a pathway for therapeutic approach.

The nociception/spinal facilitation model considers the influence of spinal facilitation on homeostasis via the neuroendocrine-immune system. The *neuroendocrine-immune system* refers to the complicated interdependency among the nervous system, hormone balance, and immune function. Basically, the human body maintains internal balance or homeostasis through rhythmic chemical secretions from the brain (neurotransmitters), immune organs (immunoregulators), and glands (hormones). The secreted chemicals interact to stimulate and suppress each other, thus coordinating the internal chemistry of the body. Potentially harmful stimuli from both external and internal sources can alter these rhythmic patterns, thus affecting the homeostasis of the internal body chemistry. Normally, once the stress is removed, the adaptive response resolves and homeostasis is reestablished. However, under long-term or severe stress, the entire physiology of the neuroendocrine-immune system can alter, creating a permanent condition of adaptive response. Brain chemistry, immune system function, and hormone balance will alter. Not only is this person more susceptible to disease, he or she will have a much harder time adapting to any new stress. Many studies have demonstrated changes in immune cells, hormone levels, and nervous system function under stress.[12,20,22,63-68] Stressful stimuli may include psychological and physiological influences. Pain or nociceptive stimuli is considered a potent stressor. From an osteopathic perspective, somatic dysfunction

or other strains in the patient's body may adversely influence the neuroendocrine-immune system.

Postural/biomechanical model. The postural/biomechanical model views the body as an integration of somatic components. Stresses or imbalances among these components result in increased energy expenditure, changes in joint structure, impediment of neurovascular function, and altered metabolic demands. In very young children, biomechanical or postural stresses may influence the development of motor skills and perhaps even cognitive processes. As the child grows, altered postural mechanics will change the weight load on joint surfaces. The increased weight load on the articular cartilage eventually causes the proteoglycans within the cartilaginous matrix to break down. This is the first stage of degenerative arthritis. Altered postural mechanics will also influence connective tissue and fascia, potentially affecting vascular and lymphatic drainage. These changes can contribute to the accumulation of cellular waste products, altered tissue pH, changes in osmotic pressure, and impediment of oxygen and nutrient delivery. This is important in cases of infection, cardiopulmonary problems, and metabolic diseases. Postural imbalances may cause irritation to paraspinal tissues including the articular tissues of the vertebrae. Irritation to these tissues will stimulate somatosympathetic fibers, resulting in sympathetically mediated changes in the involved tissues and potential changes in associated viscera through viscerosomatic reflexes. Altered joint mechanics affect proprioception and balance. This is especially important in children with chronic conditions that affect the musculoskeletal system, such as spasticity or hypotonia.

Psychosocial model. The psychosocial model views the patient within the context of his or her cultural, personal, environmental, and community issues and experiences. Although in some cases the mechanisms are poorly understood, today most people recognize the influences of emotional and social factors on physiological processes. In the 1800s, A.T. Still said "Man is triune,"[69] a combination of physical, spiritual, and emotional processes. The psychosocial model attempts to employ that philosophy by creating an amalgamation of scientific understanding with the spiritual and social milieu of the patient to establish the most appropriate therapeutic approach for the patient.

These five physiological models interweave to form the fabric of the osteopathic approach. The approach and philosophy guides how an osteopath employs manipulative techniques. Osteopaths are not as concerned with "making everything straight" as they are concerned with maximizing function. Osteopaths are not abject healers by any stretch of the imagination. The principles and techniques of osteopathy are employed to facilitate the natural healing processes within the patient's body. The osteopath uses manual techniques to support those healing changes, but the child's body and the child's homeostatic mechanisms have to make the changes.

Current Pediatric Use

Osteopathic manipulative medicine is a hands-on approach to patient care that employs manual techniques. Techniques are described as direct and indirect. Direct techniques are those that engage a restrictive barrier, such as the thrust or high-velocity manipulation commonly viewed as causing the "popping" sound in joints. Other direct techniques such as muscle energy and articulatory approaches involve patient cooperation and low-velocity movements. In general, these techniques are usually reserved for use in older children and adolescents. Gentle, direct approaches that employ a slow, gentle pressure or movement may be better suited for treating young children. These include inhibition technique, soft tissue technique, and some forms of functional and cranial technique.

Osteopathic practitioners also use indirect techniques in children and infants. These techniques do not engage a restrictive barrier, and most patients perceive them as "gentle" techniques. Indirect techniques used to treat children include the strain/counterstrain technique described by Lawrence Jones, facilitated positional release, functional techniques, balanced ligamentous and balanced membranous techniques, articular ligamentous strain techniques, visceral techniques, osteopathic cranial techniques, and osteopathy in the cranial field. In many hospitals throughout the world, osteopathic clinicians use these gentle techniques to treat newborn and premature babies.

Osteopathic practitioners choose the appropriate techniques based upon the model(s) of body function employed, the type of tissue dysfunction (articular, muscular, myofascial, or membranous); the acuity of the problem, possible comorbidities, and the child's age and ability to cooperate in the procedure.

Osteopathic physicians and osteopaths worldwide have a long history of treating children with disabilities and chronic diseases. Often osteopathic treatment is done in conjunction with other modalities to afford the child a team approach to healthcare. Many practitioners have exclusively pediatric practices, and several large osteopathic centers exist. The Osteopathic Center for Children, founded by Viola Frymann, D.O., in the late 1960s, continues to attract thousands of children from all around the world. Likewise, the Osteopathic Children's Center in London serves many U.K. children with disabilities. Dr. Still had a saying that is paraphrased by all students of osteopathy: "It is the job of the Osteopath to find Health; anyone can find disease." Ultimately, it is the goal of osteopathy to recognize and address the interrelationship between structure and function in the human body, to address imbalances and dysfunction so that the child may compensate appropriately for stress and disease states, and to facilitate the inherent health present in every patient.

Contraindications

Absolute and relative contraindications for osteopathic treatment are usually based upon the technique employed. Direct techniques such as certain types of muscle energy, thrust, and articulatory maneuvers are avoided in very young children and children with bleeding disorders, prolonged bleeding times, clotting abnormalities, and compromised bone or joint stability as might occur in metabolic disorders, suppurative arthritis, rheumatoid diseases, osteomyelitis, or fractures. In these children, indirect techniques can be used safely.

Relative contraindications to indirect techniques usually relate to the acuity of the problem. For example, cranial techniques would be avoided in children with closed head injury until the possibility of intracranial bleeding is ruled out.

A review of the published literature failed to show any documented reports of untoward effects of osteopathic treatment of children. One published report described a 5% incidence rate of adverse reactions in adults with closed head trauma who were treated with osteopathic cranial techniques.[70] Several published reviews suggest that the incidence of complications with manipulation of the cervical spine in adults is underreported. A position paper recently approved by the American Osteopathic Association included a thorough review of the literature.[71] It concluded that high-velocity/low-amplitude (HVLA) manipulative treatment is effective for neck pain and is relatively safe, especially in comparison to other common treatment modalities including nonsteroidal medications. The report went on to recommend that osteopathic physicians continue to offer this form of treatment to their patients.[71] Nevertheless, osteopathic physicians with pediatric manipulative practices rarely use HVLA and thrust technique in their pediatric patients.

Psychology

History

The notion that mind and body compose one unified system dates back to the ancients in both Eastern and Western civilizations. In modern terms, complementary and alternative medicine (CAM) postulates that the mind and body, psyche and soma, are an integrated whole. The one-dimensional, mechanistic view of human health, which treats illness as an incident-specific deviation rather than holistically as a system's malfunction or maladaptation, continues to be the prevailing medical model. Increasingly, however, a growing number of healthcare professionals are gaining fresh insight into the root causes of illness and concomitant treatment modalities. There is a growing realization that for care to be most effective—and this holds true for both adults and children—the patient must be understood in the larger context of his or her life, including biological, psychological, spiritual, and social aspects.

There is not a clear group of professionals who define themselves as CAM child psychologists. Pediatric psychology developed in the 1970s and began to focus on the connectedness and complex interaction between mind and body. Previously, child psychology emphasized only mental health. Pediatric psychology strives for short-term intervention, integrates both the child's parents and other healthcare professionals,[21] and examines the relationship between physical and mental health, especially in chronic illness.[8,22] By working directly with pediatricians, pediatric psychologists strive to identify and treat problems before they develop into severe psychopathology. At the present time, CAM pediatric psychologists are directing their efforts toward establishing scientific evidence for mind/body intervention and improving patient outcome while decreasing medical costs.

CAM Psychology Theory

CAM psychology closely examines the connection between emotions and physiology. Within the limbic system, the amygdala connects emotional responses to memories, which facilitates interpretation of current events. In essence, it determines whether something is scary or safe and signals to the hypothalamus to initiate the fight-or-flight response or the rest-and-digest response, respectively. For example, a child may view his parents' arguments as unsafe and threatening to his survival, because the parents have been the caretakers. The amygdala in this case senses danger and sends a message to the hypothalamus to initiate the fight-or-flight response. Energy stores are mobilized, and the physiological state is changed.

More specifically, stress activates the sympathetic and adrenomedullary system and the hypothalamic-pituitary-adrencortical axis. Psychological stress results in increased output of epinephrine and norepinephrine from the adrenal medulla. These adrenaline responses are part of the fight-or-flight response.[1] Because children usually can neither fight nor run away from family conflicts, their physiology can become easily overwhelmed by the outpouring of hormones. This contributes to physical or behavioral symptoms.

The research on neuropeptides has provided some of the most compelling evidence to support the link between emotions and physical symptoms. One researcher posits that the communication between the immune system and every cell in the body, including brain cells, occurs through the act of neuropeptides binding and unbinding with neuropeptide receptor sites on these cells.[6]

Many brain cells are involved in emotional regulation, such as those in the limbic system. When emotional trauma or stress occurs, the neuropeptides bind inappropriately at the receptor sites, and emotional suppression or dysfunction ensues. Studies have demonstrated that pathological binding of the neuropeptide to its receptor site occurs at brain and nonneural cellular levels as a response to stress. The cells "learn" such a response to stimuli and may bind pathologically with subsequent stimuli, which may be of lower intensity or of a different nature from the initial stimulus. With intensive and specific psychological counseling, these irreversibly bound neuropeptides may unbind, especially when the physician understands and treats the physical manifestations of the emotional disorder.

In essence, how a child interprets environmental stress determines how the body responds and what physiological action will be taken—for example, releasing hormones, shunting blood to muscles, or increasing stomach secretions.[4] If a child becomes anxious about a physical symptom, a stress response can be activated that may further exacerbate the physical condition. Similarly, if a child becomes anxious about an environmental stress, such as his parents fighting, the stress response can create physical problems (e.g., stomach pain). Therefore by helping the child adopt a different interpretation of physical symptoms or family stress, the CAM psychologist can alter the physiological reactions and reduce illness.

Even general stress has a direct impact on human physiology. In a prospective study that measured interpersonal stress, immune markers, disease activity, and pain in women with rheumatoid arthritis, it was found that interpersonal stress was related to immune changes, which were followed by increased inflammation and pain within the week.[5] This study suggests that daily stress, in addition to chronic anxiety, can affect health.

CAM psychology considers several factors that affect the child's physical and emotional health. The former President of the Society of Pediatric Psychologists summarized these factors as follows: "cultural systems, family systems, peers, school, and health care providers [all] influence the adjustment and adaptation of children with chronic illness."[24] Every child forms an integrated system with his or her environment.

This author routinely looks for physiological cues to help interpret a patient's emotional state. For example, if a child's face flushes when she talks about school, this may be a sign of problems at school. A child's tears while talking about his parents should not be dismissed as a random coincidence, but instead should be explored as a sign of deeper emotional distress, possibly caused by dysfunctional family interaction. Such signs of emotional distress are important because of the close link between emotions and physical health and between stress and physiological functions.

Evidence to Support CAM Theory

Much of the research on children with medical problems suggests a direct relationship between the physical health and emotional well-being of both the child and his or her family, supporting the theory of CAM. In a 2004 review of the literature on pediatric asthma, it was found that the parent's psychological well-being, parent-child interactions, and the child's emotional functioning strongly affected a child's asthma.[9] Another study examined children with frequent headaches to understand their emotional patterns as compared with children with infrequent headaches.[10] Both boys and girls with frequent headaches reported higher levels of depression than peers with no or infrequent headaches. Children with recurrent headaches also missed more school during a 6-month period.

For adolescents with sickle cell disease, a similar connection exists between emotional states and pain. In a 6-month study of adolescents aged 13 to 17 years, daily increases in stress and negative mood correlated with increases in same-day pain, healthcare use, and reductions in school and social activity.[11] Conversely, increases in positive mood correlated with decreased pain, less healthcare use, and participation in more activities. The authors concluded that daily variations in stress and mood were related to pain. By focusing on patients' emotional functioning, their overall heath and well-being can be significantly improved.

Studies have demonstrated that chronic illness can have a direct impact on socialization and pleasurable activity level.[10,11] Children with chronic illnesses may miss more school because of hospitalization or doctors appointments, which in turn would affect their social and emotional development. If these children then develop emotional distress, such as anxiety or depression caused by stress from illness or missing activities, their physical health may be further compromised.

The parent's psychological well-being and parent-child interactions have been found to affect the child's health and illness severity.[9] Studies have demonstrated that when mothers suffer from psychological problems, their medically ill children have more visits to the emergency room.[12] Children can also learn sick behavior from their parents. In a study that examined the genetic versus environmental risk of developing irritable bowel syndrome (IBS) among more than 6000 twin pairs, evidence suggested a social learning contribution from the parents.[13] The authors concluded that although heredity contributed to IBS, what was learned in the family environment had an equal or greater influence on developing IBS. Both biology and environment are therefore important factors for health.

Parent-child interaction problems also have a profound impact on a child's health. Among a sample of largely upper middle class children and their mothers, a prospective study of children who were at genetic risk for asthma found that parenting difficulties when infants were just 3 weeks old were predictors of asthma onset by 6 years of age.[14] Assessment of parenting difficulties included emotional availability to the child, commitment to childcare, and behavioral regulation strategies. Problems in these areas early in life predicted asthma by age 6 years. It is remarkable that the predictive ratings were made when the children were only 3 weeks old, which suggests that dysfunctional interaction even in infancy can have long-term influence on a child's health.

The literature in pediatric psychology therefore emphasizes the importance of the practitioner evaluating the larger context or system of the child. Understanding the child's environment and how that child interacts in the environment can provide useful clues for identifying the children at greatest risk. Changes made to the child's environment early on can help prevent illness or reduce complications.

Use and Contraindications of CAM Psychology Techniques

Many psychotherapy approaches follow the unified mind/body principles of CAM. The following modalities have the greatest clinical utility in treating a wide range of pediatric psychological conditions.

Neuroemotional technique

Neuroemotional technique (NET) technique integrates Eastern and Western philosophies and follows the CAM principle that the mind and body are connected. Key concepts in NET are based on traditional Chinese five-element theory and incorporate the connection among emotions, cognitions, and behavior.[20]

What distinguishes NET from traditional talk therapy is that it uses kinesiology to help identify patterns that are unconscious. Kinesiology, or muscle testing, involves manually putting pressure on muscles in a painless manner.[20] One study demonstrated that when articulating a self-referential statement with which the individual is congruent, muscle strength is stronger for a longer period of time.[15] In this study, a dynamometer measured performance of the deltoid muscle. Essentially, muscle testing functions in a similar manner to biofeedback. It registers changes in an individual's physiology when presented with stimuli. Even just the thought of something stressful can be a provocative stimulus. With the addition of kinesiology, patients are emotionally and physically engaged in therapy. The goal is to reprocess emotionally stressful events that are unresolved and may be affecting physical and mental health.

More than 4000 practitioners in more than 25 countries have been trained in NET.[16] It is appropriate for use with children and adults whose symptoms range from behavioral and emotional

afflictions to physical illness; however, it is not recommended for anyone who is psychotic or has lost touch with reality. Practitioners can become certified in NET by demonstrating a high level of proficiency in both theory and practice. Minimal research on the technique is available to date.

Hypnosis

Hypnosis is a state of mind characterized by altered brain wave patterns that are induced using deep relaxation. Although hypnosis creates a state of suggestibility, it does not weaken a person's will or control. The person must be a willing participant. A state of deep relaxation is facilitated through a series of therapist-guided suggestions. Once the hypnotic state is achieved, the therapist may explore unconscious reasons for behaviors or may attempt behavior modification. The patient typically remembers what happens during the session and develops heightened motivation for change.

One alternate form of hypnosis is autogenic training, which is a self-hypnotic procedure. By following several steps designed to relax physiology, a hypnotic trance is achieved. This has been demonstrated to help with headaches and eczema, among other conditions.[17] The autogenic technique should be taught by a therapist and practiced during a therapy session.

In traditional hypnotherapy, a session occurs in an office setting and the patient sits in a reclining chair. The therapist talks to the patient and makes suggestions, but the patient can stop the process at any point. Contrary to popular perception, no drugs or pendulums are used. For hypnosis to be effective, the patient must trust the therapist and be open to the process.

Hypnotherapy should be performed only by trained professionals with advanced study in hypnotherapy. It is safe for use with children who are experiencing a wide range of conditions from attention-deficit hyperactivity disorder (ADHD) to chronic pain. A considerable amount of literature supports the effectiveness of hypnotherapy.

Biofeedback

Biofeedback is a self-regulation technique. By monitoring a patient's physiological state through electronic devices that measure such areas as skin temperature, muscle tension, blood pressure, and brain wave activity and provide immediate feedback, the patient can learn to modify his or her physiology. Essentially, a person is trained to make involuntary physiological responses under voluntary or conscious control. Using specific monitoring devices, the patient is given immediate feedback from the therapist about any physiological changes. This allows the patient to become more sensitive to the changes in the body. Through practice, the patient can actually alter physiological responses such as muscle tension, heart rate, and blood pressure. For example, the biofeedback therapist guides the patient through strategies to regulate muscle tension and encourages the patient to independently discover what is effective or feels best.

The ultimate goal for the patient is to develop homeostasis by being more aware of the moment-to-moment changes in the body and being able to adjust his or her physiology accordingly. In biofeedback, homeostasis is considered PNS dominance. With increased arousal, the SNS dominates, which causes several hypermetabolic states that include increased heart rate and blood pressure and increased blood flow to the brain, spinal cord, and muscles (which increase muscle tone). With ongoing physical or emotional stress, a chronic state of arousal can develop. Additionally, the threshold for this fight-or-flight response can be lowered such that the body becomes overly tense with very little stimulation. In biofeedback training the patient is taught to modulate these responses.

There are several forms of biofeedback:

- Electromyographic (EMG) biofeedback compares two electrodes placed over the belly of the muscle. This reveals the small electrochemical changes that occur when the muscle contracts. Because EMG biofeedback measures muscle changes, the standard applications tend to involve muscle pain such as tension headache; neck, back, and leg pain; bruxism and temporomandibular joint syndrome; anxiety; and general muscle relaxation.
- Electroencephalographic (EEG) biofeedback measures brain wave activity and provides specific information about the patient's level of alertness, because it is able to filter out delta, theta, alpha, and beta frequency bands. Feedback about brain wave activity can be used to help a child improve concentration (e.g., with school tasks or for ADHD) or to decrease alertness (e.g., for insomnia).
- Electrodermal activity (EDA) biofeedback measures the electrical characteristics of the skin using methods such as skin conductance response (SCR), skin potential (SP), skin conductance level (SCL), and skin potential response (SPR). Training in EDA allows the patient to become more aware of stress. It is not commonly used and, when used, it is often in conjunction with other forms of biofeedback. Because EDA measures only skin changes, it does not provide feedback about more complex physiological reactions. When used for treatment, it tends to be as a monitoring system for unresolved issues in psychotherapy or for general stress.
- Skin temperature (ST) feedback training involves increasing awareness and control of hand temperature. Hand temperature is important because peripheral temperature is a reflection of sympathetic arousal. When the SNS is activated, blood is shunted away from the periphery and toward the striated muscles, spinal cord, and brain. By focusing on warming the hands, a decrease in sympathetic activity occurs. To measure hand temperature, a thermistor is taped to the hand. Limitations of this technique include the fact that the thermistor is sensitive to the temperature in the treatment room and must be applied to the same part of the hand for each treatment. Otherwise, results may not be accurate. One study that examined this procedure in children with migraines found significant improvement compared with wait-list controls in just four sessions.[18]

Regardless of the specific approach used, once the patient has been trained in biofeedback, he or she can apply what has been learned to everyday life situations without the biofeedback equipment. The goal is for the child to be able to generalize the skills learned in the therapy room.

Biofeedback is appropriate for use with children. Most children are motivated by the frequent feedback, but therapists can also use reinforcement for children who are less invested. Although the child seeking treatment is closely monitored, it is a noninvasive technique, which may explain why many children feel comfortable using biofeedback. A significant amount of empirical evidence supports the use of biofeedback with children, especially for specific medical problems.

In summary, to effectively treat a child with physical symptomatology, a pediatric CAM psychologist adopts an integrated mind/body approach and evaluates a broad spectrum of the social and emotional influences in a child's life.

References

Chiropractic

1. Palmer DD: *Three generations: a brief history of chiropractic*, Davenport, Iowa, 1967, The Palmer School of Chiropractic.
2. Palmer BJ: *The science of chiropractic*, Davenport, Iowa, 1906, The Palmer School of Chiropractic.
3. Maynard JE: *Healing hands*, ed 2, Mobile, Ala, 1977, Southeastern Graphics.
4. Palmer Chiropractic University Alumni Association, Davenport, Iowa, 2004.
5. Federation of Chiropractic Licensing Boards, Greeley, Colo, 2004.
6. National Board Chiropractic Examiners 2005 online brochure. Available at www.nbce.org.
7. Leach RA: *The chiropractic theories: a textbook of scientific research*, ed 4, Baltimore, 2004, Lippincott Williams and Wilkins.
8. ACC position papers born of consensus, *Dynamic Chiro* 15:1, 1997.
9. Lantz CA: The vertebral subluxation complex. Part 1: an introduction to the model and the kinesiological component, *CRJ* 1:23-36, 1989.
10. Tachdjian MO: *Clinical pediatric orthopedics*, Stamford, Conn, 1997, Appleton and Lange.
11. Gottlieb MS: Neglected spinal cord, brain stem and musculoskeletal injuries stemming from birth trauma, *J Manipulative Physiol Ther* 16:537-543, 1993.
12. Towbin A: Latent spinal cord and brain stem injury in the newborn infant, *Develop Med Child Neurol* 11:54-68, 1969.
13. Gasaldo TD: Labor posture, *Birth* 19:230, 1992.
14. Biedermann H: Kinematic imbalance due to suboccipital strain in newborns, *Maneulle Medizin* 6:151-161, 1992.
15. Bogduk N: Pathology of lumbar disc pain, *Manual Med* 5:72, 1990.
16. Bogduk N, Winsor M, Inglis A: The innervation of the cervical intervertebral discs, *Spine* 13:2, 1988.
17. Jiang H, Russell G, Raso VJ et al: The nature and distribution of the innervation of human supraspinal and interspinal ligaments, *Spine* 20:869, 1995.
18. Rhalmi S, Yahia LH, Newman N et al: Immunohistochemical study of nerves in lumbar spine ligaments, *Spine* 18:264, 1993.
19. Holm S, Indahl A, Solomonow M: Sensorimotor control of the spine. *J EMG Kinesiol* 12:219-234, 2002.
20. Wyke B: The neurology of joints: a review of general principles, *Clin Rheum Dis* 7:223-239, 1981.
21. Chestnut JL: *The 14 foundational premises for the scientific and philosophical validation of the chiropractic wellness paradigm*, Victoria, BC, 2003, Chestnut Wellness and Chiropractic Corporation.
22. Guyton AC: *Textbook of medical physiology*, Philadelphia, 1986, Saunders.
23. Charney DS, Deutch A: A functional neuroanatomy of anxiety and fear: implications for the pathophysiology and treatment of anxiety disorders, *Crit Rev Neurobiol* 10:419-446, 1996.
24. Byrne J: Cellular analysis of associative learning, *Physiol Rev* 76:329-439, 1987.
25. Denslow JS, Hassett CC: The central excitatory state associated with postural abnormalities, *J Neurophysiol* 2:53-58, 1942.

26. Korr IM, Thomas PE, Wright HM: Patterns of electrical skin resistance in man, *Acta Neuroveget* 17:77-96, 1958.

27. Caulfield B: Functional instability of the ankle joint, *Physiother* 86:401-411, 2000.

28. Lentell G, Bass B, Lopez D et al: The contributions of proprioceptive deficits, muscle function and anatomic laxity to functional instability of the ankle joint, *J Orthoped Sports Phys Ther* 21:206-215, 1995.

29. Slosberg M: Spinal learning: central modulation of pain processing and long-term alteration of interneuronal excitability as a result of nociceptive peripheral input, *J Manipulative Physiol Ther* 13:326-336, 1990.

30. Patterson M: The spinal cord: participant in disorder, *J Manipulative Physiol Ther* 9:2-11, 1993.

31. Solomonow M, Krogsgaard M: The sensory function of ligaments, *J EMG Kinesiol* 12:165, 2002.

32. Hooshmand H: *Chronic pain: reflex sympathetic dystrophy, prevention and management,* Boca Raton, Fla, 1993, CRC Press.

33. Bolton P: Reflex effects of vertebral subluxations: the peripheral nervous system, *J Manipulative Physiol Ther* 23:101-103, 2000.

34. Cabell J: Sympathetically maintained pain, In Willis W, editor: *Hyperalgesia and allodynia,* New York, 1992, Raven Press.

35. Sato A, Swenson RS: Sympathetic nervous system response to mechanical stress of the spinal column in rats, *J Manipulative Physiol Ther* 7:141-147, 1984.

36. Sosberg M: Effects of altered afferent articular input on sensation, proprioception, muscle tone and sympathetic reflex responses, *J Manipulative Physiol Ther* 11:400-408, 1988.

37. Nansel D, Szlazak M: Somatic dysfunction and the phenomena of visceral disease simulation: a probable explanation for the apparent effectiveness of somatic therapy in patients presumed to be suffering from visceral disease, *J Manipulative Physiol Ther* 18:379-397, 1995.

38. Budgell B: Reflex effects of subluxation: the autonomic nervous system, *J Manipulative Physiol Ther* 23:104-106, 2000.

39. Gutmann G: The atlas fixation in the baby and infant, *Manuelle Medizin* 25:5-10, 1987.

40. Kocha LE, Kochb H, Graumann-Bruntc S et al: Heart rate changes in response to mild mechanical irritation of the high cervical spinal cord region in infants, *Forensic Sci Int* 128:168-176, 2002.

41. Restak RM: *The brain: the last frontier,* New York, 1979, Warner.

42. Salter RB: *Textbook of disorders and injuries of the musculoskeletal system,* Baltimore, 1970, Williams and Wilkins.

43. Lantz CA: Immobilization degeneration and the fixation hypothesis of chiropractic subluxation, *CRJ* 1:21-46, 1988.

44. Holm S, Indahl A, Solomonow M: Sensorimotor control of the spine, *J EMG Kinesiol* 12:219-234, 2002.

45. Rahlmann JF: Mechanisms of intervertebral joint fixation: a literature review, *J Manipulative Physiol Ther* 10:177-187, 1987.

46. Liebenson C: Pathogenesis of chronic back pain, *J Manipulative Physiol Ther* 15:299-308, 1992.

47. Donatelli R, Owen-Burkhardt H: Effects of internal fixation on the articular cartilage of unfused canine facet joint cartilage, *Spine* Nov 1984.

48. Videman T: Experimental osteoarthritis in the rabbit: comparison of different periods of repeated immobilization, *Acta Orthop Scand* 53:339-347, 1982.

49. Thaxter TH, Mann RA, Anderson CE: Degeneration of immobilized knee joints in rats, *J Bone Joint Surg* 47:567-585, 1965.

50. Jirout J: Studies in the dynamics of the spine, *Acta Radiol* 46:55-60, 1956.

51. St Pierre D, Gardiner PF: The effect of immobilization and exercise on muscle function: a review, *Physiother Can* 39:29-36, 1987.

52. Palmoski M, Pericone E, Brandt KD: Development and reversal of a proteoglycan aggregation defect in normal canine knee cartilage after immobilization, *Arth Rheum* 22:508-517, 1979.

53. Evans EB, Eggers GWN, Butler JK et al: Experimental immobilization and remobilization of rat knee joints, *J Bone Joint* 42:737-758, 1960.

54. Sunderland S, Bradley L: Stress strain phenomena in human spinal roots, *Brain* 84:121, 1961.

55. Sharpless SK: Susceptibility of spinal roots to compression block, In Goldstein M, editor: *The research status of spinal manipulative therapy,* Washington, DC, 1975, National Institutes of Health/DHEW.

56. Rydevik BL: The effects of compression on the physiology of the nerve roots, *J Manipulative Physiol Ther* 15:62-66, 1992.

57. Hause M: Pain and the nerve root, *Spine* 18:2053, 1993.

58. Cole VV: Effects of the atlas lesion: preliminary report, *J Am Osteopath Assoc* 47:150-152, 1947.

59. Cole VV: The effects of the atlas lesion after six months, *J Am Osteopath Assoc* 47:399-407, 1948.

60. Cole VV: The osteopathic lesion complex: effects on the motor end plate, *J Am Osteopath Assoc* 48:14-27, 1948.

61. Cole VV: The osteopathic lesion complex: the effects of the seventh cervical vertebral lesion after ninety six hours, six weeks and six months, *J Am Osteopath Assoc* 48:281-288, 1949.

62. Cole VV: The osteopathic lesion syndrome: the effects of an experimental vertebral articular strain on the sensory unit, *J Am Osteopath Assoc* 51:381-389, 1952.

63. Sjostrand J, Rydevik B, Lundborg G et al: Impairment of intraneural microcirculation, blood nerve barrier and axonal transport in experimental nerve ischemia and compression, In Korr IM, editor: *The neurobiologic mechanisms in manipulative therapy,* New York, 1978, Plenum, pp 337-355.

64. Rydevik B, McLean WG, Sjostrand J et al: Blockage of axonal transport induced by acute, graded compression of the rabbit vagus nerve, *J Neurol Neurosurg Psychiatry* 43:690-698, 1980.

65. Callender A, Plaugher G, Anrigh CA: Introduction to chiropractic pediatrics. In Anrig C, Plaugher G, editors: *Pediatric chiropractic,* Baltimore, 1998, Williams and Wilkins.

66. Spigelblatt L, Laîné-Ammara G, Pless IB et al: The use of alternative medicine by children, *Pediatrics* 94:811-814, 1994.

67. Christensen M et al: *Job analysis of chiropractic by state,* Greeley, Colo, 2005, National Board of Chiropractic Examiners.

68. Christensen M et al: *Job analysis of chiropractic by state,* ed 2, Greeley, Colo, 2003, National Board of Chiropractic Examiners.

69. Pistolese RA: Risk assessment of neurological and/or vertebrobasilar complication in the pediatric chiropractic patient, *J Vertebr Sublux Res* 2, 1998.

70. Fysh PN: Orthopedics, In Anrig CA, Plaugher G, editors: *Chiropractic pediatrics,* Baltimore, 1998, Williams and Wilkins.

71. Dishman RW: Static and dynamic components of the chiropractic subluxation complex: a literature review, *J Manipulative Physiol Ther* 11:98-107, 1988.

72. Alvarez-Sabin J: Stroke in teenagers, *Rev Neurol* 25:919-923, 1997.

73. Khurana DS, Bonnemann CG, Dooking EC et al: Vertebral artery dissection: issues in diagnosis and management, *Pediatr Neurol* 14:255-258, 1996.

74. Zimmerman AW, Kujar AJ, Gadoth N et al: Traumatic vertebrobasilar occlusive disease in childhood, *Neurol* 28:185-188, 1978.

75. Nagle W: Vertebral artery obstruction by hyperextension of the neck: report of three cases, *Arch Phys Med Rehabil* 54:237-240, 1973.

76. Shafir, Y Daufman BA: Quadriplegia after chiropractic manipulation in an infant with congenital torticollis caused by a spinal cord astrocytoma, *J Pediatr* 120:266-269, 1992.

Massage Therapy

1. Tappan F: *Healing massage techniques: holistic, classic, and emerging methods*, Norwalk, Conn, 1988, Appleton & Lange.
2. Fritz S: *Mosby's fundamentals of therapeutic massage*, St Louis, 1995, Mosby.
3. Bohm M: *Massage: its principles and techniques*, Philadelphia, 1913, Lippincott.
4. Graham D: *A treatise on massage, its history, mode of applications and effects*, Philadelphia, 1902, Lippincott.
5. American Massage Therapy Association: States with massage therapy practice laws. Available at http://www.amtamassage.org/about/lawstate.html. Accessed: March 30, 2008
6. National Certification Board for Therapeutic Massage and Bodywork: Consumer's guide to therapeutic massage and bodywork, Oakbrook Terrace, Ill, NCBTMB. Available at http://www.ncbtmb.com/pdf/consumers_guide_brochure.pdf. Accessed: March 30, 2008
7. American Organization of Bodywork Therapies of Asia: About the American Organization for Bodywork Therapies of Asia (AOBTA). Available at http://www.aobta.org/About.php. Accessed March 30, 2008
8. Shoemaker JK, Tiidus PM, Mader R: Failure of manual massage to alter limb blood flow: measures by Doppler ultrasound, *Med Sci Sports Exerc* 29:610-614, 1997.
9. Ernst E: Does post-exercise massage reduce delayed onset muscle soreness? A systematic review, *Br J Sports Med* 32:212-214, 1998.
10. Robertson A, Watt JM, Galloway SD: Effects of leg massage on recovery from high intensity cycling exercise, *Br J Sports Med* 38:173-176, 2004.
11. Hilbert JE, Sforzo GA, Swenson T: The effects of massage on delayed onset muscle soreness, *Br J Sports Med* 37:72-75, 2003.
12. Tanaka TH, Leisman G, Mori H et al: The effect of massage on localized lumbar muscle fatigue, *BMC Complement Altern Med* 2:9, 2002.
13. Fiechter JJ, Brodeur RR: Manual and manipulation techniques for rheumatic disease, *Med Clin N Am* 86:91-103, 2002.
14. Quinn C, Chandler C, Moraska A: Massage therapy and frequency of chronic tension headaches, *Am J Public Health* 92:1657-1661, 2002.
15. Hasson D, Arnetz B, Jelveus L et al: A randomized clinical trial of the treatment effects of massage compared to relaxation tape recordings on diffuse long-term pain, *Psychother Psychosom* 73:17-24, 2004.
16. Hernandez-Reif M, Field T, Krasnegor J et al: Lower back pain is reduced and range of motion increased after massage therapy, *Int J Neurosci* 106:131-145, 2001.
17. Cherkin DC, Sherman KJ, Deyo RA et al: A review of the evidence for the effectiveness, safety, and cost of acupuncture, massage therapy, and spinal manipulation for back pain, *Ann Intern Med* 138:898-906, 2003.
18. Cherkin DC, Eisenberg DM, Sherman KJ et al: Randomized trial comparing traditional Chinese medical acupuncture, therapeutic massage, and self-care education for chronic low back pain, *Arch Intern Med* 161:1081-1088, 2001.
19. Preyde M: Effectiveness of massage therapy for subacute low-back pain: a randomized controlled trial, *CMAJ* 162:1815-1820, 2000.
20. Furlan AD, Brosseau L, Imamura I et al: Massage for low back pain: a systematic review within the framework of the Cochrane Collaboration Back Review Group, *Spine* 27:1896-1910.
21. van der Dolder PA, Roberts DL: A trial into the effectiveness of soft tissue massage in the treatment of shoulder pain, *Austr J Physiother* 49:183-188, 2003.
22. Tsao JC: Effectiveness of Massage Therapy for chronic, non-malignant pain: a review, *Evid Based Complement Alternat Med* 4165-4179, 2007.
23. Beeken JE, Parks D, Cory J et al: The effectiveness of neuromuscular release massage therapy in five individuals with chronic obstructive lung disease, *Clin Nurs Res* 7:309-325, 1998.
24. Field T, Henteleff T, Hernandez-Reif M et al: Children with asthma have improved pulmonary functions after massage therapy, *J Pediatr* 132:854-858, 1998.
25. Hernandez-Reif M, Field T, Krasnegor J et al: Children with cystic fibrosis benefit from massage therapy, *J Pediatr Psychol* 24:175-181, 1999.
26. Simons DG, Simons LS, Travell JG: *Travell and Simons' myofascial pain and dysfunction: the trigger point manual*, 2 vols, ed 2, Baltimore, 1999, Lippincott Williams and Wilkins.
27. Kaada B, Torsteinbo O: Increase of plasma endorphins in connective tissue massage, *Gen Pharmacol* 20:487-489, 1989.
28. Ferrell-Tory AT, Glick OJ: The use of therapeutic massage as a nursing intervention to modify anxiety and the perception of cancer pain, *Cancer Nurs* 16:93-101, 1993.
29. Wilkinson S: Get the massage, *Nurs Times* 92:61-64, 1996.
30. Grealish L, Lomasney A, Whiteman B: Foot massage: a nursing intervention to modify the distressing symptoms of pain and nausea in patients hospitalized with cancer, *Cancer Nurs* 23:237-243, 2000.
31. Weinrich SP, Wienrich MC: The effect of massage on pain in cancer patients, *Appl Nurs Res* 3:140-145, 1990.
32. Smith MC, Kemp J, Hemphill L et al: Outcomes of therapeutic massage for hospitalized cancer patients, *J Nurs Scholar* 34:257-262, 2002.
33. Smith MC, Reeder F, Daniel L et al: Outcomes of touch therapies during bone marrow transplantation, *Altern Ther Med* 9:40-49, 2003.
34. Post-White J, Kinney ME, Savik K et al: Therapeutic massage and healing touch improve symptoms in cancer, *Integr Cancer Ther* 2:332-344, 2003.
35. Cassileth BR, Vickers AJ: Massage therapy for symptom control: outcome study at a major cancer center, *J Pain Symptom Manage* 28:3, 2004.
36. Mehling WE, Jacobs B, Acree M et al: Symptom management with massage and acupuncture in postoperative cancer patients: a randomized controlled trial, *J Pain Symptom Manage* 33:258-266, 2007.
37. Hernandez-Reif M, Field T, Ironson G et al: Natural killer cells and lymphocytes increase in women with breast cancer following massage therapy, *Intern J Neuroscience* 115:495-510, 2005.
38. Moyer CA, Rounds J, Hannum JW: A meta-analysis of massage therapy research, *Psychol Bull* 130:3-18, 2004.
39. Field T, Peck M, Sed et al: Post-burn itching, pain, and psychological symptoms are reduced with massage therapy, *J Burn Care Rehabil* 21:189-193, 2000.
40. Field T, Hernandez-Reif M, Seligman S et al: Juvenile rheumatoid arthritis benefits from massage therapy, *J Pediatr Psychol* 22:607-617, 1997.
41. Mitchinson AR, Kim HM, Rosenberg JM et al: Acute postoperative pain management using massage as an adjuvant therapy: a randomized trial, *Arch Surg* 142:1158-1167, 2007.
42. Piotrowski MM, Paterson C, Mitchinson A et al: Massage as adjuvant therapy in the management of acute postoperative pain: a preliminary study in men, *J Am Coll Surg* 197:1037-1046, 2003.
43. Taylor AG, Galpner DI, Taylor P et al: Effects of adjunctive Swedish massage and vibration therapy on short-term postoperative outcomes: a randomized, controlled trial, *J Altern Complement Med* 9:77-89, 2003.

44. LeBlanc-Louvry I, Costaglioli B, Boulon C et al: Does mechanical massage of the abdominal wall after colectomy reduce postoperative pain and shorten the duration of ileus? Results of a randomized study, *J Gastrointest Surg* 6:43-49, 2002.

45. Richards KC, Gibson R, Overton-McCoy AL: Effects of massage in acute and critical care, *AACN Clin Issues* 11:77-96, 2000.

46. Delaney JP, Leong KS, Watkins A et al: The short term effects of myofascial trigger point massage therapy on cardiac autonomic tone in healthy subjects, *J Adv Nurs* 37:364-371, 2002.

47. Hayes J, Cox C: Immediate effects of a five-minute foot massage on patients in critical care, *Intens Crit Care Nurs* 15:77-82, 1999.

48. Fraser J, Kerr JR: Psychophysiological effects of back massage on elderly institutionalized patients, *J Adv Nurs* 18:238-245, 1993.

49. Labyak DE, Metzger BL: The effects of effleurage backrub on the physiological components of relaxation: a meta-analysis, *Nurs Res* 46:59-62, 1997.

50. Diego MA, Field T, Sanders C et al: Massage therapy of moderate and light pressure and vibrator effects on EEG and heart rate, *Int J Neurosci* 114:31-44, 2004.

51. Field T, Ironson G, Scafidi F et al: Massage therapy reduces anxiety and enhances EEG patterns of alertness and math computations, *Int J Neurosci* 86:197-205, 1996.

52. Field T, Peck M, Krugman S et al: Burn injuries benefit from massage therapy, *J Burn Care Rehabil* 19:241-244, 1998.

53. Ironson G, Field T, Scafidi F et al: Massage therapy is associated with enhancement of the immune system's cytotoxic capacity, *Int J Neurosci* 84:205-217, 1996.

54. Field T, Morrno C, Valdeon C et al: Massage reduces anxiety in child and adolescent psychiatric patients, *J Am Acad Adolesc Psychiatry* 31:125-131, 1992.

55. Field T, Sunshine W, Hernandez-Reif M et al: Chronic fatigue syndrome: massage therapy effects of depression and somatic symptoms in chronic fatigue, *J Chron Fatigue Syndr* 3:43-51, 1997.

56. Schachner L, Field T, Hernandez-Reif M et al: Atopic dermatitis decreased in children following massage therapy, *Pediatr Dermatol* 15:390-395, 1998.

57. Rexilius SJ, Mundt C, Erikson Megel M et al: Therapeutic effects of massage therapy and handling touch on caregivers of patients undergoing autologous hematopoietic stem cells, *Oncol Nurs Forum* 29:E35-E44, 2002.

58. Wilkinson SM, Love SB, Westcombe AM et al: Effectiveness of aromatherapy massage in the management of anxiety and depression in patients with cancer: a multi-center randomized controlled trial, *Journal of Clinical Oncology* 25:532-538, 2007.

59. Phipps S: Reduction of distress associated with pediatric bone marrow transplant: complementary health promotion interventions, *Pediatr Rehabil* 5:223-234, 2003.

60. Hernandez-Reif M, Ironson G, Field T et al: Breast cancer patients have improved immune and neuroendocrine functions following massage therapy, *J Psychosom Res* 57:45-52, 2004.

61. Diego MA, Field T, Hernandez-Reif M: Vagal activity, gastric motility, and weight gain in massaged preterm neonates, *J of Pediatrics* 147:50-55, 2005.

62. International Association of Infant Massage. Available at www.iaim.ws/home.html. Accessed March 30, 2008.

63. Fleming-Drehobl K, Gengler-Fuhr M: *Pediatric massage for the child with special needs*, Tucson, Ariz, 1991, Therapy Skill Builders.

64. Barlow J, Cullen L: Increasing touch between parents and children with disabilities: preliminary results from a new program, *J Fam Care* 12:7-9, 2002.

65. Cullen L, Barlow J: 'Kiss, cuddle, squeeze': the experiences and meaning of touch among parents of children with autism attending a Touch Therapy Programme, *J Child Health Care* 6:171-181, 2002.

66. Pelaez-Nogueras M, Field TM, Hossain Z et al: Depressed mothers' touching increases infants' positive affect and attention in still-face interactions, *Child Dev* 67:1780-1792, 1996.

67. Field T: Massage therapy effects, *Am Psychol* 53:1270-1281, 1998.

68. Field T: Alleviating stress in intensive-care unit neonates, *J Am Osteopath Assoc* 87:646-650, 1987.

69. Harrison LL, Williams AK, Berbaum ML et al: Physiologic and behavioral effects of gentle human touch on preterm infants, *Res Nurs Heath* 23:435-466, 2000.

70. Hart S, Field T, Hernandez-Reif M et al: Preschoolers' cognitive performance improves following massage, *Early Child Develop Care* 143:59-64, 1998.

71. Barlow J, Cullen L: Increasing touch between parents and children with disabilities: preliminary results from a new programme, *J Fam Care* 12:7-9, 2002.

72. Jay S: The effects of gentle human touch on mechanically ventilated very-short gestation infants, *Matern Child J* 11:199-257, 1982.

73. Scafidi FA, Field T, Schanberg SM: Factors that predict which preterm infants benefit most from massage therapy, *Develop Behav Pediatr* 14:176-180, 1993.

74. Dieter JNI, Field T, Hernandez-Reif M et al: Stable preterm infants gain more weight and sleep less after five days of massage therapy, *J Pediatr Psychol* 28:403-411, 2003.

75. Golstein-Ferber S, Laudon M, Kuint J et al: Massage therapy by mothers enhances the adjustment of circadian rhythms to the nocturnal period in full-term infants, *Develop Behav Pediatr* 23:410-414, 2002.

76. Field T, Lasko D, Mundy P et al: Brief report: autistic children's attentiveness and responsivity improve after touch therapy, *J Autism Develop Disord* 27:333-338, 1997.

77. Field T, Quintino O, Hernandez-Reif M et al: Adolescents with attention deficit hyperactivity disorder benefit from massage therapy, *Adolescence* 33:105-108, 1998.

78. Field T, Schanberg S, Kuhn C et al: Bulimic adolescents benefit from massage therapy, *Adolescence* 33:557-563, 1998.

79. Jones NA, Field T: Massage and music therapies attenuate frontal EEG asymmetry in depressed adolescents, *Adolescence* 34:529-534, 1999.

Osteopathy

1. Educational Council on Osteopathic Principles: Glossary of osteopathic terminology. In Ward R, editor: *Foundations for osteopathic medicine*, Philadelphia, 2002, Lippincott Williams and Wilkins.

2. Still A: *Philosophy of osteopathy*, Kirksville, Mo, 1899.

3. Sutherland WG: *The cranial bowl*, ed 2, 1939, Sutherland.

4. Magoun HIS: *Osteopathy in the cranial field*, Kirksville, Mo, 1951, The Journal Printing Co.

5. Magoun HIS: *Osteopathy in the cranial field*, ed 3, Kirksville, Mo, 1976, The Journal Printing Co.

6. Patriquin DA: *The selected writings of Beryl E. Aurbuckle, D.O., F.A.C.O.P.*, Indianapolis, 1994, American Academy of Osteopathy.

7. Frymann VM, Carney RE, Springall P: Effect of osteopathic medical management on neurological development in children, *J Am Osteopathic Assoc* 92:729-744, 1992.

8. Carreiro JE: *An osteopathic approach to children*, London, 2003, Churchill Livingstone.

9. Mills MV, Henley CE, Barnes LL et al: The use of osteopathic manipulative treatment as adjuvant therapy in children with recurrent acute otitis media, *Arch Pediatr Adolesc Med* 157:861-866, 2003.

10. Blood SD, Hurwitz BA: Brain wave pattern changes in children with ADD/ADHD following osteopathic manipulation: a pilot study, *Am Acad Osteopath J* 10:19-20, 2000.

11. Lassovetskaya L: Osteopathic treatment of schoolchildren with delayed psychic development of cerebral-organic orgin, *J Osteopath Med (Austr)* 6:38, 2003.

12. Gevitz N: The sword and the scapel—the osteopathic "war" to enter the military medical corps: 1916-1966, *J Am Osteopath Assoc* 98:279-286, 1998.

13. Dugan EP, Lemley WW, Roberts CA et al: Effect of lymphatic pump techniques on the immune response to influenza vaccine, *J Am Osteopath Assoc* 101:472, 2001.

14. Steele TF: Utilization of osteopathic lymphatic pump in the office and home for treatment of viral illnesses and after vaccine immunizations, *Fam Phys* 2:8-11, 1998.

15. Jackson KM, Steele TF, Dugan EP et al: Effect of lymphatic and splenic pump techniques on the antibody response to hepatitis B vaccine: a pilot study, *J Am Osteopath Assoc* 98:155-160, 1998.

16. Measel JW: The effect of the lymphatic pump on the immune response: I. Preliminary studies on the antibody response to pneumococcal polysaccharide assayed by bacterial agglutination and passive hemagglutination, *J Am Osteopath Assoc* 82:28-31, 1982.

17. Nelson KE: Osteopathic treatment of upper respiratory infections offers distinct therapeutic advantages, *Osteopath Fam Phys News* 2:10-12, 2002.

18. Gold P, Goodwin F: Clinical and biochemical manifestations of stress: part I, *N Engl J Med* 319:348-353, 1988.

19. Gold P, Goodwin F: Clinical and biochemical manifestations of depression: part II, *N Engl J Med* 319:413-420, 1988.

20. McEwan B: Glucocorticoid-biogenic amine interactions in relation to mood and behavior, *Biochem Pharm* 36:1755-1763, 1987.

21. Bellinger DL, Lorton D, Brouxhon S et al: The significance of vasoactive intestinal polypeptide (VIP) in immunomodulation, *Adv Neuroimmunol* 6:5-27, 1996.

22. Seeman TE, Singer BH, Rowe JW et al: Price of adaptation—allosteric load and its health consequences, *Arch Intern Med* 157:2259-2268, 1997.

23. Kiecolt-Glaser JK, Glaser R: Stress and immune function in humans, In Ader R, Felton DL, Cohen N, editors: *Psychoneuroimmunology*, ed 2, San Diego, 1991, Academic Press, pp 849-895.

24. Esterling BA, Kiecolt-Glaser JK, Glaser R: Psychosocial modulation of cytokine-induced natural killer cell activity in older adults, *Psychosom Med* 58:264-272, 1996.

25. Van Buskirk RL: Nociceptive reflexes and the somatic dysfunction: a model, *J Am Osteopath Assoc* 90:792-809, 1990.

26. Kelso AF, Grant RG, Johnston WL: Use of thermograms to support assessment of somatic dysfunction or effects of osteopathic manipulative treatment: preliminary report, *J Am Osteopath Assoc* 82:182-188, 1982.

27. Hruby RJ: Pathophysiologic models and the selection of osteopathic manipulative techniques, *J Osteopath Med* 6:25-30, 1992.

28. Hruby RJ: Pathophysiologic models: aids to the selection of manipulative techniques, *AAO J* 1:8-10, 1991.

29. Coates G, O'Brodovich H, Goeree G: Hindlimb and lung lymph flows during prolonged exercise, *J Appl Physiol* 75:633-638, 1993.

30. Pippard C, Roddie IC. The effect of acute changes in blood flow on local lymph flow in the limbs of anesthetized sheep, *Lymphology* 23:200-206, 1990.

31. McGeown JG, McHale NG, Thornbury KD: The role of external compression and movement in lymph propulsion in the sheep hind limb, *J Physiol (Lond)* 387:83-93, 1987.

32. Stranden E, Kramer K: Lymphatic and transcapillary forces in patients with edema following operation for lower limb atherosclerosis, *Lymphology* 15:148-155, 1982.

33. Ahlqvist J: On the structural and physiological basis of the influence of exercise, movement and immobilization in inflammatory joint diseases, *Ann Chir Gynaecol Suppl* 198: 10-18, 1985.

34. Bettendorf U: Lymph flow mechanism of the subperitoneal diaphragmatic lymphatics, *Lymphology* 11:111-116, 1978.

35. Blomqvist H, Berg B, Frostell C et al: Thoracic lymph drainage in the dog: evaluation of a new model, *Intens Care Med* 17:45-51, 1991.

36. Boriek AM, Wilson TA, Rodarte JR: Displacements and strains in the costal diaphragm of the dog, *J Appl Physiol* 76:223-229, 1994.

37. Boynton BR, Barnas GM, Dadmun JT et al: Mechanical coupling of the rib cage, abdomen, and diaphragm through their area of apposition, *J Appl Physiol* 70:1235-1244, 1991.

38. Brace RA: Blood volume response to drainage of left thoracic duct lymph in the ovine fetus, *Am J Physiol* 266:R709-R713, 1994.

39. Bradham RR, Parker EF: The cardiac lymphatics, *Ann Thorac Surg* 15:526-535, 1973.

40. Bull RH, Gane JN, Evans JE et al: Abnormal lymph drainage in patients with chronic venous leg ulcers, *J Am Acad Dermatol* 28:585-590, 1993.

41. Drake RE, Gabel JC: Diaphragmatic lymph vessel drainage of the peritoneal cavity, *Blood Purif* 10:132-135, 1992.

42. Eliskova M, Oldrich E: How lymph is drained away from the human papillary muscle: anatomical conditions, *Cardiology* 81:371-377, 1992.

43. Winter DA, Patia AE, Frank JS et al: Biomechanical walking pattern changes in the fit and healthy elderly, *Phys Ther* 70:340-347, 1990.

44. Rimmer KP, Ford GT, Whitelaw WA: Interaction between postural and respiratory control of human intercostal muscles, *J Appl Physiol* 79:1556-1561, 1995.

45. Norre ME: Head extension effect in static posturography, *Ann Otol Rhinol Laryngol* 104:570-573, 1995.

46. Aihara Y, Nakamura H, Sato A et al: Neural control of gastric motility with special reference to cutaneo-gastric reflexes, In Brooks C, editor: *Integrative functions of the autonomic nervous system*, New York, 1979, Elsevier, pp 38-49.

47. Garrison DW, Chandler MJ, Foreman RD: Viscerosomatic convergence onto feline spinal neurons from esophagus, heart and somatic fields: effects on inflammation, *Pain* 49:373-382, 1992.

48. Lumb BM, Lovick TA: The rostral hypothalamus: an area for the integration of autonomic and sensory responsiveness, *J Neurophysiol* 70:1570-1577, 1993.

49. Sato A, Schmidt RF: Somatosympathetic reflexes: afferent fibers, central pathways, discharge characteristics, *Physiol Rev* 53: 916-947, 1973.

50. Sato A: Somatovisceral reflexes, *J Manipulative Physiol Ther* 18: 597-602, 1995.

51. Sato A, Swenson S: Sympathetic nervous system response to mechanical stress of the spinal column in rats, *J Man Med* 7: 141-147, 1984.

52. Sato A: The reflex effects of spinal somatic nerve stimulation on visceral function, *J Man Physiol Ther* 15:57-61, 1992.

53. Beal MC, Dvorak J: Palpatory examination of the spine: a comparison of the results of two methods and their relationship to visceral disease, *Man Med* 1:25-32, 1984.

54. Beal MC: Viscerosomatic reflexes: a review, *J Am Osteopath Assoc* 85:786-801, 1985.

55. Willard FH: Autonomic nervous system, In Ward R, editor: *Foundations for osteopathic medicine*, ed 2, Philadelphia, 2003, Lippincott, Williams and Wilkins, pp 90-119.

56. Kuchera ML, Kuchera WA: *Osteopathic considerations in systemic disease*, Columbus, OH, 1994, Greydon Press.
57. Cox JM, Gorbis S, Dick L et al: Palpable musculoskelstal findings in coronary artery disease: results of a double blind study, *J Am Osteopath Assoc* 82:832-836, 1983.
58. Beal MC, Morlock JW: Somatic dysfunction associated with pulmonary disease, *J Am Osteopath Assoc* 84:179-183, 1984.
59. Fitzgerald M, Stiles E: Osteopathic hospital's solution to DRGs may be OMT, *D O* 97-101, 1984.
60. Nicholas AS, DeBias DA, Ehrenfeuchter W et al: A somatic component to myocardial infarction, *Br Med J* 291:13-17, 1985.
61. Owen C: *An endocrine interpretation of Chapman's reflexes*, ed 2, Boulder, Colo, 1963, American Academy of Osteopathy.
62. Mitchell FL Jr.: The influence of Chapman's reflexes and the immune reactions, *Osteopath Ann* 2:12, 1974.
63. Esterling B: Stress-associated modulation of cellular immunity, In Willard FH, Patterson M, editors: *Nociception and the neuro-endocrine-immune connection*, Boulder, Colo, 1992, American Academy of Osteopathy.
64. Ganong W: The stress response—a dynamic overview, *Hosp Prac* 23:155-171, 1988.
65. Sternberg EM, Wilder RL, Gold PW et al: A defect in the central component of the immune system—hypothalamic-pituitary-adrenal axis feedback loop is associated with susceptibility to experimental arthritis and other inflammatory diseases, *Ann N Y Acad Sci* 594:289-292, 1990.
66. Sternberg EM: Neuroendocrine factors in susceptibility to inflammatory disease: focus on the hypothalamic-pituitary-adrenal axis, *Horm Res* 43:159-161, 1995.
67. Sternberg EM, Licinio J: Overview of neuroimmune stress interactions—implications for susceptibility to inflammatory disease, *Ann N Y Acad Sci* 771:364-371, 1995.
68. Sternberg EM, Chrousos GP, Wilder RL et al: The stress response and the regulation of inflammatory disease, *Ann Intern Med* 117:854-866, 1992.
69. Still A: *Philosophy of osteopathy*, Kirksville, Mo, 1899.
70. Greenman PE, McPartland JM: Cranial findings and iatrogenesis from craniosacral manipulation in patients with traumatic brain syndrome, *J Am Osteopathic Assoc* 95:182-191, 1995.
71. Johnson K, Pasquarello G: *Cervical spine manipulation*, Boulder, Colo, 2003, American Academy of Osteopathy.

CHAPTER 4

Lifestyle Approaches

Nutrition: Current Understanding of Its Impact on Pediatric Health | Joy A. Weydert

Qigong in Pediatric Medicine | Effie Poy Yew Chow, Maria Choy

Nutrition: Current Understanding of Its impact on Pediatric Health

History

It is ironic that in the twenty-first century, nutrition is still considered a complementary or alternative therapy, given that food is the basic tenet for all of civilization. Since the beginning of time, food, or the lack thereof, has determined survival, and individuals have been admonished what to eat or not eat. Biblical passages give reference to what might have been the first nutritional counseling, advising the use of certain foods for their actual health benefits rather than just for survival. Later, as philosopher-scientists pondered the causation of various diseases, they recognized that illness is more than just a punishment from the gods—diet and environmental factors played an important part in human well-being. Hippocrates, who lived in the fourth century BCE, is credited with saying, "Let food be your medicine" and wrote many theses on the importance of diet.[1]

As civilization progressed a cultural change occurred in humans' relationship to food. Initially, the hunter/gatherer tribes roamed the lands in search of meats, berries, and grains for sustenance. Once the domestication of animals and the cultivation of grains came into practice, greatly increasing the available food supply, the nomadic lifestyle gave way to the development of villages and cities.[1a] As time progressed, the issues around food shifted to address not only availability but also sanitation and the prevention of nutrient deficiency diseases.[2]

With the advent of industrialization and the mass production of processed foods, availability and sanitation became lesser issues. The abundance of processed food certainly has provided greater convenience to the modern family; unfortunately, the repercussion of this abundance is the rise of obesity in children and adults. In addition, dietary excesses can also engender overall nutritional deficiencies that may affect the cognitive, behavioral, and motor development of children. These micronutrient deficiencies also appear to promote long-latency deficiency diseases such as cardiovascular disease, cancer, osteoporosis, neurodegenerative diseases, and immune dysfunction.[3]

The current understanding of nutrition's effect on health has come a long way from earlier beliefs and teachings of nutrition, which to date have been highly influenced by the agricultural industry and U.S. government policy. Through the establishment of the U.S. Department of Agriculture (USDA), the U.S. government has given official dietary advice and information on human nutrition for more than 100 years. The USDA, however, also oversees and promotes U.S. agricultural practices. This dual assignment may cause a conflict of interest, as agricultural policies may clash with the nutritional polices that promote good health.[4] This became evident in 1991, when the USDA withdrew its Eating Right Pyramid food guide in response to pressure from meat and dairy producers. This controversy focused attention on a conflict between federal protection of the rights of food lobbyists to act in their own self-interest and the federal responsibility to promote the nutritional health of the public.[5] To promote a better understanding of the role of good nutrition for good health, major changes in national dietary policies, nutritional guidance, and nutrition educational policies will be necessary.

In this new era of science and research, the study of nutrition has become more concerned with the biochemical roles of all the nutrients and their impact on health. A new field of nutrigenomics has emerged, which studies the influence of nutrition on gene expression. This field is working to provide a molecular genetic understanding for how common dietary chemicals, the nutrients, affect health by altering the expression and/or structure of an individual's genetic makeup.[6]

Macronutrients: Proteins, Carbohydrates, Fats, and Lipids

This section provides a basic review of the biochemical functions of the essential macronutrients: proteins, carbohydrates, fats, and lipids. Proper balance of these three major nutritional components is essential for optimal health. Consequences of excess and deficiencies are also discussed.

Proteins

Amino acids (AAs) are the substrates for protein synthesis, made up of carbohydrates with an amino (NH_2) group attached the α-carbon. Most AAs can be made in the body from intermediates in the metabolic pathways, but "essential" AAs have carbon structures that cannot be made and thus must come from the diet.

These essential AAs include the following:
- Histidine
- Isoleucine
- Leucine
- Lysine
- Methionine
- Phenylalanine
- Threonine
- Tryptophan
- Valine

Nitrogen can be transferred between AAs and carbohydrates through transamination, a process that requires vitamin B_6 and allows formation of all 20 AAs necessary for protein synthesis.[7] In addition, vitamin A, vitamin D, and zinc are also important substrates for the regulation of gene expression for protein synthesis.

Protein synthesis occurs through deoxyribonucleic acid (DNA) transcription and ribonucleic acid (RNA) translation. Protein structure is essential for protein function; therefore peptide bonding and protein folding of the completed AA chain is a critical step in the final protein formation of linear chains, helices, and pleated sheets or the more complex tertiary or quaternary structures such as hemoglobin.

Proteins function as enzymes, hormones, immunoproteins, transport proteins, and structural proteins.[8] When bound to other constituents, they form glycoproteins, lipoproteins, and proteoglycans necessary for cell formation. Proteins are critical for maintaining physiological functions and gene expression[9] and can be used as an energy source at a rate of 4 kcal/g. Humans require that 10% to 15% percent of their total daily energy intake be from protein. Infants and toddlers need approximately 1.5 g/kg body weight of protein, and older children need approximately 1.0 g/kg body weight. Of that, 35% of the protein needs to be in the form of the essential AAs. These requirements are increased in catabolic states such as sepsis, trauma, burns, fever, or surgery or with malabsorption states such as protein-losing enteropathy or renal disease.

Protein deficiency rarely occurs in the industrialized world. However, children at risk for inadequate protein intake are those on strict vegetarian diets, those with multiple food allergies, or those who have limited food selections due to limited access, food fads, or behavior problems.[10] Because proteins are essential for many different functions, a deficiency can result in seriously compromised immune and regulatory systems. In addition, because some of the essential AAs are necessary for neurotransmitter synthesis, the possibility that protein deficiency may affect overall mental functioning is of concern. Tryptophan is required to synthesize serotonin and melatonin. Phenylalanine converts to tyrosine and then is further metabolized to L-dopa, the precursor to dopamine, norepinephrine, and epinephrine. All of these are necessary for normal nerve functioning.

Modern diets usually include excess amounts of protein, the long-term health consequences of which are not clearly known. Excess protein consumption can increase urinary nitrogen, which can stress kidney functioning. However, the phosphorus content in protein may offset the hypercalciuric and acidic effects of protein.[8] It is possible that high-protein diets may cause immune system dysfunction, leading to allergy or autoimmune disorders, as correlations have been seen between early introduction of cow's milk with eczema and asthma and between meat intake and rheumatoid arthritis. Removal of specific proteins ameliorates symptoms.[11]

Unlike carbohydrates and fats, protein should be consumed daily because the body does not store AAs. It is important that a diet contain sufficient amounts of all essential AAs to promote adequate protein synthesis. Proteins from animal sources (meat, milk, eggs) generally have the complete complement of necessary AAs. Denaturing these proteins through heat or in the presence of salt or acids improves their digestibility by making them more available to digestive enzymes.[8] Vegetable protein is less well digested because the cell wall carbohydrates need to be broken down to expose the protein. Vegetable proteins do not have the full complement of AAs; therefore it is recommended that foods be combined to provide "complete" proteins. For example, legumes, soybeans, and nuts are typically low in methionine, but they can be combined with cereal, whole grains, or sunflower seeds to provide this essential AA. Legumes offer benefits not found with animal protein, such as fiber, isoflavones, a lower fat content, and less expense.

Carbohydrates

Carbohydrates provide the major source of energy in our diet and are consumed either as simple sugars, such as fructose, sucrose, or lactose, or in their complex forms of starch, cellulose, or dietary fiber. Many different isomers of the monosaccharides can be formed by nature; however, only three hexoses—glucose, galactose, and fructose—can be absorbed and used by humans. Each hexose differs in chemical behavior, taste, sweetness, and dietary source. When linked, they form the disaccharides sucrose (glucose + fructose), lactose (glucose + galactose), and maltose (glucose + glucose).[7]

The primary functions of carbohydrates are to provide energy, preserve proteins, and prevent ketosis. However, they are also important in providing structure and promoting cellular function in various ways. When combined with proteins as glycoproteins, they function as enzymes, hormones, immunoglobulin receptors, transport proteins, and antigens. They also play a role in cell growth and formation as well as participate in the regulation of intracellular communication.[8] As glycolipids, they make up plasma membranes, myelin sheaths, cartilage, synovial fluid, and skin and are important for the function of receptors, blood group antigens, and tumor antigens. Humans require about 45% to 50% of their total daily energy needs in the form of carbohydrates.

Glucose is converted into energy within the cell but has to be transported across cell membranes via sodium-dependent glucose transport proteins. Further transport of glucose to other organ tissues depends on the overall extracellular concentration and the presence of insulin.[11] Glucose is found naturally in fruits and vegetables and, like other carbohydrates, provides 4 kcal/g of energy.

Excess glucose is stored as glycogen in liver and muscle tissue. Glycogen from the liver can be readily converted back to glucose and used for energy when glucose levels fall. Muscle glycogen, on the other hand, is used only within the muscle tissue for energy and cannot be released into the bloodstream.

Fructose is readily absorbed in the small intestine and converted into glucose, glycogen, lactic acid, or fat. If consumed in large quantities, the excess is most commonly converted to fat. Fructose is found naturally in fruits, table sugar, and honey. It is also in high-fructose corn syrup, which is processed enzymatically by converting glucose in cornstarch to fructose.[7] High-fructose corn syrup is added to canned and frozen fruits and to soft drinks, enhancing their flavors and textures. Fructo-oligosaccharides (FOS) are naturally occurring polymers of fructose found in artichokes, onions, asparagus, tomatoes, barley, and rye. They are resistant to digestion in the upper gastrointestinal (GI) tract but are utilized by bifidobacteria in the colon.[12] When ingested chronically, they enhance intestinal flora growth, relieve constipation, improve blood lipids, and alter glucose metabolism.[13]

Complex carbohydrates are the storage forms of glucose for energy—starch from plant sources and glycogen from animal sources. Because of the larger size and configuration of these molecules, digestion takes longer, therefore slowing the rate at which glucose enters the bloodstream. The rate at which these foods are utilized is also influenced by food processing and cooking methods. Processing often removes fiber, fat, vitamins, and minerals, thus altering the health benefits of these foods.

The glycemic index is an indicator of how rapidly and to what degree blood glucose levels rise after food is eaten. The post-prandial glucose curve of a particular carbohydrate-containing food is compared with a reference food, either white bread or glucose. The glycemic index of a food is influenced by the type of sugar present, the characteristic of the starch, the amount of soluble fiber present, particle size and density, method of preparation, and the presence of protein, fat, or acid, among other factors.[14]

In general, foods with a higher glycemic index raise blood sugar levels to a greater degree after ingestion than a low-glycemic-index food. This is important, as a rapid glycemic rise triggers an insulin response, often causing a reactive hypoglycemia. When ingested chronically, high-glycemic-index foods can lead to hyperinsulinism and insulin resistance—precursors to diabetes, obesity, heart disease, and other metabolic disorders.[15] Glycemic load may be a better way of evaluating the overall effects of carbohydrate-containing foods, as it is the sum total of the amount of all foods eaten with their glycemic index. Smaller intakes of high-glycemic foods may have less of a rise in glucose and insulin levels when taken in a meal mixed with protein and fiber. Overall, however, low-glycemic meals result in lower blood glucose levels, lower insulin response, greater satiety, improved energy levels, and lower serum lipid levels.[14] In addition, sustained weight loss has been demonstrated in obese adolescents maintained on a low-glycemic-load diet compared with those on a calorie- and fat-restricted diet.[16] Lists of low-glycemic-index food (values < 55), mid-glycemic foods (55 to 70) and high-glycemic foods (70 to 100) can be found in Table 4-1.

Carbohydrate deficiency is rare in the industrialized world, except in individuals on low-carbohydrate diets, which predisposes the person to the development of ketosis. Unfortunately, overconsumption of carbohydrates is more readily seen with the end results of obesity, insulin resistance, and heart disease. Other chronic illnesses may be promoted by carbohydrate excess because of the effects of simple sugars on immune function. Consuming 3 oz of simple sugars (e.g., sucrose, fructose, honey, fruit juice) depresses white blood cell activity by 50% for 1 to 5 hours.[17]

Fats and lipids

Humans require about 35% of their total energy needs in the form of fat. Fat is energy rich and provides 9 kcal/g compared with 4 kcal/g with proteins and carbohydrates. Fats come in many forms extracted from plant and animal sources, including saturated fats from meat and dairy, monounsaturated fats from certain vegetable oils, and polyunsaturated fats obtained from various sources (see later discussion). The more saturated the fat, the more solid it is at room temperature. Of these groups of compounds, two polyunsaturated fatty acids are considered essential for human structural and metabolic needs—omega-3 and omega-6 fatty acids (FAs). Humans cannot produce carbon-carbon double bonds before the ninth carbon of an FA chain; therefore omega-3 (first double bond at carbon 3) and omega-6 FAs (first double bond at carbon 6) must be obtained from food. Each FA performs different functions. The ratio of these two FAs determines optimal functioning.[7]

FAs participate in numerous important functions: cell membrane formation and maintenance, chemical and oxygen transport, proper development of the central nervous system (CNS), energy production, and regulation of inflammation.[18] Historically early humans had diets richer in omega-3 FA, as they subsisted on marine life, plants, and grass-fed game, giving them a ratio of omega-6 to omega-3 FAs of 1:1 to 4:1. The more modern diet is richer in omega-6 FAs owing to higher intakes of grain-fed animal proteins, vegetable oils, and processed foods that have been partially hydrogenated for a longer shelf life in the grocery stores. This has shifted the current ratio of omega-6 to omega-3 FAs to 10:1 or 25:1. The significance of this is what occurs when these essential FAs are metabolized.

Omega-6 FA (linoleic acid) is the precursor to arachidonic acid, which leads to the production of prostaglandin E2 (PGE-2), thromboxanes, prostacyclins, and leukotrienes. These induce vasoconstriction, platelet aggregation, cell proliferation, inflammation, and blood clotting. Omega-3 FA (α-linolenic acid) is the precursor to eicosapentaenoic acid (EPA) and docosahexaenoic acid (DHA), which produces PGE-1, PGE-3, and leukotrienes that are less inflammatory. Omega-6 and omega-3 compete for the same enzyme for metabolism—delta-6 desaturase. Anything that shifts the production toward the omega-6 pathway (increased omega-6 intake, excessive alcohol intake, diabetes, stress) will promote inflammation.[18] Lowering the omega-6 to omega-3 ratio closer to 1:1 can potentially induce a less inflammatory state. Population studies found that the incidence of rheumatoid arthritis was significantly less in places where people ate a more "primitive" diet of whole foods, vegetables, and fiber compared with places where people consumed diets high in meat, refined carbohydrates, and fats.[17]

Omega-3 FAs are important for functioning of the human brain and CNS.[19] EPA and DHA are the main structural components of cell membranes in the brain, and their presence can change membrane structure and influence neurotransmitter functioning.[20] Depression, bipolar disorder, and postpartum depression have all been correlated with lower omega-3 intake and have been treated successfully with supplementation with omega-3 FAs.[21,22]

Increased consumption of omega-3 FAs has been linked to reduced risk of heart attack, lower triglyceride levels, and better blood clotting.[23] In children, accumulating evidence links omega-3 FA deficiency to attention-deficit hyperactivity disorder (ADHD). Supplementation with a ratio of DHA to EPA of 5:1 significantly improved blood essential FA levels and

✳ **TABLE 4-1**

Glycemic Index of Common Foods

FOODS	GLYCEMIC INDEX	FOODS	GLYCEMIC INDEX	FOODS	GLYCEMIC INDEX
Breads/Bakery Products		**Pasta**		**Beans**	
Multigrain bread	48	Spaghetti, whole wheat	37	Soybeans	16
Sourdough bread	52	Spaghetti, white	41	Lentils	29
Pound cake	54	Macaroni	45	Chickpeas	33
Angel food cake	67	Spaghetti, durum wheat	55	Kidney beans	52
White bread	70	Brown rice pasta	92	Broad beans	79
Bagel	72	**Fruits**		**Snack Foods**	
Doughnut	76			Peanuts	14
Rice cakes	77	Cherries	22	Potato chips	54
Baguette	95	Grapefruit	25	Popcorn	55
Cereals		Apple	36	Chocolate bar	64
		Pear	38	Corn chips	74
All-Bran	42	Grapes	46	Jelly beans	80
Special K	54	Mango	55	Pretzels	81
Mini-Wheats	57	Banana	56	**Beverages**	
Oatmeal	61	Raisins	65		
Shredded Wheat	69	Pineapple	66	Soy milk	30
Puffed wheat	74	Watermelon	72	Skim milk	31
Cheerios	74	**Vegetables**		Chocolate milk	34
Rice Krispies	82			Tomato juice	40
Corn flakes	83	Asparagus, cauliflower	15	Apple juice	41
Grains		Lettuce, spinach, broccoli	15	Orange juice	52
		Tomatoes, zucchini	15	Soda pop	68
Pearl barley	25	Green peas	48	Gatorade	78
Converted rice	46	Carrots	49	**Sugars**	
Bulgur	48	Sweet potato	54		
Buckwheat	54	Sweet corn	55	Fructose	43
Brown rice	55	Beets	64	Honey	58
White rice	58	Mashed potatoes	70	Table sugar (sucrose)	65
Couscous	65	Baked potato	85	Glucose	100
Taco shell	68				
Millet	71				

attention span in these children.[24] For patients with sickle cell disease, supplementation with omega-3 FAs significantly reduced red cell sickling, red cell hemolysis, anemia, and pain crisis.[25] It is theorized in sickle cell disease that omega-3 FAs can be incorporated into the red blood cell membrane, thus improving biomembrane stability and fluidity.

Increasing one's intake of omega-3 FAs has to be coupled with decreasing the intake of omega-6 FAs to effectively change this overall ratio in the diet. Sources of omega-3 FA include the following:

- Wild cold-water fish (salmon, mackerel, sardines, herring, tuna)
- Fish oils, canola oil
- Flax seeds/oil, hemp seeds/oil
- Nuts (walnuts, pecans)
- Dark green leafy vegetables
- Soybeans
- Algae
- High omega-3 eggs

Sources of omega-6 FA include the following:

- Vegetable oils (corn, soybean, safflower, cottonseed)
- Grain-fed meats (as opposed to grass-fed)
- Processed food with partially hydrogenated oils and trans fats
- Margarine
- γ-Linolenic acid (evening primrose oil, black currant oil, borage oil)

Micronutrients: Vitamins and Minerals
Vitamins

Animals cannot survive on a chemically defined diet containing only purified proteins, carbohydrates, fats, and necessary minerals. Additional factors found in natural foods, even though they are needed in minute amounts, are necessary to sustain life. These factors are called *vitamins*.[26] Vitamins were discovered more than 100 years ago when certain diseases were found to relate to deficiencies in the diet. The belief that certain factors were vital to life—"vital amines" or "vitamins"—spurred research to better understand their identities and functions. Initially vitamins were named by letters (e.g., vitamin A, vitamin B, vitamin C) and then named according to the diseases they cured (e.g., antiberiberi, antirachitic, antiscurvy). Now they are more readily classified according to their chemical structures.[27] Vitamins generally fulfill the following criteria:

- They are organic compounds different from fats, carbohydrates, or proteins.
- They are a natural component of foods.
- They cannot be synthesized in adequate amounts by the host.
- They are essential for growth, development, maintenance, and reproduction.
- They are necessary for preventing specific deficiency syndromes.[28]

Vitamins act as enzymes, antioxidants, cofactors in metabolic oxidation-reduction reactions, hormones, and membrane stabilizers. As with the macronutrients, a vitamin's structure determines function.

It was previously believed that supplying these individual nutrients in the form of dietary supplements was all that was needed to promote health. With the growing understanding of the beneficial phytochemicals in the natural food supply, more recent efforts have reoriented the focus toward consuming whole foods for health promotion and maintenance.[29]

Likewise, the amount of these nutrients that an individual needs on a daily basis is the subject of ongoing controversy. It must be understood that the recommended dietary allowances (RDA), developed in the mid-twentieth century, are amounts necessary only to prevent deficiency-related diseases in healthy people. These RDAs assume that all individuals have the same needs, metabolism, and genetic makeup and do not consider increased needs due to metabolic stress, environmental exposures, or illness. The Food and Nutrition Board is developing a newer tool, the Dietary Reference Intakes (DRI), but this also is based on the observed intake of nutrients by populations of healthy people.[30] A future goal of nutrition education should be to address the individual and his or her specific needs, taking into account genetics, lifestyle, dietary habits, environment, and level of stress. The amounts of nutrients necessary to treat specific medical conditions also must be recognized.

Vitamins are generally classified as either fat soluble or water soluble. A general overview of these various vitamins is offered here to describe their essential functions, usual food sources, and the results of excess or deficiency. In general, fat-soluble vitamins are absorbed and transported with dietary fat, stored in cells, and excreted with the feces via enterohepatic circulation. In contrast, water-soluble vitamins are absorbed by passive and active processes, transported in free solution or bound to carriers, and excreted in the urine. Water-soluble vitamins are not stored in the body in appreciable amounts.[28]

Fat-soluble vitamins

Vitamin A. Important functions of vitamin A include maintaining the integrity of internal and external epithelial tissues; regenerating rhodopsin and iodopsin (visual pigments), which are necessary for night vision; promoting growth of long bones; supporting immune function; and human reproduction. Vitamin A has been called the *antiinfective vitamin*, likely due to its role in epithelial tissue integrity.[17]

Vitamin A is a family of retinoids that includes a high-molecular-weight alcohol, retinol, retinal (the aldehyde form), and retinoic acid (the acid form). Plant pigments that can yield retinoids on metabolism are referred to as *provitamin A* and are the carotenoids. Provitamin A carotenoids are synthesized by all plants, which are then transformed into vitamin A in the liver. The most active of these is β-carotene, which yields 2 molecules of vitamin A, whereas α- and γ-carotenes yield only 1 molecule.[26]

Provitamin A carotenoids are found in dark green leafy and yellow-orange vegetables and fruit. Typically the deeper colors are associated with higher carotene levels.[28] Preformed vitamin A is found in animal sources such as fish liver oils, liver, egg yolks, butter, cream, and fortified milks.

Vitamin A in food is fairly stable in light and heat but is easily destroyed by air (oxygen) and sunlight (ultraviolet [UV] rays). This can be protected by the concurrent use of vitamin E as an antioxidant.[27]

The current RDA for children is 300 to 700 retinol equivalents (RE) per day and 800 to 1000 RE/day for adults. Lactating mothers may need as many as 1300 RE/day. High doses of vitamin A have been linked to birth defects and therefore should not be used by women who are pregnant or at risk for pregnancy. However, β-carotene, the precursor to vitamin A, is a safe and effective alternative.[17]

Vitamin A toxicity occurs with single large doses (660,000 IU/200,000 RE in adults, 300,000 IU/100,000 RE in children) or with chronic daily doses greater than 10 times the RDA.[28] Symptoms include dry mucous membranes of the eyes, nose, or mouth; dryness, redness, and scaling of the skin; hair loss; joint pain; periosteal thickening of the long bones; headaches; nausea; or vomiting. The CNS symptoms often mimic pseudotumor cerebri.

Vitamin A deficiency manifests clinically as impaired vision with night blindness; keratinization of mucous membranes and skin, increasing the susceptibility to infections; dry, rough skin; impairment of cell-mediated immunity; poor growth; anemia; or reproductive failure. Deficiencies can occur from inadequate intakes of vitamin A or the carotenoids or from malabsorption states, liver disease, or zinc deficiency.

Vitamin D. The principal action of vitamin D is to promote calcium and phosphorus homeostasis by increasing the absorption of calcium and phosphorus from the intestine, moving them out of storage in the bone, depositing them in the teeth, preventing their excretion, and maintaining their level in the blood. This is done in concert with the endocrine system, which includes parathyroid hormone (PTH), calcitonin, and estrogen. Vitamin D may also be essential for cell differentiation; maintenance of membranes, nerves, and glands; and normal functioning of the immune system.

The two most important forms of vitamin D for nutritional purposes are ergocalciferol (pro-vitamin D_2), which is derived from the plant sterol ergosterol, and cholecalciferol (pro-vitamin D_3), derived from the animal sterol 7-dehydrocholesterol. These sterols are absorbed through the intestine and are converted to pro-vitamin D_2 and pro-vitamin D_3 when skin is exposed to sunlight (UV irradiation). These pro-vitamins are further metabolized in the liver and kidneys to their active forms, 1,25 dihydroxyvitamin D_2 and 1,25 dihydroxyvitamin D_3 (calcitriol).[28] Metabolic activation to convert vitamin D to these active forms is regulated by PTH to maintain constant calcium levels. 1,25 Dihydroxyvitamin D_3 enhances active transport of Ca^{++} across the intestinal lumen, regulates mobilization and deposition of Ca^{++} and phosphorus in conjunction with PTH and estrogen, and increases reabsorption of Ca^{++} and phosphorus in the renal tubules.

Vitamin D can be readily obtained from skin exposure to sunlight for about 15 minutes per day. It has been estimated that exposing at least 6% of the body surface area to the minimal erythemal dose (MED)—the minimum quantity of UV radiation required to produce a perceptible reddening of the skin—is the equivalent of 1000 IU of vitamin D.[31] However, for those whose skin is dark pigmented, are house bound, who live in cities with dense smog, who are unable to tolerate sun exposure, or who use high–skin protection factor (SPF) sunscreen, vitamin D may need to be obtained through dietary sources. Vitamin D can be found in fish oils, butter, cream, egg yolks, liver, and fortified milk.

The current RDA/DRI for children is approximately 200 IU (5 μg) a day. For adults, 400 to 600 IU (10 to 15 μg) per day is recommended. It is not possible to "overdose" in the synthesis of vitamin D through sunlight, as the body automatically limits the amount produced.

Vitamin D toxicity can lead to hypercalcemia and hyperphosphatemia, which can manifest as calcification of the skin, kidneys, heart, lungs, and tympanic membranes. Other symptoms may include headaches, GI upset, diarrhea, and poor growth.

Vitamin D deficiency leads to rickets, which is impaired mineralization in the growing bones of children. Clinical signs and symptoms include bowing of the weight-bearing bones, deformation of the breast bone and skull, bone pain, and muscle tenderness. In severe cases, tetany can occur from hypocalcemia. Deficiency states can occur with poor exposure to sunlight, lack of food sources containing vitamin D, or malabsorption states; in survivors of severe burns; or in patients on chronic anticonvulsant therapy, which reduces the circulating 1,25 dihydroxyvitamin D_3 levels.[28]

In a recent birth-cohort study conducted in Finland, development of type 1 diabetes was associated with low intakes of vitamin D and signs of rickets in the first year of life. Children who were supplemented with at least 2000 IU daily had an 80% reduced risk of developing type 1 diabetes.[32] Osteomalacia can occur in adults, causing reduced bone density, bone tenderness, and muscular weakness. Teenage girls are at particular risk in developing this owing to low consumption of fortified milk and large consumption of phosphate-containing soft drinks, which pull calcium out of the bones. Studies have shown that people with low back pain and generalized body aches often have low circulating levels of 1,25 dihydroxyvitamin D_3; their symptoms resolved when supplemented.[33] Osteoporosis differs from osteomalacia in that actual reduction in bone mass occurs. This is more common in postmenopausal women and older men and seems to be related in part to lower hormone levels.

Vitamin E. Vitamin E is a complex of compounds made up of four tocopherols and four tocotrienols, each labeled as α, β, δ, and γ. The tocopherols and tocotrienols are asymmetrical molecules that exist in the mirror image forms—D-isomers and L-isomers; however, only the D-isomers are biologically active and are found naturally in foods.

Vitamin E is absorbed in the small intestine in the presence of dietary fat, bile acids, and pancreatic enzymes; then it is taken up by chylomicron, transported to the liver, and then incorporated into very-low-density lipoprotein (VLDL) and high-density lipoprotein (HDL). When taken up by the cell, vitamin E is located almost exclusively in the membranes so that it can easily be mobilized to reduce the oxygen-centered free radicals into harmless metabolites.[28]

The main function of vitamin E is that of free radical scavenger, protecting vitamin A and the polyunsaturated fats in the body from oxidative stress caused by the processes of metabolism and effects of the environment. This has a direct effect on all cells owing to the presence of polyunsaturated fatty acids (PUFAs) in all lipid membranes. Vitamin E works with selenium, copper, zinc, manganese, and riboflavin to augment the function of other enzymes necessary in the cellular antioxidant system and for cell metabolism.[28] This antioxidant system may be important in protecting against conditions related to oxidative stress, such as smoking, exposure to ozone, arthritis, cancer, cardiovascular disease, or other degenerative diseases.[17]

Vitamin E has been found to inhibit excessive platelet aggregation, inhibit tumor angiogenesis, promote the breakdown of fibrin, and enhance both cell-mediated immunity and humoral (antibody-related) immunity. α- and δ-tocotrienols specifically have been found to lower serum cholesterol levels by directly affecting HMG-CoA reductase,[34] and γ-tocopherol appears to have properties that help prevent certain cancers.[35] In sickle cell disease, increased intake of vitamin E leads to fewer episodes of pain crisis.[36]

Sources of vitamin E are found primarily in plant products rich in oils, such as soybean, corn, palm, and canola; wheat germ; sunflower seeds; almonds, avocado, and green leafy vegetables. Synthetically derived vitamin E typically contains both D- and L-isomers. It is important that supplementation be only with the natural forms of vitamin E, because only that form contains the mixed tocopherols and mixed tocotrienols, and that it has at least 10 mg of tocotrienols.[37]

The current RDA for children is 3 to 7 mg of D-tocopherol equivalents [TE]/day; for adults, 8 to 12 mg or about 30 IU/day. The need for vitamin E increases with the increase intake of polyunsaturated fats in the diet. Because of vitamin E's benefits in helping to prevent cell and tissue damage, higher doses (400 IU) are typically prescribed for maximal antioxidant effects.[38]

Vitamin E toxicity rarely occurs, but when taken in high doses chronically, the risk of bleeding may be increased, especially in patients on anticoagulant therapy. A recent metaanalysis revealed that intakes >400 IU vitamin E supplements may increase mortality.[39] Although not specifically stated, it is likely the supplements used in the various studies did not contain the natural and synthetic α-tocopherol, long believed to be the active components of vitamin E.

Vitamin E deficiency can occur after very prolonged periods of no intake, in lipid malabsorption states, or with lipid transport abnormalities. Newborns and premature infants are at risk because of low transplacental movement of vitamin E. Symptoms might include nervous system disturbances, increased cellular injury and necrosis, and reproductive abnormalities.

Vitamin K. Vitamin K is necessary for at least two of the many steps in the blood clotting cascade. It helps synthesize the protein prothrombin that converts to thrombin, and it changes fibrinogen into its active form, fibrin. Vitamin K also plays a role in bone formation.

The family of chemical compounds that possess vitamin K activity include the naturally occurring phylloquinones (vitamin K_1), menaquinone (vitamin K_2), and the synthetically derived menadione (vitamin K_3), which is alkylated in humans to make menaquinone. Vitamin K_3 is two to three times as potent as the naturally occurring vitamin K_1 or vitamin K_2.

Like other fat-soluble vitamins, vitamin K is absorbed across the small intestinal wall in the presence of dietary fat, bile salts, and pancreatic enzymes. Vitamin K_2 can also be synthesized by the intestinal flora and absorbed across the colon. It is taken to the liver and incorporated into VLDL and LDL before being transported to the peripheral tissues. Vitamin K drives the γ-carboxylation process of certain proteins, allowing them to bind calcium. These vitamin K–dependent proteins include four plasma clotting tissues (factors II, VII, IX, and X), four coagulation-inhibiting factors, three proteins found in calcified tissues, and one protein found in calcified atherosclerotic tissue. These processes are interrupted in the presence of anticoagulant therapy with warfarin.

Food sources of vitamin K include green leafy vegetables, green tea, liver, soybean oil, grains, and cereal. It is estimated that 50% of our daily needs are supplied via microflora synthesis in the intestines.

The current RDA for children is 5 to 30 µg/day. Newborn infants' intestinal tracts are not yet inhabited by sufficient numbers of microflora to produce vitamin K; therefore they receive a 1-mg injection of water-soluble vitamin K soon after birth to prevent hemorrhage. Adults require 45 to 80 µg/day. Large doses of vitamin K are used as an antidote to warfarin.

It is difficult to develop vitamin K toxicity unless it is given in large doses parenterally (>1000 times the RDA). This has caused hyperbilirubinemia in infants. As excess vitamin K can interfere with the action of anticoagulants, patients taking anticoagulants must be cautious of consuming large volumes of vitamin K–containing vegetables or green tea. Vitamin K deficiency leads to hypoprothrombinemia and the potential for hemorrhage. As mentioned previously, newborns are at risk for this, as are those with malabsorption syndromes or liver disease and those on chronic antibiotic therapy that disrupts the normal intestinal flora synthesizing vitamin K.[28] Undercarboxylation of osteocalcin, a vitamin K–dependent process, has been found in elderly women and is associated with an increased risk of hip fracture.[40] This may be partly due to long-term use of warfarin therapy in elderly patients. One study of osteoporotic patients in Japan demonstrated maintenance of bone mass with supplementation of vitamin K_2 compared with a 3% loss in the control group.[41]

Water-soluble vitamins. The water-soluble vitamins—the complex of B vitamins and vitamin C—are distributed widely in all tissues and are important in regulating the enzyme-mediated reactions that produce energy from carbohydrates, fats, and proteins. They are essential nutrients that need to be consumed daily from food, as the body can neither manufacture nor store these vitamins in any appreciable amounts. The B-complex vitamins are a group of biologically active compounds, closely related in that they have similar physical properties, are found in the same foods, and have similar metabolic processes. Because of their close interrelationship, however, an inadequate intake of one may impair utilization of others.[28] B vitamins function as coenzymes that combine with an inactive protein to make it an active enzyme. Vitamin C can act as a coenzyme, but it is also important as a reducing agent/antioxidant that regulates metabolic reactions. Vitamin C is also necessary for the synthesis and maintenance of connective tissue and for vascular structure and function.

Thiamin (B_1). Thiamin plays a key role in carbohydrate metabolism and is a coenzyme involved in the metabolism of pyruvate and other α-keto acids to produce energy via the Krebs cycle. Thiamin also is a coenzyme in the reactions of transketolation in the direct oxidative pathway for glucose metabolism. It is important for nerve functioning and nerve transmission, as nerves depend on carbohydrates for energy.

Food sources include lean pork, liver, yeast, legumes, green vegetables, and whole unprocessed grains. Thiamin is unstable in the presence of heat, oxygen, ionizing radiation, and alkaline pH but is heat stable in an acid solution. Thiamin is lost if the water used to cook green vegetables is discarded. Also, absorption of thiamin by the small intestine is inhibited by alcohol consumption. Raw fish and some bacteria contain thiaminases, which degrade thiamin before it can be used. The RDA for thiamin for children is 0.2 to 1.2 mg/day; for adults, 0.9 to 1.5 mg/day.

Thiamin deficiencies predominantly affect the peripheral nervous system, the GI tract, and the cardiovascular systems, causing symptoms of anorexia, weight loss, and peripheral neuropathy. A severe deficiency, beriberi, is characterized with those symptoms plus mental confusion, emaciation, arrhythmias, and cardiomegaly. Thiamin deficiency can occur in alcoholics who tend to have impaired absorption of thiamin as well as suboptimal intakes, leading to Wernicke-Korsakoff encephalopathy. Rarely, infantile beriberi can occur in infants who are fed formula not supplemented with thiamin.

Under ordinary circumstances, thiamin toxicity is not likely; however, parenteral doses greater than 100 times the RDA have produced headaches, convulsions, arrhythmias, and allergic reactions.[28]

Riboflavin (B_2). Riboflavin is essential as a coenzyme for the metabolism of carbohydrates, fats, and proteins. It provides energy for tissues that have a rapid cellular turnover and thus is essential for growth. It also supports the antioxidant mechanisms of cells. The two active coenzyme forms, flavin adenine dinucleotide (FAD) and flavin adenine mononucleotide (FMN), assist to catalyze oxidation-reduction reactions in the cells and function as hydrogen carriers in the mitochondrial electron transport system. They are also required for the biosynthesis of niacin (vitamin B_3) and the conversion of pyridoxine (vitamin B_6) into its active form.[28]

Food sources include beef liver and heart, dairy products, green leafy vegetables, meats, and enriched breads. Riboflavin is stable in heat, acid, and oxygen but is destroyed by UV radiation (sunlight) and in an alkali environment. The practice of adding baking soda to water to make cooked vegetables appear brighter and fresher destroys riboflavin and other nutrients.

The RDA of riboflavin is 0.3 to 1.3 mg/day for infants and children and 0.9 to 1.6 mg/day for adults.

Riboflavin deficiencies usually occur in combination with deficiencies of other water-soluble vitamins. Newborn infants with hyperbilirubinemia are at risk for developing riboflavin deficiency if riboflavin is not supplemented during phototherapy. Symptoms of deficiency include fissured lips; cracks in the corners of the mouth (angular stomatitis); a red, swollen tongue; capillary invasion into the corneas of the eyes; or peripheral neuropathies. Riboflavin has no known toxicities.

Niacin (B_3). Niacin (or nicotinic acid) and its active form niacinamide (or nicotinamide) are part of the coenzymes nicotinamide adenine dinucleotide (NADH) and nicotinamide adenine dinucleotide phosphate (NADPH), which are necessary to obtain energy from glucose. These two coenzymes have essential roles as co-substrates in more than 200 enzymes involved in metabolism, although each fulfills different roles. NADH-dependent reactions are involved in intracellular respirations, whereas NADPH-dependent reactions serve biosynthetic functions.[28] Large doses of niacin lower LDL cholesterol (LDL-C), triglycerides, and lipoprotein-A levels and also markedly raise HDL cholesterol (HDL-C) levels to significantly decrease cardiovascular mortality.[42]

Food sources include yeast, lean meats, liver, poultry, enriched flours, and fish. Niacin is also synthesized from the amino acid tryptophan; therefore foods rich in tryptophan, such as milk or eggs, can help produce niacin. Sixty milligrams of tryptophan equals 1 mg of niacin.

The RDA for niacin is 2 to 4 mg of niacin equivalents (NE)/day for infants, 6 to 8 mg NE/day for children, and 12 to 18 mg NE/day for adults. The upper limits are 20 to 35 mg NE/day.

Niacin deficiency symptoms include muscle weakness, anorexia, lassitude, poor digestion, and skin rash. In severe cases, called *pellagra*, further symptoms of photosensitivity, diarrhea, and mental confusion develop, causing the "three *D*s of pellagra": diarrhea, dementia, and dermatitis. This can occur in patients whose diets are lacking in both nutrients and protein.

Niacin toxicity can occur with high doses (1 to 2 g, 3 times per day), which may be given to alter blood cholesterol levels. Symptoms can include flushing, derangements in liver function tests, or severe toxic hepatitis, which is more likely to occur when supplemented with sustained-release products. A safer form of niacin is inositol hexaniacinate. When 600 to 1800 mg is taken three times a day, studies have shown an 18%

reduction in total cholesterol, 26% reduction in triglycerides, and 30% increase in HDL-C levels.[17]

Pyridoxine (B_6). Vitamin B_6 is a group of vitamins—pyridoxine, pyridoxal, and pyridoxamine—that are metabolized to the biologically active form, pyridoxal phosphate (PLP). PLP serves as a coenzyme for nearly all reactions in the metabolism of AAs, neurotransmitters, glycogen, sphingolipids, heme, and sterols.[28] More specifically, it aids in the synthesis of nonessential AAs, assists in the conversion of tryptophan to niacin, helps convert linoleic acid to arachidonic acid, plays a role in releasing glucose from glycogen for glucose stabilization, and is needed for the synthesis of the neurotransmitters serotonin, epinephrine, norepinephrine, and γ-aminobutyric acid (GABA). In addition, PLP is required for the synthesis of sphingolipids in the myelin of nerve cells and the modulation of hormone receptors.[43]

Food sources includes meats, liver, whole grains, vegetables, and nuts, although the animal forms are believed to be more bioavailable for human use.

The RDA of pyridoxine is 0.1 to 1.3 mg/day for infants and children and 1.0 to 1.5 mg/day for adults. Fetal demand for pyridoxine is high during pregnancy; therefore 1.9 to 2.0 mg/day may be necessary for pregnant and lactating women. Studies have shown that doses of 25 mg given 2 to 3 times per day can significantly reduce nausea and vomiting during the first trimester of pregnancy.[17]

Pyridoxine deficiency has been demonstrated in infants and children and is characterized by hyperirritability, an increased startle response, GI distress, and seizures. A prompt response occurs with pyridoxine therapy. When deprived of pyridoxine or when its metabolism is blocked by isoniazid (INH), patients can develop symptoms of neuropathies, weakness, insomnia, stomatitis, or impairment of cell-mediated immunity.

Pyridoxine toxicity can occur with taking several grams of pyridoxine per day. This can lead to progressive numbness, gait disturbance, and sensory changes often mistaken for multiple sclerosis.

Folic acid (folate). Folate is a group of related compounds that function as enzyme co-substrates in many metabolic reactions of AAs and nucleotides. Dietary folate is absorbed into intestinal mucosal cells and reduced into its metabolically active form, tetrahydrofolic acid (FH4). FH4 functions as a single-carbon acceptor or donor necessary for DNA synthesis and is especially important in early fetal development. It is required for the conversion of histidine to glutamic acid. In the presence of vitamin B_{12}, folate is necessary for the conversion of homocysteine to methione, therefore reducing plasma homocysteine, which is toxic to cells. Folate is also essential for the formation and maturation of both red and white blood cells.[28]

Folate is widely distributed in many foods but found in the highest concentrations in liver, green leafy vegetables, dry beans, beets, oranges, cantaloupe, corn, sweet potatoes, wheat, and milk. Some folate can be synthesized by bacteria in the intestinal tract.

The RDA of folate for infants is 65 to 80 μg/day and 150 to 400 μg for children. For adults, 300 to 400 μg/day is recommended; however, for women of childbearing age who might become pregnant, 400 to 600 µg is encouraged to prevent neural tube defects (NTDs). Studies have shown a significant reduction in the incidence of NTDs and other birth defects in women supplemented with 400 to 800 µg of folate during the periconception period.[44]

Folate deficiencies result in impaired biosynthesis of DNA and RNA and are most apparent in cells with rapid multiplication rates, such as red blood cells, white blood cells, and epithelial cells. This may occur from inadequate intake, impaired absorption, or folate antagonist drugs such as methotrexate. Symptoms might include fatigue, apathy, weakness, headaches, sore tongue, diarrhea, decreased appetite, weight loss, or irritability. A relatively low folate level may lead to homocysteinemia, which is a risk factor for cardiovascular disease.

There are no known toxicities for excessive intake of folate, but high intake may interfere with zinc absorption and may mask the findings of pernicious anemia caused by vitamin B_{12} deficiency.

Vitamin B_{12} (cyanocobalamin, cobalamin). Vitamin B_{12} is a family of compounds that contain cobalt in its nucleus and act as coenzymes for many enzymes. Most important, they work with methylmalonyl CoA mutase, required for propionate metabolism, and with methionine synthetase for the conversion of homocysteine to methionine. These reactions are necessary for normal function and metabolism of all cells, especially those of the GI tract, bone marrow, and nervous tissue.

Vitamin B_{12} is released from ingested proteins by pepsin and hydrochloric acid in the stomach; however, it must be bound to a glycoprotein (intrinsic factor) produced by the gastric mucosa before it can be absorbed through the small intestine.[8] From there it is circulated to peripheral tissues bound to plasma proteins and, unlike other water-soluble vitamins, can be stored in the liver.

Vitamin B_{12} is obtained through foods of animal origin, with particularly high levels in clams, liver, kidney, oysters, milk, eggs, and meats. Negligible amounts are found in vegetables or fermented foods, only because of contamination with bacteria that synthesize Vitamin B_{12}. However, even the minute amounts are not well absorbed.

The RDA for infants is 0.5 µg/day; for children, 0.9 to 2.4 µg/day; and for adults, 1.8 to 2.8 µg/day. Higher levels are recommended for elderly adults who may lack intrinsic factor or hydrochloric acid.

Vitamin B_{12} deficiency leads to impaired cell division, causing an arrest of DNA synthesis. This is most readily seen in the rapidly dividing cells of the bone marrow and GI mucosa. Its most common cause is a lack of intrinsic factor from atrophic gastric parietal cells, leading to pernicious anemia. Others at risk for developing vitamin B_{12} deficiency are strict vegans who do not supplement; patients with an overgrowth of bacteria in the small intestine, which absorbs the vitamin; and individuals who have had segments of their intestinal tract removed because of disease. Clinical signs and symptoms of vitamin B_{12} deficiency include megaloblastic anemia; jaundice; smooth, beefy-red tongue; and neurological symptoms such as mental confusion, generalized weakness, and peripheral neuropathies (burning, numbness, tingling). Laboratory investigations reveal increased plasma and urine levels of methylmalonic acid,

aminoisocaproate, and homocysteine with a relative loss of tetrahydrofolate. There are no known vitamin B_{12} toxicities.

Pantothenic acid (B_5). Pantothenic acid is a metabolically active component of coenzyme A (CoA) essential for the metabolism of carbohydrates, fats, and proteins and for acyl carrier protein (ACP), a component of FA synthesis. All tissues are capable of synthesizing CoA from pantothenic acid, which binds with various carboxylic acids, the most important of which is acetic acid. As acetyl-CoA, it enters the TCA cycle to produce energy or can be used to synthesize FAs, cholesterol, alcohols, amines, and AAs. It is believed to be involved in the metabolism of various drugs and the acetylation of xenobiotics.[8]

Pantothenic acid is found in all plant and animal sources and is particularly high in liver, heart, mushrooms, avocados, egg yolks, and sweet potatoes.

No RDA has been established for pantothenic acid; however, a recommended adequate intake (AI) is 1.7 to 5.0 mg/day for children and 2 to 7 mg/day for adults.

Because pantothenic acid is found so readily in many foods, its deficiency is rare. Pantothenic acid deficiency has been observed only in severely malnourished patients and in patients treated with an antagonist of pantothenic acid—omega-methylpantothenic acid. These patients experienced burning sensations of the feet, insomnia, weakness, and depression.[28]

No pantothenic acid toxicities have been reported.

Biotin. Biotin is necessary for the metabolism of fats and carbohydrates and functions as a mobile carboxyl carrier in four carboxylases in humans. Specifically, these biotin-dependent carboxylases are pyruvate carboxylase, necessary for gluconeogenesis; acetyl-CoA carboxylase, necessary for FA synthesis; proprionyl CoA carboxylase, necessary for metabolism of odd-chained FAs and the production of methylmalonyl CoA for energy; and 3-methylcrotonyl CoA carboxylase, which catabolizes the ketogenic AA, leucine.[8]

Biotin is found in small amounts in many different food sources, with milk, liver, egg yolks, wheat germ, and chocolate being the most important. Because it is bound to protein, its bioavailability varies among the different sources, as it must be released from the protein to be available. Biotin can also be synthesized by bacteria in the colon.

An RDA has not been established for biotin, but an adequate intake would be 5 to 30 µg/day for children and 20 to 35 µg for adults.

Simple deficiencies of biotin are rare because of its wide availability in many foods. It can be induced through incomplete parenteral nutrition or by eating raw egg whites containing avidin, a glycoprotein that binds to biotin, making it unavailable for absorption. Because of biotin's role in lipid metabolism and energy production, deficiencies cause hair loss, dermatitis, anorexia, weakness, glossitis, depression, hypercholesterolemia, and fatty liver.

There are no known toxicities.

Vitamin C. Vitamin C is a hexose derivative synthesized by plants from glucose and galactose and serves as an antioxidant; as a coenzyme in the synthesis of collagen, carnitine, norepinephrine, and serotonin; and as a coenzyme to reduce iron and copper, facilitating in their absorption. Vitamin C also has an indirect role as a reducing agent in producing many hormones and polypeptides. Vitamin C prevents oxidation of LDH-C, lowers total cholesterol, raises HDL-C, and inhibits platelet aggregation; therefore it is helpful in preventing atherosclerosis. Vitamin C also promotes resistance to infection through immunologic activity within leukocytes, the production of interferon, its role in the inflammatory process, and promotion of mucous membrane integrity.[28]

The best sources of vitamin C are citrus fruits, melons, strawberries, tomatoes, peppers, and potatoes. Refrigeration and quick freezing helps retain the vitamin content in these foods, but prolonged exposure to air and the cooking process destroys vitamin C. It has been estimated that as much as 45% of the vitamin is lost from prepared vegetables refrigerated for 24 hours, and as much as 52% is lost in frozen products.[45]

The RDA is 30 to 90 mg/day for children and 50 to 90 mg/day for adults. These levels may not provide acceptable reserves for this vitamin, especially for smokers and those who are under stress or with increased metabolic demands (burns), taking oral contraceptives, or being treated for certain disease processes. For these patients, doses as high as 2000 mg/day may be recommended.[37]

Vitamin C deficiency results in scurvy, the symptoms of which are swollen, bleeding gums; lethargy; fatigue; skin lesions; and psychological manifestations (depression, hysteria, hypochondria). Infants can develop this around 6 months of age if they are breastfed without maternal supplementation or do not receive any other sources of vitamin C. Moeller-Barlow disease occurs when maternal stores of vitamin C are depleted and is characterized by poor wound healing, edema, weakness of bones and connective tissue, or hemorrhages.[28]

Doses greater than 2000 mg may cause flatulence, diarrhea, and urinary frequency or urgency. Patients with a renal stone predisposition need to be cautious in taking vitamin C, as it may increase the risk of oxalate stone formation in the kidneys.

Minerals

Minerals represent a large class of micronutrients that mostly are considered essential. The macrominerals are required by humans in amounts greater than 100 mg/day. These macrominerals—sodium, potassium, calcium, chloride, phosphorus, magnesium, and sulfur—are usually found in their ionic state in the body. These electrically charged particles act to maintain water balance and acid-base balance, act as coenzymes in various enzymatic reactions, and are necessary to propagate electrical impulses along nerves, to name a few functions. The microminerals, or trace elements such as iron, zinc, fluoride, and copper, are also essential for human function in quantities of less than 100 mg/day. These microminerals, through various functions, are necessary for optimal growth, health, and development.

These elements are absorbed by the enterocytes in their ionic state within the lumen of the small intestine. Here they travel through the cytosol and are then transported across the basolateral membrane to the blood via active transport mechanisms. The bioavailability of these minerals can be influenced by other molecules in food, by gastric acidity, by stress, or by other minerals. Factors that may inhibit the bioavailability

include oxalates (found in spinach, beet, greens, rhubarb, and chard) that bind to calcium and other divalent cations; excessive zinc, which reduces the absorption of copper; non-heme iron interfering with zinc absorption; or excessive intakes of calcium that reduce absorption of iron, zinc, or magnesium.[46] On the other hand, vitamin C can enhance the absorption of non-heme iron.

A brief description of these macrominerals and microminerals and their basic functions are summarized here.

Macrominerals

Calcium. Calcium is the most abundant mineral in the body, with approximately 99% found in teeth and bones and the remaining 1% within the cells, blood, and extracellular fluids. Calcium is essential for the formation of bone, but it also regulates transmission of ions across cell membranes, is vitally important for nerve conduction, is required for muscle contraction, plays a role in blood clotting in conjunction with vitamin K, and regulates various enzymes. PTH, vitamin D, dietary glucose and lactose, estrogen, and healthy intestinal motility improve the absorption of calcium. Tannins or polyphenols in tea, excess dietary phosphorus from cola beverages, or high levels of phytic acid found in the outer coating of cereal grains can inhibit absorption. Calcium is found in dairy products, sardines, oysters, kale, turnip greens, spinach, blackstrap molasses, and tofu.[45] Daily intake should target 200 to 1300 mg/day.

Deficiencies lead to osteomalacia but may also play a role in chronic diseases such as colon cancer and hypertension. Adequate vitamin D intake is important to promote intestinal absorption and renal reabsorption of calcium.[47] Normal serum levels in children are 8.4 to 10.2 mg/dL.

Phosphorus. Phosphorus is second only to calcium in its abundance in humans, with 80% found in bones and teeth in its inorganic form bound to calcium, called *hydroxyapatite.* The remaining 20% is found in the extracellular fluid and in the intracellular compartments of every cell, where it plays a critical role in all cell functions. Phosphorus is present in nucleic acids, which are components of DNA and RNA. Phosphorus is critical in the cells' transfer of energy as part of ATP, ADP, and AMP and comprises the phospholipids in cell membranes and phosphoproteins. It is also important for maintaining intracellular acid-base balance.[8] Phosphorus is abundant in animal protein, dairy products, whole-grain cereal, legumes, and nuts. Daily intake of 100 to 1250 mg is recommended.

Deficiencies are rare but can lead to neuromuscular, skeletal, renal, or hematological abnormalities.[45] Normal serum levels in children are 4.2 to 7.0 mg/dL.

Magnesium. Magnesium is a major intracellular cation; however, about 60% of the total amount is found in bone, 26% in muscle, and the remainder in soft tissue and body fluids.[40] Magnesium bound to phospholipids stabilizes cell membranes. It also stabilizes the structure of ATP in ATP-dependent enzyme reactions important for neuromuscular transmission and activity. Magnesium is a physiological calcium channel blocker that acts as a muscle relaxant, leading to decreased reactivity of vascular and muscle cells. Magnesium is also a cofactor in more than 300 metabolic reactions, including glycolysis, nucleic acid synthesis, and AA activation.[8]

Magnesium is found in tofu, whole-grain cereals, legumes, nuts, green vegetables, and chocolate. Targeted intake is 30 to 400 mg/day. Deficiencies may lead to muscle spasms, tremors, anorexia, nausea, dysrhythmias, and hypertension. Normal serum levels in children are 1.6 to 2.3 mg/dL.

Sodium. Sodium is the major cation of the extracellular fluid responsible for regulating body fluid osmolality, pH, and fluid volume. Sodium, along with potassium and chloride, maintains gradient differentials between the intracellular and extracellular compartments, generating an electrical potential necessary for nerve and muscle function and the active transport processes in the cell. Vasopressin, atrial natriuretic hormone, renin, angiotensin II, and aldosterone regulate sodium concentration.[8]

Sodium is abundant in most foods with the exception of fruits, and normal intake should be 500 to 3000 mg/day. Relative deficiencies can occur in water intoxication, leading to hyponatremia. Otherwise, sodium deficiencies are rare. Normal serum levels in children are 132 to 142 mmol/L.

Chloride. Chloride is a major anion of the extracellular fluid involved in maintaining pH and osmotic pressure. It also serves a buffer and enzyme activator, as it is a component of hydrochloric acid present in the GI system. Chloride functions as an oxygen and carbon dioxide carrier in hemoglobin.[8]

Chloride is also readily available in a variety of foods; therefore deficiencies are rare. Normal serum levels in children are 102 to 111 mmol/L. Intakes of only 10 to 60 mg/kg/day are needed.

Potassium. Potassium is the major intracellular cation with only small amounts in the extracellular fluid. Like sodium and chloride, it is important in pH and osmolarity regulation. It is important in nerve conduction and contraction of smooth, skeletal, and cardiac muscle. It is also necessary for carbohydrate and protein metabolism.[45]

Potassium is found in fruits, cereals, meats, vegetables, and legumes. Insufficient intakes have been linked to hypertension and osteoporosis. Normal serum levels in children are 3.5 to 6.2 mmol/L. Targeted intake is 2000 mg/day.

Sulfur. Sulfur is present in all the cells and extracellular compartments as part of the AAs cystine, cysteine, and methionine. The covalent bonding of sulfhydryl groups between molecules forms disulfide bridges, which are responsible for the tertiary structure of proteins necessary for the function of certain enzymes, insulin, and other proteins. Sulfur is a component of heparin, chondroitin in bones and cartilage, thiamin, biotin, pantothenic acid, and S-adenosyl methionine (SAM-e). It also is a part of glutathione, an important antioxidant.[40]

Sources of sulfur include animal proteins, legumes, broccoli, and nuts. Sulfur levels are not monitored clinically. No recommended intake has been established.

Microminerals/trace elements

Iron. Iron found in food exists either as heme iron, found mainly in animal protein, or non-heme iron, found primarily in plant foods. Heme iron is more readily absorbed; however, non-heme absorption can be enhanced in the presence of ascorbic acid, sugars, or sulfur containing AAs. Tannins in tea and coffee, phylates in corn and whole grains, oxalic acid in vegetables and chocolate, phosvitin in egg yolks, and excess calcium, nickel, zinc, and manganese can all inhibit iron absorption.[8] Iron is a component of hemoglobin and myoglobin and is important in oxidation and reduction reactions. Because iron can interact with oxygen to form reactive intermediates, it can potentially damage cell membranes or degrade DNA. Iron is important in the function of cytochromes and for various enzymes that synthesize collagen and neurotransmitters. Iron is essential for normal brain function and normal immune function. Two iron-binding proteins, transferrin and lactoferrin, help prevent infection by withholding iron from microorganisms that require iron for proliferation.[45]

Low intakes of iron lead to iron deficiency anemia, the most common of all nutritional deficiencies. Targeted intake of 0.27 to 15 mg/day is recommended. Serum levels in children are 50 to 120 µg/dL.

Zinc. Zinc is important to many biological functions: as cofactor for more than 200 enzymes, as stabilizer for protein and nucleic acid structures, and for expression of genetic information. It also plays a role in carbohydrate metabolism and taste acuity, formation of bone and cell membranes, and normal immune functioning and is necessary for normal growth and sexual development.

Zinc in found in oysters, shellfish, herring, liver, legumes, milk, and wheat bran. Deficiencies can lead to growth retardation, poor wound healing, impaired immune functioning, and depression.[8] A recent study showed that zinc supplementation in the presence of vitamin A substantially reduced the incidence of pneumonia in children.[48]

Serum levels in children are typically 70 to 120 µg/dL. Intake of 2 to 11 mg/day is recommended.

Copper. Copper plays a role in the formation of hemoglobin and myelin, in immune function, and in gene transcription. It forms the protein ceruloplasmin, which oxidizes ferrous iron (Fe^{++}) to ferric iron (Fe^{+++}) before it can be transported in the plasma as transferrin. Copper is essential for the cross-linking of collagen and elastin and promotes the synthesis of melanin and catecholamines. Copper-dependent superoxide dismutase (SOD) protects against oxidants and free radicals.

Copper is found in liver, shellfish, legumes, dried fruits, nuts, and tofu. Recommended intake is 200 to 900 µg/day. Deficiencies can lead to anemia, neutropenia, skeletal abnormalities, and depigmentation of the skin and hair. Serum levels in children are 10 to 165 µg/dL.

Iodine. Iodine is critical for the proper functioning of the thyroid gland. It is used in the synthesis of triiodothyronine (T_3) and thyroxine (T_4) from tyrosine in the presence of selenium. These thyroid hormones are necessary for proper growth and mental development.

Iodine is found in iodized salt and seafood, but absorption can be blocked in the presence of raw food such as cabbage, turnips, peanuts, and soybeans. Recommended intake is 110 to 150 µg/day. Deficiencies can lead to hypothyroidism and goiter. Serum iodine levels are not used clinically.

Selenium. Selenium is essential for the enzyme glutathione peroxidase, which removes highly reactive hydrogen peroxide from within the cells by converting it to water.[45] Selenium works with iodine to form triiodothyronine (T_3). It also works with other enzymes to act as an antioxidant and free radical scavenger. This reduces the body's need for vitamin E.

Selenium is found in Brazil nuts, seafood, and animal protein. The amount of selenium found in grains depends on the soil content. Recommended intake is 15 to 55 µg/day.

Manganese. Manganese is concentrated in the mitochondria, where it acts as a cofactor with superoxide dismutase (SOD), which is important for the function of the respiratory chain, and as an antioxidant. It is also a cofactor for other enzymes that are important in carbohydrate and lipid metabolism and for the formation of connective tissue and skeletal muscle.

The best sources of manganese are whole grains, nuts, legumes, beet greens, and tea. Recommended intake is 30 to 400 mg/day.

Chromium. Chromium enhances the function of insulin and therefore has an impact on carbohydrate, lipid, and protein metabolism. The proposed mechanism of this is through a chromium-nicotinic acid complex called *glucose tolerance factor* (GTF). Chromium also activates the insulin receptor kinase, which increases insulin activity.[8]

Chromium is found in broccoli, brewer's yeast, oysters, potatoes, whole grains, and meats. Recommended intake is 0.2 to 35 µg/day. Deficiencies cause insulin resistance and lipid abnormalities.

Cobalt. Cobalt's essential function is as a component of vitamin B_{12} (cobalamin) necessary for the maturation of red blood cells and the function of all cells. This is found in the same sources as vitamin B_{12}—organ meats, oysters, poultry, and milk. Recommended intake is based on the intake of vitamin B_{12}: 2 to 3 µg/day.

Fluoride. Fluoride is substituted for the hydroxyl group on the hydroxyapatite molecule of bones and teeth to form fluorapatite, a stronger, harder matrix of molecules that withstands tooth decay and tooth and bone demineralization.

Sources of this mineral include fluoridated water, seafood, tea, liver, and vegetables. Recommended intake is 0.01 to 3 mg/day.

See Table 4-2 for a listing of important functions.

Qigong in Pediatric Medicine

The way to long life and health is quite simple and often escapes the attention of those who look for complicated solutions.
Dai Liu, *The Daoist Health Exercise Book*

Historical Background

The National Center for Complementary and Alternative Medicine's (NCCAM's) strategic planning efforts for the years 2005 to 2009 list Qigong as a form of "energy medicine." Energy medicine deals with energy fields of two types[1]: veritable, which can be measured, and putative (also called *biofields*), which has yet to be measured.

The veritable energies use mechanical vibrations (e.g., sound) and electromagnetic forces, including visible light, magnetism, monochromatic radiation (e.g., laser beams), and rays of specific, measurable wavelengths and frequencies to treat patients.[2] Putative energy fields, on the other hand, have defied reproducible measurement.[3] Therapies involving putative energy fields are based on the concept that the human body is infused with energy. This vital energy or life force is known

under different names in different cultures, such as *Qi* in traditional Chinese medicine (TCM), *ki* in the Japanese Kampo system, *doshas* in Ayurvedic medicine, and elsewhere as *prana, etheric energy, fohat, orgone, odic force, mana,* and *homeopathic resonance.*[4] This discussion will refer to the vital energy as *Qi*.

Qi, meaning "air, breath, or vital life force," is in everything that is living. The dead no longer have Qi. Abundant, flowing, balanced Qi is manifested as good health. It is the life energy in nature. *Gong* is the Chinese word for "work." Therefore Qigong is "working with energy." One can learn to acquire, distribute, and transform Qi to affect the health of body, mind, and soul. Qigong is an ancient philosophical system of harmonious integration of the human body with the universe.[5] TCM is based on the harmony of Qi. In the ancient TCM textbook *Huang Di Nei Jing, health* is defined as harmony of Qi, whereas *illness* is the manifestation of disharmony of Qi. Qi disharmony is manifested as illness.

Chinese philosophers believed that all living things and all of nature are interconnected within a matrix. Nature is in constant cyclical motion, and harmony within the system allows things to flourish. Humans are a "microcosm of Nature, a smaller Universe and represent the juncture between Heaven and Earth, the offspring of their union, a fusion of cosmic and terrestrial forces. The Chinese ideogram for man represents a picture of a figure rooted to the earth with arms outstretched to heaven."[6] Everything is in balance: good and evil, life and death, yin and yang. To achieve a healthy state, Qi must be in balance.

Like a garden, Qi needs to be cultivated. The term *Qigong* has been attributed to Daoist master Xu Sun (d. 374 CE).[7] However, verbalized traditional practices that resemble Qigong might date as long ago as 10,000 years, in a dance called "Da-Wu" (Big Dance) used for ceremonies and religious purposes that could cure diseases and produce a strong body. In the sixth century BCE, the scholar Laozi suggested a method of health preservation through the regulation of respiration.[5] The earliest Qigong practices probably date to the Zhou Dynasty (1028-221 BCE), with the Shamanistic animal dances.[7] In the second century CE, Hua Tuo invented a series of exercise routines called the "Frolic of Five Animals" that imitated the movements of the tiger, deer, bear, monkey, and bird, which are believed to cultivate the natural skill of the animal: strength, balance, and clarity of eyes or mind.[5] Variations of these exercises are still widely practiced today along with thousands of other styles that developed independently and served different purposes. Throughout ancient history, Qigong practices were kept secret amidst the ruling class and the elite. In the fifth century CE, martial arts application of Qigong was made famous by the Shaolin Monastery in Henan province.[5]

Medical Qigong (soft Qigong) was probably first categorized in the seventh century in the classic medical text *On the Causes and Symptoms of Diseases,* which included 260 Qigong methods used to treat 110 varieties of illness.[5]

However, the term *Qigong* was not used in its present sense ("the art of Qi cultivation") until the twentieth century.[7] The term appears in the titles of two books published in 1915 and 1929, where it "designates the force issued by working with the Qi and the martial applications of this force."[7] The medical use of this term dates to 1936, when Dong Hao published *Special*

TABLE 4-2

Important Functions

	IMPORTANT FUNCTIONS	NATURAL FOOD SOURCES	TOXICITY/EXCESS	DEFICIENCY
Macronutrients				
Proteins 10%-15% total energy needs/day 1.0-1.5 g/kg/day	Act as enzymes, hormones, immunoproteins, transport proteins, structural proteins	Animal sources: meat, milk, eggs Vegetable sources: legumes, soybeans, nuts	Increases urinary nitrogen Immune system dysfunction	Malabsorption, poor wound healing
Carbohydrates 45-50% total energy needs/day	Major source of energy, spare proteins, provide cell structure and function, regulate intracellular communication	Fruits, vegetables, honey, table sugar	Obesity, insulin resistance, heart disease, diabetes, suppressed immune function	Ketosis, hypoglycemia
Fats and lipids 35% total energy needs/day	Cell membrane maintenance and function, development of CNS, energy production, chemical and O_2 transport, regulation of inflammation	Omega-3 fatty acids: cold water fish, fish oils, nuts, dark green vegetables, soybeans, algae Omega-6 fatty acids: vegetable oils, margarine, processed foods/trans fats, borage oil, black current oil	Imbalance of omega-3: omega-6 fatty acid ratio: inflammatory states (asthma, coronary artery disease, rheumatoid arthritis, irritable bowel disease), obesity, depression, bipolar disorder, ADHD, sickle cell crisis	Omega-3 fatty acids: learning disorders, impaired vision, polydypsia, ADHD Omega-6 fatty acids: Growth retardation, dry skin, reproductive failure
Micronutrients				
Fat-soluble Vitamins				
Vitamin A 300-700 RE/day	Maintain epithelial integrity, regenerate rhodopsin/iodopsin, promote long bone growth, immune support, reproduction	Dark green leafy vegetables, yellow/orange fruits and vegetables, fish liver oils, liver, egg yolks, butter, cream, fortified milk	Birth defects; dry mucous membranes; dry, red, scaly skin; hair loss; joint pain, periosteal thickening of long bones; headache, nausea, or vomiting; pseudotumor cerebri	Impaired night vision; keratinization of skin and mucous membranes; rough, dry skin; increased infections; impaired cell immunity; poor growth, anemia; reproductive failure
Vitamin D 200 IU/day 5 μg/day	Promote calcium and phosphorus homeostasis; cell differentiation; maintenance of membranes, nerves, and glands; immune functioning	Sun exposure, fish oils, butter, cream, egg yolks, liver, fortified milk	Hypercalcemia; hyperphosphatemia; calcification of skin, heart, kidneys, lungs, tympanic membranes; headaches, GI upset, or diarrhea; poor growth	Rickets, myalgias, weakness, tetany, osteomalacia, osteoporosis
Vitamin E 7-18 IU/day 3-7 mg d-TE/day	Free radical scavenger and antioxidant, inhibit platelet aggregation, inhibit tumor angiogenesis, immune enhancement, lower serum cholesterol, protects RBCs from hemolysis	Plant oils: soybean, corn, palm, canola; wheat germ; sunflower seeds; almonds; avocado; green leafy vegetables	From supplementation: increased risk of bleeding, proximal muscle weakness, myalgias, GI disturbances	Nervous system disturbances, neuropathy/sensory loss, increased cellular injury and necrosis, reproductive abnormalities

AA, Amino acid; *ADHD,* attention-deficit hyperactivity disorder; *CNS,* Central nervous system; *DNA,* deoxyribonucleic acid; *GI,* Gastrointestinal; *HDL-C,* high-density lipoprotein cholesterol; *IU,* international units; *NE,* niacin equivalents; *N/V,* nausea, vomiting; *RBC,* red blood cell; *RE,* retinol equivalents; *SAM-e,* S-adenosyl-L-methionine; *TE,* tocopherol equivalents; *WBC,* white blood cell.

TABLE 4-2—cont'd

Important Functions

	IMPORTANT FUNCTIONS	NATURAL FOOD SOURCES	TOXICITY/EXCESS	DEFICIENCY
Vitamin K 5-30 µg/day	Blood clotting, bone formation	Green leafy vegetables, green tea, liver, soybean oil, grains and cereals; synthesized in intestinal tract	Hyperbilirubinemia, interference with anticoagulation	Hypoprothombinemia, hemorrhage, undercarboxylation of osteocalcin
Water-soluble vitamins				
Thiamin (B$_1$) 0.2-1.2 mg/day	Carbohydrate metabolism, nerve function/transmission	Lean pork, liver, yeast, legumes, green leafy vegetables, whole unprocessed grain; synthesized in intestinal tract	With >100 times the RDA: headaches, convulsions, arrhythmias, allergic reactions	Anorexia/weight loss, peripheral neuropathy, autonomic neuropathy Beriberi: Above plus mental confusion, emaciation
Riboflavin (B$_2$) 0.3-1.3 mg/day	Coenzyme for carbohydrate, fat, and protein metabolism; supports antioxidants	Beef liver and heart, dairy products, green leafy vegetables, meats, enriched breads/cereals, spelt	No known toxicities	Fissures in lips; angular stomatitis; red, swollen tongue; hypervascularized corneas; light sensitivity/tearing or burning of eyes; peripheral neuropathy
Niacin (B$_3$) 2-8 NE/day	Coenzyme for carbohydrate metabolism, intracellular respiration, biosynthetic functions, lowers serum cholesterol and triglycerides	Yeast, lean meats/poultry, liver, poultry, enriched flours/spelt, fish, milk and eggs (sources of tryptophan)	From supplementation: Flushing, derangement of liver function tests, toxic hepatitis	Muscle weakness, anorexia, lassitude, poor digestion Pellagra: diarrhea, dementia, dermatitis
Pyridoxine (B$_6$) 0.1-1.3 mg/day	Coenzyme in protein metabolism, neurotransmitter synthesis, sphingolipid synthesis, modulates hormone receptors	Meats, liver, whole grains, vegetables, nuts, legumes, egg yolk	From supplementation: Progressive numbness, gait disturbance, sensory changes/paresthesias	Hyperirritability, increased startle response, GI distress, seizure, neuropathy/weakness, insomnia, stomatitis, immune impairment
Folic acid 65-400 µg/day	Single-carbon donor/acceptor in DNA synthesis, AA synthesis, formation and maturation of RBCs and WBCs	Liver, green leafy vegetables, dry beans, beets, yellow/orange vegetables, wheat, milk, yeast	No known toxicities; may interfere with zinc absorption; may mask findings of vitamin B$_{12}$ deficiency	Neural tube defects, fatigue, apathy, weakness, headaches, sore tongue, diarrhea, irritability
Vitamin B$_{12}$ 0.5-2.4 µg/day	Biosynthesis of nucleic acids, folate and propionate metabolism, AA synthesis, metabolism of all cells, RBC formation	Oysters, seafood, clams, liver, kidney, milk/yogurt, eggs, meat	No known toxicities	Megaloblastic anemia, mental confusion, weakness/fatigue, nervousness/depression, paresthesias, postural hypotension, reduced smell/taste
Pantothenic acid (B$_5$)1.7-5 mg/day	Metabolism of proteins, fats, and carbohydrates; fatty acid synthesis; metabolism of drugs and xenobiotics	Liver/heart, sunflower seeds, mushrooms, avocados, egg yolks, sweet potatoes	No known toxicities	Peripheral neuropathy, depression, insomnia, weakness, fatigue

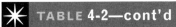 **TABLE 4-2—cont'd**

Important Functions

	IMPORTANT FUNCTIONS	NATURAL FOOD SOURCES	TOXICITY/EXCESS	DEFICIENCY
Biotin 5-30 μg/day	Gluconeogenesis, cofactor for carboxylation enzymes	Milk, liver, egg yolks, wheat germ, chocolate, mushrooms, peanuts	No known toxicities	Hair loss, dermatitis, anorexia/dysphagia, weakness/dysarthria/ataxia, depression, hypercholesterolemia, fatty liver
Vitamin C 30-90 mg/day	Antioxidant, collagen synthesis, neurotransmitter synthesis, enhances immunity and wound healing, increases non-heme iron absorption	Citrus fruits (oranges, grapefruit), tomatoes, broccoli, melons (cantaloupe), red bell peppers, strawberries, papaya, kiwi, potatoes, cauliflower	From supplementation: Flatulence, diarrhea, urinary urgency/frequency, formation of renal oxalate stones	Scurvy: swollen, bleeding gums; lethargy; fatigue; skin lesions; psychological manifestations; poor wound healing; edema; hemorrhages
Macrominerals				
Calcium 200-1300 mg/day	Bone formation, nerve conduction, muscle contraction, blood clotting	Dairy products, sardines, oysters, kale, turnip greens, spinach, blackstrap molasses, tofu	Renal stones, calcification of soft tissues, impaired absorption of other minerals, constipation	Osteomalacia, increased risk of colon cancer and hypertension
Phosphorus 100-1250 mg/day	Transfer of energy, maintenance of phospholipid bilayer, acid-base balance	Meats, dairy products, whole grain cereals, legumes, nuts	Low dietary Ca:P ratio (nutritional secondary hypoparathyroidism): increased parathyroid hormone, reduced bone mass	Neuromuscular, renal, skeletal, or hematological abnormalities
Magnesium 30-400 mg/day	Stabilize cell membranes, neuromuscular transmission, physiological Ca^{++} channel-blocker, cofactor for metabolic reactions	Tofu, whole grain cereals, legumes, nuts/seeds, green vegetables, chocolate	From supplementation: diarrhea, generalized weakness and drowsiness, decreased bone calcification	Muscle spasms/tremors, headaches, anorexia/nausea, dysrhythmias, hypertension
Sodium 500-3000 mg/day	Regulation of osmolality, pH, and fluid volumes; nerve, muscle function	All foods but fruits	Hypertension, osteoporosis	Hyponatremia
Chloride 10-60 mg/kg/day	Maintains pH and osmotic pressure	All foods	Hypertension	Metabolic alkalosis, anorexia, weakness
Potassium 2000 mg/day	pH and osmotic regulation, nerve conduction, muscle contraction	Fruits (bananas, papaya), cereals, meat, vegetables (squash, yams), legumes	Nausea/vomiting, arrhythmias	Hypertension, osteoporosis, muscle weakness, irritability/fatigue
Sulfur (not established)	Constituent for AA and protein synthesis; component of heparin, chondroitin, thiamin, biotin, pantothenic acid, SAM-e; antioxidant	Meats, legumes, broccoli, nuts	Increased Ca^{++} excretion	Poor growth, increased oxidative stress

AA, Amino acid; *ADHD,* attention-deficit hyperactivity disorder; *CNS,* Central nervous system; *DNA,* deoxyribonucleic acid; *GI,* Gastrointestinal; *HDL-C,* high-density lipoprotein cholesterol; *IU,* international units; *NE,* niacin equivalents; *N/V,* nausea, vomiting; *RBC,* red blood cell; *RE,* retinol equivalents; *SAM-e,* S-adenosyl-L-methionine; *TE,* tocopherol equivalents; *WBC,* white blood cell.

✳ **TABLE 4-2—cont'd**

Important Functions

	IMPORTANT FUNCTIONS	NATURAL FOOD SOURCES	TOXICITY/EXCESS	DEFICIENCY
Microminerals				
Iron 7-15 mg/day	Component of hemoglobin and myoglobin, important in oxidation and reduction reactions	Meats—heme iron Plants—non-heme iron	From supplementation: GI bleeding, metabolic acidosis, cardiovascular complications	Anemia, delayed development
Zinc 2-11 mg/day	Enzyme cofactor, stabilizes protein structures, promotes immune function	Oysters, shellfish, herring, liver, legumes, wheat bran	Decreased copper absorption, decreased HDL-C, GI irritation and vomiting, metallic taste in mouth	Growth retardation, poor wound healing, impaired immune function, depression, impaired sense of taste/smell
Copper 200-900 μg/day	Necessary for hemoglobin and myelin formation, immune function, gene transcription	Liver, shellfish, legumes, dried fruit, nuts/sesame seeds, tofu	Abnormal RBC formation, hepatic cirrhosis, GI irritation	Anemia, neutropenia, skeletal abnormalities, depigmentation
Iodine 110-150 μg/day	Necessary for thyroid function	Iodized salt, seafood/ sea vegetables, yogurt	From supplementation: GI mucosal irritation	Hypothyroidism, neuromuscular delay, mental deficiency, goiter
Selenium 15-55 μg/day	Antioxidant, necessary for thyroid hormone formation	Brazil nuts, seafood, meats/liver, barley	From supplementation: Nail and hair loss, gastroenteritis	Myopathy, cardiomyopathy, carcinogenesis
Manganese 30-400 mg/day	Cofactor for enzymes in carbohydrate and lipid metabolism, connective tissue and skeletal muscle formation	Whole grains, nuts, flax seeds, legumes, beet greens, tea	From supplementation/ exposure: Parkinsonlike symptoms, hallucinations, irritability, violence	N/V, poor glucose tolerance, bone loss, ataxia, reproductive problems
Chromium 0.2-35 μg/day	Enhances insulin function, activates insulin receptor kinase	Broccoli, brewer's yeast, oysters, whole grains, meat	No known toxicity	Insulin resistance, lipid abnormalities
Cobalt (2-3 μg of vitamin B_{12})	Maturation of RBCs and proper functioning of all cells	Organ meats, oysters, poultry, milk	Polycythemia, hyperplasia of bone marrow	Related to vitamin B_{12} deficiency, macrocytic anemia, pernicious anemia
Fluoride 0.01-3 mg/day	Tooth and bone mineralization	Fluoridated water, seafood, tea, liver, vegetables	Fluorosis, flaking of teeth, GI irritation, seizures, arrhythmia/cardiac arrest	Increased dental caries. decreased bone density

Therapy for Tuberculosis: Qigong in Hang Zhou.[7] Today more than 5000 different styles of Qigong are used in medical (soft Qigong) or martial arts (hard Qigong) applications. The West is already familiar with Tai Chi, a form of Qigong useful in maintaining health and energy levels.

The martial arts application of Qigong was used by ancient warriors in the technique called "Steel Body" Qigong, which provided an advantage over standard primitive weapons. However, many Qigong masters were lost during the opium wars, when they thought they could fend off bullets in the same fashion. Hard Qigong has been demonstrated by breaking bricks on one's head with a sledge hammer, balancing the body on sharp spears, and biting off hot steel and then lighting cigarettes with the red-hot rod.[5] Shaolin Qigong masters have been able to set fire to newspaper by Qi intention only, without touching. A current Qigong master from Taiwan can stand on a carton of raw eggs while painting a large watercolor piece in 2 minutes. These exhibitions indicate the level of human potential that can be achieved through the practice of Qigong and a very provocative and exciting potential of Qigong for maintaining health and curing disease.

This ancient art with its rich history was almost lost during the Cultural Revolution (1966-1976), when it was considered a vestige of the old feudal society. However, as affordable paradigms of healthcare became imperative in a runaway world of Western medicine, the leaders of the People's Republic of China began to categorize, systematize, and understand TCM. With this resurgence, Qigong masters were able to emerge from hiding and share their rich heritage. By 1979, many TCM hospitals included Qigong as an accepted treatment modality. Today, China still produces most of the bench and clinical research on Qigong. The Chinese government's attitude towards Qigong has been very positive. In some parts of China, school children are given daily breaks to practice Qigong for eyestrain to diminish the incidence of myopia.

It is hoped that researchers will be able to demonstrate both the health costs and benefits of this economical healing system.

Theory of Practice

The principle of TCM and Qigong is to enhance the underlying forces involved in health maintenance. Health is a delicate balance between the yin (female nature) and the Yang (male nature). TCM also posits that everything in nature consists of five basic elements: fire, earth, metal, water, and wood. These elements interrelate in a mutually nurturing and controlling cycle, and their balance affects meridians, or energy pathways. Qigong can balance these elements, and therefore Qi flow through the meridians results in enhancement of health and prevention of disease.

In TCM, the ideal is to determine the disharmony of the entire human system and bring it into balance. Qi has five physiological functions for maintaining system balance[9]: (1) as the Driving Force that affects the growth and development of the body and regulates the activities of all its organs, blood, and other bodily fluids; (2) as the Source of Warmth that maintains appropriate body temperature and allows organs and body fluids to function normally; (3) for resistance/prevention that protects the body against cold, heat, or external pathogens; (4) for stabilization and care (Gu and Sche), which together with the Driving Force direct the origin of the body fluids and their movements, distribution, preservation, and secretion; and (5) for transformation of all metabolic functions, such as the transformation of food into Qi.

Although more than 5000 types and styles of Qigong have evolved over the centuries, they all share the following characteristics:
1. They all involve breath exercises (spirit/soul). The literal translation of Qi is "breath" or "life force," always affecting the physical, emotion, and spirit. (The Western world also intuitively understood the importance of breath: Judeo-Christian scholars study the "breath of God," "God breathed life into man," or "breath of the Holy Spirit." Therefore breath is the essence of life—the soul.)
2. They all require consciousness and involve meditation (mind).
3. They all involve specific postures (body).

Qigong was founded upon the theory of Daoism ("right way of life"). This theory assumes a person is born perfect; must treat life preciously by eating right, sleeping right, acting right, and respecting everything in the Universe; and live in harmony with nature.

Qi has two major sources: the air and food. Therefore proper breathing—the basis of Qigong—is as important as eating proper foods. Breathing is done from the diaphragm, as a singer would do. The mind is to remain alert but relaxed (hence its usefulness in ADHD). At times, the mind may focus on a body part (e.g., the eyes in the treatment of myopia) or energy point while taking breaths. Regardless of whether meditation is performed, the mind should remain calm.

A balance and harmony of Qi means good health. Initial disharmony and imbalance or blockage of Qi are indicative of what the author refers to as "disease" of body, mind, and spirit, which may lead to full-blown diseases if the person is not capable of coping with these early imbalances. Disease conditions are classified as either yin or yang, with yin referring to deficient energy and yang being excess energy. Nature and food are also categorized accordingly. There are other considerations for the imbalances or blockages, such as stagnation, heat, cold, wind, and dampness. These concepts, along with others, have practical value because they assist in making a diagnosis of the energy disturbance that is causing an illness. After a TCM diagnosis has been made of the energy imbalance, practitioners of TCM and Qigong apply treatment steps designed to reestablish a balance and harmony of Qi in the body. Thus a healthy state is regained. These treatments may involve acupuncture, a Qigong exercise or meditation prescription, herbs, or other aspects of TCM.

Some Qigong practices focus on directing Qi to the 12 major bilateral meridians and more than 600 acupuncture points. Technology has been able to verify points and meridians with electronic instruments and radioisotopes. The points vary from a pinpoint to about 2 mm in diameter, and skin resistance at an energy point is markedly reduced. Electronic instruments can detect a point as a change in skin resistance. When an isotope is injected into an energy point, it can be tracked and found to travel up or down a channel according to the direction of flow indicated in ancient charts. However, according to Western medicine, the meridians do not correspond to any known anatomical structures such as veins, arteries, nerves, or lymphatics.

Another way of demonstrating the presence of energy is through Kirlian photography. A coronal effect occurs when the hands and feet are placed on film and exposed to 25,000 volts emanating from a Tesla transformer (at very low amperage). Scientists debate exactly what is being recorded on the photograph, but nobody doubts that the method can show changes in energy patterns from the use of drugs, mood changes, acupuncture, Qigong, or various other treatments. Photographs can be taken of the fingers, toes, or other body parts before a treatment or exercise of some kind. After the treatment, another photograph is taken to determine whether the patterns have changed. In the 1970s a researcher at the University of California–Los Angeles pioneered some of the highest-quality and most publicized work in Kirlian photography and also recorded the Kirlian effect in color on videotapes. In one tape a person placed the side of his face against the plate. Energy points were shown clearly and resembled twinkling stars. The points were located exactly where they were drawn in Chinese records more than 2000 years old. (At present, the Gas Discharge Visualization [GDV], a more sophisticated instrument developed in the former Soviet Union, is used to reliably record energy emissions during Qigong practice.)

Western medicine posits that the body senses and regulates emotion by means of approximately 60 neuropeptides. These neuropeptides have complicated feedback loops that mediate interactions among every cell throughout the body.[10]

Psychoneuroimmunology, the study of interactions among behavioral, neural, endocrine, and immune processes, coalesced as an interdisciplinary field of study in the late 1970s. Scientific research has established neuroanatomical, neurochemical, and neuroendocrine relationships between the brain and the immune system.[11]

Because TCM and Qigong have long considered the interconnectedness of body, mind, and spirit, in the near future science may be able to elucidate immune regulation as the one possible mechanism in which Qigong can prevent disease.

Current Evidence-Based Information
Scientific basis for potential mechanisms in Qigong
Medical Qigong can be classified as internal and external. Internal Qigong is the development of healthy Qi for maintaining individual health. This can be achieved by anyone who learns and practices Qigong. External Qi is the emission of Qi for the purpose of healing another person. This can best be achieved by a skilled Qigong practitioner.

Scientists have long been interested in measuring external Qi (EQ). Most of these studies have been from China. One paper studied EQ effects using five different methods: (1) physical signal detectors; (2) chemical dynamics methods; (3) detectors using biological materials; (4) detectors using life sensors; and (5) detectors using the human body. These studies have confirmed the existence of measurable EQ effects. However, current data still have not elucidated the primary nature of how EQ healing works. These studies documented some important effects of Qi healing that cannot be explained by psychological effect or the known biological processes. New methodologies, new theories, and new perspectives are urgently needed for further understanding the nature of Qigong and how EQ healing works.[12]

One study evaluated the effects of Qigong on brain function with modern neuromonitoring tools in two Qigong masters and found that Qigong increased cerebral blood flow. Another study compared the effects of internal (Qi training) and external Qi (Qi therapy) on immune cell function.[13] The data indicate that a single Qigong intervention can increase the monocyte and lymphocyte numbers and has applications for intervention in processes as complicated as human immunodeficiency virus (HIV) or as simple as the management of the common cold. The placebo had no effect.

Qigong has been scientifically demonstrated to affect physiological processes, including biomagnetic changes that may represent the flow of Qi.[14] A study using electrodermal measurements on 24 energy points found that Qigong practice improved balance of Qi and therefore improved health.[15]

Since 1986, innumerable international Qigong conferences (averaging at least two per year in various parts of the world) have heard more than 1000 papers on Qigong and the emission of Qi. For example, physicists described measuring several kinds of energies coming from the hands of Qigong masters who are emitting Qi, as well as their effects on living systems and the functions and organs of the human body. A rich database of research can be accessed through the website of The Qigong Institute of Menlo Park, California. This database lists research on the medical applications of Qigong and emitted Qi on humans, animals, cell cultures, and plants. Some of the functions and organs affected by Qigong listed in this database include the brain (electroencephalography and magnetometer); blood flow (thermography, sphygmography, and rheoencephalography); heart functions (blood pressure, electrocardiography, and ultrasonic cardiography); kidney (urinary albumin assay); biophysical (enzyme activity, immune function, sex hormone levels, laboratory analysis); eyesight (clinical); and tumor size in mice.

Qigong can improve mood, reduce side effects of treatment, improve blood pressure,[16] and increase immunity, and it may be associated with an improved outcome in cancer treatment.[17,18]

However, as interest in Qigong in China and, more recently, in the United States and Western countries continues to grow and research is undertaken in each country, the cultural gap in what is considered "scientific" has become more apparent.[19] The Western medical community considers many studies as having inadequate methodology, being not statistically significant, and not being able to be replicated in independent trials.

In the interim, new concepts for the potential mechanism of action Qigong need to be reexamined in light of new information as to how the nervous system, endocrine system, and immune system are intimately intertwined. A compelling question that also remains is whether a strict reductionist science is capable of finding conclusive evidence of Qi.[20]

Current concerns and cautions in Qigong practice
Review of the literature has revealed no contraindications to Qigong when it is taught by an experienced practitioner and not pushed beyond reasonable limits. Qigong should not be practiced under extreme weather conditions. Ideally, Qigong should be done under or near trees. Trees have life-giving, nourishing properties of Qi. Historically Qigong masters wrapped themselves around (hugged) a tree to replenish their Qi, breathing in their life-sustaining force.

When Qigong is not practiced appropriately or when it is learned from an inexperienced practitioner or from a poorly written book or video, side effects may occur infrequently, including "dizziness, headaches, nausea, chills in the body even when the weather is warm, or hot flushes... , tinnitus or hearing voices, chest or abdominal distention, shortage of breath, numbness of limbs, spasms, palpitation and restlessness."[21] For instance, some books instruct the reader to "press the tongue to the roof of the mouth to connect the Ren and Du (energy) channels." Again, when taken to extreme, pressing long and hard enough may logically lead to stiffness, pain, and dizziness.

During Qigong meditation, in which freedom of movement and sound are encouraged, resulting movements, sounds, visualization, and healing imagery may be misinterpreted to be hallucinations by observers or beginners who do not have guidance. Without explanations or guidance from experienced practitioners, these people can simply misinterpret the experience, become emotionally distraught, and develop delusions, all of which could lead to inappropriate reactions and behaviors. "Qigong psychotic reaction," which is listed in the diagnostic manual of the American Psychiatric Association,[22a] is a result of fanatical, improper, or excessive, overdone practices.

Side effects can usually be corrected by adjusting posture, breathing or meditating, consulting the master of the style being practiced, or by changing to a more suitable individual style.[21] However, if left unattended and the condition becomes chronic or severe, Qi transmission from a Qigong master may be needed.

In China, 60 to 200 million people practice Qigong[22a] and very few cases of adversity have been known. Even then, it is questionable as to whether other complex factors, not Qigong, caused the problem. As in any sport, Western or Eastern, there are inherent cautions for good training, moderation, proper nutrition, and respect for the weather.

Current pediatric application

Children can feel Qi more readily than adults. When asked to rub their hands together, then hold their palms apart about 2 to 6 inches and describe what they feel, children describe the Qi sensation as a warmth, tingling, slight breeze, coolness, or pressure, among many other sensations. Some can spread their hands several feet apart and still feel sensations of Qi.

The effect of Qigong can be maintained only through continual practice. Some Qigong exercises are very simple and can be easily learned by even young children. For example, rhythmic walking (e.g., the Guo Lin walk style), stopping, stretching, breathing, making slow movements, or standing in one position (e.g., "standing at the stake" with the feet apart and holding the arms in a circle at heart level) while performing breathing exercises all require simple movements and short periods of concentration.

In an extensive Medline search of the clinical literature, randomized clinical trials using Qigong in the pediatric population resulted in only two studies on muscular dystrophy.[23,24] However, discussion among Qigong practitioners who work with children has revealed positive results. As one practitioner states: "For children, Qigong is especially good at developing the kinesthetic sense, helping them to sense the body's relationship to the space it inhabits. Qigong, when taught patiently in small doses and with sensitivity to children's capabilities, will encourage the development of their attention spans. Qigong will also introduce children to an inner awareness of the body."[25]

Studies in adults or mixed populations may be extrapolated to children. One 10-year study through Harvard, Yale, and Emory Universities discovered that low-impact Tai Chi improved balance and coordination.[26] Similar results have been found at the Oregon Research institute.[27] Other studies found that Tai Chi offered significant cardiovascular benefits and pain relief.[26] Tai Chi burns 280 calories per hour (compared with 350 calories/hour in downhill skiing).

Because contemporary children suffer various forms of stress, often have low self-esteem or self-image problems, and have increased incidence of adult afflictions such as heart disease, hypertension, obesity, and pain syndromes, Tai Chi or Qigong can be beneficial in bringing physical and emotional well-being to the pediatric population.

A Qigong master may choose to treat children by emitting Qi. This author has successfully treated children with minor problems such as colds, flu, cuts, bruises, indigestion, colic, and more serious problems, such as brain and spinal cord injury, cerebral palsy, paralysis due to accidents, respiratory problems, cancer, and asthma, after other interventions had failed.

Contraindications

There are no contraindications to Qigong when it is practiced by an experienced, trained expert, as the foundation for Qigong is simple breathing.

References

Nutrition: Current Understanding of Its Impact on Pediatric Health

1. Lucock M: Is Folic acid the ultimate functional food component for disease prevention? *Br Med J* 328:211-214, 2004.
1a. MacLennan R, Zhang A: Cuisine: the concept and its health and nutrition implications—global, *Asia Pac J Clin Nutri* 13:131-135, 2004.
2. Schneeman B: Evolution of dietary guidelines, *J Am Diet Assoc* 103(suppl):S5-S9, 2003.
3. Hyman M: Paradigm shift: the end of "normal science" in medicine. Understanding function in nutrition, health, and disease, *Altern Ther Health Med* 10:10, 2004.
4. Gifford KD: Dietary fats, eating guides, and public policy: history, critique, and recommendations, *Am J Med* 113(suppl):89S-106S, 2002.
5. Nestle M: Food lobbies, the food pyramid, and U.S. nutritional policy, *Int J Health Serv* 23:483-496, 1993.
6. Kaput J: Nutritional genomics: the next frontier in the postgenomic era, *Physiol Genom* 16:166, 2004.
7. Ettinger S: Macronutrients: carbohydrates, proteins, and lipids. In Mahan KL, Escott-Stump S, editors: *Krause's food, nutrition, & diet Therapy*, ed 10, Philadelphia, 2000, Saunders.
8. Lockyear PLB: The biochemical functions of essential macro and micronutrients—a physician primer. Available at www.medscape.com/view/program/3259_pnt, 2004. Accessed 2005.
9. Wardlaw GM: *Perspective in nutrition*, ed 4, Boston, 1999, WCB/McGraw-Hill.
10. Lucas B: Nutrition in childhood, In Mahan KL, Escott-Stump S, editors: *Krause's food, nutrition, & diet therapy*, ed 10, Philadelphia, 2000, Saunders.
11. Coffey CJ: *Metabolism*, Madison, Conn, 1998, Fence Creek.
12. Hidaka H: Effects of fructooligosaccharides on intestinal flora and human health, *Bifidobacteria Microflora* 5:37, 1986.
13. Luo J: Chronic consumption of short-chained fructooligosaccharides by healthy subjects decreased basal hepatic glucose production but had no effect on insulin-stimulated glucose metabolism, *Am J Clin Nutr* 63:939, 1996.

14. Johnson K: The glycemic index. In Rakel D, editor: *Integrative medicine*, Philadelphia, 2003, Saunders.

15. Frost G, Leeds A, Trew G et al: Insulin sensitivity in women at risk of coronary heart disease and the effect of low glycemic diet, *Metabolism* 47:1245-1251, 1998.

16. Ebbeling CB, Leidig MM, Sinclair KB et al: A reduced-glycemic load diet in the treatment of adolescent obesity, *Arch Pediatr Adolesc Med* 157:725-777, 2003.

17. Pizzorno LU, Pizzorno JE, Murray MT: *Natural medicine: instructions for patients*, London, 2002, Churchill Livingstone.

18. Rakel D: The anti-inflammatory diet. In Rakel D, editor: *Integrative medicine*, Philadelphia, 2003, Saunders.

19. Conner WE: Essential fatty acids: the importance of n-3 fatty acids in the retina and the brain, *Nutr Rev* 50:21, 1992.

20. Pomerantz JM: Behavioral health matters: omega-3 fatty acids and mental health, *Drug Benefit Trends* 13:2, 2001.

21. Young SN: Clinical nutrition. III. The fuzzy boundary between nutrition and psychopharmacology, *Can Med Assoc J* 166:205-209, 2002.

22. Stoll AL, Severus WE, Freeman MP et al: Omega-3 fatty acids in bipolar disorder: a preliminary double-blind, placebo-controlled trial, *Arch Gen Psychiatry* 56:407-412, 1999.

22a. Ownby D: A history of Falun Gong: popular religion and chinese state since the ming dynasty, *Nova Religio* 6(2), 223-243, 2003.

23. Krauss RM, Eckel RH, Howard B et al: AHA dietary guidelines: revision 2000: a statement for healthcare professionals from the Nutrition Committee of the American Heart Association, *Circulation* 102:2284-2299, 2000.

24. Burgess JR, Stevens L, Zhang W et al: Long-chain polyunsaturated fatty acids in children with attention-deficit hyperactivity disorder, *Am J Clin Nutr* 71(1Supp):327S-330S, 2000.

25. Tomer A, Kasey S, Connor WE et al: Reduction of pain episodes and prothrombotic activity in sickle cell disease by dietary n-3 fatty acids, *Thromb Haemost* 85:966-974, 2001.

26. Harper HA: *Review of physiological chemistry*, ed 7, Los Altos, Calif, 1959, Lange Medical.

27. Hamilton EMN, Whitney EN: *Nutrition: concepts and controversies*, ed 2, St Paul, 1982, West.

28. Combs GF: Vitamins, In Mahan KL, Escott-Stump S, editors: *Krause's food, nutrition, & diet therapy*, ed 10, Philadelphia, 2000, Saunders.

29. Tucker KL: Eat a variety of healthful foods: old advice with new support, *Nutr Rev* 59:156-158, 2001.

30. Earl R, Borr ST: Guidelines for dietary planning. In Mahan KL, Escott-Stump S, editors: *Krause's food, nutrition, & diet therapy*, ed 10, Philadelphia, 2000, Saunders.

31. Holick MF: Sunlight "D"ilemma: risk of skin cancer to bone disease and muscle weakness, *Lancet (commentary)* 357:4-6, 2001.

32. Hypponen E, Laara E, Reunanen A et al: Intake of vitamin D and risk of type 1 diabetes: a birth-cohort study, *Lancet* 358:1500-1503, 2001.

33. Plotnikoff GA, Quigley JM: Prevalence of severe hypovitaminosis D in patients with persistent, nonspecific musculoskeletal pain, *Mayo Clin Proc* 78:1463-1470, 2003.

34. Chao JT, Gapor A, Theriault A: Inhibitory effect of delta-tocotrienol, a HMG CoA reductase inhibitor, on monocyte-endothelial adhesion, *J Nutr Sci Vitaminol* 48:332-337, 2002.

35. Gysin R, Azzi A, Visarius T: Gamma-tocopherol inhibits human cancer cell cycle progression and cell proliferation by downregulation of cyclins, *FASEB J* 16:1952-1954, 2002.

36. Jaja SI, Gbenebitse S, Aworinde O et al: Effect of vitamin E on arterial blood pressure, osmotic fragility and irreversibly sickled cells in sickle cell patients, *Niger Med J* 40:63, 2001.

37. Weil A: *Eating well for optimum health*, New York, 2000, Alfred A Knopf.

38. Mutter KL: Prescribing antioxidants. In Rakel D, editor: *Integrative medicine*, Philadelphia, 2003, Saunders.

39. Miller ER, Pastor-Barriuso R, Dalai D et al: Meta-analysis: high-dosage vitamin E supplementation may increase all-cause mortality, *Ann Intern Med* 142:37-46, 2005.

40. Szulc P, Chapuy MC, Meunier PJ et al: Serum undercarboxylated osteocalcin is a marker of the risk of hip fracture in older women, *J Clin Invest* 91:1769-1774, 1993.

41. Shiraki M: Vitamin K_2 [in Japanese], *Nippon Rinsho* 56:1525-1530, 1998.

42. Illingworth DR, Stein EA, Mitchel YB et al: Comparative effects of lovastatin and niacin in primary hypercholesterolemia, *Arch Intern Med* 154:1586-1595, 1994.

43. Guilarte TR: Vitamin B and cognitive development: recent research findings from human and animal studies, *Nutr Rev* 51:193, 1993.

44. Lumley J, Watson L, Watson M et al: Periconceptional supplementation with folate and/or multivitamins for preventing neural tube defects, *Cochrane Database Syst Rev* 2000:2 CD001056.

45. Carlson BL, Tabacchi MH: Loss of vitamin C in vegetables during the food service cycle, *J Am Diet Assoc* 88:65-67, 1988.

46. Anderson JJB: Minerals. In Mahan KL, Escott-Stump S, editors: *Krause's food, nutrition, & diet therapy*, ed 10, Philadelphia, 2000, Saunders.

47. Levenson DI, Ohayon KA: A practical analysis of calcium supplements, *Altern Ther Women Health* 2:28, 2000.

48. Bhandari N, Bahl R, Taneja S et al: Effect of routine zinc supplementation on pneumonia in children aged 6 months to 3 years: randomized controlled trial in an urban slum, *Br Med J* 324:1358, 2002.

Qigong in Pediatric Medicine

1. Berman JD, Straus SE: Implementing a research agenda for complementary and alternative medicine, *Ann Rev Med* 55:239-254, 2004.

2. Vallbona C, Richards T: Evolution of magnetic therapy from alternative to traditional medicine, *Phys Med Rehab Clin N Am* 10:729-754, 1999.

3. National Center for Complementary and Alternative Medicine: *U.S. Department of Health and Human Services report D235*, Washington, DC, 2004, U.S. Government Printing Office.

4. Hintz KJ, Yount GL, Kadar I et al: Bioenergy definitions and research guidelines, *Altern Ther Health Med* 9(suppl 3):A13-A30, 2003.

5. McGee C, Chow EPY: *Miracle healing from China: Qigong*, Coeur d'Alene, Idaho, 1996, MediPress.

6. Beinfield H, Korngold E: *Between heaven and earth: a guide to Chinese medicine*, New York, 1991, Ballantine Books.

7. Cohen K: *The way of Qigong*, New York, 1997, Ballantine.

8. Reference deleted in page proofs.

9. Liu Q: *Chinese fitness: a mind/body approach*, Jamaica Plain, Mass, 1997, YMAA Publication Center.

10. Pert C: *Molecules of emotion: the science of mind-body medicine*, New York, 1997, Touchstone.

11. Ader R: On the development of psychoneuroimmunology, *Eur J Pharmacol* 405:167-176, 2000.

12. Chen KW: An analytic review of studies on measuring effects of external Qi in China, *Altern Ther Health Med* 10:38-50, 2004.

13. Lee MS, Huh HJ, Jeong SM et al: Effect of Qigong on immune cells, *Am J Chin Med* 31:327-335, 2003.

14. Tiller WA, Pecci EF: *Science and human transformations: subtle energies, intentionality and consciousness*, Walnut Creek, Calif, 1997, Pavior.

15. Sancier KM: Electrodermal measurements for monitoring the effects of a Qigong workshop, *J Altern Complement Med* 9:235-241, 2003.

16. Young DR, Appel LJ, Jee SH et al: The effects of aerobic exercise and Tai Chi on blood pressure in older people: results of a randomized trial, *J Am Geriatr Soc* 47:277-284, 1999.

17. Jones BM: Changes in cytokine production in healthy subjects practicing Guolin Qigong : a pilot study, *BMC Complement Altern Med* 1:8, 2001.

18. Meares A: Regression of osteogenic sarcoma metastases associated with intensive meditation, *Med J Aust* 2:433, 1978.

19. Jonas WB: Magic and methodology: when paradigms clash, *J Altern Complement Med* 5:319-321, 1999.

20. Yount G, Qian YF, Zhang HL: Changing perspectives on healing energy in traditional Chinese medicine. In Schlitz M, Amorok T, editors: *Consciousness and healing*, London, 2005, Churchill Livingstone.

21. Wallace A: Side effects: the inside story, *Qi Magazine* May/June, 2001. Available at www.qimagazine.com/55_3article.htm. Accessed June 2001.

22. American Psychiatric Association: *Diagnostic and statistical manual of mental disorders (DSM-IV),* ed 4, Arlington, Va, 1994, American Psychiatric Association.

23. Wenneberg S, Gunnarsson LG, Ahlstrom G et al: Using a novel exercise programme for patients with muscular dystrophy. Part I: a qualitative study, *Disabil Rehabil* 26:586-594, 2004.

24. Wenneberg S, Gunnarsson LG, Ahlstrom G: Using a novel exercise programme for patients with muscular dystrophy. Part II: a quantitative study, *Disabil Rehabil* 26:595-602, 2004.

25. Yang PL. Available at www.qistar.com. Accessed June 2005.

26. Douglas B: Tai Chi & Qigong: the perfect exercise? *Sentient Times* Dec 2003/Jan 2004. Available at www.sentienttimes.com/04/dec_jan_04/tai_chi_qi_gong.htm. Accessed June 2005.

27. Li F, Harmer P, Fisher KJ et al: Tai Chi: improving functional balance and predicting subsequent falls in older persons, *Med Sci Sports Exerc* 36:2046-2052, 2004.

CHAPTER 5

Alternative Systems

Homeopathy | Janet L. Levatin*

Naturopathy | Matthew I. Baral

Homeopathy

Introduction and Historical Background

Beginnings

Homeopathy has been classified as an alternative medical system by the U.S. Department of Health and Human Services.[1] This system of medicine was developed in the late 1700s by the German physician Christian Friedrich Samuel Hahnemann (1755-1843). Hahnemann lived in the period of Western history known as "the Enlightenment" or "the Age of Reason." The Enlightenment was a time of many scientific discoveries, including advances in the field of chemistry. Medicine, however, was still a primitive practice that lacked humanism and rational principles for the treatments being used.

Raised in Meissen, Germany, Hahnemann was an outstanding student who excelled at languages, mathematics, and natural sciences. His reverence for the human body and mind, combined with his superior intelligence, led him to the study of medicine. When he began his medical practice, however, Hahnemann quickly became disillusioned with the conventional medical therapies of his day, which included bloodletting, purging of the body through the use of strong laxatives and emetics, and toxic medications that were given in large doses. He also decried the cruel, inhumane conditions to which the mentally ill were subjected. Hahnemann stood apart from most physicians of his time in advocating "fresh air, sensible diet, plenty of air, exercise and free movement," as "the preliminary conditions of well-being," in addition to sympathetic treatment for mentally ill patients.[2]

Because of his unwillingness to practice medicine using methods he considered crude and barbaric, Hahnemann withdrew from clinical practice to pursue experiments in chemistry. To support his family, he became a translator of medical texts and translated a number of major medical texts from French, Italian, and English into German. In 1788 he published an article that revealed that he was becoming interested in highly diluted medicines, an idea that later became one of the central principles of homeopathic methodology.[2]

It was while translating Dr. William Cullen's *A Treatise on Materia Medica* from English into German that Hahnemann began self-experimenting with medicines. He read that the drug cinchona (Peruvian) bark was effective against malaria because of its tonic effect on the stomach and its bitter, astringent quality. Hahnemann could not see the logic in this thinking, as he

knew that a number of substances possessed similar characteristics but were not effective against malaria.

As an experiment aimed at understanding the effects of cinchona bark, Hahnemann ingested it for several days. He found that he developed symptoms very similar to those of malaria. In his notebook he recorded, "Peruvian (cinchona) bark, which is used as a remedy for intermittent fever [malaria], acts because it can produce symptoms similar to those of intermittent fever in healthy people."[2] This discovery led him to the central concept of homeopathy, the principle of similars, which states that any substance that can cause a set of symptoms in a healthy person can also cure the same set of symptoms when they occur naturally in a sick person. Hahnemann devoted the rest of his life to exploring and expanding this principle into the science and art of homeopathic medicine.

Development of homeopathic methodology

Hahnemann continued conducting experiments, called *provings* (from the German *Prüfing*, meaning "test"), on a variety of substances. In a proving, a substance is taken and then the subject, called the *prover*, carefully records his or her experience, including physical symptoms, mental and emotional states, and dreams. To remove toxicity from the substances he was testing, Hahnemann later began diluting them to the point where deleterious side effects were removed. To heighten the action of his medicines, which had already been rendered nontoxic by dilution, Hahnemann began to vigorously shake, or succuss, his preparations after each of a series of dilutions. Hahnemann found, as a general principle, that the symptoms caused by a substance could also be cured by that substance.

Initially Hahnemann conducted his experiments on himself. Later he worked with a group of colleagues and associates who assisted him by participating in provings. Although Hahnemann wrote very little about children or infants, it is interesting to note that at least three of his own children were included in the group who volunteered to do provings for him.[2] Although they were adults at the time, one can surmise that if Hahnemann was willing to give homeopathic medicines to his own offspring, he must have believed them to be very safe.

Hahnemann's experimental methods were advanced for his time, as empiricism in medicine was virtually unknown. His methods for proving and producing medicines are still used in homeopathy today, although aspects of newer experimental methodology, such as blinding (single-blinding or, less often, double-blinding), are often employed.[3]

Hahnemann's most significant publication was his *Organon of the Medical Art*.[4] He published the first edition of the

*Dr. Levatin would like to thank the following people for reviewing the manuscript and making helpful suggestions: Jennifer Jacobs, MD, MPH; Michael Quinn, BA, RPh; and Julian Winston.

Organon in 1810 and subsequently wrote five more editions, the last of which was completed by 1842 but not published until 1921. Hahnemann also recorded the findings of his provings in the book *Materia Medica Pura.*[5] This is a catalog of medicines and the symptoms, arranged by organ system, that these medicines produced in the provers. This format has been used for most successive volumes of homeopathic materia medica (see the section on homeopathic methodology for more information on homeopathic materia medicas). Hahnemann's work was initially well accepted, and his methods were soon adopted in about 30 countries.

Homeopathy comes to America

Hans Burch Gram (1787-1840), an American physician of Danish extraction, is credited with bringing homeopathy to the United States in 1825 after being introduced to the discipline in Copenhagen.[6] Constantine Hering (1800-1880), a German physician who settled in the United States in 1833, was largely responsible for the rapid spread of homeopathy in the United States. Hering founded the Hahnemann Medical College in Philadelphia in 1848 and was one of the founders of the American Institute of Homeopathy (AIH). This professional medical organization for homeopathic physicians was founded in 1844, 3 years before the American Medical Association (AMA), and still exists today. Hering's *Domestic Physician,*[7] initially published in 1835, was one of the first books of homeopathic materia medica published in the United States. It was sold with a kit of approximately 40 homeopathic medicines and was intended to promote the spread of homeopathy by introducing it into families for use at home.[8]

Homeopathy was quickly embraced by mothers as a form of treatment that was much easier to administer to children than conventional medicines, as well as much safer. It was an important form of medicine in frontier regions where doctors were scarce and mothers often had to treat their own children's illnesses. In *Divided Legacy*, Coulter presents evidence that in the 1800s many American families employed homeopathy in the treatment of their children, even when the adults were still using allopathic medicine. Apparently the wives of a number of allopathic physicians sought treatment from homeopaths for themselves and their children.[8] A number of materia medicas on the diseases of infants and children were published in the 1800s and early 1900s, which provides evidence that homeopathy was commonly used for children at the time.[9-14] Homeopathic treatment of children was common enough that it was mentioned in popular literature written in the 1800s; for example, *Little Women*, by Louisa May Alcott, published in 1868, describes the use of homeopathic belladonna for prevention of scarlet fever in a child.[15]

Another seminal figure in the history of homeopathy was James Tyler Kent (1849-1916). Kent began his medical practice as a conventional physician and converted to homeopathy after his second wife became ill and did not respond to conventional treatments of the day. When she was cured by a homeopathic physician, Kent began to study homeopathy. Within several years he had become a leader in the field, founding a postgraduate school of homeopathy in Philadelphia and editing three homeopathic journals. Kent's lectures on materia medica and homeopathic philosophy were transcribed and published by his students and are still read by homeopaths today.[16,17] Kent's lectures on materia medica contain more than 450 references to the treatment of children and infants.[18]

Kent's most important contribution to homeopathy was his *Repertory of the Homeopathic Materia Medica.*[19] A repertory is a compilation of symptoms, arranged by organ system, along with the medicines, extracted from materia medica, that are known to treat each symptom. In homeopathic practice, repertories serve as companion books to materia medicas, facilitating efficient searching of the literature for indicated medicines. Kent began compiling his repertory in the 1890s and worked on it for the rest of his life. After his death the work was edited several times by his third wife. Kent's repertory has served as the basis for numerous other repertories that were subsequently compiled.[6]

Decline of homeopathy in the United States

The use of homeopathy peaked in the United States in the 1890s, with 22 homeopathic medical schools, more than 100 homeopathic hospitals, and 12,000 homeopathic practitioners. By the mid-1920s, however, most of these schools had closed, and by 1940 most of the hospitals had closed as well. Factors both internal and external to the profession of homeopathy contributed to the decline. The internal factors were poor organization, inadequate education of practitioners, and lack of adherence to the basic principles of homeopathy. Some homeopathic schools were started strictly as commercial ventures and offered poor-quality education. The AIH, the official organization for professional homeopaths, admitted poorly educated practitioners from these schools. Many doctors who called themselves homeopaths were not practicing in accordance with the basic principles of the method. Homeopaths were divided in terms of the homeopathic methodology they used, with some practitioners practicing polypharmacy (prescribing several medicines at once) instead of prescribing single medicines (see under Summary of Homeopathic Principles). Others combined homeopathic and allopathic medicines or routinely prescribed specific medicines for specific conditions or diagnoses in a nonhomeopathic manner. These practices caused the profession of homeopathy to crumble from within.[6]

External factors included the strong anti-homeopathic sentiments of conventional physicians toward homeopathy and the advent of modern medicine with its new pharmaceuticals that treated isolated symptoms and conditions in predictable ways. The AMA, founded in 1847, 3 years after the AIH, contained in its charter a proscription against AMA members consulting with homeopaths. All state medical societies, except that of Massachusetts, closed their doors to homeopaths. In addition, the work of homeopaths was banned from allopathic journals. Homeopathy became marginalized.

A report published by Abraham Flexner in 1910, entitled *Medical Education in the United States and Canada,*[20] proposed that all medical schools adopt a program similar to that taught at the Johns Hopkins School of Medicine at the time. Flexner was critical of most of the existing homeopathic medical schools, which he found to be lacking in scientific rigor. The Flexner report is often cited as one of the major factors that led to the decline of homeopathy in the United States. Objectively speaking, however, the schools Flexner criticized indeed offered poor-quality education.[6]

Renaissance of homeopathy

From the 1930s until the 1970s, homeopathy was kept alive in the United States by a small number of practitioners. These individuals were dedicated to the practice of homeopathy in the Hahnemannian tradition. In the 1970s more physicians became interested in homeopathy, as both doctors and patients sought ways of treating the sick with more humanism and fewer pharmaceuticals. Schools and programs that offered high-quality homeopathic education were formed.

Today U.S. homeopathic practitioners include physicians, osteopaths, dentists, nurses, advanced practice nurses, physician assistants, chiropractors, naturopaths, oriental medical doctors, and individuals who have received training as professional homeopaths but hold no other professional license. In the United Kingdom, the movement of professional homeopaths is large and well established. Homeopathy is also a thriving practice in many other parts of the world, most notably Europe and India. Current data show that homeopathy is used by approximately 2% to 3% of the U.S. and Canadian populations (see the section on current pediatric usage for more information).

Summary of Homeopathic Principles

Homeopathy is based on several principles: individualization, holism, and the minimum dose.

Individualization: the principle of similars

The cornerstone of the homeopathic method is treatment by similars. As stated by Hahnemann, "*Similia similibus curentur*," or "Likes may be cured by likes." From the homeopathic perspective, symptoms are viewed as the body's best attempt to regain homeostasis when it is out of balance. Often the body regains balance by itself, and symptoms resolve naturally; however, when the body is unable to correct an imbalance, symptoms persist, perhaps worsening with time, and the patient experiences this as illness.

Because homeopathic medicines, when correctly chosen, are similar to the patient's illness, they work with the organism's natural tendencies, rather than opposing them, as is often done in allopathic medicine (*Contraria contrariis curentur,* or "curing by contraries"). When a homeopathic medicine is chosen, the goal of the prescriber is to find the one medicine for which the proving symptoms most closely match the symptom picture and mental/emotional state of the patient. This medicine is called the *simillimum*. When the patient takes the simillimum, an energetic resonance occurs between the medicine and the patient's disease, and the medicine cures the patient's disease. The patient is then able to return to a state of homeostasis or normal health.

Holism: the totality of symptoms, the single medicine

Homeopathy is a form of holistic medicine in the sense that the whole person is considered when a homeopathic medicine is chosen. As the homeopathic practitioner takes the case from the patient, which is done in an interview setting, he or she tries to understand as much as possible about the patient's symptoms and their modalities (ameliorating and aggravating factors); emotional state; and various other characteristics, sometimes called *generalities*, such as appetite, food desires and aversions, temperature sense, and sleep habits. Traits and characteristics that are observed are often as important as what is reported verbally by the patient (or by the parent in the case of a nonverbal child).

When a medicine is chosen for the patient, its proving should contain all or many of the symptoms and characteristics of the patient. Instead of prescribing multiple medicines, one for each of a patient's complaints, the homeopath prescribes one medicine, the simillimum, that has been found in its proving to cover all or most of the patient's symptoms. The job of the homeopath is to identify what needs to be cured in the patient; to know (i.e., discover through research) what symptoms each available medicine can cure; and, finally, to match the single, correct medicine to the patient.

The minimum dose: potentized medicines

Homeopathic medicines are prepared by taking crude substances, including plants, minerals, and animal substances, and serially diluting them in alcohol. Substances are routinely serially diluted 30, 200, or 1000 or more times, yielding highly diluted solutions that often contain no trace of the original medicinal material. (See the section on homeopathic methodology for more information on preparation of medicines.) Hahnemann discovered that a diseased person is very sensitive to the correct medicine, the simillimum, and that only a minute amount of medicine is needed to stimulate a curative response. Homeopaths therefore treat the patient with the minimum amount of medicine, given the minimum number of times necessary to stimulate a curative response.

Homeopathic Methodology
Homeopathic pharmacy

Homeopathic medicines (also called *homeopathic remedies*) can be made from virtually any substance. Medicines are typically made from plants, minerals, and animal substances such as honeybee and snake venom. They are also made from products of disease, such as bacteria, viruses, and bodily discharges (these medicines are called *nosodes*), as well as "imponderables," including x-ray and the north pole of the magnet. Many of the crude substances are toxic at full strength. Plants are usually prepared as alcohol-based tinctures prior to dilution; mineral substances are usually prepared by trituration, or grinding, with milk sugar in a mortar and pestle.

After the initial extraction or trituration, the substance is diluted with water or a water/alcohol mixture in a series of 1:10 dilutions, called *X* (decimal) *potency medicines*, or a series of 1:100 dilutions, called *C* (centesimal) *potency medicines*. After each dilution in the process, the solution is vigorously shaken, or succussed. A medicine that has been diluted 12 times by a factor of 1:10 is called a *12X dilution* or *potency*; a medicine that has been diluted 30 times by a factor of 1:100 is called a *30C dilution* or *potency*. After the final dilution the solution is then incorporated into granules that contain lactose, sucrose, or both, which are administered orally or sublingually.[21]

A number of homeopathic pharmacies worldwide prepare homeopathic medicines according to exacting standards. The methods for correctly identifying substances and preparing medicines are outlined in a book of monographs, the *Homeopathic Pharmacopœia of the United States* (HPUS), which is published and regularly revised by the Homeopathic Pharmacopœia Convention of the United States (HPCUS). The HPCUS acts as a liaison between the Food and Drug Administration (FDA) and the homeopathic pharmaceutical industry.[22] It is interesting to note that the legislation forming the FDA was authored by Royal Copeland, MD, a homeopathic doctor and U.S. senator from New York. He wrote the Pure Food, Drug, and Cosmetic Act of 1938 and saw it passed into law, an effort that took much perseverance and several years. The *Homeopathic Pharmacopœia* was only one small part of this legislation.[6]

Clinical practice

The steps in homeopathic prescribing are (1) identifying what needs to be cured in the patient through case taking; (2) translating the symptoms and characteristics of the patient into homeopathic language by referring to repertories, materia medicas, provings, toxicology reports, and other sources of data about potential medicines; and (3) choosing a homeopathic medicine for the patient.[23]

Case taking. Case taking is typically done in an interview setting. The patient is asked to relate his or her concerns, including physical, mental, and emotional difficulties. This is an open, fluid process in which the patient is encouraged to talk freely. Individualizing characteristics such as concurrent symptoms or symptoms that occur at specific times or under specific conditions are particularly valuable, as they help define a person's uniqueness. In a review of systems the homeopath can elicit information about food cravings and aversions, temperature sense, sleep, and other characteristics. Dreams can give important clues to the mental or emotional state of the patient. Observation of the patient is important. Gestures, facial expressions, and voice quality are a few of the many observable attributes that may help determine the choice of medicine.[24] Relevant data can also be gathered from laboratory, radiology, and specialists' reports.

When taking the case of an infant or child, the homeopath needs to gather information in different ways. The parent or guardian will report his or her concerns to the homeopath. Clues to the choice of medicine may be found in the story of the pregnancy or birth. Family history is important; diseases of parents or earlier ancestors, such as tuberculosis, cancer, and sexually transmitted diseases, may influence a child's health. Observation is particularly important in children who are nonverbal or have limited verbal skills. Facial expression, demeanor, and behavior in the consultation room can all provide valuable information to the prescriber.

Homeopathy can treat both acute and chronic conditions. Case taking for an acute illness will usually be quicker and less involved than case taking for a chronic illness.

The patient's mental and emotional states are important in both acute and chronic cases. In all cases, the most important signs and symptoms are those that are very characteristic of the patient's state at the time.

Translating the case into homeopathic language. After fully understanding the problems of the patient, as well as his or her nature and characteristics, the practitioner then works on translating this understanding into homeopathic language. First the practitioner must decide which observations are most characteristic of the patient's illness and thus most important. Then he or she must translate these symptoms and characteristics into homeopathic language by searching the homeopathic literature for passages that contains the words, experience, symptoms, and/or pathology of the patient. A repertory may be consulted for rubrics (categories of signs and symptoms) that encapsulate a patient's symptoms or pathology. The homeopathic medicines known to treat the named symptom will be found under the rubric. These medicines can then be studied in detail in a book of materia medica. The words the patient has used are often important. Because provings are written in the language of the prover, symptoms and experiences are subjectively described. Homeopathic provings and materia medicas, which are available on computer databases, can be searched for the exact words or phrases that the patient has used.

For example, in a case of acute croup, the following rubrics might be chosen: croupy cough, frightened facial expression, and midnight occurrence (Figure 5-1).[25] The most likely homeopathic medicines, *Aconitum napellus*, *Stramonium*, and *Spongia tosta*, can then be studied in a materia medica (Box 5-1).[18]

Choosing a homeopathic medicine. After the important symptoms and characteristics of the patient's illness are understood and the homeopathic literature is studied, a homeopathic medicine is chosen for the patient. More than 2000 medicines are included in the homeopathic pharmacopoeia, any one of which may potentially be the simillimum for the patient. Some medicines have been documented frequently and are overrepresented in homeopathic materia medicas and repertories, whereas others have been written about infrequently and are therefore underrepresented in the literature. Practicing homeopaths must be aware of this imbalance, as it causes some medicines, such as sulphur and *Calcarea carbonica*, to appear frequently in repertory analyses (when they are not the simillimum) and many other medicines to be absent. Knowledge of the natural sciences can aid greatly in choosing among the many available medicines. Studying classes of substances, such as botanical or animal families or a grouping of chemical elements or compounds, may aid in finding the indicated medicine.

No science has been developed to define the potencies of medicines that are optimal for use in different situations. There are no set guidelines for dosing frequency and length of a prescription, as there are for antibiotic prescriptions, for example. As a general rule, lower-potency medicines are thought to act more on the physical plane, and higher-potency medicines are thought to act on the mental and emotional as well as the physical planes.

Homeopathic medicines are administered orally or sublingually, or they can be dissolved in water and administered as liquid solutions. They are very easy to administer to infants and children, which makes homeopathy an ideal form

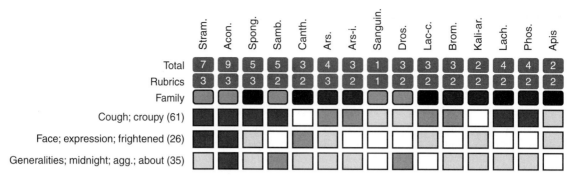

FIGURE 5-1 Repertorization for a child with croup. *From Rey L: Thermoluminescence of ultra-high dilutions of lithium chloride and sodium chloride, Physica A 323:67-74, 2002.*

✳ Box 5-1

Materia Medica of Aconitum Napellus, One of the Homeopathic Medicines Used to Treat Croup

HOMEOPATHIC—Aconite's sphere is in emergencies and acute diseases. Serous membranes and muscular tissues affected markedly. Anxiety, fright and shock. A state of fear, anxiety, anguish of mind and body. Restlessness, physical and mental. Major remedy in inflammation and fevers. Complaints and tension caused by exposure to dry, cold weather, draft of cold air, checked perspiration.

Ailments of immune system, especially if caused by suddenly checked sweat or by dry cold air, storms or cold winds. Acute, sudden and violent illness with high fever. Glands painful, hot, swollen. Neuritis with tingling. Influenza and colds. Sudden and great sinking of strength. Sudden chills or fever.

Also complaints from very hot weather, especially summer diarrhea. Localized blood congestions and inflammations. Tension of arteries, emotional and physical tension. Burning in internal parts, tingling, coldness and numbness. Does not want to be touched.

Muscular rheumatism with high fever. Joint rheumatism, much fever, restlessness and anxiety. Swellings are red and hot (Bell.), or pale, shifting from one point to another. Complaints in joints are: shooting, cramp, cracking, loss of power, drawing pain in joints and tendons.

CLINICAL—Amaurosis. Anger. Asthma. Blindness. Breast-feeding, disorders. Bronchitis. Catalepsy. Catheter fever. Chicken-pox. Chills. Cholera. Cholera infantum. Colds. Convulsions. Cough. Croup. Cystitis. Dengue fever. Dentition. Diarrhea. Dropsy. Dyspepsia. Dysentery. Dysmenorrhea. Ear disorders. Enteritis. Erythema. Esophagus inflammation. Eye disorders. Face, flushing. Fear, effects. Fever, high. Fright, ill effects. Glossitis. Gonorrhea. Headache. Heart disorders. Hemorrhages. Hemorrhoid. Hip-joint, disease. Hodgkin's disease. Influenza. Jaundiced. Labor pains. Laryngitis. Lumbago. Lungs disorders. Mania. Measles. Meningitis. Menstruation, disorders. Milk-leg. Miscarriage. Mumps. Muscle, pains. Myelitis. Nephritis. Neuralgias. Numbness. Paralysis. Peritonitis. Pleurisy, pain. Pneumonia. Puerperal fever. Purpura. Quinsy. Remittent fever. Roseola. Scarlatina. Sleeplessness. Stiff-neck. Strokes. Tetanus. Tetany. Throat disorders. Tongue disorders. Toothache. Traumatic fever. Tuberculosis. Urethra, stricture. Urethritis. Urine, retention. Uterus, prolapsed. Vaccination, effects. Vertigo. Whooping-cough. Yellow fever.

CONSTITUTIONS—Children. Plethoric persons of a lively character, bilious and nervous constitutions, high color, brown or black hair, are specially suited to Acon. Persons leading a sedentary life, plethora, etc.

MODALITIES—Better in open air from rest. better from warm sweat. Worse from fright, shock, violent emotions and vexation. Worse from being chilled by cold winds, dry weather, while sweating. Worse from pressure touch in bed, noise, light, dentition during menses, sleeping in the sun. Worse lying on affected side. Worse from music from tobacco-smoke inspiration. Worse in warm room. Worse evening and at night.

MIND—Great fear, anxiety and worry accompany every ailment. Fears the future, a crowd, crossing the street. Forebodings and fears. Fears death and believes that he will soon die, predicts the day. Never well since a fright or shock. Ailments from fright. Fear of death and dying, great anxiety. Nightmares after horror stories or movies. Nightmares, phobias, panic attacks. Tendency to be startled. Someone has a fright, sees something very frightening, and they panic and go into a shock. Panic attacks with restlessness. Agoraphobia. Fears of going to doctors and dentists. Anticaption. Fears of public speaking with panic and anxiety.

From *ReferenceWorks Pro 4.2*, San Rafael, Calif, 2008, Kent Homeopathic Associates.

---

of medicine for the pediatric population. For a simple acute case, a 12C or 3C potency medicine can be given two or three times daily, then discontinued when the patient has begun to improve. For a chronic illness or a complicated acute illness, a 30C or 200C potency medicine can be given once or twice a day, then discontinued when the patient has begun to improve. If a medicine has failed to help the patient after several doses, it is not the simillimum and should be discontinued. Another homeopathic medicine can then be administered, or another form of treatment can be tried as indicated.

✳ **TABLE 5-1**

Laboratory Evidence for Activity of Highly Diluted Solutions

INVESTIGATOR(S)	EXPERIMENTAL PROTOCOL	FINDINGS
Rey	Expose ultra-high dilutions of lithium chloride and sodium chloride to x-rays and γ-rays, and study the light emitted from the irradiated solutions	The light emitted from the solutions is specific to the chemical initially dissolved
Elia and Niccoli	Compare extremely diluted solutions with plain solvent (twice-distilled water) on the following measurements: heat of mixing with acid or basic solutions, electrical conductivity, and pH	Extremely diluted solutions show higher heat of mixing, higher electrical conductivity, and higher pH

From Rey L: Thermoluminescence of ultra-high dilutions of lithium chloride and sodium chloride, *Physica A* 323:67-74, 2002; and Elia V, Niccoli M: New physico-chemical properties of extremely diluted aqueous solutions, *J Thermal Anal Calorimetry* 75:815-836, 2004.

Legal Status of Homeopathy

Medicines

Most homeopathic medicines are classified as over-the-counter (OTC) preparations by the FDA. Any homeopathic medicine that can be used for a self-limited condition and has at least one clinical indication listed on its label can be marked as OTC.[22] It is important to remember that even though OTC homeopathic medicines are marketed with brief clinical indications on their labels, their potential uses are much broader and can be found in the homeopathic literature.

Practitioners

In the United States, licensed medical doctors, osteopathic physicians, advanced practice nurses, and dentists can legally prescribe all homeopathic medicines in the HPUS. Other healthcare professionals and "lay" homeopaths can also recommend homeopathic medicines for patients, if the medicines are classified as OTC. A few U.S. states, notably Arizona, California, Connecticut, and Nevada, have specific boards for examining and certifying professional homeopaths. Other countries such as Great Britain, India, and New Zealand have recognized homeopathy as a profession in its own right.

Theory of Homeopathy: Mechanism of Action

Homeopathy has not been well accepted by many in the medical and scientific communities because its mechanism of action has not been fully explicated. Most homeopathic medicines are so dilute that none of the original medicinal substance is contained in material form in the potentized medicine.* This fact has led basic scientists and clinicians alike to reject homeopathy despite the clinical evidence of its efficacy and laboratory evidence showing that highly diluted, succussed solutions differ from plain water. Clinical evidence is summarized later in the section on evidence-based homeopathy. Laboratory evidence from two recent experiments is summarized in Table 5-1.[25,26]

*According to a well-known principle of chemistry, if a substance is diluted by a factor of 6.02×10^{23} (Avogadro's number), there is a high statistical probability that no molecules of the original substance still exist in the solution. This dilution factor is reached when a homeopathic medicine is potentized to the 12C or 24X potency. Many homeopathic medicines are diluted well beyond this point and therefore contain no molecules of solute.[21]

Jonas has reviewed theories about the mechanism of action of homeopathy; he discusses solution dynamics, complexity science, and chaos theory, among others.[27] In 2004, Bellavite also reviewed complexity science and chaos theory.[28] Some principles of these theories are presented in brief in Table 5-2.

Most current explanations of homeopathy involve the emerging understanding of the qualities of water as a solvent and its ability to receive, hold, and transmit complex information that is specific to the solute employed. Researchers are still a long way from understanding how very diluted solutions work in the body to stimulate healing. It seems likely that the mechanism of action of homeopathy will be fully understood at some future time, after more high-quality basic and clinical research has been performed.

Evidence-Based Homeopathy

General considerations

Numerous research articles document the efficacy of homeopathy for a variety of conditions. For a comprehensive list of research articles that includes more than 90 conditions and is updated regularly, the reader is referred to *Homeopathic Family Medicine: The eBook*, by Dana Ullman, MPH.[29] Researchers investigating homeopathy have used both outcomes research and, more frequently, double-blind, placebo-controlled designs. Homeopathic research is particularly well suited to the use of placebos, as all homeopathic medicines appear similar due to the facts that they are prepared by incorporating liquid dilutions into small granules and that "blank" granules, which look and taste like active medicines, are readily available.

Homeopathy has performed well in some recently published outcome studies. When compared with conventional medicine for treatment of upper respiratory, lower respiratory, and ear complaints, homeopathy was found to provide relief more quickly, with fewer side effects and greater overall patient satisfaction.[30] A group of Scottish researchers has developed an outcome measures instrument for use in evaluating how patients perceive the impact of homeopathic interventions in their daily lives. Patients with both acute conditions (e.g., injuries, infections, allergic reactions, emotional shocks) and chronic conditions (e.g., rheumatic complaints, premenstrual tension, aftereffects of previous grief) were questioned after 1 year

TABLE 5-2

Theories Explaining the Mechanism of Action of Homeopathy and Some of Their Principles

THEORY	MECHANISM OF ACTION AND PRINCIPLES
Solution dynamics	*Clathrate (cluster) formation:* Water molecules in diluted, succussed solutions are not uniform; water molecule clusters mimic dissolved chemicals in unique and reproducible ways *Coherent excitation:* Vibrating water molecules activate other water molecules in a solution and set up similar vibration patterns
Complexity theory	*Nonlinearity:* The relationship between input and outcome is not proportional, leading to inverse, opposite, paradoxical, and biphasic events such as those seen in homeopathy *Self-organization:* Some complex systems can generate order from disorder; in fractals, for example, a minute part of the structure looks the same as the whole

From Jonas WB, Jacobs J: *Healing with homeopathy: the doctors' guide,* New York, 1996, Warner Books; and Bellavite P: Complexity science and homeopathy: a synthetic overview, *Homeopathy* 92:203-212, 2003.

TABLE 5-3

Outcome Results for 100 Sequential Patients with 80% Returns in the Glasgow Homœopathic Hospital Outcome Scale

OUTCOME MEASURE	PERCENTAGE OF PATIENTS EXPERIENCING IMPROVEMENT (%)
Improvement in presenting complaint	60
Improvement in well being	61
Sustained improvement of value in daily living	49
Sustained reduction in conventional therapy	37

From Reilly D: The evidence for homœopathy (version 9.0): a discussion of the evidence profile for homoeopathy. Available at www.adhom.com/adh_download/download.html. Updated September 2006.

of homeopathic treatment. Results for 100 sequential patients, with 80% returns, are summarized in Table 5-3.[31,32]

Numerous clinical trials have compared homeopathy with placebo or conventional treatment. These trials have been done on a variety of conditions including asthma, allergies, postoperative complications, childhood diarrhea, and rheumatic diseases. A 1997 metaanalysis of 89 well-conducted trials, covering 24 clinical conditions, showed a combined odds ratio of 2.45 in favor of homeopathy, leading to the conclusion that the therapeutic effects of homeopathy cannot be explained by the placebo effect alone.[33] Another review of 119 placebo-controlled homeopathic trials, published in 2003, revealed similar findings.[34] When high-quality studies (those with adequate sample size, randomization, blinding, and other controls of bias) are considered, homeopathic treatment has shown statistically significant positive results. No single condition has been studied comprehensively enough, however, for researchers to state unequivocally that homeopathy is a consistently effective treatment. More research on individual conditions is recommended.

Methodological considerations

Double-blind, placebo-controlled trials in homeopathy have been conducted in several ways. One method involves testing one homeopathic medicine for a given condition, as was done in a 1983 study that tested one homeopathic medicine, *Rhus toxicodendron,* against placebo for osteoarthritis.[35] It is not surprising that homeopathy performed no better than placebo, as the medicine was not individualized to the patients' symptoms. Even though a potentized medicine was used, this study should not be considered a valid test of homeopathic treatment, as homeopathic methodology was not employed. In another study testing *Rhus toxicodendron* against placebo for fibromyalgia, only patients whose symptoms were similar (related) to the characteristics of the medicine were entered into the study before randomization occurred. In this case, homeopathy performed significantly better than placebo.[36]

Other research methods have been employed, including utilization of a potentized substance closely related to the disease being studied, such as grass pollen for nasal allergies,[37] or utilization of a combination of potentized substances where each individual substance is known to sometimes be efficacious for the condition being studied. In one such study a combination of homeopathic medicines was used to treat patients with influenza.[38] Even though these experiments sometimes show the potentized medicine to be superior to placebo or conventional treatment, it should be kept in mind that such experiments are also not true tests of homeopathy, as the central principle of the method—individualization of the medicine to the patient—has not been applied.

The best design for homeopathic research is for each patient entering the study to have an individualized homeopathic medicine chosen for him or her on the basis of a homeopathic interview and analysis. Then, if the patient is randomized to the homeopathic group, he or she will receive the medicine most likely to be effective for his or her condition. This research design would test the homeopathic method, not just a specific homeopathic medicine, for a given condition. All homeopathic research papers must be read critically to assess whether proper methodology has been employed.

Homeopathic research on pediatric conditions

A small body of research exists on homeopathic treatment for two common pediatric conditions, otitis media[39-41] and diarrhea.[42-45] Otitis media is worthy of more research, as it is the most common diagnosis made in children under the age of 15 in physicians' office practices in the United States; 50% to 85% of 3-year-old children have had at least one episode of otitis media, and 39% of 7-year-old children have had three or more episodes.[46] Not surprisingly, otitis media is frequently treated by homeopaths.[47] Research findings will be summarized in the chapter on otitis media.

Acute diarrhea also merits further research, as it is the leading cause of pediatric morbidity and mortality in the world, causing an estimated 2 million deaths per year in children younger than 5 years.[48] Research findings will be summarized in the chapter on diarrhea.

Current Pediatric Use

To date there has been no large-scale survey documenting the use of complementary and alternative medical (CAM) therapies in general, or homeopathy specifically, in children. Some estimates on the use of homeopathy in children can be made, however, by generalizing from a small survey that was conducted on a pediatric population and by making some inferences from data collected on adults.

In a 1994 survey performed in a hospital-based pediatric clinic in Canada, it was found that 11% of children had been treated by a CAM practitioner, with homeopathy being the CAM therapy used second most frequently (25% of respondents), after chiropractic (36% of respondents), with a yield of 2.75% of children having received homeopathic treatment. Overall, CAM treatments, including homeopathy, were most often used for the following organ systems and conditions: respiratory, ear-nose-throat, musculoskeletal, dermatological, gastrointestinal, and allergies. Parents who included CAM in their own medical care were more likely to use it for their children.[49]

In a 1992 survey that compared practice characteristics of homeopathic physicians with those of general and family physicians, it was found that homeopathic physicians see a larger percentage of pediatric patients; among the homeopathic physicians, 23.9% of patients seen were less than 15 years old, compared with 16.6% for the conventional physicians.[47] Another survey of homeopathic (n = 42) and naturopathic (n = 23) practitioners, conducted in 2000 in Massachusetts, revealed that approximately one third of the patients seen by the respondents were children.[50] These surveys indicate that homeopathy may be used disproportionately more frequently for children than adults.

The most recent data on CAM usage in the United States were generated in a 2002 survey of 31,044 adults.[51] Of the respondents, 3.6% reported having used homeopathy in the past, with 1.7% having used it in the previous 12 months. These data were generated from individuals who used homeopathy either with professional consultation or as a form of self-treatment (most homeopathic medicines are classified as OTC and therefore can be self-administered). It is likely that a similar percentage of children in the United States were also treated homeopathically.

Contraindications and Adverse Effects Reported for Pediatric Use

There are no absolute contradictions for the use of homeopathy. Because homeopathic medicines are highly diluted, they are usually free of side effects. Homeopathy is generally safe for infants and children of all ages, as well as for women during pregnancy and lactation (this is one of the reasons homeopathy is an excellent form of therapy for children).

A systematic review of the literature on the use of homeopathic medicines found that side effects are rare.[52] A phenomenon commonly referred to as an "aggravation of symptoms" is observed in as many as 25% of patients treated with homeopathic medicines.[53] The aggravation consists of an initial worsening of symptoms, typically lasting no more than several hours, which is often followed by a decrease in or resolution of symptoms. Aggravations may represent proving symptoms that are stimulated by the potentized medicine (see earlier discussion of provings).

Because homeopathy is a form of energy therapy, it has no biochemical interactions with other medications, so it is safe to use in conjunction with allopathic medicines as well as herbs or acupuncture. As with other forms of nonstandard therapy, one of the potential dangers is that homeopathy will be used alone in cases where standard or conventional therapy is indicated, leading to a negative outcome for the patient.

Safety and Precautions for Pediatric Use

For any significant medical condition, either acute or chronic, children being treated homeopathically should be seen by a professional with expertise in both medicine and homeopathy.

Naturopathy

Historical Background

Naturopathic medicine is as much a philosophy as it is a medical practice. It is based on the use of a variety of natural therapies to treat disease. Depending on the state in which one is licensed to practice, a naturopathic physician (Naturopathic Doctor/ND/NMD) may use botanical medicine, physical medicine, homeopathy, mind/body medicine, oriental medicine, nutritional therapy, or diet and lifestyle changes to treat disease. Some states also provide prescriptive rights for naturopathic physicians. A naturopathic physician has completed a 4-year, postbaccalaureate degree at an accredited naturopathic medical school program. Currently, there are four accredited schools in the country: Bastyr University in Seattle; Southwest College of Naturopathic Medicine in Tempe, Arizona; National College of Naturopathic Medicine in Portland, Oregon; and the University of Bridgeport in Bridgeport, Connecticut.

Naturopathic physicians are a diverse group of practitioners. The U.S. naturopathic medical school system trains naturopathic medical students primarily as family practitioners. However, some practice exclusively in subspecialties, such as cardiology, women's medicine, men's health, pediatrics, and sports medicine. Other naturopathic physicians prefer to focus on certain areas of naturopathic treatment modalities, such as homeopathy, botanical medicine, or physical medicine. Although they are a diverse group, most practitioners agree on the common principles of treatment.

One of the most important tenets of naturopathy is that when the cause of disease is removed, the body will use its inherent abilities to heal itself, and the use of natural treatments can help influence these abilities. Naturopathic physicians are also trained in the conventional medical technique of clinical and laboratory diagnosis, and practitioners of naturopathy use these techniques as a regular part of their patient management. The four accredited naturopathic programs train naturopathic medical students to be family practitioners who treat adults as well as children and infants.

Naturopathy grew out of what was termed the "Nature Cure" movement that flourished in Europe in the early 1800s. Vincent Priessnitz is credited with being the first of these practitioners. He used nature's own elements such as water (termed *water cure*), fresh air, exercise, and diet to treat disease in patients of all ages, including children. The spas that populate much of Europe and America today have roots in this movement.

A description of pediatric treatment by Priessnitz is described in the book *Nature Doctors* by Kirchfeld and Boyle: A family of five children all developed scarlet fever. Four were treated by conventional medicine and died. The father entrusted the fifth child to Priessnitz, who plunged the child into ice water several times, after which the child fell asleep. When the child awoke, the fever was gone, and the child survived the illness.[1]

Naturopathic practitioners were very popular in the nineteenth century. An American newspaper reported that Father Sebastian Kneipp (1824-1897), one of the practitioners who popularized Nature Cure in Germany, was the third most popular person in the world, after the U.S. president and the German chancellor.[1a] Kneipp's influence eventually spread throughout Europe and the Americas. Another excerpt from *Nature Doctors* explains the whole-body approach in a child with a localized infection: A 9-year-old boy came to Kneipp with an undefined eye disease, along with anorexia and muscle wasting. The treatment was two warm baths per week. In addition, for 4 weeks, the boy was to wear a shirt dipped in cold salt water for 1 hour. After the 4 weeks, cold baths were given three to four times per week followed by exercise. *Hydrotherapy*, as this is termed, is thought to stimulate our innate healing abilities.

Benedict Lust (1872-1945), a patient and later a student of Father Kneipp, is credited with bringing Nature Cure to the United States. He would later coin the term *naturopathy* to describe the combination of water cure and the application of herbs, vitamins, homeopathy, diet therapy, and sun therapy. Eventually, vitamins and bodywork such as massage and physical manipulation techniques similar to chiropractic and osteopathic methods were added to this system.

Naturopathy flourished in the United States in the early 1900s. There were numerous naturopathic schools, with licensing of naturopathic physicians in most states. By mid-century, however, the trend was drastically reversed because of political and social movements, and not a single naturopathic school remained after this time.

In 1908, the Carnegie Foundation commissioned a report to evaluate U.S. medical schools, known as the Flexner Report, headed by Abraham Flexner in cooperation with leading members of the AMA. Before the report, naturopathic, homeopathic, and "conventional" medical schools had wildly divergent standards for what constituted a medical education. Medical degrees of all types could be obtained in 1 to 4 years or could even be purchased in the mail.

The report favored 4-year schools where classes were taught by professors and not by practitioners nor the use of clinical research to determine suitable treatments. At the time, most naturopathic schools did not conform to this model. The report's findings were adopted by the government, and soon only graduates of schools that were approved by the report were able to take licensing examinations. This led to the demise of not only naturopathic schools, but also of homeopathic medical education programs.

The elevation of science as the way to uncover all truth was the large social movement at the beginning of the 1900s. The application of the scientific method was changing everyday life, and the creation of medicine came out of the mind of scientists. Soon wonder drugs were discovered: antibiotics held the promise to eradicate all infectious disease, and steroids soon followed with the hope that pain and inflammation would be controlled. In this era of science, the natural approach to health became unpopular, and naturopathy was considered quackery. By the mid-1900s, no schools of naturopathy existed, and only a few states still had licensing.

Naturopathic medicine has seen a resurgence in recent years because of public demand. Many of the conventional medications that worked so well at first have lost some of their appeal. The disadvantages of conventional treatments, such as untoward side effects or decreases in effectiveness due to long-term use, have made the natural approach to pediatric care more appealing. As a result, CAM therapies are frequently used in the medical management of disease in children.[2] Another reason that families may be drawn to natural approaches is parental dissatisfaction with a child's physician,[3] whether it be due to attitudes that the physician has toward CAM therapies or the physician's inflexibility with the vaccination schedule. Parents often look into CAM therapies when conventional medicine has not cured the problem but has simply treated symptoms. For example, the constant development of new asthma medications have certainly led to a decrease in hospitalizations, but asthma rates continue to increase.[4] One might argue that this is a microcosm of modern medicine; preventing more patients from needing hospital care does not mean there is a decrease in sick patients, only a decrease in symptom severity. In the case of asthma, naturopathic medicine seeks to treat the source of the inflammation, not just to treat the inflammation itself.

Theory

The principles of naturopathic medicine form the basis for the naturopathic approach to healthcare, as follows:

- First, do no harm (*primum non nocere*): Naturopathic physicians and medical doctors share this common principle of practice. For the naturopath, this means primarily using modalities and medicines that are the least invasive and have low potential for side effects. This is an important standard when addressing infants and children, as they are a particularly sensitive population.

- The healing power of nature *(vis medicatrix naturae):* The natural state of the body is health. It is clear that when given the proper conditions, the body will heal itself, as in the example of healing a minor cut in the skin. This process may be applied to other diseases. Pediatric patients tend to recover quicker and to a fuller extent than adult patients, as they do not have to rebound from years of accumulated improper diet, lifestyle, and exposure to a toxic environment.
- Identify and treat the cause *(tolle causam):* Naturopathic physicians see symptoms as the reflection of the disease, not the disease itself. Naturopathic physicians seek to uncover the true cause of illness by removing obstacles to health and supporting the healing process. Symptoms then subside as the person becomes healthier. The current conventional medical model of disease treatment, such as in asthma, eczema, or chronic rhinitis, focuses on symptoms and not the cause. Many conditions that affect the pediatric population may be treated successfully by simply changing the diet.
- Treat the whole person *(tolle totum):* Illness may have a variety of etiologies ranging from nutritional, emotional, physical, mental, or environmental to spiritual problems. Naturopathic physicians recognize that to truly find health, a patient must be supported on all possible levels. This embodies the idea of "holism." Considerations must be given to a child's home life, school environment, and social activities, as it is clear that any of these areas can have significant effects on a child's health.
- Doctor as teacher *(docere):* The word *doctor* comes from the Latin *docere,* which means "to teach." Naturopathic physicians strive to teach first by example, and then counsel patients on diet and lifestyle. The profession prides itself on its practitioners bringing these principles into their own lives. Naturopathic physicians often focus on educating the parents of the patients, but there is an equal benefit to teaching the children as well.
- Prevention *(prevenir):* The prevention of disease is far easier than the treatment. Engaging in a healthy lifestyle has long-term effects on the patient. It only makes sense that the earlier in life the interventions are applied, the longer the duration of optimal health.

The *Therapeutic Order,* as developed by Jared Zeff, ND, is a basic approach used by naturopathic physicians to guide their treatment process using some of the principles of naturopathic medicine. The direction is from least to most invasive, as follows:

1. *Re-establish the basis for health:* Remove obstacles to cure by establishing a healthy regimen.
2. *Stimulate the healing power of nature:* Use various systems of health such as botanical medicine, homeopathy, Chinese medicine, Ayurvedic medicine, nutrition, or psychospiritual counseling.
3. *Tonify weakened systems:* Use modalities to strengthen the immune system, decrease toxicity, normalize inflammatory function, optimize metabolic function, balance regulatory systems, enhance regeneration, and harmonize life forces.
4. *Correct structural integrity:* Use therapeutic exercise, spinal manipulation, massage, and craniosacral therapy to return the body to optimal structural condition.
5. *Prescribe specific natural substances for pathology:* Use vitamins, minerals, and herbs to promote health.
6. *Prescribe pharmacological substances for pathology:* Use pharmaceutical drugs to return patient to a healthy state.
7. *Prescribe surgery, suppressive drugs, radiation, and chemotherapy:* Use aggressive therapies to attempt to maintain health.

Evidence-Based Information

The increased interest in and use of natural and alternative therapies has spurred the demand for quality research. To date, there is a paucity of literature on the specific use of naturopathic medicine in the treatment of children. However, the body of research that exists for the different therapeutic modalities employed by naturopathic physicians is much larger and continues to expand.

Along with the increase in demand for alternative and therefore naturopathic medicine comes antagonism from some in the conventional medical field.[5] The lack of double-blind, placebo-controlled studies on alternative therapies as compared with pharmaceutical drugs raises concerns among medical doctors. Opponents claim that the lack of research on alternative therapies justifies its exclusion as an effective approach to healthcare. Naturopathic medicine uses many different alternative therapies, and there is a large amount of favorable research on the individual treatments. The prevalence of studies on single therapies and medicines represents the trend in research that has been embraced by the conventional medical field, often fueled by pharmaceutical company funds.

However, naturopathy bases its approach to patient care on a holistic model, not single therapies. Conducting research on a multifaceted treatment plan is unlikely to be accepted by the general medical community, as critics would question which part of the treatment plan was effective. Powerful pharmaceutical drugs can have profound effects on symptoms and body functions, in turn producing favorable research findings in the short term. The lack of knowledge regarding the long-term effects of many pharmaceutical medications has led to severe consequences such as in the cases of Pemoline,[6] Bextra, Vioxx,[7] and recently Atomoxetine. The inclination to rely on these short-term results as the answer to health may not survive the test of time. It is in the author's opinion that the research paradigm needs to be shifted to a long-term, holistic view of medical treatment and patient care.

Current Pediatric Use

Trained as primary care physicians, naturopathic physicians may safely and successfully treat a variety of pediatric diseases. They may use standard diagnostic and traditional techniques to assess their patients' conditions, as they are educated in both natural and alternative medical theories and conventional medical theories.

Data from 1994 demonstrated the increased use of alternative medicine in the pediatric population.[8] In a recent analysis of CAM practices in this country by Cherkin et al.,

10% of children were seen by naturopathic physicians, whereas only 1% to 4% of children were seen by other CAM providers.[9] Research also shows that the interest in CAM is shared abroad.[10] The use of CAM therapies is clearly increasing among the general patient population,[11] including children.[12] Because most parents who use alternative medicine for their children also use it themselves,[13] it may be assumed that the increasing use by adults has had a significant influence on pediatric practice.

CAM therapies are slowly starting to work their way into the conventional arena, and more conventional physicians are using the treatments. Reliable research such as probiotics for antibiotic-induced diarrhea,[14] homeopathy for acute childhood diarrhea,[15,16] and riboflavin supplementation in the treatment of migraines[17] has made this an easy transition, showing the validity and value of these therapies.

Contraindications

Contraindications to naturopathic medicine are specific to the individual therapies themselves. Most dietary supplements that are used by naturopathic physicians have low toxicity and are considered safe. However, regardless of a substance being referred to as "natural," anything taken in excess can be harmful, and some medicines used in naturopathy can have considerable toxic effects. It is for this reason that discretion should be used when treating children, as would be the case with the use of any treatment, alternative or not.

Botanical medicine

Several botanical medicines should be used with caution or avoided completely by lactating mothers, because of their potential toxicity or adverse reactions. Small amounts of these herbs may be passed in the breast milk, and they may have stimulating or laxative effects, be irritating to the digestive tract, or be hepatotoxic or genotoxic[18,19] (Box 5-2).

Certain herbs and medications are thought to decrease milk production in a nursing mother and thus should be avoided. Bugleweed *(Lycopus virginicus)*, jasmine flowers *(Jasminum pubescens)*, and sage leaves *(Salvia officinalis)* may have significant effects on a mother's ability to produce adequate amounts of milk.

Decongestants such as psuedoephedrine have been implicated in decreasing milk production because of their possible suppression of prolactin secretion.[20] It would be reasonable to assume the same effects with herbs that have decongestant properties, such as ephedra/ma huang, to have similar effects.

Some botanicals should be used with caution or avoided when directly treating children. Physicians should refer to the source cited in this text to fully understand appropriate ages for administration and the effects of each herb. Several species have locally irritating effects, affect the nervous system, have a laxative effect, contain essential oils that should not be consumed, or block absorption of nutrients[19] (Box 5-3).

Specific plants such as horseradish fresh root *(Armoracia rusticana)*, watercress *(Nasturtium officinale)*, and mustard seed *(Brassica nigra, Brassica alba, Brassica juncea)* have locally irritating effects when applied to the skin, so prudence should be used when applying them to children.

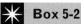

Box 5-2

Botanical Medicines That Should Be Used with Caution or Not at All in Lactating Mothers

Alkanet root (*Alkanna tinctoria*)
Aloe vera
Basil (*Ocymum basilium*)
Black cohosh (*Cimicifuga racemosa*)
Bladderwrack (*Fucus vesiculosus*)
Borage (*Borago officinalis*)
Buckthorn (*Rhamnus catharticus*)
Butterbur (*Petasites vulgaris*)
Cascara sagrada (*Rhamnus purshiana*)
Chaparral (*Larrea tridentata, Larrea divaricata*)
Cincona bark (*Cinchona spp.*)
Cocoa seeds (*Theobroma cacao*)
Coffee seeds (*Coffea arabica*)
Cola seeds (*Cola nitida, Cola acuminata*)
Colocynth (*Citrullus colocynthis*)
Coltsfoot (*Tussilago farfara*)
Comfrey (*Symphytum officinale*)
Dulse (*Rhodymenia palmetto*)
Elecampane (*Inula helenium*)
Ephedra/Ma huang (*Ephedra vulgaris*)
Frangula (*Rhamnus frangula*)
Gelsemium (*Gelsemium nitidum*)
Guarana (*Paullinia cupana*)
Hemp agrimony (*Eupatorium cannabinum*)
Joe-Pye weed (*Eupatorium purpureum*)
Kava kava (*Piper methysticum*)
Kelp thallus (*Nereocystis luetkeana*)
Licorice (*Glycyrrhiza glabra*)
Life root (*Senecio aureus*)
Ma huang (*Ephedra sinica*)
Madder root (*Rubia tinctorum*)
Male fern (*Dryopteris filix-mas*)
Mate leaves (*Ilex paraguayensis*)
Meadow saffron (*Colchicum autumnale*)
Prickly ash (*Zanthoxylum americanum, Zanthoxylum clava-herculis*)
Pulsatilla (*Anemone nemorosa*)
Queen's root/queen's delight (*Stillingia sylvatica*)
Rhubarb (*Rheum palmatum, Rheum officinale*)
Rockweed (*Fucus spp*)
Seaweed thallus (*Laminaria spp.*)
Senna (*Cassia spp.*)
Tea leaves (*Camellia sinensis*)
Tobacco leaves (*Nicotiana tabacum*)
Syrian rue (*Peganum harmala*)
Wintergreen leaves (*Gaultheria procumbens*)
Wormseed (*Artemisia cina*)
Wormwood (*Artemisia absinthium*)

Botanical Medicines That Should Be Used with Caution in Children

Aloe vera
Basil (*Ocymum basilium*)
Bitter orange peel (*Citrus aurantium* ssp. *amara*)
Buckthorn (*Rhamnus catharticus*)
Camphor tree bark (*Cinnamomum camphora*)
Cascara sagrada (*Rhamnus purshiana*)
Celandine root (*Chelidonium majus*)
Cocoa seeds (*Theobroma cacao*)
Coffee seeds (*Coffea arabica*)
Cola seeds (*Cola nitida, Cola acuminata*)
Eucalyptus leaves (*Eucalyptus* spp.)
Fennel fruit (*Foeniculum vulgare*)
Frangula (*Rhamnus frangula*)
Guarana (*Paullinia cupana*)
Horsetail plant (*Equisetum* spp.)
Ipecac root (*Cephalis ipecacuanha*)
Jamaican dogwood (*Piscidia erythrina*)
Lobelia (*Lobelia inflata*)
Ma huang (*Ephedra sinica*)
Mate leaves (*Llex paraguayensis*)
Peppermint leaves (*Mentha piperita*)
Rhubarb (*Rheum palmatum, Rheum officinale*)
Senna (*Cassia* spp.)
Tea leaves (*Camellia sinensis*)
Tobacco leaves (*Nicotiana tabacum*)
Wormseed (*Chenopodium ambrosioides, Chenopodium antihelminticum*)
Yohimbe bark (*Pausinystalia yohimbe*)

Homeopathy

When used by an experienced practitioner, homeopathy is an effective mode of treatment and very rarely has any adverse effects. There are no known contraindications to homeopathic treatment at this time.

Physical medicine

Manipulative medicine should be performed only by an experienced practitioner or one who has undergone specific training in pediatric adjustments. Contraindications to manipulation include local malignancy, local infection, fracture, inflammatory spondylitis, spondylolisthesis,[21] and vertebral artery vascular compromise. Because routine cervical radiographs taken in an emergency room setting can be unreliable in detecting fractures in patients with spinal trauma, a complete radiographic series should be performed in those patients before receiving manipulative therapy.[22] Therapeutic massage is often used as a treatment modality along with manipulative techniques. The presence of thrombosis is a contraindication to massage therapy due to the risk of dislodging.[23]

Nutritional therapy

Some vitamins and minerals provided in therapeutic doses can have detrimental effects in patients with certain disease states, as well as interact with conventional medications. When supplementing in children, the interactions of each nutrient should be considered.[24] This is by no means an all-inclusive list, but it addresses some of the most common supplements encountered in patient populations.

Vitamin C. Large doses may cause intestinal distress with gas, bloating, and osmotic diarrhea and thus should be avoided in those with diarrheal illness. Decreasing the dose, using buffered vitamin C, administering with food, or dividing the dose into smaller increments can all decrease this effect. Theoretically, high levels of vitamin C may put patients at risk for kidney stones in those that have existing renal disease, as it can increase urinary oxalate levels.[25] However, in review of the literature, doses of up to at least 2 to 4 g/day is well tolerated by healthy adults[26] and has never been shown to cause nephrolithiasis. Doses up to 10 g/day have been shown to increase urinary oxalate levels, but within a safe and normal range.[27,28] There are also reports of repeated intravenous treatments of up to 20 g/day being well tolerated. Patients with disorders of iron metabolism or iron toxicity should avoid large doses of vitamin C, as it can enhance iron absorption and keep iron in a reduced and active state.[29] In addition, patients with glucose-6-phosphate dehydrogenase deficiency may develop hemolytic anemia when supplemented with vitamin C.

Thiamin. Intakes of large doses of thiamin have not been reported to cause toxicity.[30]

Riboflavin. Intakes of large doses of riboflavin have not been reported to cause toxicity.[31]

Niacin, nicotinic acid, nicotinamide, niacinamide. Administration may cause a release of histamine, which leads to the characteristic "flushing" response as well as pruritus. Therefore caution should be used in patients with asthma or peptic ulcer disease. These effects may be avoided by gradually increasing the dosage or by taking niacin with meals. Aspirin administration may help reduce this reaction. However, it also may decrease hepatic clearance of niacin.[32] Reports of toxicity are more prevalent with sustained-release niacin and should be avoided in pediatric patients.[33-35] Niacin supplementation has been shown to have adverse effects on glycemic control in adults with and without diabetes, so the benefit of lipidemia treatment versus the risks should be weighed individually for each patient.[36,37] Niacin and its other forms should not be used in conjunction with statin drugs, as this can lead to rhabdomyolysis.[38]

Pantothenic acid. Very high doses of vitamin B$_5$ may cause intestinal distress and diarrhea. Otherwise, no adverse health reports have been reported.[31]

Pyridoxine. In this author's experience, hyperactive children may be aggravated by administration of vitamin B$_6$, but this effect may be alleviated or eliminated with coadministration of magnesium. Peripheral neuropathy has been reported with large doses of pyridoxine.

Folate. Large doses of folate may increase seizure activity in epileptic patients, either by lowering seizure threshold or by decreasing the effect of seizure medication.[39]

Vitamin A. Doses > 7500 μg vitamin A are contraindicated in patients who are of childbearing age, as supplementation has been shown to be teratogenic.[40]

Vitamin E. Oral intake of high levels of vitamin E is contraindicated in patients with vitamin K deficiency, as it can intensify blood coagulation abnormalities in those patients.[41] This contraindication should be considered especially in patients on anticoagulant therapy or with malabsorption syndromes.

Vitamin K. Supplementation can interfere with anticoagulant medications and should be avoided in these patients.

Fish oil. The administration of essential fatty acid supplements such as fish oil preparations may increase the international normalized ratio in patients on warfarin or other anticoagulant therapy.[42]

References

Homeopathy

1. United States Department of Health and Human Services: *NCCAM Five Year Strategic Plan,* NIH Publication No. 01-5001, Bethesda, Md, 2000, National Institutes of Health.
2. Cook TM: *Samuel Hahnemann: the founder of homœopathic medicine,* Wellingborough, United Kingdom, 1981, Thorsons.
3. Scherr J: *The dynamics and methodology of homœopathic provings,* ed 2, Malvern, UK, 1994, Dynamis.
4. Hahnemann S [O'Reilly WB, editor]: *Organon of the medical art,* Palo Alto, Calif, 1996, Birdcage Books.
5. Hahnemann SCF: *Materia medica pura,* vol 1-6, Dresden, 1811-1821, Arnoldischen Buchhandlung.
6. Winston J: *The faces of homœopathy: an illustrated history of the first 200 years,* Tawa, New Zealand, 1999, Great Auk.
7. Hering C: *Domestic physician,* ed 5, Philadelphia, 1851, Rademacher and Sheek.
8. Coulter HL: *Divided legacy: the conflict between homœopathy and the American Medical Association,* ed 2, Berkeley, Calif, 1982, North Atlantic Books.
9. Ruddock EH: *The diseases of infants and children and their homœopathic and general treatment,* ed 3, London, 1878, Homœopathic Publishing Company.
10. Edmond WA: *A treatise on diseases peculiar to infants and children,* London, 1881, Homœopathic Publishing Company.
11. Burnett JC: *Delicate, backward, puny and stunted children: their developmental defects, and physical, mental and moral peculiarities considered as ailments amenable to treatment by medicines,* London, 1895, Homœopathic Publishing Company.
12. Tooker RN: *The diseases of children and their homeopathic treatment: a test-book for students, colleges, and practitioners,* Chicago, 1898, Gross and Delbridge.
13. Raue CS: *Diseases of children,* Philadelphia, 1899, Boericke and Tafel.
14. Boericke W: *The management and care of children including homœopathic treatment,* 1903, San Francisco, Homœopathic Publishing Company.
15. Alcott LM: *Little women,* New York, 2004, New American Library [originally published in 1868].
16. Kent JT: *Lectures on homeopathic materia medica,* ed 3, Philadelphia, 1923, Boericke & Tafel.
17. Kent JT: *Lectures on homœopathic philosophy,* Berkeley, Calif, 1979, North Atlantic Books [originally published in 1900].
18. *ReferenceWorks Pro 4.2,* San Rafael, Calif, 2008, Kent Homeopathic Associates.
19. Kent JT: *Repertory of the homœopathic materia medica,* ed 3 (revised), Chicago, 1924, Ehrhart & Karl.
20. Flexner A: *Medical education in the United States and Canada, report to Carnegie Foundation,* Washington, DC, 1910, The Foundation.
21. Vithoulkas G: *The science of homeopathy,* New York, 1980, Grove Press.
22. Homeopathic Pharamacopoeia of the United States. Available at www.hpcus.com. Accessed June 2008.
23. Klein L: *Homeopathic master clinician course,* West Vancouver, BC, 1997-1999, Luminos Homeopathic Courses.
24. Sankaran R: *The spirit of homœopathy,* ed 2, Bombay, 1992, Homœopathic Medical Publishers.
25. Rey L: Thermoluminescence of ultra-high dilutions of lithium chloride and sodium chloride, *Physica A* 323:67-74, 2002.
26. Elia V, Niccoli M: New physico-chemical properties of extremely diluted aqueous solutions., *J Thermal Anal Calorimetry* 75:815-836, 2004.
27. Jonas WB, Jacobs J: *Healing with homeopathy: the doctors' guide,* New York, 1996, Warner Books.
28. Bellavite P: Complexity science and homeopathy: a synthetic overview, *Homeopathy* 92:203-212, 2003.
29. Ullman D: *Homeopathic family medicine: the ebook,* Berkeley, Calif, 2003, Homeopathic Educational Services.
30. Riley D, Fischer M, Singh B et al: Homeopathy and conventional medicine: an outcomes study comparing effectiveness in a primary care setting, *J Alt Comp Med* 7:149-159, 2001.
31. Reilly D, Duncan R, Bikker A et al: The clinical results of homoeopathic prescribing in primary care. Results in over 1600 cases: the development of the GHHOS (Glasgow Homoeopathic Hospital Outcome Scale), the IDCCIM action research, and the PC-HICOM project. Available at www.adhom.com/adh_download/download.html. Accessed February 2003.
32. Reilly D: The evidence for homoeopathy (version 6.0): a discussion of the evidence profile for homoeopathy. Available at www.adhom.com/adh_download/download.html. Accessed March 2004.
33. Linde K, Clausius N, Ramirez G et al: Are the clinical effects of homœopathy placebo effects? A meta-analysis of placebo-controlled trials, *Lancet* 350:834-843, 1997.
34. Jonas WB, Kaptchuk TJ, Linde K: A critical overview of homeopathy, *Ann Int Med* 138:393-399, 2003.
35. Shipley M, Berry H, Broster G et al: Controlled trial of homœopathic treatment of osteoarthritis, *Lancet* i:97-98, 1983.
36. Fisher PA, Greenwood A, Huskisson E: Effect of homœopathic treatment on fibrositis (primary fibromyalgia), *Br Med J* 299:365-366, 1989.
37. Reilly DT, Taylor MA, McSharry C et al: Is homeopathy a placebo response? Controlled trial of homœopathic potency, with pollen in hay fever as model, *Lancet* 2:881-886, 1986.
38. Maiwald L, Weinfurtner T, Mau J et al: Therapy of common cold with a homeopathic preparation in comparison with acetyl salicylic acid [in German], *Arzneim Forsch (Drug Research)* 38:578-582, 1988.
39. Friese KH, Druse S, Moeller H: Acute otitis media in children: comparison between conventional and homeopathic therapy, *HNO* 44:462-466, 1996.
40. Barnett ED, Levatin JL, Chapman EH et al: Challenges of evaluating homeopathic treatment of acute otitis media, *Pediatr Infect Dis J* 19:273-275, 2000.
41. Jacobs J, Springer DS, Crothers D: Homeopathic treatment of acute otitis media in children: a preliminary randomized controlled trial, *Pediatr Infect Dis J* 20:177-183, 2001.

42. Jacobs J, Jimenez LM, Gloyd S et al: Homeopathic treatment of acute childhood diarrhoea, *Br Homeopath J* 82:83-86, 1993.
43. Jacobs J, Jiménez M, Gloyd SS: Treatment of acute childhood diarrhea with homeopathic medicine: a randomized clinical trial in Nicaragua, *Pediatrics* 93:719-725, 1994.
44. Jacobs J, Jiménez M, Malthouse S et al: Homeopathic treatment of acute childhood diarrhea: results from a clinical trial in Nepal, *J Alt Comp Med* 6:131-139, 2000.
45. Jacobs J, Jonas WB, Jiménez-Pérez M et al: Homeopathy for childhood diarrhea: combined results and metaanalysis from three randomized, controlled clinical trials, *Pediatr Infect Dis J* 22:229-234, 2003.
46. Casselbrandt ML, Mandel EM: Epidemiology. In Rosenfeld RM, Bluestone CD, editors: *Evidence-based otitis media*, ed 2, Hamilton, Ontario, 2003, BC Decker.
47. Jacobs J, Chapman EH, Crothers D: Patient characteristics and practice patterns of physicians using homeopathy, *Arch Fam Med* 7:537-540, 1998.
48. Population Resource Center: *Executive summary: child and infant health and mortality.* Available at www.childinfo.org/diarrhoea.html.
49. Spigelblatt L, Laine-Ammara G, Pless IB et al: The use of alternative medicine by children, *Pediatrics* 94:811-814, 1994.
50. Lee ACC, Kemper KJ: Homeopathy and naturopathy, *Arch Pediatr Adolesc Med* 154:78-80, 2000.
51. Barnes PM, Powell-Griner E, McFann K et al: *Complementary and alternative medicine use among adults: United States, 2002. Advance data from vital and health statistics; No. 343*, Hyattsville, Md, 2004, National Center for Health Statistics.
52. Dantes F, Rampes H: Do homeopathic medicines provoke adverse effects? A systematic review, *Br Homeopath J* 89:S35-S38, 2000.
53. Reilly DT, Taylor MA, Beattie NGM et al: Is evidence for homeopathy reproducible? *Lancet* 344:1601-1606, 1994.

Naturopathy

1. Kirchfield F, Boyle W: *Nature doctors*, Portland, Ore, 1994, Medicina Biologica.
1a. Burghardt L: *Sebastian Kneipp: Helfer der Menschheit [Sebastian Kneipp: helper of mankind]*, Bad Worishofen, Germany, 1988, Kneipp Verlag.
2. Pitetti R, Singh S, Hornyak D et al: Complementary and alternative medicine use in children. *Pediatr Emerg Care* 17:165-169, 2001.
3. Neuhouser ML, Patterson RE, Schwartz SM et al: Use of alternative medicine by children with cancer in Washington State, *Prev Med* 33:347-354, 2001.
4. Meurer JR, George V, Subichin S et al: Asthma severity among children hospitalized in 1990 and 1995, *Arch Pediatr Adolesc Med* 154:143-149, 2000.
5. Atwood KC IV: Naturopathy: a critical appraisal, *MedGenMed* 5:39, 2003.
6. Marotta PJ, Roberts EA: Pemoline hepatotoxicity in children, *J Pediatr* 132:894-897, 1998.
7. Levesque LE, Brophy JM, Zhang B: The risk for myocardial infarction with cyclooxygenase-2 inhibitors: a population study of elderly adults, *Ann Intern Med* 142:481-489, 2005.
8. Spigelblatt L, Laine-Ammara G, Pless IB et al: The use of alternative medicine by children, *Pediatrics* 94:811-814, 1994.
9. Cherkin DC, Deyo RA, Sherman KJ et al: Characteristics of visits to licensed acupuncturists, chiropractors, massage therapists, and naturopathic physicians, *Am Board Fam Pract* 15:463-472, 2002.
10. Bensoussan A, Myers SP, Wu SM et al: Naturopathic and Western herbal medicine practice in Australia—a workforce survey, *Complement Ther Med* 12:17-27, 2004.
11. Tindle HA, Davis RB, Phillips RS et al: Trends in use of complementary and alternative medicine by US adults: 1997-2002, *Altern Ther Health Med* 11:42-49, 2005.
12. Gardiner P, Dvorkin L, Kemper KJ: Supplement use growing among children and adolescents. *Pediatr Ann* 33:227-232, 2004.
13. Yussman SM, Ryan SA, Auinger P et al: Visits to complementary and alternative medicine providers by children and adolescents in the United States, *Ambul Pediatr* 4:429-435, 2004.
14. Sullivan A, Nord CE: Probiotics and gastrointestinal diseases, *J Intern Med* 257:78-92, 2005.
15. Jacobs J, Jonas WB, Jimenez-Perez M et al: Homeopathy for childhood diarrhea: combined results and metaanalysis from three randomized, controlled clinical trials, *Pediatr Infect Dis J* 22:229-234, 2003.
16. Jacobs J, Jimenez LM, Malthouse S et al: Homeopathic treatment of acute childhood diarrhea: results from a clinical trial in Nepal, *J Altern Complement Med* 6:131-139, 2000.
17. Boehnke C, Reuter U, Flach U et al: High-dose riboflavin treatment is efficacious in migraine prophylaxis: an open study in a tertiary care centre, *Eur J Neurol* 11:475-477, 2004.
18. Brinker F: *Herb contraindications and drug reactions*, ed 2, Sandy, Ore, 1998, Eclectic Medical Publications.
19. McGuffin M, editor: *Botanical safety handbook, American Herbal Products Association*, Boca Raton, Fla, 1997, CRC Press.
20. Aljazaf K, Hale TW, Ilett KF et al: Pseudoephedrine: effects on milk production in women and estimation of infant exposure via breastmilk, *Br J Clin Pharmacol* 56:18-24, 2003.
21. de Zoete A, Assendelft WJ, Algra PR et al: Reliability and validity of lumbosacral spine radiograph reading by chiropractors, chiropractic radiologists, and medical radiologists, *Spine* 27:1926-1933; discussion 1933, 2002.
22. Crowther ER: Missed cervical spine fractures: the importance of reviewing radiographs in chiropractic practice, *J Manipulative Physiol Ther* 18:29-33, 1995.
23. Wieting JM: Massage, traction, and manipulation, *Emedicine* July 21, 2004.
24. Gropper S, Smith J, Groff JL: *Advanced nutrition and human metabolism*, ed 4, Belmont, Calif, 2005, Thompson Wadsworth.
25. Urivetzky M, Kessaris D, Smith AD: Ascorbic acid overdosing: a risk factor for calcium oxalate nephrolithiasis, *J Urol* 147:1215-1218, 1992.
26. Johnston CS: Biomarkers for establishing a tolerable upper intake level for vitamin C, *Nutr Rev* 57:71-77, 1999.
27. Tsao CS, Salimi SL: Effect of large intake of ascorbic acid on urinary and plasma oxalic acid levels, *Int J Vitam Nutr Res* 54:245-249, 1994.
28. Hughes C, Dutton S, Truswell AS: High intakes of ascorbic acid and urinary oxalate, *J Hum Nutr* 35:274-280, 1981.
29. Herbert V, Shaw S, Jayatilleke E: Vitamin C-driven free radical generation from iron, *J Nutr* 126(4 Suppl):1213S-1220S, 1996.
30. Alhadeff L, Gualtieri CT, Lipton M: Toxic effects of water-soluble vitamins, *Nutr Rev* 42:33-40, 1984.
31. Food and Nutrition Board: *Dietary reference intakes for thiamin, riboflavin, niacin, vitamin B6, folate, vitamin B12, pantothenic acid, biotin, and choline*, Washington, DC, 1998, National Academy Press.
32. Gaby A, Wright J: *Nutritional therapy in medical practice*, 1998.
33. Etchason JA, Miller TD, Squires RW et al: Niacin-induced hepatitis: a potential side effect with low-dose time-release niacin, *Mayo Clin Proc* 66:23-28, 1991.

34. Henkin Y, Oberman A, Hurst DC et al: Niacin revisited: clinical observations on an important but underutilized drug, *Am J Med* 91:239-246, 1991.

35. Henkin Y, Johnson KC, Segrest JP: Rechallenge with crystalline niacin after drug-induced hepatitis from sustained-release niacin, *J Am Med Assoc* 264:241-243, 1990.

36. Elam MB, Hunninghake DB, Davis KB et al: Effect of niacin on lipid and lipoprotein levels and glycemic control in patients with diabetes and peripheral arterial disease: the ADMIT study: a randomized trial. Arterial Disease Multiple Intervention Trial, *J Am Med Assoc* 284:1263-1270, 2000.

37. Garg A, Grundy SM: Nicotinic acid as therapy for dyslipidemia in non-insulin-dependent diabetes mellitus, *J Am Med Assoc* 264:723-726, 1990.

38. Bernini F, Poli A, Paoletti R: Safety of HMG-CoA reductase inhibitors: focus on atorvastatin, *Cardiovasc Drugs Ther* 15:211-218, 2001.

39. Berg MJ, Rivey MP, Vern BA et al: Phenytoin and folic acid: individualized drug-drug interaction, *Ther Drug Monit* 5:395-399, 1983.

40. Rothman KJ, Moore LL, Singer MR et al: Teratogenicity of high vitamin A intake, *N Engl J Med* 333:1369-1373, 1995.

41. Kappus H, Diplock AT: Tolerance and safety of vitamin E: a toxicological position report, *Free Radic Biol Med* 13:55-74, 1992.

42. Buckley MS, Goff AD, Knapp WE: Fish oil interaction with warfarin, *Ann Pharmacother* 38:50-52, 2004.

CHAPTER 6

Energy Medicine

Acupuncture | May Loo

Aromatherapy | Maura A. Fitzgerald

Laser Therapy | David Rindge, Detlef Schikora, Gerhard Litscher

Magnet Therapy | Agatha P. Colbert, Deborah Risotti

Acupuncture

History

Acupuncture dates back at least 3000 years. Archeologists have uncovered acupuncture needles and divination bones with inscriptions of medical problems from the Shang Dynasty (c. 1000 BCE). The first century BCE saw the emergence of the most important Chinese medicine classic, the *Yellow Emperor's Inner Classic*, consisting of dialogues between the Yellow Emperor and learned men of his court. The first part, *Su Wen* or *Simple Questions*, discusses general theoretical questions such as physiology, pathology, and diagnoses, whereas the second part, *Ling Shu* or *Spiritual Axis*, focuses on clinical application of acupuncture. This is the oldest Chinese medicine textbook in existence and is still being referenced by today's practitioners. During the Han dynasty (206 BCE-220 CE), the basics tenets of Chinese medical theory and practice were formulated: the concepts of Yin and Yang, the five phases, channel/meridian theory, various needling methods, an herbal pharmacopeia, and a relatively sophisticated approach to therapy.[1]

In the 1700s, missionaries brought ideas of Western medicine to China and returned to Europe with stories of "miraculous healing" with needles. During the latter part of the Manchu Qing dynasty (1644-1911), acupuncture gradually deteriorated while Western medicine gradually flourished in China. In 1882 the Qing emperor banned the teaching of acupuncture in the Royal Medical Academy. Acupuncture resurfaced in the 1940s when Mao Tse-tung reinstituted Chinese folk medicine for the massive population. Thousands of practitioners were trained using *The Barefoot Doctor's Manual*.[2] In the 1950s, China added electrical stimulation to needles for stronger surgical analgesia.

During the early twentieth century, a French diplomat, Georges Soulie de Morant, learned Chinese language and medicine and translated Chinese classics into French, which began the spread of acupuncture to Europe. American interest in acupuncture did not begin until 1971, when James Reston, a *New York Times* reporter who accompanied President Richard Nixon to China, published a report about relief of his postoperative pain by three acupuncture needles.

For decades the medical community shunned acupuncture, subscribing to the conclusions from both the American Medical Association Council (1981) and the National Council Against Health Fraud (1991) that acupuncture had no scientific basis and was "quackery" or was "Oriental hypnosis." It was not uncommon for acupuncturists to be arrested and prosecuted for practicing acupuncture.[3] However, public enthusiasm continued to explode, and acupuncture became a household word in the United States. In 1972 the National Institutes of Health (NIH) funded the first research on acupuncture, which compared hypnosis and acupuncture and concluded that the two disciplines are neurophysiologically different and that acupuncture is not hypnosis.[4-7]

In 1976, California became the first state to license acupuncture as an independent healthcare profession. In 1996 the U.S. Food and Drug Administration (FDA) promoted acupuncture needles from the investigational and experimental medical device category to the regular medical-device category.

In 1997, an NIH consensus statement indicated that acupuncture has been found to have efficacy in adult postoperative and chemotherapy nausea and vomiting and in postoperative dental pain, as well as that acupuncture may be useful as an adjunct treatment in situations such as addiction, stroke rehabilitation, headache, menstrual cramps, tennis elbow, fibromyalgia, myofascial pain, osteoarthritis, low back pain, carpal tunnel syndrome, and asthma.[8] In 1998, an acupuncture board for certification was developed.[1]

Currently, the World Health Organization (WHO) outlines 40 conditions treatable by Chinese medicine and acupuncture: 4 upper respiratory tract disorders, 2 respiratory system disorders, 4 eye disorders, 3 mouth disorders, 12 gastrointestinal (GI) disorders, and 15 neurological and musculoskeletal disorders.[9] At this time, 40 states and the District of Columbia have certification regulations for acupuncture.[10] More than 11,000 acupuncturists practice in the United States, with approximately 3000 medical doctor acupuncturists. The American Association of Oriental Medicine recommends a mandated national standard acupuncture training curriculum of more than 1500 hours, whereas some medical doctor acupuncturists receive a few hundred hours of training, and still some evidence-based acupuncture techniques are taught to physicians in a single brief session.[1,11] The number of acupuncturists is growing rapidly and is projected to quadruple by 2015.[12]

History of Pediatric Acupuncture

Although pediatric treatments were mentioned in the *Nei Jing*,[13] children were generally considered as adults until the Han dynasty in the late third century, when medical textbooks began to include separate chapters on treatment of children. In twelfth century Song dynasty (1031-1113), the famous child specialist, Qian Yi, wrote the first pediatric textbook that recognized children as unique beings with distinctive physiology and pathophysiology of diseases that merit diagnoses and treatment different from adults.

During the Ming dynasty in the fourteeth to seventeenth centuries, pediatrics flourished with formulation of specific herbal and acupuncture protocols for children and introduction of preventive measures. In 1534, Wang Luan's comprehensive text *You Ke Lei Cui (A Collection of Pediatric Cases)* described the pulse, treatment principles, acupuncture protocols, and herbal formulas for individual pediatric diseases. The distinguished imperial physician, Xue Liang-Wu, wrote *Bao Ying Cuo Yao (Essentials for the Care & Protection of Infants)* in 1556, which stressed the importance of adjusting the dosage of herbal formulas for children according to their age and size. One of the most famous Ming dynasty pediatricians, Wan Mizhai, introduced preventive pediatric measures such as exposing children to sunlight and fresh air, protecting them from being frightened, and avoiding overfeeding them or giving them too much medication.

During the last dynasty, the Qing dynasty (1644-1911), many famous pediatric textbooks were written. Some are still used as references today: *You Ke Liang Fang (Fine Formulas in Pediatrics)* and *Dou Zhen Liang Fang (Fine Formulas for Poxes & Rashes)*. The twentieth century witnessed the publication of hundreds of pediatric textbooks and the establishment of pediatric departments in Traditional Chinese Medicine (TCM) hospitals. The current trend is toward Integration of TCM with biomedicine, merging ancient wisdom with modern technology for comprehensive medical care for children.[14]

Acupuncture Theory

Acupuncture is a complex paradigm with multiple theoretic approaches that include TCM acupuncture, medical acupuncture, microsystems such as hand or ear acupuncture, Five-Element acupuncture, myofascial-trigger point acupuncture, and Japanese meridian acupuncture, among others. This text will discuss in detail the two major schools of thought: the classical TCM "Qi" model and the modern medical acupuncture model supported by neurophysiological theories.

TCM acupuncture

TCM incorporates the naturalist philosophy of Taoism, which posits that man is a microcosm, nature is a macrocosm, and human health and illnesses follow the laws of nature. The basic principles in TCM consist of Qi, Yin-Yang opposites and the Five-Element relationship of organ systems.

The fundamental notion is the flow of Qi, a vital energy or vital force that has no English equivalent, which is the physiological basis of health and disease. It circulates unidirectionally in channels called *meridians* and is also part of blood and moves within blood vessels. It permeates organs and tissues, is behind all physiological processes, and is the defining component for all four levels of being: energetic, physical, emotional, and spiritual.

Qi is the universal energy that links humans to Nature, to all living things. The two sources for Qi are air and food. Health is the harmonious, uninterrupted flow of Qi, which follows the dynamic continuum of opposites of Yin and Yang and the natural cycles of the five phases, and disease ensues when Qi flow is disrupted.

The Yin Yang theory posits that everything in humans and in the Universe can be classified as Yin or Yang. Within the human body, the Yang components are Qi, physiologic fire (called *Yang*), and the Yang organs. The Yin components are Blood, Fluid, Essence, and the Yin organs. The many universal correspondences of Yin include woman, femininity, Earth, the moon, darkness, emotions, and rest; whereas Yang represents man, masculinity, heaven, the sun, light, intellect, and activity. The Yin Yang opposites are not absolute opposites, but are complementary opposites intertwined in a continuum of change, such that within Yin there is Yang, and within Yang there is Yin. Night merges into day that merges into night; within each person are both masculine and feminine qualities with varying degrees of expression. It is the dynamic balance between the opposites that keeps all of nature in equilibrium instead of chaos. Health is defined as the balance of Yin and Yang, and the various manifestations of diseases are excess and deficiency states of Yin and Yang.

The organs in the body are grouped as six Yin Yang couplets. The Yin organs carry out physiological processes of production and transformation of Qi, and the hollow Yang organs carry out the lesser functions of storage and of transportation of Qi.

Intrinsic to the Yin Yang dualism is the theory of the Five Phases (the Five Elements)—Water, Wood, Fire, Earth, and Metal—each with numerous physical correspondences such as voice, taste, and color preferences; emotional correspondences such as joy and sadness; and metaphorical universal correspondences such as seasons, climate, and direction.

Table 6-1 shows the most common correspondences of the Five Phases.

The Five Phases interact according to the natural laws governing nurturance and destruction; therefore the internal organs interrelate in a "holistic" and not segmental manner. Each human being, whether adult or child, is intimately related to everything in the universe, the macrocosm, and yet is unique within its own universe, the microcosm (Figure 6-1).

Evaluation and treatment of children must take into consideration pediatric physiology and pathophysiology. Children's physiology is characterized by (1) "Pure Yang"/maximum Yang, which means having the maximum potential for growth and development; (2) Young Yang and Young Yin, meaning that the child has immature physiology and a weak immune system such that blood and fluids can easily become out of balance; and (3) clear visceral Qi, meaning that the Qi within the organs and channels is pure and strong, uncontaminated by improper diet and emotions. Unfortunately, because of medications, improper diet, environmental toxins, and increasing emotional stress, the "visceral Qi" in the modern child is becoming less "clear," as evidenced by increased incidence in children of adult illnesses such as cardiovascular disease and type 2 diabetes.

Pediatric pathophysiology is characterized by the following:
1. Easy onset of childhood illnesses: Pathogenic influences can easily enter fragile and immature organs.
2. Rapid transformation: Disease processes can progress quickly in the immature, underdeveloped physiological state and can lead to exhaustion of both Yin and Yang.

✳ **TABLE 6-1**

Correspondences of the Five Elements

	FIRE	EARTH	METAL	WATER	WOOD
Yin organs	Heart/pericardium	Spleen	Lung	Kidney	Liver
Yang organs	Small Intestine Triple Energizer	Stomach	Large intestine	Bladder	Gallbladder
Sense organs	Tongue	Mouth	Nose	Ears	Eyes
Tissues	Vessels	Muscles	Skin	Bone	Tendons
Tastes	Bitter	Sweet	Pungent	Salty	Sour
Colors	Red	Yellow	White	Blue/black	Green
Sounds	Laughing	Singing	Crying	Groaning	Shouting
Odor	Scorched	Fragrant	Rotten	Putrid	Rancid
Emotions	Joy	Worry/Pensiveness	Grief/Sadness	Fear	Anger
Seasons	Summer	Late summer	Autumn	Winter	Spring
Environment	Heat	Dampness	Dryness	Cold	Wind
Direction	South	Center	West	North	East
Body types and personal characteristics	Pointed features, small hands, quick, energetic	Large features, strong legs, calm, generous	Triangular features, strong voice, meticulous, strong willed	Round features, strong digestion, loyal, enjoys movement	Tall, slender, strong bones and joints, hard worker

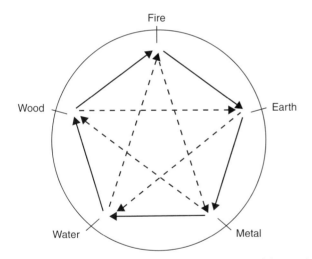

FIGURE 6-1 The Five Element cycle: the nurturing and destructive cycles combined. *From Loo M:* Pediatric acupuncture, *Edinburgh, 2002, Churchill Livingstone.*

3. Lingering pathogenic Qi: In TCM, even after symptoms of an illness resolve, pathogenic energy may still linger in the body, causing further injury to and transformation in the child. For example, persistent dry cough or recurrent sore throat with negative streptococcal cultures points to the energetic residuals of pathogens.
4. Rapid recovery: Fortunately, the majority of pediatric conditions are acute illnesses that tend to involve more superficial responses without complex organ or emotional involvement that, coupled with relatively clear visceral Qi, enable children to recuperate quickly.[14]

Treatment is directed toward elimination of pathogenic influences (e.g., heat, cold, dampness), restoring harmony of Qi, yin-yang, and the five elements in the organs. The classical theory in *Nei Jing* recognizes approximately 365 points located on 14 main meridians, or channels, that connect the body in a weblike interconnecting matrix.[15] These channels are not detectable by ordinary scientific methods.[15] Additional acupuncture points (both on and off the channel) have been added through the millennia, and the total universe of points has increased to at least 2000.[16] In practice, however, the repertoire of a typical acupuncturist may be only 100 to 150 points. (See Appendix B for general pediatric treatment protocols and acupuncture meridians.)

Five Element developmental theory

Loo has proposed an original theory of evaluating childhood development according to the Five Elements,[14] which integrates TCM with conventional developmental theories of Piaget and Freud, for the purpose of identifying vulnerable organs in different age groups, and the organ of origin of chronic illnesses.

Childhood can be divided approximately into four developmental stages that correlate with the Five Elements, with one element being predominant in each phase, and gradually transitions into the next Element in the Five Element cycle.
1. Infancy to early childhood: birth to 2-3 years
   Metal (mother of Water) transition into Water phase
2. Early childhood: 2-3 years to 6-7 years
   Water transition into Wood Phase
3. Young child to preteen: 6-7 years to 12 years
   Wood Phase, transition into Fire Phase
4. Teenage and early adulthood (early 20s)
   Fire Phase, transition into Earth Phase
5. Adulthood
   Earth Phase, transition into Metal Phase (Middle Age), Water Phase (Old Age)

Infancy to early childhood
Metal transition into Water phase. Infancy to early childhood is Piaget's sensorimotor phase of development,[117,118] when children perceive reality by what they can see, grab, touch, or put in their mouths. The mother is perceived as part of the self. Psychologically, Freud defines this stage as a closed monadic, psychological system—a symbiosis,[119] with the child's identity firmly attached to the mother. The child is in the oral phase of development, with the Id driven by instinct and impulses.[119] In Chinese medicine, this stage can be characterized metaphorically as the Metal transition to the Water phase of development. Birth marks the entry of the Corporeal Soul, which resides in the Lung—the Metal organ. Crying with tears and sadness corresponds to the Lung. The vulnerable organs during this phase are the Lung and Kidney, manifesting as frequent respiratory illnesses and sensitivity of the brain and nervous system to insults.

Early childhood
Water transition to Wood phase. Piaget's Preoperational or Preconcrete stage describes the child from approximately 2 to 6-7 years of age, embodying specific cognitive characteristics: egocentrism, illogical transformations, vivid imagination, and animism.[117,118,120] This description correlates to the Freudian anal stage, when basic psychological energy and libido begins to be invested in the anus.[121,122] Toilet training—the most important developmental milestone—can have psychological ramifications that can persist into adulthood.[119] The neo-Freudian Dr. Margaret Mahler characterizes the toddler as struggling with separation-individuation issues.[119] Much of this behavior can be explained by instinctual fear: fear of separation, fear of abandonment, fear of losing the mother's love. Fear is the underlying emotion of enuresis—persistent bedwetting when toilet training fails.

The preoperational child, like a seed and young sprout, metaphorically corresponds to many characteristics of both the Water and Wood Elements, with fear as the corresponding emotion of Kidney. The vulnerable organs in this Water to Wood phase are the Kidney and the Liver.

Early child to preteen
Wood phase, transition to fire. The early child to preteen is Piaget's operational child, who is capable of rationalization, of learning right from wrong, and of relating to the world on a more realistic level defined by time and space.[117,118,120] Psychologically, the Freudian Ego—the reality-oriented facet of the personality—matures.[117,119,122] The child has a sense of self-awareness, a separate physical identity from the mother and others so that he is now capable of describing himself or comparing himself to others. From the Five Element perspective, the operational child is a young tree, growing above the ground with a distinct physical identity. The tree is the Taoist symbol for man: rooted in Earth, reaching upward toward sky, coming into being between Heaven, the father, the Yang; and Earth, the mother, the Yin. The corresponding Wood organ is the Liver. The emotions associated with Liver are frustration, irritability, smoldering anger, and anxiety—the emotions of an impatient, operational child, of Ego. The Liver Yin houses Hun, the Ethereal (eternal) Soul, that influences thinking, reasoning, mental abilities, and emotions.[123]

Adolescence and early adulthood
Fire phase, transition into Earth phase. Adolescence and early adulthood is Piaget's stage for Formal operation, when the child progresses from linear to abstract thinking and can make plans for the future.[117,118,120] Psychologically, the child enters Freud's Genital phase of development, discovering his sexual identity.[122] Accompanying dramatic hormonal and bodily changes are drastic, with fearless behavior manifesting as driving recklessly and freely experimenting with sex, drugs, and alcohol. The Fire element predominates in this phase, with the Shen, the Spirit, and the Mind "housed" in the Heart, enabling the young adult to perceive the infinite, the eternal, and the universal. The predominant emotion is the "fiery passion" that can consume a teenager while he separates from both father and mother, following his own directions and at times scorching the Earth.

Adulthood
Earth phase, transition into Metal phase (middle age), Water phase (old age). Adulthood is the Earth phase, when the adult can become the nurturer. The middle years correspond to the Metal phase, while old age declines into the Water phase, and the life cycle begins again.

The Five Element Developmental Theory is also summarized in Table 6-2.

Application of the Five Element developmental approach. The importance of the Five Element developmental phase in chronic disorders is twofold: first, it identifies the vulnerable Element according to the age and development of the child; second, it provides a means to trace the Element associated with the *origin* of chronic illness. This is especially helpful in sorting out which Element to treat in complex disorders with multiple symptoms, such as attention deficit hyperactivity disorder.

The protocol for using the Five Element phases is as follows:
1. Identify and treat the vulnerable Element that corresponds to the phase of development (e.g., Wood in the school-aged child).
2. Identify and treat the *origin* of the disorder according to the developmental age of onset. For example, a child who develops asthma as an infant needs to have Water points treated along with Lung points, whereas a school-aged child needs to have Liver points treated along with Lung points (Liver-Lung in controlling cycle relationship).
3. Identify the corresponding Element during a time of trauma.
4. Preventive and well-child care can be carried out by prophylactically balancing the element of the next phase of development.

Medical acupuncture–neurophysiological theories

Medical acupuncture explains the effects of acupuncture in terms of complex and dynamic neurophysiological changes supported by evidence-based information. The most prominent theories revolve around acupuncture analgesia, acupuncture effect on inflammation, immunity, and blood flow; on the autonomic nervous system (ANS); and regional and functional specificity of acupoints. Acupuncture has also been found to affect emotions and may even affect health and diseases at the human genetic level.

✳ TABLE 6-2

Five Element Developmental Correspondences to Cognitive and Psychoemotional Phases

AGE	COGNITIVE	PSYCHOEMOTIONAL	FIVE ELEMENT DEVELOPMENTAL PHASE	VULNERABLE ORGANS	TAOIST CORRELATION
Birth to 2 years	Sensorimotor Object Permanence	Oral stage Symbiotic relation w/mother	Metal—Corporeal Soul: senses, limbs, movement, "Mother" of Water Water—beginning of life (seed) Strong attachment to Mother (Earth) = identity of one mother/child	**LU** **KI** SP	One
2 to 6 years	Preoperational—one-dimensional thinking Egocentric Illogical transformations Vivid imagination Animism	Anal stage Separation/individuation Id—instinctual, pleasure principle Fear: letting go, holding on	Water Child: distorted perception of reality; fear Water-Earth junction: to-and-fro, push-pull, letting go–holding on Identity of one (seedling still under water) = mother/child Water transition into Wood	**KI** **LR** LU SP	One begets
6 years to preteen	Concrete operational rationalization, two-dimensional, linear cause-effect thinking	Ego formation Reality principle Gradually more independent; needs guidance Still has strong identification with mother Looks to father for advice/guidance	Wood Child—Taoist tree symbolic of man: rooted in earth, reach upward toward sky Heaven and Earth = father/mother, right/wrong, Yin/Yang decision making Identity of two = mother/child, father Hun—Ethereal Soul, resides in Liver Yin Wood transition into Fire	**LR** HT SP	Two begets
Teenage to young adult	Formal operational abstract thinking	Genital phase, sexual identity Drastic changes: hormonal, physical, emotional Preference for peers Fearless, reckless, rebellious behavior Sexual identity; passion	Fire Child—coming into own identity Identity of three: father, mother, self Shen—Mind, through Ethereal Soul—perceives infinity Fiery passion Reckless sparks Rebellious—scorches earth, follows own direction Fire transition into Earth	**HT** SP LR	Three begets
Adult			Earth = center, mother = own nurturer and nurturer of others Identity = everything Transition into Metal = declining years Water = old age	**SP** **HT** LR KI, LU	Everything

From Loo M: *Pediatric acupuncture,* Edinburgh, 2002, Churchill-Livingstone.

General effects of acupuncture

De-Qi. De-Qi, the characteristic needle manipulation sensation of acupuncture, usually manifests as numbness, heaviness, distention, soreness, or a spreading sensation. It is traditionally considered to be the sine qua non of achieving clinical acupuncture therapeutic effect.[17] However, recent evidence indicates that even gentle, painless acupuncture without the De-Qi sensation also can be neurophysiologically effective, probably working through a local tissue healing effect and central antistress mechanisms.[18,19]

Acupuncture analgesia

Acupuncture has been most widely used for treatment of both acute and chronic pain, and voluminous research has demonstrated several neurophysiological mechanisms for induction of acupuncture analgesia.

Gate theory. The gate theory is one of the earliest explanations of acupuncture analgesia.[20,21] The nociceptive signal from the acupuncture needle is transmitted rapidly via small myelinated type II and III afferent nerve fibers, inhibiting or blocking (i.e., "closing the gate") pain signals that move more slowly along larger nerve fibers in the same segment of the spinal cord,[1,22] thus inhibiting the brainstem reticular formation from receiving the other pain signals.[22-25]

Biomechanics of acupuncture. The mechanical explanations of needle acupuncture analgesia suggest that needling produces minute tissue damage, resulting in changes in circulation or temperature or chemical effects.[1,26] Although the precise biomechanics of acupuncture action remain largely unknown, the local and distal responses can be explained by both ancient theory and modern scientific findings. Acupuncture effect may be carried out through counterirritation—an old medical art of causing local tissue irritation to trigger a local response that can be transmitted to a distal area.[27] A recent randomized controlled trial showed that De-Qi is a measurable biomechanical phenomenon in that the pullout force used to remove the needles was greater at acupuncture points than at control points.[28] The same researcher used B-scan ultrasonic imaging of 12 human subjects to show mechanical tissue displacement during acupuncture manipulation.[29] Furthermore, the De-Qi or "needle grasp" sensation is due to the winding of tissue around the needle during needle rotation; this needle manipulation transmits a mechanical signal to connective tissue cells via mechanotransduction, which explains mechanically the local, remote, and long-term effects of acupuncture.[30]

Acupuncture and central nervous system analgesia pathway. Functional magnetic resonance imaging (fMRI), which is sensitive to cerebral blood flow and cerebral oxygenation as indices of neuronal activity, and transcranial Doppler sonography and single photon emission computed tomography (SPECT) have been widely used to map the effect of acupuncture on the human brain.[17]

The analgesic impulses from acupuncture follow a specific pathway, continuing from the afferent spinal nerves to the brainstem (periaqueductal gray area), then along the descending antinociceptive system, including hypothalamic (arcuate) neurons, the nucleus accumbens, and the mesencephalon, to the dorsal horn of the spinal cord.[12,31] In addition, several areas of the limbic system have been found to participate in the nervous system circuit for acupuncture analgesia. Because it has long been hypothesized that limbic areas encode the affective-cognitive aspects of pain, the limbic system may be as important as the descending antinociceptive pathway for the central nervous system (CNS) mechanism of acupuncture analgesia.[12,17]

Acupuncture and neurotransmitters

Opiods. Currently, it is widely accepted that acupuncture acts as a neuromodulating input into the CNS that activates multiple analgesia systems and stimulates release of endogenous opioid neuropeptides, resulting in increased plasma and cerebrospinal fluid (CSF) levels of opioids.[17,27,32,33] The endogenous opioid peptides or endorphins are grouped into three classes: enkephalins, β-endorphins, and dynorphin. Antibody injection technique showed that enkephalins and β-endorphin are mediators for acupuncture analgesia in the brain, whereas dynorphins[1,34] are responsible for blocking incoming painful signals to the spinal cord.[35] Many studies have demonstrated support for the opioid theory. In one study, pain relief induced by electroacupuncture (EA) on ST36 and BL60 was diminished by microinjection of antiserum against β-endorphin.[7,36] Intrathecal instillation of antidynorphin and antienkephalin has also produced blockade of acupuncture analgesia.[35,37] In an animal study from China showing that acupuncture analgesia is transferable, the CSF from an acupuncture-treated rabbit was transferred to a nontreated rabbit, and the recipient rabbit demonstrated pain relief, thus giving further support to the idea that the analgesia is induced by neurochemical transmitters released from the CNS into the CSF.[38]

Other animal studies from China indicate that acupuncture stimulates nuclei accumbens, amygdala, habenula, and periaqueductal gray area, the strategic sites for endogenous opioids and for morphine analgesia.[39] Therefore acupuncture analgesia is mediated through a similar mechanism as morphine. One study demonstrated that EA on Zusanli ST36 and Sanyinjiao SP6 produced similar pain relief as morphine, as well as cross-tolerance between acupuncture and morphine.[1,40] Furthermore, acupuncture analgesia can be blocked by naloxone, a morphine antagonist.[1,31,40-43]

Other neurotransmitters. Acupuncture's numerous effects beyond pain control suggest that β-endorphin is not the only neuropeptide affected by acupuncture. Acupuncture needling also causes the pituitary to release adrenocorticotropic hormone (ACTH), a biological precursor to cortisol, such that blood cortisol levels increase with acupuncture treatment,[35,44] which explains the efficacy of acupuncture in treating arthritis and asthma.[1,45] Research has now demonstrated increased levels of vasoactive intestinal peptide (VIP), calcitonin gene-related peptide (CGRP), and neuropeptide Y (NPY) in saliva after acupuncture stimulation.[27] fMRI studies demonstrated that EA results in significantly increased concentrations in the rat brain (specifically, the occipital cortex and hippocampus) of NPY, neurokinin A, and substance P.[12,46] Acupuncture also affects catecholamines. In a study of both children and adults, serum and urine catecholamine metabolites were detected after acupuncture. The needling of Tai Chong LR3 alone showed a clear increase in indolamine metabolism.[47] Animal studies demonstrate that acupuncture leads to secretion of serotonin and norepinephrine.[48]

Effects on inflammation, immunity, and blood flow

Acupuncture has been found to activate the defense systems. It influences specific and nonspecific cellular and humoral immunities; activates cell proliferation, including blood, reticuloendothelial, and traumatized cells; and activates leukocytosis, microbicidal activity, antibodies, globulin, complement, and interferon. It modulates hypothalamic-pituitary control of the autonomic and neuro-endocrine systems, especially microcirculation, response of smooth and striated muscle, and local and general thermoregulation.[49]

Current research points to two possible mechanisms through which acupuncture exerts antiinflammatory effects: a decrease in vascular permeability and the modulation of proinflammatory neuropeptides. Initial inflammation is due to the deposition of immune complexes in tissues or vessel walls, leading to vascular permeability changes that result in edema and leukocyte extravasation. Acupuncture may inhibit early-phase vascular permeability, impair leukocyte adherence to vascular endothelium, and suppress exudative reaction equivalent to that of orally administered aspirin and indomethacin.[12,50]

Recent information demonstrates that acupuncture modulates mediators of inflammation via common pathways as analgesia[51]: the release of pituitary β-endorphin and ACTH.[52]

Acupuncture treatment has been demonstrated to stimulate humoral immune factors.[53-57] Clinical research has demonstrated that acupuncture decreases blood eosinophil and serum immunoglobulin (Ig) E in allergic conditions.[57] Animal studies demonstrated that when acupuncture points corresponding to human CV2 and HT8 were stimulated, an active humoral response ensued.[58] Acupuncture also significantly enhanced T-cell population and activities in both clinical and animal studies.[54,59-63] There can be an increase in lymphocyte proliferation,[63] in phagocytosis,[64,65] or in enhanced killer cell cytotoxicity.[66] There may be a close relationship between the Stomach meridian and mast cell population, because stimulation of many stomach points seem to result in an increase in mast cells.[67] An animal study using a point that corresponds to BL23, the human Kidney Shu point, demonstrated increased T-cell activities.[60] Acupuncture can improve immune function in trauma-induced immunosuppression.[63,68] Noninvasive laser acupuncture, which is well tolerated by children, was demonstrated to positively affect both humoral and cellular immunity.[54,69] Immune response may also be mediated via the ANS,[70] through the release of acetylcholine from the parasympathetic nerve endings, or through stimulation of the sympathetic nervous system,[71] resulting in activation of the release of helper T cells from the bone marrow.[72] In fact, stimulation of Kidney Shu point BL23 has been demonstrated to stimulate T cells.[60]

Although acupuncture stimulates immune response as a protective mechanism, it also appears to exert regulatory effect on hyperinflammation. Acupuncture seems to be able to modulate the synthesis and release of proinflammatory mediators through a common pathway that connects opioids and the immune system.[27,48,49,73,74] Acupuncture-released β-endorphin interacts with some cytokines by diminishing proinflammatory cytokines such as IL-1β and tumor necrosis factor (TNF)-α

and by increasing levels of antiinflammatory interleukins such as IL-e2, IL-2, IL-4, IL-6, and IL-10 levels and plasma IFN-γ.[27] Clinical findings of the antiinflammatory effect includes increasing IL-10 in allergic rhinitis and IL-2 in arthritis[35,36] and inhibiting the expression of proinflammatory cytokines IL-1β in ulcerative colitis.[27]

Acupuncture helps tissue healing by increasing blood flow centrally and peripherally, thereby carrying oxygen and nutrients to tissues.[75] Modern neuroimaging methods have shown that acupuncture increases cerebral blood flow and cerebral oxygen supply[24,76] and increases visceral and intestinal blood flow.[77] Unilateral needling of a single point, Hoku (LI4), immediately led to an increase in skin blood perfusion and to segmental temperature increases that decrease in a cranial-to-caudal direction.[76,77]

Acupuncture and Autonomic Nervous System

Acupuncture also induces ANS functions. β-Endorphin, in addition to its analgesic effect, is important in regulation of blood pressure and body temperature. Experimental and clinical evidence suggest that acupuncture may affect the sympathetic system via mechanisms at the hypothalamic and brainstem levels and that the hypothalamic β-endorphinergic system has inhibitory effects on the vasomotor center (VMC).[78,79]

Acupoint regional and functional specificity

Research has demonstrated that useful acupuncture points are mostly motor points or areas adjacent to nerve fibers and nerve roots.[1,7] Recent studies have demonstrated that acupoints can be linked to specific cerebral regions. One study using fMRI found that stimulation of a specific acupuncture point located on the lateral aspect of the foot, traditionally related to vision, activated an occipital lobe region that was the same area activated by stimulation of the eye using direct light. Stimulation of nearby sham points did not result in similar activation.[80] An fMRI study showed that stimulation of ST36/SP6 specifically activated the orbital frontal cortex and deactivated the hippocampus, whereas GB34/BL57 activated the dorsal thalamus and inhibited those of the primary motor area and premotor cortex.[81] Other studies show that specific acupuncture points, but not controls, activate structures of descending antinociceptive pathways and deactivate multiple limbic areas that participate in pain processing.[17,82] The neural activation also appears to be time dependent. An animal study using manganese-enhanced fMRI showed that EA on Zusanli (ST36) resulted in activation of the hippocampus, whereas stimulation on Yanglingquan (GB34) resulted in activation of the hypothalamus, insula, and motor cortex. Activation became less specific after 20 minutes.[83]

fMRI of nine healthy subjects during acupuncture stimulation of acupoints ST36 (on the leg) and LI4 (on the hand) resulted in bradycardia, activation of the hypothalamus and nucleus accumbens, and deactivation of the rostral part of the anterior cingulate cortex, amygdala formation, and hippocampal complex (i.e., it activates structures of descending antinociceptive pathway and deactivates multiple limbic areas subserving pain association).[17] EA stimulation of Zusanli ST36 resulted in increased activities in the nucleus raphe magnus (NRM). Studies show that NRM is an important position in EA analgesia.[84]

An fMRI animal study found EA on Hegu (LI4) increased activity in pain-modulation areas in the hypothalamus.[85] An fMRI study on Hegu (LI4) needling in normal subjects on either hand produced prominent decreases of fMRI signals in the nucleus accumbens, amygdala, hippocampus, parahippocampus, hypothalamus, ventral tegmental area, anterior cingulate gyrus (BA24), caudate, putamen, temporal pole, and insula, with increases primarily in the somatosensory cortex, suggesting that acupuncture exerts its complex multisystem effects through differential modulation of the activity of the limbic system and subcortical structures.[82]

A study of 15 healthy adults showed EA at real analgesic point Gallbladder 34 (Yanglinquan) resulted in significantly higher activation than sham EA over the hypothalamus and primary somatosensory-motor cortex, leading to the conclusion that the hypothalamus-limbic system was modulated by acupoints rather than at nonmeridian points.[86]

Manual acupuncture versus electroacupuncture. Since the introduction of EA, studies have found that analgesic effects of EA are greater and more effective than manual manipulation[7,87,88] and that manual acupuncture and EA appear to stimulate different CNS areas. An fMRI study of normal adults found that stimulation with EA at a frequency of 3 Hz on LI4, Hegu, produced fMRI signal increases in the precentral gyrus, postcentral gyrus/inferior parietal lobule, and putamen/insula, whereas manual needle manipulation of the same point produced prominent decreases of fMRI signals in the posterior cingulate, superior temporal gyrus, and putamen/insula.[89] EA also increases the tissue content of endorphins.[44] When EA was compared with transcutaneous nerve stimulation (TENS) without needles, the effects were similar, which suggests that needles are not necessary to produce an acupuncture effect.[1,87]

Frequency specificity of electroacupuncture. Further studies have shown that EA exerts frequency-specific effects on regions of the CNS, on the types of neuropeptides released, and on genetic expressions.

Low-frequency EA stimulates neurons of the arcuate nucleus of the hypothalamus (ARH) not found with high-frequency EA.[90] Low-frequency EA (e.g., 2 Hz) accelerates the release of enkephalin, endorphin, and endomorphin, whereas 100-Hz EA selectively increases the release of dynorphin. A combination of the two frequencies produces a simultaneous release of all four opioid peptides, resulting in a maximal therapeutic effect. This finding has been verified in animal studies[7,91] and in clinical studies of patients with various kinds of chronic pain, including low back pain and diabetic neuropathic pain.[92] Low-frequency EA resulted in a significant rise of CSF β-endorphin[93] and seems to be able to confer long-term pain relief.[94]

Acupuncture and emotions

For thousands of years, acupuncture has successfully treated emotional conditions based on the Five Elements' emotional correspondences to the organs and meridians. Current biomedicine hypothesizes functional impairment of the monoamine systems in CNS as the causative factor for the development of depression. Pharmacological manipulations of the monoaminergic neuronal system using tricyclics and monoamine oxidase inhibitors produced promising therapeutic effects as well as certain unwanted side effects, which urged the search of a physiological means to activate the central monoamine systems. Evidence from animal experiments show that acupuncture or EA is capable of accelerating the synthesis and release of serotonin (5-HT) and norepinephrine in the CNS. Clinical data indicate that EA is effective in treating depressive patients and is at least as effective as and has a higher therapeutic index than tricyclic amitriptyline.[95] Studies of acupuncture treatment of patients with chronic pain syndrome demonstrated improvement in both pain and psychiatric symptoms that correlated with higher plasma concentrations of plasma metenkephalin.[96]

Genetic effects of acupuncture

The variation in opioid release by acupuncture may occur at the genetic level,[1,12] as animal studies have demonstrated that 2-Hz EA induced a more extensive preproenkephalin (PPE) messenger ribonucleic acid (mRNA) expression than 100-Hz EA but had no effect on preprodynorphin (PPD) mRNA expression, which was significantly increased by 100-Hz EA stimulation.[97,98]

Pediatric Acupuncture: Evidence-Based Information

Numerous surveys show that, of all the CAM therapies, acupuncture has the largest body of literature and has the most credibility in the medical community.[12,99-101] During the past decade, there has been a worldwide increase of studies on acupuncture treatment of children. An entry of "acupuncture, children" on Medline resulted in 220 citations between 1995 and 2005 and 432 citations in the 35 years between 1960 and 1994. However, many are clinical reports or studies with poor methodologies that are not accepted by the medical community. The majority of the studies are conducted in China, and some are from Europe and the Middle East, with very few studies or reviews from the United States. Even randomized clinical trials (RCTs) are often considered inadequate because of insufficient sample size, poorly defined or imprecise outcome measures, vague enrollment criteria leading to heterogeneous study groups, and inadequate follow-up.

Acupuncture faces numerous specific research difficulties that include (1) blinding the acupuncturist; (2) sham versus control treatments; (3) assessment of placebo effects; (4) bias of the acupuncturist in expecting positive results; (5) variety of acupuncture modalities (e.g., EA versus manual acupuncture, laser, moxa); (6) correlation of uniform conventional diagnosis and treatment with varying TCM diagnoses and treatment (e.g., 100 patients with asthma may have numerous different TCM interpretations, necessitating individualized treatments); and (7) level of experience and competence of acupuncturists performing the studies. Despite these difficulties, there is still strong continual interest in acupuncture research, as acupuncture has measurable physiological effects that can be replicated clinically and in the laboratory. The multitude of research data presented in the previous section is applicable to adults and children. Most likely the coming years will witness increasing evidence-based support for acupuncture treatment of childhood illnesses. Currently available data will be presented with each condition.

Current Pediatric Use of Acupuncture

In China and in many Asian countries, acupuncture is used to treat an entire spectrum of childhood illnesses, ranging from mild respiratory ailment to neurological disorders such as seizures and autism to affective disorders. Acupuncture and TCM are often integrated into biomedical pediatric care. Pediatric acupuncture is slowly being introduced to Europe and the United States. The only mention in the current *Nelson Textbook of Pediatrics* is improvement of pain with acupuncture.[101a]

In 1998, Children's Hospital Boston established the first Center for Holistic Pediatric Education and Research (CHPER), a CAM multidisciplinary team that provides clinical services, education, and research. Acupuncture and massage therapies were incorporated into a clinical practice guideline.[102] Other university centers have gradually established pediatric integrative centers, although referrals to acupuncture may be tentative. One explanation for this hesitancy is the concern of pediatricians that children would not accept acupuncture. A recent study of 50 adolescents with chronic, severe pain indicated that the patients found needle acupuncture treatment to be pleasant and helpful.[103] Furthermore, with the increasing usage of non-needle, noninvasive acupuncture such as magnets and laser acupuncture, which are well accepted by even young children,[14] pediatric acupuncture can be widely applied to children of all ages with a wide range of conditions. Recent studies indicate that U.S. children have begun to seek acupuncture treatments for a broad spectrum of illnesses beyond pain and musculoskeletal disorders.[104]

Contraindications

Acupuncture is usually considered to be a reliable safe modality with few side effects when practiced by an experienced practitioner who follows strict hygiene precautions.[105,106] Mild side effects to needle acupuncture include pain during insertion or after withdrawal of the needle; minor bleedings or hematomas; and nausea. Syncope, or orthostatic dysregulation, occurs in about 1% of patients and can be prevented by treating the patient in a supine position, especially in the first treatment session.[107-109] Ear acupuncture with permanent needles can cause chondritis or perichondritis.[107] It has been estimated that 3% of the world population is infected with the hepatitis C virus.[110] Needle acupuncture with inadequate hygiene is a risk factor for the infrequent development of hepatitis.[107-109] Acupuncture can mask symptoms of cancer and tumor progression, so it is very important for the acupuncturist to have full knowledge of the clinical stage of the disease and the status of chemotherapy.[111] Pneumothorax, septicemia, and severe injuries of peripheral nerves and blood vessels are very rare.[107,109,112,113] Most serious adverse events caused by acupuncture reported in journals seem to be due to negligence.[114]

Contraindications for acupuncture include valvular heart disease (the potential for development of endocarditis), wound-healing disorders, immune deficiency (including patients on cytotoxic drugs), coagulation defects, an unstable spine, and lymphedema.[107,109,111] When treating an adolescent girl, it is important to make sure she is not pregnant. Although pregnant women frequently receive acupuncture in China, pregnancy is considered a contraindication in the Western world.[109]

Laser light should not be used on bony-growth endplates in growing children, fontanelles of infants, warts or any rapidly growing skin lesions such as cancerous growths, or the eyes because laser can cause retinal damage. Laser acupuncture should not be use in children taking cytotoxic drugs.[115]

There are several precautions with placement of magnets on acupoints. A child wearing magnets should not come into close contact with an adult with a pacemaker. It is also important to avoid magnet contact with credit cards and computers. When parents apply magnets for home treatments, it is very important that there be *no* possibility of accidental ingestion of magnets, which can result in intestinal fistula.[116]

Aromatherapy

Aromatherapy, as with many other CAM therapies, stems from ancient practices that are now being applied to modern circumstances. Aromatherapy refers to the use of plant extracts, known as *essential oils,* for their action on the body, mind, and spirit, and has been used in a wide range of situations including esthetics, cosmetics, spiritual practices, and healthcare (Table 6-3). The term *aromatherapy* was coined by Gattefosse, a French cosmetic chemist, because all the essential oils are volatile and therefore aromatic.[1] Although many people infer that smell or inhalation is the method of administration, essential oils are also delivered by topical application and oral ingestion. To separate the modern use of essential oil for therapeutic purposes from other uses, the terms *clinical aromatherapy, medical aromatherapy,* and *essential oil therapy* have been proposed.[2,3] Because aromatherapy involves the use of a plant product, others consider it to be a type of herbal medicine.[1] This discussion covers the history and current practices in the field of aromatherapy.

Historical Background

For thousands of years plants and their extracts, including essential oils, have been used in religious rites, perfumery, hygiene, and medicine. Historical records have established the use of essential oils from ancient civilizations through the Middle Ages to the modern era. There is evidence of the distillation of essential oils in Egyptian temples. Documents from ancient Greece, China, and India refer to medicinal uses of essential oils.[1,2] Records indicate that the twelfth-century Benedictine abbess Hildegard of Bingen used lavender essential oil, and European herbal texts from the sixteenth century refer to the use of essential oils.[1,4]

Modern aromatherapy developed with a focus on the treatment of wounds and infectious diseases. In the late 1800s it was noted that the incidence of tuberculosis was lower among the workers who processed plants in the flower-growing districts of France.[1] This led to investigation of the antimicrobial and wound-healing properties of essential oils in the late nineteenth and early twentieth centuries.[1,2,4,5] Gattefosse used

✳ TABLE 6-3

Essential Oils Commonly Used for Children

COMMON NAME	PLANT NAME	USES
Bergamot	*Citrus bergamia*	Sedative, mentally uplifting, and antiseptic. Used for relaxation. Bergamot may cause reaction with sun; use bergapten-free product.
Chamomile, Roman	*Chamaemelum nobile*	Sedative and antispasmodic. Children often do not like the smell. It can be blended with bergamot, lavender, or mandarin.
Eucalyptus	*Eucalyptus* sp.	There are many species of eucalyptus. Globulus (blue gum) and smithii (gully gum) have analgesic, antibacterial, and decongestant properties.
Frankincense	*Boswellia carteri*	Soothing and an expectorant. Used for respiratory conditions.
Geranium	*Pelargonium graveolens*	Balances the nervous system. Useful for skin conditions and has been used as an insecticide.
Ginger	*Zingiber officinalis*	Stimulant, digestive aid, and analgesic. Although peppermint and spearmint are more often chosen by children to use to control nausea, ginger is also useful.
Lavender	*Lavandula angustifolia*	Sedative, analgesic, and antiseptic. Lavender is considered to be one of the most useful essential oils. It is gentle with a pleasing smell and helpful in many situations.
Lemon	*Citrus limon*	Stimulating, alerting, and antiseptic. It is a pleasing scent to most children and can serve to decrease nausea.
Lemongrass	*Cymbopogon citratus*	Stimulating, alerting, and analgesic. Lemongrass feels warm when placed on the skin and is useful for musculoskeletal pain.
Mandarin	*Citrus reticulata*	Sedative, relaxing, and antiseptic properties. Improves digestion.
Marjoram, sweet	*Origanum majorana*	Analgesic, antiinflammatory, and balances the nervous system. Especially good topically for musculoskeletal pain.
Orange, sweet	*Citrus sinensis*	Relaxing, antispasmodic, and antiseptic. This is a pleasant and familiar smell that appeals to many children.
Peppermint	*Mentha piperita*	Stimulating and alerting, analgesic and digestive. It is often recommended for headache pain and nausea. Some texts suggest that it may be overstimulating in children younger than 7.
Rosemary	*Rosmarinus officinalis*	Stimulating and alerting, analgesic, and antiseptic. It often feels warms when placed on the skin and is good for musculoskeletal pain and tension headaches.
Rose otto	*Rosa damascena* *Rosa centifolia*	Antiseptic, antiinflammatory, and a hormone balancer. Rose is also thought to have spiritual qualities. In its pure form rose is often quite expensive.
Sandalwood	*Santalum album*	Sedative, antiseptic, expectorant, and decongestant. Its woody odor is sometimes more appealing to boys.
Tea tree	*Melaleuca alternifolia*	Antiseptic and stimulant. Its primary use is for prevention and treatment of infection. Because the smell is medicinal, it is often combined with other essential oils such as bergamot, lavender, lemon, or rosemary.
Spearmint	*Mentha spica*	Stimulating and digestive. Helpful for nausea, especially in younger children in whom peppermint might be too stimulating.
Thyme, sweet	*Thymus vulgaris*	Antiseptic, antispasmodic, expectorant, and stimulant. It is useful for respiratory infections. Some texts caution against its use in individuals with high blood pressure.
Ylang ylang	*Cananga odorata*	Sedative and soothing. it has a strong, sweet smell that is very appealing to some and overwhelming to others.

From Battaglia S: *The complete guide to aromatherapy*, Virginia, Queensland, Australia, 1995, The Perfect Potion; Keville K, Green M: *Aromatherapy: a complete guide to the healing art*, Berkeley, Calif, 1995, The Crossing Press; Price S, Parr PP: *Aromatherapy for babies and children*, San Francisco, 1996, Thorsons; Price S, Price L: *Aromatherapy for health professionals*, Edinburgh, 1995, Churchill Livingstone.

essential oils in the treatment of injured soldiers in World War I, and Dr. Jean Valnet used them in the French Indochina war (1948-1959).[1] The antimicrobial properties of essential oils continue to be a source of interest and are undergoing resurgence with the increase of antibiotic-resistant bacteria.[2] The clinical or medical use of aromatherapy was pioneered by Dr. Paul Belaiche, a professor of phytotherapy at the University of Paris Nord, leading to its use by conventionally trained physicians in France. Additionally, Henri Viaud, an essential oil distiller, established the first guidelines for purity, which also opened greater options for clinical use.[5]

The practice of aromatherapy in Europe and the United States varies. In France, aromatherapy developed as a part of accepted medical practice and is largely used within the context of general medicine and medical specialties. Medical professionals are trained in aromatherapy as part of their practice, and there is no separate aromatherapy profession. Oral use by prescription is common.[6] In the United Kingdom and other English-speaking countries including the United States, the practice of aromatherapy developed with a focus on external applications such as aromatherapy massage and inhalation techniques. Instead of treatment of specific disease processes, the primary concern has been on symptoms such as pain, nausea, and anxiety and general well-being. Although health professionals, primarily nurses, have incorporated aromatherapy into their practice, a separate profession of aromatherapists has developed.[6] In the United States, aromatherapy has expanded to include a variety of physical, emotional, and spiritual states.[7] The National Association for Holistic Aromatherapy (NAHA) is a U.S. organization that brings together individuals practicing aromatherapy by offering education and training and publishing the *Aromatherapy Journal*. International journals on aromatherapy include the *International Journal of Aromatherapy*, *Aromatherapy Today*, and the *International Journal of Clinical Aromatherapy*.

Theory

Essential oils are complex mixtures comprising more than 100 organic chemical compounds.[5,8] Most of these compounds are terpenes or phenylpropanes including alcohols, aldehydes, phenols, esters, and oxides.[2,4,5] Categories of essential oils share similar properties based on their chemical components. For example, essential oils higher in esters such as rosemary *(Rosmarinus officinalis)* or clary sage *(Salvia sclarea)* are antispasmodic and calming, whereas those higher in monoterpenic phenols and alcohols such as thyme *(Thymus vulgaris),* oregano *(Origanum vulgaris),* or geranium *(Pelargonium graveolens)* are antimicrobial.[2,5,6]

In plants, essential oils are chemical messengers that serve to both protect the plant and restore balance after injury. The various combinations of organic molecules that compose a single essential oil lead to unique traits (such as either attracting or repelling insects) that are needed for the plant in which they function. In clinical use, the essential oils have been found to have qualities that are useful for humans, including analgesic, antiseptic, sedative, alerting, antispasmodic, mucolytic, and insecticidal properties.[2-4] Because each essential oil is composed of a number of compounds in different proportions, a single essential oil may have a range of physiological effects. The alcohol portion of an essential oil is antiseptic, gentle to the skin, and calming, whereas the phenol can be a skin irritant, antibacterial, and mentally stimulating.[2] An example is the essential oil true lavender *(Lavandula angustifolia),* which is an analgesic, antibacterial, and antiinflammatory as well as a sedative.[4,9,10]

The plants from which essential oils are obtained are grown worldwide under a variety of conditions. There is always some variation in the chemical profile of an essential oil because of changes in climate, growing conditions, and the age of the plant when harvested.[8] There may also be a variation in chemical composition of a plant resulting in different wild strains known as *chemotypes*.[8,11] Chemotypes of some plants vary substantially in the chemical composition of the essential oil. A prominent example of this is rosemary *(Rosmarinus officinalis),*

of which there are three chemotypes. The borneol type, which contains a higher amount of camphor, is grown in Spain and the former Yugoslavia; the cineole type has a high cineole content and is grown in Africa; and the verbenone type is high in verbenone and is grown in France and Corsica (Schnaubelt). Another concern is adulteration of products due to inorganic fertilizers and pesticides; organic cultivation is recommended but not yet common.

A source of confusion to many users of aromatherapy is that a single common name may be applied to more than one plant type. For example, there are many types of eucalyptus, including globulus, radiata, and citridora, all of which have different profiles. True lavender *(Lavendula angustifolia)* may be confused with spike lavender *(Lavendula spica),* two very different essential oils. True lavender is used for calming and analgesia, whereas spike lavender is stimulating and used as an expectorant.

Once the plants have been harvested, the essential oil is extracted by means of steam distillation, expression, solvent extraction, or enfleurage (transfer of the essential oil from flower petals to fat). Of these methods, steam distillation is the most common overall, and expression is most commonly used to obtain essential oils from the peels of citrus fruit. When the essential oil has been extracted, quality-control testing is done by gas chromatography. The percentage of each constituent in the tested essential oil creates a chemical signature, which is then compared with a standard for that particular essential oil.[4,5,8] Each batch of essential oil should approximate the standard; however, a degree of variation is expected.

Essential oils can be applied topically, ingested, or inhaled. In the United States, most clinical aromatherapy is applied topically or inhaled. In many countries oral administration is limited to healthcare providers with prescribing authority.[2] When applied topically, the essential oil has a direct action at the site and is absorbed into the local tissue. When applied to wounds or infections, the essential oils exert surface antimicrobial effects. Because the essential oils are lipid soluble, they are readily absorbed through the skin, resulting in a deeper local effect (e.g., reduction of muscle spasm) and are absorbed into the bloodstream. At any given time, essential oil absorption will be affected by local and systemic circulation, condition of the skin, surface area of the application site, and application methods (e.g., use of massage or heat).[2,12] Because the skin of infants and young children is more permeable and more susceptible to irritation, dilution of topical essential oils to 0.05% to 1% is recommended.[12]

Inhaled essential oils have a direct action and are absorbed systemically. When inhaled, the essential oil exerts an action on the mucous membranes of the nasopharynx, trachea, and lungs, resulting in the opening of airways and nasal passageways, drainage of the sinuses, and an antimicrobial effect on mucous membranes. Additionally, CNS function is affected, which forms the primary bases for the use of essential oils for mental calming or stimulation. The exact mechanism for the CNS response is unclear, but two schools of thought exist.[8] The first is indirect: the essential oil molecules are thought to trigger the olfactory nerves, which in turn send chemical messages to the brain. The second is direct: the essential oil is absorbed into the bloodstream through the olfactory membranes. In either case, the primary action in the CNS is thought to be on the limbic system, where the essential oils exert an influence on the amygdala, hippocampus, thalamus, and hypothalmus, which are key structures in the modulation of emotion, arousal, and memory. Additionally, independent of the specific essential oil, smell evokes memories and associations. An individual's response to specific essential oils is often varied based on experience with or reaction to a specific smell. Because of the volatile nature of the essential oils, some element of inhalation is always present, even in topical application.

Measurement of the level of absorption of essential oils into the systemic circulation has been attempted, but true bioavailability is not known.[8] Analysis of the absorption of essential oils is complicated by the heterogeneous chemical structure, as each essential oil is composed of many compounds. Usually the analysis is done by choosing the two or three constituents that comprise the bulk of an essential oil. For example, in an analysis of the absorption of true lavender (*Lavandula angustafolia),* plasma concentrations of two components, linalool and linalyl, were measured (which together comprise 54% of lavender). After application to the skin in a 2% solution, blood samples were drawn at intervals up to 90 minutes. A peak level of 120 ng/mL for linalool and 90 ng/mL for linalyl was reached at 20 minutes. Neither component was detected at 90 minutes.[8] This analysis indicates that components of essential oils are absorbed systemically, at least in low levels.

Predicting the level of absorption for an individual essential oil is difficult. Individual characteristics (e.g. skin condition, circulation), size of the area of application, and the dilution of the essential oil are all factors. Additionally, the carrier oil in which the essential oil is diluted may affect the absorption rate. Finally, once the essential oil is absorbed, it may be affected by or may have an effect on other medications or herbal remedies, but little information on those potential interactions is available.

Evidence-Based Information

A substantial number of articles and books are devoted to the use of aromatherapy, but there is a lack of clinical trials in adults and still fewer in children. The effort to conduct aromatherapy research is growing but shares the same problems that plague other CAM studies: lack of funding, difficulty in developing a placebo, and difficulty in obtaining an adequate sample and in minimizing variables.[13] Additionally the variation in aromatherapy products, methods of administration, and dosing creates another level of complexity. The problems associated with aromatherapy research were demonstrated in a review of 12 aromatherapy research trials on reduction of anxiety.[14] Although all of the studies suggested positive effects, the sample sizes were small and aromatherapy interventions were sometimes mixed with a massage intervention. It was also difficult to compare the trials because of the variation in methodologies. Without a wide body of research data, aromatherapy is largely based on experiential and anecdotal evidence. This does not discount its use, but clearly more controlled studies are needed and would be of benefit in delineating those conditions for which aromatherapy is most beneficial.

Aromatherapy is recommended for many conditions owing to the large number of essential oils and the variety of properties attributed to each oil. These include promoting comfort and relieving pain, fostering relaxation and decreasing anxiety, improving mental function and alertness, managing symptoms such as nausea and insomnia, and treating infection and disease states. Aromatherapy is used to enhance wellness, as well as for chronic and palliative care. In order to describe which therapies are appropriate for treatment of specific medical conditions, a survey was conducted on professional organizations that represented a single CAM therapy. Ten aromatherapy professional organizations responded and rated the top five conditions most appropriate for aromatherapy as being anxiety/stress, musculoskeletal conditions, insomnia, headaches/migraine, and hormonal problems.[15]

Aromatherapy, either alone or coupled with massage, has been used for the management of many types of pain, including arthritis, headaches, and musculoskeletal pain.[2,15-17] When used for pain management, the essential oils are applied topically and those oils with either antispasmodic or rubefacient properties are considered the most effective agents. A rubefacient effect is one in which mild local skin irritation results in vasodilation; rubefacients often feel warm or tingly when placed on the skin. Essential oils that have this effect include rosemary (*Rosmarinus officinalis),* black pepper (*Piper nigrum),* and sweet marjoram (*Origanum majorana).* Other essential oils useful for pain management include peppermint (*Mentha piperita),* true lavender (*Lavandula angustifolia),* and Roman chamomile (*Chamaemelum nobile).*

Aromatherapy has long been used for its effect on mental and emotional states. Based on chemical composition and individual reaction, some essential oils are anxiolytic or sedating whereas others are mentally stimulating. When used for this purpose, the essential oil is administered by inhalation. This is achieved either by inhaling the essential oil from the bottle, placing a few drops on a tissue or cotton ball to allow passive vaporization, or mixing the oil in a solution and diffusing it with a spray bottle. Additionally, diffusion devices that aerosolize the essential oils with either heat or puffs of air may be used. A number of essential oils are described as having calming or sedative properties, including true lavender (*Lavandula angustifolia),* bergamot (*Citrus bergamia),* ylang-ylang (*Cananga odorata),* and sweet orange (*Citrus sinensis).* Essential oils that are alerting include peppermint (*Metha piperita),* lemon (*Citrus limon),* ginger (*Zingiber officinalis),* and basil (*Ocimum basilicum).*

Studies of aromatherapy are often conducted in settings in which it is difficult to control variables and in which more than one outcome is evaluated, such as the impact of an essential oil on pain, anxiety, and sleep. Many such studies have been carried out in adult cancer care and palliative or hospice care. In these settings the focus is primarily on comfort and symptom reduction, and results have been mixed. Ten studies of aromatherapy massage in cancer and palliative care were reviewed recently. The 10 studies were either RCTs, controlled before-and-after studies, or interrupted time-series studies that measured patient-reported levels of physical or psychological distress or quality of life.[18] The reviewers concluded that massage and aromatherapy confer short-term benefits on psychological and physical symptoms, but evidence is not clear whether the addition of aromatherapy offers an advantage over massage alone.

In a single study conducted on 103 adults in palliative care, a comparison was done between massage with and massage without the addition of Roman chamomile *(Chamaemelum nobile)* essential oil. Subjects were randomly assigned to either the massage alone or the aromatherapy massage group, and there was no blinding for the smell of the aromatherapy, nor was there a control group. Measures included a symptom checklist and an anxiety scale. Anxiety was reduced for both groups, but improvement of the symptom scores reached statistical significance for only the aromatherapy massage group.[19] Another study of 46 subjects at a palliative-care day center compared subjects receiving standard care with those who also received aromatherapy massage. Subjects rated mood, quality of life, and physical symptoms. The measures improved in both groups, with no statistical significance between groups.[20] Finally, 42 subjects in a hospice setting were enrolled in an RCT of the effects of massage and lavender essential oil on pain, depression, anxiety, quality of life, and sleep. Subjects were randomly assigned to one of three groups: massage, massage with lavender essential oil, and no intervention. There were no group differences for pain, anxiety, or quality of life. Sleep scores improved with both massage and aromatherapy massage, and depression scores improved with massage.[21]

Essential oils for the treatment of GI problems including functional dyspepsia, irritable bowel syndrome (IBS), and nausea have also been topics for research, including pediatric studies. Essential oil of peppermint is an important constituent of a number of OTC products for GI problems. Pittler and Ernst did a review and metaanalysis of eight randomized studies of the peppermint's effects on individuals with IBS.[22] They concluded that many studies had design issues and the results were mixed. Results were more favorable in a randomized, double-blind, control trial of 50 children older than 8 years. All subjects met the Manning or Rome criteria for IBS and received either peppermint oil in an enteric capsule or a placebo for a period of 2 weeks. The children receiving the peppermint showed significant improvement in severity of pain and no significant difference in other GI symptoms such as abdominal rumbling, distention, belching, or gas. No adverse drug reactions were reported. The investigators concluded that peppermint oil is useful for the treatment of IBS-related pain in children.[23]

Nausea is seen frequently in the clinical setting and is most often associated with recovery from surgery and anesthesia or is related to other medications such as analgesics or chemotherapy. Essential oils that have been described as helpful for the relief of nausea include peppermint *(Mentha piperita),* ginger *(Zingiber officinalis),* spearmint *(Mentha spicata),* and fennel *(Foeniculum vulgaris).*[1,2,5] In two studies of postoperative nausea in adults, the results were mixed. An RCT of 18 patients undergoing gynecological surgery were divided into three groups: control, placebo (peppermint essence), and experimental (peppermint essential oil). There was a statistically significant reduction in nausea in the group that received

peppermint essential oil; however, this study had a small sample size and the type of surgical procedure was not controlled.[24] Peppermint essential oil, isopropyl alcohol, and normal saline placebo were compared for their effects on 33 adults in a postanesthesia recovery unit. Subjects were randomized into intervention groups after they reported nausea. All subjects' nausea decreased, with no difference among groups. The authors postulated that controlled breathing patterns used with the administration of the intervention may have provided a beneficial effect on nausea that was greater that any effect from the essential oil.[25]

Current Pediatric Use

As the trend for increasing use of CAM continues, it would follow that the use of aromatherapy will also increase. The use of CAM therapies for children in general pediatric care as well as those with chronic conditions continues to rise. Recently, in three separate studies, the use of CAM for children was reported as 33% by parents in a primary care setting, 56% by parents of a child with cerebral palsy, and 32% by parents of children with cancer. Additionally, parents reported that they are more likely to use CAM for their children if they use it for themselves. Aromatherapy massage was one of the commonly used therapies for children with cancer, whereas massage without indication of aromatherapy was high for the other two groups.[26-28]

Although there is more clinical research on aromatherapy in adults, practitioners of aromatherapy have recommended essential oils for children for many years.[1,2,4] Authors of aromatherapy texts suggest lower doses for children and some restrict the use of specific oils, but generally aromatherapy is used across the lifespan.[30] Aromatherapy has been found to be useful for comfort and symptom reduction in chronic pain and in pediatric palliative care.[2,16,31] Essential oils considered to be particularly gentle and appropriate for young children are true lavender *(Lavandula angustifolia),* Roman chamomile *(Chamaemelum nobile),* neroli *(Citrus aurantium),* mandarin *(Citrus reticulata),* sandalwood *(Santalum album),* palmarosa *(Cymbopogon martinii),* geranium *(Pelargonium graveolens),* and sweet orange *(Citrus sinensis).*[1,31]

Contraindications and Safety

Although essential oils are generally considered to be relatively safe, a number of issues should be considered, especially when working with children. Allergic reactions and sensitivity are possible, skin reactions can occur, and accidental ingestion and poisoning is a concern. Potential interaction with medications are not well researched or understood but should be considered for children with chronic illness. As with many CAM therapies, there is the danger that parents assume the products are completely safe and therefore do not use reasonable discretion.

Safety data with essential oils is somewhat limited. Most of the testing has been on determining the LD_{50}, the point at which 50% of subjects die from either oral or dermal exposure. This is based on animal testing, largely rodents, who have different skin and internal characteristics than humans.[32] LD_{50} for most essential oils exceeds the quantity in a bottle of essential oil and is much higher than dosage recommendations. Essential oil safety can also be evaluated by studying case reports of poisoning in humans. Based on this data, most of the essential oils have been found to be safe in the small quantities (1 to 5 drops) in which they are usually suggested. However, aromatherapists will sometimes use novel essential oils. These are essential oils of new chemotypes for which there may not be a safety analysis.[11]

Severe reactions for some oils have been reported in both children and adults when larger quantities of essential oil were ingested, in some cases as little as 10 to 15 mL. There are many recorded cases of accidental poisoning in children, usually those between 1 and 3 years of age.[8] Key factors in childhood poisoning are: the curiosity of young children coupled with the alluring smell of some of the oils, caregivers not being fully aware of the danger posed by ingesting large quantities, and bottles that were not childproofed or did not have an internal dropper limiting the amount dispensed. Any essential oil in large quantities should be considered dangerous, and poison control should be contacted if ingestion occurs.

Safety precautions for children include:
1. Treat essential oils like a medication, and keep them out of the reach of young children.
2. Buy essential oils that have integral drop dispensers rather than open-mouth bottles.
3. Buy essential oils that are clearly labeled with all ingredients, including addition of carrier oils, and all essential oils (if blended).

Three types of cutaneous reactions may occur with essential oils: irritation, allergic reaction, and phototoxic reaction. Skin irritation occurs because some essential oils, especially those higher in aldehydes or phenols, are caustic and more likely to cause skin reactions or contact dermatitis.[4,8] Essential oils with higher risk include cinnamon (*Cinnamomum zeylanicum*), lemongrass (*Cymbopogon citratus*), oregano (*Origanum vulgare*), clove (*Eugenia caryophyllata*), and thyme (*Thymus vulgaris*), but skin irritation is possible with any essential oil.[4] The skin irritation is reduced and usually eliminated by diluting essential oils in carrier oil or lotion. Carrier oils are vegetable-based fatty oils such as grapeseed oil or sweet almond oil. For infants and young children, the dilution should be no greater than 2% and usually 0.5% to 1% is recommended. For adolescents and adults, the recommended range is a 2% to 5% solution (Table 6-4).

Any carrier oil can be used; however, other allergies should be considered (e.g., peanut oil should be avoided if a child is allergic to peanuts). If an irritation occurs, it should be treated by thoroughly washing the site with soapy water and applying a mild hydrocortisone ointment if redness persists.[8]

Allergic sensitivity is a greater concern. As with any allergic reaction, this is more likely to occur with multiple exposures but has been demonstrated on an initial exposure. Two cases of allergic sensitivities that developed over time were recently reported. In the first case, a student who was learning aromatherapy massage experienced swollen, tingling, and reddened hands, which progressed to tracheal edema and shortness of breath. She was treated with antihistamines and recovered. The second case involved a student who experienced lightheadedness, tachycardia, and nausea after inhaling an essential

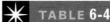

TABLE 6-4

Dilutions of Essential Oils

DROPS OF ESSENTIAL OIL PLACED IN 5 ML OF CARRIER OIL OR LOTION	AMOUNT OF CARRIER OIL OR LOTION	% SOLUTION
1 drop	5 mL	1%
2 drops		2%
3 drops		3%
4 drops		4%
5 drops		5%
1 drop	10 mL	0.05%
1 drop	20 mL	0.25%

Modified from Buckle J: *Monographs for clinical aromatherapy I*, Minneapolis, 2000, University of Minnesota Center for Spirituality and Healing.

oil. This student was removed from the source and monitored; no other treatment was necessary. The author notes that these are the only two cases that have occurred in this educational setting during a 10-year period.[34] A third type of skin reaction is phototoxicity. Some essential oils contain furanocoumarins, which, when placed on the skin, result in an increased sensitivity to ultraviolet light. Phototoxicity is a concern with essential oils of lemon (*Citrus limonum*), lime (*Citrus medica*), bitter orange, and bergamot (*Citrus bergamia*). Some preparations of bergamot will be marked "bergaptene free" or "FCF (furanocoumarin free)," indicating that the furanocoumarin has been removed.[8] This is especially important to consider when children are out in the sun, have skin tones that make them more prone to sunburn, and/or are taking medications that increase sensitivity to the sun.

A significant amount of anecdotal, and sometimes contradictory, information in the aromatherapy literature suggests that certain essential oils should not be used in particular disease states. For example, it is often suggested that essential oils of rosemary (*Rosmarinus officinalis*) or sage (*Salvia sclarea*) should not be used for patients with high blood pressure, or that fennel (*Foeniculum vulgaris*) should not be used in patients with epilepsy. Much of this seems to be based on toxic doses rather than the usual recommended dilution.[35] The relative safety of aromatherapy was highlighted in an 8-year observational study. In this study, 8058 women in a childbirth unit were offered aromatherapy by topical application or inhalation. Only 1% of this sample attributed side effects to the aromatherapy: nausea and vomiting was reported in 0.8% of cases, rash/itching in 0.2%, hay fever/watery eyes in 0.03%, and precipitous labor in 0.1%.[36]

The following steps are recommended to increase the safe use of essential oils: Limit oral use to medical providers who can prescribe. Topical and inhalation doses should be in the range of 1-5 drops. Essential oils for topical application should always be diluted in a carrier oil or lotion. When determining the dosage, the size and condition of the child should be considered: smaller doses should be given to small children and children who are medically fragile (e.g., those in palliative care).

If patients are seriously ill or taking a number of medications, it is prudent to begin with smaller doses. For patients with a higher index of suspicion for sensitivity, such as children with multiple allergies or taking multiple medications, practitioners should do a patch test before using an essential oil.[1,2] The patch test is as follows:

1. Dilute essential oil in carrier oil at double the dose desired.
2. Apply 2 drops to an adhesive bandage, and place bandage on the inner aspect of the arm for 24 hours.
3. At end of the time frame, observe for cutaneous reactions. Do not use if skin is reddened or raised.

Aromatherapy is a complementary and alternative therapy that has a long history of use for patients of all ages. Although the body of scientific evidence is still developing, it has been shown to be a relatively safe and gentle therapy appropriate for use with children. Aromatherapy can be especially useful for management of symptoms such as pain, nausea, stress-related anxiety, and insomnia. Additionally there is developing research and documentation for the use of aromatherapy in a number of other conditions, including abdominal pain and infectious disease. It is hoped that continued investigation will lead to a better understanding of the role of aromatherapy in pediatric care.

Laser Therapy

Laser Therapy* in Pediatrics

Laser acupuncture is emerging as a painless, effective treatment modality that is readily accepted by children. In this discussion, three contributors present background information on laser therapy: David Rindge on current U.S. applications using single laser probes, and Dr. D. Schikora and Dr. G. Litscher on the latest laser needle acupuncture treatment used in Europe and Asia.

History

The biostimulative properties of laser light at low intensities were first observed and described by Endre Mester in 1966 and 1967.[1] Perhaps because he published his findings in his native Hungarian in a regional medical journal, laser therapy spread rapidly throughout the former Soviet Union and China while remaining virtually unknown in the West.

By the early 1970s, laser therapy was well established throughout the Soviet bloc. There was great interest in the effects of therapeutic lasers and other energetic modalities, and Russian researchers developed techniques for intravenous blood irradiation and specialized apparatus to deliver laser energy for many applications.

Laser therapy was introduced to Western Europe on a large scale in the 1980s as inexpensive, solid-state diodes became available. It is now widely practiced throughout much of Europe and Asia both as a primary treatment and as an adjunct to other modalities. Although laser therapy's classification by the FDA as investigational has restricted its expansion in the United States, a growing number of devices are now being cleared for marketing, and clinical research and practitioner awareness are increasing rapidly.

Theory and current evidence-based information

(Also see the following section on laserneedle acupuncture.) Four effects are commonly cited in the literature, as follows:

1. Biostimulation/tissue regeneration
2. Reduction of inflammation
3. Analgesia
4. Virustatic/bacteriostatic

Laser therapy adds energy to living systems. Currently, understanding of this mechanism is limited. Photon absorption energizes mitochondria, stimulating the production of adenosine triphosphate (ATP), which then serves to fuel deoxyribonucleic acid (DNA), RNA, and protein synthesis within the cell. As a result, cellular respiration, metabolism, and reproduction are all accelerated.

At the tissue level, blood and lymphatic vessels dilate, increasing circulation and reducing edema. Over time, new blood and lymphatic vessels form. The inflammatory phase of healing is shortened significantly. The numbers of fibroblasts increase, and these cells step up their production of collagen, providing the means for accelerated structural repair. The activity of many other formative cells is enhanced. Laser therapy's positive effects to regenerate nerve, connective tissue, muscle, and bone are well documented.

There are many reasons for laser therapy's analgesic effects. Pain is relieved as fresh, oxygenated blood perfuses tissue to correct acidosis and ischemia. Improved lymphatic circulation reduces edema, taking pressure off nerves. Elevated endorphin levels, cell membrane hyperpolarization, and the complex electrolytic blockade of nerve fibers are other pain alleviating factors.[1-4]

Current pediatric use

Laser therapy is most commonly given in contact via a hand-held probe at visible, red to near infrared wavelengths.* It may be administered to areas of local pathology in contact with increasing pressure for deeper treatment. Laser therapy may also be given to acupuncture points, above organs, or by scanning over wounds and burns without contact and treating along their margins in contact.

The power of most lasers in clinical use varies between a few milliwatts and 500 milliwatts. The trend is toward higher power, and some devices with much greater output powers have recently been reported to be cleared for use in laser therapy.

Delivering a dosage within the therapeutic range at the target is the key to success. Too low a dosage will have no effect, and giving too much energy may be suppressive and cause discomfort. Although it is easy to measure the energy given at the skin, determining how much is actually delivered to a target deep within the body is impractical. Response to laser therapy is individual, and dosages should be adjusted according to the patient.

---

*Laser therapy is the most common term used to describe the therapeutic application of laser light at intensities below the threshold of thermal damage. Low-level laser therapy, low-intensity laser therapy, and laser photobiostimulation are other terms that have been used. The devices themselves have been called *therapeutic lasers, low-level lasers, soft lasers,* and *cold lasers.*

---

*Wavelengths between 630 and 1100 nm are referred to as the *optical window.* The longer the wavelength within these parameters, the greater the depth of penetration until water begins to absorb laser light at approximately 1100 nm.

In laser therapy the unit of dosage is joules, determined by the power of the laser (in watts) × the time (in seconds). However, to express dosage meaningfully, reference to the surface area treated must be included whenever possible. Dosage is calculated by:

$$\text{Dosage (joules/cm}^2) = \frac{\text{Power (watts)} \times \text{Time (seconds)}}{\text{Area (cm}^2)}$$

The main difference between the treatment of children and adults is that lower dosages should be administered to younger patients (Table 6-5). The recommendations in Table 6-5 are conservative in this writer's view, but they also provide a good starting place. Higher dosages may be necessary and very appropriate depending upon the patient's response as determined by a qualified and well-trained practitioner.

The library of related scientific literature now includes nearly 4000 titles, and conditions in which positive results have been reported include the following:

- Acne
- Allergic purpura
- Alopecia
- Arteriosclerosis/atherosclerosis
- Arthritis
- Back pain
- Carpal tunnel syndrome
- Cerebral palsy
- Dental applications
- Diabetes
- Fibromyalgia
- Headaches/migraines
- Hearing disorders
- Herpes
- Hypertension
- Hyperlipidemia
- Lymphedema
- Maxillofacial disorders
- Nerve regeneration
- Neuropathy
- Pain (musculoskeletal, myofascial, nerve)
- Pancreatobiliary disease
- Peyronie's disease
- Prostatitis
- Reflex sympathetic dystrophy
- Respiratory disorders (asthma, bronchitis, pleurisy, pneumonia, sinusitis, tuberculosis)
- Scars
- Skin disorders
- Sports injuries
- Tendonitis
- Tinnitus
- Wound healing

Many of these conditions are applicable for children, with treatment dosages adjusted for pediatric patients.

Treatment should always be explained to both the child and parent. Laser therapy should be performed only by qualified, licensed individuals and with informed parental consent. Good rapport between the practitioner and child will help to ensure cooperation and is likely to enhance clinical outcomes.

 TABLE 6-5

Dosage of Laser

AGE (YEARS)	MAXIMUM AT SKIN SURFACE	MAXIMUM AT MUCOUS MEMBRANES
3-6	3 J/cm^2	1 J/cm^2
6-9	6 J/cm^2	2 J/cm^2
9-14	9 J/cm^2	3 J/cm^2
>14	Treat as adults	Treat as adults

From Simunovic Z: Lasers in medicine and dentistry: basic science and up-to-date clinical application of low energy-level laser therapy (LLLT), London, 2000, Springer.

Intravenous laser blood irradiation is a highly specialized technique, and transcutaneous irradiation over blood or lymphatic vessels may also enhance systemic effects noninvasively.[1-4]

Contraindications*

Therapeutic lasers have an outstanding safety record. Unlike surgical lasers, which may operate at much higher powers and carry greater risks, laser therapy is almost always administered below the threshold of damage to tissue by heat. An adverse reaction has never been documented in more than 35 years of clinical and research use. Because it is painless, laser therapy is well accepted by children. The following contraindications apply:

1. *Laser should not be shone directly into the eyes.* This is particularly dangerous at near-infrared wavelengths, those most commonly used in laser therapy. As the beam is imperceptible, there will be no blink reflex, and the lens of the eye could potentially focus laser light to intensities damaging to the retina. Protecting vision is the primary safety consideration in laser therapy. Goggles may be important and knowledge more so. Measures to protect vision should be taken whenever one is administering laser therapy near the face and eyes.
2. *Laser should not be applied on malignancies.* Lasers have been found to stimulate cancer cell growth in vitro in studies. On the other hand, in other studies laser therapy appears to have shrunk small tumors in vivo. Laser therapy in cancer may be administered distally and for pain relief in terminal illness.
3. *Contraindications in photosensitive individuals:* Specific guidelines need to be established.[2]

Relative contraindications, precautions, and other considerations

Relative contraindications, precautions, and other considerations are as follows:

- Laser therapy should not be given over the fetus or uterus in pregnancy.
- Steroids have been found to diminish or even block the effects of laser therapy.

---

*These three absolute contraindications are those established by the North American Association for Laser Therapy.

- Pacemakers, metal implants, stitches, and plastics will be un-affected by laser therapy or other light therapy as long as it is given below the threshold of thermal damage.
- Treating over the thyroid gland is considered a relative contraindication by the North American Association for Laser Therapy, and high dosages should be avoided.
- Administering laser therapy over tattoos will usually cause localized heating and is not recommended.
- Treating over dark hair may cause localized heating, but this effect can usually be overcome by moving the laser more frequently to administer the total dosage in parts.
- A transient increase in pain may occur following laser treatment. This is more likely in chronic, longstanding conditions and is *not* an adverse reaction. In fact, this demonstrates that laser therapy is working. This pain will usually pass within 24 hours. Patients should always be advised of this possibility *before* treatment.
- At the other extreme, patients (particularly those with sport injuries or other acute trauma) may report complete relief of pain after the first laser treatment and may believe that the underlying causes have been addressed. These patients should always be advised in advance of treatment that it will be necessary to complete the recommended course of therapy and to refrain from stressful activity to the injured area.[2]

Laserneedle Acupuncture

History

The initial idea of laserneedles resulted from a critical analysis of laser acupuncture which developed and spread throughout Europe in the 1990s. With the existing handheld laser acupuncture devices, a simultaneous stimulation of indicated acupuncture point combinations is not possible. The points can be stimulated only one after the other (e.g., in a serial manner). However, this is not in accordance with traditional and fundamental principles of the Chinese acupuncture, which require a simultaneous stimulation of any given acupoint combination. Moreover, at present no significant evidence exists that the serial stimulation of acupoints by such handheld laser devices leads to any acupuncture-relevant physiological effects.

Laserneedle acupuncture was invented at the University of Paderborn[5] (Germany) and scientifically developed at the Medical University of Graz[6,14] (Austria).

Laserneedles are basically noninvasive medical devices. They do not puncture the skin. Laserneedles are placed on the skin above the acupuncture points. The laserneedles emit red laser radiation of 685-nm wavelength, which is supplied by an optical fiber cable. This principle allows stimulation of the acupuncture points simultaneously, as shown in Figure 6-2.

The activated laserneedle radiation cannot be felt by the patient and does not generate any micromorphological changes or damage in the skin tissue.[7] As shown in Figure 6-2, the laserneedles are fixed on the skin by means of a special taping technique. This allows the patient to move a little bit during the treatment without changing the positions of the laserneedles, a significant advantage in the treatment of children. Laserneedle acupuncture was successfully applied in many thousands of treatments of children during 2001 to 2005 in Europe and Asia. To date, no side effects have been reported. The intensity

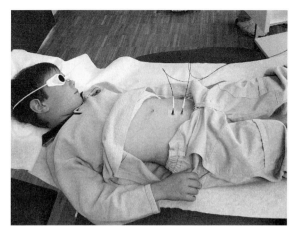

FIGURE 6-2 Acupuncture treatment of a 12-year-old child using laserneedles. *Courtesy Detlef Schikora.*

of the laserneedle radiation is optimized in such a way that a sufficiently high stimulus strength is generated at the acupuncture point, but a moderate radiation dosage is transferred into the body. Even babies can be treated with laserneedle acupuncture.

Theory and evidence-based information

Basically the laserneedle acupuncture can be performed in the same way as the classic metal needle acupuncture. The diagnostic principles of Chinese acupuncture, the selection rules of acupoints, and all the methodological experiences of the traditional metal needle acupuncture are preserved and can be fully applied to the laserneedle acupuncture.

Specific effects. When red laser light illuminates an acupuncture point, two different effects occur, which must be carefully distinguished. The first effect is the specific acupuncture effect. Owing to the interaction of photons with relevant nociceptive molecules, an action potential is generated by the light in peripheral, nociceptive nerves and transducted via the afferent paths of spinal cord to the brain. One of the first scientific evidences of this specific effect was published in 1985 by Walker and Akhanjee,[8] who showed that the illumination of the median nerve by red laser light of about 10-mW power evokes somatosensory potentials in the nerve fibers.

It should be pointed out that the insertion of a metal needle into the tissue at an acupuncture point also generates action potentials in peripheral nerve fibers, which are transducted to the brain.[9]

Acupuncture is basically a stimulation therapy. It is widely accepted that the therapeutic efficacy of classic needle acupuncture depends first of all on the stimulation strength. In particular in acupuncture analgesia the stimulation strength is a deciding parameter. De-Qi sensations, which obviously play a significant role in acupuncture analgesia, can be induced only by intense stimulation. The same arguments are valid for laser acupuncture. The stimulus strength of laser acupuncture depends on the power density of the light at the acupuncture point. One needs to distinguish carefully between the power density of the laser light and the light power of the laser source.

The stimulus strength of laser acupuncture does not depend on the power of the laser source. Rather, the power density of the light at the acupuncture point determines the stimulus strength. The *power density* is defined as the laser power per unit area and usually given in mW per cm². A variation of the power density of laserneedles results in a characteristic variation of specific physiological parameters that are relevant for the particular acupoint combination used. Figure 6-3 illustrates this dependency.

The blood flow velocity in the ophthalmic artery (OA) and its changes during stimulation of an eye-specific acupuncture scheme were studied in these experiments using a randomized, crossover study design,[10] showing that acupuncture of seven eye-specific acupoints leads to a significant increase in blood flow velocity in the OA. Metal needle acupuncture of the same scheme results also in a significant increase.

It is obvious that changes in the blood flow velocity depend on the optical power densities applied. From the experimental determined relationship between the power density and the blood flow in the ophthalmic artery, two conclusions can be made.

1. The dependence between the stimulus strength in laser acupuncture and the resulting specific physiological effects obviously follow the well-known dosage-effect relationship according to the Weber-Fechner rule.
2. The power density of any laser acupuncture device must exceed a critical "threshold" value to obtain an acupuncture-relevant physiological effect. In Figure 6-3 this critical "threshold" value is in the order of about 1 W/cm²; no acupuncture-relevant effects occur below this value.

A significant advantage of laser acupuncture compared to metal needle acupuncture is that the stimulus strength can be exactly quantified. Therefore scientific correlations become possible between the acupuncture stimulus strength and the resulting acupuncture efficacy. Because of this threshold characteristic, laser acupuncture cannot be reduced to dosage discussions only. The dosage as a parameter in laser acupuncture becomes relevant only when it has been proved that the critical "threshold" value of the power density of the light is exceeded at the acupuncture points. The average stimulus strength in laserneedle acupuncture is in the order of 5 W/cm², the dosage applied during a laserneedle acupuncture treatment of 20 minutes' duration is in the order of about 300 J. The energetic equivalent of 300 J is about 80 calories, which is less than a half-teaspoon of yogurt. The laserneedle treatments induce De-Qi sensations, indicating the analgetic efficacy of laserneedle acupuncture.

Nonspecific effects of laser acupuncture. In addition to the generation of action potentials in peripheral nerve fibers, the photons of the laser source interact with other cells and molecules of the human tissue. Three different effects result from this interaction, which occur independent of the localization and meaning of the acupuncture points and therefore are nonspecific in nature:

1. The increase of the adenosine diphosphate (ADP)-ATP conversion in mitochondria
2. The increase of the microcirculation of blood in peripheral vessels

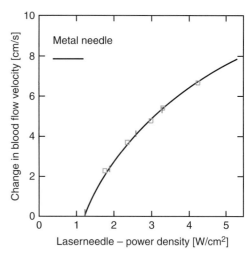

FIGURE 6-3 Alteration of the blood flow in the opthalmic artery is dependent on the power density during the laserneedle stimulation of a visual acupuncture scheme (Yan Dian, Zanzhu, Yuyao, E2, Liver and Eye point in the ear).

3. The increase of oxygen metabolism in the brain and in the tissue

Laser photons that are transferred into the organism adsorb at different molecules of the cell membranes and add energy to the living systems.

These processes are investigated in detail in particular for the mitochondria. The adsorption of a photon creates a proton gradient over the cell membrane, which enhances the phosphorization of the ADP. The production of ATP is increased, which then serves to fuel DNA, RNA, and protein synthesis within the cell. As a result, cellular respiration, metabolism, and reproduction are enhanced.

The Austrian group of researchers at the Medical University of Graz have investigated experimentally the influence of the laser radiation emitted by laserneedles on the microcirculation of blood in peripheral vessels using laser Doppler flowmetry technique.[11] This experiment revealed that the flux, which is the product of the mean flow velocity and the concentration of red blood cells, is significantly enhanced during the laserneedle exposure and increases in average by about 10%. These data are in agreement with the observations reported in literature about the efficacy of red laser radiation in reducing edema and inflammations.[12]

The illumination of acupuncture points and neighborhood tissue leads to significant changes in oxygen metabolism in the body. Cerebral near-infrared spectroscopy (NIRS) can show that oxygen metabolism in the brain is significantly increased during laserneedle acupuncture and metal needle acupuncture. Interestingly this effect is persistent even after the treatment ends.[13]

In conclusion, in addition to the direct stimulation of peripheral sensory nerve fibers at the acupoints, the laser photons also generate some positive accompanying effects in the surrounding tissue, blood vessels, and lymphatic system. These nonspecific effects have to be considered in laser acupuncture to explain the therapeutic efficacy of acupuncture treatments.

Current pediatric use

Laserneedle acupuncture has been well established in almost all European countries, in Asia, and in Middle Eastern countries for 4 years. A total of approximately 850,000 treatments have been performed, and no side effects have been reported to date.

In particular pediatricians use laserneedle acupuncture because it is a completely painfree treatment, it has outstanding therapeutic efficacy, and its scientific basis is well developed. The most frequently treated conditions are allergies, in particular allergic conjunctivitis and allergic rhinitis, asthmatic disorders, colic, headache, attention-deficit hyperactivity disorder (ADHD), childhood depressions, conjunctivitis, enuresis, pertussis, and pharyngitis.

Two conditions, colic and asthma, are discussed in this book. As mentioned previously, laser acupuncture can be used to stimulate acupoints used in any needle acupuncture protocol.

Contraindications

Contraindications include the following:

- Laserneedle acupuncture should not be used over the unclosed fontanelles of an infant or in children with immature fontanelles.
- Patients with head injuries, in particular involving an unclosed cranium, should not be treated with laser radiation.
- Direct illumination of the eyes must be avoided; therefore patients have to wear laser safety goggles during the laserneedle treatments.
- Laserneedle therapy should not be given to patients with known photosensitivity.

It has to be considered that the absorption relationships of the laser photons are strongly influenced by dark skin, dark hair, or artificially colored skin (tattoos), which reduce the penetration depth of the laser radiation and possibly the efficacy of the acupuncture treatment.

Summary

Laserneedle acupuncture is a new method that allows for the first time a simultaneous stimulation of any acupuncture point combination by laser light. Therefore laserneedle acupuncture is a painfree and robust method particularly suited for the treatment of children. The therapeutic efficacy of this method has been demonstrated in 850,000 treatments in Europe and Asia. Laserneedles emit red laser light of optimized dosage and stimulus strength. The activated laserneedles cannot be felt by the patients; therefore randomized, controlled, double-blind clinical acupuncture studies have been performed for the first time.[14]

Magnet Therapy

Historical Perspective

Magnetic products in the form of neck, shoulder, elbow, knee, and ankle wraps; shoe insoles; heel inserts; belts; headbands; mattress pads; pillows; and seat cushions are widely popular, commercially available, and not currently under FDA regulation. Therapeutic magnets have been used for more than 4000 years in China.[1] Although acupuncturists continue to apply magnets to acupuncture points either in conjunction with or as an alternative to needling, magnets are also being used increasingly by other CAM practitioners. Although this author could find only two specific references[2,3] describing the application of therapeutic magnets to children, magnets have historically been used to treat rheumatism, arthritic swelling of the limbs, bronchial asthma, paraplegia, deafness, and epilepsy,[4] conditions occurring in children as well as adults.

Although therapeutic magnets seem to have had continuous usage in China, practice in the Western world has been marked by what may be interpreted as a waxing and waning of interest characterized by an initial unsophisticated public acceptance, followed by medical disdain, investigation, and finally a failure to find objective evidence of efficacy.[5] Famous proponents of magnet therapy include Paracelsus (1493-1542), who investigated the effects of magnets on epilepsy, diarrhea, and hemorrhage; William Gilbert (1544-1603), who wrote the seminal book on magnetism and the use of therapeutic magnets; and Franz Anton Mesmer (1734-1815), who worked in the realm of neuropsychiatric diseases.[5]

In what appears to be a reaction to years of "heroic medicine" (bleeding, purging, blistering, and other aggressive treatments), Shealy[6] notes that the late nineteenth century witnessed a renewed interest in gentler alternatives such as homeopathy, naturopathy, and magnet therapy. As electrotherapeutics and radiology were developing into legitimate medical specialties, the marketplace was being flooded with untested devices that generated static magnetic fields (SMFs) and/or electromagnetic fields (EMFs). By the early twentieth century, although electrical cardioversion and electroconvulsive therapy were established treatments in mainstream medicine, the Flexner report of 1910 delayed further investigation of static magnetic therapies until the late twentieth century. A recent surge in the publication of scientific texts edited by biophysicists, physiologists, electrical engineers, bioengineers, and clinical researchers attests to a revived interest in researching the field of applied low-frequency EMFs and SMFs.[1,7-10] Additionally, rigorous clinical trials are now demonstrating a high margin of safety and some evidence of therapeutic effectiveness associated with the application of SMFs in specific clinical situations[3,11-29] (Tables 6-6 and 6-7).

SMFs versus EMFs

Electrical and magnetic fields are inextricably linked.[30] Electricity in motion produces a magnetic field, just as magnetism in motion produces an electrical field. If a wire is exposed to a magnetic field, a current is induced in the wire, and conversely a wire with an electrical current flowing through it becomes a magnet. SMFs are generated by permanent magnets, designated as such because they retain their magnetization once magnetized. Most permanent magnets available today are composed of aluminum, nickel, and cobalt (alnicos); iron (ferrites); or rare earth metals such as neodymium or samarium. Electromagnets, unlike permanent magnets, are easily demagnetized once the magnetizing field is removed. The two main distinguishing features of EMFs and SMFs are the maximum field strengths that can be built in each and their ability to be turned on and off. Electromagnets can generate magnetic fields up to 30,000 gauss (G) or 3 Tesla (T), such as in an MRI unit, whereas

Text continued on p. 95.

✳ TABLE **6-6**

Clinical Trials Using Permanent Magnets on Different Areas of the Body

REFERENCE	NUMBER OF SUBJECTS	DIAGNOSIS	RESEARCH DESIGN	MAGNET FIELD STRENGTH	POLARITY	EXPOSURE TIME AND APPLICATION	RESULTS
Hong et al.[11] (1982)	52	Neck and shoulder pain	Double blind	1300 G	Unspecified	24 h/day × 3 weeks; necklace	Both sham and real improved; no statistical difference between groups
Holcomb et al.[12] (1991)	54	Chronic knee or back pain	Randomized double-blind crossover	200 mT	Alternative neg/pos	24 hrs on back or knee	Statistically significant improvement in pain; no change in sedimentation rate
Segal et al.[13] (2001)	64	Knee pain; rheumatoid arthritis	Double blind	72 mT	Alternating neg/pos	Applied to 4 points around knee × 1 wk	Both real and control improved significantly from baseline; no significant difference between groups
Wolsko et al.[15] (2004)	29	Osteoarthritis of knee	Randomized double blind, placebo-controlled	Active magnet 40-850 G Placebo magnet <0.5 G	Checkerboard array sewn into latex knee sleeve	4 hr in monitored setting and self-treated for 6 hr/day × 6 weeks at home	Significant improvement at 4 hours in experimental group; improvement in both groups at 6 weeks; no significant difference between groups
Harlow et al.[66] (2004)	194	Osteoarthritis of hip or knee	Randomized, placebo-controlled	Standard magnet 1700-2000 G Weak magnet 210-300 G Nonmagnetic steel washer	Bipolar	Bracelet worn daily × 12 weeks	Mean pain score reduced more in standard magnet group than in sham control group; mean difference 1.3 points on WOMAC
Segal et al.[67] (1999)	18	Inflammatory arthritis with knee pain	Observational; no placebo	190 mT	Alternating neg/pos	Continuous × 1 week	Change in pain intensity from 24.1 to 14.7 points

WOMAC, Western Ontario and McMaster University osteoarthritis index.

TABLE 6-6—cont'd

Clinical Trials Using Permanent Magnets on Different Areas of the Body

REFERENCE	NUMBER OF SUBJECTS	DIAGNOSIS	RESEARCH DESIGN	MAGNET FIELD STRENGTH	POLARITY	EXPOSURE TIME AND APPLICATION	RESULTS
Holcomb et al.[3] (2000)	2	Chronic abdominal and low back pain in 2 pediatric patients	Case study reports	190 mT	Alternating neg/pos	Continuous × >1 year	Dramatic pain reduction with 10 minutes of application; complete relief after 1 year
Collacott et al.[31] (2000)	20	LBP with DJD HNP, radiculopathy, spinal stenosis, spondylolisthesis, S/P laminectomy, ankylosing spondylitis, fibromyalgia	Randomized, double-blind, placebo crossover	300 G	Alternating neg/pos	6 hr/day, 3 days/week × 1 week	No statistical difference between sham and real groups
Valbona et al.[16] (1997)	50	Postpolio pain syndrome	Double blind	300-500 G	Alternating neg/pos	45 minutes on trigger point	Significant improvement, 76% (real) versus 19% (sham)
Weintraub[19] (1999)	19	Foot pain, peripheral neuropathy	Randomized double placebo crossover	475 G	Alternating neg/pos	Insoles worn 24 hr/day × 4 mos.	90% of diabetics and 33% of nondiabetics improved
Weintraub et al.[18] (2003)	259	Diabetic neuropathy	Randomized, placebo controlled	450 G	Triangular array	Continuous × 4 months	Decreases in burning, numbness, tingling, and exercise-induced foot pain in third and fourth months
Caselli et al.[17] (1997)	34	Plantar heel pain syndrome	Randomized, placebo controlled	500 G	Alternating neg/pos	Daily × 4 wks; shoe insoles	Both real and sham improved, not statistically significant
Simoncini et al.[69] (2001)	20	Hallux pain after surgery	Randomized, double blind, placebo controlled	100-150 G	Not described	Inserted inside surgical dressing	Reduced edema, but no pain reduction at 2 days; reduction of pain but not edema at 1 and 2 months

LBP, Low back pain; *DJD*, degenerative joint disease; *HNP*, herniated nucleus pulposus; *S/P*, status post.

Continued

✳ **TABLE 6-6—cont'd**

Clinical Trials Using Permanent Magnets on Different Areas of the Body

REFERENCE	NUMBER OF SUBJECTS	DIAGNOSIS	RESEARCH DESIGN	MAGNET FIELD STRENGTH	POLARITY	EXPOSURE TIME AND APPLICATION	RESULTS
Winemiller et al.[71] (2003)	101	Plantar heel pain	Randomized, double blind, placebo controlled	192 G	Bipolar, multicircular array	4 hr/day x 4 days/week	Both real and sham improved significantly over 8 weeks; no difference between groups
Brown et al.[20] (2002)	132	Chronic pelvic pain	Double blind, placebo controlled	500 G	Bipolar	Two active abdominal trigger points × 4 or 6 weeks continuous	SMF improves disability and may improve pain when magnet worn × 4 weeks
Eccles[70] (2005)	17	Dysmenorrhea	Double blind	Active = 2000 G, placebo = 150 G	Unipolar	Applied over pelvis 2 days before menses; removed at end of menses	Significant reduction in pain in magnet group compared with placebo group
Carter et al.[72] (2002)	30	CTS	Double blind, placebo controlled	1000 G	Not specified	Carpal tunnel × 45 min	Significant pain reduction in both groups; no statistical difference between groups
Pope and McNally,[73] 2002	14	Wrist pain on typing	Randomized, double blind	2450 G	Unipolar	Magnetic wrist bracelet, 30-minute application	Significant improvement in both sham and active groups; no difference between groups
Colbert et al.[21] (1999)	25	Fibromyalgia	Randomized, double blind	100 G at magnet surface; 200-600 G to skin	Negative	Mattress pad nightly × 4 mos	Statistically significant improvement in pain, fatigue trigger points, and pain distribution drawings

SMF, Static magnetic field; *CTS,* carpal tunnel syndrome.

✳ TABLE 6-6—cont'd

Clinical Trials Using Permanent Magnets on Different Areas of the Body

REFERENCE	NUMBER OF SUBJECTS	DIAGNOSIS	RESEARCH DESIGN	MAGNET FIELD STRENGTH	POLARITY	EXPOSURE TIME AND APPLICATION	RESULTS
Alfano et al.[22] (2001)	119	Fibromyalgia	Double blind, placebo-driven	Mattress pad A: 3950 G (6-3 G to target tissue)	Negative	Matress pad nightly × 6 months	Statistically significant improvement in pain perception; no significant change in function or trigger point tenderness
				Mattress pad B: 750 G (33-9 G to target tissue)	Alternating neg/pos	Mattress pad nightly x 6 months	Symptoms improved in all measures, but no statistically significant difference between groups
Man et al.[23] (1999)	20	S/P liposuction	Prospective double blind	150-400 G	Negative	Postoperative × 14 days	Statistically significant improvement in pain, edema, and ecchymosis
Borsa et al.[78] (1998)	45	Induced muscle microinjury	Single blind, placebo controlled	700 G	Alternating neg/pos	Magnetic disk applied 24 hours after injury	No significant change in pain perception or dysfunction
Chaloupka et al.[79] (2002)	35	Strength improvement	Double-blind, randomized crossover	700 G	Not specified	FDP and FDS then FPB and opponens × 3 min	No increase in muscle strength with either intervention

neg/pos, Negative/positive; *FDS*, flexor digitorum superficialis; *FPB*, flexor pollicis brevis.

the highest magnetic fields produced by permanent magnets made from rare earth elements are in the order of 15,000 G or 0.15 T. For comparison, the earth's magnetic field is approximately 0.5 G (5 µT).

Discussion in this chapter will be limited to the therapeutic use of SMFs generated by permanent magnets. Interventions such as EMFs to enhance bone healing and transcranial repetitive stimulation to treat depression are established therapeutic modalities in the armamentarium of conventional orthopedists and neurologists respectively and are not generally considered part of CAM. Permanent magnets that generate SMFs, on the other hand, are ideally suited as a self-help modality and can be safely applied with minimal oversight from a CAM practitioner.

Dosing Regimens of SMFs

Just as the dosing regimen of a particular medication must be specified by the treating physician, the dosage of the SMF should be prescribed for individuals in accordance with the clinical condition being treated. Unfortunately, essential elements of the dosing are frequently unreported in clinical trials. Tables 6-6 and 6-7 point out the diversity of dosing regimens used with no justification for one set of parameters over another. Basic questions to be addressed when applying a SMF via a permanent magnet are: What tissue do you intend to treat? What field strength is produced by the magnet being used? To what depth does the SMF penetrate? What is an ideal duration and frequency of SMF application for the condition being treated?

✳ **TABLE 6-7**

Clinical Trials Using Permanent Magnets on Acupuncture Points

REFERENCE	NUMBER OF SUBJECTS	DIAGNOSIS	RESEARCH DESIGN	MAGNETIC FIELD STRENGTH	POLARITY	EXPOSURE TIME AND APPLICATION	RESULTS
Li et al.[25] (2003)	40 healthy subjects	Autonomic nervous system changes in heart rate variability and mental fatigue	Randomized, double blind	250 mT	Not specified	Acupuncture points GV 14 and MH 6; magnets on control non-acupoints 1.5 cm from real points	Significant differences in heart rate variability and symptoms of mental fatigue between groups
Liu Shaozing et al.[26] (1991)	206	Cisplatinum-induced nausea and vomiting	Clinical observations comparing 3 groups (magnetic, nonmagnetic disks, and point compression)	60 mT	Not specified	6-8 hours while receiving IV cisplatinum on acupoint PC 6	Effective in 89% with active magnet, 22% with sham, and 0% with point compression
Suen et al.[27] (2002)	60	Insomnia	Controlled prospective trial	6.8 mT	Negative	3 weeks on ear acupuncture points	Significant improvement in nocturnal sleep time and sleep efficiency
Colbert[28] (2000)	10	Depression	Case series	200 G	Alternating negative/positive, connected with ion-pumping cords	Sishencong and GV 20 acupoints × 20-40 min, 5-7 times/week × 6-8 weeks	Significant improvement in symptoms of depression in 7 patients
Chen[29] (2002)	1	Type 2 diabetes	N of 1 controlled trial; placebo disks used × 7 days; active disks used × 7 days	2500 G	Not specified	Auricular acupuncture points, right and left thalamus points, and left pancreas point	Fasting blood sugar decreased from 194 ± 15 mg/dL with placebo to 136 ± 10 mg/dL with magnetic disks; continued magnet wear × 5 years with continued normal fasting blood sugars and improved retinopathy

Targeted tissue

Musculoskeletal pain syndromes are the most common condition for which magnet therapy is used. A practical problem arising when treating patients with *chronic pain syndromes* is that the origin of the pain is often unknown. This results in a tendency to place the magnet "where it hurts" or over an area with demonstrated radiological abnormalities, neither of which may be the source of the patient's symptoms. Such a nonspecific approach is unlikely to result in therapeutic benefit, as was evidenced in one frequently quoted report.[31] The patient population treated by Collacott et al.[31] included patients with at least eight different medical diagnoses associated with low back pain. Despite the diversity of diagnoses and the lack of a specified targeted tissue, all patients were treated in exactly the same manner with the placement of a 300-G (surface field strength) alternating polarity magnet over the lumbosacral spine. The SMF generated by this particular permanent magnet penetrates to a maximum depth of approximately 1 cm. Consequently, if the source of pain was a deep structure such as a nerve root, a facet joint, a spinal ligament, or even a distant trigger point, the SMF generated by this magnet could not be expected to reach that tissue. On the other hand, when Vallbona's group[16] applied the same type of magnet to active trigger points (located in skin, muscle and superficial connective tissue) in patients with postpolio pain syndrome, the pain reduction in those treated with the real magnet versus those treated with a sham magnet was highly statistically significant.

Strength and depth of penetration of permanent magnets

Misleading information about gauss strength is sometimes given by manufacturers of magnetic products. Considerable discrepancies between the claimed field flux density (surface field strength) of particular commercially available magnets and actual gauss meter measurements have been reported.[32] The strength of an SMF is denoted in three ways: the manufacturer's gauss rating, the surface field strength (magnetic flux density), and the magnetic field delivered to the target tissue. The *manufacturer's gauss rating* is an indication of the field strength at the core of the magnet and is dependent on the intensity of the electrical current and the number of coils used when making the magnet. This gauss rating is sometimes quoted by distributors as the "strength" of a particular magnet, but such a description is incorrect and tells us nothing about the SMF at the surface of the magnet or the actual dose of SMF reaching the target tissue. *Surface field strength* or *flux density*, a more relevant gauge, is the strength of the SMF measured by a gauss meter at the surface of the magnet. Of primary importance, however, is the *magnetic field delivered to the target tissue*. The intensity of the SMF reaching the target tissue is generally an estimated value dependent on several factors including the surface field strength of the magnetic device, its size, its volume (bulky or flat) and weight, the directionality of poles, and, most important, its distance away from the target tissue. It should be remembered that it is not the magnet itself that is the therapeutic intervention, but rather the SMF generated from the magnet. SMF decreases exponentially with distance from the magnetic device. However, it should also be noted that unlike electrical fields, which are stopped at any surface, SMFs penetrate all biological tissue including bone, cartilage, muscle, nerve, fat, and other soft tissues almost equally.

The available literature suggests that when magnets of adequate surface field strength are applied over relevant trigger points or on appropriate acupuncture points in the correct dosing regimen,[2-4,16,20,26-28] a substantial therapeutic effect occurs. Because magnets placed on acupuncture points appear to have a more powerful effect than when placed on nonspecific body points, "overtreating" the patient is a very real possibility. The study by Carpenter et al.[33] highlights this potential complication. The acupuncture points used in this study, although

unnamed, are reportedly highly influential in the management of hot flashes. Magnets with a surface field strength of 2000 G were left in place on these clinically relevant acupuncture points for 72 hours. In women on whom active magnets were applied to these acupuncture points, hot flashes increased compared with those receiving the sham device. A less intensive dosing regimen composed of applying 800-G (surface field strength) magnets to *one* or *two* of the six acupuncture points (instead of all six treated in the acupuncture session) for 3-4 days would have been recommended by experienced magnet therapists.

Polarity of permanent magnets

Controversy and confusion abound in the magnet therapy literature with regard to descriptions and recommendations of polarity of applied SMFs. All magnets are by nature bipolar, having a north and a south pole, usually located on opposite sides of the magnet. SMFs are sometimes likened to electrical fields and described as having a positive (+) or negative (−) charge corresponding to their south and north poles, respectively. This concept is inaccurate. Gauss meters (devices used to measure the strength of a magnetic field) read negative or positive depending on the orientation of the measuring probe toward the surface of the magnet, not on the actual polarity of a particular side of the magnet. As the gauss meter probe turns 180 degrees, the negative reading will become positive and vice versa.

To add to this confusion, two contradictory conventions are used for naming *south* and *north* poles. The scientific/engineering community designates the south pole as the side of the magnet that rotates toward the geographical South Pole (south seeking) when the magnet is hung freely from a string. Practitioners of bioenergetic medicine, however, use a reverse notation, labeling that same pole *bionorth* (because it seeks the geographical South Pole) and call it negative (−). Although claims of differential therapeutic effects resulting from the application of a *bionorth* versus a *biosouth* pole are recounted in popular books on magnet therapy[34-37] and in acupuncture texts,[38,39] biophysicists assert that there is no scientific foundation for differing biochemical, physiological, or biological effects as a result of applying either the north, south, or both poles of a magnet to the body.

Clinicians, however, particularly acupuncturists, have repeatedly observed opposite therapeutic effects when different poles face the skin, maintaining that the side of the magnet that seeks the geographical South Pole (bionorth) has a sedating effect and that the opposite side of the magnet, called *biosouth*, has a stimulating effect.[34,35,37-39] Acupuncturists who wish to enhance energy flow in a particular meridian (i.e., to tonify the kidney meridian) might apply the bionorth side of the magnet to acupuncture point KD7 and the biosouth side of the magnet to KD10. On the other hand, if the acupuncturist is trying to alleviate an excess condition or sedate a meridian such the large intestine, he or she would place the magnets so as to reverse the meridians's energetic flow (e.g., bionorth on LI11 and biosouth on LI5). Ion pumping cords (described by Matsumoto and Euler[38]) may be attached to magnets in order to enhance a treatment effect and encourage energy flow in the desired direction. Specific treatment protocols using magnets and ion pumping cords are delineated in Section 2.

Practitioners further caution that the bionorth pole should be applied only when treating painful or "excess" conditions and the biosouth pole applied for conditions of "deficiency." Of clinical relevance is their strongly held contention that the biosouth pole should not be applied when treating areas with possible infection or tumor. To date, no RCTs have been reported in the peer-reviewed scientific literature that authenticate or negate these clinical testimonials. Nevertheless, based on the experience of respected acupuncturists, it seems prudent to refrain from applying the biosouth pole to areas of suspected infection or tumor.

Manufacturers of magnetic devices arrange the poles of the incorporated magnets in different configurations and classify them as unipolar, bipolar, multipolar, triangular, quadripolar, or concentric arrays. Strictly speaking, SMFs should be designated as "unidirectional" if the magnets are configured such that only one pole is identified on a single surface or "bidirectional" if the magnets are configured in such a way that the magnetic field on a single surface alternates between north and south polarities.

Concepts and Theories for Mechanism of Action of Magnetic Fields

Although it is somewhat frustrating and disappointing that a mechanism of action for SMFs has yet to be defined, consolation may be taken in the knowledge that a mechanism for general anesthesia, despite its practice for more than 150 years, also eludes scientific inquiry.

It is well known that living organisms produce subtle yet detectible EMFs.[40] These very weak fields emanate from all tissues in the human body and have been quantified by magnetoencephalograms,[41] magnetocardiograms,[42] and magneto-retinograms.[43] Evidence from preclinical studies supports the influence of SMFs at the biochemical[44] and neuronal levels.[45-47] Whole-organism studies have yielded mixed results. McLean et al.[48] found that an SMF modulated the severity of audiogenic seizures and the anticonvulsant effects of phenytoin in mice. Okano and Ohkubo[49] demonstrated a similar modulatory effect of SMF (1 mT × 30 minutes) on pharmacologically altered blood pressure in healthy rabbits. Morris and Skalek also found that that a SMF of 70 mT modulated microvascular tone depending on the initial diameter of the vessels.[50] However, other investigators[51,52] who tested magnetic device manufacturers' claims that SMFs elicit their effect through modifying blood flow found no evidence that the application of an SMF increased blood flow in the hand or forearm of healthy young subjects with normal unstressed circulations. Findings of modulatory physiological effects highlight the difficulties of demonstrating change in healthy subjects versus subjects in whom a physiological dysfunction needs to be corrected. If, as postulated, SMFs exert a regulatory effect on the organism's homeostatic processes, it is quite possible that the response elicited is bidirectional. For example, in healthy individuals with high-normal blood pressure, the effect may be a reduction in systolic blood pressure, whereas in healthy subjects with low-normal blood pressure, the effect may be just the opposite. This bidirectional effect is difficult to detect using standard statistical analyses.

Free radicals

A thought-provoking hypothesis to explain the interaction at the molecular level between SMFs and biological systems has been advanced by the late Ross Adey.[53] Paraphrasing his elegant logic and summary of the literature, he states that the collective evidence points to the cell membrane as the probable site of first tissue interactions with magnetic fields. The medium of *free radicals* offers an important possible explanation for biomolecular interactions with both static and oscillating magnetic fields. Chemical bonds are magnetic bonds, formed between adjacent atoms through paired electrons that have opposite spins and thus are magnetically attracted to each other. The breaking of chemical bonds is an essential step in virtually all chemical reactions, with each atomic partner reclaiming its electron and moving away as a free radical to seek another partner with an opposite electron spin. During the brief lifetime of a free radical (about a nanosecond or less) an applied magnetic field may delay the return to the singlet pair condition, thus influencing the amount of product of an ongoing chemical reaction. This model predicts a potentially enormous effect on chemical reactions for SMFs in the low millitesla range.

Adey further states that signaling from cell to cell occurs as biomolecules travel through the intercellular space (ICS), a network of narrow fluid channels, not more than 150 Å wide, to reach binding sites on the cell membrane receptors. These tiny low-impedance pathways or "gutters" are the preferred pathways for induced currents of intrinsic and environmental EMFs. Electrical impedance in the ICS is lower by 5 to 6 orders of magnitude than transmembrane impedances, as in conduction along nerves. The fact that electrical impedance at acupuncture points is reported to be significantly lower than in surrounding areas of skin[54-64] provides a theoretical explanation for a greater clinical response to SMFs when they are placed on acupuncture points.

Evidence-Based Information

Evidence-based medicine as used for making specific treatment decisions for an individual patient is hierarchically ordered.[65] The so-called N of 1 trials in which a single subject undergoes treatment with both an active and a placebo intervention, applied in a double-blinded fashion, in random order, ranks highest in this hierarchy for clinical decision making. Systematic reviews of RCTs are second in the hierarchical order, followed by single RCTs, systematic reviews of observational studies, single observational studies, physiological studies and finally unsystematic clinical observations including individual case studies and case series.

The available SMF literature, including an N of 1 study, observational studies, and RCTs, assessing the effectiveness of SMFs applied to body points and acupuncture points are summarized in Tables 6-6 and 6-7.

The single N of 1 trial describes a 78-year-old woman with a 13-year history of insulin-dependent type 2 diabetes mellitus, diabetic retinopathy, and open-angle glaucoma who underwent a 2-week trial in which placebo discs were placed on relevant ear acupuncture points for 7 days followed by placement of 2500-G (surface field strength) magnetic discs on the same acupuncture points for 7 days. Her fasting blood sugars were assessed during this 2-week period. The results were impressive, with the patient experiencing a significant drop in fasting blood sugar while wearing the active magnets compared with the week spent wearing the placebo discs. Over a 4.5-year follow-up, this patient's insulin dosage was decreased, fasting blood sugars remained in the range of 132 ±20 mg/dL, her diabetic retinopathy was inactive, and her intraocular pressure decreased from 25-27 mm Hg in 1996 to 15 mm Hg in 1997 without changing eyedrops.

Twenty clinical trials considered the effects of SMFs on painful conditions including neck and shoulder, low back, knee, heel, and foot pain; pelvic pain, dysmenorrheal pain; carpal tunnel syndrome; postpolio pain syndrome; and fibromyalgia (Table 6-5). Eight other studies assessed diverse conditions including wound healing after liposuction, insomnia, depression, tinnitus, hot flashes after breast cancer, effect on reducing mental fatigue from driving, effect on strength training, functional disability after an experimentally induced microinjury to the biceps brachii muscle, effect on blood flow, and effect on skin and intramuscular temperature. Eighteen of 28 reported trials* had positive outcomes. An inexplicable finding in seven of the "negative" trials was substantial improvement in both the sham and the experimental groups.[11,13,15,17,71-73] In only one trial were adverse effects noted.[33] In this study, alternating-polarity magnets were left in place on six highly influential acupuncture points for 72 hours with resultant worsening of hot flash symptoms in the experimental group of patients compared with the placebo group.

Two of the published studies describe the application of SMFs in pediatric patients.[2,3] Children with ascariasis who drank magnetized water and had magnets placed on relevant abdominal points showed a significant increase in expulsion of live worms and ova and improved subjective symptoms compared with both a piperazine-treated group and the placebo group.[2] In the second trial, Holcomb et al. treated one male patient and one female patient (ages 15 and 17) for chronic abdominal pain radiating to the genitals.[3] Both patients experienced substantial improvement when magnets were placed at sites along the thoracolumbar spine, thought to be the radicular source of the pain.

It is noteworthy that all studies, with the exception of one,[33] in which placement of magnets was on relevant trigger points or appropriate acupuncture points resulted in positive outcomes.†

Current Pediatric Use

Information about the incidence of magnet use in children is sparse. In a qualitative report on pediatric patients with chronic pain who received acupuncture, the authors state that magnets on acupoints constituted 26% of the non-needle acupuncture techniques utilized in their clinic.[74]

Although not specifically directed at pediatric patients, Hsu and Fong[4] provide specific magnet treatment recommendations

for conditions such as musculoskeletal pain, enuresis, diarrhea, insomnia, asthma, and skin lesions. This author, in collaboration with consultant Deborah Risotti, RN, has successfully used magnets on acupuncture points, with and without ion pumping cords, to treat a number of chronic conditions such as cerebral palsy and its associated symptoms (e.g., drooling, spasticity, gastroesophageal reflux, constipation, neurologic impairment), autism, ADHD, headache, warts, eczema, allergies, and asthma. Dr. Loo also discusses magnet use in her *Pediatric Acupuncture* book.[75]

Adverse Events

The most common adverse events associated with the use of topically applied magnets are itching and/or skin rash, which may be related to either the adhesive holding the magnets in place or the material of which magnets are made.[4] Few patients have reported feeling lightheaded.[4,28] Occasionally patients complain of nausea; have a weak, rapid pulse; or are tired or sleepy when the therapy is started.[4]

Contraindications

Reaction to the magnetic field itself precautions against use in gravely ill or weakened patients.[76] Of extreme importance is a cautionary note with regard to the maturity of the child treated. Serious problems have resulted when multiple magnets were swallowed.[77] Because of the propensity for magnets to attract each other, loops of bowel caught between two magnets have led to necrosis resulting in bowel obstruction. There are also reports of two magnets attracting each other and compressing intervening tissue such as the nasal septum or the penis, with detrimental effect.

Additional contraindications are pregnancy, because of possible unknown effects on the fetus, and lactating women. Magnets are not recommended for people using medical devices such as pacemakers, defibrillators, or insulin pumps because of the possible effect on electronic controls.[76] Precautions should also be taken not to place magnets close to credit cards, watches, or computers. Credit cards, ATM cards, and some drivers' licenses have strips of magnetic material that may become demagnetized when exposed to a strong magnet; conversely, these items may become magnetized with a stronger magnetic field and result in loss of readability.

Conclusion

SMFs as therapeutic modalities have a historical precedent of several thousand years. The scientific evidence base documenting successful outcomes when treating a wide variety of clinical disorders with SMFs is expanding at a rapid rate. The available literature, however, reveals an obvious need for establishing appropriate dosing regimens specific to the conditions being treated and a standardized method of reporting in order to replicate clinical trials. Bench scientists continue to study SMF effects at the molecular, cellular, and histological levels to define a mechanism of action.

Finally, from the available evidence it appears that the application of therapeutic magnets on acupuncture points, trigger points, or relevant areas of the body results in no serious adverse events and offers some promise of clinical benefit.

---

*References 3, 12, 16, 19-23, 25-29, 66-70.

†References 3, 16, 20, 25, 27-29, 67.

References

Acupuncture

1. Ulett GA, Han J, Han S: Traditional and evidence-based acupuncture: history, mechanisms, and present status, *South Med J* 91:1115-1120, 1998.
2. *Barefoot doctor's manual: the English translation of the official Chinese paramedical manual*, Philadelphia, 1977, Running Press, p 942.
3. State of California Department of Consumer Affairs Acupuncture Board: *History.* Available at www.acupuncture.ca.gov./about_us/history/htm. Accessed June 2004.
4. Parwatikar S, Brown M, Stern J et al: Acupuncture, hypnosis and experimental pain. I. Study with volunteers, *Acupunct Electrother Res Int J* 3:161-190, 1979.
5. Ulett G, Parwatikar S, Stern J et al: Acupuncture, hypnosis and experimental pain: II. Study with patients. Acupuncture and electrotherapeutics, *Res Int J* 3:191-201, 1979.
6. Ulett G: Acupuncture is not hypnosis, *Am J Acupunct* 11:5-13, 1983.
7. Ulett G, Han S, Han JS: Electroacupuncture: mechanisms and clinical application, *Biol Psychiatry* 44:129-138, 1998.
8. National Institutes of Health Consensus Development Conference Statement, *Acupuncture* November 1997.
9. Traditional Chinese Medicine and Acupuncture Health Information Organization: *Acupuncture research: World Health Organization.* Available at www.tcm.health-info.org/WHO-treatment-list.htm. Accessed June 2005.
10. National Institutes of Health: *NIH panel issues consensus statement on acupuncture.* Available at www.nih.gov/news/pr. Accessed June 2005.
11. Ulett G: *Beyond Yin and Yang: how acupuncture really works*, St Louis, 1992, Warren H Green.
12. Kaptchuk TJ: Acupuncture: theory, efficacy, and practice, *Ann Intern Med* 136:374-383, 2002.
13. Veith I translator: *Nei Jing (The Yellow Emperor's classic of internal medicine)*, Berkeley, Calif, 1949, University of California Press.
14. Loo M: *Pediatric acupuncture*, London, 2002, Elsevier.
15. Shang C: The past, present, and future of meridian system research. In Stux G, Hammerschlag R, editors: *Clinical acupuncture: scientific basis,* Berlin, 2001, Springer.
16. Huai LS, Broffman MD: *Acupuncture points: 2001—a comprehensive textbook*, Taipei, Taiwan, 1976, China Acupuncture and Moxibustion Supplies (Translated by SU Pei).
17. Wu MT, Hsieh JC, Xiong J et al: Central nervous pathway for acupuncture stimulation: localization of processing with functional MR imaging of the brain—preliminary experience, *Radiology* 212:133-141, 1999.
18. Carlsson C: Acupuncture mechanisms for clinically relevant long-term effects—reconsideration and a hypothesis, *Acupunct Med* 20:82-99, 2002.
19. Abad-Alegria F, Pomaron C. About the neurobiological foundations of the De-Qi—stimulus-response relation, *Am J Chin Med* 32:807-814, 2004.
20. Melzac R, Wall P: Pain mechanisms; a new theory, *Science* 150:971-973, 1965.
21. Ceniceros S, Brown GR: Acupuncture: a review of its history, theories, and indications, *South Med J* 91:1121-1125, 1998.
22. Melzack R: Myofascial trigger points: relation to acupuncture and mechanisms of pain, *Arch Phys Med Rehabil* 62:114-117, 1981.
23. Melzack R: Acupuncture and pain mechanisms [in German], *Anaesthesist* 25:204-207, 1976.
24. Jellinger KA: Principles and application of acupuncture in neurology [in German], *Wien Med Wochenschr* 150:278-285, 2000.
25. Man PL, Chen CH: Mechanism of acupunctural anesthesia. The two-gate control theory, *Dis Nerv Syst* 33:730-735, 1972.
26. Peng A, Greenfield WA: Precise scientific explanation of acupuncture mechanisms: are we on the threshold? (editorial review), *Acupunct Sci Int J* 1:28-29, 1990.
27. Bonta IL: Acupuncture beyond the endorphin concept? *Med Hypotheses* 58:221-224, 2002.
28. Langevin HM, Churchill DL, Fox JR et al: Biomechanical response to acupuncture needling in humans, *J Appl Physiol* 91:2471-2478, 2001.
29. Langevin HM, Konofagou EE, Badger GJ et al: Tissue displacements during acupuncture using ultrasound elastography techniques, *Ultrasound Med Biol* 3:1173-1183, 2004.
30. Langevin HM, Churchill DL, Cipolla MJ: Mechanical signaling through connective tissue: a mechanism for the therapeutic effect of acupuncture, *FASEB J* 15:2275-2282, 2001.
31. Pomeranz B, Stux G, editors: Scientific bases of acupuncture, New York, 1989, Springer-Verlag.
32. Hokfelt T: Neuropeptides in perspective: the last ten years, *Neuron* 7:867-879, 1991.
33. Cao X: Scientific bases of acupuncture analgesia, *Acupunct Electrother Res* 27:1-14, 2002.
34. Chen QS, Xie CW, Tang J et al: Effect of electroacupuncture on the content of immunoreactive beta endorphin in the rat's brain regions, *Kexue Tong* 28:312-319, 1983.
35. Ceniceros S, Brown GR: Acupuncture: a review of its history, theories, and indications, *South Med J* 91:1121-1125, 1998.
36. Xie GX, Han JS, Hollt V: Electroacupuncture analgesia blocked by microinjection of anti-beta-endorphin antiserum into periaqueductal gray of the rabbit, *Int J Neurosci* 18:287-291, 1983.
37. Han JS, Xie GX, Zhou ZF et al: Enkephalin and beta-endorphin as mediators of electro-acupuncture analgesia in rabbits: an antiserum microinjection study, *Adv Biochem Psychopharmacol* 33:369-377, 1982.
38. Research Group of Acupuncture Anesthesia, Peking Medical College: The effect of acupuncture on the human skin pain threshold, *Chin Med J* 3:151-157, 1973.
39. Zhou ZF, Du MY, Wu WY et al: Effect of intracerebral microinjection of naloxone on acupuncture and morphine analgesia in the rabbit, *Sci Sin* 24:1166-1178, 1981.
40. Han JS: *The neurochemical basis of pain relief by acupuncture. A collection of papers*, Beijing, 1987, Beijing Medical University Press.
41. Ulett GA, Han J, Han S: Traditional and evidence-based acupuncture: history, mechanisms, and present status, *South Med J* 91:1115-1120, 1998.
42. Cheng RS, Pomeranz BH: Electroacupuncture analgesia is mediated by stereospecific opiate receptors and is reversed by antagonists of type I receptors, *Life Sci* 26:631-638, 1980.
43. David J, Townsend S, Sathanathan R et al: Effect of acupuncture on patients with rheumatoid arthritis: a randomized placebo-controlled cross-over study, *Rheumatology (Oxford)* 38:864-869, 1999.
44. Chen XH, Han JS: All three types of opioid receptors in the spinal cord are important for 2/15 Hz electroacupuncture analgesia, *Eur J Pharmacol* 211:203-210, 1992.
45. Stux G, Pomeranz B: *Acupuncture: textbook and atlas*, Heidelberg, 1989, Springer-Verlag.
46. Bucinskaite V, Lundeberg T, Stenfors C et al: Effects of electroacupuncture and physical exercise on regional concentrations of neuropeptides in rat brain, *Brain Res* 666:128-132, 1994.

47. Riederer P, Tenk H, Werner H et al: Manipulation of neurotransmitters by acupuncture? (A preliminary communication), *J Neural Transm* 37:81-94, 1975.

48. Han JS, Terenius L: Neurochemical basis of acupuncture analgesia, *Annu Rev Pharmacol Toxicol* 22:193-220, 1982.

49. Rogers PA, Schoen AM, Limehouse J: Acupuncture for immune-mediated disorders. Literature review and clinical applications, *Probl Vet Med* 4:162-193, 1992.

50. Sun YM: Acupuncture and inflammation, *Int J Chin Med* 1:15-20, 1984.

51. Gollub RL, Hui KK, Stefano GB: Acupuncture: pain management coupled to immune stimulation, *Zhongguo Yao Li Xue Bao* 20:769-777, 1999.

52. Samuels N: Acupuncture for cancer patients: why not? [in Hebrew] *Harefuah* 141:608-610, 666, 2002.

53. Sato T, Yu Y, Guo SY et al: Acupuncture stimulation enhances splenic natural killer cell cytotoxicity in rats, *Jpn J Physiol* 46:131-136, 1996.

54. Dong L, Yuan D, Fan L et al: Effect of HE-NE laser acupuncture on the spleen in rats [in Chinese], *Zhen Ci Yan Jiu* 21:64-67, 1996.

55. Ketiladze ES, Krylov VF, Ershov FI et al: Interferon and other immunological indices of influenza patients undergoing different methods of treatment [in Russian], *Vopr Virusol* 32:35-39, 1987.

56. Liu WG, Zhao JC: Relationship between acupuncture-induced immunity and the regulation of central neurotransmitters in the rabbit: VI. The influence of NDR stimulation on acupuncture regulation of immune function in rabbit, *Acu Electrother Res* 14:197-203, 1989.

57. Lau BH, Wong DS, Slater JM: Effect of acupuncture on allergic rhinitis: clinical and laboratory evaluations, *Am J Chin Med* 3:263-270, 1975.

58. Sakic B, Kojic L, Jankovic BD et al: Electro-acupuncture modifies humoral immune response in the rat, *Acu Electrother Res* 14:115-120, 1989.

59. Joos S, Schott C, Zou H et al: Immunomodulatory effects of acupuncture in the treatment of allergic asthma: a randomized controlled study, *J Altern Complement Med* 6:519-525, 2000.

60. Okumura M, Toriizuka K, Iijima K et al: Effects of acupuncture on peripheral T lymphocyte subpopulation and amounts of cerebral catecholamines in mice, *Acu Electrother Res* 24:127-139, 1999.

61. Liu X, Sun L, Xiao J et al: Effect of acupuncture and point-injection treatment on immunologic function in rheumatoid arthritis, *J Trad Chin Med* 13:174-178, 1993.

62. Zhai D, Din B, Liu R et al: Regulation on ACTH, beta-EP and immune function by moxibustion on different acupoints [in Chinese], *Zhen Ci Yan Jiu* 21:77-81, 1996.

63. Du L, Jiang J, Cao X: Time course of the effect of electroacupuncture on immunomodulation of normal rat [in Chinese], *Zhen Ci Yan Jiu* 20:36-39, 1995.

64. Zhao R, Ma C, Tan L et al: The effect of acupuncture on the function of macrophages in rats of immunodepression [in Chinese], *Zhen Ci Yan Jiu* 19:66-68, 1994.

65. Petti F, Bangrazi A, Liguori A et al: Effects of acupuncture on immune response related to opioid-like peptides, *J Trad Chin Med* 18:55-63, 1998.

66. Yu Y, Kasahara T, Sato T et al: Enhancement of splenic interferon-gamma, interleukin-2, and NK cytotoxicity by S36 acupoint acupuncture in F344 rats, *Jpn J Physiol* 47:173-178, 1997.

67. Deng Y, Zeng T, Zhou Y et al: The influence of electroacupuncture on the mast cells in the acupoints of the stomach meridian [in Chinese], *Zhen Ci Yan Jiu* 21:68-70, 1996.

68. Cheng XD, Wu GC, He QZ et al: Effect of continued electroacupuncture on induction of interleukin-2 production of spleen lymphocytes from the injured rats, *Acu Electrother Res* 22:1-8, 1997.

69. Yuan D, Fu Z, Li S: Effect of He-Ne laser acupuncture on lymphnodes in rats [in Chinese], *Zhen Ci Yan Jiu* 17:54-58, 1992.

70. Lundeberg T, Eriksson SV, Theodorsson E: Neuroimmunomodulatory effects of acupuncture in mice, *Neurosci Lett* 128:161-164, 1991.

71. Zhao J: The effects of C-fibers of primary afferent on immune responses regulated by EA in mice [in Chinese], *Zhen Ci Yan Jiu* 21:36-41, 1996.

72. Fujiwara R, Tong ZG, Matsuoka H et al: Effects of acupuncture on immune response in mice, *Int J Neurosci* 57:141-150, 1991.

73. Ma Z, Wang Y, Fan Q: The influence of acupuncture on interleukin 2 interferon-natural killer cell regulatory network of kidney-deficiency mice [in Chinese], *Zhen Ci Yan Jiu* 17:139-142, 1992.

74. Yan WX, Wang JH, Chang QQ: Effect of leu-enkephalin in striatum on modulating cellular immune during electropuncture [in Chinese], *Sheng Li Xue Bao* 43:451-456, 1991.

75. Liu Q: Effects of acupuncture on hemorrheology, blood lipid content and nail fold microcirculation in multiple infarct dementia patients, *J Trad Chinese Med* 24:219-223, 2004.

76. Litscher G: Cerebral and peripheral effects of laser needle-stimulation, *Neurol Res* 25:722-728, 2003.

77. Zijlstra FJ, van den Berg-de Lange I, Huygen FJ et al: Anti-inflammatory actions of acupuncture, *Mediators Inflamm* 12:59-69, 2003.

78. Kuo TC, Lin CW, Ho FM: The soreness and numbness effect of acupuncture on skin blood flow, *Am J Chin Med* 32:117-129, 2004.

79. Andersson S, Lundeberg T: Acupuncture—from empiricism to science: functional background to acupuncture effects in pain and disease, *Med Hypotheses* 45:271-281, 1995.

80. Cho ZH, Chung SC, Jones JP et al: New findings of the correlation between acupoints and corresponding brain cortices using functional MRI, *Proc Natl Acad Sci U S A* 95:2670-2673, 1998.

81. Zhang WT, Jin Z, Luo F et al: Evidence from brain imaging with fMRI supporting functional specificity of acupoints in humans, *Neurosci Lett* 354:50-53, 2004.

82. Hui KK, Liu J, Makris N et al: Acupuncture modulates the limbic system and subcortical gray structures of the human brain: evidence from fMRI studies in normal subjects, *Hum Brain Mapp* 9:13-25, 2000.

83. Chiu JH, Cheng HC, Tai CH et al: Electroacupuncture-induced neural activation detected by use of manganese-enhanced functional magnetic resonance imaging in rabbits, *Am J Vet Res* 62:178-182, 2001.

84. Fan T, Li J, Kong T: Relationship between acupuncture analgesia and neurotransmitters in nucleus raphe magnus [in Chinese], *Zhen Ci Yan Jiu* 18:168-171, 1993.

85. Chiu JH, Chung MS, Cheng HC et al: Different central manifestations in response to electroacupuncture at analgesic and non-analgesic acupoints in rats: a manganese-enhanced functional magnetic resonance imaging study, *Can J Vet Res* 67:94-101, 2003.

86. Wu MT, Sheen JM, Chuang KH et al: Neuronal specificity of acupuncture response: a fMRI study with electroacupuncture, *Neuroimage* 16:1028-1037, 2002.

87. Wang J, Mao L, Han JS: Antinociceptive effects induced by electroacupuncture and transcutaneous electrical nerve stimulation in the rat, *Int J Neurosci* 65:117-129, 1992.

88. Saletu B, Saletu M, Brown M et al: Hypnosis and acupuncture analgesia: a neurophysiological reality? *Neuropsychobiology* 1:218-242, 1975.

89. Kong J, Ma L, Gollub RL et al: A pilot study of functional magnetic resonance imaging of the brain during manual and electroacupuncture stimulation of acupuncture point (LI-4 Hegu) in normal subjects reveals differential brain activation between methods, *J Altern Complement Med* 8:411-419, 2002.

90. Wang Q, Mao L, Han J: The arcuate nucleus of hypothalamus mediates low but not high frequency electroacupuncture analgesia in rats, *Brain Res* 513:60-66, 1990.

91. Fei H, Xie GX, Han JS: Differential release of met-enkephalin and dynorphin in spinal cord by electroacupuncture of different frequencies, *Kexue Tongbo* 31:1512-1515, 1986.

92. Han JS: Acupuncture and endorphins, *Neurosci Lett* 361:258-261, 2004.

93. Clement-Jones V, McLoughlin L, Tomlin S et al: Increased beta-endorphin but not met-enkephalin levels in human cerebrospinal fluid after acupuncture for recurrent pain, *Lancet* 2:946-949, 1980.

94. Thomas M, Lundberg T: Importance of modes of acupuncture in the treatment of chronic nociceptive low back pain, *Acta Anaesthesiol Scand* 38:63-69, 1994.

95. Han JS: Electroacupuncture: an alternative to antidepressants for treating affective diseases? *Int J Neurosci* 29:79-92, 1986.

96. Kiser RS, Khatami MJ, Gatchel RJ et al: Acupuncture relief of chronic pain syndrome correlates with increased plasma metenkephalin concentrations, *Lancet* 2:1394-1396, 1983.

97. Guo HF, Tian J, Wang X et al: Brain substrates activated by electroacupuncture (EA) of different frequencies (II): role of Fos/Jun proteins in EA-induced transcription of preproenkephalin and preprodynorphin genes, *Brain Res Mol Brain Res* 43:167-173, 1996.

98. Gao M, Wang M, Li K, He L: Changes of mu opioid receptor binding sites in rat brain following electroacupuncture, *Acupunct Electrother Res* 22:161-166, 1997.

99. Astin JA, Marie A, Pelletier KR et al: A review of the incorporation of complementary and alternative medicine by mainstream physicians, *Arch Intern Med* 158:2303-2310, 1998.

100. Vickers AJ: Bibliometric analysis of randomized trials in complementary medicine, *Complement Ther Med* 6:185-189, 1998.

101. Klein L, Trachtenberg AI, National Library of Medicine. Reference Section. Acupuncture: January 1970 through October 1997. (Series: Current Bibliographies in Medicine.) Bethesda, Md, 1997, US Department of Health and Human Services.

101a. Behrman RE, Kliegman RM, Jenson HB et al, editors: *Nelson textbook of pediatrics*, ed 17, Philadelphia, 2004, Saunders.

102. Highfield ES, McLellan MC, Kemper KJ et al: Integration of complementary and alternative medicine in a major pediatric teaching hospital: an initial overview, *J Altern Complement Med* 11:373-380, 2005.

103. Kemper KJ, Sarah R, Silver-Highfield E et al: On pins and needles? Pediatric pain patients' experience with acupuncture, *Pediatrics* 105:941-947, 2000.

104. Bellas A, Lafferty WE, Lind B et al: Frequency, predictors, and expenditures for pediatric insurance claims for complementary and alternative medical professionals in Washington State, *Arch Pediatr Adolesc Med* 159:367-372, 2005.

105. MacPherson H, Thomas K, Walters S et al: A prospective survey of adverse events and treatment reactions following 34,000 consultations with professional acupuncturists, *Acupunct Med* 19:93-102, 2001.

106. White A, Hayhoe S, Hart A et al: British Medical Acupuncture Society and Acupuncture Association of Chartered Physiotherapists: Survey of adverse events following acupuncture (SAFA): a prospective study of 32,000 consultations, *Acupunct Med* 19:84-92, 2001.

107. de Groot M: Acupuncture: complications, contraindications and informed consent [in German], *Forsch Komplementarmed Klass Naturheilkd* 8:256-262, 2001.

108. Chung A, Bui L, Mills E: Adverse effects of acupuncture. Which are clinically significant? *Can Fam Physician* 49:985-989, 2003.

109. Strzyz H, Ernst G: Adverse reactions to acupuncture [in German], *Schmerz* 11:13-19, 1997.

110. Strauss E: Hepatitis C [in Portuguese], *Rev Soc Bras Med Trop* 34:69-82, 2001.

111. Filshie J: Safety aspects of acupuncture in palliative care, *Acupunct Med* 19:117-122, 2001.

112. Peuker E, Gronemeyer D: Rare but serious complications of acupuncture: traumatic lesions, *Acupunct Med* 19:103-108, 2001.

113. Morrone N, Freire JA, Ferreira AK et al: Iatrogenic pneumothorax caused by acupuncture [in Portuguese], *Rev Paul Med* 108:189-191, 1990.

114. Yamashita H, Tsukayama H, White AR et al: Systematic review of adverse events following acupuncture: the Japanese literature, *Complement Ther Med* 9:98-104, 2001.

115. Naeser MA, Wei XB: *Laser acupuncture, an introductory textbook for treatment of pain, paralysis, spasticity, and other disorders*, Boston, 1994, Boston Chinese Medicine.

116. McCormick S, Brenan P, Yassa J et al: Children and minimagnets: an almost fatal attraction, *Emerg Med J* 19:71-73, 2002.

117. Lecture notes taken by author during postdoctoral fellowship in behavioral and developmental pediatrics, 1989, University of California–San Francisco Medical Center.

118. Piaget J: *The child's conception of physical causality*, New York, 1951, Harcourt Brace.

119. Mahler MS: *On human symbiosis and the viscissitudes of individuation*, New York, 1970, International Universities Press.

120. Flavel JH: *The developmental psychology of Jean Piaget*, Princeton, NJ, 1963, D Van Nostrand.

121. Freud S: Character and anal eroticism. In *The standard edition of the complete psychological works of Sigmund Freud*, London, 1962, Hogarth Press.

122. Kline P: *Facts and fantasy in freudian theory*, London, 1972, Methuen and Company.

123. Maciocia G: *The practice of chinese medicine: the treatment of diseases with acupuncture and chinese herbs*, London, 1994, Churchill Livingstone.

Aromatherapy

1. Battaglia S: *The complete guide to aromatherapy*, Virginia, Queensland, Australia, 1995, The Perfect Potion.

2. Buckle J: *Clinical aromatherapy: essential oils in practice*, ed 2, Edinburgh, 2003, Churchill Livingstone.

3. Halcon L: Aromatherapy: therapeutic applications of plant essential oils, *Minn Med* November 2002. Available at www.mmaonline.net/publications/MNMed2002/November/Halcon.html.

4. Price S, Price L: *Aromatherapy for health professionals*, Edinburgh, 1999, Churchill Livingstone.

5. Schnaubelt, K. *Advanced aromatherapy: the science of essential oil therapy* [US edition], Rochester, Vt, 1998, Healing Arts Press. [Translation of *Neue Aromatherapie*, Cologne, 1995, Verlag.]

6. Penoel D: A global introduction to medical aromatherapy, *Eur Nurse* 3:64-76, 1998.

7. Buckle J: Aromatherapy in the USA, *Int J Aromather* 13:42-46, 2003.

8. Tisserand R, Balacs T: *Essential oil safety*, Edinburgh, 1995, Churchill Livingstone.

9. Sugano H: Effects of odours on mental function, *Chem Senses* 14:303, 1989.

10. American Botanical Council: *Lavender flower*. Available at www.herbalgram.org.

11. Lis-Balchin M: Possible health and safety problems in the use of novel plant essential oils and extracts in aromatherapy, *J Roy Sci Promo Health* 119:240-243, 1999.

12. Buck P: Skin barrier function: effect of age, race and inflammatory disease, *Int J Aromather* 14:70-76, 2004.

13. Westcombe AM, Gambles MA, Wilkinson SM et al: Learning the hard way! Setting up an RCT of aromatherapy massage for patients with advanced cancer, *Palliative Med* 17:300-307, 2004.

14. Cooke B, Ernst E: Aromatherapy: a systematic review, *Br J Gen Pract* 50:493-496, 2000.

15. Long L, Huntley A, Ernst E: Which complementary and alternative therapies benefit which conditions? A survey of the opinions of 223 professional organizations, *Complement Ther Med* 9:178-185, 2001.

16. Buckle J: Use of aromatherapy as a complementary treatment for chronic pain, *Altern Ther* 5,1999.

17. Hirsch AR: Aromatherapy for headache: evidence pro and con, *Natur Pharm* September/October, 2003.

18. Fellowes D, Barnes K, Wilkinson S: Aromatherapy and massage for symptom relief in patients with cancer, *Cochrane Database Syst Rev* 2:CD002287, 2004.

19. Wilkinson S, Aldridge J, Salmon I et al: An evaluation of aromatherapy massage in palliative care, *Palliative Med* 13:409-417, 1999.

20. Wilcock A, Manderson C, Weller R et al: Does aromatherapy massage benefit patients with cancer attending a specialist palliative care day centre? *Palliative Care* 18:287, 2004.

21. Soden K, Vincent K, Craske S et al: A randomized controlled trial of aromatherapy massage in a hospice setting, *Palliative Med* 18:87-92, 2004.

22. Pittler M Ernst, E: Peppermint oil for irritable bowel syndrome: a critical review and meta-analysis, *Am J Gastroenterol* 93:1131-1135, 1998.

23. Kline RM, Kline JJ, Di Palma J et al: Enteric-coated, pH-dependent peppermint oil capsules for the treatment of irritable bowel syndrome in children, *J Pediatr* 138:125-128, 2001.

24. Tate S: Peppermint oil: a treatment for postoperative nausea, *J Adv Nurs* 26:543-549, 1997.

25. Anderson LA, Gross JB: Aromatherapy with peppermint, isopropyl alcohol, or placebo is equally effective in relieving postoperative nausea, *J Perianesthesia Nurs* 19:29-35, 2004.

26. Loman DG: The use of complementary and alternative health care practices among children, *J Pediatr Health Care* 17:58-63, 2003.

27. Hurvitz EA, Leonard C, Ayyangar R et al: Complementary and alternative medicine use in families of children with cerebral palsy, *Dev Med Child Neurol* 45:364-370, 2003.

28. Molassiotis A, Cubbin D: Thinking outside the box: complementary and alternative therapies use in paediatric oncology patients, *Eur J Oncol Nurs* 8:50-60, 2004.

29. Price S, Parr PP: *Aromatherapy for babies and children*, San Francisco, 1996, Thorsons.

30. Keville K, Green M: *Aromatherapy: a complete guide*, Berkeley, Calif, 1995, Crossing Press.

31. Styles JL: The use of aromatherapy in hospitalized children with HIV disease, *Complement Ther Nurs* 3:16-20, 1997.

32. Guba R: Toxicity myths: the actual risks of essential oil use. Part I, *Aromather Today* 11:28-34, 1999.

33. Buckle J: Monographs for cinical aromatherapy I. Minneapolis, 2000, University of Minnesota Center for Spirituality and Healing.

34. Maddocke-Jennings W: Critical incident: idiosyncratic allergic reactions to essential oils, *Complement Ther Nurs Midwife* 10:58-60, 2004.

35. Guba R: Toxicity myths: the actual risks of essential oil use. Part II, *Aromatherapy Today* 12:16-22, 1999.

36. Burns E, Blamey C, Lloyd AJ et al: The use of aromatherapy in intrapartum midwifery practice: an observational study, *Complement Ther Nurse Midwife* 6:33-34, 2000.

Laser Therapy

1. Ohshiro T, Calderhead RG: *Low level laser therapy: a practical introduction*, Chichester, UK, 1988, John Wiley & Sons.

2. Blahnik JA, Rindge DW: *Laser therapy: a clinical manual*, Melbourne, Fla, 2003, Healing Light Seminars.

3. Tuner J, Hode L: *Low level laser therapy—clinical practice and scientific background*, Grängesberg, Sweden, 1999, Prima Books.

4. Simunovic Z: *Lasers in medicine and dentistry: basic science and up-to-date clinical application of low energy-level laser therapy (LLLT)*, Locarno, Switzerland, 2000.

5. Schikora D: European Patent EP 1 337 298.

6. Litscher G, Schikora D, editors: *Laserneedle-acupuncture: science and practice*, Lengerich, Germany, 2005, Pabst Science Publishers.

7. Litscher G, Nemetz W, Smolle J et al: Histological investigations regarding micromorphological effects of laserneedle illumination. Results of an animal experiment, *Biomed Technik* 49:2-5, 2004.

8. Walker JB, Akhanjee LK: Laser-induced somatosensory evoked potentials: evidence of photosensitivity in peripheral nerves, *Brain Res* 344:281-285, 1985.

9. Pommeranz B, Berman B: Scientific basics of acupuncture. In Stux G, Berman B, Pomeranz B, editors: *Basics of acupuncture*, ed 5, Berlin, 2003, Springer Verlag.

10. Litscher G, Schikora D: Cerebral vascular effects of non-invasive laserneedles measured by transorbital and transtemporal Doppler sonography, *Lasers Med Sci* 17:289-295, 2002.

11. Litscher G, Wang L, Huber E: Effects of laserneedle stimulation on microcirculation and skin temperature. In Litscher G, Schikora D, editors. *Laserneedle-acupuncture. Science and practice*, Lengerich, Germany, 2005, Pabst Science Publishers, pp 64-72.

12. Tuner J, Hode L: *Low level laser therapy—clinical practice and scientific background*, Grängesberg, Sweden, 1999, Prima Books.

13. Litscher G, Schikora D: Near-infrared spectroscopy for objectifying cerebral effects of needle and laserneedle acupuncture, *Spectroscopy* 16:335-342, 2002.

14. Litscher G, Petz P, Litscher D: High-tech acupuncture [in German]. Available at http://litscher.info. Accessed April 2, 2008.

Magnet Therapy

1. Rosch PJ, Markov MS: *Bioelectromagnetic medicine*, New York, 2004, Marcel Dekker.

2. Wu J: Further observations on the therapeutic effect of magnets and magnetized water against ascariasis in children–analysis of 114 cases, *J Trad Chin Med* 9:111-112, 1989.

3. Holcomb RR, Warthington WB, McCullough BA et al: Static magnetic field therapy for pain in the abdomen and genitals, *Pediatr Neurol* 23:261-264, 2000.

4. Hsu M, Fong C: The biomagnetic effect: its application in acupuncture therapy, *Am J Acupuncture* 6:289-296, 1978.

5. Basford JR: A historical perspective of the popular use of electric and magnetic therapy, *Arch Phys Med Rehabil* 82:1261-1269, 2001.

6. Shealy CN, Liss S, Liss BS: Evolution of electrotherapy: from TENS to cyberpharmacology. In Rosch PJ, Markov MS, editors: *Bioelectromagnetic medicine*, New York, 2004, Marcel Dekker.

7. Blank M, editor. *Electromagnetic fields: biological interactions and mechanisms*, Washington, DC, 1995, American Chemical Society.

8. Brighton CT, Pollack SR, editors: *Electromagnetics in medicine and biology*, San Francisco, 1991, San Francisco Press, p 365.

9. Polk C, Postow EP, editors: *Biological effect of electromagnetic fields*, ed 2, Boca Raton, Fla, 1995, CRC Press, p 618.

10. O'Connor ME, Bentall RHC, Monahan JC, editors: *Emerging electromagnetic medicine*, New York, 1990, Springer-Verlag.

11. Hong CZ, Lin JC, Bender LF et al: Magnetic necklace: its therapeutic effectiveness on neck and shoulder pain, *Arch Phys Med Rehabil* 63:462-466, 1982.

12. Holcomb RR, Parker RA, Harrison MS: Biomagnetics in the treatment of human pain—past, present, future, *Envir Med* 8:24-60, 1991.

13. Segal NA, Toda Y, Huston J et al: Two configurations of static magnetic fields for treating rheumatoid arthritis of the knee: a double-blind clinical trial, *Arch Phys Med Rehabil* 82:1453-1460, 2001.

14. Hinman MR, Ford J, Heyl H: Effects of static magnets on chronic knee pain and physical function: a double-blind study, *Altern Ther Health Med* 8:50-55, 2002.

15. Wolsko PM, Eisenberg DM, Simon LS et al: Double-blind placebo-controlled trial of static magnets for the treatment of osteoarthritis of the knee: results of a pilot study, *Altern Ther Health Med* 10:36-43, 2004.

16. Vallbona C, Hazlewood CF, Jurida G: Response of pain to static magnetic fields in postpolio patients: a double-blind pilot study, *Arch Phys Med Rehabil* 78:1200-1203, 1997.

17. Caselli MA, Clark N, Lazarus S et al: Evaluation of magnetic foil and PPT insoles in the treatment of heel pain, *J Am Podiatr Med Assoc* 87:11-16, 1997.

18. Weintraub MI, Wolfe GI, Barohn RA et al: Static magnetic field therapy for symptomatic diabetic neuropathy: a randomized, double-blind, placebo-controlled trial, *Arch Phys Med Rehabil* 84:736-746, 2003.

19. Weintraub MI: Magnetic bio-stimulation in painful diabetic peripheral neuropathy: a novel intervention—a randomized, double-placebo crossover study, *Am J Pain Manage* 9:8-17, 1999.

20. Brown CS, Ling FW, Wan JY et al: Efficacy of static magnetic field therapy in chronic pelvic pain: a double-blind pilot study, *Am J Obstet Gynecol* 187:1581-1587, 2002.

21. Colbert A, Markov BS, Banerji M et al: Magnetic mattress pad use in patients with fibromyalgia: a randomized double-blind pilot study, *J Back Musculoskel Rehab* 13:19-31, 1999.

22. Alfano AP, Taylor AG, Foresman PA et al: Static magnetic fields for treatment of fibromyalgia: a randomized controlled trial, *J Altern Complement Med* 7:53-64, 2001.

23. Man D, Man B, Plosker H: The influence of permanent magnetic field therapy on wound healing in suction lipectomy patients: a double-blind study, *Plast Reconstr Surg* 104:2261-2266; discussion 2267-2268, 1999.

24. Coles R, Bradley P, Donaldson I et al: A trial of tinnitus therapy with ear-canal magnets, *Clin Otolaryngol Allied Sci* 16:371-372, 1991.

25. Li Z, Jiao K, Chen M et al: Effect of magnitopuncture on sympathetic and parasympathetic nerve activities in healthy drivers–assessment by power spectrum analysis of heart rate variability, *Eur J Appl Physiol* 88:404-410, 2003.

26. Liu S, Chen Z, Hou J et al: Magnetic disk applied on Neiguan point for prevention and treatment of cisplatin-induced nausea and vomiting, *J Trad Chin Med* 11:181-183, 1991.

27. Suen LKP, Wong TKS, Leung AWN: Auricular therapy using magnetic pearls on sleep: a standardized protocol for the elderly with insomnia, *Clin Acup Oriental Med* 3:39-50, 2002.

28. Colbert AP: Magnets on Sishencong and GV 20 to treat depression: clinical observations in 10 patients, *Med Acupunct* 12:20-24, 2000.

29. Chen Y: Magnets on ears helped diabetics, *Am J Chin Med* 30:183-185, 2002.

30. Livingston JD: *Driving force: the natural magic of magnets*, Cambridge, Mass, 1996, Harvard University Press.

31. Collacott EA, Zimmerman JT, White DW et al: Bipolar permanent magnets for the treatment of chronic low back pain: a pilot study, *J Am Med Assoc* 283:1322-1325, 2000.

32. Blechman AM, Oz MC, Nair V et al: Discrepancy between claimed field flux density of some commercially available magnets and actual gaussmeter measurements, *Altern Ther Health Med* 7:92-95, 2001.

33. Carpenter JS, Wells N, Lambert B et al: A pilot study of magnetic therapy for hot flashes after breast cancer, *Cancer Nurs* 25:104-109, 2002.

34. Santwani MT: *Magnetotherapy for common diseases*, Delhi, 1992, Hind Pocket Books.

35. Birla GS, Hemlin C: *Magnet therapy: the gentle & effective way to balance the body*, Rochester, Vt, 1999, Healing Arts Press.

36. Schiegl H: *Healing magnetism*, London, 1987, Century.

37. Rose P: *The practical guide to magnet therapy*, New York, 2001, Sterling.

38. Matsumoto K, Euler D: *Kiiko Matsumoto's clinical strategies: in the spirit of Master Nagano*, vol 1, Natick, Mass, 2002, Kiiko Matsumoto International.

39. Manaka Y, Itaya K, Birch S: *Chasing the dragon's tail*, Brookline, Mass, 1995, Paradigm Press.

40. Cohen D, Palti Y, Cuffin BN et al: Magnetic fields produced by steady currents in the body, *Proc Natl Acad Sci U S A* 77:1447-1451, 1970.

41. Reite M, Zimmerman JE, Edrich J et al: The human magnetoencephalogram: some EEG and related correlations, *Electroencephalogr Clin Neurophysiol* 40:59-66, 1976.

42. Saarinen M, Siltanen P, Karp PJ et al: The normal magnetocardiogram: I. Morphology, *Ann Clin Res* 10(supply 21):1-43, 1978.

43. Armstrong RA, Janday B: A brief review of magnetic fields from the human visual system, *Ophthalmic Physiol Opt* 9:299-301, 1989.

44. Engstrom S, Markov MS, McLean MJ et al: Effects of non-uniform static magnetic fields on the rate of myosin phosphorylation, *Bioelectromagnetics* 23:475-479, 2002.

45. McLean MJ, Holcomb RR, Wamil AW et al: Blockade of sensory neuron action potentials by a static magnetic field in the 10 mT range, *Bioelectromagnetics* 16:20-32, 1995.

46. Hong CZ: Static magnetic field influence on human nerve function, *Arch Phys Med Rehabil* 68:162-164, 1987.

47. Hong CZ, Harmon D, Yu J: Static magnetic field influence on rat tail nerve function, *Arch Phys Med Rehabil* 67:746-749, 1986.

48. McLean MJ, Engström S, Holcomb RR et al: A static magnetic field modulates severity of audiogenic seizures and anticonvulsant effects of phenytoin in DBA/2 mice, *Epilepsy Res* 55:105-116, 2003.

49. Okano J, Ohkubo C: Modulatory effects of static magnetic fields on blood pressure in rabbits, *Bioelectromagnetics* 22:408-418, 2001.

50. Morris C, Skalak T: Static magnetic fields alter arteriolar tone in vivo, *Bioelectromagnetics* 26:1-9, 2005.

51. Mayrovitz HN, Groseclose EE, Markov M et al: Effects of permanent magnets on resting skin blood perfusion in healthy persons assessed by laser Doppler flowmetry and imaging, *Bioelectromagnetics* 22:494-502, 2001.

52. Martel GF, Andrews SC: Roseboom CG: Comparison of static and placebo magnets on resting forearm blood flow in young, healthy men, *J Orthop Sports Phys Ther* 32:518-524, 2002.

53. Adey WR: Potential therapeutic applications of nonthermal electromagnetic fields: ensemble organization of cells in tissue as a factor in biological field sensing. In Rosch PJ, Markov MS, editors: Bioelectromagnetic medicine, New York, 2004, Marcel Dekker, pp 4-7.

54. Hyvarinen J, Karlsson M: Low-resistance skin points that may coincide with acupuncture loci, *Med Biol* 55:88-94, 1977.

55. Jakoubek B, Rohlicek V: Changes of electrodermal properties in the "acupuncture points" on men and rats, *Physiol Bohemoslov* 31:143-149, 1982.

56. Johng HM, Cho JH, Shin HS: Frequency dependence of impedances at the acupuncture point Quze (PC3), *IEEE Eng Med Biol Mag* 21:33-36, 2002.

57. Barlea N-M, Ciupa SH: *Electrical detection of acupuncture points.* Available at www.cs.utcluj.ro/~mbirlea/m/04m.htm.

58. Ahn AC, Wu J, Badger GJ et al: Electrical impedance along connective tissue planes associated with acupuncture meridians, *BMC Complement Altern Med* 5:10, 2005.

59. Cho SH, Chun SI: The basal electrical skin resistance of acupuncture points in normal subjects, *Yonsei Med J* 35:464-474, 1994.

60. Comunetti A, Laage S, Schiessl N et al: Characterisation of human skin conductance at acupuncture points, *Experientia* 51:328-331, 1995.

61. Reichmanis M, Marino AA, Becker RO: Laplace plane analysis of transient impedance between acupuncture points Li-4 and Li-12, *IEEE Trans Biomed Eng* 24:402-405, 1977.

62. Reichmanis M, Marino AA, Becker RO: Laplace plane analysis of impedance on the H meridian, *Am J Chin Med* 7:188-193, 1979.

63. Reichmanis M, Becker RO: Physiological effects of stimulation at acupuncture loci: a review, *Comp Med East West* 6:67-73, 1978.

64. Becker RO et al: Electrophysiological correlates of acupuncture points and meridians, *Psychoenergetic Systems* 1:105-112, 1976.

65. Guyatt G, Rennie D: *User's guide to medical literature: essentials of evidence based practice*, Chicago, 2002, American Medical Association Press.

66. Harlow T, Greaves C, White A et al: Randomised controlled trial of magnetic bracelets for relieving pain in osteoarthritis of the hip and knee, *Br Med J* 329:1450-1454, 2004.

67. Segal N, Houston J, Fuchs H et al: Efficacy of a static magnetic device against knee pain associated with inflammatory arthritis, *J Clin Rheumatol* 5:302-305, 1999.

68. Weintraub MI: Splinting vs surgery for carpal tunnel syndrome, *J Am Med Assoc* 289:422, 2003; author reply 422–423.

69. Simoncini L, Giuriati L, Giannini S: Clinical evaluation of the effective use of magnetic fields in podology, *Chir Organi Mov* 86:243-247, 2001.

70. Eccles NK: A randomized, double-blinded, placebo-controlled pilot study to investigate the effectiveness of a static magnet to relieve dysmenorrhea, *J Altern Complement Med* 11:681-687, 2005.

71. Winemiller MH, Billow RG, Laskowski ER et al: Effect of magnetic vs sham-magnetic insoles on plantar heel pain: a randomized controlled trial, *J Am Med Assoc* 290:1474-1478, 2003.

72. Carter R, Aspy CB, Mold J: The effectiveness of magnet therapy for treatment of wrist pain attributed to carpal tunnel syndrome, *J Fam Pract* 51:38-40, 2002.

73. Pope KW, McNally RJ: Non-specific placebo effects explain the therapeutic benefits of magnets, *Sci Rev Altern Med* 6:13-16, 2002.

74. Kemper KJ, Sarah R, Silver-Highfield E et al: On pins and needles? Pediatric pain patients' experience with acupuncture, *Pediatrics* 105:941-947, 2000.

75. Loo M: *Pediatric acupuncture*, London, 2002, Elsevier.

76. NCCAM: *Questions and answers about using magnets to treat pain*, NCCAM Publication No D208, Washington, DC, 2004, US Department of Health and Human Services.

77. McCormick S, Brenan P, Yassa J et al: Children and mini-magnets: an almost fatal attraction, *Emerg Med J* 19:71-73, 2002.

78. Borsa PA, Liggett CL: Flexible magnets are not effective in decreasing pain perception and recovery time after muscle microinjury, *J Athlet Train* 33:150-155, 1998.

79. Chaloupka EC, Kang J, Mastrangelo MA: The effect of flexible magnets on hand muscle strength: a randomized, double-blind study, *J Strength Cond Res* 16:33-37, 2002.

CHAPTER 7

Herbs and Biological Agents

Herbs—Chinese Catherine Ulbricht, Jennifer Woods, Mark Wright

Herbs—Western Alan D. Woolf, Paula M. Gardiner, Lana Dvorkin-Camiel, Jack Maypole

Probiotics Russell H. Greenfield

Herbs—Chinese

Historical Background

Chinese medicine is believed to be a complete medical system that has diagnosed, treated, and prevented illness for more than 23 centuries. It is one of the earliest forms of holistic medicine and is still widely used today. Chinese herbal medicine, which dates back to 3400 BCE, uses plants, minerals, and sometimes animal products prepared in specific ways and combinations to develop therapeutic prescriptions. This form of alternative medicine can be administered in oral, topical, or injectable forms.[1] Of the more than 2000 different kinds of herbs, about 400 are commonly used.

Chinese medicine continued to evolve over the centuries. Herbal medicine reached a high point during the Ming dynasty (1368-1644), which is considered one of the most prosperous time periods for China. The Ming dynasty was the last native Chinese dynasty to rule the empire. Significant advances in the arts and sciences were made during this era.

For example, it was during this time period that pediatrics became a subspecialty of Chinese herbal medicine. Healthcare professionals began to create herbal remedies especially for children because their immune systems are not completely developed yet and they are more susceptible to sickness and other health ailments than adults.

A major contributor to herbal medicine during the Ming dynasty was Li Shizhen, a physician and pharmacologist. He conducted research and investigated thousands of plants for medicinal qualities. Shizhen compiled his research findings in a book titled *Compendium of Materia Medica,* which lists 1892 medicines and more than 10,000 prescriptions. His book is still consulted today.

Shen Nong is accredited with being the mythical forefather of Traditional Chinese Medicine (TCM). He taught individuals how to raise crops, rear domestic animals, and recognize herbal plants.[2]

Huang Ti, also known as the "Yellow Emperor," and Chi Po, who worked closely with Huang, are considered pioneers of Chinese medicine because they created the basis of Chinese medical knowledge. They recorded the *Huang Ti Nei Jing,* or the *Yellow Emperor's Classic,* which is a text documentation of the primary understanding of Chinese medicine dated at about 3000 BCE.[2]

The Ching dynasty, also known as the Qing dynasty or Manchu dynasty, was founded by the Manchu clan and lasted from 1644 to 1911. During the Ching dynasty, prosperity diminished as China suffered economic strife and a dramatic population increase. China experienced significant influence from the West, especially from Britain and the United States, which forcibly gained special commercial privileges within China. Chinese medicine was one area that was influenced by the West, and the Ching dynasty was the beginning of the integration of Western and Chinese medicine.

The Cultural Revolution in China, which began in 1966 and lasted until 1976, also had a major effect on Chinese medicine. The Cultural Revolution was launched because the Chinese Communist Party Chairman Mao Zedong was concerned that China would develop along the line of the Soviet model. The revolution threw the country into turmoil. One area that suffered significantly was the medical field. During the 10-year revolution, medical schools ceased to exist and did not admit new students. No formal medical training was given to students. When medical schools reopened in 1970, a new philosophy emerged. Students were subsequently trained based on a curriculum that focused primarily on political ideology and practical training over basic science.[3]

According to the World Health Organization (WHO), TCM is fully integrated into the Chinese health system, as 95% of Chinese hospitals have special units for traditional medicine. Chinese herbal medicine is used alongside Western medicine. For example, in regard to pediatrics, many hospitals treat children having serious infections with intravenous antibiotics. At hospitals where Chinese medicine is integrated, the children also receive Chinese herbs. The Chinese herbs are injected at the same time in order to counteract the side effects of the antibiotic and boost the child's immune system.

Theory

The strategy of Chinese medicine is to restore harmony, and the goal of treatment is to balance Yin and Yang, which represent the opposite forces or attributes such as wet and dry, cold and hot, inner and outer, body and mind. Yin (negative, dark, and feminine) and Yang (positive, bright, and masculine) are the underlying principles of Chinese philosophy and medicine. According to TCM, the imbalance of Yin and Yang is one of the basic causes of disease. Preponderance of yang will lead to "heat" manifestations such as thirst, dark scanty urine, dryness of the throat, and constipation. Harmony is achieved by the regulation of Qi (vital energy) and of moisture and blood in the organ networks.[4]

Pediatrics is one of the oldest specialties within Chinese medicine. In TCM pediatrics, children are not considered miniature adults. Instead, children are believed to be immature both physically and functionally, and most of the common pediatric complaints are thought to be due to this immaturity. Chinese medicine promotes the idea that children are susceptible to diseases that affect the lungs, spleen (digestion), and liver because their bodies are immature and therefore inherently weak. This belief is used to explain why children have upper respiratory tract complaints such as colds, coughs, allergies, and asthma, as well as digestive disorders such as colic, vomiting, diarrhea, indigestion, and stomachache.

Chinese herbal medicine applies herbs to the body both externally and internally. Dried herbs may be mixed with water and used as poultices to treat arthritis, rheumatism, sprains, bruises, abscesses, and strained backs. A distinctive technique is the use of moxibustion, which is the application of heat to an area of skin directly over a meridian by burning a wick made of herbs (usually mugwort) a slight distance above the skin. Moxibustion is used to treat many conditions, including mumps, vaginal bleeding, pulled nerves, arthritis, and chronic nosebleeds.

Chinese herbs are always used in a combination to create a formula to maximize therapeutic effect and minimize side effects. TCM practitioners treat the patient rather than the disease and use several herbs in different combinations based on the individual needs of patients.[1]

The principal active herb in a formula is called the "emperor" or "king" herb. This herb is aimed at the root cause of the ailment or symptom and is usually the most potent herb in the formula. A "minister" herb is then added to assist and complement the emperor herb, often bringing the formula broader efficacy. "Assistant" herbs often play an important role by counteracting any toxins or potentially negative side effects of either the emperor or minister herbs. Finally, the "servant" herbs are added to harmonize and balance the actions of the other herbs, promote rapid absorption, and help prolong the effects of the formula.

For example, bai tou went tang, which is used to relieve the body of toxins and cool the blood, consists of pulsatilla, huang lian, huang bai and qing pi. Pulsatilla is considered the emperor drug and stops dysentery, relieves heat and toxins. Huang lian, which removes damp heat from the body, is the minister herb. The assistant herb, huang bai, also clears damp heat. Finally, qing pi, which works to clear heat and stop diarrhea, is considered the servant drug.[5]

Each herb has its own medicinal qualities that are either enhanced or reduced when used in combination with other herbs. For example, TCM regards acne as generally being a result of the environmental force of heat. The typical name for acne in Chinese medicine is *fei feng fen ci*, or "lesion of the lung wind." In the theory of Chinese medicine, skin is closely related to the lung organ as it depends upon the lungs to supply the essential substances of water and grains. The skin in turn can affect the normal process of respiration, as in the case when feng (evil wind) and coldness gain access into the body through the sweat pores.

The active ingredients of Chinese herbs are usually the root and bark of the plants, whereas herbs in the west are usually made from the leaves and flowers of the plant. In order to extract the active ingredients, the herbs need to be cooked for an extended period of time. Because the strongest medicinal ingredients are in the root and bark of the plants, Chinese herbs tend to be much more potent in the raw form than in the manufactured form and often taste bitter.[6]

Channels or medians run along through the human body, and in Chinese medicine, certain herbs are meant to affect each of these channels. According to TCM philosophy, the body is composed of the Five Elements: Fire, Earth, Metal, Water, and Wood. Chinese herbs are categorized into five tastes: sweet, salty, bitter, pungent, and sour, which correspond to the Five Elements. TCM is also based on the idea that each internal organ and body system is related to an element. For example, the skin, which is considered a metal element Yang organ, is treated with a pungent herb.

Chinese herbal therapy is rooted in the same traditional theory as acupressure, in that it incorporates the theory of the Five Basic Elements. The symptoms of the patient are seen from an expanded paradigm using the eight principles of Chinese medicine (internal/external, cold/hot, deficient/excess, yin/yang).

Recent Evidence-Based Information

Chinese herbal remedies have been used to treat a variety of medical ailments including allergies, dermatitis, diarrhea, motion sickness, and the common cold.

Bupleurum, which resembles dill and fennel, has been used in Chinese medicine for more than 2000 years as a liver tonic with spleen and stomach toning properties, purportedly efficacious in treating fevers, flu-like syndromes, cough, gynecological disorders, and inflammation. Its root is an important ingredient in Xiao-chai-hu-tan/Sho-saiko-to, a combination of nine herbs, including ginseng, ginger, and licorice, which is used in traditional Chinese and Japanese herbal medicine for hepatitis and cirrhosis.

Preliminary evidence from animal and in vitro studies suggests that bupleurum improves liver function and serum markers in patients with chronic hepatitis B and may reduce hepatic fibrosis in cirrhosis.

Bupleurum may help treat thrombocytopenia, a blood disorder that results in difficulty clotting. Researchers studied a decoction of bupleurum consisting of radix bupleuri, radix ginseng, radix codonopsis pilosulae, radix scuellariae, radix glycyrrhizae, herba equiseti hiemalis, herba verbenae, and radix rehmanniae fructus ziziphi on patients with severe hemorrhage and found the therapy to be effective. Radix bupleuri, the emperor herb in the decoction, is used to reduce fever and inflammation.

Seasonal allergic rhinitis (SAR), also known as *hay fever*, is an allergic reaction to airborne substances that are able to get into the upper respiratory system. Chinese herbal medicine is widely used to treat SAR. Studies in adults have shown that Chinese herbal therapy may reduce the symptoms and increase the quality of life in patients with SAR.

The Chinese herb echinacea, which is also frequently used in the West, is one of the most common herbs used for the early treatment of colds. Studies suggest that the herb may reduce the symptoms and duration of the common cold.[7] However, long-term use of echinacea as a preventative measure has not been proven effective.[8]

Ligusticum, ginseng, schizandrae, and astragalus, four commonly used Chinese herbs, may boost the human immune system, according to the results from several human and animal research studies.[9]

Respiratory infection is a common illness that is treated primarily with antibiotic therapy. However, drug-resistant pathogenic microbes make antibiotic therapy challenging. Chinese herbs may warrant further research and exploiture because studies have found evidence that some herbs have antimicrobial function and the potential effects of immunoregulation.[10]

Current Pediatric Use

With the steady rise in antibiotic-resistant bacteria, many people are seeking alternative therapies instead of conventional medicine. According to the Centers for Disease Control and Prevention, more than 50% of all antibiotics prescribed are unnecessary. Many parents are turning to Chinese herbal therapy to treat their children's ailments.

The U.S. Food and Drug Administration (FDA) guidelines that went into effect on March 23, 1999, require herbal manufacturers to list a serving size and directions for use on the label. However, TCM is based on individualized herbal formulas.

Today, Chinese herbs are manufactured in ways that are conducive to pediatric consumption. Herbs are available in the form of liquid, tablets, and concentrated drops, for example. The manufacturing makes it easier for children to consume while at the same time decreasing the potency of the herb.

Diet, Chinese herbal medicine, Chinese pediatric massage, and acupuncture are commonly used in traditional Chinese medicine to treat children. Herbal therapy is generally regarded as a safe method of medical treatment for children because it is associated with limited risks and minimal adverse effects.[11] Herbal therapy is fairly common among children. For example, one study found that 12% of children in Detroit used complementary and alternative medicine (CAM). Of the 12% who used CAM therapy, 41% used herbs as their form of therapy.[12] Studies show that adults are even more likely to use herbs. In one study, 61.2% of adults surveyed in the Minneapolis-St. Paul area said they had used herbs in the last year.[13] Another study that surveyed adults in England found that 12.8% of people took herbs on a regular basis.[14]

In addition, diet is especially important in the health of children and can be used to treat or prevent many diseases that afflict children.[11]

Contraindications and Adverse Effects

Because Chinese herbal formulas consist of several different herbs, consumers must be very conscious of potential side effects and dangerous interactions with other herbs, supplements, and drugs.

Studies on the Chinese herb ma huang, which is the main active ingredient in the weight-loss drug ephedra, indicate that use of the substance is associated with serious health complications. Acute hepatitis has been associated with the herb.[15] There have been more than 800 reports of serious toxicity, including at least 22 deaths, in adolescents and young adults using ma huang.[16]

Based on numerous cases of heart attack, seizure, and stroke reported by the FDA, ephedra is likely unsafe when used in children. It is not safe to consume the herb in doses greater than recommended or for longer than 7 days. Scientific evidence also suggests that ephedra is not safe when used by patients with anorexia/bulimia, anxiety, benign prostatic hypertrophy, cerebrovascular disease, history of stroke or transient ischemic attack, closed-angle glaucoma, depression, diabetes, heart disease, hypertension, hyperthyroidism, hypovolemia, insomnia, pheochromocytoma, or tremor. Ma huang should not be used in combination with other stimulants such as caffeine. Pregnant and lactating women should not use ma huang.[16]

Panax ginseng, one of the most common over-the-counter herbs taken by the general public, is generally safe when taken as recommended. Ginseng does not have dosage standards, as it is often found in supermarkets in teas. About 24% of Americans take ginseng on a regular basis. However, based on limited evidence, long-term use may be associated with skin rash or spots, itching, diarrhea, sore throat, loss of appetite, excitability, anxiety, depression, or insomnia. Less commonly reported side effects include headache, fever, dizziness, blood pressure abnormalities (increases or decreases), chest pain, heart palpitations, rapid heart rate, leg swelling, nausea/vomiting, or manic episodes in people with bipolar disorder. Human research suggests that ginseng may lower blood sugar levels. Caution is advised for patients with diabetes or hypoglycemia. There is also evidence in humans of ginseng reducing the effectiveness of the blood-thinning medication warfarin. Caution is advised in patients with bleeding disorders. Several cases of severe drops in white blood cell counts were reported in people using a combination product containing ginseng in the 1970s and may have been a result of contamination. Ginseng may have estrogen-like effects and has been associated with menstrual abnormalities or breast tenderness, erectile dysfunction, or increased "sexual responsiveness." A severe life-threatening rash known as *Stevens-Johnson syndrome* occurred in one patient and may have been a result of contamination. A case report describes liver damage (cholestatic hepatitis) after taking a combination product that contained ginseng. High doses of ginseng have been associated with rare cases of temporary inflammation of blood vessels in the brain (cerebral arteritis), abnormal dilation of the pupils of the eye, confusion, or depression. There is preliminary evidence that ginseng, at doses of 200 mg of extract daily, may increase the QTc interval (thus increasing the risk of abnormal heart rhythms) and decrease the diastolic blood pressure 2 hours after ingestion in healthy adults.[16]

Pregnant or lactating women should not take ginseng because its safety has not been clearly established.

Echinacea may cause allergic reactions in atopic patients. Some experts discourage use in patients with cancer, tuberculosis, leukocytosis, collagenosis, multiple sclerosis, acquired immune deficiency syndrome (AIDS), human immunodeficiency virus (HIV) infection, or autoimmune diseases, although this is based on theory rather than human data, and there are no case reports of adverse events in such patients. The risk of rash in children may outweigh potential benefits in indications for which efficacy is not clearly demonstrated, such as treatment of the common cold. Echinacea may cause allergic reactions in patients with allergies to members of the Asteraceae (Compositae) plant family (e.g., ragweed, chrysanthemum, marigold, daisy).[16]

One small preliminary study suggests that echinacea is safe for pregnant women and children if taken as directed, although further evidence is warranted in this area.[16]

Dong quai is commonly used to regulate women's menstrual cycles and reduce menopausal symptoms and as a general blood tonic. Although dong quai, an aromatic Chinese herb made from the root of *Angelica sinensis*, is considered a safe food additive in the United States and Europe, its safety in medicinal doses is not known. Components of dong quai may increase the risk of bleeding owing to anticoagulant and antiplatelet effects, although there are no reliable reports of clinically significant bleeding in humans. Caution is advised in patients with bleeding disorders or who are taking drugs that may increase the risk of bleeding. Use should be discontinued prior to surgical or major dental or medical procedures. It remains unclear whether dong quai has the same effects on the body as estrogens, blocks the activity of estrogens, or has no significant hormonal effects. Results of animal studies are conflicting, and one human trial found no short-term estrogenlike effects on the body. It remains unclear whether dong quai is safe in individuals with hormone-sensitive conditions such as breast cancer, uterine cancer, or ovarian cancer. It is not known whether dong quai possesses the beneficial effects that estrogen is believed to have on bone mass or has potential harmful effects such as increased risk of stroke or hormone-sensitive cancers. Increased sun sensitivity with a risk of severe skin reactions (photosensitivity) may occur because of chemicals in dong quai (furocoumarins, psoralen, and bergapten). Prolonged exposure to sunlight or ultraviolet light should be avoided while taking dong quai. It is reported that steam-distilled oils of the root and seed may not possess the phototoxic chemicals. Safrole, a volatile oil in dong quai, may be carcinogenic (cancer causing). Long-term use should therefore be avoided, and suntan lotions that contain dong quai often limit the amount of dong quai to less than 1%.

Dong quai has traditionally been associated with gastrointestinal symptoms (particularly with prolonged use), including laxative effects/diarrhea, upset stomach, nausea, vomiting, loss of appetite, burping, or bloating. Published literature is limited in this area. Dong quai preparations may contain high levels of sucrose and should be used cautiously by patients with diabetes or glucose intolerance. Various other side effects have rarely been reported with dong quai. However, side effects have not been evaluated in well-designed studies. These include headache, lightheadedness/dizziness, sedation/drowsiness, insomnia, irritability, fever, sweating, weakness, abnormal heart rhythms, blood pressure abnormalities, wheezing/asthma, hot flashes, worsening premenstrual symptoms, reduced menstrual flow, increased male breast size (gynecomastia), kidney problems (nephrosis), or skin rash. The safety of dong quai injected into the skin, muscles, or veins is not known and should be avoided. Essential oil of dong quai injected under the skin of dogs has stopped breathing.[16]

Dong quai is not recommended during pregnancy because of possible hormonal and anticoagulant/antiplatelet properties. Animal research has noted conflicting effects on the uterus, with reports of both stimulation and relaxation. Dong quai is traditionally viewed as increasing the risk of abortion. There is insufficient evidence regarding the safety of dong quai during breastfeeding.[16]

Seijyo-bofu-to, Jumi-haidoku-to, and Toki-shakuyaku-san effectively suppressed acne rashes as well as incidental symptoms. The synergistic activities of the ingredients in the Kampo formulations might produce these effects. In contrast, distinct suppression of incidental symptoms was not found with antimicrobials. The cause of adverse effects in antimicrobials has not yet been clarified, and different degrees of suppression of incidental symptoms among the Kampo formulations exist.[17]

Some *Astragalus* species have caused poisoning in livestock, although these types are usually not used in human preparations (which primarily include *Astragalus membranaceus*). *Astragalus* spp. used alone and in recommended doses is traditionally considered to be safe, although its safety is not well studied. Overall, the side effects or toxicity of *Astragalus* spp. is difficult to determine because it is most commonly used in combination with other herbs. There are numerous reports of side effects ranging from mild to deadly in the FDA's computer database, although most of these are with multiple-ingredient products and cannot be attributed to *Astragalus* spp. specifically. The most common side effects appear to be mild stomach upset and allergic reactions. Based on preliminary animal studies and limited human research, *Astragalus* spp. may decrease blood sugar levels. Caution is advised in patients with diabetes or hypoglycemia and in those taking drugs, herbs, or supplements that affect blood sugar. Serum glucose levels may need to be monitored by a healthcare professional.

Based on anecdotal reports and preliminary research, *Astragalus* spp. may increase the risk of bleeding. Caution is advised in patients with bleeding disorders or taking drugs that may increase the risk of bleeding. Preliminary reports of human use in China have noted decreased blood pressure at doses <15 g and increased blood pressure at doses >30 g. Animal research suggests possible blood pressure–lowering effects. Because of a lack of well-designed studies, no firm conclusions can be drawn. Patients with abnormal blood pressure or taking blood pressure medications should use caution and be monitored by a qualified healthcare professional. Palpitations have been noted in human reports in China. Based on an animal study, *Astragalus* spp. may act as a diuretic and increase urination. In theory, this may lead to dehydration or metabolic abnormalities. There is one report of pneumonia in an infant after breathing in an herbal medicine powder including *Astragalus sarcocolla*. *Astragalus* spp. may increase growth hormone levels.[16]

Few side effects have been reported from bupleurum taken orally at recommended doses. The recommended dose for adults is 1.5 to 9 g/day orally for burpleurum root and 1.5 to 3 mL/day of the fluid extract. Dosing and safety in children has not been studied. Bupleurum is usually taken to reduce fever and symptoms associated with hepatitis. The most common complaints include sedation, drowsiness, and lethargy.[16]

Decreased appetite, nausea, heartburn (reflux), abdominal distention, flatulence (gas), and increased bowel movements have been reported after taking large doses of bupleurum.

Among patients using herbal combination products containing bupleurum, least one case of eosinophilic pneumonia and pulmonary edema (fluid in the lungs) has been published, and several cases of pneumonitis (inflammation of the lungs) have been reported. It is not clear whether these effects were caused by bupleurum or other ingredients in the preparations. Hepatitis has been reported.[16]

Bupleurum may increase blood sugar levels and stimulate the adrenal gland. Individuals with diabetes, high blood pressure, or other chronic health conditions should consult their healthcare provider before taking bupleurum.[16]

Bupleurum cannot be recommended during pregnancy or breastfeeding because of a lack of scientific information.[16]

Ginger supplements should be avoided by individuals with a known allergy to ginger or other members of the Zingiberaceae family, including *Alpinia formosana*, *Alpinia purpurata* (red ginger), *Alpinia zerumbet* (shell ginger), *Costus barbatus*, *Costus malortieanus*, *Costus pictus*, *Costus productus*, *Dimerocostus strobilaceus*, or *Elettaria cardamomum* (green cardamom). Allergic contact rashes and an allergic eye reaction have also been reported.[16] Few side effects have been associated with ginger at low doses. No studies confirm the safety of long-term use of ginger supplements. The most commonly reported side effects of ginger involve the stomach and intestines. Irritation or bad taste in the mouth, heartburn, belching, bloating, gas, and nausea are reported, especially with powdered forms of ginger. There are several reports that fresh ginger swallowed without enough chewing can result in blockage of the intestines. Individuals who have had ulcers, inflammatory bowel disease, or blocked intestines should use caution when taking ginger supplements and should avoid large quantities of fresh cut ginger. People with gallstones should use ginger with caution. In theory, ginger can cause abnormal heart rhythms, although reports in humans are lacking. Some publications suggest that ginger may raise or lower blood pressure, but limited scientific information is available. In addition, ginger may prevent blood clotting by preventing the clumping of platelets. This raises a concern that individuals who are treated with medications that slow blood clotting or who undergo surgery may have a high risk of excessive bleeding if they take ginger supplements. Ginger is traditionally said to reduce blood sugar levels at high doses, but no scientific evidence is available. In one study, two of eight participants reported an intense urge to urinate 30 minutes after ingesting ginger.[16]

Some authors suggest that pregnant women should not take ginger in amounts greater than found in food (or more than 1 gram dry weight per day). Ginger has been reported to increase discharge from the uterus in menstruating women and possibly lead to abortion, mutations of the fetus, or increased risk of bleeding. However, other reports state that there is no scientific evidence that ginger endangers pregnancy. Little scientific study is available in this area to support either perspective, although ginger has been studied in a small number of pregnant women (to assess effects on nausea), without reports of adverse pregnancy outcomes. Notably, this matter is sometimes confused because the use of ginger in pregnancy is discouraged in TCM, in which much higher doses of ginger may be used.[16]

Safety and Precautions

TCM is a popular method of alternative therapy, yet many clinicians and patients have some misconceptions about the therapy. There is a strong need for stricter regulation and monitoring of TCM herbs, especially those at risk for contamination.[2] The Dietary Supplement Health and Education Act (DSHEA) of 1994 requires that all herb and supplement manufacturers label their products with information that is accurate and not misleading and also requires producers to comply with Good Manufacturing Practice (GMP) guidelines. The guidelines for herbal evaluation in Europe are based on the WHO's Guidelines for the Assessment of Herbal Medicines. When scientific evidence is lacking for a substance, historical use is a valid way to document the safety and efficacy of the product.

Consumers should be fully aware of the risks and benefits of taking raw herbs. Raw herbs are herbal plants that are in their natural state and have not been manufactured. As there are more than 2000 different kinds of herbs (of which about 400 are commonly used), raw herbs are subject to misidentification, substitution, adulteration, and environmental contamination. Raw herbs also require long hours of extraction by decoction. The industry lacks a central mechanism of quality control of raw herbs.[18]

Although raw herbs are much weaker than pharmaceutical drugs, they are usually stronger than manufactured herbs. Concentrated herbs, however, are typically easier to ingest than raw herbs. The basic difference is a matter of convenience. Raw herbs need to be cooked, whereas the concentrated forms do not.[19] On average, Chinese herbs take about 1.5 hours to cook. Overcooking them can make the herbs less effective. In addition, raw herbs often have a distinct smell and a bitter taste, which can deter individuals from using them.

Many Chinese herbs are available over the counter, which makes them easily accessible to consumers. However, it also increases the chances that consumers will take herbs not suited for them, because they are not required to seek advice from qualified healthcare professionals.

Herbs—Western

History

Introduction

Medicinal herbs existed long before human beings had discovered their healing power. Some historic sites in Iraq show that Neanderthals used herbs more than 60,000 years ago. It appears that even then our ancestors were noticing herbal use by animals during their illnesses. Later herbs were incorporated into prehistoric shamanism and then into medicine.[1]

Healing herbs have not changed since the time they were first used by physicians, who were expected to know uses for each specific herb in order to correctly apply their knowledge. The information was passed down from generation to generation. Many men and women deserve recognition for their sacrifices to this science.

Several of the reasons why early humans used herbs include repelling insects, hiding their human odor from animals they were hunting, and pleasing their mates. Later, they began to use herbs (or what we call today *culinary spices*) to mask the foul smell of spoiling foods. An ability to store food with the help of herbs was essential for prehistoric households. Major herbal effects such as vomiting or hallucinations made very big impressions on our ancestors, but they had also recognized the more subtle benefits of plants discovered through trial and error.

There are four major herbal healing traditions: Chinese, Ayurvedic (in India), European (including Egyptian), and Native American, and the similarities among the cultures separated by land and sea are simply amazing. During the nineteenth century, herbs were used in the discovery of the first pharmaceuticals. More than 120 prescription medications have been derived from plants, almost three fourths of which were discovered because of their traditional uses.

In most articles on the history of herbalism, discoveries are attributed to such great men as Hippocrates, the father of medicine; Alexander Fleming, discoverer of penicillin; and others. Their place in history should always be remembered, but the role of women healers (midwives, wise women, green women, witches, old wives, and nurses) should never be underestimated. Many physicians have dismissed the work of the women who had introduced a large number of therapies currently used in our medical practice. An example is the discovery of foxglove, the plant containing such cardiac glycosides as digoxin and digitoxin, by a woman folk healer in Great Britain, whose name was not recorded.[2-4]

Chinese tradition

The origins of Chinese herbalism are lost, but we know today that around 3400 BCE the mythological emperor and sage Shen Nung had invented agriculture and started to experiment with medicinal properties of different plants. He authored China's first great herbal text, the *Pen Tsao Ching (The Classic of Herbs)*. This publication described 237 herbal prescriptions containing dozens of herbs. Each of the following emperors continued with this tradition, and by 1590 Li Shin-Chen published 52 volumes of *Pen Tsao Kang Mu (The Catalogue of Medicinal Herbs)*. This publication listed 1094 medicinal plants and more than 11,000 diverse medicinal formulas.

In modern China, Western and Chinese systems coexist peacefully. In 1972, after President Nixon's visit to China, several broadcasts and publications about TCM helped the U.S. public to cautiously accept Chinese herbalism.[5-8]

Ayurvedic tradition

In ancient India, medicine was called *Ayurveda* (in Sanskrit, *ayur* means "life" and *veda* means "knowledge"). Ayurvedic medicine was based on four *Vedas*, books of classic wisdom. The oldest book, *Rig Veda*, includes descriptions of very modern procedures such as amputation and eye surgeries, as well as descriptions of 67 different herbs. Some herbs mentioned are ginger, cinnamon, and senna. Later, in 600 CE, Indian herbal healing was influenced by Arabic medicine. The British brought more conventional Western medicine to India in the nineteenth century, but today the majority of Ayurvedic doctors still rely on herbal prescriptions.[2,7-9]

European tradition

Western herbalism has its roots in Egypt. In 1874, a 65-foot papyrus dating back to approximately 1500 BCE was discovered by the German egyptologist Georg Ebergs. The Ebergs Papyrus contains information about 1000 years of medical practice in Egypt and describes 876 herbal formulations made from more than 500 plants, many of them listed in today's Western pharmacopeia. In 500 BCE Egyptian herbalists were considered to be the best practitioners in the Mediterranean region, and many European physicians traveled to Egypt to learn the art of herbalism.

The first botanist identified by name is Pedanius Dioscorides, a physician who practiced in Rome during the time of Nero. In the fifteenth century, Dioscorides published the first European herbal text, *De Materia Medica (On Medicines)*, a publication describing 600 plants, 90 of which are still in use. *De Materia Medica* was one of the first books printed after the development of the printing press. Roman herbalists of that time were not only healers, but were also fascinated with poisoning people with herbal substances. Roman emperors constantly sought new antidotes to the poisons.

After the fall of Rome, the Catholic Church did not believe in using herbs for the treatment of illnesses. Instead the Church believed in prayer, but herbal remedies remained alive owing to the efforts of monks copying the ancient texts. Some of the most avid herbalists were Benedictines. They adopted the Arabic practice of using alcohol to extract the power of herbs, which led to development of what is known today as a *liqueur*. The most notable Benedictine herbalist was Hildegard of Bingen, whose book *Hildegard's Medicine* combed Catholicism and early German folk medicine with her experience with herbs. She also left us with recommendations of a good balanced diet, toothbrushing, and a number of other beneficial techniques.

From 1300 to 1650, many women who practiced medicine and herbalism were burned as witches for reasons that are not entirely clear. The witch hunt failed to eradicate women's herbalism, but it was successful in forcing the practice underground.[2,4,5,9-11]

In 1652 the invention of the printing press, mentioned previously, allowed one of the most influential herbalists of the time, Nicholas Culpeper, to publish *The Complete Herbal and English Physician*. This revolutionary action gave equal weight to the official herbalism and to the folk wisdom of England's "country people." Culpeper was a very unique herbalist of his time, as he read Greek and Latin and was trained as a classical physician at Cambridge University. Culpeper considered almost every herb to be a panacea, exaggerating its healing powers. He even has some modern followers. He should definitely be remembered as one of the first European herbalists, but some of Culpeper's herbal claims must be examined with caution.[2,9]

Native American and modern American traditions

The last tradition of herbal medicine described here was developed on the shores of the New World. The Europeans who came to America were amazed by the health and physical strength of the native peoples. The European settlers slowly started to work with native healers, although some were criticized by university-trained physicians. Native Americans were able to introduce European settlers to many valuable herbs such as black and blue cohosh, black haw, boneset, cascara sagrada, echinacea, chaparral, goldenseal, lobelia, Oregon grape, sarsaparilla, slippery elm, wild cherry, and witch hazel.[2]

The herbal history of the United States had several trends. Samuel Thomson, a leading herbalist of his time, was inspired by the traditions of European herbalism and mineral bathing and by Native American herbalism and sweat lodges. Thomson became famous for developing a medical system based on herbs and hot baths, and in 1839 he claimed to have close to 3 million followers. His system, Thomsonianism, fell out of fashion after his death in 1843. In the 1820s, a number of Thomsonians and Native American–trained herbalists organized a group that was later called the *Eclectics*. Their herb-based approach to the medicine combined European, Asian, Native American, and African American traditions. During its height of popularity, more than 8000 practitioners worked in this field. The Eclectics were scientific herbalists who analyzed herbs chemically, extracted their active ingredients, published articles in scientific journals, and were an important part of the early pharmaceutical industry. Two naturopathic medical schools, the National College of Naturopathic Medicine in Portland, Oregon, and Bastyr University in Seattle, are examples of modern representatives of this herbal legacy.

Herbal medicine was almost lost between the 1920s and 1960s, when medical schools stopped teaching the discipline and pharmaceutical companies developed new synthetic medications. In 1970s the WHO stated that herbal remedies have a definite role in modern healthcare. Today, herbalism is actively practiced by physicians in a number of foreign countries such as Germany, France, Great Britain, Australia, and India. U.S. laws addressing the role of herbal therapies are changing as well.[2,3,5]

Epidemiology

Rates of pediatric use of herbs

Many parents routinely give their children dietary supplements to preserve their health or to treat disease. Previous studies have shown that more than 50% of all young children and more than 30% of all adolescents in the United States have used a dietary supplement, such as multivitamins and minerals, vitamin C with iron, and/or ergogenic aids.[12-14] In one survey of 348 parents in primary care practices in Washington, D.C., 21% had treated their child with CAM during the previous year; of those, 50% reported specific vitamin supplementation, 40% used herbal therapies, and 25% used other nutritional supplements or elimination diets.[15] In another survey of 142 families in an emergency department, 45% of caregivers reported giving their child an herbal product such as aloe plant/juice, echinacea, or sweet oil.[16] Pediatric practitioners should be aware of the likelihood that children under their care are taking herbs and/or other dietary supplements. They should be well informed about such products and prepared to counsel families about their use.

Special groups

Children and adolescents with chronic or recurrent medical conditions will frequently use CAM modalities to treat the condition or otherwise improve their health. Examples include children with attention-deficit hyperactivity disorder,[17] asthma,[18] atopic dermatitis,[19] cancer,[20] inflammatory bowel disease,[21] and rheumatoid arthritis.[22] Because some herbs may interact with pharmaceutical products, routine inquiry into what herbs and/or dietary supplements children with chronic health problems may be using should be a standard part of care.

Diversion

Unfortunately children and adolescents may also use herbs and dietary supplements for questionable, nontherapeutic indications. Caffeine, guarana, citrus aurantium, ephedra, and others can act as stimulants and/or appetite suppressants. Such herbs can be misused by adolescents who want to lose weight, stay alert during school tests, or improve their athletic performance. Some herbal products are touted by unscrupulous companies over the Internet and elsewhere as "herbal ecstasy" or "just like marijuana," capable of producing a safe "legal high" for the drug-abusing consumer.

Definitions/Terms

According to the *Dictionary of Natural Products*, an herb is the aboveground part of a nonwoody plant that does not persist through the winter. It is also known as a crude drug or as a flavoring used in cooking.[25] Other terms might be used interchangeably for herbs or herbal products, such as *botanical*, *nutraceutical*, and *phytopharmaceutical*.

Botanicals

A botanical drug product is intended for use in the diagnosis, cure, mitigation, treatment, or prevention of disease in humans. A botanical drug product consists of vegetable materials, which may include plant materials, algae, macroscopic fungi, or combinations of these. These products may be available in a variety of forms, including a solution (e.g., tea), powder, tablet, capsule, elixir, topical, or injection. Alternatively fermentation products (e.g., alcohol) and highly purified or chemically modified botanical substances are not considered botanical drug products.[23]

Dietary supplements

The Dietary Supplement Health and Education Act of 1994 defines a dietary supplement as a product (other than tobacco) that is taken in addition to the normal diet. Furthermore, dietary supplements must contain one or more dietary ingredients, including vitamins, minerals, herbs or other botanicals, amino acids, and other substances such as enzymes, organ tissues, glandular materials, and metabolites. The FDA characterizes botanicals and other dietary agents according to their use, not according to their composition.[24] If the intended use is to "promote health," the agent is viewed as a dietary supplement; if the intended use is to treat or prevent a disease, the agent is considered a drug. To meet labeling requirements, a dietary supplement must be intended to be taken by mouth as a pill, capsule, tablet, or liquid.

Dietary Supplements Health and Education Act of 1994

The Federal Government regulates the sale and manufacture of herbal and dietary supplement products through the FDA. Per DSHEA legislation, herbs and dietary supplements are regulated as foods rather than drugs, which places herbs and dietary supplements under a much less rigorous standard. Herbs and dietary supplements differ from pharmaceutical products primarily in terms of the regulation regarding their safety, effectiveness, and quality.

Safety. It is not required that research establish an herb or dietary supplement's safety for consumers prior to its release in the market. By contrast, a pharmaceutical product's safety must be rigorously reviewed and researched prior to its being brought to market.

Effectiveness. Manufacturers do not have to prove an herb or dietary supplement to be effective. Rather, the manufacturer can say that the product addresses a nutrient deficiency, supports health, or reduces the risk of developing a health problem, if that is true. If the manufacturer does make a claim regarding the structure/function potential of an herb or dietary supplement product, it must be labeled clearly as follows: "This statement has not been evaluated by the Food and Drug Administration. This product is not intended to diagnose, treat, cure, or prevent any disease."[26]

Quality. The manufacturer does not have to prove an herb or dietary supplement's purity or caliber. The FDA is not required to analyze the content of herbal or dietary supplement products. Because they are considered "food products" under the DSHEA, manufacturers must meet a lesser standard under the FDA's GMPs for foods. Some manufacturers voluntarily follow the FDA's stricter GMPs for drugs, but this is not required.

The FDA provides further caveats in this area: Some manufacturers use the term *standardized* to describe efforts to make their products consistent. However, U.S. law does not define standardization. Therefore the use of this term (or similar terms such as *verified* or *certified*) does not guarantee product quality or consistency. If the FDA finds a supplement to be unsafe once it is on the market, only then can it take action against the manufacturer and/or distributor, such as by issuing a warning or requiring the product to be removed from the marketplace. In March 2003, the FDA published new proposed guidelines for supplements that would require manufacturers to avoid contaminating their products with other herbs, pesticides, heavy metals, or prescription drugs. In 2007, the FDA established good manufacturing practice requirements for dietary supplements. This ruling helps to ensure that Americans are able to purchase accurately labeled and properly manufactured dietary supplements.

The U.S. Trade Commission also oversees advertising of herbs and dietary supplements. It requires that all information about supplements be truthful and without "misleading information." However, because companies can disseminate claims and advertising over innumerable media outlets, enforcement resources available are widely thought to be underequipped for the task.

Mechanisms for reporting adverse events

MedWatch. The MedWatch system has been used in limited fashion for adverse event reporting for herb/dietary supplement use. A more specific adverse event reporting system is being developed by the FDA.[27] Other surveillance systems include the American Association of Poison Control Centers (AAPCC) incident database known as the Toxic Exposure Surveillance System (TESS).

Theoretical and Practical Concepts

Pharmacokinetic considerations in pediatrics: developmental aspects of herbal consumption

Pharmacokinetic and pharmacodynamic characteristics (absorption, distribution, metabolism, and elimination) of children change significantly at different stages of development. Table 7-1 demonstrates how these characteristics vary in neonates, infants, and children.

Definitions and applications of herbal products

Applications of herbs have been divided into several different categories. These categories explain the physiological processes in which the herb will assist (Table 7-2).

Route of Administration

Toxicities of herbs: general considerations in analyzing herbal risks and toxicities

There are some general concerns regarding herbal products and their ability to produce toxicity and adverse effects. As with other therapeutic agents, herbs and dietary supplements may produce unwanted side effects and other toxic reactions. Unlike drugs, herbal products are not regulated by the FDA. Variable and unpredictable concentrations, ingredients, and contaminants are of concern, especially when such products are used in children. The lack of industrywide standards of purity creates a "buyer beware" approach to confidence in an herbal product.

Natural toxicants. Herbal products may be inherently unsafe. Table 7-3 references some examples of potent chemicals present in certain herbs and the toxic effects they can produce when these herbs are used as remedies. *Aconitum* species, including *Aconitum napellus* (monk's-hood) and *Aconitum vulparia* (wolfsbane), are herbs widely used in Asian remedies and elsewhere, despite the fact that they can produce life-threatening cardiac and neurological toxicity. Aconite's actions are mediated through its effects on sodium channels in nerve, muscle, baroreceptors, and Purkinje fibers. Increasing sodium influx in the heart's conduction system results in increased automaticity and uncontrolled afterdepolarizations and accompanying cardiac dysrhythmias, torsades de pointes, and sometimes death.[28]

Some herbal products contain pyrrolizidine alkaloids, which can be extremely hepatotoxic, causing a Budd-Chiari–type veno-occlusive pattern. It is likely that the pyrrolizidine alkaloids form reactive pyrrole adducts that are injurious to cells in the small vessels of the liver. Pediatric veno-occlusive

TABLE 7-1

Comparison of Pediatric Pharmacokinetic Differences

	NEONATE	INFANT	CHILD
Absorption			
Gastric acidity	Birth achloridia: 10-30 days after birth	pH 2-3 at age 2-3 years, then settles to adult level	
Gastrointestinal motility, intestinal transit time	Highly variable Influenced by the presence/absence of food		
Gastric emptying	Slower in pediatric population		
Pancreatic enzyme activity	Decreased	Full activity capacity dependent on specific enzyme	
Gastrointestinal surface area	More sensitive to chemicals that may cause nausea, vomiting, diarrhea		
Dietary components	Acidic/alkaline foods will alter gastric pH		
Skin permeability	Thinner stratum corneum More surface area/body weight	Thinner stratum corneum	
Distribution			
Total body water	Increased		Same as adult
Albumin	Lower concentrations Lower binding affinity	Plasma protein reaches adult levels by 1 year	
Blood-brain barrier	More permeable	Similar to adult	
Fat composition	Lower than adult; lipid-soluble drugs stored to a lesser degree		Adolescent boys lose fat; adolescent girls accumulate fat
Metabolism			
Liver	Liver metabolism immature at birth Some hepatic enzymes reduced; most metabolize drugs at a rate several times lower than adults		Most enzyme systems mature by 2-4 years
Excretion			
Renal blood flow	Reduced	9 months: reaches adult levels	
Glomerular filtration	Decreased	9 months: reaches adult levels	
Tubular function	Decreased	>9 months: reaches adult levels	Decrease in renal tubular clearance with the onset of adolescence

disease occurred in near-epidemic proportions in Jamaica after ingestion of "bush tea" brewed from pyrrolizidine-containing plants, such as *Crotolaria fulva*.[29] Exposure to pyrrolizidine alkaloids in herbal teas has led to acute liver failure and death in infants and toddlers, as well as in newborns whose mothers consumed the tea during pregnancy. In older children, the effects may be less dramatic, presenting as mild elevations in liver enzymes that may lead to progressive liver dysfunction with chronic use.

Mistaken identity. On occasion, foragers who seek herbal remedies will mistakenly collect a toxic plant, confusing it for another edible one. For example, consumption of water hemlock, confused with wild ginseng, has resulted in death.[30]

Variable potencies. The concentration of active ingredients as well as other chemicals in plants varies by the part of the plant harvested and sold as a remedy, the maturity of the plant at the time of harvest, the time of year during harvest, the geography and soil conditions where the plant is grown, soil composition and its contaminants, and annual variations in soil acidity, water, weather conditions, and other growth factors.

Dose and duration. Because of the variability in herbal product ingredients, the actual dose of active ingredients being consumed is often variable, unpredictable, or simply unknown. Although some commercial herbal manufacturers attempt to standardize the concentration of the active ingredient as listed on the product label, others do not follow such GMPs. Children are particularly susceptible to dosage considerations by virtue of their smaller size, their greater vulnerability to developmental toxicity, and their lowered capacity for

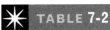 **TABLE 7-2**

Applications of Herbs

APPLICATIONS OF HERBS	DEFINITION
Adaptogenic herbs (adaptogens)	Used to increase resistance and resilience to stress, enabling the body to adapt around the problem and avoid reaching collapse; work by supporting the adrenal glands
Alternative herbs	Used to gradually restore proper functioning of the body, increasing health and vitality
Anticatarrhal herbs	Used to reduce the rate of production of mucus; primarily used for disorders of respiratory system
Antihelminthic herbs	Used to destroy or expel intestinal worms
Antiinflammatory herbs	Used to directly reduce inflammatory response of the affected tissues without inhibiting the natural inflammatory reaction
Antimicrobial herbs	Used to destroy pathogenic microorganisms by enhancing natural immunity of the body
Antispasmodic herbs	Used to alleviate the tension by relieving cramps of smooth and skeletal muscles; can also ease psychological tension
Astringent herbs	Used to allow wounds and burns to heal by reducing irritation and inflammation of mucous membranes, skin, and other tissues and creating a barrier against infection
Bitter herbs	Used to stimulate appetite, increase flow of bile and digestive juices, aid in liver detoxification, and motivate gut self-repair; responses triggered by stimulating central nervous system; have a special role in preventive medicine
Carminative herbs	Used to reduce inflammation of the gut, decrease pain, and assist in removal of gas from gastrointestinal tract
Cholagogues	Used to stimulate the secretion of bile; are commonly bitters; have a slight laxative action
Demulcent herbs	Used to reduce irritation and inflammation of the entire bowel; decrease sensitivity to gastric acids; help to prevent diarrhea and reduce muscle spasms responsible for colic
Diaphoretic herbs	Used to promote sweating; historically some of earliest herbs referenced
Diuretic herbs	Used to increase the production and elimination of urine, therefore supporting the process of inner cleansing
Emmenagogues	Used to stimulate menstrual flow
Expectorant herbs	Used to aid the removal of mucous from the lungs; subdivided into two categories: (1) stimulating expectorants "irritate" the bronchioles, causing expulsion of mucus; (2) relaxing expectorants soothe bronchial spasm and loosen mucous secretions, helping in dry, irritating coughs
Hepatic herbs	Used to tone and strengthen the liver and enhance the bile flow; maintain health by facilitating digestion and removing toxins
Hypnotic herbs	Used to induce normal sleep and relieve anxiety without exhibiting highly addictive properties (in most situations)
Hypotensive herbs	Used to lower abnormally elevated blood pressure
Laxative herbs	Used to promote bowel movements; subdivided into three major categories: (1) bulk laxatives, (2) laxatives stimulating production and enhancing the release of bile, and (3) laxatives directly triggering peristalsis
Nervine herbs	Subdivided into three groups: (1) nervine tonics strengthen and restore the nervous system; (2) nervine relaxants ease anxiety and tension by soothing both body and mind; and (3) nervine stimulants directly stimulate nerve activity
Stimulating herbs	Thought to quicken and invigorate the physiological and metabolic activity of the body
Tonic herbs	Used to nurture the body; primarily used for maintenance of health in traditional Chinese and Ayurvedic medicine; thought to build vital energy
Vulnerary herbs	Used to assist in wound healing; an old-fashioned herbal term used to describe few overlapping categories of herbs such as astringents, demulcents, and others

detoxifying certain chemicals compared with adults. The duration of use is another consideration, with longer courses of herbal therapy exposing the patient to a higher risk of both acute and subacute cumulative or chronic adverse effects. For some herbs, such as those containing pyrrolizidine alkaloids, there may be no safe dose for children.

Product-related issues

Lack of standardization

Quality control. The FDA does not regulate the manufacturing, purity, concentration, or labeling claims of herbal remedies and dietary supplements. Errors in labeling may be inadvertent; however, intentional mislabeling has also been problematic.

✳ **TABLE 7-3**

Common Herbal Dosage Forms

INTERNAL PREPARATIONS		EXTERNAL PREPARATIONS
Liquid Dosage Forms	**Solid Dosage Forms**	
Water Extractions	*Solid Extracts*	
Infusions	Granules	Creams
Decoctions	Uncoated tablets	Ointments
	Coated tablets	Salves
	Capsules	Balms
	Lozenges	Poultices
Solvent or Hydroalcoholic Extractions		
Tinctures		
Glycerites		
Fluid extracts		
Syrups		
Other		
Medicinal oils		
Medicinal spirits		
Plant juices		

Modified from Schultz V, Hansel R, Tyler V: *Rational phytotherapy: a physicians' guide to herbal medicine*, ed 3, New York, 1998, Springer; Rotblatt M, Ziment I: *Evidence-based herbal medicine*, Philadelphia, 2001, Hanley and Belfus.

For example, one study revealed that some products sold as ginseng actually contained such substitutes as scopolamine and reserpine.[31] In another case, a Chinese proprietary medicine was adulterated with phenytoin, valproate, and carbamazepine, resulting in a child's intoxication and coma.[32]

Nomenclature. There are no international conventions in naming plants, but there are many confusing synonyms. The common names of plants and herbal remedies can be archaic and variable depending on geography. For example *cohosh* refers to one species of plant in New England and a different plant in Southern Appalachia.

Admixtures. Plants have complex mixtures of terpenes, alkaloids, saponines, and other chemicals, increasing the risk of adverse reactions to any one of them or to the additive or synergistic effects of chemical interactions. For example, more than 100 different chemicals have been identified in tea tree oil. Some herbs are inducers or inhibitors of the cytochrome P450 system of metabolism, which may act to affect the blood concentrations of other herbs or drugs concurrently taken, leading to intoxication or, conversely, less than expected therapeutic efficacy.

Contaminants/Adulterants. Contaminants and adulterants of herbal products can be pharmacologically active and responsible for unexpected toxicity. Herbal plants may be harvested from contaminated soils or cleaned improperly, such that they contain illness-producing microorganisms. Ayurvedic medications have been known to cause lead poisoning in children because of their contamination with this heavy metal, as well as others such as arsenic and mercury. An analysis of 260 imported traditional Chinese medicines found that almost half had high levels of contaminants.[33] Adulterated Chinese "herbal" medications have caused adverse effects in both adults and children. These medications may contain drugs such as barbiturates, aminopyrine, diazepam, and phenylbutazone; coumadin-like compounds; and/or metals such as lead, mercury, and cadmium. In one case, a 12-year-old child developed aplastic anemia from ingesting Chinese herbal pills that were later found to contain phenylbutazone, chlorpheniramine, and diclofenac.[34] Treatment of a child with severe cerebral palsy, refractory seizures, aphasia, and retardation with an herbal medication that the mother bought in Eastern Europe resulted in deep coma and respiratory depression. The remedy was shown to contain both bromides and phenobarbital, which together intoxicated the child.[35]

Adverse reactions and interactions

Adverse effects resulting from consumption of dietary supplements may involve one or more organ systems. In some cases a single ingredient can have multiple adverse effects. More than one dietary supplement product may be consumed concurrently, and many products may contain more than one physiologically active ingredient.

Interactions. Active ingredients in herbs and dietary supplements can cause unexpected reactions when used with other herbs or with medications. Effects on the distribution, metabolism, or excretion of drugs may be pronounced and lead to drug toxicity. For example, sassafras and St. John's wort reportedly inhibit microsomal enzymes and can increase the half-life of those drugs metabolized by the liver.

Sensitization/anaphylaxis. The allergic potential of plants is well known. Infants and young children may be particularly sensitive to their first introduction to chemicals in herbs and dietary supplements. Some plants cause contact dermatitis, whereas others may produce wheezing, rhinitis, conjunctivitis, itchy throat, and other allergic manifestations. Chamomile, for example, can cause anaphylaxis in patients who are allergic to members of the Compositae family of plants (e.g. ragweed, chrysanthemum, chamomile). Echinacea is also capable of inducing allergic reactions in sensitive individuals. Photosensitization can occur with some herbs, such as St. John's wort or Angelica and rue, which contain psoralen-type furocoumarins.[36]

Other pediatric-related issues

Therapeutic use. Many herbal remedies are self-administered without any guidance from knowledgeable sources as to their indications, efficacy, or safety. Herbal products are now ubiquitous in their distribution. Parents may be tempted to give the herbs to their children based on advertising, information in popular magazines, online (Internet) availability, or advice from friends or relatives. Such experimentation is expensive and risks exposure of the child to unwanted adverse effects. Infants and young children are more vulnerable than adults to certain side effects of herbs. For example, some herbs such as buckthorn, senna, and aloe are known cathartics, and some herbal teas and juniper oil contain powerful diuretic compounds. These actions may cause clinically significant dehydration and electrolyte disturbances quickly in an infant or young child, whereas adults would more easily make up for such fluid losses.

Pediatric differences. Children differ from adults in their absorption, distribution, metabolism, and excretion of some substances. They have a relatively larger liver and thus in some respects are more efficient at detoxification. However, they also have developing nervous and immune systems that may make them more sensitive to the adverse effects of herbs. Differences in metabolism may make some products more toxic in children. Gum assafoetida, *Ferula* can be consumed by adults with no apparent adverse effects, but infants may demonstrate a severe methemoglobinemia due to the oxidizing effect on fetal hemoglobin.[37]

Excessive use. Herbal products are misused in excessive doses or in combinations without any known rationale. Multi-ingredient products may contain mixtures of 10 or more different plants, vitamins, or minerals. The consumption of many different herbs increases the risk of toxicity from any one of them or from their interactions with each other.

Inappropriate use. Herbal products are marketed over the Internet and elsewhere as "safe" ecstasy alternatives, delivering a "natural" high. Caffeine, guarana, citrus aurantium, and ephedra are popular as nonprescription products promoted as dietary aides or as mild stimulants. Adolescents and young adults may be more than willing to experiment with such herbs to improve their alertness before a test in school or to improve their athletic performance.

Teratogens. *Mutagenesis.* Toxic effects of herbs on the male or female reproductive systems are of concern. Some essential oils, for example, have cytotoxic properties or cause cellular transformation in in vitro cell culture studies.[38] Many herbs have not been adequately tested for mutagenicity.

Fetotoxicity. The effects of herbs on the embryo and fetus are not known in many cases. It is possible that herbal chemicals may be transported through the placenta to cause toxic effects on the sensitive growing fetus.[39] For example, Roulet and his associates in Switzerland reported the case of a new-born whose mother drank senecionine-containing herbal tea daily for the duration of her pregnancy.[40] The infant was born with hepatic vaso-occlusive disease and died; senecionine is one of the pyrrolizidine alkaloids associated with hepatic venous injury. Animal studies have suggested the teratogenicity of some herbs,[14] but the implications of such findings remain unclear, and more research is necessary.

Carcinogens. Although the chemicals in herbs may have carcinogenic effects, this concern has not been adequately investigated. Some chemicals found in plants are known carcinogens or tumor promoters. For example, chaparral has been linked to renal cell carcinoma.[42] Aristolochic acid has been associated with the development of urothelial carcinoma.[43,44] Children, by virtue of their longer life expectancy, are particularly vulnerable to those herbs whose chemicals may have a long latency before their toxic activity becomes manifest as tumors later in life.

Herbs and lactation. The excretion of herbs into breast milk is a concern to pediatricians, and many herbs have lipophilic chemicals, which would be expected to concentrate in breast milk. However, there is little in the way of scientific studies of this issue. The question of whether the active chemicals or excipients in herbal products can be passed into breast milk, inadvertently exposing the young infant, remains an issue for further investigation.

Safety-related recommendations

The care of children whose parents may be considering medical options such as herbal remedies requires the use of strategies that promote the therapeutic interaction among physician, parent, and child. Some key questions need to be answered by the care provider as he or she counsels the family through the decision-making process, as follows:

1. Is the herbal therapy likely to confer a benefit for this child's condition?
2. Will the herbal therapy subject the child to unreasonable risk?
3. How will I follow up with the family and keep its trust?

The following are some tips for counseling parents who seek advice about the use of herbal remedies for their children:

- They should not equate "natural" with "safe."
- There may be important differences in potency and contents between herbal products purportedly containing the same ingredients ("buyer beware").
- They should seek expert guidance when considering the use of CAM practices, including herbal remedies, and avoid self-medication.
- Herbs and plants (just like drugs) may have beneficial effects, as well as expected adverse effects and sometimes unanticipated toxicity.
- Parents should always inform physicians of *any* herb or dietary supplement they are giving their children.

Contraindications and reporting herbal adverse effects

Some situations may contraindicate the use of herbal remedies. A recent review of herbal side effects and the surgical care of patients concluded that there exists a considerable risk of intra-operative or postoperative complications when patients do not inform physicians of herbal use prior to surgery.[45] Families and pediatric care providers must freely communicate concerning the use of herbs and dietary supplements in children. It is also incumbent upon pediatric care providers to report adverse effects of herbs and dietary supplements, just as they would report adverse effects from pharmaceuticals, to the MED-WATCH program.

Overview of Herbal Pharmacotherapy
Evaluating the Efficacy of Herbs

The Natural Standard (Cambridge, Mass.) has created a template for evaluating evidence in the literature available to date. They have used the criteria of Jadad et al. to indicate methodological quality of information.[46] The following is Natural Standard's gradation for each category of evidence available (strong scientific evidence, good scientific evidence, unclear or conflicting scientific evidence, fair negative scientific evidence, strong negative scientific evidence, and lack of evidence)[47] :

- In strong scientific evidence (grade A), statistically significant evidence of benefit is obtained from > 2 properly randomized trials (RCTs), *or* evidence from one properly conducted RCT *and* one properly conducted metaanalysis, *or* evidence from multiple RCTs with a clear majority of the properly conducted trials showing statistically significant evidence of benefit *and* with supporting evidence in basic science, animal studies, or theory.
- In good scientific evidence (grade B), statistically significant evidence of benefit is obtained from 1 or 2 properly randomized trials, *or* evidence of benefit from ≥1 properly conducted metaanalysis *or* evidence of benefit from > 1 cohort/case control/nonrandomized trial *and* with supporting evidence in basic science, animal studies, or theory.
- In unclear or conflicting scientific evidence (grade C), evidence of benefit is obtained from ≥ 1 small RCT without adequate size, power, statistical significance, or quality of design by objective criteria, *or* conflicting evidence from multiple RCTs without a clear majority of the properly conducted trials showing evidence of benefit or ineffectiveness, *or* evidence of benefit from >1 cohort/case-control/nonrandomized trial *and* without supporting evidence in basic science, animal studies, or theory, *or* evidence of efficacy only from basic science, animal studies, or theory.
- In fair negative scientific evidence (grade D), statistically significant negative evidence (i.e., lack of evidence of benefit) is obtained from cohort/case control/nonrandomized trials, *and* evidence in basic science, animal studies, or theory suggesting a lack of benefit.
- In strong negative scientific evidence (grade F), statistically significant negative evidence (i.e., lack of evidence of benefit) is obtained from ≥ 1 properly randomized adequately powered trial of high-quality design by objective criteria.
- Finally, lack of evidence is usually described when, based on the literature, we are unable to evaluate efficacy owing to lack of adequate available human data.

Examples of therapeutic efficacies at each level

To understand how the evidence can be evaluated, a specific example of a plant is used. The same plant can have different grades of evidence depending on its indications. For example, aloe used as a laxative receives grade A; when the plant is used for seborrheic dermatitis, psoriasis vulgaris, and genital herpes, it receives grade B; aloe use for skin burns, aphthous stomatitis, diabetes (type 2), HIV infection, and cancer prevention has grade C evidence; and, finally, evidence on infected surgical wounds, pressure ulcers, and radiation dermatitis has grade D.

Probiotics

History and Definition

Experience with the use of probiotics can be traced to ancient times. The Roman historian Plinius noted that fermented foods could be of benefit to those with signs and symptoms compatible with what would now be termed *gastroenteritis*.[1]

The modern use of microbial interference therapy (MIT), or probiotics, is tied to the late nineteenth-century observation by microbiologists that the resident bacterial flora of people who were healthy differed from the flora of those symptomatically ill.[2,3] They proposed that illness could be attributed to disruption of the "normal" intestinal flora and that establishing a more favorable microbial balance would enhance health and prevent illness. In the early twentieth century, the Russian scientist and Nobel laureate Elie Metchnikoff posited that ingestion of *Lactobacillus* spp. in fermented foods contributed to the longevity of Bulgarian peasants.[4,4a]

During the past 20 years there has been a veritable explosion of interest in altering the enteric flora (or as some refer to it, an individual's microbiota), not only to maintain a balance away from pathogens, but also to promote overall health. From recent successful experience with supplements has come an ever-widening array of functional foods that purposely contain microbes in the hope of offering specific health benefits. Yet it is worth remembering that only within the past 5 to 10 years has the word *probiotic* entered consistently into both the medical and lay lexicons. The word was first introduced 40 years ago,[5] but its very definition has, until recently, remained elusive. Most experts would now agree in principle that probiotics are living microorganisms that, upon ingestion in sufficient numbers, exert health benefits beyond basic nutrition.[2,6]

Historically, in order for a food or supplement to be considered a probiotic, the following certain specifications had to be met:

1. Live organisms capable of multiplying, adhering to, and providing short-term colonization of the gastrointestinal (GI) tract must be present.
2. The microbes must be able to withstand exposure to gastric acid and bile salts to successfully implant and colonize.
3. The agent should improve the health and well-being of the host.
4. The organisms contained therein should not be pathogenic (generally recognized as safe [GRAS]).
5. Host-specific strains of organisms should be used (human versus animal),

It has traditionally been believed that a health benefit is more likely to occur if the microbes are present in sufficient number, if they are administered repeatedly, and if, once ingested, the organisms remain viable for a significant period of time. Recent data have called some of these basic claims into question, specifically those addressing the requirement for viability. One study examining the effect of probiotic organisms on a murine model of colitis found that nonviable organisms were just as effective as live microbes. Even more interesting was evidence presented by the researchers that the beneficial effects of probiotics were attributable not to microbial colonization and generation of metabolic byproducts as long held, but through toll-like receptor signaling mediated by microbial DNA.[7] If proven true, the finding that probiotic therapy need not employ live organisms to offer health benefits would have a significant effect on both worldwide access to such treatment and the supplement industry, if for no other reasons than with respect to shelf life and means of product delivery. Research now focuses not only on the therapeutic use of specific live microbes, but also explores the clinical potential of bacterial fragments and genetically modified bacteria.[8] That stated, the majority of experts continue to believe that live microorganisms have the greatest potential for positive health benefits as probiotics.

Prebiotics, also known as "probiotic enhancers" or "colon food," are nondigestible nutrients that selectively stimulate the growth and activity of one or more colonic microbes that, theoretically, then act to promote the optimal health of the host.[9] Presently available prebiotics are mainly nondigestible oligosaccharides that traditionally have been used to add fiber to foods without also adding bulk, such as inulin (a chicory fructan), and fructooligosaccharides, which occur naturally in onions, asparagus, chicory, bananas, and artichokes.[9] Inulin and oligofructose have been shown to specifically stimulate growth of *Bifidobacterium* spp. at the expense of *Bacteroides* spp., *Clostridium* spp., or coliforms.[9,10] Maltose, xylose, and mannose are other oligosaccharides that may yet prove effective as prebiotics.

One area where research into the use of prebiotics is gaining momentum is chemoprevention of colon cancer. In vitro studies suggest that prebiotics and probiotics together could reduce the incidence of aberrant crypt foci.[11-13] Synbiotics represent a new area of clinical investigation, wherein a probiotic and a prebiotic are combined within in a single product. The combination may improve the chances for microbial colonization while also selectively stimulating the growth of beneficial microbes found as residents of the GI tract and those within the supplement itself.

Theory

The intestinal mucosa has a very large surface area and is the main site of interaction with foreign substances and microorganisms.[6] Aside from the digestion and absorption of nutrients critical to survival, the digestive tract also represents a potent line of defense against disease that is composed of three distinct components: mucosal barrier, local immune system, including gut-associated lymphoid tissue (GALT), and microflora.

In healthy persons, the transit time from mouth to anus is between 55 and 72 hours, of which 4 to 6 hours is from the mouth to the cecum and 54 to 56 hours is in the colon.[14] Bacteria are not evenly distributed throughout the GI tract because of the variety of physiological conditions with which the bacteria have to contend.[6] The much longer transit time in the colon allows for significant bacterial growth.

Some have posited that the intestines are in fact the primary immune organ of the body as represented by GALT through innate and acquired immunity.[6] The argument gains steam in consideration of estimates that place the largest pool of immunocompetent cells, more than 60% of total immunoglobulins, within the intestinal tract.[6] Considering the concentration of immune activity within the GI tract, it becomes easy to see the theoretical underpinnings of probiotic therapy: the microbiota of the GI tract play an integral role in human health by helping to resist colonization by pathogens and by enhancing activity of the immune system. Thus gut health is one of the

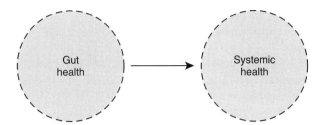

FIGURE 7-1 A broader view of the digestive system.

more important determinants of overall health and wellness (Figure 7-1).

The mucosal system that begins in the mouth and ends at the anus is a permeable one, such that a wide variety of molecules and microbes regularly pass into and out of the GI tract. In considering this, one is left with the realization that what people eat can significantly affect health, the development of disease, and symptom severity directly as a consequence of exposure to microorganisms (microbial translocation) and other antigens that leach from the GI tract into the systemic circulation and tissues.

Enteric bacteria make up 95% of the total number of cells in the human body, and the composition of intestinal microflora is unique to a given individual. Many billions of bacteria representing hundreds of different species make their homes in our intestines, but only 30 to 40 species comprise the majority of microbes. The organisms generate intense metabolic activity, especially in the colon, where transit time is slow. Data also suggest that significant communication among bacteria takes place at this level, known as *quorum sensing*,[7] as well as "dialogue" between bacteria and host.[15] A qualitative and quantitative balance among the gut microbes appears critically important to the promotion of health.

It has been suggested that gut bacteria play a crucial role in the development of a person's immune and digestive systems. One paper[15] presented data showing that intestinal microbes directly and indirectly affect the expression of genes critical to the proper development and function of the intestines, including nutrient absorption and metabolism, integrity of mucosal barrier, metabolism of toxic compounds, and blood vessel formation and gut maturation.

The makeup of an individual's microflora then has a significant impact on gut maturation, including the development of both local and systemic immunity. It could be said that the composition of intestinal microflora actually helps shape individual physiology.[16] However, the species that comprise the intestinal flora do not all have the same effects on host physiology.

Each person's unique microbiota is significantly affected at birth, specifically by the mode of delivery. A newborn's gut is sterile, and a baby delivered vaginally will have its GI tract seeded by organisms from the mother's vagina, whereas that of a child delivered via cesarean section will largely be populated by microbes from the surrounding environment.[17-19] These initial gut organisms prime the immune system and are recognized by the immune system as self. Other factors

in the neonatal period play a role in the individual composition of gut microbiota that ultimately takes hold, include the following:
- Type of feeding: breast versus bottle (A higher concentration of beneficial *Bifidobacterium* spp. are present in the gut of breastfed babies, as are fewer potential pathogens.[20])
- Term versus preterm birth
- Antibiotic administration
- Degree of sanitation of surrounding environment
- Socioeconomic status
- Geographic factors

An extremely important fact to remember is that, once in place, the intestinal microbiota is relatively constant and very difficult to alter over the long term. Firmly established over a brief time, the now indigenous bacteria fend off new colonization, including that of pathogens, except under extreme challenge. However, extreme challenges to the microbial balance of the GI tract are both common and varied and include the following:
- Poor eating habits
- Chronic stress, both physical and emotional
- Lack of exercise
- Insufficient rest
- Antibiotic use, chemotherapy, or radiation therapy
- Geography
- Unique host physiology

In theory, then, when stressors affect the dynamic equilibrium of the gut microbiota, judicious introduction of health-promoting microbes in sufficient numbers may help offset physiological impairment and promote overall systemic health. The addition of "good" bacteria does not alter the long-term makeup of the gut bacterial population, but instead temporarily limits colonization by pathogens and theoretically optimizes both metabolic and immune processes.

Hypotheses abound, but as yet no firm consensus exists regarding the mechanism of action of probiotics. A number of processes, both direct and indirect, are likely at work and include the following:
- Stimulation of host immune response
- Competition with pathogens for a limited number of receptor sites and nutrients
- Increased production of mucin, thereby blocking mucosal adhesion of pathogens
- Interference with bacterial toxins
- Production of antimicrobial substances
- Neutralization of dietary carcinogens
- Modulation of cytokines and mediators
- Production of a physiologically restrictive environment (low pH, production of toxic metabolites or hydrogen sulfide)

The suggested benefits derived from the use of probiotics are equally varied, as follows:
- Maintenance of balance between "friendly" organisms and pathogens (especially in association with antibiotic therapy)
- Decreased intestinal inflammation and enhanced mucosal integrity (normalization of gut permeability)
- Lessened systemic antigenic exposure/allergic sensitization (Nonallergic children have higher concentrations of *Lactobacillus* spp. and *Bifidobacterium* spp.)

- Increased local, and perhaps systemic, immune activity (immunoglobulin [Ig] A, GALT, interferon)
- Possible cancer chemoprotective effect

Probiotics are intended to be used for the prevention and, in some instances, the treatment of specific maladies and likely optimize immune system function when this is not being achieved by the resident intestinal flora.[6] Toward this end, the World Health Organization recommends the use of MIT (or simply "bacterial interference") as an alternative to antibiotic therapy whenever possible.

When appraised at the research and clinical level, therapeutic benefits noted for probiotic therapy include the following:
- Reduced incidence, duration, and severity of rotavirus-related diarrhea (stimulates anti-rotavirus IgA antibodies)
- Prevention of antibiotic-associated diarrhea
- Treatment of recurrent *Clostridium difficile*
- Protective role against traveler's diarrhea (not firmly established)
- Prevention and treatment of atopic dermatitis
- Treatment of cow's-milk allergy, lactose intolerance (improved digestion)
- Treatment of *Helicobacter pylori* infection
- Treatment of inflammatory disorders (juvenile rheumatoid arthritis, Crohn's disease, ulcerative colitis)

Therapeutic benefits might also be expected in the following areas, but supportive data are lacking in some instances (Box 7-1):
- Colon cancer chemoprevention
- Irritable bowel syndrome
- Dyslipidemia and elevated triglycerides
- Adjunctive use with vaccines
- Desired weight gain (improved nutrient absorption)
- Genitourinary health

From Theory to Pediatric Practice

Sustained therapy using adequate numbers of specifically chosen microorganisms can temporarily alter the gut microbiota in a manner beneficial to the health and well-being of the host. Research supports the use of probiotics in preventing and treating rotaviral infectious diarrhea, diarrhea due to *C. difficile* infection, antibiotic-associated diarrhea, traveler's diarrhea,

---

✳ **Box 7-1**

Organisms Researched and Used for Probiotic Potential*

Lactobacillus GG (best studied)
Lactobacillus casei
Lactobacillus acidophilus
Lactobacillus plantarum
Lactobacillus reuteri
Bifidobacterium bifidum/longum
Streptococcus thermophilus
Saccharomyces boulardi (yeast)

*All strains do not act equally well for specific situations. For pediatric care, the majority of research has been done using lactobacilli.

and allergic colitis. There is suggestion of benefit for patients with inflammatory bowel disease, rheumatic disorders, constipation, recurrent vaginitis, and urinary tract infections and even for children with cystic fibrosis.[21,22] Again, however, it is important to remember that the health benefits ascribed to probiotic therapy are *strain specific*. Data comparing the numerous strains with one another in terms of clinical efficacy for specific maladies are in short supply at this time. With numerous studies using different strains in varying doses for a wide variety of illnesses in dissimilar populations over disparate time courses using different experimental models, one can see how generalizations regarding probiotic therapy must be avoided.

Dosage Regimen

At this time there are no standard recommendations to be offered with regard to specific dosing instructions for specific illnesses. Supplements should contain at least 100 million colony forming units (CFUs). Daily doses used in clinical settings vary widely, anywhere from 1 million to 20 billion CFUs, but recommendations tend to be 1 billion to 10 billion CFUs for infants and 10 billion to 20 billion CFUs for children and adults. To achieve and maintain a therapeutic effect, probiotics must be administered repeatedly to ensure a sufficient and consistent population level over time.

Although some manufacturers disagree, most experts recommend taking probiotics on an empty stomach to minimize exposure to gastric acid. When taken during a course of antibiotic therapy, probiotics should be started as soon as possible and continued for 7 to 14 days after completion of therapy. Separating the times of ingestion of antibiotic and probiotic does not appear to be necessary.

Food Alternatives

European, Asian, and African consumers have long enjoyed the benefits of probiotics found in functional foods, most commonly in fermented and nonfermented dairy products including yogurt, buttermilk, sauerkraut, kefir, and kim chi. However, the organisms typically found within these foods are often not the same microbes for which significant supportive research data exist regarding health benefits. For example, the live cultures in yogurt products frequently emphasize *Lactobacillus bulgaricus* and *Streptococcus thermophilus*, two organisms that may not survive passage through gastric acid and bile to colonize the gut mucosa. An area of concern specific to dairy products is the potential for high saturated fat intake, the presence of insulin growth factor 1, cow estrogens and perhaps xenoestrogens, and a perceived association with increased morbidity with certain illnesses (e.g., atopic disorders).

Refrigeration is recommended for most products to promote the greatest number of viable probiotic bacteria. Although the breakdown products of dead microorganisms may provide some probiotic benefit, adequate refrigeration ensures the greatest number of viable organisms and thus the greatest potential for therapeutic benefit. Consumers should be sure to purchase products in which the probiotic organisms are added after pasteurization; otherwise the bacteria will be killed during the process. Using products that clearly state "contains active cultures" or "living yogurt cultures" is best.[23]

Probiotic Safety

Diets high in fermented foods are popular worldwide, and little, if any, risk has been identified with such a practice. Probiotic use appears to be extremely safe.[24-28] The American Academy of Pediatrics Provisional Committee on Quality Improvement, Subcommittee on Acute Gastroenteritis noted in 1996 that significant toxic effects are unlikely with probiotics.[29] However, bacteria do translocate and case reports of bacteremia and liver abscess do exist.[30-32] Caution is advised regarding probiotic use in the following settings:

- Immunocompromised patients
- Premature infants
- Patients with central venous access in place
- Use of an untested probiotic strain

References

Herbs—Chinese

1. Koo J, Arain S: Traditional Chinese medicine for the treatment of dermatologic disorders, *Arch Dermatol* 134:1388-1393, 1998.
2. Keane J: *Traditional Chinese medicine: herbal heat pouch,* 2003. Available at www.earlyspring.com.au.
3. Reynolds TA, Tierney LM: Medical education in modern China, *J Am Med Assoc* 291:2141, 2004.
4. Hsu CH, Yu MC, Lee CH et al: High eosinophil cationic protein level in asthmatic patients with "heat" Zheng, *Am J Chin Med* 31:277-283, 2003.
5. *Theory of Chinese herbal medicine,* 2005. Available at www.chinesemedicinesampler.com/herbmedtheory.html. Accessed October 2000.
6. Bainbridge M: *An introduction to Chinese herbal medicine.* Available at www.naturalstandard.com. Accessed October 2005.
7. Yale SH, Liu K: *Echinacea purpurea* therapy for the treatment of the common cold: a randomized, double-blind, placebo-controlled clinical trial, *Arch Intern Med* 164:1237-1241, 2004.
8. Block KI, Mead MN: Immune system effects of echinacea, ginseng, and stragalus: a review, *Integr Cancer Ther* 2:247-267, 2003.
9. Sinclair S: Chinese herbs: a clinical review of Astragalus, Ligusticum, and Schizandrae, *Altern Med Rev* 3:338-344, 1998.
10. Wang YY: New strategy for treatment of respiratory infection and the predominance of traditional Chinese medicine, *Zhong Xi Yi Jie He Xue Bao* 2:167-171, 2004.
11. Wilkowski R: *Creating healthy children with Chinese medicine,* 2003. Available at www.lightworks.com/monthlyaspectarian/2000/september/900-22.htm. Accessed October 2005.
12. Sawni-Sikand A, Schubiner H, Thomas RL: Use of complementary/alternative therapies among children in primary care pediatrics, *Ambul Pediatr* 2:99-103, 2002.
13. Harnack LJ, Rydell SA, Stang J: Prevalence of use of herbal products by adults in the Minneapolis/St Paul, Minn, metropolitan area, *Mayo Clin Proc* 76:688-694, 2001.
14. Harrison RA, Holt D, Pattison DJ et al: Who and how many people are taking herbal supplements? A survey of 21,923 adults, *Int J Vitam Nutr Res* 74:183-186, 2004.
15. Nadir A, Agrawal S, King PD et al: Acute hepatitis associated with the use of a Chinese herbal product, ma-huang, *Am J. Gastroenterol* 91:1436-1438, 1996.
16. Natural Standard Research Collaboration: *Bupleurum,* 2005. Available at www.naturalstandard.com. Accessed October 2005.

17. Higaki S, Toyomoto T, Morohashi M et al: Toki-shakuyaku. Suppress rashes and incidental symptoms in acne patients, *Drugs Exp Clin Res* 28:193-196, 2002.

18. *Traditional Chinese Medicine*, 2005. Available www.39clinic.com/english/TCM/default.asp?fname=herbal_medicines. Accessed October 2005.

19. Wu ES: *Chinese herbs*, 2005, The Holistic HealthCenter. Available at www.holisticland.com/chineseherbs.html. Accessed October 2005.

Suggested Reading for Herbs—Chinese

Anastasi JK, McMahon DJ: Testing strategies to reduce diarrhea in persons with HIV using traditional Chinese medicine: acupuncture and moxibustion, *J Assoc Nurses AIDS Care* 1:28-40, 2003.

Chen KJ, Li CS, Zhang GX: Clinical and experimental studies of royal made ping an dan on treatment of motion sickness, *Zhongguo Zhong Xi Yi Jie He Za Zhi* 12:452, 469-472, 1992.

Ho YL, Chang YS: Studies on the antinociceptive, anti-inflammatory and antipyretic effects of *Isatis indigotica* root, *Phytomedicine* 9:419-424, 2002.

Ho YL, Kao KC, Tsai HY et al: Evaluation of antinociceptive, anti-inflammatory and antipyretic effects of *Strobilanthes cusia* leaf extract in male mice and rats, *Am J Chin Med* 31:61-69, 2003.

Holtmann S, Clarke AH, Scherer H et al: The anti-motion sickness mechanism of ginger. A comparative study with placebo and dimenhydrinate, *Acta Otolaryngol* 108:168-174, 1989.

Hon KL, Leung TF, Wong Y et al: A pentaherbs capsule as a treatment option for atopic dermatitis in children: an open-labeled case series, *Am J Chin Med* 32:941-950, 2004.

Hsiang CY, Hsieh CL, Wu SL et al: Inhibitory effect of anti-pyretic and anti-inflammatory herbs on herpes simplex virus replication, *Am J Chin Med* 29:459-467, 2001.

Kong XT, Fang HT, Jiang GQ et al: Treatment of acute bronchiolitis with Chinese herbs, 68:468-471, 1993.

Lebedev VA: The treatment of neurogenic bladder dysfunction with enuresis in children using the SKENAR apparatus (self-controlled energy-neuroadaptive regulator), *Vopr Kurortol Fizioter Lech Fiz Kult* Jul-Aug:25-26, 1995.

Lien HC, Sun WM, Chen YH et al: Effects of ginger on motion sickness and gastric slow-wave dysrhythmias induced by circular vection, *Am J Physiol Gastrointest Liver Physiol* 284:G481-G489, 2003.

Li FC, Zhou XL, Mao HL: A study of paeonol injection on immune functions in rats, *Zhongguo Zhong Xi Yi Jie He Za Zhi* 14:37-38, 1994.

Li ZL, Dai BQ, Liang AH et al: Pharmacological studies of nin jion pei pa koa, *Zhongguo Zhong Yao Za Zhi* 19:362-365, 384, 1994.

Liu Z, Li H, Peng Z et al: 239 cases of high fever in viral upper respiratory infection (URI) treated with xiang shi qing jie (XSQJ) bag tea, *J Tradit Chin Med* 16:101-104, 1996.

Makino T, Ito Y, Sasaki SY et al: Preventive and curative effects of Gyokuheifu-san, a formula of traditional Chinese medicine, on allergic rhinitis induced with Japanese cedar pollens in guinea pig, *Biol Pharm Bull* 27:554-558, 2004.

Nishida T, Kusakai Y, Ogoshi R: Four cases of cystitis induced by the anti-allergic drug tranilast, *Hinyokika Kiyo* 31:1813-1817, 1985.

Pei JS, Tong BL, Chen KJ et al: Experimental research on antimotion sickness effects of Chinese medicine "pingandan" pills in cats, *Chin Med J (Engl)* 195:322-327, 1992.

Stewart JJ, Wood MJ, Wood CD et al: Effects of ginger on motion sickness susceptibility and gastric function, *Pharmacology* 42:111-120, 1991.

Tai CJ, Chien LY: The treatment of allergies using Sanfujiu: a method of applying Chinese herbal medicine paste to acupoints on three peak summer days, *Am J Chin Med* 32:967-976, 2004.

Tan BK, Vanitha J: Immunomodulatory and antimicrobial effects of some traditional Chinese medicinal herbs: a review, *Curr Med Chem* 11:1423-1430, 2004.

Tian WX, Li LC, Wu XD et al: Weight reduction by Chinese medicinal herbs may be related to inhibition of fatty acid synthase, *Life Sci* 74:2389-2399, 2004.

Wang T: Effects of Chinese medicine zhenxianling in 239 cases of epilepsy, *J Tradit Chin Med* 16:94-97, 1996.

Wang WJ. Prevention and treatment of metabolic syndrome with integrated traditional Chinese and western medicine, *Zhong Xi Yi Jie He Xue Bao* 2:3905, 2004.

Wang Y: Clinical therapy and etiology of viral diarrhea in children, *Zhong Xi Yi Jie He Za Zhi* 10:25-26, 1990.

Wood CD, Manno JE, Wood MJ et al: Comparison of efficacy of ginger with various antimotion sickness drugs, *Clin Res Pr Drug Regul Aff* 6:129-136, 1988.

Xie QM, Shen WH, Wu XM: Anti-tussive and expectorant effects of Liangyuan Pipagao, a Chinese medicine, *Zhejiang Da Xue Xue Bao Yi Xue Ban* 31:131-134, 2002.

Xue CC, Thien FC, Zhang JJ et al: Effect of adding a Chinese herbal preparation to acupuncture for seasonal allergic rhinitis: randomised double-blind controlled trial, *Hong Kong Med J* 9:427-434, 2003.

Zhu HH, Chen YP, Yu JE et al: Therapeutic effect of Xincang Decoction on chronic airway inflammation in children with bronchial asthma in remission stage, *Zhong Xi Yi Jie He Xue Bao* 3:23-27, 2005.

Herbs—Western

1. Griggs B: *A history of herbal medicine*, New York, 1982, Viking Press.

2. Castleman M: *The healing herbs: the ultimate guide to the curative power of nature's medicines*, Emmaus, Pa, 1991, Rodale Press.

3. Clark CC: *Encyclopedia of complementary health practice*, New York, 1999, Springer.

4. Samuelson G: *Drugs of natural origin: a text book of pharmacognosy*, ed 4, Stockholm, Sweden, 1999, Swedish Pharmaceutical Press.

5. Sumner J: *The natural history of medicinal plants*, Portland, Ore, 2000, Timber Press.

6. Huang KC: *The pharmacology of Chinese herbs*, Boca Raton, Fla, 1993, CRC Press.

7. Ody P: *The complete medicinal herbal*, New York, 1993, Dorling Kindersley.

8. Micozzi MS: *Fundamentals of complementary and alternative medicine*, ed 2, Philadelphia, 2001, Churchill Livingstone.

9. Van Wyk BE, Wink M: *Medicinal plants of the world*, Portland, Ore, 2004, Timber Press.

10. Anderson FJ: *An illustrated history of the herbals*. New York, 1977, Columbia University Press.

11. Eldin S, Dunford A: *Herbal medicine in primary care*, Burlington, Mass, 1999, Butterworth-Heinemann.

12. Stang J, Story MT, Harnack L et al: Relationships between vitamin and mineral supplement use, dietary intake, and dietary adequacy among adolescents, *J Am Diet Assoc* 100:905-910, 2000.

13. Yu SM, Kogan MD, Gergen P: Vitamin-mineral supplement use among preschool children in the United States, *Pediatrics* 100:E4, 1997.

14. Martin KJ, Jordan TR, Vassar AD et al: Herbal and nonherbal alternative medicine use in northwest Ohio, *Ann Pharmacother* 36:1862-1869, 2002.

15. Ottolini MC, Hamburger EK, Loprieato JO et al: Complementary and alternative medicine use among children in the Washington, DC area, *Ambul Pediatr* 1:122-125, 2001.

16. Lanski SL, Greenwald M, Perkins A et al: Herbal therapy use in a pediatric emergency department population: expect the unexpected, *Pediatrics* 111:981-985, 2003.

17. Cala S, Crismon ML, Baumgartner J: A survey of herbal use in children with attention-deficit-hyperactivity disorder or depression, *Pharmacother* 23:222-230, 2003.

18. Andrews L, Lokuge S, Sawyer M et al: The use of alternative therapies by children with asthma: a brief report, *J Paediatr Child Health* 34:131-134, 1998.

19. Johnston GA, Bilbao RM, Graham-Brown RA: The use of complementary medicine in children with atopic dermatitis in secondary care in Leicester, *Br J Dermatol* 149:566-571, 2003.

20. Friedman T, Slayton WB, Allen LS et al: Use of alternative therapies for children with cancer, *Pediatrics* 100:E1, 1997.

21. Heuschkel R, Afzal N, Wuerth A et al: Complementary medicine use in children and young adults with inflammatory bowel disease, *Am J Gastroenterol* 97:382-388, 2002.

22. Hagen LE, Schneider R, Stephens D et al: Use of complementary and alternative medicine by pediatric rheumatology patients, *Arthritis Rheumatism* 49:3-6, 2003.

23. U.S. Food and Drug Administration: *What is a botanical drug?* Available at www.fda.gov/cder/Offices/ODE_V_BRT/botanicalDrug.htm. Accessed July 6, 2004.

24. *Considerations for NCCAM Clinical Trial Grant Applications.* Available at nccam.nih.gov/research/policies/clinical-considerations.htm#skipnav. Accessed June 30, 2004.

25. Djerassi D, Connolly JD, Faulkner DJ et al: *Dictionary of natural products*, New York, 1997, Chapman & Hall/CRC.

26. U.S. Food and Drug Administration: *Dietary supplement health and education act of 1994, sec 3, defitions.* Available at www.fda.gov/opacom/laws/dshea.html#sec3. Accessed February 11, 2008.

27. ASHP Statement on the use of dietary supplements, *Am J Health System Pharm* 61:1707-1711, 2004.

28. Furbee B, Wermuth M: Life-threatening plant poisoning, *Crit Care Clin* 13:849-888, 1997.

29. Huxtable RJ: Herbal teas and toxins: novel aspects of pyrrolizidine poisoning in the United States, *Perspect Biol Med* 24:1-14, 1980.

30. Centers for Disease Control & Prevention: Water hemlock poisoning—Maine, 1992, *MMWR Morbidity Mortality Weekly Report* 43:229-231, 1994.

31. Siegel R: Kola, ginseng, and mislabeled herbs, *J Am Med Assoc* 237:25, 1978.

32. Lau KK, Lai CK, Chan AW: Phenytoin poisoning after using Chinese proprietary medicines, *Human Exper Toxicol* 19:385-386, 2000.

33. Kaltsas HJ: Patent poisons, *Altern Med* Nov:24-28, 1999.

34. Nelson L, Shih R, Hoffman R: Aplastic anemia induced by an adulterated herbal medication, *Clin Toxicol* 33:467-470, 1995.

35. Boyer EW, Kearney S, Shannon MW et al: Poisoning from a dietary supplement administered during hospitalization, *Pediatrics* 109:49, 2002.

36. Toxic reactions to plant products sold in health food stores, *Med Lett Drugs Therapeutics* 21:29-32, 1979.

37. Kelly KJ, Neu J, Camitta BM et al: Methemoglobinemia in an infant treated with the folk remedy glycerated asafetida, *Pediatrics* 73:717-719, 1984.

38. Soderberg TA, Johansson A, Gref R: Toxic effects of some conifer resin acids and tea tree oil on human epithelial and fibroblast cells, *Toxicology* 107:99-109, 1996.

39. Pecevski J, Savkovic N, Radivojevic D et al: Effect of oil of nutmeg on the fertility and induction of meiotic chromosome rearrangements in mice and their first generation, *Toxicol Lett* 7:239-243, 1981.

40. Roulet M, Laurini R, Rivier L et al: Hepatic veno-occlusive disease in newborn infant of a woman drinking herbal tea, *J Pediatr* 112:433-436, 1988.

41. Pages N, Fournier G, Chamorro G et al: Teratogenic effects of *Plecanthus fruticosus* essential oil in mice, *Planta Medica* 54:296-298, 1988.

42. Smith AY, Feddersen RM, Gardner KD Jr et al: Cystic renal cell carcinoma and acquired renal cystic disease associated with consumption of chaparral teas: a case report, *J Urol* 152:2089-2091, 1994.

43. Arlt VM, Stibrova M, Schmeiser H et al: Aristolochic acid as a probable human cancer hazard in herbal remedies: a review, *Mutagenesis* 342:1686-1692, 2002.

44. Nortier JL, Martinez MC, Schmeiser HH, et al: Urothelial carcinoma associated with the use of a Chinese herb, *Aristolochia fangchi*, *N Engl J Med* 342:1686-1692, 2000.

45. Ang-Lee MK, Moss J, Yuan CS: Herbal medicines and perioperative care, *J Am Med Assoc* 286:208-216, 2001.

46. Jadad AR, Moore RA, Carroll D et al: Assessing the quality of reports of randomized clinical trials: is blinding necessary? *Control Clin Trial* 17:1-12, 1996.

47. Natural Standard: Health and Wellness database. Available at www.naturalstandard.com. Accessed: February 11, 2008.

48. Schwartz R: Enhancing children's satisfaction with antibiotic therapy: a taste of several antibiotic suspensions, *Arch Pediatr Adolesc Med* 151:599-602, 1997.

49. Schultz V, Hansel R, Tyler V: *Rational phytotherapy: a physicians' guide to herbal medicine*, ed 3, New York, 1998, Springer.

50. Rotblatt M, Ziment I: *Evidence-based herbal medicine*, Philadelphia, 2001, Hanley and Belfus.

Probiotics

1. Schrezenenmeir J, de Vrese M: Probiotics, prebiotics, and synbiotics—approaching a definition, *Am J Clin Nutr* 73:361S-364S, 2001.

2. Vanderhoof J: Preface, *Am J Gastroenterol* 95(suppl):1, 2000.

3. Pasteur L et al: Charbon et septicemia, *C Roy Soc Biol* 85:101, 1877.

4. Sanders ME: Considerations for use of probiotic bacteria to modulate human health, *J Nutr* 130:384S-390S, 2000.

4a. Metchnikoff E: *The prolongation of life: optimistic studies*, London, 1907, William Heinemann.

5. Lilley DM, Stillwell RH: Probiotics: growth promoting factors produced by microorganisms, *Science* 147:747-748, 1965.

6. Bourlioux P, Koletzko B, Guarner F et al: The intestine and its microflora are partners for the protection of the host: report on the Danone Symposium "The Intelligent Intestine," held in Paris, June 14, 2002, *Am J Clin Nutr* 78:675-683, 2003.

7. Gorbach SL: Efficacy of *Lactobacillus* in treatment of acute diarrhea, *Nutr Today* 31:19S-23S, 1996.

8. Isolauri E, Juntunen M, Rautanen T et al: A human *Lactobacillus* strain (*Lactobacillus casei* sp. strain GG) promotes recovery from acute diarrhea in children, *Pediatrics* 88:90-97, 1991.

9. Marteau PR, de Vrese M, Cellier CJ et al: Protection from gastrointestinal diseases with the use of probiotics, *Am J Clin Nutr* 73(suppl):430S-436S, 2001.

10. Shornikova A-V et al: *Lactobacillus reuteri* as a therapeutic agent in acute diarrhea in young children, *J Pediatr Gastroenterol Nutr* 24:399-404, 1997.

11. Ribiero H et al: Reduction of diarrheal illness following administration of *Lactobacillus plantarum* 299V in a daycare facility (abstract), *J Pediatr Gastroenterol Nutr* 265:561, 1998.

12. Chapoy P: Treatment of acute infantile diarrhea: controlled trial of *Saccharomyces boulardii*, *Ann Pediatr (Paris)* 32:561-563, 1985.

13. Cetina-Saurig et al: Evaluacion terapeutica de *Saccharomyces boulardii* en ninos con diarrea aguda, *Tribuna Medica* 56:111-115, 1989.

14. Shornikova AV, Casas IA, Isolauri E et al: *Lactobacillus reuteri* as a therapeutic agent in acute diarrhea in young children, *J Pediatr Gastroenterol Nutr* 24:399-404, 1997.

15. Guarino A, Canani RB, Spagnuolo MI et al: Oral bacteria therapy reduces the duration of symptoms and of viral excretion in children with mild diarrhea, *J Pediatr Gastroenterol Nutr* 25:516-519, 1997.

16. Saavedra J: Probiotics and infectious diarrhea, *Am J Gastroenterol* 95(suppl):S16-S18, 2000.

17. Saavedra J, Bauman NA, Oung I et al: Feeding of *Bifidobacterium bifidum* and *Streptococcus thermophilus* to infants in hospital for prevention of diarrhea and shedding of rotavirus, *Lancet* 344:1046-1049, 1994.

18. Majamaa H, Isolauri E, Saxelin M et al: Lactic acid bacteria in treatment of acute rotavirus gastroenteritis, *J Pediatr Gastroenterol Nutr* 20:333-339, 1995.

19. Van Niel CW, Feudtner C, Garrison MM et al: *Lactobacillus* therapy for acute infectious diarrhea in children: a meta-analysis, *Pediatrics* 109:678-684, 2002.

20. Rosenfeldt V, Michaelsen KF, Jakobsen M et al: Effect of probiotic *Lactobacillus* strains on acute diarrhea in a cohort of non-hospitalized children attending day-care centers, *Pediatr Infect Dis J* 21:417-419, 2002.

21. Huang S, Bousvaros A, Lee JW et al: Efficacy of probiotic use in acute diarrhea in children: a meta-analysis, *Dig Dis Sci* 47:2625-2634, 2002.

22. Guandalini S, Pensabene L, Zikri MA et al: *Lactobacillus* GG administered in oral rehydration solution to children with acute diarrhea: a multicenter European trial, *J Pediatr Gastroenterol Nutr* 30:54-60, 2000.

23. www.drweil.com. Accessed August 18, 2003.

24. Isolauri E, Sütas Y, Kankaanpää P et al: Probiotics: effects on immunity, *Am J Clin Nutr* 73(suppl):S444-S450, 2001.

25. Vanderhoof JA, Whitney DB, Antonson DL et al: *Lactobacillus* GG in the prevention of antibiotic-associated diarrhea in children, *J Pediatr* 135:564-568, 1999.

26. Arvola T, Laiko K, Torkkeli S et al: Prophylactic *Lactobacillus* GG reduces antibiotic-associated diarrhea in children with respiratory infections: a randomized study, *Pediatrics* 104:e64, 1999.

27. Gorbach SL, Chang TW, Goldin B et al: Successful treatment of relapsing *Clostridium difficile* colitis with *Lactobacillus* GG [letter], *Lancet* 2:1519, 1987.

28. McFarland LV: Biotherapeutic agents for *Clostridium difficile*-associated disease. In Elmer GW, McFarland LV, Surawicz CM, editors: *Biotherapeutic agents and infectious diseases*, Totowa, NJ, 1999, Humana Press, pp 159-193.

29. Pochapin M: The effect of probiotics on *Clostridium difficile* diarrhea, *Am J Gastroenterol* 95(suppl 1):511-513, 2000.

30. Biller JA, Katz AJ, Flores AF et al: Treatment of recurrent *Clostridium difficile* colitis with Lactobacillus GG, *J Pediatr Gastroenterol Nutr* 21:224-226, 1995.

31. McFarland LV, Mulligan ME, Kwok RY et al: Nosocomial acquisition of *C. difficile* infection, *N Engl J Med* 1989; 320:204-210, 1989.

32. Kelly CP, Pothoulakis C, LaMont JT: *Clostridium difficile* colitis, *N Engl J Med* 330:257-262, 1994.

Probiotics Suggested Readings

Agerholm-Larsen L, Raben A, Haulrik N et al: Effect of 8 week intake of probiotic milk products on risk factors for cardiovascular diseases, *Eur J Clin Nutr* 54:288-297, 2000.

Bazzochi G: Intestinal microflora and oral bacteriotherapy in irritable bowel syndrome, *Dig Liver Dis* 34(suppl 2):S48-S53, 2002.

Biller JA, Katz AJ, Flores AF et al: Treatment of recurrent *Clostridium difficile* colitis with *Lactobacillus* GG, *J Pediatr Gastroenterol Nutr* 21:224-226, 1995.

Brady LJ, Gallaher DD, Busta FF: The role of probiotic cultures in the prevention of colon cancer, *J Nutr* 130(2S Suppl):410S-414S, 2000.

Campieri M et al: Probiotics in inflammatory bowel disease: new insight into pathogenesis or a possible therapeutic alternative? *Gastroenterology* 116:1246-1249, 1999.

Colombel JF, Cortot A, Neut C et al: Yoghurt with *Bifidobacterium longum* reduces erythromycin-induced gastrointersinal effects [letter], *Lancet* 2:43, 1987.

Cremonini F, Di Caro S, Covino M et al: Effect of different probiotic preparations on anti-*Helicobacter pylori* therapy-related side effects: a parallel group, triple blind, placebo-controlled study, *Am J Gastroenterol* 97:2744-2749, 2002.

Cummings JH et al: Fecal weight, colon cancer risk and dietary intake of non-starch polysaccharides (dietary fiber), *Gastroenterology* 103:1408-1412, 1992.

Dani C, Biadaioli R, Bertini G et al: Probiotics feeding in prevention of urinary tract infection, bacterial sepsis and necrotizing enterocolitis in preterm infants, *Biol Neonate* 82:103-108, 2002.

Davidson GP, Butler RN: Probiotics in pediatric gastrointestinal disorders, *Curr Opin Pediatr* 12:477-481, 2000.

Delzenne NM, Kok N: Effects of fructans-type prebiotics on lipid metabolism, *Am J Clin Nutr* 73(suppl):456S-458S, 2001.

de Vrese M et al: Probiotics—compensation for lactase insufficiency, *Am J Clin Nutr* 73(suppl):421S-429S, 2001.

Faber SM: Are probiotics useful in irritable bowel syndrome? *J Clin Gastroenterol* 37:93-94, 2003.

Felley C, Michetti P: Probiotics and *Helicobacter pylori*, *Best Pract Res Clin Gastroenterol* 17:785-791, 2003.

Floch M: Probiotics, irritable bowel syndrome, and inflammatory bowel disease, *Curr Treat Options Gastroenterol* 6:283-288, 2003.

Gibson GR, Roberfroid MB: Dietary manipulation of the human colonic microbiota: introducing the concept of prebiotics, *J Nutr* 125:1401-1412, 1995.

Gionchetti P, Rizzello F, Venturi A et al: Probiotics in infective diarrhea and inflammatory bowel diseases, *J Gastroenterol Hepatol* 15:489-493, 2000.

Gionchetti P et al: Maintenance therapy of chronic pouchitis: a randomized, placebo-controlled, double blind trial with a new probiotic preparation, *Gastroenterology* 114:A4037, 1998.

Gionchetti P et al: Microflora in the IBD pathogenesis. Possible therapeutic use of probiotics, *Gastroenterol Int* 11:108-110, 1998.

Gionchetti P et al: Prophylaxis of pouchitis onset with probiotic therapy: a double-blind placebo-controlled trial, *Gastroenterology* 124:1202-1209, 2003.

Gionchetti P et al: Oral bacteriotherapy as maintenance treatment in patients with chronic pouchitis: a double-blind, placebo-controlled trial, *Gastroenterology* 119:305-309, 2000.

Goldin BR, Gualtieri LJ, Moore RP: The effect of *Lactobacillus GG* on the initiation and promotion of dimethylhydrazine-induced intestinal tumors in the rat, *Nutr Cancer* 25:197-204, 1996.

Grönlund MM, Lehtonen OP, Eerola E et al: Fecal microflora in healthy infants born by different methods of delivery: permanent changes in intestinal flora after cesarean section, *J Pediatr Gastroenterol Nutr* 28:19-25, 1999.

Guarino A: Effects of probiotics in children with cystic fibrosis, *Gastroenterol Int* 11:91, 1998.

Hamilton-Miller JM: The role of probiotics in the treatment and prevention of *Helicobacter pylori infection,* Int J Antimicrob Agents 22:360-366, 2003.

Harmsen HJ, Wildeboer-Veloo AC, Raangs GC et al: Analysis of intestinal flora development in breastfed and formula-fed infants by using molecular identification and detection methods, *J Pediatr Gastroenterol Nutr* 30:61-67, 2000.

Hilton E, Kolakowsi P, Singer C et al: Efficacy of *Lactobacillus GG* as a diarrheal preventive in travelers, *J Travel Med* 4:41-43, 1997.

Hooper LV, Gordon JI: Commensal host-bacterial relationships in the gut, *Science* 292:1115-1118, 2001.

Hooper LV, Wong MH, Thelin A et al: Molecular analysis of commensal host-microbial relationships in the intestine, *Science* 291:881-884, 2001.

Hughes VL, Hillier SL: Microbiologic characteristics of *Lactobacillus* products used for colonization of the vagina, *Obstet Gynecol* 75:244-248, 1990.

Ishibashi N, Yamazaki S: Probiotics and safety, *Am J Clin Nutr* 73(suppl):465S-470S, 2001.

Isolauri E, Joensuu J, Suomalainen H et al: Improved immunogenicity of oral DxRRV reassortment rotavirus vaccine by *Lactobacillus casei GG, Vaccine* 13:310-312, 1995.

Isolauri E et al: Probiotics in the management of atopic eczema, *Clin Exp Allergy* 30:1605-1610, 2000.

Isolauri E, Majamaa H, Arvola T et al: *Lactobacillus casei* strain GG reverses increased gastrointestinal permeability induced by cow milk in suckling rats, *Gastroenterology* 105:1643-1650, 1993.

Kabir AM, Aiba Y, Takagi A et al: Prevention of *Helicobacter pylori* infection by lactobacilli in a gnotobiotic murine model, *Gut* 41:49-55, 1997.

Kalliomaki M, et al: Probiotics in primary prevention of atopic disease: a randomized placebo-controlled trial, *Lancet* 357:1076-1079, 2001.

Kim HJ: A randomized controlled trial of a probiotic, VSL#3, on gut transit and symptoms in diarrhoea-predominant irritable bowel syndrome, *Aliment Pharmacol Ther* 17:895-904, 2003.

Kim HS, Gilliland SE: *Lactobacillus acidophilus* as a dietary adjunct for milk to aid lactose digestion in humans, J Dairy Sci 66:959-966, 1983.

Kolars JC, Levitt MD, Aouji M et al: Yogurt—an autodigesting source of lactose, N Engl J Med 310:1-3, 1984.

Kollaritch H et al: Prophylaxe der Reis-diarrhoe mit Saccharomyces boulardii, *Fortschr Med* 111:153-156, 1993.

Linsalata M, Russo F, Berloco P et al: The influence of *Lactobacillus brevis* on ornithine decarboxylase activity and polyamine profiles in *Helicobacter pylori*-infected gastric mucosa, *Helicobacter* 9:165-172, 2004.

Lodinová-Zádníková R, Cukrowska B, Tlaskalova-Hogenova H: Oral administration of probiotic *Escherichia coli* after birth reduces frequency of allergies and repeated infections later in life (after 10 and 20 years), *Int Arch Allergy Immunol* 131:209-211, 2003.

Madsen K, Cornish A, Soper P et al: Probiotic bacteria enhance murine and human intestinal epithelial barrier function, *Gastroenterology* 121:580-591, 2001.

Majamaa H, Isolauri E: Probiotics: a novel approach in the management of food allergy, *J Allergy Clin Immunol* 99:179-185, 1997.

Malin M, Suomalainen H, Saxelin M et al: Promotion of IgA immune response in patients with Crohn's disease by oral bacteriotherapy with *Lactobacillus GG, Ann Nutr Metab* 40:137-145, 1996.

Malin M, Verronen P, Mykkänen H et al: Increased bacterial urease activity in faeces in juvenile chronic arthritis: evidence of altered intestinal microflora? *Brit J Rheumatol* 35:689, 1996.

McGroarty JA: Probiotic use of lactobacilli in the human female urogenital tract, *FEMS Immunol Med Microbiol* 6:251-264, 1993.

Naidu AS et al: Probiotic spectra of lactic acid bacteria. In Clydesdale FM, editor: *Critical reviews in food science and nutrition,* Boca Raton, Fla, 1999, CRC Press.

Nenonen MT, Helve TA, Rauma AL et al: Uncooked, lactobacilli-rich, vegan food and rheumatoid arthritis, *Brit J Rheumatol* 37:274-281, 1998.

Niedzielin K, Kordecki H, Birkenfeld B: A controlled, double-blind, randomized study on the efficacy of *Lactobacillus plantarum* 299V in patients with irritable bowel syndrome, *Eur J Gastroenterol Hepatol* 13:1143-1147, 2001.

Notario R, Leardini N, Borda N et al: [Hepatic abscess and bacteremia due to *Lactobacillus rhamnosus*], *Rev Argent Microbiol* 35:100-101, 2003.

Oksanen PJ, Salminen S, Saxelin M, et al: Prevention of diarrhea by *Lactobacillus GG, Ann Med* 22:53-56, 1990.

Rachmilewitz D, Katakura K, Karmeli F et al: Toll-like receptor 9 signaling mediates the anti-inflammatory effects of probiotics in murine experimental colitis, *Gastroenterology* 126:520-528, 2004.

Rautava S, Kalliomäki M, Isolauri E et al: Probiotics during pregnancy and breastfeeding might confer immunomodulatory protection against atopic disease in the infant, *J Allergy Clin Immunol* 109:119-121, 2002.

Rautio M et al: Liver abscess due to a *Lactobacillus rhamnosus* strain indistinguishable from *L. rhamnosus* strain GG, *Clin Infect Dis* 28:1159-1160, 1998.

Reddy BS: Prevention of colon cancer by pre- and probiotics: evidence from laboratory studies, *Br J Nutr* 80(suppl 2):S219-S223, 1998.

Reddy BS, Hamid R, Rao CV: Effect of dietary oligofructose and inulin on colonic preneoplastic aberrant crypt foci inhibition, *Carcinogenesis* 18:1371-1374, 1997.

Reid G: Probiotic agents to protect the urogenital tract against infection, *Am J Clin Nutr* 73(suppl):437S-443S, 2001.

Reid G, Bruce AW, Taylor M: Influence of three-day antimicrobial therapy and *Lactobacillus* suppositories on recurrence of urinary tract infections, *Clin Ther* 14:11-16, 1992.

Reid G et al: Instillation of *Lactobacillus* and stimulation of indigenous organisms to prevent recurrence of urinary tract infections, *Microecol Ther* 65:3763-3766, 1995.

Roberfroid MB: Functional effects of food components and the gastrointestinal system: chicory fructooligosaccharides, *Nutr Rev* 54:S38-S42, 1996.

Robinson EL, Thompson WL: Effect on weight gain and the addition of *Lactobacillus acidophilus* to the formula of newborn infants, *J Pediatr* 41:395-398, 1952.

Rowlands IR, Rumney CJ, Coutts JT et al: Effect of *Bifidobacterium longum* and inulin on gut bacterial metabolism and carcinogen-induced crypt foci in rats, *Carcinogenesis* 19:281-285, 1998.

Saavedra JM, Abi-Hanna A, Moore N et al: Long-term consumption of infant formulas containing live probiotic bacteria: tolerance and safety, *Am J Clin Nutr* 79:261-267, 2004.

Saggioro A: Probiotics in the treatment of irritable bowel syndrome, *J Clin Gastroenterol* 38(6 suppl):S104-S106, 2004.

Salminen MK, Tynkkynen S, Rautelin H et al: *Lactobacillus* bacteremia during a rapid increase in probiotic use of *Lactobacillus rhamnosus* GG in Finland, *Clin Infect Dis* 35:1155-1160, 2002.

Salminen S, von Wright A, Morelli L et al: Demonstration of safety of probiotics—a review, *Int J Food Microbiol* 44:93-106, 1998.

Schultz M, Linde HJ, Lehn N et al: Immunomodulatory consequences of oral administration of *Lactobacillus rhamnosus* strain GG in healthy volunteers, *J Dairy Res* 70:165-173, 2003.

Schultz M, Sartor RB: Probiotics and inflammatory bowel diseases, *Am J Gastroenterol* 95(suppl):S19-S21, 2000.

Sen S: Effect of *Lactobacillus plantarum* 299v on colonic fermentation and symptoms of irritable bowel syndrome, *Dig Dis Sci* 47:2615-2620, 2002.

Sgouras D, Maragkoudakis P, Petraki K et al: In vitro and in vivo inhibition of *Helicobacter pylori* by *Lactobacillus casei* strain Shirota, *Appl Environ Microbiol* 70:518-526, 2004.

Shanahan F: Probiotics and inflammatory disease: is there a scientific rationale? *Inflamm Bowel Dis* 6:107-115, 2000.

Sheu BS, Wu JJ, Lo CY et al: Impact of supplement with *Lactobacillus*- and *Bifidobacterium*-containing yogurt on triple therapy for *Helicobacter pylori* eradication, *Aliment Pharmacol Ther* 16:1669-1675, 2002.

Silva M, Jacobus NV, Deneke C et al: Antimicrobial substance from a human *Lactobacillus* strain, *Antimicrob Agents Chemother* 31:1231-1233, 1987.

Smith S et al: Quorum sensing within the gut, *Microbiol Ecol Health Dis* 2(suppl):81-92, 2000.

Taranto MP, Medici M, Perdigon G et al: Evidence for hypocholesterolemic effect of *Lactobacillus reuteri* in hypercholesterolemic mice, *J Dairy Sci* 81:2336-2340, 1998.

Taylor GR, Williams CM: Effects of probiotics and prebiotics on blood lipids, *Br J Nutr* 80(suppl 2):S225-S230, 1998.

Ushiyama A, Tanaka K, Aiba Y et al: *Lactobacillus gasseri* OLL2716 as a probiotic in clarithromycin-resistant *Helicobacter pylori* infection, *J Gastroenterol Hepatol* 18:986-991, 2003.

Vanderhoof JA: Probiotics and intestinal inflammatory disorders in infants and children, *J Pediatr Gastroenterol Nutr* 30:S34-S38, 2000.

Wagner RD, Warner T, Roberts L et al: Colonization of congenitally immunodeficient mice with probiotic bacteria, *Infect Immun* 65:3345-3351, 1995.

Wendakoon CN, Thomson AB, Ozimek L: Lack of therapeutic effect of a specially designed yogurt for the eradication of *Helicobacter pylori* infection, *Digestion* 65:16-20, 2002.

Wheeler JG, Shema SJ, Bogle ML, et al: Immune and clinical impact of *Lactobacillus acidophilus* on asthma, *Ann Allergy Asthma Immunol* 79:229-233, 1997.

Wollowski I, Rechkemmer G, Pool-Zobel BL: Protective role of probiotics and prebiotics in colon cancer, *Am J Clin Nutr* 73(suppl):451S-455S, 2001.

Young RJ, Huffman S: Probiotic use in children, *J Pediatr Health Care* 17:277-283, 2003.

Clinical Application of Chinese Herbal Products in Children*

Chinese herbs can be given to children of all ages, including newborns. The herbal products are available as pills, tablets, powder, liquid, and syrup. At the present time, pills are the most common form. Between 7 and 13 years of age, when children can swallow pills, the dose can be given as follows: age 7 to 10 years, ½ adult dose; 11+ years, full adult dose.

For children who are unable to swallow pills, the pills can be prepared as a liquid as follows:

1. Grind the pills into a powder in a small household coffee grinder.
2. Mix ½ to 1 tsp of the powder with enough boiling water to yield 3 tsp of syrupy liquid.
3. Administer every 3 hours:
   Infants <1 year: 1 mL
   Age 1 to 4 years: 1 mL for every year plus 1 mL (e.g., 3 mL for a 2 year old)
   Age 5 and older: 1 tsp

It is best to follow the dose administration recommended by the practitioner treating the child.

This author and consultants recommend using herbal products made under Good Manufacturing Practice (GMP) standards. The following companies meet GMP standards:

Bio Essence Brand, manufactured by Bio Essence Corp., Richmond, Calif.

Herbal Times Brand manufactured by Nuherbs, Inc., Oakland, Calfi.

Plum Flower Brand, manufactured by Mayway, Oakland, Calif.

Evergreen, La Puente, Calif.

Honso, Phoenix, Ariz.

KPC, distributed by Golden Flower Chinese Herbs, Placitas, N.M.

Mintong, distributed by Bio Essence Corp., Richmond, Calif.

Qualiherb, Santa Fe Springs, Calif.

Sunten Products, distributed by Brion Corporation, Irvine, Calif.

Blue Poppy, Boulder, Colo.

Golden Flower, Placitas, N.M.

Health Concerns, Oakland, Calif.

Kan Herb Company, Scotts Valley, Calif.

---

*Dr. Loo would like to thank Jake Paul Fratkin and Randall Neustaedter for consulting on this section.

Toxicity of Selected Herbs and Dietary Supplements

LATIN NAME	COMMON NAME(S)	TOXIC COMPONENT(S)	TOXIC EFFECTS IN HUMANS
Aconitum napellus, Aconitum columbianum[1-3]	Monk's-hood	Aconite	Cardiac dysrhythmias, hemodynamic instability, seizures, coma, weakness, nausea, emesis, paresthesias
Anthmis nobilis, Matricaria chamomilia, Compositae spp.[4]	Chamomile	Chamomile	Anaphylaxis, allergic reactions, contact dermatitis
Aristolochia spp.[5-10]	Wild ginger	Aristolochic acid	Acute renal failure, uroepithelial carcinoma
Artemesia spp.[11,12]	Wormwood	Thujone	Headache, tremors, ataxia, seizures, dementia, renal failure
Cinnamomum spp.[13-15]	Cinnamon oil	Cinnamaldehyde	Dermatitis, abuse syndrome, stomatitis venenata
Crotalaria spp.[16,20,22-24,26]	Rattle box, rattlepods	Pyrrolizidine alkaloids	Hepatic veno-occlusive disease
Digitalis purpurea[31]	Foxglove	Cardiac glycosides	Dysrhythmias, cardiac arrest, hypotension, hyperkalemia, coma
Ephedra sinica, Ephedra hebra, Ephedra intermedia, Ephedra equisetina[32-55]	Ephedra	Phenylethylamine compounds	Hypertension, stroke, seizures, psychiatric disorders
Ferula assafoetida[56]	Gum asafetida		Methemoglobinemia
Glycyrrhiza glabra[57]	Licorice	Glycyrrhetic acid	Hypertension, hypokalemia, dysrhythmias
Heliotropium spp.[16,20,22-24,26]	Heliotrope, turnsole	Pyrrolizidine alkaloids	Hepatic veno-occlusive disease
Larrea divericata, Larrea tridentate[58-69]	Chaparral	Nordihydroguaiaretic acid (NDGA)	Nausea, emesis, lethargy, hepatitis, hepatic carcinoma
Lobelia inflata[70]	Lobelia, Indian tobacco	Nicotine	Sweating, nausea, emesis, abdominal pain, dizziness, lethargy
Lycopodium serratum[71-74]	Jin Bu Huan	Levo-tetrahydropalmatine	Acute and chronic hepatitis
Mentha pulegium, Hedeoma spp.[78-80]	Pennyroyal	Pulegone	Hepatitis, fulminant hepatic necrosis, seizures, hemodynamic instability, spontaneous abortion
Myristica fragrans[81-86]	Nutmeg	Myristacin, eugenol	Hallucinations, emesis, headache
Nux vomica[87]	Solang nut	Strychnine	Seizures, abdominal pain, respiratory arrest
Piper methysticum[88-95]	Kava	Kava lactones	Hepatitis, cognitive impairment
Prunus spp.[96,97]	Amygdalin, laetrile	Cyanide	Hypotension, coma, respiratory failure, arrhythmias, cardiac arrest
Senecio jaconaea, Senecio aureus, Senecio echium, Senecio longilobus, Echium spp.[16,20,22-24,26]	Ragwort, groundsel, golden ragwort	Pyrrolizidine alkaloids	Hepatic veno-occlusive disease
Symphytum officinale[16,20,22-24,26]	Comfrey	Pyrrolizidine alkaloids	Hepatic veno-occlusive disease
Teucrium chamaedrys[98-101]	Germander	Diterpinoids	Hepatitis
Tussilogo farfara[16,20,22-24,26]	Coltsfoot	Pyrrolizidine alkaloids	Hepatic veno-occlusive disease

References

1. Fatovich DM: Aconite: a lethal Chinese herb, *Ann Emerg Med* 21:309-311, 1992.
2. Chan TYK, Tse LKK, Chan JCN et al: Aconitine poisoning due to Chinese herbal medicines: a review, *Vet Human Toxicol* 36:452, 1994.
3. Shan TYK, Tomlinson B, Critchley JAH: Aconitine poisoning following the ingestion of Chinese herbal medicines: a report of eight cases, *Austr N Z J Med* 23:268, 1993.
4. Benner MH, Lee HJ: Anaphylactic reaction to chamomile tea, *J Allerg Clin Immunol* 53:307-308, 1973.
5. Abt A, Oh JY, Huntington RA et al: Chinese herbal medicine induced acute renal failure, *Arch Intern Med* 155:211-212, 1995.
6. Arlt VM, Stiborova M, Schmeiser HH: Aristolochic acid as a probable human cancer hazard in herbal remedies: a review, *Mutagenesis* 17:265-277, 2002.
7. Nortier JL, Martinez MC, Schmeiser HH et al: Urothelial carcinoma associated with the use of a Chinese herb, *Aristolochia fangchi, N Engl J Med* 342:1686-1692, 2000.
8. Stiborova M, Frei E, Wiessler M et al. Human enzymes involved in the metabolic activation of carcinogenic aristolochic acids: evidence for reductive activation by cytochromes P450 1A1 and 1A2, *Chem Res Toxicol* 14:1128-1137, 2001.

9. Vanhaelen M, Vanhaelen-Fastre R, But P et al. Identification of aristolochic acid in Chinese herbs, *Lancet* 343:174, 1994.

10. Vanherweghem JL, Depierreux M, Tielemans C et al. Rapidly progressive interstitial renal fibrosis in young women: association with slimming regimen including Chinese herbs, *Lancet* 341: 387-391, 1993.

11. Weisbord SD, Soule JB, Kimmel PL: Poison online—acute renal failure caused by oil of wormwood purchased through the Internet, *N Engl J Med* 337:825-827, 1997.

12. Arnold WN: Vincent van Gogh and the thujone connection, *J Am Med Assoc* 260:3042-3044, 1988.

13. Krenzelok EP, Dean BS: Cinnamon oil abuse by adolescents, *Vet Human Toxicol* 32:162-164, 1990.

14. Miller RL, Gould AR, Bernstein ML: Cinnamon-induced stomatitis venenata, *Oral Surg Oral Med Oral Pathol* 73:708-716, 1992.

15. Pilapil VR: Toxic manifestations of cinnamon oil ingestion in a child, *Clin Pediatr* 28:276, 1989.

16. Abbott PJ: Comfrey: assessing the low-dose health risk, *Med J Austr* 149:678-682, 1988.

17. Anderson PC, McLean AEM: Comfrey and liver damage, *Human Toxicol* 8:68-69, 1989.

18. Awang DVC: Comfrey update, *Herbalgram* 25:20-23, 1991.

19. Bach N, Thung SN, Schaffner F: Comfrey herb tea-induced hepatic veno-occlusive disease, *Am J Med* 87:97-99, 1989.

20. Centers for Disease Control and Prevention: Self-treatment with herbal and other plant derived remedies—rural Mississippi, 1993, *MMWR Morbid Mortal Wkly Rep* 44:204-207, 1995.

21. Hirono L, Mori H, Haga M et al: Carcinogenic activity of *Sympytum officinale*, *J Natl Cancer Inst* 61:865-868, 1978.

22. Huxtable RJ: Herbal teas and toxins: novel aspects of pyrrolizidine poisoning in the United States, *Perspect Biol Med* 24:1-14, 1980.

23. Mattocks AR: Toxicity of pyrrolizidine alkaloids, *Nature* 217: 723-728, 1968.

24. Ridker PM, Ohkuma S, McDermott WV et al: Hepatic venocclusive disease associated with the consumption of pyrrolizidine-containing dietary supplements, *Gastroenterology* 88:1050-1054, 1985.

25. Ridker PM, McDermott WV: Comfrey herb tea and hepatic veno-occlusive disease, *Lancet* 1:657-658, 1989.

26. Robins DJ: Pyrrolizidine alkaloids, *Natur Prod Rep* 12:413-418, 1995.

27. Rode D: Comfrey toxicity revisited, *Trends Pharmacol Sci* 23: 497-499, 2002.

28. Roulet M, Laurini R, Rivier L et al: Hepatic veno-occlusive disease in newborn infant of a woman drinking herbal tea, *J Pediatr* 112:433-436, 1988.

29. Weston CF, Cooper BT, Davies JD, et al. Veno-occlusive disease of the liver secondary to ingestion of comfrey. *Br Med J* 295:183, 1987.

30. Winship KA: Toxicity of comfrey, *Adv Drug React Toxicol Rev* 10:47-59, 1991.

31. Woolf A, Wenger T, Smith TW et al: Use of digoxin-specific Fab fragments for severe pediatric digitalis poisoning: report of a multi-center experience, *N Engl J Med* 326:1739-1744, 1992.

32. Bruno A, Nolte KB, Chapin J: Stroke associated with ephedrine use, *Neurol* 43:1313-1316, 1993.

33. Chua SS, Benrimoj SI: Non-prescription sympathomimetic agents and hypertension, *Med Toxicol* 3:387-417, 1988.

34. Centers for Disease Control and Prevention: Adverse events associated with ephedrine-containing products—Texas, December 1993-September 1995, *MMWR Morbid Mortal Wkly Rep* 45: 689-693, 1996.

35. Cockings JGL, Brown MA: Ephedrine abuse causing acute myocardial infarction, *Med J Austr* 167:199-200, 1997.

36. Doyle H, Kargin M: Herbal stimulant containing ephedrine has also caused psychosis, *Br Med J* 313:756, 1996.

37. Emmanuel NP, Jones C, Lydiard RB: Use of herbal products and symptoms of bipolar disorder, *Am J Psychiatr* 155:1627, 1998.

38. Haller CA, Benowitz NL: Adverse cardiovascular and central nervous system events associated with dietary supplements containing ephedra alkaloids, *N Engl J Med* 343:1833-1838, 2000.

39. Herridge CF, A'brook MF: Ephedrine psychoses, *Br Med J* 2: 160-161, 1968.

40. Hirsch MS, Walter RM, Hasterlik RJ: Subarachnoid hemorrhage following ephedrine and MAO inhibitor, *J Am Med Assoc* 194: 201-202, 1965.

41. Jacobs KM, Hirsch KA: Psychiatric complications of Ma-Huang, *Psychosomatics* 41:58-62, 2000.

42. Kaberi-Otarod J, Conetta R, Kundo KK et al: Ischemic stroke in a user of Thermadrene: a case study in alternative medicine, *Clin Pharmacol Therapeut* 72:343-346, 2002.

43. Kane FJ, Florenzano R: Psychosis accompanying use of bronchodilator compound, *J Am Med Assoc* 215:2116, 1971.

44. Morgenstern LB, Viscoli CM, Kernan WN et al: Use of ephedra-containing products and risk for hemorrhagic stroke, *Neurology* 60:132-135, 2003.

45. Samenuk D, Link MS, Homoud MK et al: Adverse cardiovascular events temporally associated with Ma Huang, an herbal source of ephedrine, *Mayo Clin Proc* 77:12-16, 2002.

46. Shekelle P, Hardy M, Morton SC et al: Ephedra and ephedrine for weight loss and athletic performance enhancement: clinical efficacy and side effects. Evidence report/technology assessment no. 76 (prepared by Southern California Evidence-Based Practice Center, RAND, under contract no. 290-97-0001, task order no. 9). AHRQ Publication No. 03-E022, Rockville, MD, 2003, *Agency for Healthcare Research and Quality.*

47. Stoessl AJ, Young GB, Feasby TE: Intracerebral haemorrhage and angiographic beading following ingestion of catecholaminergics, *Stroke* 16:734-736, 1985.

48. Theoharides TC: Sudden death of a healthy college student related to ephedrine toxicity from a ma huang-containing drink, *J Clin Psychopharmacol* 17:437-439, 1997.

49. To LB, Sangster JF, Rampling D et al: Ephedrine-induced cardiomyopathy, *Med J Austr* 2:35-36, 1980.

50. Traub SJ, Huyek W, Hoffman RS: Dietary supplements containing ephedra alkaloids, *N Engl J Med* 344:1096, 2001.

51. Van Mieghem W, Stevens E, Cosemans J: Ephedrine-induced cardiopathy, *Br Med J* 1:816, 1978.

52. Weesner KM, Denison M, Roberts RJ: Cardiac arrhythmias in an adolescent following ingestion of an over-the-counter stimulant, *Clin Pediatr* 21:700-701, 1982.

53. Whitehouse AM, Duncan JM: Ephedrine psychosis rediscovered, *Br J Psychiatr* 150:258-261, 1987.

54. Wooten MR, Khangure MS, Murphy MJ: Intracerebral hemorrhage and vasculitis related to ephedrine abuse, *Ann Neurol* 13:337-340, 1983.

55. Yin PA: Ephedrine-induced intracerebral hemorrhage and central nervous system vasculitis, *Stroke* 21:1641, 1990.

56. Kelly KJ, Neu J, Camitta BM et al: Methemoglobinemia in an infant treated with the folk remedy glycerated asafetida, *Pediatrics* 73:717-719, 1984.

57. Walker BR, Edwards CRW: Licorice-induced hypertension and syndromes of apparent mineralocorticoid excess, *Endocrinol Metabol Clin N Am* 23:359-377, 1994.

58. Alderman S, Kailas S, Goldfarb S et al: Cholestatic hepatitis after ingestion of chaparral leaf: confirmation by endoscopic retrograde cholangiopancreatography and liver biopsy, *J Clin Gastroenterol* 19:242-247, 1994.

59. Batchelor WB, Heathcote J, Wanless IR: Chaparral-induced hepatic injury, *Am J Gastroenterol* 90:831-833, 1995.

60. Brinker F: *Larrea tridentata* (DC) Coville (chaparral or creosote bush), *Br J Phytother Res* 3:10-29, 1993.

61. Clark F, Reed R: Chaparral-induced toxic hepatitis—California and Texas, 1992. *MMWR Morbid Mortal Wkly Rep* 41:812-814, 1992.

62. Gordon DW, Rosenthal G, Hart J et al: Chaparral ingestion: the broadening spectrum of liver injury caused by herbal medications, *J Am Med Assoc* 273:489-490, 1995.

63. Grant KL, Boyer LV, Erdman BE: Chaparral-induced hepatotoxicity, *Integr Med* 1:83-87, 1998.

64. Heron S, Yarnell E: The safety of low-dose *Larrea tridentata* (DC) Coville (creosote bush or chaparral): a retrospective clinical study, *J Altern Complement Med* 7:175-185, 2001.

65. Katz M, Saibil F: Herbal hepatitis: subacute hepatic necrosis secondary to chaparral leaf, *J Clin Gastroenterol* 12:203-206, 1990.

66. Pritchard D, Obermeyer W, Bradlaw J et al: Primary rate hepatocyte cultures aid in the chemical identification of toxic chaparral *(Larrea tridentata), In Vitro Cell Develop Biol* 30A:91-92, 1994.

67. Sheikh NM, Philen RM, Love LA et al: Chaparral-associated hepatotoxicity, *Arch Intern Med* 157:913-919, 1997.

68. Smith AY, Feddersen RM, Gardner KD Jr et al: Cystic renal cell carcinoma and acquired renal cystic disease associated with consumption of chaparral teas: a case report, *J Urol* 152:2089-2091, 1994.

69. Smith BC Desmond PV: Acute hepatitis induced by ingestion of the herbal medication chaparral, *Austr N Z J Med* 23:526, 1993.

70. Curry S, Bond R, Kunkel D: Acute nicotine poisonings after ingestions of tree tobacco, *Vet Human Toxicol* 30:369, 1988.

71. Horowitz RS, Dart RC, Gomez H et al. Jin Bu Huan toxicity in children—Colorado 1993, *MMWR Morbid Mortal Wkly Rep* 42:633-636, 1993.

72. Horowitz RS, Feldhaus K, Dart RC et al: The clinical spectrum of Jin Bu Huan toxicity, *Arch Intern Med* 156:899-903, 1996.

73. Woolf GM, Petrovic LM, Rojter SE et al: Acute hepatitis associated with the Chinese herbal product Jin Bu Huan, *Ann Intern Med* 121:729-735, 1994.

74. Woolf GM, Rojter SE, Villamil FG et al: Jin Bu Huan toxicity in adults—Los Angeles 1993, *MMWR Morbid Mortal Wkly Rep* 42:920-922, 1993.

75. Anderson IB, Mullen WH, Meeker JE et al: Pennyroyal toxicity: measurement of four metabolites in two cases and review of the literature, *Ann Intern Med* 124:726-734, 1996.

76. Bakerink J, Gospe S, Dimand R et al: Multiple organ failure after ingestion of pennyroyal oil from herbal tea in two infants, *Pediatr* 98:944-947, 1996.

77. Gordon WP, Forte AJ, McMurtry RJ et al: Hepatotoxicity and pulmonary toxicity of pennyroyal oil and its constituent terpenes in the mouse, *Toxicol Appl Pharmacol* 65:413-424, 1982.

78. Gordon WP, Huitric AC, Seth CL et al: The metabolism of the abortifacient terpene, (R)-(+)-Pulegone, to a proximate toxin, menthofuran, *Drug Metabol Dispos* 15:589-594, 1987.

79. Madyastha KM, Moorthy B: Pulegone mediated hepatotoxicity: evidence for covalent binding of R(+)-^{14}C pulegone to microsomal proteins in vitro, *Chem Biol Interact* 72:325-333, 1989.

80. Sullivan JB, Rumack BH, Thomas H et al: Pennyroyal oil poisoning and hepatotoxicity, *J Am Med Assoc* 242:2873-2874, 1979.

81. Abernathy MK, Becker LB: Acute nutmeg intoxication, *Am J Emerg Med* 10:429-430, 1992.

82. Brenner N, Frank OS, Knight E: Chronic nutmeg psychosis, *J R Soc Med* 86:179-180, 1993.

83. Pecevski J, Savkovic N, Radivojevic D et al: Effect of oil of nutmeg on the fertility and induction of meiotic chromosome rearrangements in mice and their first generation, *Toxicol Lett* 7:239-243, 1981.

84. Sangalli BC, Chiang W: Toxicology of nutmeg abuse, *J Toxicol Clin Toxicol* 38:671-678, 2000.

85. Shulgin AT: Possible implication of myristicin as a psychotropic substance, *Nature* 210:380-384, 1966.

86. Weil AT: Nutmeg as a psychoactive drug, *J Psyched Drug* 3:72, 1971.

87. Katz J, Prescott K, Woolf AD: Strychnine poisoning from a traditional Cambodian remedy, *Am J Emerg Med* 14:475-477, 1996.

88. Hepatic toxicity possibly associated with kava-containing products—United States, Germany, Switzerland, 1999-2002, *MMWR Morbid Mortal Wkly Rep* 51:1065-1067, 2002.

89. Cairney S, Maruff P, Clough AR et al: Saccade and cognitive impairment associated with kava intoxication, *Human Psychopharmacol* 18:525-533, 2003.

90. Escher M, Desmeules J, Giostra E et al: Hepatitis associated with kava, a herbal remedy for anxiety, *Br Med J* 322:139, 2001.

91. Gow PJ, Connelly NJ, Hill RL et al: Fatal fulminant hepatic failure induced by a natural therapy containing kava, *Med J Austr* 178:442-443, 2003.

92. Humberston CL, Akhtar J, Krenzelok EP: Acute hepatitis induced by kava kava, *J Toxicol Clin Toxicol* 41:109-113, 2003.

93. Mathews JD, Riley MD, Fejo L et al: Effects of the heavy usage of kava on physical health: summary of a pilot survey in an Aboriginal community, *Med J Austr* 148:548-555, 1988.

94. Russmann S, Lauterburg BH, Helbling A: Kava hepatotoxicity, *Ann Intern Med* 135:68-69, 2001.

95. Spillane PK, Fisher DA, Currie BJ: Neurological manifestations of kava intoxication, *Med J Austr* 167:172-173, 1997.

96. Hall AH, Linden CH, Kulig KW et al: Cyanide poisoning from laetrile ingestion: role of nitrite therapy, *Pediatr* 78:269-272, 1986.

97. Wallace KL, Gerkin R, Mitchell RB: Acute cyanide toxicity due to apricot kernel ingestion, *J Toxicol Clin Toxicol* 34:599, 1996.

98. Fau D, Lekehal M, Farrell G et al: Diterpenoids from germander, an herbal medicine, induce apoptosis in isolated rat hepatocytes, *Gastroenterology* 113:1334-1346, 1997.

99. Laliberte L, Villenueve JP: Hepatitis after the use of germander, an herbal remedy, *Can Med Assoc J* 154:1689-1692, 1996.

100. Larrey D, Vial T, Pauwels A et al: Hepatitis after germander *(Teucrium chamaedrys)* administration. Another instance of herbal medicine hepatotoxicity, *Ann Intern Med* 117:129-132, 1992.

101. Mostefa-Kara N, Pauwels A, Pines E et al: Fatal hepatitis after herbal tea, *Lancet* 340:674, 1992.

Suggested Readings

Bensky D, Barolet R: *Chinese herbal medicine: formulas and strategies*, Seattle, 1990, Eastland Press.

Fratkin JP: *Chinese herbal patent medicines: the clinical desk reference*, Boulder, Colo, 2001, Shya Publications.

Ellis A: *Notes from South Mountain*, Berkeley, Calif, 2003, Moon Publishing.

CHAPTER 8

Abdominal Pain

Acupuncture | May Loo

Aromatherapy | Maura A. Fitzgerald

Chiropractic | Anne Spicer

Herbs—Chinese | May Loo, Harriet Beinfield, Efrem Korngold

Homeopathy | Janet L. Levatin

Magnet Therapy | Agatha P. Colbert, Deborah Risotti

Mind/Body | Timothy Culbert, Lynda Richtsmeier Cyr

Nutrition | Joy A. Weydert

Osteopathy | Jane Carreiro

✳ PEDIATRIC DIAGNOSIS AND TREATMENT

Abdominal pain can be a perplexing problem for the pediatrician. It accounts for the majority of visits made by children and adolescents to pediatricians as well as gastroenterologists,[1] and it is the most common complaint for pediatric hospital admission.[2] It can range from having no significant pathology to being a life-threatening, surgical emergency. The presenting symptoms are further complicated by discrepancy in the child's maturity and sensitivity to pain and by the caretaker's subjective interpretation based on the child's behavior (especially in infants and young children). Differential diagnoses vary according to age and sex of the child and to the timing of onset of symptoms as acute or chronic. Western evaluation consists of a comprehensive physical examination; laboratory studies that include blood, urine, or stool tests; and radiographic studies. Recently, ultrasonography has been shown to be beneficial in evaluating children with abdominal pain.[3-5] An integrated approach can use Western technology to precisely identify the structural pathology and complementary and alternative medicine (CAM) therapies to function in a complementary fashion for identifying and treating energetic disturbances and alleviating pain.

Acute Abdominal Pain

It is important for both Western and CAM pediatric practitioners to be familiar with the common acute abdominal presentations and to differentiate those that require surgery referral for either routine or emergency evaluations.

Acute abdominal pain in children is distinguished both in clinical manifestations and in age of presentation. Gastroenteritis and constipation are common causes of acute onset of abdominal pain at any age. Colic usually presents in infants who are younger than 3 months. Intussusception should be suspected in slightly older infants (6 to 24 months old) who present with sudden, severe abdominal pain. Appendicitis usually affects children between 2 and 18 years of age. Abdominal pain secondary to renal disorders usually presents in the preschooler, and mittelschmerz and pelvic inflammatory disease enter the differential for a menstruating adolescent girl.

Nonsurgical Acute Abdominal Pain

Colic

In babies younger than 3 months, the most common cause of "abdominal pain" is colic, described by the mother as crying episodes with flexion of the legs and distended abdomen (see Chapter 23).

Gastroenteritis

Gastroenteritis is one of the most common presentations of acute abdominal pain in children of all ages. The predominant symptom is diarrhea, sometimes also vomiting, with accompanying generalized, nonspecific abdominal pain. The majority of cases are caused by viruses—correlates with external pathogenic invasion—with rotavirus being the most prevalent. Heat pathogens correlate with bacterial agents, which include the genera *Shigella, Salmonella, Campylobacter, Giardia*, and invasive *Escherichia coli*. Most viral diarrheal illnesses last between 3 and 7 days. Children whose symptoms last longer should have stool cultures to identify nonviral pathogens. Treatment is directed toward the specific stage or level of invasion, with the primary focus on prevention of dehydration (see Chapter 30).

Constipation

Constipation is high on the list of causes of abdominal pain in children. In infants, recurrent episodes should lead to suspicion of Hirschsprung's disease. In breastfed infants, periods of 7 to 10 days without stools can be normal. Abdominal pain is often accompanied by straining when attempting to defecate. This is often seen in the school-aged child who is fearful of using the public toilet. Encopresis is a condition that results when a child holds enough stool in the colon to cause abnormal stretching of the bowel, resulting in decreased motility. Leakage of loose bowel contents with staining of the underwear is common (see Chapter 26).

Urological causes of abdominal pain

Urological causes of abdominal pain include urinary tract infections, congenital genitourinary tract anomalies, kidney stones, and ureteropelvic junction obstruction.[6-9] (See Chapter 61, Urinary Cystitis.)

Ulcer disease

In children younger than 6 years, stress ulcers are most common. Children older than 10 years can more verbally describe the ulcer symptoms, which usually consists of epigastric pain occurring after meals and may be accompanied by nausea and abdominal distention. The correlation of duodenal ulcerations and antral gastritis has been shown in children.[10] An Italian report of four adult patients treated with acupuncture demonstrated complete resolution of symptoms and healing of lesions demonstrated by gastroscopy.[11] Suspicion of ulcer in children should be appropriately diagnosed with endoscopic evaluation and treatment coordinated with the gastroenterologist.

Pancreatitis

Pancreatitis, inflammation of the pancreas, is rare but may occur at any age in childhood. It may be idiopathic with familial predisposition. The most common cause of pancreatitis in children is mumps infection. Trauma and drugs such as steroids can lead to pancreatic symptoms.[12] Ultrasonography usually shows an abnormal, nonspecific swelling of the pancreas.

Acute surgical abdomen such as appendicitis, intussusception, and intestinal obstruction and nonacute conditions such as pyloric stenosis, inguinal hernia, and gallstones should be referred to surgery.

Chronic Recurrent Abdominal Pain

Children and adolescents with chronic abdominal pain are challenging both for their caregivers and their pediatricians. The daily lives and activities of affected children and their families are interrupted by the distressing symptoms. For the past 40 years, the definition of chronic abdominal pain denotes at least three pain episodes over at least 3 months interfering with function.[1] In clinical practice, it is generally believed that pain exceeding 1 or 2 months in duration can be considered chronic.[13,14]

Previously, chronic abdominal pain in children was referred to as "recurrent abdominal pain" (RAP) and classified as either organic RAP, which applied to 5% to 10% of children,[15-18] or functional abdominal pain, which affected 90% to 95% of children with chronic abdominal pain.[19,20]

In March 2005, the American Academy of Pediatrics (AAP) and the North American Society for Pediatric Gastroenterology, Hepatology, and Nutrition issued a policy statement recommending that the term "recurrent abdominal pain" no longer be used: "Functional abdominal pain is the most common cause of chronic abdominal pain. It is a specific diagnosis that needs to be distinguished from anatomic, infectious, inflammatory, or metabolic causes of abdominal pain."[13,14] Functional abdominal pain should be categorized as one or a combination of functional dyspepsia, irritable bowel syndrome (IBS), abdominal migraine, or functional abdominal pain syndrome.

Functional abdominal pain

Functional abdominal pain consists of abdominal pain without demonstrable evidence of a pathological condition, such as anatomical, metabolic, infectious, inflammatory, or neoplastic disorder. Functional abdominal pain may present with symptoms typical of functional dyspepsia, IBS, abdominal migraine, or functional abdominal pain syndrome.

Functional dyspepsia

Functional dyspepsia is usually epigastric or upper abdominal pain that is temporally related to eating, with associated symptoms such as nausea, vomiting, heartburn, abdominal bloating, regurgitation of food, early satiety, excessive hiccups, and excessive belching. There may be altered bowel patterns such as diarrhea, constipation, or a sense of incomplete evacuation with bowel movements.[12-14]

Irritable bowel syndrome

Irritable bowel syndrome is typically periumbilical pain that varies in intensity, has inconsistently alternating pain and painfree periods, and is usually associated with irregular bowel movements and pain relief with defecation, sense of urgency, and feeling of bloating or abdominal distention.[12-14]

Abdominal migraine

Previously considered controversial,[21] AAP now categorizes abdominal migraine as a definitive functional abdominal pain with features of migraine (paroxysmal abdominal pain associated with anorexia, nausea, vomiting, or pallor as well as a maternal history of migraine headaches).[12,13] The abdominal component will often cease by adolescence and be replaced with more classical migrainous headaches.[22,23]

Functional abdominal pain syndrome

Functional abdominal pain syndrome consists of functional abdominal pain without the characteristics of dyspepsia, IBS, or abdominal migraine.[12,13]

The pathophysiology of functional abdominal pain is thought to be due to dysregulation or dysfunction in the bidirectional communication between the enteric nervous system (ENS), a rich and complex nervous system that envelops the entire gastrointestinal (GI) tract, and the central nervous system.[24] Recent data dispute the previous tenet that functional abdominal pain is due to a baseline motility disturbance. Instead, these children may have an abnormal bowel reactivity to physiological stimuli (meal, gut distention, hormonal changes), noxious stressful stimuli (inflammatory processes), or psychological stressful stimuli (parental separation, anxiety).[12,25]

Increasing evidence suggests that functional abdominal pain may be associated with visceral hyperalgesia, a decreased threshold for pain in response to changes in intraluminal pressure.[26,27]

Mucosal inflammatory processes attributable to infections, allergies, or primary inflammatory diseases may cause sensitization of afferent nerves and have been associated with the onset of visceral hyperalgesia.[28] Genetic predisposition—family history of nonspecific abdominal illnesses, IBS, peptic ulcer, or migraine headaches that are emotionally or stress related—also contribute to the development of functional abdominal pain in children.[12]

Currently, the AAP posits that functional abdominal pain can be diagnosed correctly by the primary care clinician in children 4 to 18 years of age when there are no alarm symptoms or signs, the physical examination is normal, and the stool sample tests are negative for occult blood, without additional diagnostic evaluation. The presence of alarm symptoms or signs, such as involuntary weight loss, linear growth deceleration, GI blood loss, significant vomiting, chronic severe diarrhea, persistent right upper or right lower quadrant pain, unexplained fever, family history of irritable bowel disease, or abnormal physical findings, should have further diagnostic testing for specific anatomical, infectious, inflammatory, or metabolic etiologies.

Although children with chronic abdominal pain and their parents are more often anxious or depressed, the presence of anxiety, depression, behavior problems, or recent negative life events does not distinguish between functional and organic abdominal pain.[29]

Treatment should be a multimodal, biopsychosocial approach with education of the family as an important part of treatment of the child with functional abdominal pain. Reasonable treatment goals should aim at returning the child to normal function rather than complete disappearance of pain. Medications for functional abdominal pain are best prescribed judiciously, although the AAP considers time-limited use of medications reasonable to help decrease the frequency or severity of symptoms.[13,14]

✳ CAM THERAPY RECOMMENDATIONS

Acupuncture

Acute Abdominal Pain

Acupuncture has been recorded as a therapeutic measure for acute abdominal pain as early as the *Nei Jing*, the *Yellow Emperor's Canon of Medicine*. Although it is widely used today for adults in China,[1] its efficacy has not been adequately demonstrated in children, who are much more fragile in acute situations and who can change and clinically deteriorate much more rapidly than adults. Most likely, at least for the present, Chinese medicine can provide specific treatments for some nonemergent pediatric conditions and can be an adjunctive, palliative therapy for pain and other symptoms prior to and after surgery.

Acupuncture has been shown to be effective in reducing pain and vomiting in adult patients undergoing various GI procedures. Because the treatment is benign and without side effects, usually stimulating only a few points, this use of acupuncture can be extrapolated for pediatric patients. One clinical report used four acupuncture points—Hegu (LI4), Neiguan (P6), Zusanli (ST36), and Gongsun (SP4) bilaterally—and demonstrated pain reduction during colonoscopy.[2] A study from Taiwan revealed electroacupuncture stimulation of Neiguan (P6) alone was as effective as anesthetic medication in reducing postoperative emesis in patients who underwent laparoscopy[3] (see also Chapter 62). Acupuncture can be used in fiberoptic gastroscopy,[4] possibly by just needling

Zusanli (ST36).[5] A success rate as high as 88.2% has been reported for acupuncture as analgesia for upper GI tract endoscopy.[6] Endoscopy was found to be much easier for the practitioner and better tolerated by the patient after acupuncture analgesia was administered.[7]

Nonsurgical Acute Abdominal Pain

Colic

Gastroenteritis

See Chapter 30, Diarrhea.

Constipation

See Chapter 26, Constipation.

Urological causes of abdominal pain

See Chapter 61, Urinary Cystitis.

Abdominal migraine

Acupuncture treatment can be directed at alleviating headaches (see Chapter 40, Headache), relieving stress, and diminishing abdominal pain.

Ulcer disease

An Italian report of four adult patients treated with acupuncture demonstrated complete resolution of symptoms and healing of lesions demonstrated by gastrocopy.[8] There are no current data on acupuncture treatment of ulcer in children.

Suspicion of ulcer in children should be appropriately diagnosed with endoscopic evaluation and treatment coordinated with the gastroenterologist. Acupuncture may be instituted for pain relief.

Pancreatitis

Adult studies indicate a treatment protocol that integrates Chinese medicine with Western medicine reduced mortality in recently diagnosed severe pancreatitis. Chinese medicine interprets pancreatitis as heat in the spleen/pancreas. A four-point Heat-dispersing treatment can be used[9]:

Tonify SP9, KI10; sedate SP2, HT8.

General treatment of acute abdominal pain

When surgical emergencies and serious abdominal disorders are ruled out or are being treated, acupuncture can be used to treat pain by regulating and tonifying the stomach and spleen[9]:

ST36, CV12, and P6.

Chronic Recurrent Abdominal Pain/Functional Abdominal Pain

In general, most of the functional abdominal pain is due to spleen/stomach imbalance and Spleen Qi deficiency, often with excess cold. Emotions such as anxiety, resentment, frustration, and anger are associated with liver Qi stagnation or Liver Yang rising. Strong family history corresponds to Kidney Qi and Jing deficiency.

A recent controlled randomized study from Korea applied hand acupuncture therapy to 40 children with intermittent abdominal pain. The experimental group received treatment on hand points A8, A9, A10, A11, A12, E22, and E45 for 20 minutes and manifested significant pain reduction.[10]

The following general recommendation can be applied to all functional abdominal pain. More specific treatments require a thorough TCM evaluation to elucidate precise imbalances.

- Disperse both internal Cold and Coldness in the Spleen, tonify spleen, and alleviate pain.
- Diminish exposure to environmental Cold. Apply warmth to CV8.
- KI3, KI7 to disperse cold globally.
- Disperse spleen cold with the four-point protocol: Tonify SP2, HT8; sedate SP9, KI10.
- Tonify spleen with the four-point protocol (after dispersing spleen Cold): Tonify SP2, HT8; sedate SP1, LR1.
- ST36, CV12, P6 to regulate stomach/spleen and alleviate pain.
- SP6, ST36 to tonify SP and ST Qi.
- Supplementary dietary management: Decrease or eliminate excess energetically Cold foods, excess sweets, or dairy products.

For emotional symptoms:

- LR3, LR13 to move LR Qi; LR3 to tonify LR Yin and diminish LR Yang.
- LR14 to harmonize Liver and Stomach.
- Teach the child self-calming techniques.
- For children with familial predisposition: Tonify kidney yin and Kidney Qi with the Five Element protocol: Tonify KI7, LU8; sedate KI3, SP3.[9]

Aromatherapy

Essential oils, especially peppermint essential oil, have traditionally been used for abdominal conditions such as irritable bowel, constipation, and nonspecific abdominal pain.[1] Texts on aromatherapy prescribe a number of essential oils for use with abdominal conditions. Generally these oils include those that are classified as either antispasmodics or carminatives. Carminatives are essential oils that are thought to relax the stomach muscles and support peristalsis. Essential oils with both of these properties include black pepper *(Piper nigrum)*, roman chamomile *(Chamaemelum nobile)*, sweet fennel *(Foeniculum vulgaris)*, peppermint *(Mentha piperita)*, ginger *(Zingiber officinalis)*, and rosemary *(Rosmarinus officinalis)*. Essential oils used for relaxation, such as lavender *(Lavandula angustifolia)*, frankincense *(Boswellia carteri)*, and mandarin *(Citrus reticulata)*, are also recommended.[1,2]

Essential oils for abdominal pain are administered by inhalation or topical (massage and compress) or oral routes. Generally it is recommended that oral administration be done under the direction of a licensed healthcare provider with prescriptive authority or medical herbalists. Either provider should have specific training in clinical aromatherapy.[1,3] Essential oil of peppermint is commonly recommended for abdominal pain and is available over the counter in an enteric coated form. In a randomized, placebo-controlled, double-blind study of 96 adults diagnosed with functional dyspepsia, enteric capsules of peppermint oil (90 mg) and caraway oil (50 mg) resulted in a statistically significant reduction in pain, pressure, heaviness, and fullness and in an increase in ratings of clinical improvement.[4] Oral peppermint comes in enteric-coated capsules. Each capsule usually contains 0.2 mL of oil of peppermint and is administered up to three times daily.

Chiropractic

The causes of abdominal pain are widely varied, and therefore identification of the underlying cause will provide a necessary direction in management to the chiropractor. Acute conditions require urgent diagnosis and commensurate management. Methods used by chiropractors in the course of assessment of abdominal pain include history of the condition and any digestive, environmental, or psychological stressors. Examination would include vitals as well as observation, auscultation, percussion, and palpation of the abdomen. A genital examination may help identify genitourinary-related conditions contributing to abdominal pain, such as testicular torsion. Blood, urine, and stool tests may help identify underlying pathology. Plain radiographs can identify bowel obstruction or other abdominal mass.

Owing to vagal influence of the upper GI tract, the chiropractor would carefully evaluate the upper cervical spine for signs of vagal interference. Hemidiaphragm spasm causing referred pain to the right flank and shoulder as well as local upper abdominal pain may be due to a subluxation complex (SC) in the cervical spine, and symptoms may be relieved with adjustments to the cervical spine from C3 caudally.[1] Specific conditions of the GI tract will also relate neurologically to varied areas of the thoracolumbar spine. These subluxations are identified, managed, and monitored concomitantly with any GI symptom. Spinal somatic origin is more likely to be present when there is tissue texture change at the costotransverse junction between T5 and T12.[2] Another screening test used by chiropractors is the Carnett maneuver. This test has the patient tighten the abdominal muscle wall through a supine "crunch" hold or sustained deep inhalation that fixes the abdominal wall. If abdominal pain increases or stays the same with palpation of this taut wall, then the pain is more likely of somatic origin.[3] Abdominal wall somatic pain typically will not change with diet or bowel activity and tends to be more postural in nature.[4] Muscular injury or discreet trigger points are often found in patients with a positive Carnett's sign. This author has identified persistent abdominal pain originating from a subluxation of the pubic symphysis in an infant. If visceral origin is identified, medical co-management of the patient is recommended.

Recurrent Abdominal Pain

Those children that respond with reduced symptoms of RAP after chiropractic intervention may have an autonomic dysfunction affecting motility.[5] This is substantiated by the work of Jorgenson, who found that children with RAP demonstrate higher basal parasympathetic activity than those with an identifiable organic source of abdominal pain,[6] and by Olafdottir, who found an impairment of the relaxation response to a meal at the proximal stomach.[7] Relaxation techniques may reduce symptoms for these children[7] and for those with psychological stress reaction RAP.

Chiropractic adjustments to the cervical spine have demonstrated effectiveness in reducing symptoms of abdominal dysfunction in infants[5] and may be productive in addressing abdominal pain such as RAP in older children.

Some children with abdominal pain may be experiencing referred symptomatology from an inflamed lumbar disc.[8] Although this is an uncommon pediatric occurrence, a thorough chiropratic spinal examination including advanced imaging would be diagnostic.

Transabdominal stimulation of the colon may be useful when motility is diminished. This process is performed at five points on the abdomen by vigorous and focal digital stimulation. The first point is midway between the umbilicus and the xiphoid process. The second point is midway between the umbilicus and the pubic ramus. The third and fourth points are at the nipple line just inferior to the lower rib margin on the left and right, respectively. Point five is overlying the ileocecal valve. Pressure is applied at each point sequentially with a single digit until tissue resistance is just met. At the point of resistance, the point is vigorously stimulated for a period of 5 to 10 seconds each. This process is repeated approximately four times per day. It should be noted that this process has also been successful in reducing constipation.

Reflexive stimulation to the dorsum of the foot may reduce symptoms of abdominal distress and pain. This is performed by using broad thenar pad pressure from the heel across the lateral margin of the sole and across the metatarsal-phalangeal (MTP) joints to the great toe. The pressure is then applied in a circular pattern over each MTP joint from the great toe to the fifth toe. This is repeated three times consecutively on each foot several times per day.

Herbs—Chinese

TCM posits that the central issue underlying most ailments of infants and young children is the limited capacity of the developing digestive system, which is responsible for the rapid assimilation of nutrients and many important immunological mechanisms that are mediated via interactions across the membrane of the intestines. Because the Qi of the Stomach is so active in the early years and because the organs are so sensitive, it is easy for the smooth peristaltic movement of the gut to become disturbed, resulting in reflux of food and fluid, the creation of gas, and the onset of diarrhea or constipation.[1]

The Tummy Tamer (Gentle Warrior Pediatric Formula, Kan Herb Company, Scotts Valley, Calif.) is based on the fourteenth century prescription *Bao He Wan*. It strengthens and regulates functions of the digestive system, ensuring the ability of the stomach and intestines to move food and waste through the gut in a smooth and rhythmic fashion.

Herbal formulations: hawthorn fruit (shan zha), citrus peel (chen pi), radish seed (lai fu zi), aurantium fruit (zhi ke), aucklandia root (mu xiang), fennel seed (xiao hui xiang), and perilla fruit (zi su ye) aid the digestion of proteins, fats, and starches by toning and activating the stomach and small intestine while dispersing and descending the Stomach Qi, thus promoting the proper movement of digestate through the gut. Pogostemon herb (huo xiang), perilla fruit (zi su ye), and forsythia bud (lian qiao) dispel the Heat and

Dampness that collect in the Stomach and Intestines due to food accumulation, as well as expel the external invasion of pathogenic influences such as Wind, Cold, Dampness, and Heat (pathogenic organisms) that cause food poisoning or gastroenteritis. Atractylodes rhizome (bai zhu), jujube fruit (da zao), poria fungus (fu ling kuai), alisma rhizome (ze xie), and licorice root (gan cao) strengthen the Spleen, eliminate Dampness, and enhance assimilation of nutrients. Cardamon seed (sha ren), fennel seed (xiao hui xiang), citrus peel (chen pi), perilla fruit (zi su ye), aucklandia rhizome (mu xiang), and radish seed (lai fu zi) warm the Qi of the Stomach and Spleen, dispel phlegm, eliminate gas, and counter reflux and nausea.[1]

Caution and contraindications: None.[1]

Dosage: 1 to 2 droppers as needed before or after meals.[1]

Dispersing Cold in the Abdomen

Abdominal pain results from ingestion of cold food and drink or dairy products. External heat compresses, hot water, or tea can be simple treatments for an acute attack. Often an infusion of fresh ginger root (grated, steeped in boiling water, and strained) can often provide immediate relief. In chronic, recurrent cases, the recommended formula is *Fu Zi Li Zhong Wan* ("Aconite Benefit the Center Pills"), which warms the stomach and increases spleen and stomach Qi. Another formula known as *Xiao Jian Zhong Wan* ("Minor Strengthen the Center Pills") can tonify spleen Yang and Qi.[2]

Obstruction by Heat or Damp-Heat

Abdominal pain caused by Heat or Damp-Heat is often accompanied by constipation with hard stools, although on occasion hard stools may alternate with loose and foul-smelling stools. Herbal treatment aims at purging the intestines of Heat using a cool purgative. Several formulas are available, particularly *Da Cheng Qi Tang* ("Major Regulate *Qi* Decoction") or *Ma Zi Ren Wan* ("Linum Seed Pills").[2]

Food Stagnation

Acute or chronic abdominal pain caused by food stagnation is precipitated by overeating. The herbal formulas break up food stagnation and help to descend Stomach Qi. Two formulas are commonly used: *Bao He Wan* ("Preserve Harmony Pill") and *Kang Ning Wan* ("Curing Pill"). Often one or two doses will relieve the symptoms.[2]

Stagnation of Liver Qi

Chronic abdominal pain caused by the stagnation of Liver Qi is usually accompanied by emotional distress or depression. Belching could be a key symptom, as stagnation of the liver inhibits the stomach's ability to descend Qi. The formula of choice is *Chai Hu Shu Gan San,* "Bupleurum Soothe Liver Powder."[2]

Abdominal pain caused by blood stasis as seen in postsurgical trauma and acute appendicitis should be referred for emergency treatment.

Standard herbal formulas can be obtained from Chinese herbal pharmacies.

Dosage for powdered herbs or granular extracts:

- Mix ½ to 1 teaspoon of herbal powder with boiling water to make syrup.
- Give 1 mL + 1 mL for every year under 6 years of age. For example, a 2 year old received 3 mL; maximum 6 mL, given every 2 hours for acute pain, every 3 to 4 hours for chronic, recurrent pain.[2]

Homeopathy

Abdominal pain is classified into two practitioner expertise categories, as follows.

Category 1, Acute Abdominal Pain

With the understanding that each case is unique and must be evaluated fully at the time of presentation, category 1 conditions usually can be treated homeopathically with a reasonable degree of safety and a reasonable chance of success by *clinicians who have only introductory training and limited experience in homeopathy*. Category 1 conditions include acute conditions of low to moderate severity and chronic or recurrent conditions of low severity.

Category 2, Chronic Abdominal Pain

With the understanding that each case is unique and must be evaluated fully at the time of presentation, category 2 conditions usually can be treated homeopathically with a reasonable degree of safety and a reasonable chance of success by *clinicians who have a moderate amount of training and some clinical experience in homeopathy*. Category 2 conditions include acute conditions of moderate to high severity and chronic or recurrent conditions of low to moderate severity. (See Appendix A, Homeopathy, for more information on practitioner expertise categories.)

There are no controlled clinical trials of homeopathic treatment for abdominal pain, although the homeopathic literature contains much evidence for its use in the form of accumulated clinical experience.[1] Abdominal pain has many causes, some acute and some chronic. Both acute and chronic causes of abdominal pain often require laboratory and/or radiological diagnostic procedures to determine the cause and appropriate treatment.

For abdominal pain that is acute and relatively minor (nonsurgical), particularly infant colic or pain associated with diarrhea, it is safe to try homeopathic treatment. For acute abdominal pain caused by more serious conditions, such as that due to early appendicitis, administering a homeopathic remedy early in the course, as the patient is on the way to seek emergency care, may avert the need for surgery. Chronic abdominal pain can also be treated homeopathically, but successful treatment usually requires extensive training in the science and art of homeopathy. Homeopathy can and should be used in conjunction with dietary changes and/or other treatment modalities, either alternative or conventional.

The goal in treating abdominal pain homeopathically is to determine the single homeopathic medicine whose description in the materia medica most closely matches the symptom picture of the patient. Often mental and emotional states, in addition to physical symptoms, are considered. Once the medicine has been selected, it can be given in the 30C potency two to three times daily. If it has not helped after four to five doses,

then another homeopathic medicine should be tried or another form of therapy should be instituted as needed. Once symptoms have begun to resolve, the medicine can be given less frequently or stopped. It can be repeated again for a relapse of symptoms. See Appendix A, Homeopathy, for further information on prescribing and administering homeopathic medicines.

The following is a list of homeopathic medicines commonly used to treat patients with abdominal pain. It must be emphasized that this list is partial and represents some of the probable choices from the homeopathic materia medica. If the symptoms of a given patient are not represented here, a search of the homeopathic literature would be needed to find the simillimum. For more homeopathic medicines that may treat abdominal pain, see Chapter 23, Colic, and Chapter 30, Diarrhea.

The materia medica in this chapter was adapted in part from Morrison's *Desktop Companion to Physical Pathology*[2] and other sources found in *Referenceworks*.[1]

Arsenicum album

Arsenicum album treats abdominal pain that is paroxysmal and burning in nature. Diarrhea (possibly secondary to food poisoning) that feels hot and leaves the patient feeling weak may occur. The patient is restless, anxious, and very chilly. Symptoms are worse from midnight to 1 or 2 AM.

Chamomilla vulgaris

Chamomilla vulgaris is a remedy that is frequently used for colicky pain, particularly neonatal colic. The infant is angry, crying, red, and hot. He or she may arch the back. Symptoms are worse at 9 AM or 9 PM. If diarrhea is present, it may be green and slimy.

Lycopodium clavatum

Lycopodium clavatum is a remedy for abdominal pain that is located mainly in the right upper quadrant. Bloating and distention are accompanied by gurgling in the intestines and passage of gas, which only ameliorates the symptoms for a brief time. Symptoms are worse from 4 to 8 PM because of eating until full and the pressure of tight clothing.

Nux vomica

Nux vomica is a remedy for spasmodic abdominal pain. The patient may have difficult, painful stools, either hard or soft. After passing a stool the patient feels better. The patient is chilly and irritable and may be overly sensitive to light and noise.

Magnet Therapy

The child's abdomen and low back should be palpated for 3 to 5 distinct areas that are most tender. The ¾-inch Neodymium Spot Magnets with fused nylon coating may be placed in a pattern of alternating bionorth/biosouth polarity on the abdomen (up to three points) and the back (up to four points) for 1 to 2 hours twice a day. Neodymium Spot Magnets may be obtained from Painfree Lifestyles, 800-480-8601.

Mind/Body

Recurrent abdominal pain is a common presenting complaint among children and adolescents. An integrative approach combines conventional medical assessment with self-regulation skills training (e.g., hypnosis, guided imagery, biofeedback, meditation, cognitive-behavioral therapy) aimed at balancing the autonomic nervous system. In a recent review of the literature, Weydert and colleagues concluded that children with nonspecific RAP respond positively to cognitive-behavioral therapy and biofeedback.[1] Another recent study evaluated the efficacy of treatment protocols that included mind/body skills training as a core component.[2] In this prospective, randomized study of children with recurrent abdominal pain (mean age 9.75 years), thermal biofeedback and cognitive/behavioral therapy were both effective components in an overall treatment approach that also included diet modifications and parent support. Sanders and colleagues[3,4] provided one of the first studies that demonstrated self-regulation skills training (e.g., distraction techniques, progressive muscle relaxation, coping statements) combined with family intervention improved patients' pain and coping skills, and the subjects were more painfree at follow-up and had lower rate of relapse than the control group that received standard pediatric care. Banez and Bigham[5] stated that heart rate variability biofeedback is a promising approach for RAP; however, controlled research studies are still needed. Yoga may also be beneficial for children and adolescents with abdominal pain.[6] Finally, clinical experience supports the use of mental imagery (self-hypnosis) for abdominal pain in pediatric patients; however, published studies have been limited to date.[7]

The authors' clinical approach to children with RAP includes a variety of components. First, children must have had a full, appropriate medical workup to rule out organic causes of pain. The authors normally deal with functional abdominal pain (see the 2005 AAP *Clinical Report on Chronic Abdominal Pain in Children*),[8] although the approach to functional dyspepsia is similar. All RAP patients are taught biofeedback-based relaxation with a goal of reducing excess sympathetic nervous system activity. If significant comorbid anxiety or depression is present, a short course of a selective serotonin reuptake inhibitor and/or psychotherapy may be initiated concurrently with the biofeedback training. Peripheral temperature, heart rate variability, and breathing (pneumographic) biofeedback are the preferred modalities, typically delivered as four to six 45-minute sessions spaced 1 to 2 weeks apart. Mental imagery involving visualizations about healing the GI tract and also about general health and wellness are often added. If constipation is a concern, then the use of an appropriate laxative/softening agent along with a bowel training program is utilized as well. The authors also consider IBS in the spectrum of RAP, and in a recent study in the adult literature, Taneja and colleagues[9] report that yogic intervention improves bowel symptoms, anxiety, gastric activity, and general autonomic functions in IBS patients receiving conventional treatment.

Nutrition

Discussion

Diet manipulation has been attempted for years as a treatment for RAP either through the elimination of certain foods (i.e., lactose-containing products) or the addition of others (i.e., high fiber). Research of these dietary interventions has had varying results. One study looked at the effects of adding 10 g of insoluble fiber to children's diets daily for 6 weeks. They reported a 50% decrease in pain reports compared with only a 27% decrease in the placebo group.[1] Another study compared the use of 165 g of fiber given daily versus placebo (5 g given daily) for 7 weeks to children with a diagnosis of RAP. There was no reported difference in the mean number of pain episodes between groups.[2] Although the studies were small and the evidence is weak, additional fiber may be beneficial to some children, especially those with constipation.

Lactose avoidance was studied in children, some who were identified as lactose malabsorbers and others identified as lactose absorbers. Each child received, in random order, a normal diet containing lactose, a lactose-free diet plus a formula with 400 mL/day of lactose, and a lactose-free diet plus a lactose-free formula. Each diet period lasted 6 weeks. Approximately 48% in the malabsorber group reported an increase of abdominal pain with the lactose formula, but only 33% had increased pain on the nonlactose diet. Of the absorbers, that percentage was 24% for each diet. When followed for 12 months on a lactose-free diet, 40% of the malabsorbers and 38% of the absorbers were painfree.[3] In another study, children were given a lactose-free diet, supplemented with either 2 g/kg of lactose or a placebo tonic. During the trials there were no differences in the reports of pain, regardless of whether the subjects were lactose intolerant or not. After a 3-month follow-up, 44% of the intervention group and 44% in the control group reported improvement.[4]

Food allergy has been implicated in abdominal pain; however, attempts to test for this via the presence of immunoglobulin (Ig) E–mediated antibody responses has not been helpful. A recent study focused on food elimination based on IgG antibodies detected by enzyme-linked immunosorbent assay (ELISA). In a randomized control trial, there was a 26% greater reduction in symptoms for those compliant patients who were on a food elimination diet based on IgG antibodies compared with those on a sham elimination diet.[5]

Other studies[6,7] showed that ingestion of various sugars, such as lactose, fructose, sorbitol, or fructose plus sorbitol, caused an increase in measured breath hydrogen and clinical symptoms in patients with functional abdominal pain when compared with the ingestion of sucrose. Subsequently, with restriction of the offending sugars, 40% to 60% experienced improvement. Fructose is readily available in sweetened soft drinks and juices. Sorbitol is the leading sweetener used in "sugar-free" foods.

Treatment of Abdominal Pain

If certain foods seem to exacerbate abdominal pain, they should be avoided. If it is uncertain that certain foods are the culprit, a 4-week elimination of that particular food can be initiated, with any symptoms recorded in a pain diary. After 4 weeks, the food in question should be reintroduced and symptoms should be recorded. If the person is intolerant to that food, symptoms will greatly increase when reintroduced.

Food allergy/intolerance can be tested through IgG antibody to certain foods. If antibodies are present, those foods should be eliminated. Again, symptoms can be monitored using a symptom/pain diary. It is theorized that once the body is cleared of these identified foods and antibody levels decrease, the foods can be eaten again, but only on an infrequent basis to prevent recurrence of GI symptoms and antibody formation.

Sources of excess carbohydrates that might promote malabsorption or excess fermentation in the GI tract should be eliminated. Sweetened beverages containing fructose, sorbitol, and sucrose and sugar-free foods should be avoided.

Elimination of chronic constipation can be achieved through dietary measures by increasing daily fiber and water intake. Leading food sources of fiber include figs, brown rice, peas, dried beans, prunes, raisins, and whole grains. Consuming at least 8 glasses of water per day will help move the fiber through the colon.

Osteopathy

Many etiologies exist for nonsurgical abdominal pain. The osteopathic approach to specific functional problems such as colic, constipation, and gastroesophageal reflux will be discussed in Chapters 23, 26, and 38, respectively. Within the osteopathic tradition, most abdominal complaints and gastrointestinal pathologies may be related to imbalances in the function of the autonomic nervous system and/or dysfunction in the low-pressure circulatory system (i.e., the venous and lymphatic systems). These imbalances and dysfunctions may represent the underlying conditions that fostered the pathology, the actual pathophysiology of the condition, or the body's attempt to compensate for the pathology. In all cases, these components should be addressed to facilitate healing. Conditions thought to be related to autonomic imbalance are divided into two categories; sympathetic dominant complaints and parasympathetic dominant complaints.[1] Autonomic imbalances influence the vascular autoregulatory reflexes of the gut. Sympathetic activity affects the entire gut, causing vasoconstriction of the arterioles. Parasympathetic stimulation increases blood flow to the stomach and lower colon and also increases secretory gland activity in these areas.[2,3] These sympathetic and parasympathetic effects are taken into consideration in the diagnosis and management of the child's condition. Pharmaceutical, herbal, dietary, and lifestyle changes may also be addressed within the context of the autonomic imbalance.

Children with sympathetic dominant complaints have boring, poorly localized abdominal pain accompanied by constipation, flatulence, and/or bloating. Osteopathic findings include somatic dysfunction at the thoracolumbar junction, Chapman's points related to the colon, myofascial strain in the abdomen and visceral tissues, and paraspinal muscle hypertonicity in the lower thoracic and upper lumbar areas.[1,4] Depending on the specific findings, osteopathic treatment might consist of inhibition and visceral techniques as well as techniques to address the junctional areas of the spine. Parents can be taught to provide gentle inhibition or massage to alleviate some of their child's discomfort. In children with parasympathetic dominant complaints, the abdominal pain is usually cramping and may be associated with nausea, vomiting, or diarrhea. Somatic dysfunction is typically found in the anatomical areas related to the parasympathetic nerves, especially the vagus. Tissue texture changes are found at the craniocervical junction and suboccipital area, occipitomastoid area, sacroiliac joints, lumbosacral junction, and/or pelvic diaphragm. Treatment

is directed at these areas using indirect or direct approaches depending on the child's age. The somatic findings associated with abdominal pain are usually compensatory and are reinforcing the autonomic imbalance. Indirect and gentle, direct techniques such as rib raising, inhibition, soft tissue, and balancing techniques are most often employed.

Alternatively, abdominal pain may be associated with dysfunction of the low-pressure circulatory system. The *low-pressure circulatory system* refers to the venous and lymphatic systems responsible for removal of cellular waste products and extravasated fluids. Dysfunction of the low-pressure circulatory system leads to venous and lymphatic congestion. This in turn affects tissue health by prolonging the presence of cellular waste products, altering tissue pH, and decreasing nutrient and oxygen delivery. Lymphatic lacunae lining the undersurface of the diaphragm are responsible for removing fluid that normally extravasates into the peritoneal cavity. Consequently, proper respiratory mechanics are important in children with abdominal complaints related to lymphatic congestion. When the low-pressure circulatory system is involved, children may present with signs of mild illness such as fatigue and low-grade fever in addition to their abdominal complaints. Evaluation and treatment of the rib cage, thoracic and lumbar spine, scalene muscles, and thoracic and pelvic diaphragms are all important in addressing dysfunction of the low-pressure circulatory system. Visceral, myofascial, lymphatic, and balancing techniques are typically used in these children.

Although there are no pediatric studies, reports of two examples of autonomic dysfunction in adults, IBS and postoperative ileus, suggest a role for osteopathic manipulative treatment in the care of these patients. An older study[5] and a more recent one[6] suggest that the previously mentioned techniques can improve bowel function in patients with postoperative paralytic ileus. Several published articles discuss the efficacy of osteopathic manipulative therapy in treating IBS[7-9]; however, none of these meet the criteria for an evidence-based study.

References

Pediatric Diagnosis and Treatment

1. Antonson DL: Abdominal pain, *Gastrointest Endosc Clin N Am* 4:1-21, 1994.
2. Reynolds SL, Jaffe DM: Diagnosing abdominal pain in a pediatric emergency department, *Pediatr Emerg Care* 8:126-128, 1992.
3. Ruddy RM: Pain—abdomen. In Fleisher GR, Ludwig S, editors: *Textbook of pediatric emergency medicine*, ed 3, Baltimore, 1993, Williams and Wilkins, pp 340-347.
4. Quillin SP, Siegel MJ: Color Doppler US of children with acute lower abdominal pain, *Radiographics* 13:1281-1293, 1993.
5. Laing FC: Ultrasonography of the acute abdomen, *Radiol Clin N Am* 30:389-404, 1992.
6. Belman AB: Ureteropelvic junction obstruction as a cause for intermittent abdominal pain in children, *Pediatrics* 88:1066-1069, 1991.
7. Ross AJ: Intestinal obstruction in the newborn, *Pediatr Rev* 15: 338-347, 1994.
8. Swischuk LE: Acute abdomen with right lower quadrant pain, *Pediatr Emerg Care* 8:241-242, 1992.
9. Swischuk LE: Sudden onset right side abdominal pain, *Pediatr Emerg Care* 8:51-53, 1994.

10. Macarthur C, Saunders N, Feldman W: *Helicobacter pylori*, gastroduodenal disease, and recurrent abdominal pain in children, *J Am Med Assoc* 273:729-734, 1995.

11. Salvi E, Pistilli A, Romiti P et al: Duodenal ulcer. Gastroscopic aspects before and after acupuncture treatment [in Italian], *Minerva Med* 74:2541-2546, 1983.

12. Boyle TJ: Recurrent abdominal pain: an update, *Pediatr Rev* 18:310-321, 1997.

13. American Academy of Pediatrics Subcommittee on Chronic Abdominal Pain: Chronic abdominal pain in children, *Pediatrics* 115:812-815, 2005.

14. American Academy of Pediatrics Subcommittee on Chronic Abdominal Pain; North American Society for Pediatric Gastroenterology, Hepatology, and Nutrition: Chronic abdominal pain in children, *Pediatrics* 115:e370-e381, 2005.

15. Turck D: Chronic abdominal pain in children [in French], *Rev Prat* 48:369-375, 1998.

16. Lake AM: Chronic abdominal pain in childhood: diagnosis and management, *Am Fam Phys* 59:1823-1830, 1999.

17. Croffie JM, Fitzgerald JF, Chong SK: Recurrent abdominal pain in children—a retrospective study of outcome in a group referred to a pediatric gastroenterology practice, *Clin Pediatr (Philadelphia)* 39:267-274, 2000.

18. Buller HA: Problems in diagnosis of IBD in children, *Neth J Med* 50:S8-S11, 1997.

19. Hyams JS: Functional gastrointestinal disorders, *Curr Opin Pediatr* 11:375-378, 1999.

20. Thompson WG, Longstreth GF, Drossman DA et al: Functional bowel disorders and functional abdominal pain, *Gut* 45(Suppl 2):43-47, 1999.

21. Axon AT, Long DE, Jones SC: Editorial: abdominal migraine: does it exist? *J Clin Gastroenterol* 13:615-616, 1991.

22. Mason JD: The evaluation of acute abdominal pain in children. Gastrointestinal emergencies, part I, *Emerg Med Clin N Am* 14:629-643, 1996.

23. Singer HS: Migraine headaches in children, *Pediatr Rev* 15:94-101, 1994.

24. Cooke HJ: Role of the "little brain" in the gut in water and electrolyte homeostasis, *FASEB J* 3:127-138, 1989.

25. Drossman DA, Camilleri M, Mayer EA et al: AGA technical review on irritable bowel syndrome, *Gastroenterol* 123:2108-2131, 2002.

26. Van Ginkel R, Voskuijl WP, Benninga MA et al: Alterations in rectal sensitivity and motility in childhood irritable bowel syndrome, *Gastroenterol* 120:31-38, 2001.

27. Di Lorenzo C, Youssef NN, Sigurdsson L et al: Hyperalgesia in children with functional abdominal pain, *J Pediatr* 139:838-843, 2001.

28. Talley NJ, Spiller R: Irritable bowel syndrome: a little understood organic bowel disease? *Lancet* 360:555-564, 2002.

29. Di Lorenzo C, Colletti RB, Lehmann HP, et al; American Academy of Pediatrics Subcommittee on Chronic Abdominal Pain; NASPGHAN Committee on Abdominal Pain: Chronic abdominal pain in children: a clinical report of the American Academy of Pediatrics and the North American Society for Pediatric Gastroenterology, Hepatology and Nutrition, *J Pediatr Gastroenterol Nutr* 40:245-248, 249–261, 2005.

Acupuncture

1. Zheng XL, Chen C, Wu XZ: Acupuncture therapy in acute abdomen, *Am J Chin Med* 13:127-131, 1985.

2. Li CK, Nauck M, Loser C, Folsch UR et al: Acupuncture to alleviate pain during colonoscopy [in German], *Dtsch Med Wochenschr* 116:367-370, 1991.

3. Ho RT, Jawan B, Fung ST et al: Electro-acupuncture and postoperative emesis, *Anaesthesia* 45:327-329, 1990.

4. Chu H, Zhao SZ, Huang YY: Application of acupuncture to gastroscopy using a fiberoptic endoscope, *J Tradit Chin Med* 7:279, 1987.

5. Cheng YQ, Wang ZQ, Zhang SY et al: The use of needling Zusanli in fiberoptic gastroscopy, *J Tradit Chin Med* 4:91-92, 1984.

6. Sodipo JO, Ogunbiyi TA: Acupuncture analgesia for upper gastrointestinal endoscopy: a Lagos experience, *Am J Chin Med* 9:171-173, 1981.

7. Cahn AM, Carayon P, Hill C et al: Acupuncture in gastroscopy, *Lancet* 1:182-183, 1978.

8. Salvi E, Pistilli A, Romiti P et al: Duodenal ulcer. Gastroscopic aspects before and after acupuncture treatment [in Italian], *Minerva Med* 74:2541-2546, 1983.

9. Loo M: *Pediatric acupuncture*, London, 2002, Elsevier.

10. Hong YR: The effects of hand-acupuncture therapy on intermittent abdominal pain in children [in Korean], *Taehan Kanho Hakhoe Chi* 35:487-493, 2005.

Aromatherapy

1. Battaglia S: *The complete guide to aromatherapy*, Virginia, Queensland, Australia, 1995, The Perfect Potion.

2. Price S, Parr PP: *Aromatherapy for babies and children*, San Francisco, 1996, Thorsons.

3. Buckle J: *Clinical aromatherapy: essential oils in practice*, ed 2, Edinburgh, 2003, Churchill Livingstone.

4. May B, Kohler S, Schneider B: Efficacy and tolerability of a fixed combination of peppermint oil and caraway oil in patients suffering from functional dyspepsia, *Aliment Pharmacol Ther* 14:1671-1677, 2000.

Chiropractic

1. Homewood AE: *The neurodynamics of the vertebral subluxation*, St Petersburg, Fla, 1997, Valkyrie Press.

2. Beal MC: Viscerosomatic reflexes: a review, *J Am Osteopath Assoc* 85:786, 1985.

3. Schaefer RC: *Symptomatology and differential diagnosis: a conspectus of clinical semeiographies*, Arlington, VA, 1986, American Chiropractic Association, p 783.

4. Suleiman S, Johnston D: Abdominal wall: an overlooked source of pain, *Amer Fam Physician* 64:431-444, 2001.

5. Fysh P: *Chiropractic care of the pediatric patient*, Arlington, VA, 2002, International Chiropractors Association Council on Chiropractic Pediatrics.

6. Jorgenson LS, Christiansen P, Raundahl U et al: Autonomic nervous system function in patients with functional abdominal pain: an experimental study, *Scan J Gastoenterol* 28:63-68, 1993.

7. Olafdottir E Gilja OH, Aslaksen A et al: Impaired accommodation of the proximal stomach in children with recurrent abdominal pain, *J Pediatr Gastroenterol Nutr* 30:157-163, 2000.

8. Leahy AL, Fogarty EE, Fitzgerald RJ et al: Discitis as a cause of abdominal pain in children, *Surgery* 94:412-414, 1984.

Herbs—Chinese

1. Beinfield H, Korngold E: *Chinese medicine works clinical handbook*, San Francisco, 2007, www.chinesemedicineworks.com.

2. Fratkin J: Personal communication, 2006.

Homeopathy

1. ReferenceWorks Pro 4.2, San Rafael, Calif, 2008, Kent Homeopathic Associates.

2. Morrison R: *Desktop companion to physical pathology*, Nevada City, Calif, 1998, Hahnemann Clinic Publishing.

Mind/Body

1. Weydert JA, Ball TM, Davis MF: Systematic review of treatments for recurrent abdominal pain, *Pediatrics* 111:e1-e11, 2003.
2. Humphreys PA, Gevirtz RN: Treatment of recurrent abdominal pain: components analysis of four treatment protocols, *J Pediatr Gastroenterol Nutr* 31:47-51, 2000.
3. Sanders M, Rebgetz M, Morrison M et al: Cognitive-behavioral treatment of recurrent nonspecific abdominal pain in children: an analysis of generalization and maintenance side effects, *J Consult Clin Psychol* 57:294-300, 1989.
4. Sanders M, Shepherd R, Cleghorn G et al: The treatment of recurrent abdominal pain in children: a controlled comparison of cognitive-behavioral family intervention and standard pediatric care, *J Consult Clin Psychol* 62:305-314, 1994.
5. Banez G, Bigham E: Recurrent abdominal pain in children and adolescents: conventional and alternative treatments, *Biofeedback* 31:23-29, 2003.
6. Kuttner: Personal communication, June 2003.
7. Anbar R: Self-hypnosis for the treatment of functional abdominal pain in childhood, *Clin Pediatric* 40:447-451, 2001.
8. American Academy of Pediatrics, Subcommittee on Chronic Abdominal Pain, North American Society for Pediatric Gastroenterology and Nutrition: Chronic abdominal pain in children, *Pediatrics* 115:e370-e381, 2005.
9. Taneja I, Deepak K, Poojary G et al: Yogic versus conventional treatment in diarrhea-predominant irritable bowel syndrome: a randomized control study, *Appl Psychophysiol Biofeed* 29:19-32, 2004.

Nutrition

1. Feldman W, McGrath P, Hodgeson C et al: The use of dietary fiber in the management of simple, childhood, idiopathic, recurrent abdominal pain, *Am J Dis Child* 9:1216-1218, 1985.
2. Christiansen MF: Recurrent abdominal pain and dietary fiber, *Am J Dis Child* 140:738-739, 1986.

3. Lebenthal E, Rossi TM, Nord KS et al: Recurrent abdominal pain and lactose absorption in children, *Pediatrics* 67:828-832, 1981.
4. Dearlove J, Dearlove B, Pearl K et al: Dietary lactose and the child with abdominal pain, *Br Med J* 286:1936, 1983.
5. Atkinson W, Sheldon TA, Shaath N et al: Food elimination based on IgG antibodies in irritable bowel syndrome: a randomized controlled trial, *Gut* 53:1459-1464, 2004.
6. Fernandez-Baneres F, Esteve-Pardo M, deLeon R et al: Sugar malabsorption in functional bowel disease: clinical implications, *Am J Gastorenterol* 88:2044-2050, 1993.
7. Goldstein R, Braverman D, Stankiewicz H: Carbohydrate malabsorption and the effect of dietary restriction on symptoms of irritable bowel syndrome and functional complaints, *Isr Med Assoc J* 2:583-587, 2000.

Osteopathy

1. Kuchera ML, Kuchera WA: *Osteopathic considerations in systemic disease*, Columbus, Ohio, 1994, Greydon Press.
2. Guyton AC: *Textbook of medical physiology*, ed 9, Philadelphia, 1996, Saunders.
3. Crissinger K, Granger DN: Gastrointestinal blood flow. In Yamada T, editor: *Textbook of gastroenterology*, Philadelphia, 1995, Lippincott.
4. *Louisa Burns, DO: Memorial*, Indianapolis, 1994, American Academy of Osteopathy.
5. Herrmann E: Post-operative ileus prevention, *The D O* 163-164, 1965.
6. Douglas J: *OMT in Post-operative ileus*, residency research presentation, Maine Osteopathic Association, 2000.
7. Masterson EV: Irritable bowel syndrome: an osteopathic approach, *Osteopathic Annals* 12:12-18, 1984.
8. Denslow J: Functional colitis: etiology, *AAO Yearbook* 1:192-197, 1965.
9. McBain R: Treatment of functional colon, *AAO Yearbook* 1: 190-191, 1965.

CHAPTER 9

Acne

Acupuncture | May Loo

Aromatherapy | Maura A. Fitzgerald

Chiropractic | Anne Spicer

Herbs—Chinese | Catherine Ulbricht,
Jennifer Woods, Mark Wright

Herbs—Western | Alan D. Woolf, Paula M. Gardiner,
Lana Dvorkin-Camiel, Jack Maypole

Homeopathy | Janet L. Levatin

Magnet Therapy | Agatha P. Colbert, Deborah Risotti

Naturopathy | Matthew I. Baral

✳ PEDIATRIC DIAGNOSIS AND TREATMENT

Acne affects 80% to 95% of all adolescents, making it the most common skin disease in the world.[1-3] Although it is an expected physiological phenomenon that peaks in the age range of 14 to 17 years in girls and 16 to 19 years in boys,[4] the potential physical disfigurement can engender enormous psychosocial impact in teenagers[5,6] that can have long-term sequelae.[7-10]

Acne is a disease of the sebaceous glands. Its pathogenesis is multifactorial and can differ significantly among patients. The sebaceous glands are located in the face, neck, and upper trunk, the most common areas affected by acne. Before puberty, the sebaceous glands are generally atrophic. The increase in androgen levels triggers hypertrophy of the sebaceous glands, resulting in increased sebum production,[1] which usually begins around age 9 years with adrenarche and continues until age 17 years, when the adult level is reached.[11] Factors influencing sebum production include free fatty acids, dihydrotestosterone, and 5-α reductase. Patients with severe acne may have sebaceous glands that are hyperresponsive to normal levels of androgen.[1] In addition to sebum excretion, other sebaceous gland functions associated with acne development include sebaceous proinflammatory lipids; various cytokines produced locally; periglandular peptides and neuropeptides such as corticotrophin-releasing hormone, which is produced by sebocytes; and substance P, which is expressed in the nerve endings in the vicinity of healthy-looking glands of patients with acne.[11]

Microcomedones, the earliest lesions of acne, appear at adrenarche, followed by comedones, which appear about 2 years later when androgens of gonadal origin are produced and colonization of follicles by *Propionibacterium acnes* increases.[12]

Current thinking considers acne vulgaris as primarily an inflammatory disease.[11] Inflammatory lesions such as pustules, papules, and nodules are the result of the host's immune responses to *P. acnes*; the proinflammatory cytokines are released by immunocompetent leukocytes that are recruited in response to this bacterium and its metabolic byproducts.[12] Acne is a well-known side effect of systemic steroids. Western diet does not appear to play a significant role in the pathogenesis of acne.[4]

Acne can be predominantly broadly classified into four basic types of lesions: open and closed comedones, papules, pustules, and nodulocystic lesions.[13] Although new modalities are being developed every day, a cure for acne has not yet been discovered.[14] Treatment is directed toward controlling the progression of the inflammatory process and preventing scarring.[7,8,10]

Nonmedically, one of the most effective ways to limit the severity of acne is proper hygiene, which consists of gentle washing (not vigorous scrubbing) of the face twice daily and patting the face dry with a towel. Topical medication (retinoids, azelaic acid, benzoyl peroxide, and topical antibiotics) should be the first-line treatment, whereas oral medications (systemic antibiotics, hormone replacement, oral contraceptives, and especially isotretinoin) should be used for severe acne if initial treatment fails.[15] However, all medications have some degree of side effects, from local erythema, irritation, and sun sensitivity of topical retinoids to pseudotumor cerebri (PTC)[16] and controversial association with depression in patients taking oral isotretinoin.[15,17,18]

Currently, the U.S. Food and Drug Administration (FDA) is strengthening a program to prevent pregnancy among women taking isotretinoin because of teratogenic effect of the drug.[19] Laser surgery has recently been used for management of acne and treatment of acne scars.[20]

✳ CAM THERAPY RECOMMENDATIONS

Acupuncture

In Chinese medicine, acne is due to accumulation of Phlegm and Heat, which correlate well to the Western concept of obstructive and inflammatory types of comedones and pustules. The physiological changes during puberty results in imbalances primarily in the Stomach and Lung channels but may also involve Liver and Gallbladder channels.[2,3] The face is the most affected because many channels pass through the face and because it is the most exposed area of the body to Wind Heat. Other common areas are the chest and upper back.[3] Because the skin corresponds to the lung, excess Lung Heat can manifest as acne. Children in the Wood phase of development would be more prone to Liver and Gallbladder Heat (see Chapter 6, under Acupuncture), with distribution of acne lesions more prevalent along lateral aspects of the face and body.

Although diet does not appear to influence the pathophysiology or treatment in Western medicine, Chinese medicine posits that energetically Hot and Phlegm-containing foods are significant in acne. One Traditional Chinese Medicine (TCM) explanation for the efficacy of antibiotics is that antibiotics are antiinflammation drugs and therefore are considered energetically Cold. Similar effects may be achieved by increasing Cold foods in the diet. Acupuncture treatment using body and auricular points seems to work synergistically in balancing the viscera and harmonizing Yin and Yang.[2]

Acupuncture Recommendations

Recommendations for acupuncture treatment of acne include the following[1]:

- Avoid Heat- and Phlegm-producing foods in the diet.
- Increase energetically Cold foods.
- Use local points on the face and back, and connect them with an ion-pumping cord to a distal point on the corresponding channels or to BL60. For example, if acne lesions are on the forehead around Stomach points, use a local ST point on the face and a distal Stomach point (e.g., ST45), or use BL 60 as the distal point. Connect with an ion-pumping cord—black on the ST face point and red on the distal ST point or BL60. If using magnets, place the bionorth (–) pole facing down on the local point and biosouth (+) pole facing down on the distal point, and connect with an ion-pumping cord as previously described.
- ST40, SP6 to resolve Phlegm.
- GV14, LI11 to clear Heat; this has been shown to be effective against acne pustules.[4]
- For more chronic or severe acne, especially with pustules, use a stronger treatment to clear Heat from the channels, such as the two-point or four-point protocols (see Appendix B):
  - Clear Heat from Lung channel: tonify LU5, KI10; sedate LU10, HT8; or use two points: tonify LU5, sedate LU10.
  - Clear Heat from Stomach channel: tonify ST44, BL66; sedate ST41, SI5; or use two points: tonify ST44, sedate ST41.
  - Clear Heat from Liver channel: tonify LR2, KI10; sedate LR8, HT8; or use two points: tonify LR2, sedate LR8.
  - Clear Heat from Gallbladder channel: tonify GB43, BL66; sedate GB38, SI5.
- Auricular points: Shenmen, Point Zero, Master Skin point, Endocrine Hormone point, Lung points.[5]
- Kidney, Spleen, and Heart if pustules are present.[2]

Aromatherapy

A number of essential oils are recommended for acne including bergamot (*Citrus bergamia*), geranium (*Pelargonium graveolens*), juniper (*Juniperus communis*), palmarosa (*Cymbopogon martinii*), and tea tree (*Melaleuca alternifolia*).[1] When used for acne, essential oils are added to light oils such as apricot kernel oil or are mixed into cleansing creams in a 3% to 5% solution and applied with facial massage.

Of this group, only tea tree oil has been studied. In a single blind study of 124 subjects, a 5% solution of tea tree oil (*M. alternifolia*) in a water-based gel was compared with a commercially available 5% solution of benzoyl peroxide in a water-based lotion. Subjects applied the preparations topically to the face for 3 months. Improvement was measured by number of inflamed and non-inflamed lesions. Both preparations reduced mild to moderate acne to a significant degree. The benzoyl peroxide group improved faster and to a greater degree, but side effects of scaling, pruritus, and dryness were also greater.[2] The authors also note that a 5% solution of tea tree oil is fairly dilute and that stronger solutions might result in stronger effects.

Chiropractic

The chiropractic approach to the patient with acne is to carefully assess the sympathetic nervous system. This input arises from the spinal levels of T1 to L2. Irritation of the sympathetics may cause increase in activity at the sweat and sebaceous glands, resulting in overload at the pores.[1] During puberty, a normal hormone-induced increase in sebum, enlarged sebaceous glands, narrowing of the duct lumen, and massive neutrophil infiltration occur, along with an increase in the normally benign bacteria on the surface of the skin.[2] A facilitated sympathetic nervous system clearly compounds the normal developmental changes that precipitate acne in many teenagers.

Supportive measures often used by chiropractors include nutritional support in the form of skin support nutrients such as vitamins A and C and zinc.[3] Also of benefit are those supplements that enhance bowel function, including microflora, and addition of fresh fruit and vegetable fibers to the diet. Improved hydration, as well as elimination of sugars, hydrogenated fats, and caffeine, may bring about noticeable change. Referral to an acupuncturist may be fruitful.

One chiropractor reported a 17-year-old boy who presented to her private practice with a chief complaint of acne. The history revealed that he also had hyperhydrosis, weakness in the neck, dizziness, and poor bowel elimination. After 12 chiropractic visits in a 4-week span, his acne had resolved and his bowel function had normalized. By the eighth week of care, the hyperhydrosis was reduced and the dizziness was resolved. By the twelfth week of care, the weakness was resolved in the neck.[4]

Herbs—Chinese

Seijyo-bofu-to, Jumi-haidoku-to, and *Toki-shakuyaku-san* have been reported to suppress acne rashes and incidental symptoms. The synergistic activities of the ingredients in the Kampo formulations might produce these effects. Among the Kampo formulations there are different degrees of suppression of incidental symptoms.[1,3] Because incidental symptoms are variously suppressed, the determination of the herbal prescription is not based solely on treatment of a single symptom, but rather upon a constellation of signs and symptoms leading to an understanding of the "root" of the disharmony, in traditional terms (e.g., Heat, Dampness). Although the condition being treated might receive an obvious emphasis in treatment, improvement of the associated symptoms (from the Oriental diagnostic viewpoint) would be expected and possibly unavoidable.

Glycyrrhiza glabra L. has shown a remarkable antibacterial activity against *Proprionibacterium acnes,* resulting in negligible induction of resistance, compared with a marked development of resistance in the bacteria treated with erythromycin.*

---

*TCM usually uses Gan Cao, which is the root of *Glycyrrhiza uralensis* Fisch. Extrapolation of pharmacological effects among congeneric species is not reliable.

Researchers concluded that a formulation containing root of *Angelica dahurica* (Hoffm.) Franch. & Sav. *(Bai Zhi)*, rhizome of *Coptis chinensis* Franch. *(Huang Lian)*, and *G. glabra* L. may help prevent and treat acne lesions.[2,3]

TCM posits that acne may be rooted in the Stomach, Spleen, and Intestines as Heat or Damp Heat. This flows up onto the Face, in particular. Bai Zhi clears heat from the Stomach and is traditionally considered useful in treating pyogenic conditions, especially those of the upper body. Huang Lian is said to clear Damp Heat from the Spleen, Stomach, and Intestines. Acne can have underlying TCM subtypes (Blood-heat type, toxic-heat type, phlegm-heat type), which would all be treated slightly differently, would mostly involve the use of Huang Lian, but would also likely include flower of *Lonicera japonica* Thunb., (Jin Yin Hua) and Lian fruit of *Forsythia suspensa* (Thunb.) Vahl. (Qiao). If a case of acne does not respond to treatment, or only partially responds to a particular formulation, then a practitioner of TCM or Kampo might suspect that the formulation did not correspond precisely to the subtype.

Huang Lian and its berberine extract have been shown to be strongly bacteriostatic to *Streptococcus hemolyticus, Meningoccus* spp., *Diplococcus pneumoniae, Vibrio cholerae, Bacillus anthracis,* and *Staphylococcus aureus;* it also inhibitive to *Bacillus dysenteriae, Bacillus diptheriae, Bacillus subtilis,* and *Pseudomonas aeruginosa,* and it is active against *Haemophilus pertussis, Clostridium tetani, Bacillus pestis,* and *Bacillus tuberculosis.*[4] No specific documentation pertaining to inhibition of *P. acnes* is noted.

Similarly, aqueous decoction of Bai Zhi in vitro is antibiotic against *Escherichia coli, Bacillus paratyphi, Bacillus typhi, Shigella dysenteriae, Pseudomonas aeruginosa, Proteus* spp., *Vibrio cholerae,* and *Vibrio comma.* It is also inhibitive to *Mycobacterium tuberculosis* var. *hominis* and dermal mycoses.[4]

The three Kampo formulations listed are made into two decoctions: *to* is an aqueous decoction of raw herbs, and *san* is raw herb that is ground into a powder and given with warm water. Both are taken internally. The formulation containing Bai Zhi, Huang Lian, and licorice root is not stated. However, it is unlikely that a Huang Lian preparation would be used topically in a visible area—except in an extremely stubborn or acute case—because the principal active compound, berberine (7% to 9%), is intensely yellow-staining. In TCM, Bai Zhi and Huang Lian are mostly used internally.

Herbs—Western

Good facial hygiene and a healthy balanced diet can be of benefit in the management of acne. Benzoyl peroxide–containing lotions, creams, and gels are the mainstay of therapy, and oral and topical antibiotics are also beneficial. Mild acne may respond to the daily supplementation of the diet with some oral herbal preparations. Both flaxseed oil and evening primrose oil (containing γ-linoleic acid) are excellent sources of essential fatty acids, which can dilute sebum and help unclog skin pores.[1] An excellent antioxidant, vitamin C, which is present in rose hips or other sources, can enhance immune function and help keep acne-causing skin bacteria in check. A single 8-oz glass of orange juice contains 124 mg of vitamin C. (Children are recommended to not use doses above the tolerable

upper intake level [UL] of 400 mg/day for children ages 1 to 3 years, 650 mg/day for children 4 to 8 years, 1200 mg/day for children 9 to 13 years, and 1800 mg/day for adolescents 14 to 18 years.[2]) Tea tree oil comes from the leaves of the Australian tree *M. alternifolia* and has been used topically to treat mild acne. Terpenes in the essential oil can kill bacteria that cause acne and even *Candida* yeast and other fungi.[3-5] Even antibiotic-resistant *Staphylococcus* may be susceptible to tea tree oil.[6] In an Australian single blind randomized controlled study of 124 teenagers with mild to moderate acne, 5% tea tree oil gel was as effective as 5% benzoyl peroxide in reducing open and closed comedones.[7] Although the action of the tea tree oil was slower, fewer side effects such as dryness, irritation, stinging, burning, itching, and redness occurred in the tea tree group.[8] However, severe skin allergies have developed while using tea tree oil appropriately to treat ringworm and acne.[9,10]

Homeopathy

Before using this section, please see Appendix A, Homeopathy, for definitions of practitioner expertise categories and general information on prescribing homeopathic medicines.

Practitioner Expertise Category 2

There are no controlled clinical trials of homeopathic treatment for acne, although the homeopathic literature contains evidence for its use in the form of accumulated clinical experience.[1] Acne is difficult to treat homeopathically for the following reasons: the condition may be long-standing and chronic, and thus resolution will take time and follow-up; and the problem occurs in adolescents who may not fully agree to or be compliant with treatment. Additionally, because the condition is chronic, successful homeopathic treatment usually requires extensive training in the art and science of homeopathy.

The goal in treating acne homeopathically is to determine the single homeopathic medicine whose description in the materia medica most closely matches the symptom picture of the patient. Usually the mental and emotional state of the patient will be important indicators for the simillimum. Once the medicine has been selected, it can be given orally or sublingually in the 30C potency two to three times weekly. In more serious cases of acne, patients may benefit from utilizing a higher potency, such as 200C, on the same schedule.

If a patient is being treated conventionally before initiating homeopathic treatment, it is advisable to maintain that treatment for at least 1 month after the introduction of the homeopathic medicine. At that time, if improvements are noted from the homeopathic treatment, conventional treatment can be slowly reduced or withdrawn.

Other measures such as topical care with natural skin care products and/or dietary measures are appropriate adjuncts to homeopathic treatment. A variety of such skin care products are on the market. One of the best-quality product lines is the Dr. Hauschka Holistic Face Care system (WALA, Eckwälden, Germany), which is available at many natural food stores. Homeopathy can also be used in conjunction with conventional topical skin care products.

The following is a list of homeopathic medicines sometimes used to treat patients with acne. It must be emphasized that this list is partial and represents some of the probable choices from the homeopathic materia medica. If the symptoms of a given patient are not represented here, a search of the homeopathic literature would be needed to find the simillimum.

The materia medica in this chapter was adapted in part from Morrison's *Desktop Companion to Physical Pathology*[2] and other sources found in *ReferenceWorks*.[1]

Calcarea sulphurica

Calcarea sulphurica is indicated for severe acne that oozes pus, often for a long period of time. The lesions may be cystic and are slow to heal. The patient is usually warm-blooded and may have a jealous, aggressive nature.

Hepar sulphuris calcareum

Hepar sulphuris calcareum is indicated for painful, small pimples. The skin is slow to heal. The patient is chilly and intolerant of the cold. He or she is anxious, irritable, and very sensitive to pain and other stimuli.

Lachesis muta

Patients needing *Lachesis muta* have a large number of pimples that may be a purplish color and leave purplish scars when they resolve. The acne is worse before the menses. The patient is often intense and talkative and may be jealous and suspicious. The patient usually feels hot.

Silica terra

The acne is diffuse, and the lesions are hard and located under the skin. As the lesions absorb, they may leave a pitting scar. The patient is quiet and refined. Often there are immune system problems with recurrent infections of various sorts.

Sulphur

Sulphur is a remedy for acne vulgaris and acne rosacea when the skin is very oily. The lesions are large and superficial and the skin is red, itchy, and aggravated by heat.

Magnet Therapy

9000-Gauss rare earth magnets (0.06 × 0.16 inch) should be taped directly on individual pimples and may be left in place for up to 24 hours. The designated bionorth side (marked with a small indentation) should face the skin. These magnets may be obtained from OMS (800-323-1839) or AHSM (800-635-7070).

Naturopathy

Typical naturopathic approaches for acne treatment would include the following measures.

Diet

- Simplify the diet by eating food as close to the way it comes from nature. This means the elimination of food additives such as flavorings, colorings, and preservatives. Foods should be minimally processed; whole grains are better than breads made from the same grains.
- Avoid common food triggers such as sugar, alcohol, chocolate, or fried foods.

- Increase vegetable intake. Ideally, vegetables should account for 30% to 50% of the diet. Fruits are often good additions if used in moderation, but too much fruit sugar can be just as bad as too much refined sugar.
- The replacement of trans-fatty acids and hydrogenated oils with essential fatty acids from fish and flax oils seems to be of benefit.
- A high-protein diet is often recommended on the belief that lower blood glucose will contribute to less acne. The association among blood sugar, insulin, and acne has been investigated in some studies.[1,2]
- For severe acne, an allergy elimination diet is often recommended. This diet removes most common food allergies including dairy, soy, eggs, chocolate, nuts, citrus fruits, wheat, and corn. This is an extreme diet for most adolescents and can be used for only the most committed of patients.

Herbs

- Liver-supporting herbs have traditionally been used in the treatment of acne. These include burdock (*Arctium lappa*) and dandelion root (*Taraxacum officinalis*). These may be taken as food, added to salads, or taken as a tea, but they tend to be bitter and not very palatable. The use of liquid extracts or pills is usually preferred.
- Guggul (*Commiphora mukul*), an herb found in traditional Aryvedic medicine that is commonly used for dysglycemic conditions, has shown some efficacy in reducing inflammatory lesions in a small, randomized trial. Using the equivalent of 25 mg of gugulsterone, a 68% reduction in the number of inflammatory lesions was demonstrated after 3 months of use. It demonstrated a 65% reduction in inflammatory lesions[3] and compared favorably with 500 mg of tetracycline.
- Topical Oregon grape (*Mahonia aquifolia*) cream has demonstrated some efficacy in a small observational study in which patients were followed for 4 to 12 weeks. The trial was poorly constructed and preliminary, but most participants reported good results.[4]
- A 5% topical solution of tea tree oil was effective in treating acne vulgaris in a trial of 124 patients. Although frequency of treatment was not mentioned, improvement in the numbers of inflamed lesions, noninflamed lesions, and skin oiliness was similar for both benzoyl peroxide and tea tree oil groups. Skin tolerance was much better for the tea tree oil group (p < 0.05). Patients reported fewer unwanted effects with the use of tea tree oil (44% versus 79% for those treated with benzoyl peroxide).[5]
- Vitex (*Vitex agnus-castus*) demonstrated positive results in the treatment of acne in 117 males and females aged 16 to 40 years. Patients took 20 drops twice daily orally of 0.2% dried extract of *V. agnus-castus* fruit for 4 to 6 weeks, then 15 drops twice daily for 1 to 2 years. Patients also treated their faces with a topical disinfectant.[6]

Supplements

- In a metaanalysis of phosphatidylcholine (usual formulation is a liposomal cream containing 10% lecithin fraction with 80% phosphatidylcholine) applied topically for 8 weeks in adolescents (ages 14 to 17), there was a 65% reduction of comedones and a 75% reduction of efflorescences by the end of the treatment period.[7]

- A topical vitamin B_5 (pantothenic acid) in combination with oral vitamin B_5 was effective in controlling acne in 100 patients. Patients were given 10 g oral vitamin B_5 in 4 divided doses along with the topical application four to six times per day. Moderate cases improved in 8 weeks, with more severe cases taking 6 months to clear. Maintenance doses between 1 and 5 g oral daily were needed in subjects followed for 18 months.[8]

- Vitamin A (retinol) and its derivatives have shown effectiveness in a variety of clinical settings. Dosing from 300,000 to 500,000 IU have been shown to be effective.[9] Any patient on such high doses should have routine chemistry screens with attention to liver indices. No patient who is pregnant or has the possibility of becoming pregnant should be taking more than 8000 IU of vitamin A per day.[10]

Other

- Naturopathic physicians will commonly recommend exercise. Although no direct evidence supports exercise as a treatment for acne, anecdotal evidence suggests that it may be helpful and is certainly not harmful to the patient.
- Sun exposure, including light lamps and sauna exposure, seems to be of benefit to acne patients.
- Both biofeedback and hypnosis have shown some promise for reducing acne lesions.[11]

References

Pediatric Diagnosis and Treatment

1. Eichenfield L: Acne pathophysiology: a biological view. Advances in the treatment of teenage acne, *Infect Dis Child Suppl* X:4-5, 2004.
2. Jacob CI, Dover JS, Kaminer MS: Acne scarring: a classification system and review of treatment options, *J Am Acad Dermatol* 45:109-117, 2001.
3. Fyrand O: Treatment of acne [in Norwegian], *Tidsskr Nor Laegeforen* 117:2985-2987, 1997 (abstract).
4. Nelson WE, Behrman RE, Kliegman RM et al, editors: *Nelson textbook of pediatrics*, ed 15, Philadelphia, 1996, Philadelphia.
5. Sanfilippo AM, Barrio V, Kulp-Shorten C et al: Common pediatric and adolescent skin conditions, *J Pediatr Adolesc Gynecol* 16:269-283, 2003.
6. Smolinski KN, Yan AC: Acne update: 2004, *Curr Opin Pediatr* 16:385-391, 2004.
7. Krowchuk DP: Managing acne in adolescents, *Pediatr Clin N Am* 47:841-857, 2000.
8. Krowchuk DP: Treating acne. A practical guide, *Med Clin N Am* 84:811-828, 2000.
9. Goodman GJ: Post-acne scarring: a short review of its pathophysiology, *Australas J Dermatol* 42:84-90, 2001.
10. Usatine RP, Quan MA: Pearls in the management of acne: an advanced approach, *Primary Care* 27:289-308, 2000.
11. Zouboulis CC: Acne and sebaceous gland function, *Clin Dermatol* 22:360-366, 2004.
12. Bergfeld WF: The pathophysiology of acne vulgaris in children and adolescents, Part 1, *Cutis* 74:92-97, 2004.
13. Behrman RE, Kliegman RM, Jenson HB, editors: *Nelson's textbook of pediatrics*, ed 17, Philadelphia, 2004, Saunders.
14. Kimball AB: *Putting your best face forward*. Presented at the 63rd Annual Meeting of the American Academy of Dermatology, New Orleans, 2005.
15. Honig PJ: Treating acne: choosing the right agent. Advances in the treatment of teenage acne, *Infect Dis Child Suppl* X:7-9, 2004.
16. Friedman DI: Medication-induced intracranial hypertension in dermatology, *Am J Clin Dermatol* 6:29-37, 2005.
17. Phillips TJ: An update on the safety and efficacy of topical retinoids, *Cutis* 75(2 Suppl):14-22, 24; discussion 22-23, 2005.
18. Acne: isotretinoin and depression, *Drug Ther Bull* 41:76-78, 2003.
19. U.S. Food and Drug Administration: FDA alert: patient information sheet, Isoretinoin (marked as Accutane), *AAP News* February 2005.
20. Cantatore JL, Kriegel DA: Laser surgery: an approach to the pediatric patient, *J Am Acad Dermatol* 50:165-184; quiz 185-188, 2004.

Acupuncture

1. Loo M: *Pediatric acupuncture*, London, 2002, Elsevier.
2. Xu Y: Treatment of facial skin diseases with acupuncture, *J Tradit Chin Med* 10:22-25, 1990.
3. Dai GQ: Advances in the acupuncture treatment of acne, *J Tradit Chin Med* 17:65-72, 1997.
4. Liu J: Treatment of adolescent acne with acupuncture, *J Tradit Chin Med* 13:187-188, 1993.
5. Oleson TD: *Auriculotherapy manual, Chinese and Western Systems of ear acupuncture*, Los Angelese, 1992, Health Care Alternatives.

Aromatherapy

1. Battaglia S: *The complete guide to aromatherapy*, Virginia, Queensland, Australia, 1995, The Perfect Potion.
2. Bassett IB, Pannowitz DL, Barnetson RS: A comparative study of tea-tree oil versus benzoyl peroxide in the treatment of acne, *Med J Austr* 153:455-458, 1990.

Chiropractic

1. Aikenhead KJ: Dermatological disorders. In Lawrence D, editor: *Fundamentals of chiropractic diagnosis and management*, Baltimore, 1991, Williams and Wilkins.
2. Plewig G, Kigman AM: The dynamics of inflammatory acne; immunologic factors. In *Acne and rosacea*, Berlin, 1993, Springer-Verlag.
3. Schachner L, Eaglstein W, Kittles C et al: Topical erythromycin and zinc therapy for acne, *J Am Acad Dermatol* 22:489-495, 1990.
4. Ninno-Wiltsie L: Autonomic nervous system dysfunction, primarily hyperhydrosis in an adolescent male, *ICA Rev* 77-80, 1997.

Herbs—Chinese

1. Higaki S, Toyomoto T, Morohashi M et al: Seijo-bofu-to, Jumi-haidoku-to and Toki-shakuyaku suppress rashes and incidental symptoms in acne patients, *Drugs Exp Clin Res* 28:193-196, 2002.
2. Nam C, Kim S, Sim Y et al: Anti-acne effects of Oriental herb extracts: a novel screening method to select anti-acne agents, *Skin Pharmacol Appl Skin Physiol* 16:84-90, 2003.
3. Natural Standard Research Collaboration. Available at www.naturalstandard.com. Accessed October 2005.
4. Anonymous: Xin Bian Zhong Yao Da Ci Dian [*Newly Compiled Chinese Official Dictionary*], Tapei, Taiwan, 1984, Xin Wen Feng Chu Ban Gong Si.

Herbs—Western

1. Frondoza CG, Sohrabi A, Polotsky A et al: An in vitro screening assay for inhibitors of proinflammatory mediators in herbal extracts using human synoviocyte cultures, *In Vitro Cell Dev Biol Anim* 40:95-101, 2004.
2. Food and Nutrition Board, Institute of Medicine: DRI dietary reference intakes for vitamin C, vitamin E, selenium, and carotenoids, Washington, DC, 2000, National Academy Press. Available at: www.nap.edu/books/0309069351/html/. Accessed: January 24, 2008.
3. Carson CF, Riley TV, Cookson BD: Efficacy and safety of tea tree oil as a topical antimicrobial agent, *J Hosp Infect* 40:175-178, 1998.
4. Carson CF, Riley TV: The antimicrobial activity of tea tree oil, *Med J Austr* 160:236, 1994.
5. Raman A, Weir U, Bloomfield SF: Antimicrobial effects of tea-tree oil and its major components on *Staphylococcus aureus, Staph. epidermidis* and *Propionibacterium acnes, Lett Appl Microbiol* 21:242-245, 1995.
6. Carson CF, Hammer KA, Riley TV: Broth micro-dilution method for determining the susceptibility of *Escherichia coli* and *Staphylococcus aureus* to the essential oil of *Melaleuca alternifolia* (tea tree oil), *Microbios* 82:181-185, 1995.
7. Bassett IB, Pannowitz DL, Barnetson RS: A comparative study of tea-tree oil versus benzoylperoxide in the treatment of acne, *Med J Austr* 153:455-458, 1990.
8. Selvaag E, Eriksen B, Thune P: Contact allergy due to tea tree oil and cross-sensitization to colophony, *Contact Derm* 31:124-125, 1994.
9. Apted JH: Contact dermatitis associated with the use of tea-tree oil, *Australas J Dermatol* 32:177, 1991.
10. Sharquie KE, Al-Turfi IA, Al-Salloum SM: The antibacterial activity of tea tree oil *in vitro* and *in vivo* (in patients with impetigo contagiosa), *J Dermatol* 27:706-710, 2000.

Homeopathy

1. *ReferenceWorks Pro 4.2*, San Rafael, Calif, 2008, Kent Homeopathic Associates.
2. Morrison R: *Desktop companion to physical pathology*, London, 1998, Hahnemann.

Naturopathy

1. Kader MM, Hafiez AA, El-Mofty AM et al: Glucose tolerance in blood and skin of patients with acne vulgaris, *Indian J Dermatol* 22:139-149, 1977.
2. Semon H, Herrmann F: Some observations on the sugar metabolism in acne vulgaris, and its treatment by insulin, *Br J Dermatol* 52:123-128, 1940.
3. Thappa DM, Dogra J: Nodulocystic acne: oral gugulipid versus tetracycline, *J Dermatol* 21:729-731, 1994.
4. Farrant E, Lampert N: Chinese herbal uropathy and nephropathy, *Lancet* 368:1417, 1995.
5. Bassett IB, Pannowitz DL, Barnetson RS: A comparative study of tea-tree oil versus benzoyl peroxide in the treatment of acne, *Med J Austral* 53:455-458, 1990.
6. Amann W: Acne vulgaris and *Agnus castus* (Agnolyt) [in German], *Z Allgemeinmed* 51:1645-58, 1975.
7. Ghyczy M, Nissen HP, Biltz H: The treatment of acne vulgaris by phosphatidylcholine from soybeans, with a high content of linoleic acid, *J Appl Cosmetol* 14:137-145, 1996.
8. Leung L: Pantothenic acid deficiency as the pathogenesis of acne vulgaris, *Med Hypotheses* 44:490-492, 1995.
9. Kligman AM, Mills OH Jr, Leyden JJ et al: Oral vitamin A in acne vulgaris, *Int J Dermatol* 20:278-285, 1981.
10. Hall JG: Vitamin A: a newly recognized human teratogen. Harbinger of things to come? *J Pediatr* 105:583-584, 1984.
11. Shenefelt PD: Hypnosis in dermatology, *Arch Dermatol* 136:393-399, 2000.

CHAPTER 10

Allergies

Chiropractic | Anne Spicer

Herbs—Chinese | Catherine Ulbricht, Jennifer Woods,
Mark Wright

Herbs—Western | Alan D. Woolf, Paula M. Gardiner,
Lana Dvorkin-Camiel, Jack Maypole

Homeopathy | Janet L. Levatin

Magnet Therapy | Agatha P. Colbert, Deborah Risotti

Osteopathy | Jane Carreiro

✳ PEDIATRIC DIAGNOSIS AND TREATMENT

Allergy can be defined as an adverse physiologic event resulting from a complex, immunologically mediated response. The symptom or illness is due to an antigen-induced immune response, such as to medications, environmental allergens, foods, or foreign proteins. In contrast, an atopic disease is a chronic disorder that has a strong genetic predisposition, such as asthma, allergic rhinitis, atopic dermatitis, and food allergies. These conditions can be both immunoglobulin (Ig) E-mediated and non–IgE-mediated responses. Some allergic diseases, such as contact dermatitis, are primarily T cell–mediated responses to environmental triggers without IgE involvement.

It is often difficult to determine the precise mechanism of an allergic response, as it may be the result of a complex interplay of genetic predisposition, environmental influences, cultural differences in lifestyle, and dietary habits.

The most common pediatric allergic conditions are allergic rhinitis, allergic conjunctivitis, asthma, eczema, urticaria, and food allergies. See each specific condition for more detailed discussion of conventional pediatric and various CAM perspectives.[1,2]

✳ CAM THERAPY RECOMMENDATIONS

Chiropractic

To date, there are no case studies recorded in peer-reviewed journals identifying chiropractic management of allergies. However, evidence exists that the chiropractic adjustment has influence over natural killer cell production and autonomic balance[1]; immunoglobulin (Ig) A, G, and M levels, and B-cell lymphocyte count[2]; polymorphonuclear neutrophils and monocytes[3]; and even CD4 counts.[4] Because allergies are considered an excessive immune-mediated physiological response to environmental substances, clearly the chiropractic adjustment, as well as its capacity to enhance immunological function, may have an important role in the management of allergies. If possible, avoidance of identified allergens is a common-sense measure that is sometimes overlooked.

The chiropractic approach to allergies is to remove interference to normal function of the nervous system. Therefore the chiropractor would adjust indicated findings, keeping in mind that facilitation of the sympathetics is associated with an increased inflammatory response and that increased vagal activity would reduce this response.[5] Recommendation is made to specifically assess C6 to T3 and T7 to T12 for adrenal involvement, as well as L4 to L5.[6]

Diet also plays an extremely important role in body physiology.[7,8] Breastfeeding is the best source of nutrition for the infant and reduces allergic reactivity.[12,13] Wherever possible, the chiropractor recommends organic foods that minimize the toxic load on the body from substances such as pesticides, herbicides, chemical ripening agents, food additives, preservatives, artificial flavorings, and colorings. Any foods that enhance antiinflammatory function should be added to or increased in the daily diet, particularly nonallergenic fresh fruits and vegetables.

Ninety percent of food allergies in children younger than 3 years come from milk, eggs, peanuts, soy, fish, and wheat. In children between 3 and 12 years of age, the allergens that account for most reactions include peanuts, tree nuts, eggs, milk, soy, fish, seafood, and chicken.[9] Although all of these foods can produce anaphylaxis, delayed sensitivity reactions are also possible and make the identification of allergy more challenging.

Skin scratch and blood immunoglobulin testing is not always adequate in identifying those elements responsible for allergic-type symptoms but are nonetheless useful tools for the chiropractor.

Applied kinesiology muscle testing correlates with more than 90% of items found on radioallergosorbent (RAST) testing, IgE, and IgG and may also find items unidentified by conventional allergy testing.[10] This chiropractic technique is particularly useful when conventional laboratory testing is inadequate or unobtainable.

For those with pollen allergies, it may be useful to consume locally produced bee pollen.[11]

Eicosapentaenoic acid/docosahexapentaenoic acid (EPA/DHA) supplementation has been shown to enhance antiinflammatory activity in the body.[14]

Hair analysis, comprehensive blood profile, and digestive stool analysis may provide insight into systemic chemical imbalances that predispose to allergic-type symptoms. Consumption of foods high in these omega-3 fats has been found to be associated with a lower incidence of allergic rhinitis.[15,16]

Herbs—Chinese

One study found that Gyokuheifu-san (GHS; *Yu Ping Feng San*), an herbal formula that consolidates the superficial resistance to protection from invasion by external pathogenic influences, appears to have nonsymptomatic and nonallopathic effects on allergic rhinitis.[1,2] The formulation comprises root of *Astragalus membranaceus* (Fisch.) Bunge *(Huang Qi)*, rhizome of *Atractylodes macrocephala* Koidz. *(Bai Zhu)* and root of *Saposhnikovia divaricata* (Turcz.) Schischk. (Fang Feng). The classical source text[3] indicates Huang Qi 30 g, with Bai Zhu and Fang Feng both at 60 g, to be ground into a powder and given in doses of 6 g, 2 to 3 times daily. Variation in relative levels of the three herbs would depend upon the individual being treated.

Another study in adults found that Bi Min Kang mixture, which mainly consists of the Kazak folk herb *Artemisia* spp., may effectively treat seasonal allergic rhinitis (SAR) because it plays a role in resisting histamine, inhibiting allergic reaction I, and stabilizing the cell membrane of mastocytes.[3]

However, one study found that administering a Chinese herbal formula to adult SAR patients who were receiving acupuncture did not provide additional symptomatic relief or improvement in quality of life.[2,5]

Sanfujiu is a method of applying herbal drug paste onto acupoints Fengmen (B12, 1½ inches on either side of the lower border of the spinous process of the 2nd thoracic vertebra) and Feishu (B13, 1½ ins. either side of the lower border of the spinous process of the 3rd thoracic vertebra) during the three hottest summer days to treat patients with allergies using Traditional Chinese Medicine (TCM). More than 80% of the patients reported having reactive symptoms after using the Sanfujiu treatment. Younger subjects (≤ 16 years of age) were more likely to have reactive symptoms. Patients with rhinitis were more likely to have runny noses and nasal congestion after the treatment. Patients with allergic eczema were more likely to have skin itching all over the body. The perceived efficacy of Sanfujiu treatment was not related to the patients' age, sex, or diagnosis. Symptoms reactive to the treatment were common but usually mild.[2,6]

In the context of TCM, allergies are regarded mostly as being caused by either Spleen Qi deficiency, which tend to manifest as liquid/runny allergic responses, or Yin deficiencies, which tend to manifest with redness, itching and dryness. Allergic rhinitis is considered to arise from Spleen Qi deficiency. The formula Bu Zhong Yi Qi Tang, which is a long-established classical prescription generally available in pill form, often forms the basis of treatment for allergic rhinitis. The formula comprises the following:

- Root of *Astragalus membranaceus* (Fisch.) Bunge *(Huang Qi)*
- Root of *Panax ginseng* C.A. Mey. *(Ren Shen)*
- Rhizome of *Atractylodes macrocephala* Koidz. *(Bai Zhu)*
- Root of *Bupleurum chinense* DC. *(Chai Hu)*
- Rhizome of *Cimicifuga foetida* L. *(Sheng Ma)*
- Root of *Angelica sinensis* (Oliv.) Diels *(Dang Gui)*

- Mature pericarp of *Citrus reticulata* Blanco *(Chen Pi)*
- Fresh rhizome of *Zingiber officinale* (Willd.) Roscoe *(Sheng Jiang)*
- Ripe fruit of *Ziziphus jujuba* Mill. var. *inermis* (Bunge) Rehder *(Da Zao)*
- Root of *Glycyrrhiza uralensis* Fisch. *(Gan Cao)*

Ren Shen is often replaced by root of *Codonopsis pilosula* (Franch.) Nannf. (Dang Shen), which is cheaper, but considered adequate in the main. This formulation would theoretically provide treatment of the "root" of the condition and might convey sufficient support to relieve symptoms. In the event of symptoms not being adequately controlled, it might be administered along with fruit of *Xanthium sibiricum* Patr. (Cang Er Zi) and flower of *Magnolia liliflora* Desr. (Xin Yi Hua), which are considered to keep open the nose and sinus. No scientific evidence based information was found to substantiate this application, but Mark Wright *(pers. comm.)* has found it to be generally successful as the core of treatment for the condition.

Herbs—Western

Ginger tea has also been used to relieve the symptoms of colds and allergies. Parents should be cautious about the use of chamomile tea, lotions, ointments, or other chamomile-containing products for children who have allergies. Chamomile, a member of the Compositae family of plants along with ragweed, aster, and chrysanthemum, can cause allergic reactions in sensitive individuals and should be avoided.

Other multi-ingredient preparations, such as minor blue dragon from TCM providers, may include ephedra and other mushrooms and herbs. Minor blue dragon's effectiveness has not been established in adults or children. Japanese herbal formulations, including Ryo-Kan-Kyomi-Sin-Ge-Nin-To-Sho-Seiryu-To (*Pinellia* tuber, *Glycyrrhiza* root, cinnamon bark, *Schisandra* fruit, asiari root, peony root, ephedra herb, and dried ginger root), Bakumondo-To, Syo-Saiko-To (*Bupleurum* root, *Pinellia* tuber, *Scutellaria* root, jujube, ginseng, *Glycyrrhiza*, and ginger), Sairei-To (*Bupleurum* root, *Pinellia* tuber, *Scutellaria* root, alisma rhizome, ginseng, *Glycyrrhiza*, ginger, *Atractylodes lancea* rhizome, *Zizyphus*, licorice, hoelen, *Polyporus umbellatus*, and cinnamon bark) and Saiboku-To. Although sometimes applied for allergic rhinitis, their effectiveness has not been established in adults or children.

Quercetin and nettle have been used to inhibit histamine release and reduce nasal congestion and swelling associated with hay fever. In adults, 600 mg of nettle was found possibly effective in the treatment of seasonal allergic rhinitis in a small study[1]; however, there are no studies in children.

Homeopathy

Before reading this section, please see Appendix A, Homeopathy, for definitions of practitioner expertise categories and general information on prescribing homeopathic medicines.

Practitioner Expertise Category 1 or 2

Category 1 and 2 include acute allergy symptoms.

Practitioner Expertise Category 2 or 3

Category 2 and 3 include chronic allergic conditions.

A small amount of research evidence supports the use of homeopathy for treatment of allergies. A survey conducted in Mexico of more than 400 people with respiratory allergies revealed that 34.4% of people used at least one type of alternative medicine for their allergies, with homeopathy, used by almost 27% of survey respondents, being the most popular.[1]

Linde et al. reviewed nine placebo-controlled studies of homeopathic treatment for allergies and found that all showed statistically significant findings in favor of homeopathy.[2] Reilly et al. conducted three of those nine trials[3-5] and subsequently conducted another randomized, double-blind, placebo-controlled study of homeopathic treatment for perennial allergic rhinitis.[6] When the data from the four studies were pooled and analyzed, homeopathy was found to have different effects than placebo, the most clinically significant being an objectively measured improvement in nasal inspiratory peak flow. It should be noted that these studies did not utilize the classical homeopathic approach for choosing the homeopathic medicine (as described in Chapter 5 and Appendix A). Instead the researchers used a homeopathically prepared (diluted and succussed) mix of pollens[3] or a diluted and succussed preparation of the patient's main allergen, as determined by skin testing.[4,5] This method could be compared with allergy desensitization because an attenuated dose of the offending substance is given to the patient, which is intended to provoke a curative response.

In a retrospective outcome study by an Israeli research group, the use of prescription and nonprescription conventional medicines (including antihistamines, bronchodilators, decongestants, steroids, and antibiotics) was examined in 48 allergy sufferers before and after homeopathic treatment with individualized homeopathic medicines. It was found that of the 31 patients who were using conventional medicines prior to homeopathic treatment, 27 had reduced use of these medicines after homeopathic treatment, 2 had increased use, and 2 had no change. Of the 17 patients who were non-users of conventional medicine before the study period, 13 remained non-users. An average of $8 per patient was saved in medication costs.[7]

These findings suggest that homeopathy can be a useful form of therapy for allergies. Larger, more rigorous trials are needed to confirm this hypothesis. In addition to the aforementioned research evidence, the homeopathic literature contains much evidence in the form of accumulated clinical experience to support the use of homeopathic treatment for allergies.[8]

The goal in treating allergies homeopathically is to determine the single homeopathic medicine whose description in the materia medica most closely matches the symptom picture of the patient. Often mental and emotional states, in addition to physical symptoms, are considered. Once the medicine has been selected, it can be given orally or sublingually in the 30C potency two to three times daily, depending on the severity of the symptoms. For more severe symptoms, a 200C potency can be given two to three times daily. If the medicine has not helped within a few days, then another homeopathic medicine should be tried, or some other form of therapy should be instituted, as needed. Once symptoms have begun to resolve, the medicine can be given less frequently or stopped. It can be repeated again for a relapse of symptoms. Homeopathic medicines can be used in conjunction with other forms of therapy including conventional medications, herbs, nutritional supplements, and acupuncture.

The following is a list of homeopathic medicines commonly used to treat patients with allergies. It must be emphasized that this list is partial and represents some of the probable choices from the homeopathic materia medica. If the symptoms of a given patient are not represented here, further research in the homeopathic literature would be needed to find the simillimum.

Allium cepa

If the patient's symptom picture fits the description, *Allium cepa* is a useful medicine to try for cases of acute allergic rhinitis, as it will successfully treat a significant percentage of cases. The patient has profuse, nonirritating eye discharge and watery nasal discharge that may burn the upper lip. The throat may feel raw. The symptoms are worse in the later afternoon and evening, from exposure to flowers, and in a warm room and are better in the open air.

Euphrasia officinalis

Euphrasia officinalis is used to treat allergies with bland nasal discharge and profuse watery eye discharge that is irritating (the opposite of *Allium cepa*). The eyes feel quite irritated, and the patient experiences photophobia and blinking. Coughing is accompanied by watering of the eyes. The reaction can progress to asthma (patients with asthma will need conventional medical diagnosis and treatment in addition to homeopathic treatment).

Natrum muriaticum

Consider *Natrum muriaticum* when the allergy sufferer is serious, introverted, or even depressed. The discharge resembles eggwhite. There may be vesicular lesions of the intraoral or perioral tissues. The patient has allergic "shiners" under the eyes. The patient is generally warm blooded and aggravated by becoming overheated. The symptoms may be worse or better near the ocean and worse around 10 AM.

Sabadilla officinalis

The patient needing *Sabadilla officinalis* has marked paroxysmal sneezing. The sneezing may be aggravated when the patient becomes cold or from various odors. The inside of the nose itches and tingles. There is a thin discharge that is frequently irritating. A sore throat and/or a dry cough may also be present. There may also be asthma triggered by seasonal allergens (patients with asthma will need conventional medical diagnosis and treatment in addition to homeopathic treatment).

Sanguinaria canadensis

The patient needing *Sanguinaria canadensis* is sensitive to flowers, pollen, and odors. He or she has a watery nasal discharge, frequent sneezing, and a burning sensation in the mouth, nose, and throat. There may also be asthma that is aggravated by exposure to allergens (patients with asthma will need conventional medical diagnosis and treatment in addition to homeopathic treatment).

Wyethia helenioides

The allergy patient who needs *Wyethia helenioides* has great itching of the mouth, throat, and palate, which may extend to the ears. He or she may also have an irritated throat. The patient feels compelled to swallow frequently and rub the tongue over the palate in an effort to scratch it.

Magnet Therapy

Palpate bilateral TH16 and, if tender apply the bionorth side of the Accu-Band 800 magnet (the side with the tiny protrusion). Next, palpate the area around acupuncture Points LI11 and TH10.[1] This point, known as *Master Nagano's Immune Point*, is used by Kiiko Matsumoto to treat several allergic/immune system problems. The Immune Point is found while the child is lying in a supine position with arms placed along the side of the body, dorsal side up and slightly bent at the elbow. The point in this area that is most tender should have the smooth side (biosouth side) of the Accu-Band 800 magnet taped to the skin. The bionorth magnet on TH16 and the biosouth magnet on the Immune Point may be left in place for up to 48 hours. These magnets may be obtained from OMS (800-323-1839) or AHSM (800-635-7070).

Food Allergies

Apply an Accu-Band 800 magnet, the side with the tiny protrusion (bionorth) facing the skin, to a point at the proximal crease under the second toe bilaterally. Leave the magnets in place for 12 hours. Treatment may be repeated three times per week. These magnets may be obtained from OMS (800-323-1839) or AHSM (800-635-7070).

Osteopathy

Children with symptoms of allergic rhinitis, chronic allergic dermatitis, and hay fever may benefit from osteopathic treatment. Traditionally, the osteopathic perspective views allergic rhinitis and hay fever as symptoms of an imbalance in sympathetic and parasympathetic function. The pterygopalatine ganglion, which is located between the pterygoid process of the sphenoid bone and the palatine bone, may be susceptible to altered hemodynamics when the surrounding muscles or connective tissues become tense.[1-3] Delayed or slowed drainage of the facial sinuses may prolong or exacerbate the child's symptoms of congestion.

The nose and sinuses are part of the respiratory tract and are lined with pseudostratified columnar epithelium having cilia that form a mucociliary transport system. The mucociliary transport system is dependent upon proper ciliary function and mucous viscosity. The secretory cells provide a thin coating of mucous gel through which the cilia may move debris and antigenic particles. The character of nasal and sinus secretions is influenced by autonomic control of the secretory cells. Sympathetic influence is thought to increase the viscosity of the secretions, whereas parasympathetic influences are thought to increase the quantity of the secretions. Alterations in the consistency or biochemical components of this gel layer impede

normal drainage. This results in nasal and sinus congestion, prolonged exposure to antigens, and altered intrasinus pressures. Additionally, obstruction of the sinus ostia or impaired function of the cilia will impede this mechanism and lead to symptoms of chronic sinusitis.

Rudimentary sinuses are present at birth and develop slowly over the next 12 to 14 years to reach their adult size. The sinus ostia are quite small throughout life and lined with respiratory mucosa. They are most commonly obstructed by mucosal swelling. Most often partial obstruction is present, which leads to delayed removal of secretions and inadequate aeration. Facial mechanics are typically restricted in children with chronic or recurrent rhinitis or sinusitis. The tissues of the pterygopalatine area are edematous and tender. The space between the pterygoid muscles and the connective tissues of the fossa is often quite narrow, and congestion exists in the surrounding facial tissues.[4] Techniques addressing the face and cranium have been reported to be effective in the osteopathic management of allergies and sinus congestion.[1,4-6] Hoyt describes techniques to stimulate the sphenopalatine ganglion, which result in a thinning of the nasal secretions and a symptomatic relief of congestion.[5] One study reported decreased workload on the nasal passages as measured by rhinomanometry after osteopathic treatment.[7] Somatic dysfunction, tender points, and tissue strain are also commonly found in the suboccipital muscles of children with allergies. This may be due to facilitation from irritated tissues in the paranasal sinuses via the trigeminal-cervical reflex,[8] a somatovisceral reflex involving the sinuses and suboccipital muscles.[9-11]

In children with viral or allergic conditions, osteopathic treatment to resolve the associated biomechanical dysfunction may help to facilitate mucociliary clearance of the sinuses and promote overall health. In addition to the traditional osteopathic description of the role of articular and soft tissues in sinus drainage and aeration,[1,2,6,12,13] tissue edema may also play a role in persistent rhinitis and sinusitis through the activation of local primary afferents in the area that secrete proinflammatory substances.

Newborns are obligate nose breathers for the first 2 or 3 months of life. Airway obstruction results in cyanosis and even apnea. Although allergies are not common in this age group, nasal congestion in the newborn can be a real worry for parents. The baby is typically described as snuffling and snorting during feeding. Physical examination is normal except for mucus in the nasal passages, and occasionally the mucosa is erythematous. Congenital abnormality including deviated nasal septum must be ruled out. In the majority of cases of chronic neonatal congestion, no causative etiology can be found and the congestion is explained away by the infant's undersized nasal passages. Theoretically the sinuses are too small to be involved. Osteopathic examination of these children usually reveals altered mechanics and tissue restriction through the face. Biomechanical restriction and altered tissue tensions at the frontosphenoidal area, the ethmoid notch, and the cranial base may be present in some infants.[14] Empirically, vertical strain patterns at the SBS and intraosseous strains in the sphenoid between the lesser wings and the body also appear to be associated with chronic congestion. Osteopathic physicians typically use gentle, indirect approaches including cranial osteopathy, biodynamic, and balancing techniques to treat neonates with chronic congestion.

References

Pediatric Diagnosis and Treatment

1. Nelson WE, Berhman RE, Kliegman RM, editors: *Nelson textbook of pedeiatrics*, ed 17, Philadelphia, 2004, WB Saunders.
2. Stiehm ER et al, editors: *Immunologic disorders in infants and children*, ed 5, Philadelphia, 2004, Elsevier.

Chiropractic

1. Neuroimmune hypothesis. In Leach RA, editor: *The chiropractic theories*, Baltimore, 2004, Lippincott Williams and Wilkins.
2. Brennan PC, Kokjohn K, Triano J et al: Immunologic correlates of reduced spinal mobility: preliminary observations in a dog model. In Wold S, editor: *Proceedings of the 1991 International Conference on Spinal Manipulation* Arlington, Va, 1991, Foundation for Chiropractic Education and Research.
3. Brennan PC, Kokjohn K, Kaltinger CJ, et al: Enhanced phagocytic cell respiratory burst induced by spinal manipulation: potential role of substance P, *J Manipulative Physiol Ther* 14:399-408, 1991.
4. Hightower B, Pfleger B, Selano JL et al: The effects of specific upper cervical adjustments on the CD4 counts of HIV positive patients, *Chiro Res J* 3:32, 1994.
5. Zeichner A, Boczkowski JA: Clinical application of biofeedback techniques for the elderly, *Clin Gerontol* 5:457-473, 1996.
6. Buerger MA: History and physical assessment. In Anrig C, Plaugher G, editors: *Chiropractic pediatrics,* Baltimore MD, 1998, Williams and Wilkins.
7. Isolaure E, Slaminen S, Sandholm-Mattila T: New functional foods in the treatment of food allergy, *Ann Med* 31:299-302, 1999.
8. Isolauri E, Ribeiro Hda C, Gibson G et al: Functional foods and probiotics: working group report of the First World Congress of Pediatric Gastroenterology, Hepatology and Nutrition, *J Pediatr Gastroenterol Nutr* 35(Suppl 2):S106-S109, 2002.
9. Farchi S, Forastiere N, Agabiti G et al: Dietary factors associated with wheezing and allergic rhinitis in children, *Eur Respir J* 22: 772-780, 2003.
10. Schmitt WH JR, Leisman G: Correlation of applied kinesiology muscle testing findings with serum immunoglobulin levels for food allergies, *Int J Neurosci* 96:237-244, 1998.
11. Buerger MA: History and physical assessment. In Anrig C, Plaugher G, editors: *Chiropractic pediatrics,* Baltimore, Md, 1998, Williams and Wilkins.
12. Maldonado J, Gil A, Narbona E et al: Special formulas in infant nutrition: a review, *Early Hum Dev* 53 Suppl:S23-S32, 1998.
13. Beaudry M, Dufour R, Marcoux S: Relation between infant feeding and infections during the first six months of life, *J Pediatr* 126:191-197, 1995.
14. Hall BS: Allergy, endocrine and metabolic diseases in childhood. In Davies NJ, editor: *Chiropractic pediatrics*, London 2000, Churchill Livingstone.
15. Miyake Y, Sasaki S, Tanaka K et al: Fish and fat intake and prevalence of allergic rhinitis in Japanese females: the Osaka Maternal and Child Health Study, *J Am Coll Nutr* 26:279-287, 2007.
16. Hoff S, Seiler H, Heinrich J et al: Allergic sensitisation and allergic rhinitis are associated with n-3 polyunsaturated fatty acids in the diet and in red blood cell membranes, *Eur J Clin Nutr* 59:1071-1080, 2005.

Herbs—Chinese

1. Makino T, Ito Y, Sasaki SY et al: Preventive and curative effects of Gyokuheifu-san, a formula of traditional Chinese medicine, on allergic rhinitis induced with Japanese cedar pollens in guinea pig, *Biol Pharm Bull* 27:554-558, 2004.
2. Natural Standard Research Collaboration. Available at www. naturalstandard.com. Accessed August 2005.
3. Bao L, Sun QW, Hu L: Clinical and experimental study for allergic rhinitis with treatment of biminkang mixture [in Chinese] *Zhongguo Zhong Xi Yi Jie He Za Zhi* 17:70-72, 1997.
4. *The heart and essence of Dan-Xi's methods of treatment: a translation of Zhu Dan-Xi's Zhi Fa Xin Yao*, Boulder, Colo, 1993, Blue Poppy Press (translated by Yang Shou-Zhong).
5. Xue CC, Thien FC, Zhang JJ, et al: Effect of adding a Chinese herbal preparation to acupuncture for seasonal allergic rhinitis: randomised double-blind controlled trial, *Hong Kong Med J* 9:427-434, 2003.
6. Tai CJ, Chien LY: The treatment of allergies using Sanfujiu: a method of applying Chinese herbal medicine paste to acupoints on three peak summer days, *Am J Chin Med* 32:967-976, 2004.

Herbs—Western

1. Mittman P: Randomized, double-blind study of freeze-dried *Urtica dioica* in the treatment of allergic rhinitis, *Planta Med* 56:44-47, 1990.

Homeopathy

1. Felix Berumen JA, Gonzalez Diaz SN, Canseco Gonzalez C et al: Use of alternative medicine in the treatment of allergic diseases [in Spanish], *Rev Alerg Mex* 51:41-44, 2004.
2. Linde K, Clausius N, Ramirez G et al: Are the clinical effects of homoeopathy placebo effects? A meta-analysis of placebo-controlled trials, *Lancet* 350:834-843, 1997.
3. Reilly DT, Taylor MA: Potent placebo or potency? *Br Hom J* 74: 65-75, 1985.
4. Reilly DT, Taylor MA, McSharry C et al: Is homoeopathy a placebo response? Controlled trial of homoeopathic potency, with pollen in hayfever as model, *Lancet* 2:881-885, 1986.
5. Reilly D, Taylor MA Beattie NGM et al: Is evidence for homoeopathy reproducible? *Lancet* 344:1601-1606, 1994.
6. Taylor MA, Reilly D, Llewellyn-Jones RH et al: Randomised controlled trial of homoeopathy versus placebo in perennial allergic rhinitis with overview of four trial series, *Br Med J* 321:471-476, 2000.
7. Frenkel M, Hermoni D: Effects of homeopathic intervention on medication consumption in atopic and allergic disorders, *Alt Ther* 8:76-79, 2002.
8. *ReferenceWorks Pro 4.2,* San Rafael, Calif, 2008, Kent Homeopathic Associates.

Magnet Therapy

1. Loo M: *Pediatric acupuncture*, London, 2002, Elsevier.

Osteopathy

1. Magoun HIS: *Osteopathy in the cranial field*, ed 3, Kirksville, Mo, 1976, The Journal Printing Co.
2. Sutherland WG: *Teachings in the science of osteopathy*, Portland, Ore, 1990, Rudra Press.
3. Sutherland WG: *Contributions of thought*, ed 2, Portland, Ore, 1998, Rudra Press.
4. Sept KE: AAO case study—"sinusitis," *AOA J* 4:20-21, 1994.

5. Hoyt W: Current concepts in the management of sinus disease, *J Am Osteopath Assoc* 90:913-919, 1990.

6. Paul FA, Buser BR: Osteopathic manipulative treatment applications for the emergency department patient, *J Am Osteopath Assoc* 96:403-409, 1996.

7. Kaluza CL, Sherbin M: The physiologic response of the nose to osteopathic manipulative treatment, *J Am Osteopath Assoc* 83:654-660, 1983.

8. Carreiro JE: Neurology. In *An osteopathic approach to children,* London, 2003, Churchill Livingstone.

9. Sato A: Somatovisceral reflexes, *J Manipulative Physiol Ther* 18:597-602, 1995.

10. Carreiro JE: Nervous system. In *An osteopathic approach to children,* London, 2003, Churchill Livingstone.

11. Willard FH: Autonomic nervous system. In Ward R, editor: *Foundations for osteopathic medicine,* ed 2, Philadelphia, 2003, Lippincott Williams and Wilkins.

12. Ward RC, Hruby RJ, Jerome JA et al: *Foundations for osteopathic medicine,* St Louis, 2002, Lippincott.

13. Lum WH: Serous otitis media, *J Am Osteopath Assoc* 67:440-444, 2004.

14. Carreiro JE: Otolaryngology. In *An osteopathic approach to children,* Edinburgh, 2003, Elsevier.

CHAPTER 11

Arthritis

Acupuncture | May Loo

Aromatherapy | Maura A. Fitzgerald

Chiropractic | Anne Spicer

Herbs—Western | Alan D. Woolf, Paula M. Gardiner, Lana Dvorkin-Camiel, Jack Maypole

Homeopathy | Janet L. Levatin

Magnet Therapy | Agatha P. Colbert, Deborah Risotti

Massage Therapy | Mary C. McLellan

Nutrition | Joy A. Weydert

Osteopathy | Jane Carreiro

✳ PEDIATRIC DIAGNOSIS AND TREATMENT

Juvenile rheumatoid arthritis (JRA) refers to a group of disorders characterized by chronic arthritis. It is the most common chronic rheumatic illness in children and is a significant cause of short- and long-term disability.[1,2] The incidence of JRA is approximately 13.9/100,000 children/year among children 15 years or younger, with an overall prevalence of approximately 113/100,000 children.[3]

The clinical characteristic is an idiopathic synovitis of the peripheral joints, associated with soft tissue swelling and effusion. The American College of Rheumatology (ACR) classifies JRA as a category of diseases with three principal types of onset: (1) oligoarthritis, fewer than five inflamed joints; (2) polyarthritis, five or more inflamed joints; and (3) systemic-onset disease, arthritis with characteristic fever. Nine distinct course subtypes have also been identified. Additional criteria include: age < 16 years at onset; arthritis (swelling or effusion, or presence of two or more of the following signs: limitation of range of motion, tenderness or pain on motion, and increased heat) in one or more joints; duration of disease 6 weeks or longer; and onset type defined by type of disease in the first 6 months and exclusion of other forms of juvenile arthritis.[4,5]

The precise etiology for JRA is unknown, but it is generally thought to occur in immunogenetically susceptible children exposed to an external, presumably environmental, trigger.[3,6] Specific HLA subtypes have been identified in at-risk children: HLA-DR4 is associated with polyarticular disease; pauciarticular JRA has been associated with HLA alleles at the DR8 and DR5 loci, the strongest associations with the HLA-DRB1 alleles.[7] Possible external triggers for JRA include certain viruses (e.g., parvovirus B19, rubella, Epstein-Barr virus), host hyperreactivity to specific self-antigens (type II collagen), and enhanced T-cell reactivity to bacterial or mycobacterial heat shock proteins. T-cell activation results in a cascade of events leading to release of proinflammatory cytokines, resulting in tissue damage in joints.[3]

The diagnosis of JRA is based on the ACR classification criteria with the exclusion of other articular diseases. There is no single pathognomonic finding for these diseases in children.[4,5]

The diagnosis is based on a history of inflammatory joint disease, physical examination that confirms the presence of arthritis, and characteristic laboratory abnormalities for inflammation that include an elevated erythrocyte sedimentation rate (ESR) and C-reactive protein (CRP), leukocytosis, thrombocytosis, and the anemia of chronic disease.[3] Elevated antinuclear antibody (ANA) titers are present in at least 40% to 85% of all children with pauciarticular or polyarticular JRA but are unusual in children with systemic-onset disease. Detectable ANA, usually with homogeneous or speckled pattern, is associated with increased risk for the development of chronic uveitis, but the precise specificities for various ANA patterns have not been determined. A positive rheumatoid factor (RF) may be associated with onset of the disease in an older child with polyarticular involvement (approximately 8%) and the development of rheumatoid nodules, with a poor overall prognosis and eventual functional disability.[3]

Early radiographic changes include soft tissue swelling, osteoporosis, and periostitis around the affected joints. Characteristic late radiographic changes of JRA are seen in the hands and cervical spine, most frequently in the neural arch joints at C2-C3.[3] The wide variety of imaging modalities are crucial for the diagnosis and follow-up of arthritis.[8,9] Quantitative computed tomography can show decreased muscle mass and abnormal bone geometry.[10] Magnetic resonance imaging allows direct visualization of the inflamed synovium and pannus and may detect early cartilage changes.[8,10]

Although the disorder is chronic and not life-threatening, early institution of treatment is crucial, as poorly controlled JRA can profoundly affect growth, development, and quality of life in children.[11] Medication treatment should follow a pyramid approach beginning with a combination of the least toxic medications (usually nonsteroidal antiinflammatory drugs [NSAIDs]) and proceeding through sulfasalazine, methotrexate, and possibly etanercept or immunosuppressive or experimental drugs. Azathioprine and cyclophosphamide are reserved for the very few children who do not respond to less aggressive therapy, whereas glucocorticoids are used for overwhelming inflammatory or systemic illness.[3] Routine slit-lamp ophthalmological examination is important for all patients with JRA to monitor for development of asymptomatic uveitis, a common extraarticular manifestation that occurs in 20% to 30% of JRA patients.[12,13] Parental education, dietary evaluation to ensure appropriate calcium intake, physical and occupational therapy, and psychotherapeutic intervention to help families cope with the stress of a debilitating chronic illness are also important to implement in the treatment regimen.[2,3]

Prognosis varies according to the type, age of onset, laboratory findings, and other factors as summarized in Table 11-1.

Currently, there is active international interest in advancing clinical studies in pediatric rheumatology. A number of collaborative groups have formed, the best known of which are the Pediatric Rheumatology Collaborative Study Group in North America and the Paediatric Rheumatology International Trials Organization in Europe, South America, and Asia.[15]

✳ CAM THERAPY RECOMMENDATIONS

Acupuncture

Chinese medicine explains arthritis as an "obstruction syndrome," meaning that the pain and swelling is due to an obstruction of flow of Qi and Blood through the channels, usually associated with or secondary to a pathogenic influence such as Wind, Cold, and/or Dampness. Oligoarthritis is usually due to Dampness or Cold blockage, whereas polyarthritis with symptoms that appear at different joints at different times is more compatible with wind blockage.[1]

In TCM, joints are important areas of entry, convergence, and exit of Qi and Blood; a meeting place of Yin and Yang-Qi. The predisposing factors for development of arthritis are genetic vulnerability, the child's Qi, underlying Blood or Yin deficiency, overuse, and emotional problems. Genetic vulnerability suggests that the strength of the Kidney Qi can affect the physiology of the joints. When the child's Qi is weak relative to the force of pathogenic influence, Wind, Cold, or Damp can accumulate in the joints. Blood or Yin deficiency leads to malnourishment of the channels and joints such that they become more vulnerable to external pathogenic factors. Overuse (e.g., excessive sports) can lead to arthritic symptoms. Emotional problems can lead to Qi stagnation and Qi and Blood depletion. Persistent obstruction in the joints can lead to muscle atrophy and bony deformities. Acupuncture treatment is directed toward eliminating or expelling the pathogenic factors, alleviating pain, and treating the root cause of the arthritic or obstructive symptoms.[1,2]

The analgesic effect of acupuncture is discussed in detail in Chapter 6. The various mechanisms include biomechanical tissue response, "blocking" pain signals by rapid transmission of signals along small myelinated type II and III afferent nerve fibers, by stimulating the release of opioids and other neurotransmitters to modulate pain, and by influencing immune response. Acupuncture also increases blood flow both centrally and peripherally,[3] thereby augmenting the supply of oxygen and nutrients to arthritic joints. Acupuncture further helps

✳ TABLE 11-1

Prognosis of Juvenile Rheumatoid Arthritis by Type of Onset

ONSET TYPE	COURSE SUBTYPE	SUBSEQUENT CLINICAL MANIFESTATIONS	OUTCOME
Polyarthritis	RF-seropositive	Female	Poor
		Older age	
		Hand/wrist	
		Erosions	
		Nodules	
		Unremitting	
	ANA-seropositive	Female	Good
		Young age	
	Seronegative	—	Variable
Oligoarthritis	ANA-seropositive	Female	Excellent (except eyes)
		Young age	
		Chronic anterior uveitis (iridocyclitis)	
	RF-seropositive	Polyarthritis	Poor
		Erosions	
		Unremitting	
	HLA-B27-positive	Male	Good
		Older age	
	Seronegative	—	Good
Systemic disease	Oligoarthritis	—	Good
	Polyarthritis	Erosions	Poor

From Cassidy JT, Petty RE, editors: *Textbook of pediatric rheumatology*, ed 4, Philadelphia, 2001, Saunders.

ANA, Antinuclear antibody; *RF*, rheumatoid factor.

arthritis through modulation of the inflammatory response, with a decrease in vascular permeability and modulation of proinflammatory neuropeptides. Recent information demonstrates that acupuncture modulates mediators of inflammation via common pathways as analgesia.[4] Acupuncture released β-endorphin interacts with some cytokines by diminishing proinflammatory cytokines, such as IL-1β and tumor necrosis factor (TNF)-α, and by increasing levels of antiinflammatory interleukins, such as interleukin (IL)-2, IL-4, IL-6, and IL-10 levels, and (24±27)[5] plasma interferon (IFN)-γ.[5] Clinical application of the antiinflammatory effect includes increasing IL-2 in arthritis.[6]

Rheumatoid Arthritis Evidence-Based Information

Although there is extensive evidence of acupuncture efficacy in pain relief, the utility and efficacy of acupuncture in treating rheumatoid arthritis (RA) has not been demonstrated in large, randomized controlled trials (RCTs) in adults or children.[7] Clinical reports indicate that as much as 70% successful pain elimination or modulation can occur in patients with various chronic pain syndromes, including arthritis.[8,9]

ST36 and LI4 are the two most widely used acupoints in experimental studies for acupuncture analgesia.[10,11] A clinical report from Taiwan indicates that needling at Hoku (LI4) resulted in increase of regional blood flow and increase in temperature.[12] Acupuncture at Hoku point produced analgesia that peaked at 20 to 40 minutes after the needle insertion and diminished 45 minutes after the needles were removed, with a half-life of 16.2 ± 1.9 minutes. A greater increase in pain threshold was produced when both Hoku and Zusanli points were stimulated simultaneously than when either was stimulated alone.[11]

A clinical study from China of 12 adults with RA demonstrated modulation of immunoglobulins by decreasing IgG, IgA, and IgM.[13] A small randomized controlled grial from China showed that the IL-2 levels—a very important signal for regulating immune response—were lower in patients with RA. After acupuncture treatment, the IL-2 level increased significantly.[14] A clinical trial from Russia demonstrated that multimodal treatment including acupuncture was found to be effective in treating adult RA.[15] Another Russia study using laser therapy produced insignificant effect on 82 children with active JRA, whereas adults with moderate RA responded well.[16]

An animal study from China demonstrated laser acupuncture treatment on ipsilateral Kun-Lun BL60 point for 10 minutes every day for 5 days reduced pain and swelling in the ankle.[17]

An animal study from China applied electroacupuncture (EA) at 100 Hz and 15 Hz on bilateral Yanglingpuan GB34 acupoints and demonstrated 15-Hz EA was effective for analgesia and significantly lowered spinal glutamic acid content, which suggests that modulation of spinal glutamic acid may be an analgesic effect of EA.[18]

Suggestions for Acupuncture Treatment of Arthritis

Specific acupuncture treatment for JRA should be carried out by a practitioner experienced in assessing the underlying predisposing factor, the specific channel(s) involved with the joints, and the pathogenic influences. The following suggestions are for simple, general pain relief.

General pain relief

Use ST36 and LI4 for general pain relief. A word of caution in applying LI4 in children: Because LI4 is a very strong dispersing (sedating) point, it would not be advisable to use it alone, especially in children who are deficient. ST36 and LI4 together can be a potent combination for stimulating immunity as well.

General points according to pathogenic etiology:
- Wind: BL17
- Cold: GV14, BL23
- Dampness: BL20[2]

Regional pain relief

For local treatment of affected areas:
Fingers: Ba Xie, TE5, SI5[2]
Wrist: TE4, TE5, SI4, P7, LI5[1]
Hip: GB30—the most important local point
   SP12—use in addition to GB30 when pain extends to the groin[2]
Knee: local points: ST34, GB33, ST36, SP10, LR8, SP9[1]
Ankle: SP5,[2] BL60[17]
Immunostimulant points: LI4, LI11, ST36, SP6, BL11, BL20, BL23, CV12[19]

Aromatherapy

Analgesic and antiinflammatory essential oils are recommended to aid in the reduction of symptoms in RA.[1,2] These include German chamomile (*Matricaria recutita*), rosemary (*Rosmarinus officinalis*), black pepper (*Piper nigrum*), eucalyptus (*Eucalyptus* sp.), lavender (*Lavandula angustifolia*) and lemongrass (*Cymbopogon citratus*). Essential oils are applied by massage, in a warm or cold compress over a painful area, or in the bath. In a small pilot study, nine adults with RA were randomly assigned to one of three groups: control, treatment with massage, and treatment with lavender aromatherapy massage. The results were contradictory: Although self-assessment by visual analog scale revealed no change in pain or sleep, interview data indicated that subjects in the aromatherapy massage group reported a reduced intake of analgesics and improvement in sleep.[3]

Chiropractic

A single case is found in the literature referring to chiropractic management of arthritis: a 51-year-old female, who did not respond to a wide variety of pharmaceuticals and dietary modifications, underwent chiropractic care and had complete elimination of pain within 8 weeks of her initial visit.[1]

It is important to note that arthritic conditions commonly lead to subluxation complex (SC) in affected individuals. The medical subluxation is commonly understood to result from arthrides.[2,3] The spine (especially cervical) of the person with arthritis will likely require more frequent attention.[4] Brainstem compression may follow upper cervical subluxation resulting from translocation of the odontoid secondary to arthritic changes.[5,6] Cord compression may lead to the development of quadriplegia, headache, paresthesia, and perhaps even sudden death.[3]

The chiropractor must take care to identify such extreme subluxation and modify any corrective technique accordingly.

Adjustments are specifically recommended in cases of juvenile chronic arthritis.[7]

Stretches and exercises that endeavor to maintain normal ranges of motion at affected joints may diminish degenerative changes.[8]

Omega-3 fatty acids (EPA/DHA) may inhibit cartilaginous degeneration.[9] It is also advisable to eliminate trans fats, as they compete for essential fatty acid sites and establish a proinflammatory process.

Glucosamine sulfate has been shown to enhance joint function and cartilaginous resilience.[10]

Chiropractors recommend avoidance of NSAIDs because of the destructive effects on joints and other organ systems.[11]

A trial of gluten elimination may reduce symptoms.[12]

Hair analysis, comprehensive blood profile, digestive stool analysis, and urine analysis may be productive in identifying a particular agent, deficiency, or condition contributing to the problem.

Herbs—Western

JRA is a chronic disease that may require an integrative approach of therapy including nonsteroidal and/or steroidal antiinflammatory medications as well as antirheumatic drugs. Providers are urged to use caution with patients identified as using herbal therapies in light of potential interactions or side effects of drugs or herbal products.

Turmeric *(Curcuma longa)* may be applied topically or orally. It is a common ingredient in foods and is believed to be safe.[1] Turmeric's major active constituents include curcumin (diferuloylmethane), a yellow pigment for which a single study suggested may have some effects in adult individuals with RA.[2] There is no evidence to establish its effectiveness in children with RA.

The root and rhizome of ginger *(Zingiber officinale)* are thought to possess antiinflammatory properties that make it an oral treatment for individuals with RA. Active ingredients such as gingerol, gingerdione, and shogaol are believed to be active in suppressing inflammation via the cyclooxygenase pathway[3] and other cytokine pathways. Although generally regarded as safe by the Food and Drug Administration, there are no studies to gauge its effectiveness for children with RA and little evidence to support its use for adults with symptoms of RA.

When administered orally, the ingredients found in evening primrose oil *(Oenothera biennis)*—γ-linoleic acid, linoleic acid, and vitamin E—are thought to possess antiinflammatory properties. There is no evidence to support its effectiveness in children. Limited evidence in adult studies also shows no clear benefit regarding symptoms of RA in children.[4-6]

Evaluation of the extract of willowbark (see Chapter 39, Headache, discussion of salicin) in a double-blind controlled trial of adult patients with RA did not find it to be effective for pain control or arthritis symptoms (dose 240 mg/day).[7] Salicylates are sometimes used for RA in children. Willowbark

is a natural source for this herbal ingredient, but there is no evidence for its use and efficacy in children. Owing to concerns about Reye's syndrome and associated fatty hepatitis and encephalopathy, families should consult a physician regarding ongoing use of willowbark.

Recent double-blind studies have shown some benefit of borage oil in treatment in adults of rheumatoid arthritis.[8,9] In RCTs of adults, 1.4 g/day γ-linolenic acid in borage seed oil was necessary to derive the expected benefits.[8] TNF-α has been shown to be a central mediator of inflammatory and joint destructive processes in rheumatoid arthritis.[10] There are no studies regarding the effectiveness of this therapy in children.

Homeopathy

Before using this section, please see Appendix A, Homeopathy, for definitions of practitioner expertise categories and for general information on prescribing homeopathic medicines.

Practitioner Expertise Category 3

There are no controlled clinical trials of homeopathic treatment for arthritis, although the homeopathic literature contains evidence for its use in the form of accumulated clinical experience. Homeopathic treatment can be used safely for arthritis, either alone or in combination with other treatment modalities. Because arthritis is a complex medical problem, often involving autoimmune processes or infectious agents, successful homeopathic treatment usually requires extensive training in the art and science of homeopathy. Any one of many homeopathic medicines may be used to treat arthritis, depending on the characteristics of the patient being treated. Sophisticated homeopathic analysis and long-term follow-up are required. For these reasons, specific medicines for treating arthritis are not presented here. Interested readers are referred to the homeopathic literature for further study.

Magnet Therapy

When only one joint is involved, the labeled bionorth side of a 3950-gauss ceramic block magnet should be applied to one side of the joint and the opposite (biosouth) side of a similar magnet to the other side of the involved joint. The size of the magnets used should be proportionate to the size of the child's involved joint. The two magnets should be positioned so as to attract each other, creating a concentrated field within the joint. Magnets can be secured in position with an elastic wrap and left in place for up to 48 hours, and the treatment may be repeated two times per week. Magnets may be obtained from Painfree Lifestyles (800-480-8601) or AHSM (800-635-7070).

Massage Therapy

Studies have concluded that massage is an effective therapy for the management of chronic and acute pain. Research has shown elevated plasma β-endorphin levels following massage therapy,[1] which may explain some of its pain-reducing properties. Theorists have postulated that massage therapy may decrease substance P levels during massage treatment, but controlled studies have yet to be done. A systematic review of

22 articles on the effects of massage therapy on relaxation and comfort indicated significantly decreased anxiety or perception of tension in 8 of 10 studies; physiological relaxation was produced in 7 of 10 studies, and massage effectively reduced pain in 3 studies.[2] The efficacy of massage therapy to decrease pain scores in acute postoperative pain management has also been demonstrated.[3-7]

A randomized controlled study in children with JRA who received 15 minutes daily parental massage reported lower parental and child anxiety scores, lower salivary cortisol levels, decreased self-reported pain, parental reports of decreased pain, and physician reports of less pain and morning stiffness compared with a control group who received relaxation interventions.[8]

Swedish massage is an effective, gentle treatment for children with arthritic pain; it is also relatively easy to teach parents and caregivers. It is recommended not to massage directly over areas of acute inflammation; however, massage can be performed on areas of chronic inflammation. Effleurage and petrissage to the long, broad muscles of the body can help relieve pain in the joints associated with these muscle groups, as massage directly on the affected joints may be uncomfortable for children. For example, both massage strokes could be applied to the quadriceps and the hamstrings to help relieve hip pain; for knee pain, both of these muscle groups plus the lower leg muscles (the peroneals, dorsiflexors, soleus, and gastrocnemius) should be massaged. If a child is affected by knee pain, massage to the arches of the feet can help relax the peroneal and dorsiflexor muscles, which insert into the knee. Massage should never be done on the back of the knee, as this is considered an endangerment site.

Similarly, for joint involvement of the upper extremities, the same approach should be used. For shoulder pain, massage to the upper arm muscles (triceps and biceps) and the shoulder muscles (latissimus dorsi, deltoid, and pectorals) using effleurage and petrissage may be helpful. Care should be taken not to put the shoulder into hyperextension, which puts an inflamed joint at risk for dislocation. Care should also be taken not to massage in the axillae, as this is an endangerment site. In older children, areas of breast tissue should be avoided when trying to massage the pectoral muscles, as these areas may be tender for both genders. Avoidance may be accomplished by using localized effleurage strokes directly along the sternum and just below the clavicle out toward the shoulder joint. Some older children may prefer to do this stroke themselves for improved comfort levels.

Elbow pain may be relieved by the mentioned massage strokes applied to the muscles of the upper arm (biceps and triceps) as well as brachioradialis. Massage specifically to the brachioradialis is best accomplished using flat, broad effleurage, as deeper strokes may be uncomfortable for that muscle grouping.

Massage to the digits can best be done with a distal to proximal and back motion ("give me the money sign" gesture) along each bicep muscle of the fingers or toes. This will help avoid the joint areas and have the most impact. It will also help massage the muscles of the digits rather than the tendons and tissue located in the lateral aspects of the digits.

If a child does not have symmetrical joint involvement, an alternative to massaging near affected areas is to massage the mirror opposite of the area. For example, if the right knee is acutely inflamed and the leg is painful to touch, massage to the muscles of the left leg can help reduce pain on the right (see Chapter 3). For children who suffer from morning stiffness, parental massage to the affected extremities prior to the child arising in the morning may help to warm up the body tissues and decrease immediate pain caused by movement and stiffness.

Nutrition

Discussion

As RA is caused by a pathological immune response to some environmental insult, a link to food triggers has been studied. It is theorized that certain food allergies may trigger an antibody response forming immune complexes that damage the intestinal wall, causing increased permeability. This increased permeability allows for the absorption of microbial antigens similar to protein found in the joint tissues. The body recognizes these antigens as foreign and attacks these proteins, but it also attacks the protein in joint tissues.[1] Studies have shown that dietary changes can decrease the symptoms of arthritis.

Fasting from food, followed by a vegetarian diet, has been studied extensively in patients with RA. A systematic review of controlled studies that lasted for at least 3 months showed a statistically and clinically significant long-term beneficial effect to this dietary approach.[2] This review concluded that fasting for 7 to 10 days followed by a vegetarian diet might be a useful treatment for RA. Further study into the mechanism of this strategy found that a vegetarian diet produced a reduction in the level of proteus antibody.[3] High anti-proteus antibodies in serum and proteus found in urine are isolated in higher numbers in patients with RA and are thought to play an etiopathogenic role.[4]

Supplementing the diet with fish oil fatty acids (omega-3 combination of EPA/DHA) demonstrated a decrease in symptoms of RA and a reduction in neutrophil leukotriene B-4 production.[5] A subsequent study found greater effects with higher doses of EPA and DHA, with no increase of side effects. This second study also demonstrated a decrease in macrophage IL-1 production as well as improved clinical measures.[6]

A more recent study investigated the effects of a vegetarian diet (considered an antiinflammatory diet [A-ID] providing an arachidonic acid intake of less than 90 mg/day) alone or in combination with supplemental fish oil capsules. This was compared with a conventional western diet (WD) (considered high in arachidonic acid) with and without fish oil supplementation. A-ID patients had a 14% reduction of tender and swollen joints during the fish oil placebo phase when compared with the WD. This change increased to 34% when fish oil was added to the A-ID. Compared with baseline, a 34% decrease in leukotriene B formation, 15% decrease in 11-dehydro-thromboxane-B level, and 21% decrease in prostaglandin metabolites were observed. This study concluded that an antiinflammatory diet augmented the beneficial effects of fish oil supplementation.[7]

Other studies have considered the effects of allergic foods on RA. The most common offenders are wheat, corn, milk, beef, and foods from the night shade family (e.g., tomato, potato, eggplant, pepper, tobacco). RA patients with a positive skin-prick test to food extracts were compared with patients with negative tests. Both groups fasted from the most common allergenic foods for 12 days and were then challenged with various allergenic foods for 12 days. Re-elimination was carried out before the next challenge. Results of this study found significant increases in pain, stiffness, and number of tender swollen joints and increases in TNF-α, IL-β, ESR, and CRP levels with the food challenges in the patients with positive skin prick tests. No significant change in any of the variables except pain was found in the skin prick–negative group. The researchers conclude that individualized diet revisions may regulate TNF-α and IL-1β levels in selected patients with RA.[8]

Treatment

Nutritional management for RA might include the following recommendations:

- Fasting is not generally recommended for children and adolescents; however, a medically supervised antiinflammatory diet could be started to lower the intake of arachidonic acids. A diet high in fresh fruits and vegetables provide the best sources of dietary antioxidant, which neutralizes free radicals involved in the inflammatory process. Pineapple is a rich source of bromelain, a mixture of enzymes that block the production of the inflammatory kinins. Bromelain also breaks down immune complexes that cause tissue destruction.
- Supplement the diet with fish oil capsules using approximately 54 mg/kg of EPA and 36 mg/kg of DHA per day.
- The diet should also be supplemented with vitamin B$_{12}$, as this is not present in a vegetarian diet.
- Investigate for food allergies, and eliminate foods that test positive in that individual.

Osteopathy

Arthritis in children has typically been described as inflammatory, metabolic, or infectious. Recently the incidence of functional musculoskeletal pain syndromes including fibromyalgia and chronic fatigue has increased in older children, teenagers, and young adults. In all of these conditions, musculoskeletal pain and stiffness are primary complaints. General osteopathic management includes appropriate medical care where indicated, complemented by osteopathic procedures to address the pain and lost mobility. The pain of arthritis is twofold: the inflammation within the articular compartment activates joint nociceptors, which in turn generate a reflexive contraction of the muscle stabilizers of the involved joint. The maintained contraction produces irritation of the muscle afferents, alters joint mechanics, and increases unit load across the articular surface. As a result the child has pain from the primary etiology of the arthritis in addition to pain from the compensatory responses of the surrounding tissues. Although different pathologies require slightly different approaches and goals of treatment, in general osteopathic manipulation is used to decrease the nociceptive drive from the surrounding tissues and

normalize joint mechanics. The choice of techniques employed depends upon the etiology of the problem, the child's age, and associated comorbidities. Usually the child is encouraged to practice age-appropriate postural rebalancing exercises to reinforce the changes made in the treatment. Examples of postural rebalancing or core stabilization activities might include martial arts, yoga, or horseback riding for an older child. A younger child might benefit from a "gymboree" program.

Infectious arthropathies need to be treated with appropriate antibiotics. In the acute phase, the osteopathic practitioner employs the respiratory-circulatory model as a framework for the use of osteopathic manipulation to improve lymphatic and venous drainage from the area and perfusion and antibiotic delivery to the involved tissues. Lymphatic, myofascial, and most indirect techniques are appropriate in these children. Once appropriate tissue levels of the antibiotics are obtained and the condition is stable, osteopathic management is directed at maintaining range of motion and preventing intraarticular adhesions. In all cases, articulatory and direct techniques are avoided in the acute phase. Reports on the efficacy of osteopathic manipulation in the management of infectious arthritis are anecdotal.

Metabolic arthritis is usually painful and involves joint stiffness. Needless to say, the underlying pathology must be addressed. Osteopathic treatment is directed at improving fluid mechanics and venous and arterial flow to the area, decreasing nociceptive drive, and rebalancing abnormal compensatory patterns in the surrounding tissue. There is only one published case study on the efficacy of osteopathic manipulative therapy in metabolic arthritis. The patient was an adult, and although the report[1] had a positive outcome, it is rather out of date and poorly written by today's standards.

Inflammatory arthritis in children may be part of a rheumatological disorder, a spondyloarthropathy, or a reactive process to an infection or other antigen exposure. In all cases, the problem can be viewed as dysregulation of the immune system. Treatment goals include decreasing the nociceptive drive from the surrounding tissues and normalizing joint mechanics. In addition, the pathology of rheumatoid disease requires that the osteopath also address tissue dysfunction in areas that might be contributing to neuroendocrine imbalance or an increased allostatic load.[2] Alterations in the neuroendocrine-immune (NEI) network are associated with rheumatological diseases.[3-5] Nociceptive or pain input plays a role in the modulation of the hypothalamic-pituitary-adrenal axis[6-8] and consequently in the function of the NEI network. Consequently, the osteopathic approach to a child with RA would take into consideration all the possible influences on the NEI network. Physical stress in the form of pain is only one of the possible drives on this system; social and emotional stress that may or may not be related to the child's diagnosis may also influence neuroendocrine balance. In the case of reactive arthritis, the underlying condition needs to be addressed. Osteopathic manipulation may be used in conjunction to decrease pain, improve range of motion, and facilitate lymphatic function. Spondyloarthropathies, particularly ankylosing spondylitis and psoriatric arthritis, require a long-term treatment plan aimed at minimizing pain and prolonging maximum mobility. All inflammatory arthritic conditions may benefit from interdisciplinary approaches in which pharmaceutical, homeopathic, herbal, and osteopathic interventions are used concurrently. Although there are no published data, many osteopaths find combining osteopathic treatment with homeopathy or acupuncture to be beneficial for patients with inflammatory diseases.

Musculoskeletal pain syndromes involve the articular and myofascial tissues and are usually multifocal or diffuse. Tender points and trigger points are often present. The symptoms are usually accompanied by fatigue, and the child may also have headaches. Osteopathic management includes emphasis on decreasing nociceptive activity and improving functional mobility. However, because of their suspected roles in the etiology of these conditions, stress and the NEI need to be addressed. Gentle direct techniques and indirect techniques are usually employed.

There are no randomized controlled studies evaluating the efficacy of osteopathic manipulation in children with arthritis. A recent small randomized controlled adult study reported significant improvement in measures of pain threshold, perceived pain, attitude toward treatment, activities of daily living, and perceived functional ability in fibromyalgia patients treated with osteopathic manipulative therapy.[9] There are also several case reports and articles in the older osteopathic literature. However, none would meet criteria for publication today.

References

Pediatric Diagnosis and Treatment

1. Weiss JE, Ilowite NT: Juvenile idiopathic arthritis, *Pediatr Clin North Am* 52:413-442, vi, 2005.
2. Cakmak A, Bolukbas N: Juvenile rheumatoid arthritis: physical therapy and rehabilitation, *South Med J* 98:212-216, 2005.
3. Behrman R, Kliegman RM, Jenson HB, editors: *Nelson's textbook of pediatrics*, Philadelphia, 2004, Saunders.
4. Cassidy JT, Levinson JE, Bass JC et al: A study of classification criteria for a diagnosis of juvenile rheumatoid arthritis, *Arthritis Rheum* 29:274-281, 1986.
5. *Juvenile rheumatoid arthritis (JRA): criteria for JRA.* Available at www.reheumatology.org. Accessed December 2004.
6. Manners PJ: Epidemiology of the rheumatic diseases of childhood, *Curr Rheumatol Rep* 5:453-457, 2003.
7. Nepom BS, Glass DN: Juvenile rheumatoid arthritis and HLA: report of the Park City III workshop, *J Rheumatol Suppl* 33:70-74, 1992.
8. Azouz EM: Arthritis in children: conventional and advanced imaging, *Semin Musculoskelet Radiol* 7:95-102, 2003.
9. Babyn P, Doria AS: Radiologic investigation of rheumatic diseases, *Pediatr Clin North Am* 52:373-411, vi, 2005.
10. Lovell DJ, Ruth NM: Pediatric clinical research, *Curr Opin Rheumatol* 17:265-270, 2005.
11. Reiff AO: Developments in the treatment of juvenile arthritis, *Expert Opin Pharmacother* 5:1485-1496, 2004.
12. Kotaniemi K, Savolainen A, Karma A et al: Recent advances in uveitis of juvenile idiopathic arthritis, *Surv Ophthalmol* 48:489-502, 2003.
13. Petty RE, Smith JR, Rosenbaum JT: Arthritis and uveitis in children. A pediatric rheumatology perspective, *Am J Ophthalmol* 135:879-884, 2003.
14. Cassidy JT, Petty RE: Juvenile rheumatoid arthritis. In *Textbook of pediatric rheumatology*, ed 4, Philadelphia, 2001, Saunders.
15. Feldman BM: Treating children with arthritis: towards an evidence-based culture, *J Rheumatol Suppl* 72:33-35, 2005.

Acupuncture

1. O'Connor J, Bensky D, editors: *Acupuncture, a comprehensive text,* Seattle, 1981, Eastland Press.
2. Maciocia G: *The practice of Chinese medicine, the treatment of diseases with acupuncture and Chinese herbs,* London, 1994, Churchill Livingstone.
3. Liu Q: Effects of acupuncture on hemorheology, blood lipid content and nail fold microcirculation in multiple infarct dementia patients, *J Tradit Chin Med* 24:219-223, 2004.
4. Gollub RL, Hui KK, Stefano GB: Acupuncture: pain management coupled to immune stimulation, *Zhongguo Yao Li Xue Bao* 20:769-777, 1999.
5. Bonta IL: Acupuncture beyond the endorphin concept? *Med Hypotheses* 58:221-224, 2002.
6. Lau BHS, Wong DS, Slater JM: Effect of acupuncture on allergic rhinitis: clinical and laboratory evaluations, *Am J Chin Med* 3:263-270, 1975.
7. Berman BM, Swyers JP, Ezzo J: The evidence for acupuncture as a treatment for rheumatologic conditions, *Rheum Dis Clin North Am* 26:103-115, ix-x, 2000.
8. Ulett GA, Han J, Han S: Traditional and evidence-based acupuncture: history, mechanisms, and present status, *South Med J* 91:1115-1120, 1998.
9. Ng DK, Chow PY, Ming SP et al: A double-blind, randomized, placebo-controlled trial of acupuncture for the treatment of childhood persistent allergic rhinitis, *Pediatrics* 114:1242-1247, 2004.
10. Wu MT, Hsieh JC, Xiong J et al: Central nervous pathway for acupuncture stimulation: localization of processing with functional MR imaging of the brain—preliminary experience, *Radiology* 212:133-141, 1999.
11. Ulett G, Han S, Han JS: Electroacupuncture: mechanisms and clinical application, *Biol Psychiatry* 44:129-138, 1998.
12. Kuo TC, Lin CW, Ho FM: The soreness and numbness effect of acupuncture on skin blood flow, *Am J Chin Med* 32:117-129, 2004.
13. Guan ZJ, Zhang J: Effects of acupuncture on immunoglobulins in patients with asthma and rheumatoid arthritis, *Tradit Chin Med* 15:102-105, 1995.
14. Xiao J, Liu X, Sun L et al: Experimental study on the influence of acupuncture and moxibustion on interleukin-2 in patients with rheumatoid arthritis [in Chinese], *Zhen Ci Yan Jiu* 17:126-128, 132, 1992.
15. Zherebkin VV: The use of acupuncture reflexotherapy in treating patients with rheumatoid arthritis [in Russian], *Lik Sprava* Nov-Dec:175-177, 1997.
16. Polushina ND, Grinzaid IuM, Shliapak EA et al: A clinical and experimental analysis of the effects of laser therapy [in Russian], *Vopr Kurortol Fizioter Lech Fiz Kult* Jul-Aug:14-16, 1997.
17. Zhu L, Li C, Ji C et al: The effect of laser irradiation on arthritis in rats [in Chinese], *Zhen Ci Yan Jiu* 15:71-76, 1990.
18. Cao W, Deng Y, Dong X et al: Effects of electroacupuncture at different frequencies on the nociceptive response and central contents of GABA and glutamic acid in arthritic rats [in Chinese], *Zhen Ci Yan Jiu* 18:48-52, 1993.
19. Rogers PA, Schoen AM, Limehouse J: Acupuncture for immune-mediated disorders. Literature review and clinical applications, *Probl Vet Med* 4:162-193, 1992.

Aromatherapy

1. Battaglia S: *The complete guide to aromatherapy*, Virginia, Queensland, Australia, 1995, The Perfect Potion.
2. Buckle J: *Clinical aromatherapy: essential ols in practice*, ed 2, Ediburgh, 2003, Churchill Livingstone.
3. Brownfield A: Aromatherapy in arthritis: a study, *Nurs Stand* 13:34, 1998.

Chiropractic

1. Nelson WA: Rheumatoid arthritis: a case report, *Chiro Tech* 2: 17-19, 1990.
2. Matthews JA: Atlanto-axial subluxation in rheumatoid arthritis: a five-year follow-up study, *Ann Rheum Dis* 33:526-531, 1974.
3. Robinson HS: Rheumatoid arthritis—atlanto-axial subluxation and its clinical presentation, *Can Med Assoc J* 94:470-477, 1966.
4. Lantz CA: Inflammation hypothesis. In Leach RA, editor: *The chiropractic theories,* Baltimore, 2004, Lippincott Williams and Wilkins.
5. Leach RA: Instability hypothesis. In Leach RA, editor: *The chiropractic theories,* Baltimore, 2004, Lippincott Williams and Wilkins.
6. Davidson RC, Horn JR, Herndon JH et al: Brain stem compression in rheumatoid arthritis, *J Am Med Assoc* 238:2633-2634, 1977.
7. Perussi RM, Rubin BR, Blackwell D: Juvenile rheumatoid arthritis, *J Am Osteopath Assoc* 96:298-301, 1996.
8. Koes BW, Bouter LM, van Mameren H et al: A randomized clinical trial of manual therapy and physiotherapy for persistent low back and neck complaints: subgroup analysis and relationship between outcome measure, *J Manipulative Physiol Ther* 16: 211-219, 1993.
9. Curtis CL, Hughes CD, Falnnery CR et al: n-3 fatty acids specifically modulate catabolic factors involved in articular cartilage degradation, *J Biol Chem* 275:721-724, 2000.
10. Gottlieb MS: Conservative management of spinal osteoarthritis with glucosamine sulfate and chiropractic treatment, *J Manipulative Physiol Ther* 20:400-414, 1997.
11. Leach RA, Lantz CA: Immobilization degeneration hypothesis. In Leach RA, editor: *The chiropractic theories,* Baltimore, 2004, Lippincott Williams and Wilkins.

Herbs—Western

1. U.S. Food and Drug Administration: *EAFUS: a food additive database.* Available at http://vm.cfsan.fda.gov/~dms/eafus.html. Accessed January 25, 2005.
2. Deodhar SD, Sethi R, Srimal RC: Preliminary study on antirheumatic activity of curcumin (diferuloyl methane), *Indian J Med Res* 71:632-634, 1980.
3. Srivastava KC, Mustafa T: Ginger *(Zingiber officinale)* and rheumatic disorders, *Med Hypoth* 29:25-28, 1989.
4. Belch JJ, Ansell D, Madhok R et al: Effects of altering dietary essential fatty acids on requirements for non-steroidal anti-inflammatory drugs in patients with rheumatoid arthritis: a double blind placebo controlled study, *Ann Rheum Dis* 47:96-104, 1988.
5. Belch J, Hill A: Evening primrose oil and borage oil in rheumatologic conditions, *Am J Clin Nutr* 71:352S-356S, 2000.
6. Hansen TM, Lerche A, Kassis V et al: Treatment of rheumatoid arthritis with prostaglandin E1 precursors cis-linoleic acid and gamma-linolenic acid, *Scand J Rheumatol* 12:85-88, 1983.
7. Biegert C, Wagner I, Ludtke R et al: Efficacy and safety of willow bark extract in the treatment of osteoarthritis and rheumatoid arthritis: results of 2 randomized double-blind controlled trials, *J Rheumatol* 31:2121-2130, 2004.
8. Leventhal LJ, Boyce EG, Zurier RB: Treatment of rheumatoid arthritis with gammalinolenic acid, *Ann Intern Med* 119:867-873, 1993.
9. Kremer JM: n-3 Fatty acid supplements in rheumatoid arthritis, *Am J Clin Nutr* 71(Suppl):349S-351S, 2000.
10. Kast RE: Borage oil reduction of rheumatoid arthritis activity may be mediated by increased cAMP that suppresses tumor necrosis factor-alpha, *Int Immunopharmacol* 1:2197-2199, 2001.
11. Blumenthal M, editor: *The complete German Commission E monographs: therapeutic guide to herbal medicines,* Boston, 1998, American Botanical Council (Translation by S Klein).
12. Frondoza CG, Sohrabi A, Polotsky A et al: An in vitro screening assay for inhibitors of proinflammatory mediators in herbal extracts using human synoviocyte cultures, *In Vitro Cell Dev Biol Anim* 40:95-101, 2004.
13. Yoshida S, Takayama Y: Licorice-induced hypokalemia as a treatable cause of dropped head syndrome, *Clin Neurol Neurosurg* 105:286-287, 2003.

Homeopathy

1. *ReferenceWorks Pro 4.2,* San Rafael, Calif, 2008, Kent Homeopathic Associates.

Massage Therapy

1. Kaada B, Torsteinbo O: Increase of plasma endorphins in connective tissue massage, *Gen Pharmacol* 20:487-489, 1989.
2. Field T, Hernandez-Reif M, Seligman S et al: Juvenile rheumatoid arthritis benefits from massage therapy, *J Pediatr, Psychol* 22:607-617, 1997.
3. LeBlanc-Louvry I, Costaglioli B, Boulon C et al: Does mechanical massage of the abdominal wall after colectomy reduce postoperative pain and shorten the duration of ileus? Results of a randomized study, *J Gastrointest Surg* 6:43-49, 2002.
4. Piotrowski MM, Paterson C, Mitchinson A et al: Massage as adjunctive therapy in the management of acute postoperative pain: a preliminary study in men, *J Am Coll Surg* 197:1037-1046, 2003.
5. Taylor AG, Galpner DI, Taylor P et al: Effects of adjunctive Swedish massage and vibration therapy on short-term postoperative outcomes: a randomized, controlled trial, *J Altern Complement Med* 9:77-89, 2003.
6. van der Dolder PA, Roberts DL: A trial into the effectiveness of soft tissue massage in the treatment of shoulder pain, *Aust J Physiother* 49:183-188, 2003.
7. Mitchinson AR, Kim HM, Rosenberg JM et al: Acute postoperative pain management using massage as an adjuvant therapy: a randomized trial, *Arch Surg* 142:1158-1167, 2007.
8. Field T, Hernandez-Reif M, Seligman S et al: Juvenile rheumatoid arthritis benefits from massage therapy, *J Pediatr Psychol* 22: 607-617, 1997.

Nutrition

1. Pizzorno LU, Pizzorno JE, Murray MT: *Natural medicine: instructions for patients,* London, 2002, Churchill Livingstone.
2. Muller H, deToledo FW, Resch KL: Fasting followed by vegetarian diet in patients with rheumatoid arthritis: a systematic review, *Scand J Rheumatol* 30:1-10, 2001.
3. Kjeldsen-Kragh J, Rashid T, Dybwad A et al: Decrease in anti-*Proteus mirabilis* but not anti-*Escherichia coli* antibody levels in rheumatoid arthritis patients treated with fasting and a one year vegetarian diet, *Ann Rheum Dis* 54:221-224, 1995.
4. Wilson C, Thakore A, Isenberg D et al: Correlation between anti-Proteus antibodies and isolation rates of *P. mirabilis* in rheumatoid arthritis, *Rheumatol Int* 16:187-189, 1997.
5. Kremer JM, Jubiz W, Michalek A et al: Fish-oil fatty acid supplementation in active rheumatoid arthritis. A double-blinded, controlled, crossover study, *Ann Intern Med* 106:497-503, 1987.
6. Kremer JM, Lawrence DA, Jubiz W et al: Dietary fish oil and olive oil supplementation in patients with rheumatoid arthritis. Clinical and immunologic effects, *Arthritis Rheum* 33:810-820, 1990.

7. Adam O, Beringer C, Kless T et al: Anti-inflammatory effects of a low arachadonic acid diet and fish oil in patients with rheumatoid arthritis, *Rheumatol Int* 23:27-36, 2003.

8. Karatay S, Erdem T, Yildirim K et al: The effect of individualized diet challenges consisting of allergenic foods on YNF-alpha and IL-1 beta levels in patients with rheumatoid arthritis, *Rheumatol (Oxford)* 43:1429-1433, 2004.

Osteopathy

1. DeShazer JD, Davis LB: Gout, *J Osteopath* 9:126, 1902.

2. Seeman TE, Singer BH, Rowe JW et al: Price of adaptation—allosteric load and its health consequences, *Arch Intern Med* 157: 2259-2268, 1997.

3. Sternberg EM, Chrousos GP, Wilder RL et al: The stress response and the regulation of inflammatory disease, *Ann Intern Med* 117:854-866, 1992.

4. Sternberg EM: Neuroendocrine factors in susceptibility to inflammatory disease: focus on the hypothalamic-pituitary-adrenal axis, *Horm Res* 43:159-161, 1995.

5. Sternberg EM, Licinio J: Overview of neuroimmune stress interactions—implications for susceptibility to inflammatory disease, *Ann NY Acad Sci* 771:364-371, 1995.

6. Donnerer J: Nociception and the neuroendocrine-immune system. In Willard FH, Patterson M, editors: *Nociception and the neuroendocrine-immune connection*, Indianapolis, 1992, American Academy of Osteopathy.

7. Esterling B: Stress-associated modulation of cellular immunity. In Willard FH, Patterson M, editors: *Nociception and the neuroendocrine-immune connection*, Indianapolis, 1992, American Academy of Osteopathy.

8. Vaccarino AL, Couret LC Jr: Relationship between hypothalamic-pituitary-adrenal activity and blockade of tolerance to morphine analgesia by pain: a strain comparison, *Pain* 63: 385-389, 1995.

9. Gamber RG, Shores JH, Russo DP et al: Osteopathic manipulative treatment in conjunction with medication relieves pain associated with fibromyalgia syndrome: results of a randomized clinical pilot project, *J Am Osteopath Assoc* 102:321-325, 2002.

Asthma

Acupuncture | May Loo

Aromatherapy | Maura A. Fitzgerald

Chiropractic | Anne Spicer

Herbs—Chinese | May Loo, Catherine Ulbricht,
Jennifer Woods, Mark Wright, Harriet Beinfield,
Efrem Korngold

Herbs—Western | Alan D. Woolf, Paula M. Gardiner,
Lana Dvorkin-Camiel, Jack Maypole

Magnet Therapy | Agatha P. Colbert, Deborah Risotti

Massage Therapy | Mary C. McLellan

Mind/Body | Timothy Culbert, Lynda Richtsmeier Cyr

Naturopathy | Matthew I. Baral

Nutrition | Joy A. Weydert

Probiotics | Russell H. Greenfield

Psychology | Anna Tobia

Qigong | Effie Poy Yew Chow, Maria Choy

❋ PEDIATRIC DIAGNOSIS AND TREATMENT

Asthma is the most common chronic illness in childhood, with more than 9 million children currently carrying this diagnosis in the United States.[1] Asthmatic children miss more than 14 million school days per year.[1] Incidence varies worldwide, with the highest rates in the United Kingdom, Australia, and New Zealand and the lowest in Eastern Europe, China, and India.[2,3] In recent years, the prevalence of asthma has increased in the United States and in all other countries, especially in children younger than 12 years.[4-7]

Although asthma can have onset at any age, 80% of asthmatic children have their first symptoms before 6 years of age.[7] Children 4 years of age or younger have distinctive symptoms and require special consideration.[8] They have increased health service utilization including a higher annual rate of hospitalization,[9] which has nearly doubled in the United States from 1980 to 1992 for children 1 to 4 years of age.[4] The same trend is observed by other nations worldwide.[10] Among U.S. children aged 5 to 14 years, asthma death rates almost doubled from 1980 to 1995.[4,11] New Zealand and Canada have observed a similar increase in severity and mortality.[12,13] One of every 20 asthmatic children will be hospitalized at least once during childhood.[14] Although the cause of childhood asthma has not been pinpointed, contemporary research implicates an interplay between genetic and environmental factors. The strong association of common childhood asthma with concomitant allergies suggests that environmental factors influence immune development toward the asthmatic phenotype in susceptible individuals.[7]

Asthma is a diffuse, reversible, obstructive lung disease with three major features: bronchial smooth muscle spasm, edema and inflammation of the mucous membrane lining the airways, and intraluminal mucus plugs.[7,15,16] During the last 2 decades, chronic airway inflammation, rather than smooth muscle contraction alone, has been recognized as playing the key role in the pathogenesis of asthma in adults.[17-19] Although this association is less well established in children, recent guidelines for managing asthma in the pediatric population have nonetheless emphasized that treatment be directed toward the inflammatory aspects of the disease.[20-22] Chronic inflammation is due to the local production of inflammatory mediators and an increase in recruitment of inflammatory cells, predominantly eosinophils and mast cells. Studies in young adults suggest that the chronic inflammation may be responsible for long-term pulmonary changes including bronchial hyperresponsiveness, airway remodeling, and irreversible airflow obstruction. Because of difficulties in conducting studies in infants and young children, information about them is incomplete.[23] Limited studies have detected increases in inflammatory cells and thickening of the lung basement membrane in infants and young children and have found asthmatic children to have significantly lower lung function at 6 years of age compared with non-wheezers when both groups of children began with the same baseline at age 6 months. These data support the fact that asthma-like inflammation can be present at a very early age and is associated with nonreversible impairment of lung function.[24]

The excessive inflammatory changes indicate that asthma is a disorder due to an "immunological runaway response" that was poorly regulated such that, instead of protecting the host, the hyperactive immune response destroyed normal structure. Increased concentrations of proinflammatory mediators such as histamine and leukotrienes are found in the airways, as well as in the blood and urine, of asthmatics[18] during an acute attack and after allergen and exercise challenge.[25] Cysteinyl leukotrienes are proinflammatory mediators that play an especially important role in the pathophysiology of asthma.[25] Lymphocytic and eosinophilic submucosal infiltrates appear to correlate with severity of disease.[17] In addition to inflammatory changes, epithelial destruction occurs at all levels of the tracheobronchial tree with exposure of the nerve endings, rendering the airways of the asthmatic patient hyperirritable.[26] The chronically inflamed and hyperirritable airway hinder mucociliary clearance and become susceptible to acute obstruction by numerous triggers such as infections,[7] allergens,[27] environmental irritants[28] including secondhand smoke,[29] dust mites,[7] exercise,[30] emotional stress,[31] drugs,[32] and even laughter.[33]

Strong evidence correlates asthma with respiratory syncytial virus infection; children who enter day nursery before age 12 months become exposed to viruses early in life and can build up immunity, resulting in decreased development of allergies.[34] In most children whose asthma is triggered mainly by respiratory infections at a younger age, asthma symptoms appear to remit by the adolescent years.[24] In older children and teenagers, emotions play a significant role both as the cause of symptoms and as the result of interplay of a chronic illness affecting the child's self-image and family dynamics.[7] A strong genetic predisposition, an atopic diathesis,[1] low birth weight, tobacco smoke exposure, and male gender are risk factors for development of childhood asthma.

The National Asthma Education & Prevention Program (NAEPP) guidelines classify pediatric asthma into four groups of severity: mild intermittent, mild persistent, moderate persistent, and severe persistent.[35,36] A major objective of this approach is to identify and treat all "persistent" asthma with antiinflammatory controller medications. The "3 strikes" rule helps determine which child should receive controller therapy based on the NAEPP guidelines: a child with asthma symptoms requires quick-relief medication >3 times per week, awakens at night owing to asthma >3 times per month, or requires a medication refill >3 times per year. Low-dose inhaled glucocorticoids, leukotriene pathway modifiers, or cromolyn/nedocromil are the recommended controllers for mild persistent asthmatics; sustained-release theophylline is an alternative. The recommended controller medication for patients with moderate persistent asthma is medium-dose inhaled glucocorticoids or low-dose inhaled glucocorticoids in combination with a long-acting β-agonist or a leukotriene pathway modifier; sustained-release theophylline or long-acting oral β-agonists are alternatives. Severe persistent asthmatics should receive high-dose inhaled glucocorticoids, a long-acting bronchodilator, and routine oral glucocorticoids if needed. Mild intermittent asthma is the only level for which daily controller therapy is not recommended; short-acting inhaled β-agonists are recommended as needed for symptoms and for pretreatment in exercise-induced bronchospasm. Short-acting β-agonists are the recommended reliever medication for all severity levels as needed for acute symptoms.[35,36] The U.S. Food and Drug Administration (FDA) has approved leukotriene receptor antagonists for use in asthmatic children younger than 4 years.[37] These agents counteract the hyperimmune response such that there are diminished airway inflammation and decreased eosinophilia in the airway mucosa and peripheral blood.[20] Because infections that trigger asthma attacks are mostly viral,[38] antibiotics are not routinely indicated. Concomitant with any medication management are avoidance of allergens, which is a complex problem in view of the increasing number of pollutants and chemicals in the environment that are potential allergens for children,[39] and parental education, especially in regard to smoking.[40] Status asthmaticus requires aggressive treatments with multiple drugs. Efforts should be made to avoid mechanical ventilation as much as possible, as hyperinflation will worsen with positive-pressure ventilation.[15]

It has been suggested that asthma may be overdiagnosed and that some practitioners have a tendency toward more aggressive

treatment of children with mild persistent asthma. A study conducted by the Childhood Asthma Management Program (CAMP) found that inhaled corticosteroids decrease inflammation but do not cure asthma. If controller therapy is stopped, inflammation recurs.[41] The concern with any long-term medication regimen for children is the development of adverse effects (e.g., tremor and elevated heart rate with β-agonists) and the numerous side effects of inhaled glucocorticoids, ranging from local (e.g., oral candidiasis, dysphonia) to systemic, notably growth suppression and other metabolic and endocrinological effects; dermatological effects such as increased skin fragility and acne; suppression of immunity; and various hematological, cardiovascular, and psychoneurological effects.[7]

✳ CAM THERAPY RECOMMENDATIONS

Acupuncture

Current Data

Acupuncture is among the most popular alternative medical treatments for asthma. It is currently available in major population centers in the United States. Clinical response from patients remains favorable because of its efficacy, low risk, and relatively low cost.[1]

Many reports on acupuncture treatment of asthma, most of them published in the Chinese and Russian literature, are based on uncontrolled clinical observations whose results are usually dismissed by the medical community. In the past 25 years, fewer than 20 controlled clinical trials of real versus sham acupuncture in asthma have been published. The majority of research studies have been criticized as having methodological shortcomings such as lack of double-blinding, randomization, or both; small sample of patients; and inadequate description of statistical analysis, rendering the studies invalid and unacceptable. Recently, numerous metaanalyses and systematic reviews have been conducted in the United States and in Europe; almost all conclude that the efficacy of acupuncture for asthma has not yet been convincingly supported by adequately designed clinical trials and urgently call for properly conducted studies.[2-8] The National Institutes of Health (NIH) Consensus Conference on Acupuncture in 1997 stated that acupuncture may be useful as an adjunct treatment or an acceptable alternative or may be included in a comprehensive management program for treatment of asthma.[9]

Asthma epitomizes the Chinese medicine concept of "winter disease, summer cure." In China, many asthmatic children who were treated with herbal patches applied to acupoints during the summer had minimal or no symptoms during asthmatic seasons.[10,11] The few clinical reports on acupuncture treatment of children with asthma in general are favorable.[10,12,13] Empirical results using a simple acupuncture regimen yielded good results in asthmatic children in Germany.[14] One study demonstrated that although acupuncture did not affect the basal bronchomotor tone, when administered 20 minutes before exercise, acupuncture was shown to be effective in attenuating exercise-induced asthma,[15] which is common in children. One possible mechanism of acupuncture is in reducing the reflex component of bronchoconstriction, but not in influencing direct smooth muscle constriction caused by histamine.[16] For children who are fearful of or who cannot tolerate needles, non-needle treatments such as cupping and auricular press pellets[12] and massage of acupuncture points[13] have also been found to be effective.

Adult studies indicate that acupuncture was successful in treatment of allergic rhinitis accompanying allergic asthma and significantly affected serum immunoglobulin (Ig) E and lymphocyte count.[17] Even with treatment of just the master immunity point, Zusanli (ST36) acupuncture was found to reduce the eosinophil count.[18] Two points on the Lung channel, LU6 and LU10, produced immediate effect in acute asthma attacks of the "Cold" type according to traditional Chinese medicine (TCM) diagnosis. Needle retention for 40 minutes produced long-term benefits.[19] Combined electrical stimulation and topical herbal patches were synergistic—more effective in both acute and maintenance situations.[10] When both auricular and body acupuncture points were used, steroid-dependent patients with asthma were able to taper the use of steroid doses.[12]

The most interesting future role for acupuncture in asthma lies in its potential both in stimulating an immune response and, more important, in regulating or modulating a hyperimmune response. At this time, there is ample biochemical support in the literature to indicate that acupuncture activates both the humoral and cellular immune system to protect the host.[20-25] Studies have also demonstrated that acupuncture can modulate the synthesis and release of proinflammatory mediators,[24,26,27] so that the efficacy of acupuncture in asthma can be based on its antiinflammatory actions.[28,29] Current hypotheses suggest that this is most likely mediated through a common pathway connecting the immune system and the opioids,[30-32] which has been well known to be associated with analgesic effects of acupuncture.

Acupuncture is frequently used for Chinese asthmatic outpatients.[33] A case report from China of 217 adults with chronic bronchitis and asthma treated with preventive therapy combining electrical stimulation with topical application of herbs on acupoints during symptom-free summer months indicated that the combined therapy has both short- and long-term curative effect.[34] A clinical report from China treated 23 adults and 2 children with steroid-dependent asthma using body points (GV14, BL13, BL20, BL23) (children were treated with cupping instead of needles) and pressing with *Vaccaria* seeds on five auricular points selected from Shenmen, Lung, Large Intestine, Sensitive Point, Pingchuan, Subcortex, and Kidney revealed reduction of medications and marked decrease in symptoms after 15 treatments. The clinicians recommended another 10 treatments for curative effect.[35] A double-blind, placebo-controlled, crossover study using laser acupuncture concluded that a single laser acupuncture treatment offers no protection against exercise-induced bronchoconstriction in children and adolescents with exercise-induced asthma.[36] Acupuncture performed by an experienced practitioner is generally considered safe for asthma. A review of 320 cases showed only 23 (7%) manifested side effects, most of which were mild (e.g., vasovagal reactions, earache, gastrointestinal symptoms).[37]

Acupuncture Recommendations

Chinese medicine classifies pediatric asthma as acute external pathogenic Wind-Cold (viral) or Wind-Heat (bacterial) invasions; or as chronic internal Kidney, Spleen, or Liver imbalances. A careful history would decipher the etiology and facilitate a treatment plan. The history needs to evaluate age of onset, diet (Phlegm-producing foods, sweets, excess energetically Cold or Hot foods); family history; history of previous other illnesses; history of emergency visits and hospitalizations for asthma (frequency and duration are indications of severity of illness that may be more difficult to treat); precipitating factors such as Wind-Cold, Wind-Heat, external allergens, diet, and emotions; and current and previous medication(s), especially steroids.

The following are basic and general recommendations.[38] An asthmatic child should be thoroughly evaluated by an experienced acupuncturist for more comprehensive and individualized acupuncture treatment regimen.

Acute episodes due to external pathogens

Wind-Cold invasion (viral infection). During an acute attack:
- Dingchuan: special point for stopping wheezing
- BL12, BL13, P6, CV17, LU1[35]

During the Wind-Cold illness, sequential treatments need to be instituted to shorten the course of illness:
- First dispel Cold from the Lung, then tonify the Lung, and then tonify the immune system.

Because the Spleen is also directly or indirectly involved, similar treatment of the Spleen would be beneficial:
- Dispel Cold: KI3, KI7
- Use the Four-Point protocol to dispel Cold (see Appendix B):
  - Lung Cold: Tonify LU10, HT8; sedate LU5, KI10
  - Spleen Cold: Tonify SP2, HT8; sedate SP9, KI10
  - (HT8 and KI10 are common points, so six points would disperse Cold from both LU and SP.)
  - For infants and young children, only the LU or SP points need to be stimulated.
- Tonification: Use the Four-Point protocol for tonification:
  - LU tonification: Tonify LU9, SP3; sedate LU10, HT8
  - SP tonification: Tonify SP2, HT8; sedate SP1, LU1
  - Use only LU or SP points for infants and young children.
- Tonify and modulate the immune system:
  - ST36; back Shu points: BL13, 18, 20, 21, 23
- Modify diet:
  - Decrease energetically Cold drinks and foods. Decrease sweet foods.
  - Avoid Phlegm-producing foods: dairy products, sugar, honey, peanuts, almonds, or pork. Choose foods that tend to thin Phlegm: mushrooms, papaya, potatoes, pumpkin, radishes, strawberries, or string beans.

Wind-Heat invasion (bacterial infection). During an acute attack:
- Dingchuan, BL12, BL13, P6, CV17, LU1
- GV14, LI11 to disperse Heat

During the course of Wind-Heat illness, treatment needs to first dispel Heat from the Lung and Spleen, then vigorously tonify the Lung and Spleen with additional tonification of Lung and Spleen Yin, followed by tonification of the immune system.

- Disperse Heat: GV14, LI11 to disperse Heat
- Use the Four-Point protocol to disperse Heat (see Appendix B):
  - Lung Heat: Tonify LU5, KI10; sedate LU10, HT8
  - Spleen Heat: Tonify SP9, KI10; sedate SP2, HT8
  - HT8 and KI10 are common points, so six points would tonify both LU and SP.
  - Use only the LU and SP points for infants and young children.
  - Use the Four-Point protocols listed previously to tonify LU and SP.
- Tonify Yin: KI6 and SP6
- Tonify and modulate the immune system.
- Decrease energetically Hot drinks and foods. Decrease Phlegm-producing and sweet foods.
- For thick and yellow "hot" Phlegm, white fungus is the most healing food. If it is not available, choose asparagus, apples, carrots, celery, pear, or mango; and avoid Hot foods such as garlic and ginger.

Chronic asthma: constitutional weaknesses

Lung deficiency/Kidney deficiency. These children often have a strong family history of asthma.
- Acute attack: same as external pathogen
- Tonification treatments:
  - Dispel Lung Cold.
  - Tonify Lung.
  - Tonify Kidney with the Four-Point protocol (see Appendix B): Tonify KI7, LU8; sedate KI3, SP3.
  - Decrease Cold foods.
  - Decrease spicy and salty foods that are harmful to the Lung and Kidney.
  - Minimize exposure to environmental allergens such as smoke.

Spleen deficiency. These children tend to have digestive symptoms and a tendency for buildup of Phlegm.
- Acute attack: same as external pathogen
- Tonification treatments:
  - ST40 to transform Phlegm
  - Warm CV8— moxa or heated ginger
  - Vigorous tonification of Lung and Spleen with tonification of the meridians, or Two-Point or Four-Point Five-Element tonification protocols.
  - Decrease spicy foods, Phlegm-producing foods, and artificially sweetened foods.
  - For school-aged children, make sure they have a balance of studies, physical activities, and rest.

Liver Yin deficiency/Liver Yang rising. These tend to be school-aged patients with asthma, with attacks often precipitated by emotions or stress.
- Acute attack: same as external pathogen
- Balance Liver:
  - LR3 tonifies LR Yin, subdues LR Yang, moves LR Qi
  - LR13 moves LR Qi
  - Tonify Lung
  - Tonify Spleen

- Decrease sour-tasting foods, fried foods, and medications.
- Help the child explore factors that precipitate emotional stress and find ways to minimize them. Teach the child calming techniques.

Maintenance Treatment for All Forms of Asthma
"Summer cure"

A prophylaxis treatment described in the literature consists of massaging BL points for 3-5 minutes followed by application of an herbal mixture.[39] The TCM pediatric staff at the Xinhua Hospital in Shanghai stimulates CV22 and BL points.[11] This author had success in stimulating CV22 and ST36 and teaching parents to massage the Bladder meridian in the direction of flow during the summer when the asthma is in remission.

Tapering of Medications

It would be best for the acupuncturist to work with the physician in tapering medications, especially steroids, because of possible hypothalamo-pituitary-adrenal axis suppression with chronic steroid administration. Chinese medicine posits that steroids can cause Kidney deficiency.[40] Therefore it would be reasonable to tonify the Kidney while the child is on steroids. The tapering of bronchodilators most likely would occur naturally, as the child would automatically require less medication with less wheezing.

Aromatherapy

Use of essential oils in asthma should be monitored to first establish that the child does not have sensitivity to essential oils that could trigger or worsen an asthma episode. When using essential oils for asthma, inhalation is the primary route of administration. This includes inhalation directly from a bottle, applying a few drops to a tissue, using a diffuser, or applying a topical solution (1% to 5%) to the back and upper chest. Essential oils that are calming such as lavender (*Lavandula angustifolia*) may be used to allay emotional concerns during an asthma episode. When an asthma episode is accompanied with an upper respiratory tract infection with increased secretions, essential oils that are expectorants are useful. These include frankincense (*Boswellia carteri*), sweet fennel (*Foeniculum vulgaris*), eucalyptus globulus (*Eucalyptus globulus*), and peppermint (*Mentha piperita*).[1,2]

In two unpublished exploratory studies, frankincense was tested for use in asthma. Frankincense combined with spike lavender (*Lavandula spica*) and true lavender (*Lavandula angustifolia*) in a 3% solution applied to the back and chest was found to improve peak flow in one study of eight subjects (ages 14-70).[3] In a second study subjects reported decreased anxiety and decreased use of inhalers when inhaling pure essential oil of frankincense from the bottle at the start of an asthma episode.[3] Frankincense is an ideal agent for asthma, as it is both calming and supportive to the respiratory tract.

Chiropractic

The chiropractor would assess the spine for subluxations (disruption of normal functional alignment leading to interference in neurological integrity). Because the medulla encompasses a portion of the respiratory control and exits the skull at the foramen magnum, coursing the spinal canal at the level of C1, a subluxation at this level may induce irritation to the medulla or cervical cord, thereby disrupting normal neural function to primary respiration. Also, the phrenic nerve exits the cervical plexus of C3-C5. Subluxation at these levels, as well as the lower thoracic spine, may potentially alter proper diaphragmatic excursion. Accessory muscles for respiration also have their neurological origin in the cervical spine, as with the platysma (cervical branch of the facial nerve) and the sternocleidomastoid (spinal branch of the accessory and anterior rami of C2 and C3). Primary lung and respiratory musculature innervation arises from the middle thoracic spine, including intercostals, anterior serratus, scalenes, and abdominals.

During an acute asthmatic episode, musculature is recruited into excessive function, potentially resulting in muscle injury. Also, strain of the thoracic musculature secondary to an asthmatic episode can result in fixation of the ribcage and further limit movement at the diaphragm.

The sympathetic system largely regulates systemic inflammatory processes[3]; it also controls mucus secretions and edema in the lungs, along with bronchodilation and cholinergic status. Sympathetic suppression or parasympathetic facilitation may establish a trophic disturbance associated with the development of asthma.[1] T1 to T6 is the area most commonly adjusted for patients with asthma.[2] Adjustments may also be applied to the costovertebral junction,[4] where strain injuries and subluxations occur during acute episodes of asthma.

Whereas "wet" asthma (production of mucus) is commonly associated with subluxation within the parasympathetic system (especially C0-C5, the sacrum, and the ilia[5]), "dry" asthma is commonly associated with subluxation within the sympathetic system (especially C6-T3 and T7-T12[6]).

Multiple case studies have demonstrated elimination or reduction in asthma symptoms following chiropractic adjustments.[7-19]

A randomized controlled trial (RCT) was conducted comparing active and simulated chiropractic adjustments in the management of childhood asthma. There was substantial improvement in symptoms and quality of life and reduction in β-agonist usage in both the active and simulated groups.[20] This study population was composed of children who had been treated medically for long periods without improvement. The active group responses varied, with many individuals showing remarkable improvements. Discussion suggests that the study group was a population likely to have low response rates and that averaging the responses decreased the appearance of the actual improvements of the participants and that the simulated adjustments may not have been as inert as anticipated.

A pilot study with emphasis on patient-rated outcomes found significant improvements in quality of life and improvements in asthma severity.[21]

A Danish survey of parents reports that 90% of children received benefit from chiropractic management of chronic asthma.[22]

A retrospective study of a 63-year-old individual with asthma found that the patients most likely to respond favorably to chiropractic management were the youngest patients on the fewest medications.[23]

A case series of children with asthma who were treated with chiropractic care found that all but one patient was able to reduce the need for medication and that lung capacity increased.[24]

A study of 81 children with asthma reported that 90% of subjects had statistically significant improvements after 60 days of chiropractic care.[25]

Also used in the management of the patient with asthma are Chapman's neurolymphatic reflexes. The lung points are found at the third and fourth intercostal space adjacent to the sternum on the anterior body, and posteriorly they are found bilaterally midway between the spinous process and transverse process of the second, third, and fourth thoracic vertebrae.

The chiropractor, family members, and school nurse can use percussion of the thoracic spine during asthmatic episodes and peak seasons. This technique involves "thumping" the thoracic spine with the palm of the hand or a closed fist. This sympathetic stimulation may decrease the duration or severity of an acute episode.

Respiratory exercises and stretches are recommended.

In support of the chemical status of the body, chiropractors often recommend nutritional supplementation to accommodate deficiencies or increased need on an individual basis. Common recommendations include vitamin A/β-carotene and gut microflora to support the immune function, omega-3 fats for their antiinflammatory actions, vitamin C for its inhibition of histamine reactions and its ability to thin mucus, vitamin E for antioxidant as well as antiinflammatory properties,[26] selenium for its strong oxidative stress management and because higher levels of this elements are associated with fewer breathing abnormalities.[27-29] For children using theophylline, supplementation of vitamin B_6 is essential.[30,31]

Identification of food triggers is a priority. Most food triggers also give rise to dermal or gastrointestinal symptoms. However, a trial reduction or elimination is recommended for dietary products containing artificial additives, cow's milk, chocolate,[32] bananas,[28] and citrus,[33] because these are some more common triggers. Low sodium intake may reduce the hyperreactivity of the lungs.[34,35]

Herbs—Chinese

In TCM, asthma consists of Xiao (bronchial wheezing) and Chuan (dyspnea). One study suggests that the Chinese cough syrup, King To Nin Jiom Pei Pa Kao (for constituents, see Chapter 15) may effectively relieve asthma symptoms because of its antiinflammatory effects.[1,2]

Xincang decoction, composed of flower of *Magnolia liliflora* Desr. (Xin Yi Hua) and fruit of *Xanthium sibiricum* Patr. (Cang Er Zi) has been tested on children with asthma. Researchers found that the herb decreases the levels of peripheral eosinophils (EOS), which is the eosinophil white blood cell count, and improves the pulmonary function in treating chronic airway inflammation in children with bronchial asthma in remission stage.[1,3] Further research is needed to confirm these results.

Another study found that drug acupoint application was more effective in treating allergic asthma patients in the short-term rather than crude drug moxibustion.[1,4]

Allergic asthma, especially childhood asthma associated with atopic eczema, is often related to underlying Kidney Yin deficiency. The classical formulation Mai Wei Di Huang Wan (also known as *Ba Xian Chang Shou Wan*), which is available in pill form, can often be helpful. A typical preparation might contain the following:

- steamed root of *Rehmannia glutinosa* (Gaertn.) Libosch. (Shu Di Huang)
- rhizome of *Dioscorea opposita* Thunb. (Shan Yao)
- sclerotium of *Poria cocos* (Schw.) Wolf (Fu Ling)
- root-bark of *Paeonia suffruticosa* Andrews (Mu Dan Pi)
- rhizome of *Alisma plantago-aquatica* L. var. *orientale* Samuels. (Ze Xie)
- sarcocarp of *Cornus officinalis* Siebold & Zucc. (Shan Zhu Yu)
- tuber of *Ophiopogon japonicus* (Thunb.) Ker Gawl. (Mai Men Dong)
- and fruit of *Schisandra chinensis* (Turcz.) Baill. (Wu Wei Zi).

As a raw herb prescription, these herbs would likely be present in the following levels:

- Shu Di Huang, 24 g
- Shan Yao and Fu Ling, each 12 g
- Mu Dan Pi, Ze Xie, Shan Zhu Yu, Mai Men Dong, and Wu Wei Zi, each 9 g

This prescription might be administered as a decoction in three equal doses per day. The first six herbs listed form a commonly used basic formula (Liu Wei Di Huang Wan), which originated in a Song dynasty pediatrics text, and around which are a number of prescription variations. One clinician has found Mai Wei Di Huang Wan to be a good base prescription in the treatment of childhood asthma of the type described. No evidence based research was found.

Dose Variations: Dose for newborns is generally ⅙ that for adults. Dose for babies is ⅓ to ½ that for adults. Dose for children aged 2 to 5 years is ½ to ⅔ that for adults. Children above school age normally take an adult dose.

Caution: In patients who are prone to loose stools, diarrhea may result. The prescription would need to be modified to prevent dehydration.

The Chinese herbal treatments can help Qi descend from the chest, due to various causes that include excessive mucus, dryness, cold or hot air, wind, physical strain and fatigue, emotional upset, or exposure to toxins.[5]

Open Air (Gentle Warrior Pediatric Formula, Kan Herb Company, Scotts Valley, Calif.) is a variation of the famous Perilla Seed Decoction (Su Zi Jiang Qi Tang) that employs perilla (zi su zi) as the leading ingredient for dispersing and descending congested Lung Qi. Unlike ephedra (ma huang), the foremost anti-asthma herb in the Chinese materia medica, perilla will not cause undue strain on the heart or nervous system and is therefore a safer medicinal agent. Perilla is joined by herbs that ventilate the Lung and descend the Qi, expel Phlegm, replenish Moisture, and support the Spleen and Kidneys.[5]

Herbal formula: *Perilla* seed (zi su zi), *Lepidium* seed (ting li zi), apricot seed (xing ren), mulberry bark (sang bai pi), and *Platycodon* root (jie geng) combine to descend the Lung Qi, clear Lung Heat, expel Wind-Heat from the Lung, dispel Phlegm, ameliorate coughing, and relieve wheezing. Aster root (zhi zi wan), *Stemona* root (zhi bai bu), anemarrhena rhizome (zhi mu), and citrus peel (chen pi) replenish moisture in the Lung, loosen Phlegm, and aid expectoration. Cardamon seed (sha ren) soothes the Stomach and aids digestion and warms the Spleen and Kidneys, countering any Dampness induced by the moisturizing ingredients, and together with schisandra fruit (wu wei zi) aids the Kidneys in anchoring the descending Lung Qi and retaining Moisture and Essence. Licorice root (gan cao) gently tonifies the Qi of Stomach and Spleen and assists in arresting the cough, neutralizing Heat and Toxins (reducing inflammation) and harmonizing all of the ingredients.[5]

Dosage: 1 to 2 droppersful as needed every 2 to 4 hours.[5]

Caution: Use with caution in children with extreme weakness, lethargy, high body temperature (102° F or greater), dehydration, or bronchial infection.[5,6]

Chronic Asthma

Deep Breath (Gentle Warrior Pediatric Formula, Kan Herb Company, Scotts Valley, Calif.) supplements the underlying deficiencies of chronic asthma, namely depleted Qi, Blood, Moisture, and Essence of the Spleen, Lung, and Kidney (the three sources of Qi). It also contains some herbs that disperse and purge (Qi and Phlegm) to counter the potential stagnation that can result from tonifying Qi and Moisture in the midst of stagnation: coexisting Phlegm, Cold, Heat, and congested Qi.[5]

Open Air and Deep Breath can be used together in patients with chronic asthma with persistent mild cough and wheezing.

Herbal formula: Cynanchum rhizome/root (bai qian), *Platycodon* root (jie geng), aster root (zhi zi wan), *Stemona* root (zhi bai bu), *Inula* flower (xuan fu hua), and coltsfoot flower (kuan dong hua) combine to warm and moisten the Lung, ventilate and descend the stagnant Qi, inhibit coughing, and stop wheezing. *Peucedanum* root (qian hu), mulberry root bark (sang bai pi), and mulberry leaf (zhi sang ye) assist the primary herbs in descending the Lung Qi while also expelling Wind-Cold and Wind-Heat from the Lung. Schisandra fruit (wu wei zi), black plum (wu mei), angelica tang kwei root (dang gui shen), and ginseng root (bai ji li ren shen) replenish Essence and Blood, tonify Qi, astringe the Essence and Moisture of the Lung, and, together with ginger rhizome (shen jiang), strengthen the Root by warming and consolidating the Qi and Essence of the Kidneys. Licorice root (gan cao) aids in ameliorating the cough, neutralizing Heat and Toxins (reducing inflammation), tonifying Qi, and harmonizing all of the ingredients.[5]

Dosage: 1 to 2 droppersful as needed 3 to 4 times per day.

Caution: Use with caution in children with acute asthma, common cold, or flu with fever.

Lung Qi Jr. (Blue Poppy Enterprises, Boulder, Colo.) is a modified version of classical formulas Zhi Sou San and Xiao

Chai Hu Tang designed to treat asthmatic wheezing, cough, and croup. It is a formula of 15 herbs in a 9:1 extract in a glycerine base that clears Heat and transforms Phlegm, supplementing the Spleen and fortifying Qi.

Dosage: 1 to 2 droppersful for younger children, and 3 to 4 droppersful for older children. During an acute asthmatic episode, doses can be given every hour or more frequently, and three times per day during remission.

Herbs—Western

A recent review of medical databases evaluated the clinical efficacy of herbal preparations for the treatment of asthma symptoms; 17 RCTs were described, including traditional Indian medicine, Japanese Kampo, Chinese herbal medicines, and others. No definitive evidence for any herbal preparations were found.[1] Regarding ivy leaf extract, some evidence from small-scale study demonstrates that drops may improve respiratory functions of children with mild to moderately severe chronic bronchial asthma, but only one placebo control trial has been noted.[2]

Kampo, or tusmorua saibuko-to, TJ-96, is a combination of 10 mushroom and herbal products and is used safely and extensively in China, as well as in Japan with government approval. Kampo is applied orally and has steroid-sparing effects that have been described in adults with steroid-dependent asthma. In part, this preparation is thought to have an antiinflammatory action in suppressing eosinophilic activation.[3] There are no clinical trials regarding the use of this product in children, and its use is not recommended.

Ephedra *(Ephedra sinica)*, also known as *ma huang* in TCM, has been a mainstay of treatment for asthma for thousands of years. However, a growing body of research and adverse events associated with this use of this herbal product for weight loss and sport supplementation suggests it poses unacceptable short- and long-term risks including hypertension, arrhythmias, seizures, stroke, and sudden death.[4-6] Although this herbal product may be available in imported products, it has been banned from sale in for weight loss and sport supplements in the United States since March 2004. Its use for children for symptoms of asthma is strongly contraindicated.

Magnet Therapy

Magnets can be applied as routine health maintenance with twice-weekly 15-minute sessions in children who experience intermittent asthmatic attacks. Four Accu-Band 9000 magnets are used, two on each side of the body. Ask the child or observe whether the child has more difficulty breathing in (inhalation) or breathing out (exhalation). If the child has more difficulty on the inhalation phase, place the designated bionorth side of the magnet (the side with the indentation) on KD3 and the biosouth (opposite side of the magnet) on LU5 bilaterally.[1] If the child has more difficulty with exhalation, place the designated bionorth side of the magnet (side with the indentation) on SP4[1] and the designated south side (opposite side) on LU5. These magnets may be obtained from OMS (800-323-1839) or AHSM (800-635-7070).

Massage Therapy

Children with asthma and their parents report high CAM use in self-reported surveys.[1-3] Respondents to the surveys indicated they felt CAM was as effective as pharmacological measures (59%)[1,2] and indicated massage as one of the CAM modalities that were used.[1-3]

Massage therapy may help improve respiration when applied to the accessory muscles of breathing as well as reduce anxiety and promote relaxation (see Chapter 3), which could make it a helpful adjunct to asthma symptom management. A 1-month RCT that compared nightly massage therapy by parents with progressive muscle relaxation in children with asthma demonstrated decreased anxiety levels, improved activity, improved vocalization, and decreased cortisol levels in the massage group.[4] In addition, the 4- to 8-year-old children had improved peak air flows and pulmonary function tests.[4] Some massage practitioners have cited reflexology, which is an acupressure technique applied to the feet and/or hands, as being a helpful therapy for individuals with asthma. However, two blinded controlled trials of adult asthma patients who received either placebo or therapeutic reflexology demonstrated no difference between the treatment and placebo group on peak air flows or asthma symptoms.[5,6]

Parents could readily use massage therapy as an additional tool to help their children cope with their asthma symptoms. Massage could promote relaxation, reduce anxiety, and possibly improve respiration. If children are experiencing dyspnea or orthopnea but would like massage, it is best to keep the child in an upright position so as not to exacerbate symptoms. This can best be accomplished by having the child sit in a chair and lean forward onto the tabletop with a pillow or while sitting on the parent's lap with the patient's head on the parent's shoulder. Another method of offering massage at this time is to provide slow Swedish massage to the hands or feet to help soothe the child while not interfering with his or her respiratory pattern.

Mind/Body

Numerous studies have supported mind/body connections in children with asthma and the impact of emotional functioning on the severity and frequency of asthma symptoms.[1,2] Therefore a number of mind/body interventions can play an important role in conventional asthma and some related pulmonary conditions including vocal cord dysfunction, habitual cough, and exercise-induced asthma.

Controlled diaphragmatic breathing (relaxation breathing) training can be of great benefit to children and adolescents with asthma and, in the case of exercise-induced asthma, may replace or significantly reduce the need for bronchodilators.[3]

Outcome literature reviewed by Lehrer[1] support that bifrontal electromyography (EMG), thermography, air flow feedback (pneumography or capnography), and heart rate variability biofeedback training all appear to have potential beneficial effects on children and adolescents with asthma. In a prospective, randomized controlled study, Kotses and colleagues[4] found that the facial relaxation subjects exhibited higher pulmonary scores, more positive attitudes toward asthma, and lower chronic anxiety at follow-up. In a multiple case study report, Lehrer and colleagues[2] taught 20 pediatric asthma patients with mild disease a specific breath control technique (Smetankin breathing) while tracking heart rate variability. Significant improvements were noted in two spirometric measures following treatment intervention.

A growing body of literature supports the benefits of yoga for asthma as well.[5] A study of 46 subjects with childhood asthma demonstrated benefits of yoga training as measured by improvements in resting pulmonary functions and exercise tolerance over a 2-year period.[6] A 1986 study by Nagendra and Nagarthna[7] supported benefits, including reductions in medication usage, over a 3- to 54-month period for 570 asthmatic children who were trained in yoga practices including yogasanas, pranayama, meditation, and kriyasana. A specialized yoga breath control technique called "Buteyko" breathing method was also reported in one randomized trial to be helpful in reducing symptoms of asthma and successful in reducing the use of bronchodilators, but not successful in changing lung function in patients with asthma.[8]

Autonomic nervous system dysregulation has been proposed as a mediating variable in precipitating asthmatic episodes. In a 1993 study, Henry et al.[9] demonstrated autogenics training to be a successful adjunct to conventional asthma therapy with improvements of more than 15% seen compared with pretreatment levels in a variety of spirometric measures. No significant change in respiratory function was observed for the matched control group.

Mental imagery is also a potential useful adjunct as described by Kohen in his case series.[10] Anbar[11] also reports success in 80% of children with persistent asthma seen in a pulmonary center who were taught hypnosis.

In a 2002 systematic review of RCTs that studied relaxation strategies in asthma, Huntley et al.[12] concluded there is some evidence that muscular relaxation improves lung function in patients with asthma but that evidence for efficacy of other relaxation techniques was lacking. In summary, further controlled studies are needed to support the efficacy of mind/body approaches for patients with asthma.

In the authors' clinical experience, mind/body skills including the teaching of diaphragmatic breathing and stress management skills can significantly reduce the need for asthma medications in many children. It is important to coordinate medication needs with the appropriate primary care or specialty provider. Typically, children with asthma are taught paced diaphragmatic breathing. The typical sequence involves having the individual breathe in to the count of 2 to 3 seconds through the nose and exhale through the mouth to the count of 4 to 6 seconds while relaxing the neck and shoulder muscles and allowing effortless abdominal movement. Positive self-talk statements and stress management strategies are also offered. For children who have tight upper body muscles, a home-trainer surface EMG biofeedback unit is sometimes loaned to them to assist in practice each day at home for a few weeks, which seems to enhance progress. Self-hypnosis training using suggestions about "opening up the airways" and mastering and controlling "easy" breathing is also blended into treatment strategies. These same techniques are also very effective with

vocal cord dysfunction, a problem that is commonly confused with asthma.

Naturopathy

Dietary Evaluation of Allergenic Food

Asthma is characterized by a hyperreactivity of lung tissue, and the naturopathic approach is to target this reaction both by calming the immune system and removing any aggravating factors to which the patient is exposed, as follows:

Completely remove any foods from the diet to which the child is reacting for at least 2 weeks, including any foods with reactive ingredients. The most commonly offending foods are those that are standard in the U.S. diet, such as dairy, wheat, eggs, nuts, citrus, corn, and soy. After the elimination period, the patient introduces the food at every meal for 1 day, and parents observe for symptoms for the following 2 days. This will allow enough time for a delayed response to show.

Identification of reactive foods his may be determined by observation or by specific lab testing. Several laboratories offer blood tests for IgG levels to certain foods. The author has found this testing method more reliable than the conventional IgE skin testing, because the extracts that are used may degrade and show false-negative results.[1] Foods that score high on skin-prick tests are often those that show a more immediate-type reaction. IgE and IgG enzyme-linked immunosorbent assay (ELISA) testing seems to be more sensitive than skin testing for reactivity to foods,[2] and IgG testing provides the added benefit of detecting delayed-type hypersensitivities.

Address Increased Intestinal Permeability and Necessary Flora

In certain conditions, the integrity of the intestinal mucosal lining is compromised, especially in chronic inflammatory states such as in atopic individuals. The result is larger antigenic molecules passing into the luminal bloodstream, called *increased intestinal permeability*, and is often seen in patients with asthma.[3] This results in increased antibody and immune complex production.

- Solid food introduction should be postponed at least until 6 months of age, and allergenic foods should definitely be avoided until 18 months to 2 years of age. Use of antibiotics can give way to pathogenic bacteria and *Candida albicans* overgrowth, also known as *dysbiosis*, and these imbalances can exacerbate intestinal permeability.

- Evaluate by means of laboratory testing: levels of urinary organic acids (this author favors the use of Great Plains Laboratory, Lenexa, Kan., 913-341-8949) represent byproducts of *C. albicans* and *Clostridium difficile*. Some physicians feel that this test is more of an evaluation of intestinal permeability than biological overgrowth. However, either of these perceptions will be helpful for case evaluation, as floral imbalance can lead to or exacerbate increased intestinal permeability. Intestinal permeability can be determined with a simple lactulose/mannitol test, which is provided by several laboratories.

- Trial of oral Nystatin up to a duration of 1 month. A gradual dosing schedule may be a more gentle approach to treatment, because patients occasionally experience flulike symptoms, including fatigue, headache, nausea, gas, bloating, diarrhea, and constipation. An example of gradual dosing would be 50,000 units for day 1; 50,000 units twice for day 2; 100,000 units twice for day 3; and 200,000 units twice for day 4. After that time, 400,000 to 500,000 units several times per day may be then used for the remaining days of the treatment. After 1 month of treatment, if organic acid levels still resemble dysbiosis, the schedule may be repeated or other medications may be used. Fluconazole (Diflucan) is another option to treat resistant *Candida* spp., and a duration of 3 weeks is recommended, at 3 mg/kg per day. Liver enzymes should be evaluated before and after using fluconazole. Some physicians use fluconazole for as long as several months in some patients, and liver enzymes should be checked monthly if this is the case.

- During antifungal treatment, probiotic supplementation should be provided. Probiotics can help prevent early atopic disease,[5] and this may carry through into asthma prevention later in life. Lactobacilli's ability to produce antioxidants[6] is another reason for its usefulness in treating asthma, as these patients are under a significant amount of oxidative stress. The *Lactobacillus* GG strain has a large amount of research supporting its use. There is currently no published dose standard, but the general trend seems to be between 5 and 10 billion colony-forming units (CFUs) per day. Fortunately, probiotics are a safe treatment, so the chance of adverse reactions is very rare. The yeast species *Saccharomyces boulardii* has also been shown to prevent translocation of *Candida* spp. from gut to intestinal lymph tissue in animal models and therefore may also be helpful to add into the treatment regimen. A dose of 250 mg of *S. boulardii* per day is recommended.
- Supplement with the amino acid glutamine. Glutamine serves as the primary fuel source for enterocytes. It is commonly used in patients with increased intestinal permeability to increase mucosal thickness and the integrity of the intestinal barrier.[7] It also helps promote secretory IgA secretion, which can further aid in modulating the immune system. A dose of 1 to 4 g per day in several daily doses is adequate to promote gut healing. Glutamine is available in either capsule or powder form.

General Antioxidant, Vitamin, and Mineral Supplementation

Asthma patients have increased levels of oxidative stress,[8] so children who are either at risk or have already developed asthma should consume foods high in antioxidants and supplement with antioxidant vitamins and minerals. Other studies show that increases in serum levels of β-carotene, selenium, vitamin C, and magnesium have favorable effects in asthma patients.[9-11]

- Provide the asthma patient with a multivitamin that has adequate amounts of the antioxidant nutrients. In some cases, higher, more therapeutic levels of the previously mentioned nutrients can provide benefit.
- Vitamins B_6 and B_{12} have been shown to be at lower levels in asthma patients and may help decrease attack frequency. Doses of 50 to 100 mg of B_6 has been well tolerated and

shown to decrease frequency of wheezing and asthma attacks.[12] Both zinc[13] and selenium[14] are other minerals also shown to be lower in asthmatics, and supplementation may be beneficial.[15] Selenium may be dosed at 50 to 100 μg per day for children 1 year old to adolescence, and 200 μg per day for teens. Zinc may be dosed 15 mg per day for patients 1 to 10 years old and 30 to 60 mg per day for adolescents and teens. Zinc should always be taken with food to avoid stomach upset. Liquid forms of these nutrients are available by several manufacturers.

Nutrition

Eliminating certain allergenic foods has been a practice thought to decrease chronic asthma symptoms and its severity. The dietary triggers may be foods themselves, such as dairy products, eggs, soy, or wheat, or they may be the components of various foods such as yeast in bread, cheeses, or mushrooms; sulfites in dried fruits; pesticide residues on foods; or food additives such as tartrazine (yellow dye No. 5), citric acid, benzoates, or aspartame.[1] Children with atopic skin symptoms are more likely to have asthma symptoms, rhinitis, urticaria, or gastrointestinal symptoms when exposed to these foods additives.[2] Although it may be exhaustive and difficult (and not particularly healthy) to do a full elimination diet in children to assess their responses, doing this on a small scale may be of benefit for some. One recent pilot study eliminated only eggs and milk for a period of 8 weeks in a group of children with asthma. Peak expiratory flow rates (PEFR), total IgE, and serum IgG antibody levels to milk and egg protein were measured. During the study period, those in the experimental group not only had reduced atopic symptoms when compared with controls, but also had increased PEFR. Anti-IgG antibody levels to egg and milk were significantly reduced in the experimental groups, whereas anti-IgG antibody levels to egg (but not milk) were increased in the control group. The IgE values were unchanged in either group.[3]

Other studies have implicated more strongly the role of dietary factors beyond food allergens in the increasing incidence of asthma. Asthmatic subjects were more likely to eat fast foods and consume less fruits and vegetables and thus less vitamins, minerals and fiber than the controls.[4] Low levels of vitamin C and other antioxidants have been associated with a higher risk of asthma,[5] as has the increased intake of trans-fatty acids.[6] Trans-fatty acids occur in dairy products, saturated animal fats, and industrially hydrogenated vegetable fats used in processed and fried foods. The "Western diet" with its prevalence of highly processed foods and lack of whole foods rich in the essential nutrients, vitamins, and fatty acids likely is contributing to the increased incidence of asthma worldwide.

Omega-3 fatty acids have antiinflammatory effects, and low dietary levels are associated with inflammatory diseases. In a randomized controlled study, subjects with asthma received either fish oil capsules containing 84 mg EPA and 36 mg DHA or olive oil capsules for 10 months. Asthma symptoms scores and responsiveness to acetylcholine decreased in the fish oil group but not the olive oil group, suggesting that dietary supplementation with omega-3 fatty acids is beneficial for children with asthma.[7]

Treatment

- Increase daily intake of fresh fruits and vegetables, preferably free of pesticides and herbicides. This practice will reduce exposure to toxins and increase the amount of the natural antioxidants—vitamin C, vitamin E, vitamin A, selenium, flavones, and flavonoids—which reduce the oxidative stress and damage to lungs. Onions have nine different constituents found to inhibit leukotrienes synthesis and therefore decrease inflammation. Vitamin C also has antihistamine properties.

- Follow an antiinflammatory diet with less saturated fats, trans-fats, refined and processed foods; and increased intake of omega-3 fatty acids such as from cold-water fish, fish oil, flax seed/oil, or walnuts.

- Eliminate food allergens from the diet, the most common being dairy, wheat, eggs, corn, soy, citrus, peanuts, fish, food coloring, and additives. Food elimination diet is the gold standard; however, IgG ELISA food allergy testing may be used to narrow the number of foods to be eliminated.

- Supplementation with individual nutrients such as magnesium or any of the B vitamins has been implicated due to its theoretical effects on bronchial reactivity; however, current studies have not supported this when single nutrients were given orally. Whole foods rather than individual nutrients should be encouraged, as it is likely the combined effect of several nutrients that provides benefit.

- Probiotics, such as those found in yogurt, may have a role in treating asthma. Daily consumption of 450-g yogurt with live cultures increased interferon (IFN)-γ levels fivefold. It is theorized probiotic supplementation may attenuate asthma as IFN-γ inhibits IgE synthesis.[8]

Probiotics

Although research data are scanty at best, a trial of probiotic therapy may prove beneficial for a subset of patients with asthma, especially for those who have been exposed to antibiotics. Because the pathophysiology of asthma is inflammatory in nature, the reported antiinflammatory actions of probiotic therapy may help ameliorate processes that drive symptoms.[1] That stated, few studies have evaluated the use of probiotic therapy in this situation, and no definitive guidelines regarding dose or choice of specific microbe(s) have been published.

Support for probiotic therapy in the setting of asthma is largely extrapolated from data pertaining to eczema, allergic rhinitis, and immune system function. In theory, specific microbial strains may impact the modification/degradation of antigens, optimize mucosal barrier function, regulate secretion of inflammatory mediators, and promote proper immune system function.[2,3] Data also suggest that probiotic therapy may help lessen activation of cells important to an inflammatory response. A study of 14 consecutive subjects, aged 6 to 48 years, with clinical symptoms of asthma and/or conjunctivitis, rhinitis, urticaria, atopic dermatitis, food allergy, and irritable bowel syndrome was published in 2004. The subjects were given a daily mixture of *Lactobacillus acidophilus, Lactobacillus delbrueckii,* and *Streptococcus thermophilus* (a total of 1 billion live bacteria) for 30 days. Circulating CD34+ cell values decreased significantly after the treatment.[4] Based upon early research, some experts now recommend probiotic therapy, specifically *Lactobacillus* GG in a dose of 10 billion CFU, as preventive therapy for mothers during late third trimester and when breastfeeding when there is a family history of atopic disorder.[5] One published study of children with perennial allergic rhinitis using 2 billion CFU daily of *Lactobacillus paracasei-33* (LP-33) reported significant improvements in quality of life and frequency of symptoms after 30 days of treatment compared with controls.[6] Not all reports, however, have been positive. A study comparing respiratory and eye symptoms and use of medications in two groups of 18 people with allergic rhinitis found no effect with *Lactobacillus rhamnosus* when subjects were given an open oral challenge test with a slice of apple before, during, and after the birch-pollen season. The authors did note, however, that the small sample size limited the significance of their results.[7] One adult asthma study has been published and reported on the effects of live cultures of *L. acidophilus* in yogurt (225 g twice daily) on 15 patients in a crossover, double-blind trial. No clinically significant differences between the two groups were found for results of pulmonary function testing or quality of life indices.[8] There was a trend, however, toward decreased eosinophilia and increased IFN-γ.

Guidance with respect to choice of specific organisms and duration of therapy is sorely lacking. To further complicate matters, there seems little rationale behind the variety of dosages or combination of microbes employed in published studies. Often similar dosages have been utilized for distinct microbes, whereas widely disparate dosages have been employed by researchers studying the same probiotic. At this time, dosage recommendations are far from set in stone.

Although supportive data are scanty at best, this author recommends using a 2 to 3 month trial of probiotic therapy for patients with asthma that includes well-studied organisms shown to be safe, such as *Lactobacillus* GG (the microbe associated with the most supportive data), *Lactobacillus plantarum, Lactobacillus paracasei, Lactobacillus reuteri,* or *L. acidophilus.* Dosing guidelines to consider are 10 billion CFU for children weighing < 12 kg and 20 billion CFU for children > 12 kg. Treatment is extremely well tolerated, and palatability is an infrequent issue, as the capsules can be opened and mixed into drinks or soft foods. Sometimes the agents are available as a powder as well. If effective, treatment can continue indefinitely. Use with extreme caution, if at all, for those children at risk for infectious complications (e.g., immunosuppression or use of immunosuppressive agents, presence of central venous catheter, prematurity).

Psychology

There is a strong relationship between emotional functioning and asthma onset and outcome. In a 2004 review of the literature on pediatric asthma, it was found that parent's psychological well-being, parent-child interactions, and child's emotional functioning strongly affected a child's asthma.[1] More specifically, emotional regulation is a skill that develops through parent modeling of effective ways to manage feelings.

Poor emotional regulation is associated with behavior problems and the development of psychopathology. Less effective emotional regulation was found to be a significant predictor of asthma symptoms, even after controlling for asthma severity. Families characterized as high in conflict are at greatest risk for nonadherence. Interestingly, among adolescents hospitalized with asthma, high parental criticism was associated with greater noncompliance. However, when separated from their parents, adolescents had a significantly better response to treatment.

Parents' psychopathology can also have a negative impact on children's health. Mothers with high levels of depressive symptoms were 40% more likely to take their children with asthma to the emergency room over a 6-month period with to mothers with low levels of depressive symptoms.[2] Caregivers' ability to handle daily stress and their own emotional difficulties may affect their response to health concerns in their sick children.

Parent-child interaction difficulties can also profoundly affect asthma onset. In a prospective study for children at genetic risk for asthma, parenting difficulties such as emotional availability to the child and commitment to childcare at 3 weeks of age predicted asthma onset by 6 years.[3] The children that developed asthma at age 6 were also rated as being at greater psychological risk than were the children without asthma.

The literature on children with asthma suggests they are vulnerable to stress in their environment. Parent psychopathology and parent-child conflict can influence the development of asthma, as well as affect hospitalization and medical compliance. CAM psychological treatment for children with asthma should involve focusing on family dynamics and how such dynamics work to undermine health. Multidisciplinary programs that involve family members are recommended. One study examined the impact of a pediatric day treatment program that, in addition to intensive medical care, included group therapy several times per week as well as individual and family counseling.[4] At 1- and 2-year follow-up, there was significant improvement in severity, corticosteriod use, perceived competence in asthma management, and quality of life for caregiver and child.

Treatment Recommendations

A CAM psychologist would begin with an initial interview to explore every family member's emotional well-being with a specific focus on the child with asthma and the primary caregiver. How the parent feels about the treatment regimen, caretaking responsibility, and even parenthood in general are important to discuss in a manner that is as nonjudgmental and nonthreatening as possible. The child's perspective should also be understood; for example, does she feel her parents are supportive and helpful in managing the disease or critical and demanding? The CAM psychologist would explore how the child is coping with the limitations imposed by the disease (e.g., limited participation in sports, frequent absences from school). If the caretaker is overwhelmed, perhaps more frequent contact from a nurse or regular appointments with a doctor might be helpful. It may be possible to identify other family members who can contribute, or respite care may be available to the family.

Developing a consistent reinforcement program may help the child feel more positive about the condition. For example, playing video games during pulmonary treatment or earning rewards for remembering to take medication can improve compliance and create a positive outlook. From an early age, children should be encouraged to participate in their medical program. When possible, have the child pick a consistent time for treatment or taking medication. This will help prevent enforcement of treatment from becoming a power struggle with parents.

The psychologist should ask the child about the aspects of the disease that are creating anxiety or sadness. Whenever possible, the psychologist triesto help the child and family find solutions (e.g., if the child is worried about school work, can parents can find a tutor or arrange for regular visits with a teacher?). A child may feel stressed if she is isolated from peers due to hospitalization for an illness. Parents can try to arrange for visits from friends or phone calls. For younger children, teachers are often be willing to have the class write "get well" cards that can help decorate a dreary hospital room or lonely bedroom. If parents are feeling overwhelmed and children are stressed, everyone will have more difficulty with effective problem-solving. Helping families find a few simple solutions will create a sense of empowerment and provide hope for change.

Poor psychological and family functioning can influence asthma management and course. Psychological treatment should involve teaching both parent and child healthy ways to regulate emotions. Treatment will typically be most effective when its focus includes not only the child and parents, but also the family environment and outside stressors. Current literature does not support one specific treatment approach for children with asthma. However, by using a psychological treatment that aims to enhance emotional stability, both the children and parents may be better able to navigate the stress and complexity of medical illness and its treatment.

Qigong

An NIH grant application posits that one possible mechanism of medical Qigong is through achieving yin-yang equilibrium, which translates in biochemical terms as a balance of cyclic adenosine monophosphate (cAMP) and cyclic guanosine monophosphate (cGMP), which in turn regulate hormones, balance the autonomic nervous system, and enhance circulation, thus improving the oxygen distribution and relaxing the bronchi, alleviating asthma.[1] Conventional hormone therapy using prednisone, hydrocortisone or adrenocorticotropic hormone can cause excessive water retention and moon facies and may lead to long-term side effects, such as atrophy of the adrenal glands, atrophy of the thymus, risk of osteoporosis, yeast infections, and memory impairment possibly caused by the atrophy of the hippocampal dendrites. The indiscriminate uses of drugs that enhance cAMP can also cause an overactive sympathetic nervous system, which might lead to heart and blood vessel problems.[1]

In a German clinical study, 30 asthma patients with varying degrees of severity practiced Qigong for 6 months showed improvement in peak-flow measurements, use of medication, and asthma-relevant symptoms (sleeping through the night, coughing, expectoration, dyspnea, and general well-being). When comparing the study year with the previous year, additional improvements included reduced hospitalization rate, less sickness leave, reduced antibiotic use, and fewer emergency consultations resulting in reduced treatment costs. The researchers concluded that an improvement in airway capability and a decrease in illness severity can be achieved by regular, self-conducted Qigong exercises. Therefore Qigong, under professional supervision, could be used for asthma patients.[2] This study can be extrapolated to pediatric patients.

Qigong assessment of chronic asthma usually reveals Lung insufficiency with Dampness and habitual poor posture and breathing.

Qigong treatment can consist of intensive diaphragmatic breathing and proper posture at all times. Qigong exercises are practiced two times a day (or as often as necessary), usually for less than 30 minutes (although longer practices are fine), with meditation and gentle brushing of energy away from the center line of the body outward around the lung area, then inward brushing to give energy. Qipressure (adapted acupressure with intense breathing by both person) is applied to LI4 (between the thumbs and forefingers), LI11 (at the crook of the elbows), ST36 (4 inches down from the knee on the lateral side of the tibia), SP6 (on the inner edge of the tibia, 4 inches up from the upper edge of the ankle bones), BL11 and 12 (1.5 inches lateral to the first and second thoracic vertebra), and CV22 (center of the suprasternal fossa, 0.5 inch above the sternal notch). A positive mental attitude is also advocated. Therapy may vary at different occasions of assessment.

This author has seen more than 50 cases and has had excellent results. Improvements consist of decreasing frequency of use and dosage of medications.

References

Pediatric Diagnosis and Treatment

1. Nield LS, Markman L, Kamat DM: Asthma update: pearls you may have missed, *Consult Pediatr* May:219-226, 2005.
2. National Center for Health Statistics: Asthma—United States, 1980-1987, *MMWR Morbid Mortal Wkly Rep* 39:493-497, 1990.
3. Warner JO: Worldwide variations in the prevalence of atopic symptoms: what does it all mean? *Thorax* 54:S46-S51, 1990.
4. Asthma mortality and hospitalization among children and young adults—United States, 1980-1993, *MMWR Morbid Mortal Wkly Rep* 45:350-353, 1996.
5. Sly RM: Changing prevalence of allergic rhinitis and asthma, *Ann Allerg Asthma Immunol* 82:233-248, 1999.
6. Mannino DM, Homa DM, Akinbami LJ et al: Surveillance for asthma—United States, 1980-1999, MMWR CDC Surveill Summ 51:1-6, 2002.
7. Behrman RE, Kliegman RM, Jenson HB, editors: *Nelson's textbook of pediatrics*, ed 17, Philadelphia, 2004, Saunders.
8. Blessing-Moore J: Asthma affects all age groups but requires special consideration in the pediatric age group especially in children less than five years of age, *J Asthma* 31:415-418, 1994.
9. Neville RG, McCowan C, Hoskins G et al: Cross-sectional observations on the natural history of asthma, *Br J Gen Pract* 51:361-365, 2001.
10. Asthma–United States, 1980–1987, *MMWR Morbid Mortal Wkly Rep* 39:493-497, 1990.
11. Mannino DM, Homa DM, Pertowski CA et al: Surveillance for asthma—United States, 1960-1995, *MMWR CDC Surveill Summ* 47:1-27, 1998.
12. Crane J, Pearce N, Flatt A et al: Prescribed fenoterol and death from asthma in New Zealand, 1981-83: case control study, *Lancet* 1:917-922, 1989.
13. Spitzer WO, Suissa S, Ernst P et al: The use of β-agonists and the risk of death and near death from asthma, *N Engl J Med* 326:501-506, 1992.
14. Meurer JR, George V, Subichin S et al: Asthma severity among children hospitalized in 1990 and 1995, *Arch Pediatr Adolesc Med* 154:143-149, 2000.
15. Werner HA: Status asthmaticus in children: a review, *Chest* 119:1913-1929, 2001.
16. Settipane RA: National Asthma Education and Prevention Program (NAEPP). Defining the effects of an inhaled corticosteroid and long-acting beta-agonist on therapeutic targets, *Allergy Asthma Proc* 24:85-89, 2003.
17. Chung KF: Non-invasive biomarkers of asthma, *Pediatr Pulmonol Suppl* 18:41-44, 1999.
18. Gaston B: Managing asthmatic airway inflammation: what is the role of expired nitric oxide measurement? *Curr Prob Pediatr* 28:245-252, 1998.
19. Jarjour NN, Kelly EA: Pathogenesis of asthma, *Med Clin North Am* 86:925-936, 2002.
20. Szefler SJ, Nelson HS: Alternative agents for anti-inflammatory treatment of asthma, *J Allergy Clin Immunol* 102:S23-S35, 1998.
21. Weisberg SC: Pharmacotherapy of asthma in children, with special reference to leukotriene receptor antagonists, *Pediatr Pulmonol* 29:46-61, 2000.
22. Kemp JP: Role of leukotriene receptor antagonists in pediatric asthma, *Pediatr Pulmonol* 30:177-182, 2000.
23. Larsen GL: Differences between adult and childhood asthma, *Dis Mon* 47:34-44, 2001.
24. Martinez FD: Links between pediatric and adult asthma, *J Allergy Clin Immunol* 107(Suppl):449S-455S, 2001.
25. Bisgaard H: Pathophysiology of the cysteinyl leukotrienes and effects of leukotriene receptor antagonists in asthma, *Allergy* 56(S66):7-11, 2001.
26. Laitinen LA, Heino M, Laitinen A et al: Damage of airway epithelium and bronchial reactivity in patients with asthma, *Am Rev Respir Dis* 131:599-606, 1985.
27. Platts-Mills TA, Rakes G, Heymann PW: The relevance of allergen exposure to the development of asthma in childhood, *J Allergy Clin Immunol* 105:503-508, 2000.
28. Pilotto LS, Smith BJ, Nitschke M et al: Industry, air quality, cigarette smoke and rates of respiratory illness in Port Adelaide, *Aust N Z J Public Health* 23:657-660, 1999.
29. Wahlgren DR, Hovell MF, Meltzer EO et al: Involuntary smoking and asthma, *Curr Opin Pulmonary Med* 6:31-36, 2000.
30. Avital A, Springer C, Bar-Yishay E et al: Adenosine, methacholine, and exercise challenges in children with asthma or paediatric chronic obstructive pulmonary disease, *Thorax* 50:511-516, 1995.
31. Vamos M, Kolbe J: Psychological factors in severe chronic asthma, *Aust N Z J Psychiatry* 33:538-544, 1999.
32. Covar RA, Macomber BA, Szefler SJ: Medications as asthma triggers, *Immunol Allergy Clin North Am* 25:169-190, 2005.
33. Liangas G, Morton JR, Henry RL: Mirth-triggered asthma: is laughter really the best medicine? *Pediatr Pulmonol* 36:107-112, 2003.
34. Dubus JC, Bosdure E, Mates M et al: Virus and respiratory allergy in children [in French], *Allergy Immunol (Paris)* 33:78-81, 2001.

35. National Asthma Education & Prevention Program: *Expert Panel report II: Guidelines for the diagnosis and management of asthma*, Bethesda, MD, 1997, National Institutes of Health, National Heart, Lung, and Blood Institute, 1997.

36. National Heart, Lung, and Blood Institute; National Asthma Education and Prevention Program: *Expert panel report 3: guidelines for the diagnosis and management of asthma*, Washington, DC, 2007, US Department of Health and Human Services. Available at www.nhlbi.nih.gov/guidelines/asthma/asthgdln.pdf. Accessed September 2007.

37. Skoner DP: Management and treatment of pediatric asthma: update, *Allergy Asthma Proc* 22:71-74, 2001.

38. Bibi H, Shoychet E, Shoseyov D et al: Evaluation of asthmatic children presenting at emergency rooms [in Hebrew], *Harefuah* 137:383-387, 430, 1999.

39. Helfaer MA, Nichols DG, Rogers MCL: Lower airway disease: bronchiolitis and asthma. In Rogers M, Nichols D, editors: *Textbook of pediatric intensive care*, ed 3, Baltimore, 1996, Williams and Wilkins, pp 127-164.

40. Woodcock A, Custovic A: Allergen avoidance: does it work? *Br Med Bull* 56:1071-1086, 2000.

41. Irani AM: *The challenges of mild persistent asthma.* Presented at the 17th Annual Infectious Diseases in Children Symposium, Nov 20-21, 2004, New York.

Acupuncture

1. Ziment I, Tashkin DP: Alternative medicine for allergy and asthma, *J Allergy Clin Immunol* 106:603-614, 2000.

2. Davis PA, Chang C, Hackman RM et al: Acupuncture in the treatment of asthma: a critical review, *Allergol Immunopathol (Madr)* 26:263-271, 1998.

3. Martin J, Donaldson AN, Villarroel R et al: Efficacy of acupuncture in asthma: systematic review and meta-analysis of published data from 11 randomised controlled trials, *Eur Respir J* 20:846-852, 2002.

4. Linde K, Jobst K, Panton J: Acupuncture for chronic asthma, *Cochrane Database Syst Rev.* (2):CD000008, 2000. Update in: Cochrane Database Syst Rev (1):CD000008, 2004.

5. Linde K, Vickers A, Hondras M et al: Systematic reviews of complementary therapies—an annotated bibliography. Part 1: acupuncture, *BMC Complement Altern Med* 1:3, 2001.

6. McCarney RW, Lasserson TJ, Linde K et al: An overview of two Cochrane systematic reviews of complementary treatments for chronic asthma: acupuncture and homeopathy, *Respir Med* 98:687-696, 2004.

7. McCarney RW, Brinkhaus B, Lasserson TJ et al: Acupuncture for chronic asthma, *Cochrane Database Syst Rev* (1):CD000008, 2004.

8. Birch S, Hesselink JK, Jonkman FA et al: Clinical research on acupuncture. Part 1. What have reviews of the efficacy and safety of acupuncture told us so far? *J Altern Complement Med* 10:468-480, 2004.

9. *National Institutes of Health consensus development conference statement,* Washington, DC, 1997, National Institutes of Health. Available at www.consensus.nih.gov/1997/1997Acupuncture107html.htm. Accessed May 2004.

10. Chen K, Li S, Shi Z et al: Two hundred and seventeen cases of winter diseases treated with acupoint stimulation in summer, *J Tradit Chin Med* 20:198-201, 2000.

11. Personal observation: TCM Pediatric Ward, Xinhua Hospital, Shanghai, China, 1999.

12. Yan S: 14 cases of child bronchial asthma treated by auricular plaster and meridian instrument, *J Tradit Chin Med* 18:202-204, 1998.

13. Hossri CM: The treatment of asthma in children through acupuncture massage, *J Am Soc Psychosom Dent Med* 23:3-16, 1976.

14. Haidvogl M: Alternative treatment possibilities of atopic diseases [in German], *Padiatr Padol* 25:389-396, 1990.

15. Fung KP, Chow OK, So SY: Attenuation of exercise-induced asthma by acupuncture, *Lancet* 2:1419-1422, 1986.

16. Yu DY, Lee SP: Effect of acupuncture on bronchial asthma, *Clin Sci Mol Med* 51:503-509, 1976.

17. Zhou RL, Zhang JC: An analysis of combined desensitizing acupoints therapy in 419 cases of allergic rhinitis accompanying asthma [in Chinese], *Zhongguo Zhong Xi Yi Jie He Za Zhi* 17:587-589, 1997.

18. Chen LL, Li AS, Tao JN: Clinical and experimental studies on preventing and treating anaphylactic asthma with Zusanli point immunotherapy [in Chinese], *Zhongguo Zhong Xi Yi Jie He Za Zhi* 16:709-712, 1996.

19. Zang J: Immediate antiasthmatic effect of acupuncture in 192 cases of bronchial asthma, *J Tradit Chin Med* 10:89-93, 1990.

20. Rogers PA, Schoen AM, Limehouse J: Acupuncture for immune-mediated disorders. Literature review and clinical applications, *Prob Vet Med* 4:162-193, 1992.

21. Sato T, Yu Y, Guo SY et al: Acupuncture stimulation enhances splenic natural killer cell cytotoxicity in rats, *Jpn J Physiol* 46:131-136, 1996.

22. Dong L, Yuan D, Fan L et al: Effect of HE-NE laser acupuncture on the spleen in rats [in Chinese]. *Zhen Ci Yan Jiu* 21:64-67, 1996.

23. Sakic B, Kojic L, Jankovic BD et al: Electro-acupuncture modifies humoral immune response in the rat, *Acupunct Electrother Res* 14:115-120, 1989.

24. Joos S, Schott C, Zou H et al: Immunomodulatory effects of acupuncture in the treatment of allergic asthma: a randomized controlled study, *J Altern Complement Med* 6:519-525, 2000.

25. Okumura M, Toriizuka K, Iijima K et al: Effects of acupuncture on peripheral T lymphocyte subpopulation and amounts of cerebral catecholamines in mice, *Acupunct Electrother Res* 24:127-139, 1999.

26. Ma Z, Wang Y, Fan Q: The influence of acupuncture on interleukin 2 interferon-natural killer cell regulatory network of kidney-deficiency mice [in Chinese], *Zhen Ci Yan Jiu* 17:139-142, 1992.

27. Yan WX, Wang JH, Chang QQ: Effect of leu-enkephalin in striatum on modulating cellular immune during electropuncture [in Chinese], *Sheng Li Xue Bao* 43:451-456, 1991.

28. Miller AL: The etiologies, pathophysiology, and alternative/complementary treatment of asthma, *Altern Med Rev* 6:20-47, 2001.

29. Zijlstra FJ, van den Berg-de Lange I, Huygen FJ et al: Anti-inflammatory actions of acupuncture, *Mediators Inflamm* 12:59-69, 2003.

30. Sato T, Yu Y, Guo SY et al: Acupuncture stimulation enhances splenic natural killer cell cytotoxicity in rats, *Jpn J Physiol* 46:131-136, 1996.

31. Petti F, Bangrazi A, Liguori A et al: Effects of acupuncture on immune response related to opioid-like peptides, *J Tradit Chin Med* 18:55-63, 1998.

32. Bianchi M, Jotti E, Sacerdote P et al: Traditional acupuncture increases the content of beta-endorphin in immune cells and influences mitogen induced proliferation, *Am J Chin Med* 19:101-104, 1991.

33. Xu X: Acupuncture in an outpatient clinic in China: a comparison with the use of acupuncture in North America, *South Med J* 94:813-816, 2001.

34. Chen K, Li S, Shi Z et al: Two hundred and seventeen cases of winter diseases treated with acupoint stimulation in summer, *J Tradit Chin Med* 20:198-201, 2000.

35. Hu J: Clinical observation on 25 cases of hormone dependent bronchial asthma treated by acupuncture, *J Tradit Chin Med* 18:27-30, 1998.

36. Gruber W, Eber E, Malle-Scheid D et al: Laser acupuncture in children and adolescents with exercise induced asthma, *Thorax* 57:222-225, 2002.

37. Jobst KA: A critical analysis of acupuncture in pulmonary disease: efficacy and safety of the acupuncture needle, *J Altern Complement Med* 1:57-85, 1995. Erratum in: *J Altern Complement Med* 1:219, 1995.

38. Loo M: *Pediatric acupuncture*, London, 2002, Elsevier.

39. Sun Y: External approach to the treatment of pediatric asthma, *J Tradit Chin Med* 15:290-291, 1995.

40. Maciocia G: *The practice of Chinese medicine, the treatment of diseases with acupuncture and Chinese herbs*, London, 1994, Churchill Livingstone.

Aromatherapy

1. Battaglia S: *The complete guide to aromatherapy*, Virginia, Queensland, Australia, 1995, The Perfect Potion.

2. Price S, Price L: *Aromatherapy for health professionals*, Edinburgh, 1995, Churchill Livingstone.

3. Buckle J: *Clinical aromatherapy: essential oils in practice*, ed 2, Edinburgh, 2003, Churchill Livingstone.

Chiropractic

1. Gatterman MI: *Chiropractic management of spine related disorders*, Baltimore, 1990, Williams and Wilkins.

2. Wiles MR: *Visceral disorders related to the spine*, Baltimore, 1990, Williams and Wilkins.

3. Waddell SC, Davison JS, Befus AD et al: Role for the cervical sympathetic trunk in regulating anaphylactic and endotoxic shock, *J Manipulative Physiol Ther* 15:10-15, 1992.

4. Vallone S, Fallon J: Treatment protocols for the chiropractic care of common pediatric conditions: otitis media and asthma, *J Clin Chiropractic Pediatr* 2:113-115, 1997.

5. Plaugher G, Lopes MA, Konlande JE et al: Spinal management for the patient with a visceral concomitant. In Plaugher G, editor: *Textbook of clinical chiropractic: a specific biomechanical approach*, Baltimore, 1993, Williams and Wilkins.

6. Plaugher G, Anrig C: *Pediatric chiropractic*, Baltimore, 1998, Williams and Wilkins.

7. Green A: Chronic asthma and chiropractic spinal manipulation: a case study, *Br J Chiropractic* 4:32-35, 2000.

8. Vernon LF, Vernon GM: A scientific hypothesis for the efficacy of chiropractic manipulation of the pediatric asthmatic patient, *Chiropractic Pediatr* 1:7-8, 1995.

9. Bachman TR, Lantz CA: Management of pediatric asthma and enuresis with probable traumatic etiology, *ICA Int Rev Chiropractic* 51:37, 1995.

10. Brunier A: The side effects of the chiropractic adjustment, *Chiropractic Pediatr* 1:22, 1995.

11. Garde R: Asthma and chiropractic, *Chiropractic Pediatr* 1:9, 1994.

12. Amalu WC: Autism, asthma, irritable bowel syndrome, strabismus and illness susceptibility: a case study in chiropractic management, *Today's Chiropractic* Sept/Oct:32, 1998.

13. Killinger LZ: Chiropractic care in the treatment of asthma, *Palmer J Res* 2930:74-77, 1995.

14. Fysh PN: Childhood asthma, *ICA Rev* Sept/Oct: 36-39, 1996.

15. Gioia AV: Chiropractic treatment of childhood asthma: a case history, *J Am Chiropractic Assoc* Oct:35-36, 1996.

16. Cohen E: Case history: an eight-year old asthma patient, *Today's Chiropractic* 17:81, 1988.

17. Mega JJ: Bronchial asthma, *Am Chiropractor* Jan/Feb:26, 1982.

18. Mega JJ: Eliminating toxic conditions in the treatment of bronchial asthma, *J Natl Chiropractic Assoc* 30:11-12, 1960.

19. Arbiloff G: Bronchial asthma: a case report, *J Clin Chiropractic* 2:40-42, 1969.

20. Balon J, Aker PD, Crowther ER et al: A comparison of active and simulated chiropractic manipulation as adjunctive treatment for childhood asthma, *N Engl J Med* 339:1013-1020, 1998.

21. Bronfort G, Evans R, Kubic P et al: Chronic pediatric asthma and chiropractic spinal manipulation: a prospective clinical series and randomized clinical pilot study, *J Manipulative Physiol Ther* 24:369-377, 2001.

22. Bronfort G: *Childhood and adolescent asthma: the scientific basis for chiropractic management*, World Federation of Chiropractic 6th Biennial Congress, Paris, May 2001.

23. Nilsson N, Christiansen B: Prognostic factors in bronchial asthma in chiropractic practice, *J Austr Chiropractic Assoc* 18:85-87, 1988.

24. Peet JB, Marko SK, Piekarczyk W: Chiropractic response in the pediatric patient with asthma: a pilot study, *Chiropractic Pediatr* 1:9-13, 1995.

25. Graham RL, Pistolese RA: An impairment rating analysis of asthmatic children under chiropractic care, *Chiropractic Pediatr* 1:41, 1997.

26. Heffner JE, Repine JE: Pulmonary strategies of antioxidant defense, *Am Rev Resp Dis* 140:531-554, 1989.

27. Krueger A: Alternative remedies, *Altern Med* Jan/Feb: 71, 2003.

28. Leviton R: Asthma—breathe easily again, *Altern Med* 25:60, 1998.

29. Huntley A, White A, Ernst E: Complementary medicine for asthma, *Focus Altern Complement Ther* 5:111-116, 2000.

30. Collipp P, Godzier S, Weiss N et al: Pyridoxine treatment of childhood bronchial asthma, *Ann Allergy* 35:93-97, 1975.

31. Shimizu T, Maeda S, Arakawa H et al: Relation between theophylline and circulating vitamin levels in children with asthma, *Pharmacology* 53:384-389, 1996.

32. Plaugher G, Anrig C: *Pediatric chiropractic*, Baltimore, 1998, Williams and Wilkins.

33. Swenson RL: Pediatric disorders. In Lawrence D, editor: *Fundamentals of chiropractic diagnosis and management*, Baltimore, 1991, Williams and Wilkins.

34. Kemper K: Alternative asthma therapies: an evidence-based review, *Contemp Pediatr* 16:162-165, 1999.

35. Kemper K: Chronic asthma: an update, *Pediatr Rev* 17:11-147, 1996.

Herbs—Chinese

1. Natural Standard Research Collaboration. Available at www.naturalstandard.com. Accessed August 2005.

2. Li ZL, Dai BQ, Liang AH et al: Pharmacological studies of nin jion pei pa koa, *Zhongguo Zhong Yao Za Zhi* 19:362-365, 384, 1994.

3. Zhu HH, Chen YP, Yu JE et al: Therapeutic effect of Xincang decoction on chronic airway inflammation in children with bronchial asthma in remission stage, *Zhong Xi Yi Jie He Xue Bao* 3:23-27, 2005.

4. Lai X, Li Y, Fan Z, Zhang J et al: An analysis of therapeutic effect of drug acupoint application in 209 cases of allergic asthma, *J Tradit Chin Med* 21:122-126, 2001.

5. Beinfield H, Korngold E: *Chinese medicine works clinical handbook*, San Francisco, 2007, www.chinesemedicineworks.com.

6. Neustaedter R: Personal communication, 2006.

Herbs—Western

1. Huntley A, Ernst E: Herbal medicines for asthma: a systematic review, *Thorax* 57:127-131, 2002.

2. Hofmann D., Hecker M., Volp A.: Efficacy of dry extract of ivy leaves in children with bronchial asthma—a review of randomized control trials, *Phytomedicine* 10:213-220, 2003.

3. Urata Y., Yoshida S., Irie Y. et al: Treatment of asthma patients with herbal medicine TJ-96: a randomized controlled trial, *Respir Med* 96:469-474, 2002.

4. Hsieh K.H.: Evaluation of efficacy of traditional Chinese medicines in the treatment of childhood bronchial asthma: clinical trial, immunological tests and animal study, Pediatr Allergy Immunol 7:130-140, 1996.

5. *Dietary supplements containing ephedrine alkaloids: final rule summary.* Available at: www.fda.gov/oc/initiatives/ephedra/february 2004/finalsummary.html. Accessed: January 18, 2005.

6. Zhang J: TCM treatment of bronchial asthma, *J Tradit Chin Med* 20:101-103, 2000.

Magnet Therapy

1. Loo M: *Pediatric acupuncture*, London, 2002, Elsevier.

Massage Therapy

1. Braganza S, Ozuah PO, Sharif I: The use of complementary therapies in inner-city asthmatic children, *J Asthma* 40:823-827, 2003.

2. Reznik M, Ozuah PO, Franco K et al: Use of complementary therapy by adolescents with asthma, *Arch Pediatr Adolesc Med* 156:1042-1044, 2002.

3. Andrews L, Lokuge S, Sawyer M et al: The use of alternative therapies by children with asthma: a brief report, *J Paediatr Child Health* 34:131-134, 1998.

4. Field T, Henteleff T, Hernandez-Reif M et al: Children with asthma have improved pulmonary functions after massage therapy, *J Pediatr* 132:854-858, 1998.

5. Brygge T, Heinig JH, Collins P et al: Reflexology and bronchial asthma, *Respir Med* 95:173-179, 2001.

6. Peterson LN, Faurschou P, Olsen OT et al: Foot zone therapy and bronchial asthma—a controlled clinical trial, *Ugeskr Laeger* 155:329-331, 1992.

Mind/Body

1. Lehrer P, Sargunaraj D, Hochron S: Psychological approaches to the treatment of asthma, *J Consult Clin Psychol* 60:639-643, 1992.

2. Lehrer P, Smetankin A, Potapova T: Respiratory sinus arrhythmia biofeedback therapy for asthma: a report of 20 unmedicated pediatric cases using the Smetankin method, *Appl Psychophysiol Biofeed* 25:193-200, 2000.

3. Peper E: Hope for asthmatics: biofeedback systems teaching the combination of self-regulation strategies and family therapy in the self-healing of asthma, *Somatics* 2:56-62, 1988.

4. Kotses H, Harver A, Segreto J et al: Long-term effects of biofeedback induced facial relaxation on measures of asthma severity in children, *Biofeed Self-Reg* 16:1-21, 1991.

5. Singh V: Kunjal: a nonspecific protective factor in management of bronchial asthma, *J Asthma* 24:183-186, 1987.

6. Jain S, Rai L, Valecha A et al: Effect of yoga training on exercise tolerance in adolescents with childhood asthma, *J Asthma* 28:437-442, 1991.

7. Nagendra H, Nagarathna R: An integrated approach of yoga therapy for bronchial asthma: a 3-54-month prospective study, *J Asthma* 23:123-37, 1986.

8. Cooper S, Osorne J, Newton S et al: Effect of two breathing exercises (Buteyko and Pranayama) in asthma: a randomized controlled trial, *Thorax* 58:674-679, 2003.

9. Henry M, de Rivera JL, Gonzalez-Martin I, et al: Improvement of respiratory function in chronic asthmatic patients with autogenic therapy, *J Psychosom Res* 37:265-270, 1993.

10. Kohen D, Wynne E: Applying hypnosis in preschool family asthma education program: uses of storytelling, imagery, and relaxation, *Am J Clin Hypnosis* 39:169-181, 1997.

11. Anbar R: Hypnosis in pediatrics: applications at a pediatric pulmonary center, *BMC Pediatr* 2:11, 2002.

12. Huntley A, White A, Ernst E: Relaxation therapies for asthma: a systematic review, *Thorax* 57:127-131, 2002.

Naturopathy

1. Onorato J, Merland N, Terral C et al: Placebo-controlled double-blind food challenge in asthma, *J Allergy Clin Immunol* 78:1139-1146, 1986.

2. Campbell DE, Ngamphaiboon J, Clark MM et al: Indirect enzyme-linked immunosorbent assay for measurement of human immunoglobulins E and G to purified cow's milk proteins: application in diagnosis of cow's milk allergy, *J Clin Microbiol* 25:2114-2119, 1987.

3. Benard A, Desreumeaux P, Huglo D et al: Increased intestinal permeability in bronchial asthma, *J Allergy Clin Immunol* 97:1173-1178, 1986.

4. Shaw W: *Biological treatments for autism and PDD,* Vancouver, 1998, Sunflower.

5. Kalliomaki M, Salminen S, Arvilommi H et al: Probiotics in primary prevention of atopic disease: a randomised placebo-controlled trial, *Lancet* 357:1076-1079, 2001.

6. Saide JA, Gilliland SE: Antioxidative activity of lactobacilli measured by oxygen radical absorbance capacity, *J Dairy Sci* 88:1352-1357, 2005.

7. Miller A: The pathogenesis, clinical implications, and treatment of intestinal hyperpermeability, *Altern Med Rev* 2:330-345, 1997.

8. Nadeem A, Chhabra SK, Masood A et al: Increased oxidative stress and altered levels of antioxidants in asthma, *J Allergy Clin Immunol* 111:72-78, 2003.

9. Rubin RN, Navon L, Cassano PA: Relationship of serum antioxidants to asthma prevalence in youth, *Am J Respir Crit Care Med* 169:393-398, 2004.

10. Gilliland FD, Berhane KT, Li YF et al: Dietary magnesium, potassium, sodium, and children's lung function, *Am J Epidemiol* 155:125-131, 2002.

11. Dominguez LJ, Barbagallo M, Di Lorenzo G et al: Bronchial reactivity and intracellular magnesium: a possible mechanism for the bronchodilating effects of magnesium in asthma, *Clin Sci (Lond)* 95:137-142, 1998.

12. Reynolds RD, Natta CL: Depressed plasma pyridoxal phosphate concentrations in adult asthmatics, *Am J Clin Nutr* 41:684-688, 1985.

13. Kadrabova J, Mad'aric A, Podivinsky F et al: Plasma zinc, copper and copper/zinc ratio in intrinsic asthma, *J Trace Elem Med Biol* 10:50-53, 1996.

14. Kadrabova J, Mad'aric A, Kovacikova Z et al: Selenium status is decreased in patients with intrinsic asthma, *Biol Trace Elem Res* 52:241-248, 1996.

15. Gazdik F, Kadrabova J, Gazdikova K: Decreased consumption of corticosteroids after selenium supplementation in corticoid-dependent asthmatics, *Bratisl Lek Listy* 103:22-25, 2002.

Nutrition

1. Mark J: Asthma. In Rakel D, editor: *Integrative medicine*, St Louis, 2003, Saunders.

2. Fuglsang G, Madsen G, Jalken S et al: Adverse reactions to food additives in children with atopic symptoms. *Allergy* 49:31-37, 1994.

3. Yusoff NA, Hampton SM, Dickerson JW et al: The effects of exclusion of dietary egg and milk in the management of asthmatic children: a pilot study, *JR Soc Health* 124:74-80, 2004.

4. Hijazi N, Abalkhail B, Seaton A. Diet and childhood asthma in a society in transition: a study in urban and rural Saudi Arabia, *Thorax* 55:775-779, 2000.
5. Harik-Khan RI, Muller DC, Wise RA: Serum vitamin levels and the risk of asthma in children, *Am J Epidemiol* 159:351-357, 2004.
6. Weiland SK, von Mutius E, Husing A et al: Intake of trans fatty acids and the prevalence of childhood asthma and allergies in Europe, *Lancet* 353:2040-2041, 1999.
7. Nagakura T, Matsuda S Shichijyo K et al: Dietary supplementation with fish oil rich in omega-3 polyunsaturated fatty acids in children with bronchial asthma, *Eur Respir J* 16:861-865, 2000.
8. Hackman RM, Stern JS, Gershur ME: Asthma and allergies. In Spencer JW, Jacobs JJ, editors: *Complementary and alternative medicine: an evidence-based approach*, St Louis, 2003, Mosby.

Probiotics

1. Stanaland BE: Therapeutic measures for prevention of allergic rhinitis/asthma development, *Allergy Asthma Proc* 25:11-15, 2004.
2. Isolauri E: Dietary modification of atopic disease: use of probiotics in the prevention of atopic dermatitis, *Curr Allergy Asthma Rep* 4:270-275, 2004.
3. Isolauri E: Probiotics in the prevention and treatment of allergic disease, *Pediatr Allergy Immunol* 12(Suppl):56-59, 2001.
4. Mastrandrea F, Coradduzza G, Serio G et al: Probiotics reduce the CD34+ hemopoietic precursor cell increased traffic in allergic subjects, *Allerg Immunol (Paris)* 36:118-122, 2004.
5. Kalliomaki M, Salminen S, Arvilommi H et al: Probiotics in primary prevention of atopic disease: a randomized placebo-controlled trial, *Lancet* 357:1076-1079, 2001.
6. Wang MF, Lin HC, Wang YY et al: Treatment of perennial allergic rhinitis with lactic acid bacteria, *Pediatr Allergy Immunol* 15:152-158, 2004.
7. Helin T, Haahtela S, Haahtela T: No effect of oral treatment with an intestinal bacterial strain, *Lactobacillus rhamnosus* (ATCC 53103), on birch-pollen allergy: a placebo-controlled double-blind study, *Allergy* 57:243-246, 2002.
8. Wheeler JG, Shema SJ, Bogle ML et al: Immune and clinical impact of *Lactobacillus acidophilus* on asthma, *Ann Allergy Asthma Immunol* 79:229-233, 1997.

Psychology

1. Kaugars AS, Klinnert MD, Bender BG: Family influences on pediatric asthma, *J Pediatr Psychol* 29:475-491, 2004.
2. Bartkett SJ, Kolodner KB, Butz AM et al: Maternal depressive symptoms and emergency department use among inner-city children with asthma, *Arch Pediatr Adolesc Med* 155:347-353, 2001.
3. Klinnert MD, Nelson HS, Price MR et al: Onset and persistence of childhood asthma: predictors from infancy, *Pediatrics* 108:E69, 2001.
4. Bratton DL, Price M, Gavin L et al: Impact of a multidisciplinary day program on disease and healthcare costs in children and adolescents with severe asthma: a two-year follow-up study, *Pediatric Pulmonol* 31:177-189, 2001.

Qigong

1. Chu JHK: A study of treating asthma with wai qi and qigong training by affecting adrenocortical hormone, cAMP and cGMP. Available at www.alternativehealing.org/ENGLISHNI3.htm. Accessed April 2, 2008.
2. Reuther I, Aldridge D: Qigong Yangsheng as a complementary therapy in the management of asthma: a single-case appraisal, *J Altern Complement Med* 4:173-183, 1998.

CHAPTER 13

Attention-Deficit Hyperactivity Disorder

Acupuncture | May Loo

Aromatherapy | Maura A. Fitzgerald

Chiropractic | Anne Spicer

Herbs— Chinese | May Loo, Catherine Ulbricht, Jennifer Woods, Mark Wright, Harriet Beinfield, Efrem Korngold

Herbs—Western | Alan D. Woolf, Paula M. Gardiner, Lana Dvorkin-Camiel, Jack Maypole

Homeopathy | Janet L. Levatin

Massage Therapy | Mary C. McLellan

Mind/Body | Timothy Culbert, Lynda Richtsmeier Cyr, Karen Olness

Nutrition | Joy A. Weydert

Osteopathy | Jane Carreiro

Probiotics | Russell H. Greenfield

Psychology | Anna Tobia

Qigong | Effie Pow Yew Chow, Maria Choy

✳ PEDIATRIC DIAGNOSIS AND TREATMENT

Attention-deficit hyperactivity disorder (ADHD) is the most common neurobehavioral disorder of children.[1-5] The broad constellation of hyperactive, inattentive, and impulsive symptoms combined with the multiple comorbid conditions makes the definition and ADHD itself controversial[6] and its diagnosis flawed.[7] The incidence in school-aged children ranges from 4% to 12%, averaging around 8% to 10%.[1,5,7,8-11] ADHD more commonly affects boys,[8] although with *Diagnostic and Statistical Manual of Mental Disorders*, fourth edition, (DSM-IV) criteria, more females have been diagnosed with the predominantly inattentive type.[12,13]

ADHD is a chronic, heterogeneous condition with academic, social, and emotional ramifications.[1,14] It has generated a great deal of public and media interest.[5,15,15a] The disabling symptoms persist into adolescence in approximately 65%[16] to 85% of children[17] and into adulthood in approximately 50%.[8,9,11,17-19] A developmental pattern[20] is observed in the primary symptoms of the disorder: hyperactivity diminishes while attentional deficits persist or increase with age.[1] Adolescents with ADHD often seem immature, display excessive affect, tend to procrastinate, and continue to be easily distracted.[21]

The precise etiology is still not well understood,[7] but the complex debate of nature versus nurture continues to bring up multifactorial causes[6] and polarizing views.[22] It is generally agreed that ADHD has a strong genetic predisposition.[2,11,18,20,23-26] The risk of developing ADHD in first-degree relatives is about five times higher than in the general population.[18,19] Molecular genetic studies implicate at least three genes in ADHD: the D4 dopamine receptor gene, the dopamine transporter gene, and the D2 dopamine receptor gene.[19] Neurobiological and neuroimaging studies suggest that both neuroanatomical and neurotransmitter defects contribute to ADHD symptomatology. Various dysfunctional central nervous system (CNS) structures include prefrontal cortex,[27] frontal lobe,[19] and corticostriatal pathway defect.[2,19,23,28,29] Neurobiological abnormality involves dysregulation of neurotransmitters, especially dopamine and catecholamines.[30] Many ADHD experts posit that the central disability is impaired motor and behavioral inhibition, which leads to inability to manifest self-control, acquire appropriate social skills, and organize time, all of which in turn lead to hyperactivity, learning disability, aggression, anxiety, and other primary and comorbid characteristics.[31-33] Currently, researchers are also studying the correlation between infant/child temperament, such as low frustration tolerance and low adaptability, with development of ADHD.[34]

Nongenetic "nurture" etiologies include prematurity, when hypoxia and ischemia can cause varying degrees of injury to a vulnerable CNS.[27,28] Various foods, including excess sugar, artificial colors, additives, and preservatives, have been implicated in influencing the behavior and mood of children with ADHD.[2,35,36] Environmental chemicals, molds and fungi, and neurodevelopmental toxins such as heavy metals and organohalide pollutants have all been found to correlate with ADHD symptoms.[2] Thyroid hypofunction[2] and abnormalities of fatty acid phospholipid metabolism[6] have also been implicated as potential causes of ADHD. On the other hand, there does not appear to be conclusive correlation of traumatic brain injury with development of ADHD.[37]

ADHD remains a clinical diagnosis based on specific criteria and clinical impression. It is important to use a structured, systematic approach to evaluate these children instead of relying on clinical judgment alone. Evaluation of the child with ADHD consists of a comprehensive history, physical and neurological examination, and hearing and vision screen.[4] The American Academy of Pediatricians (AAP) guidelines for diagnosis recommend that the minimum sources of information include parents and teachers.[5] School observation, various rating scales, and neurodevelopmental tests can be incorporated to assess whether the child meets the DSM-IV criteria for ADHD. Precise assessment is difficult because of a lack of specific biological or psychological test or marker for the disorder,[3,14,23,29,38] because of subjectivity in answers to questionnaires, sometimes even a child's parents might disagree on the child's level of hyperactivity or ability to concentrate, and because the DSM-IV diagnostic characteristics occur along a continuum that can be applicable to the normal population—for example, everyone can be impatient at times, such as when waiting in line—or can be associated with other neurodevelopmental and psychiatric disorders. The evaluation of the preschooler is even more difficult, as high activity level, impulsivity, and short attention span are (to a certain extent) age-appropriate characteristics of young children.[39] The 18 DSM-IV criteria are classified into three categories: inattention, hyperactivity, and impulsivity. Diagnosis is categorized as inattentive type, hyperactive type, or combined type that has both inattentive and hyperactive characteristics.

DSM-IV Diagnostic Criteria for ADHD[40]

A. Either (1) or (2):
1. Six (or more) of the following symptoms of inattention have persisted for at least 6 months to a degree that is maladaptive and inconsistent with developmental level:
   Inattention:
   a. Often fails to give close attention to details or makes careless mistakes in schoolwork, work, or other activities
   b. Often has difficulty sustaining attention in tasks or play activities
   c. Often does not seem to listen when spoken to directly
   d. Often does not follow through on instructions and fails to finish schoolwork, chores, or duties in the workplace (not due to oppositional behavior or failure to understand instructions)
   e. Often has difficulty organizing tasks and activities
   f. Often avoids, dislikes, or is reluctant to engage in tasks that require sustained effort (such as schoolwork or homework)
   g. Often loses things necessary for tasks or activities (e.g., toys, school assignments, pencils, books, tools)
   h. Often is easily distracted by extraneous stimuli
   i. Often is forgetful in daily activities
2. Six (or more) of the following symptoms of *hyperactivity/impulsivity* have persisted for at least 6 months to a degree that is maladaptive and inconsistent with developmental level:
   Hyperactivity:
   a. Often fidgets with hands or feet or squirms in seat
   b. Often leaves seat in classroom or in other situations in which remaining seated is expected
   c. Often runs about or climbs excessively in situations in which it is inappropriate (in adolescents or adults, may be limited to subjective feelings of restlessness)
   d. Often has difficulty playing or engaging in leisure activities quietly
   e. Often "on the go" or often acts as if "driven by a motor"
   f. Often talks excessively

   Impulsivity:
   g. Often blurts out answers before questions have been completed
   h. Often has difficulty awaiting turn
   i. Often interrupts or intrudes on others (e.g., butts into conversations or games)
B. Some hyperactive-impulsive or inattentive symptoms that caused impairment were present before age 7 years.
C. Some impairment from the symptoms is present in two or more settings (e.g., at school or work and at home).
D. There must be clear evidence of clinically significant impairment in social, academic, or occupational functioning.
E. The symptoms do not occur exclusively during the course of a Pervasive Developmental Disorder, Schizophrenia, or other Psychotic Disorder and are not better accounted for by another mental disorder (e.g., Mood Disorder, Anxiety Disorder, Dissociative Disorder, or a Personality Disorder).

In addition to the DSM–IV characteristics, this complex disorder also has numerous comorbid conditions: oppositional defiant disorder (ODD), conduct disorder (CD), antisocial personality disorder, tic disorder, and depression, anxiety, and other mood disorders.[3,4,8,18,41-46] About 20% to 25% of children with ADHD have learning disability (LD).[41,47] The most common LD is reading disability or dyslexia,[48] but other difficulties include auditory processing disability,[49] communicative disorders,[50] motor and perceptual output problems,[51] executive dysfunction,[52] inability to understand causal relations,[47] and difficulties in organizing, preparing, and inhibiting responses.[29] Between 25% and 75% of adolescents with ADHD have oppositional or conduct disorder.[31]

Some studies have demonstrated differences in baseline electroencephalogram (EEG) abnormalities in the parietal region for on-task conditions.[53] Currently, routine EEG is not recommended for children with ADHD. Academic problems lead to further behavioral problems, lack of peer acceptance, interpersonal difficulties,[29] low self-esteem,[1] and high levels of alcohol and/or drug abuse.[8,54] The troublesome child with ADHD generates more complications, as families coping with these children tend to experience more stress and have more problems,[17] and the disruptive ADHD adolescent with chemical dependence is difficult to maintain in a treatment facility.[55] The child with ADHD tends to be more self-destructive and is more prone to injuries.[56]

Because of the chronic, pervasive effects of the multiplicity of symptoms, ADHD management needs to be multifaceted and prolonged.[29] Medication continues to be the mainstay of treatment, with psychostimulants, especially methylphenidate (Ritalin), still being the AAP-recommended[57] and most widely used drug.* Although these drugs seem effective for improving attention and diminishing hyperactivity, their potential benefit on cognition and academic performance, conduct, and social behavior remain controversial.[1,60] The tricyclic antidepressants were added as an alternative medication in the 1970s,[61] with clonidine, buspirone (Buspar), and other antidepressants and neuroleptics added in the 1980s.[62,63] These medications are currently recommended for stimulant nonresponders

---
*References 1, 3, 18, 23, 58, 59.

and children with more than one psychiatric disorder. Combined pharmacotherapy is sometimes prescribed for more complex cases of ADHD.[18]

Although it is generally agreed that drugs are beneficial on a short-term basis, there is a paucity of data on the long-term efficacy and safety of medications,[57,60,64,65] especially in children younger than 3 years of age.[39] Children with ADHD on medication should be monitored closely.[23,66] There is mounting controversy over the widespread use of Ritalin[2] because of concern of possible long-term side effects that include poor weight gain and development of tic disorder, especially in children with family history of Tourette syndrome. Pemoline, which is associated with possible increased risk of acute hepatic failure,[67] is no longer used. Clonidine is associated with many side effects and has an increased risk of overdose.[68,69]

In addition to pharmacotherapy, a multimodal approach using a combination of drugs and other methods such as cognitive behavioral therapy (CBT), psychotherapy, social skills training, and school interventions is frequently prescribed for ADHD. CBT represents the most widely used alternative to pharmacotherapy. Previous studies showed disappointing effects.[70-73] A long-term multicenter study by the National Institues of Health Multimodal Treatment Study of Children with ADHD (NIH MTA) demonstrated slightly better results in children treated with a combination of medication and behavioral therapy.[64]

Psychotherapy can be an effective adjunct to medication[1,14] but usually requires a long-term commitment to several years of treatment. Concerns about side effects of medication, treatment acceptability, and compliance[74-76] are additional factors that complicate management of the child with ADHD. There is increasing interest in more natural, holistic integrative approaches to ADHD.[2]

✳ CAM THERAPY RECOMMENDATIONS

Acupuncture

Traditional Chinese medicine (TCM) also considers ADHD a complex disorder that affects all levels of the child's being: energetic, physical, emotional, and even spiritual. The following discussion is based on the author's 20-year experience in working with children with ADHD, integrating Western pediatrics with acupuncture to help unravel the complexities enveloping the ADHD child.

A close TCM evaluation of ADHD indicates that ADHD is in fact a complicated state of deficiencies. The Mind, Shen, resides in Heart Yin and is intimately related to the Ethereal Soul, Hun, which resides in the Liver Yin. Both Shen and Hun are needed for thinking, consciousness, insight, memory, intelligence, and cognition. It is also the Ethereal Soul that provides the Mind with the spiritual "movement" between self-recognition and introspection and the ability for the child to relate to other people and the world.[1] The outward manifestation of "hyperactivity," often interpreted as a symptom of excess, is in reality also due to Liver Yin deficiency. Whereas activity is Yang, inhibition is Yin. The out-of-control motor activity is due to a lack of inhibition, a Yin deficiency, specifically Liver yin deficiency

with disturbance of the Ethereal Soul, resulting in behavior that alienates others. Being constitutionally Yin deficient and Liver vulnerable,[2] children, especially boys (who are less Yin than girls), are prone to developing the hyperactive type of ADHD.

Children are also constitutionally Spleen deficient,[2] with resultant poor transformation and transportation of body fluids that can lead to accumulation of Phlegm. The word *Phlegm* in Chinese medicine connotes both the "mucous" form associated with lung conditions and an "unseen" or "nonsubstantial" form that circulates in channels and can obstruct organs. It is the latter Phlegm that can cause obstruction in the Heart, termed "Phlegm misting the Mind" that can manifest as "unclear, foggy, unfocused thinking, mental sluggishness, and confusion." The child is not hyperactive but tends to be quiet. This correlates well with the inattentive type of ADHD, which affects girls more than boys. The type of ADHD can vary with genetic predisposition, which involves Kidney Essence/Yin and Kidney Qi. As the foundation of marrow, the Kidney is the basis of all brain (marrow in TCM) functions.

TCM interpretation of ADHD can also be approached using the Five-Element developmental theory, which evaluates types of ADHD according to the child's age and stage of development (see Appendix B).[2]

There are no published research data on acupuncture treatment of ADHD. The author conducted a prospective, randomized, double-blind pilot study funded by the NIH that integrated DSM-IV diagnostic criteria and conventional theories of frontal lobe dysfunction, and neurotransmitter abnormalities with traditional Chinese theories of energetic imbalances. Laser acupuncture was used in the treatment of 7- to 9-year-old children newly diagnosed with ADHD. Preliminary data showed promise in reducing signs and symptoms of ADHD with improvement in behavior and cognitive function in children who are mild to moderately affected with ADHD.[3] An Israeli retrospective study, a U.S. survey, and two Australian surveys all revealed that very few children with ADHD turn to acupuncture treatment.[4-7] A South Korean animal study revealed acupuncture treatment of HT7 decreased morphine induced behavioral hyperactivity.[8] Because acupuncture has been shown to affect neurotransmitters, including dopamine, catecholamines, and serotonin, research should be able to demonstrate neurophysiological effects of acupuncture on ADHD. There is a dire need for clinical studies of acupuncture and other complementary and alternative medicine (CAM) treatments for this disorder.

This author has treated ADHD by integrating conventional developmental pediatrics training with evaluation and treatment practices from acupuncture textbooks. The following are very basic and general treatment recommendations extracted from protocols in the clinic. Experienced practitioners who can assess and monitor the ADHD child clinically should carry out more comprehensive evaluations and treatments.

General Treatment for ADHD

- GV20 and Sishenchong: raises clear Qi to the Mind
- A special point for the frontal lobe: 0.5 cm lateral to midpoint of forehead
- SP6 nourishes Yin and strengthens LR, SP, KI
- Yintang point for calming

For Liver Yin deficiency:
- LR8 nourishes LR Yin
- KI3, CV4 nourishes KI Yin
- BL18, BL47 to tonify LR Yin, root the Ethereal Soul
- LR3 to subdue Liver Yang, nourish Liver Yin

For Heart:
- HT7 nourishes Heart
- BL15, BL44 stimulates Mind's intellect, stimulates Shen
- HT7, CV15 to regulate and nourish the Heart, calm the Shen
- BL44 Shentang to strengthen and calm the Mind, stimulate clarity and intelligence
- BL49 Yishe, "Thought shelter," to stimulate memory and concentration

For KI Yin/Essence deficiency:
- CV4, CV7 nourish Essence
- KI3, KI6, SP6 to nourish KI Yin
- CV4 nourishes KI Yin, calms Mind
- BL23 strengthens KI

For Spleen:
- ST40 to resolve Phlegm
- CV12, ST36, SP6, BL20 to tonify Stomach and Spleen[1,9-11]

Aromatherapy

Although effects of aromatherapy on attention has been a subject of research, there are little data on ADHD specifically. One author notes from her personal experience that alerting essential oils are more beneficial than calming or sedating essential oils.[1] Alerting essential oils include lemon *(Citrus limon)*, rosemary *(Rosmarinus officinalis)*, grapefruit *(Citrus paradisi)*, peppermint *(Mentha piperita)*, and basil *(Ocimum basilicum)*. The essential oil is administered by inhalation for a prompt response. However, application through massage might also be useful for calming hyperactive children. If using massage it is important to understand that slow, firm strokes are calming whereas light or rapid stroking are stimulating.

In one study on cognitive function, 144 subjects were randomly assigned to three groups: control, rosemary or lavender, *(Lavandula angustifolia)* and blinded.[2] Each subject completed a computerized cognitive assessment battery while in a cubicle that contained the essential oil or no oil. Analysis demonstrated that lavender resulted in a decrease in performance of working memory and impaired reaction time, whereas rosemary produced an increase in memory and secondary memory factors but a decrease in speed of memory. Subjects were asked to assess their level of alertness and mood on visual analog scales at the start and finish of the testing. At the end of the testing, lavender and control groups were rated less alert than the rosemary group and the control group was rated less content than the rosemary and lavender groups.

Essential oils of peppermint, jasmine *(Jasminum grandiflorum),* and ylang-ylang *(Cananga odorata)* were compared with a control of water in a study on motor reaction time.[3] The study was conducted as a series of six trials in which subjects (ages 16 to 67) were randomized and blinded (they were not told which group they were in, but there was no blinding for the odor of the essential oil). In the first four trials, 20 subjects were in the control group (water) and 20 were in the experimental group (essential oil). In the last two trials, 30 subjects were in each group. Comparison between experimental and control groups did not reach statistical significance. However, motor time reaction decreased when subjects rated the control as a pleasant smell and the essential oil as unpleasant. The authors postulated that change in attentional behavior is psychological.

In a randomized comparison study (no control group), 40 adult subjects were exposed to rosemary and lavender essential oil.[4] Pre- and post-measures were self-reported measures of state anxiety, profile of mood, visual analog mood scale, math computation, and EEG. The lavender group self-reported increased state of relaxation and less depressed mood; the EEG was consistent with increased drowsiness and math computations were completed more quickly and more accurately after aromatherapy. The rosemary group reported feeling more relaxed and alert and had a decrease in state anxiety score and an EEG consistent with alertness; speed of math computation increased but accuracy did not.

In an observational study of 10 children with special needs (ages 7 to 9), changes in behavior were rated before and after inhalation of rosemary (2 drops were placed on a porous stone that allows for diffusion in the space in which the child was being observed). Occupational therapists rated the child's ability to stay in his or her chair, the need to have directions repeated, how often the child engaged in self-stimulating behavior (rocking), and how long the child was able to sustain attention. Exposure to rosemary resulted in improved behavior in 7 children, no change in 2 children, and worsening of behavior in 1 child. In a second observational study, 11 children with ADHD (ages of children and type of ADHD not reported) were exposed to a mixture of three essential oils, which each child selected. This mixture was applied topically to the wrist and also used (diffused) at home in the bath. Parents reported that their children were generally calmer, but one parent reported increased hyperactivity.[1]

Chiropractic

Chiropractors look first to three primary factors affecting behavior: neurological integrity of the musculoskeletal system, proper nutritional intake, and level of physical acivity. Afferent stimulation of the brain provides for self-regulation, making control of behavior more attainable. This afferent stimulation can be accomplished by chiropractic adjustment, cranial therapies, and physical exercise. Regular gross motor activity and dietary intake of nutrients necessary for neurological processing can often accomplish great strides in behavioral control, as can elimination of dietary toxins. Supportive therapies may include behavior modification and brain retraining exercises. An assessment to rule out the presence of learning disabilities would assist in the direction of management, because learning disabilities may underlie or accompany ADD/ADHD symptoms.

In 1989 a single-subject research design evaluated chiropractic adjustments for changes in overt behavior, electrodermal conduction, and parental ratings in a group of seven children diagnosed as hyperkinetic. Each child (ages 7 to 13) had shown previous success with stimulant medications but was on a pharmaceutical hiatus at the time of the study. The data were collected on the children while they were medicated and again after a 2-week waiting period from the point of cessation of pharmaceuticals. The children underwent 2 weeks of placebo treatments in which a mechanical device that made a "popping" sound was placed against the skin of the neck. This placebo phase was followed by an active phase. During the active phase of the study, adjustments were given three times per week and weekly evaluations of electrodermal conduction and overt motor behavioral activity levels were conducted. After the chiropractic intervention, 71.4% of the subjects showed decreased overt activity, 57% showed positive change in electrodermal conduction, and 57% had improved parental report of hyperactivity.[1]

One study compared chiropractic care with pharmaceutical therapy in 37 children with behavioral impairments and learning disabilities. One group underwent chiropractic adjustments with cross-crawl exercises. A second group was given only the chiropractic adjustment, and the third group was given only the medication. The chiropractic care was found to be 24% more effective than the pharmaceuticals over 13 measured areas while affecting a broader range of symptoms and without side effects.[2]

Multiple case reports suggest a correlation between reduction of the chiropractic subluxation complex (SC) and decreased hyperactivity.[3-14] Adjustments, when identified in the studies, were most often applied to the upper cervical spine, and a specific listing of anterior/superior (AS) occiput was identified as common.

Studies demonstrating reduction of attention problems with deep pressure[15] and massage[16,17] may actually support the deep pressure effect of the chiropractic adjustment on the central and peripheral nervous system.

Cranial therapies, which are used by many chiropractors, may also diminish hyperactive behaviors in children.[18,19]

Recommendations to minimize overt stimulation of the nervous system through television and electronic games[19a] reduces nervous system irritation and encourages physical activity, which helps to diminish inappropriate hyperactivity through afferent stimulation of the brain. Motor activity that employs the postural muscles is particularly influential in the development of the brain, and imbalance in the posture creates imbalance of brain activity. The chiropractic adjustment, which removes segmental postural imbalance, directly affects the brain's ability to process information.[20]

Also of interest to the chiropractor is the chemical/nutritional balance of the individual. The foundation for better body and brain function for all children is a wholesome, unprocessed diet of fresh fruits and vegetables, whole grain products, lean meats, and fish. Organic products, where available, will reduce toxic chemical exposure from pesticides, herbicides, and chemical ripening agents.

Although many different foods are associated with behavioral abnormalities, a list of the most common culprits includes dairy products, gluten, soy, corn, oranges, eggs, and chocolate.[21-23] Chiropractors also recommend eliminating or decreasing hydrogenated fats and additives such as artificial food coloring, flavoring, and preservatives, all of which have been associated with adverse reactions.[24] Feingold also reported adverse reactions to naturally occurring salicylates in foods such as apricots, berries, tomatoes, and bell peppers.[25]

Although individual nutritional recommendations are made based on the child's current nutrient status, some common deficiencies are associated with behavior irregularities. Magnesium is essential for normal neurological processing and catecholamine homeostasis. Supplementation with magnesium, which is deficient in 95% of children with ADHD, has been shown to decrease hyperactive behavior.[26] (Avoiding soft drinks may reduce magnesium loss.)

Clinical iron deficiency may result in lowered attention and is the most common of all nutritional deficiencies.[27] Supplementation subsequently improved behavior ratings in a group of ADHD children.[28] Because iron is also the most common supplement toxicity, laboratory assessment is a wise starting point.

Zinc, an important neurotransmitter cofactor, is also found to be lower than normal in children with ADHD.[29]

Studies also correlate incidence of recurrent ear infections with later development of hyperactivity.[30] The use of antibiotics for the recurrent ear infections disrupts the gut flora, and therefore use of probiotics restores flora to allow for more normal food digestion and improved nutrient absorption status.[31,32] Digestive enzyme supplementation may also enhance normal digestion.

Omega-3 fatty acids (particularly eicosapentaenoic/acid/docosahexopentoenoic acid [EPA/DHA]) are necessary for normal brain synaptic function.[33,34] Lack of EPA/DHA may lead to ADHD.[35-42] If the diet is not rich in EPA/DHA, it should be supplemented.

The child may also have a toxicity or an amino acid imbalance that interferes with behavioral control.[43] For instance, tyrosine is a precursor to dopamine and is better absorbed in the presence of B vitamins; supplementation of both may improve ADHD.

Hair analysis, comprehensive blood analysis, digestive stool analysis, and urine analysis may be productive in identifying a particular agent, deficiency, or condition contributing to the problem.

Referral to a chiropractic neurologist (a chiropractor with a diplomate degree in identification and treatment of neurological disturbances without drugs or surgery) would serve to address many of the symptoms that do not resolve with adjustments and nutritional changes alone.[44]

Some intriguing evidence has shown that use of an interactive metronome may reestablish normal brain synaptic function and diminish symptoms of ADHD.[45]

Behavioral modification techniques as outlined in a series of books by David B. Stein have been found to be exceedingly beneficial. Stein has written protocols for physicians, for teachers, and for parents to use in the home environment. Although Stein largely refutes neurological and biochemical discovery with ADHD, his protocals remain useful.[46-48] Referral to a psychologist or behavioral therapist trained in this work would also be a prudent measure for a chiropractor.

Vision therapy has been noted to increase IQ and improve behavior in 2500 delinquent youth.[46] An assessment by a qualified professional of the need for vision therapy would be advisable.

Herbs—Chinese

One possible herbal formula that can help in ADHD is Quiet Calm (Gentle Warriors Pediatric Formula, Kan Herb Company, Scotts Valley, Calif.), which cultivates children's self-regulating capacities. It calms the mind, relaxes the muscles, clears Heat, dispels Phlegm, focuses the Mind, and elevates the Spirit. It does not sedate or tranquilize, but instead nurtures the Brain and Marrow and harmonizes Kidneys, Liver, and Heart. It can complement other TCM treatments such as acupuncture.[1]

Herbal formula: This formula is a melding of Wild Jujube Seed Decoction (Suan Zao Ren Tang) for allaying agitation, insomnia, and anxiety and Gastrodia and Uncaria Decoction (Tian Ma Gou Teng Yin) for relieving nervous tension, reducing pressure, and countering spasm. Together they combine the principles of soothing nerves, relaxing the Liver, taming the Mind/Hun, quieting the Heart and enfolding the Mind/Spirit, and subduing the "uprising of Liver Yang" (also known as the "stirring of Internal Wind").

Jujube seed (suan zao ren), *Polygala* root (yuan zhi), acorus rhizome (shi chang pu), *Polygonum* stem (ye jiao teng), lotus seed (lian zi), *Albizia* stem/flower (he huan pi/hua), amber (hu po), and poria fungus/pine root (fu shen) soothe the Mind/Spirit (Shen), stabilize the Mind/Hun, clarify the senses (clear Heat and Phlegm from the Upper Orifices), and relieve pain and spasm. *Uncaria* stem (gou teng), gastrodia rhizome (tian ma), silkworm (jiang can), and gardenia bud (zhi zi) subdue Liver Yang and Internal Wind, clear Heat, counter spasm, and allay irritability and restlessness. Lily bulb (bai he), anemarrhena rhizome (zhi mu), and *Schisandra* fruit (wu wei zi) clear deficiency Heat by replenishing and consolidating Moisture, relieving restless fatigue and melancholy. Pummelo peel (ju hong) and licorice root (gan cao) aid digestion and harmonization of the herbal ingredients while toning Stomach Qi, preventing congestion and stagnation due to the excessive accumulation of Moisture (retention of Dampness).

Dosage: 1 to 3 droppersful as needed, every 2 to 4 hours.

Caution: Monitor closely when combining with over-the-counter or prescription medications including antihistamines, cough medicines, antiemetics, opiate analgesics, psychotropics (e.g., sleeping pills, sedatives, tranquilizers, antipsychotics, anxiolytics, antidepressants), and antiseizure drugs.[1]

Root of *Bupleurum chinense* DC. (Chai Hu) has been assessed in the treatment of attention-deficit hyperactivity disorder.[2] One study involving 80 ADHD patients, compared the safety and effectiveness of Chinese medicine and Western medicine. Twenty participants received 5 to 15mg of methylphenidate hydrochloride (Ritalin) twice daily for one month. The effects were evaluated after 1 to 3 courses of treatment. The study found that a combination of *B. chinense*, root of *Scutellaria baicalensis* Georgi (Huang Qin), root of *Astragalus membranaceus* (Fisch.) Bunge (Huang Qi), root of *Codonopsis pilosula* (Franch.) Nannf. (Dang Shen), fruit of *Ligustrum lucidum* Aiton (Nu Zhen Zi), stem and leaf of *Lophatherum gracile* Brongn. (Dan Zhu Ye), and thread of ivory was as effective as Ritalin. However, the Chinese herbal therapy had fewer side effects. Further research is needed before a recommendation can be made.[3]

Herbs—Western

A number of herbs with a variety of proposed mechanisms of action have been applied for attention deficit in children. Overall, there is insufficient evidence and research to suggest any single herbal approach has proven effective.[1]

Patients may apply a number of combinations of herbs and/or pharmaceutical agents, which suggests that consumers and providers need to be aware of potential interactions or adverse effects. There is preliminary evidence that ginkgo leaf extract *(Ginkgo biloba)*, in combination with American ginseng *(Panax quinquefolius)*, might help improve symptoms in children with ADHD (b.i.d. dosing of a combination herbal product containing American ginseng extract, *P. quinquefolium* [200 mg] and *G. biloba* extract [50 mg]).[2] St. John's wort *(Hypericum perforatum)* may be safe when used orally and appropriately short-term; however, evidence is insufficient to support the use of St. John's wort alone for ADHD.[3] St. John's wort herb may interact with digitalis (thus elevating levels) and antiretroviral medications and may enhance serotonergic effects of other pharmacoactive dietary agents.

Pycnogenol *(Pinus pinaster* ssp. *atlantica)* is an extract of the bark of the French maritime pine tree; the flavonoid ingredients are anecdotally reported to help in the treatment of ADHD in children. However, there are no research or data to support this claim. Investigations in adults, including a double-blind, placebo-controlled, crossover study of Pycnogenol and methylphenidate suggest that there is no effect on its use for ADHD either.[4] Brahmi *(Bacopa monnieri)*, popular in India, is an Ayurvedic herb that may increase cognitive performance in adults with ADHD. However, although it is likely safe to use, there is insufficient evidence regarding this herbal's effectiveness for ADHD in children.[3]

Of note, concern for toxicity make some herbs potentially unsafe, and they are not recommended: borage seed oil (may be safely tolerated in children, but has associated liver and kidney toxicity with potential unsaturated pyrrolizidine alkaloids in some preparations)[5-8] and blue-green algae (heavy metal contamination and microcystins, plant produced toxins).[9]

Homeopathy

Before using this section, please see Appendix A, Homeopathy, for definitions of practitioner expertise categories and general information on prescribing homeopathic medicines.

Practitioner Expertise Category 3

There are no controlled clinical trials of homeopathic treatment for ADHD, although the homeopathic literature contains evidence for its use in the form of accumulated clinical experience.[1] Homeopathic treatment can be used safely for ADHD, either alone or in combination with other treatment modalities, both alternative and conventional. Because ADHD is a complex and multifaceted developmental problem, successful homeopathic treatment usually requires extensive training in the art and science of homeopathy. Any one of many homeopathic medicines may be used to treat ADHD, depending on the characteristics of the patient being treated; sophisticated homeopathic analysis and long-term follow-up are required. For these reasons, specific medicines for treating ADHD will not be presented here. Interested readers are referred to the homeopathic literature for further study.[1] Of particular interest is Reichenberg-Ullman and Ullman's *Ritalin-Free Kids*.[2]

Massage Therapy

In a randomized controlled trial, adolescents with ADHD who received daily massage therapy for 10 days rated themselves as happier than the controls. Blinded observers rated the massaged adolescents as having less fidgeting after treatments, and teachers reported more on-task behaviors and lower hyperactivity scores.[1]

Providing massage therapy to very active children can be challenging even if they do not have ADHD. Those children who do have ADHD that is not effectively managed can be just as challenging. The method in which they are massaged, rather than the locations being massaged, may make a difference. Swedish massage is the more relaxing therapy, whereas trigger point therapy and sports massage can produce a stimulating effect during treatment. Light touch during massage can also produce a stimulating effect, so moderate, slow, rhythmic pressure and strokes may be more helpful to this patient population. Parents could try to massage "a la carte" to utilize times when the child is less active; for example, offering a shoulder massage while the child watches television. Some therapists have found it helpful to induce a still point when a child is beginning to escalate. Inducing a still point is a craniosacral technique; it is a difficult technique for a practitioner or parent to perform without craniosacral training, as it requires focused attention to a very subtle craniosacral rhythm.

Mind/Body

Peripheral Biofeedback and Relaxation Training

Electromyographic (EMG) biofeedback as well as other basic relaxation techniques can play a helpful role in the management of children with ADHD.[1-3] One recent study described four sessions of heart rate variability biofeedback (as a marker for autonomic nervous system activity) in 19 subjects meeting the DSM-IV criteria for ADHD as being effective in lowering Parent Child Behavior Checklist and Conner's Teacher questionnaires ratings in a statistically meaningful fashion. A recent controlled study from Germany utilized autogenic training techniques with a group of 50 children and adolescents who had various internalizing and externalizing disorders including ADHD. Compared with a control group, children trained with autogenic procedures showed statistically significant improvements on the Child Behavior Checklist, and more than 50% of parents and children reported goal attainment. The authors concluded that autogenic training is effective as a broadband method.[4]

In the authors' clinical experience, various forms of self-regulation skill training to promote relaxation and calming have been clinically useful for many children with ADHD. Children are taught progressive muscle relaxation (an exercise in which children alternately squeeze and then relax various muscle groups throughout the body) as well as relaxation breathing as ways to self-calm and reduce motoric restlessness and impulsivity. Coordinating the use of these techniques in the classroom can be arranged by communicating with the teacher, and a reinforcement program can be designed with the cooperation of appropriate school personnel. Children can also be coached to develop mental imagery strategies including therapeutic suggestions for enhanced learning, improved interest and attention, and a calm body during school hours.

Neurofeedback

A number of clinical trials of EEG biofeedback (neurofeedback) in children and adolescents have suggested possible benefit in children with ADHD subtypes. However, the literature to date has contained serious methodological flaws, and therefore the use of neurofeedback as a front-line treatment for ADHD has not received endorsement by pediatric professional organizations or in evidence-based guidelines. Nevertheless, EEG biofeedback is likely beneficial for many children with ADHD. It generally involves learning to identify and voluntarily control the ratio of β-waves or a subset (sensorimotor rhythm) to theta waves in certain key areas of the brain. Training usually requires 20 to 40 sessions over several weeks. The duration and generalizability of the effects have been questioned, but many children do seem to receive some benefit, with little risk of any adverse effects. A recent nonrandomized, controlled study[5] looked at the benefits of a 3-month training sequence of neurofeedback as compared with stimulant medication therapy in 34 children with ADHD ages 8 to 12 years (patients were assigned to treatment groups based on informed parental choice). Both neurofeedback and stimulant medication resulted in significant benefits as rated by teachers and parents on the IOWA Conners scales. In a smaller controlled study, Linden and colleagues[6] reported clinically significant improvements in intellectual functioning and attention for an experimental group who received 40 EEG biofeedback sessions over 6 months compared with a wait-list control group.

Other Mind/Body Approaches

A variety of psychosocial and cognitive/behavioral treatments play a role in the multimodality treatment of ADHD. These include parent training, child behavior management methods, and academic interventions.[7] Other complementary approaches, such as meditation, are showing promise in pilot studies with adults.[8]

In the authors' experience, children can be exposed to a variety of mind/body self-management options and then be allowed to choose and practice these techniques at home and school, often with good benefit. Cueing and positive reinforcement from adult caregivers can increase the likelihood of the child's using such mind/body techniques. These techniques are useful for anger or frustration management as well. Children may still need to continue with conventional treatments such as stimulant medications and behavioral therapies, but relaxation strategies including yoga, imagery, biofeedback, and meditation can all be useful adjuncts.

Nutrition

Although ADHD is likely a culmination of environmental, genetic, and metabolic factors, there are indications that nutritional management may offer benefit to these children. Many of these children have been found to have food and food additive sensitivities,[1,2] imbalances of neurotransmitters[3] and fatty acid levels,[4,5] vitamin and mineral deficiencies,[6] gut dysbiosis, or heavy metal toxicities.[7] Correction of these underlying problems seems to help behavior for some children.

One study of hyperactive children found that 82% responded favorably to an elimination diet and, when given a food challenge in a double-blind, placebo-controlled fashion, they responded negatively.[8] This has been repeated by other researchers with similar results.[2,9,10] Although food sensitivities are highly individualized, they need to be considered systematically when evaluating behavior problems.

Another study found that patients with ADHD had significantly lower plasma levels of phenylalanine, tyrosine, tryptophan, histidine, and isoleucine compared with controls.[11] As many of these "essential" amino acids are necessary for neurotransmitter production, a deficiency in the intake of complete proteins or a problem with absorption may also play a role in ADHD, which has a dysregulated central norepinephrine system.[3]

Noticeable improvement was seen in children with ADHD who were supplemented with the various fatty acids in which they were found to be deficient. Red cell membrane analysis revealed imbalances in EPA and DHA (omega-3 fatty acid) and in α-linolenic acid and arachadonic acid (omega-6 fatty acid).[12]

An outcome-based comparison was made between Ritalin and a dietary supplement with a mix of vitamins, minerals, phytonutrients, amino acids, essential fatty acids, phospholipids, and probiotics. Similar outcomes were seen in each group using various measurements, which suggests that food supplement treatment of ADHD may be as effective as Ritalin treatment.[13]

Treatment

Any treatment needs to be based on the individual child.
- Provide a diet of whole unprocessed, preferably organic foods (fruits, vegetables, whole grains, beans, nuts, cold-water fish) to lessen the exposure to toxins and provide the best source of essential nutrients. If not allergic, increase the consumption of garlic, onions, and eggs in the diet, which are high in sulfur, to chelate any heavy metals. Decrease intake of refined and processed foods, and have a balanced intake of proteins, carbohydrates, and fats.
- Identify and eliminate food allergens.
- Consider supplementing with a high-potency multivitamin with minerals.
- Encourage foods high in calcium, magnesium, and zinc, such as dark-green leafy vegetables, whole grains, legumes, shellfish, nuts, and blackstrap molasses.
- Replace and balance the essential fatty acids by increasing the intake of omega-3 fatty acids (found in cold-water fish, fish oils, walnuts, flax seeds/oil, and hemp seeds/oil) and decreasing intake of omega-6 fatty acids and trans fats (e.g., partially hydrogenated vegetable oils, margarine, processed foods). If choosing to supplement, use a balanced ratio of omega-6 to omega-3 fatty acids, such as 4:1. Some children benefit from omega-3 replacement only.[14] Also, the ratio of DHA to EPA can be 2:1 to 5:1, although ratios may be variable.
- Use probiotics to correct intestinal dysbiosis if the child also has allergic, atopic, or asthma symptoms.

Osteopathy

The three types of ADHD are predominantly inattentive, predominantly hyperactive-impulsive, and combined type. Within varying degrees of each type, the child exhibits problems with executive function, behavior inhibition, and attention control. From an osteopathic perspective, children with ADHD can be divided into two groups: (1) children with a preponderance of

structural findings suggestive of irritability of the peripheral tissues and altered proprioceptive mechanisms and (2) children with findings suggestive of CNS irritability. From an osteopathic perspective, both of these clusters of findings have the potential to produce the symptoms associated with ADHD.

One group of children with ADHD typically have repetitive stimulation behaviors, usually involving vestibular stimulation. They might be viewed as predominantly hyperactive-impulse type. These children can be thought of as having a form of sensory integration dysfunction. Anecdotally, osteopathic examination often reveals areas of tissue dysfunction that would be expected to be painful or tender but are not. It is as though the child's ability to perceive the nociception is dampened. These children also tend to have multiple areas of dysfunction in the lumbar, pelvic, cervical, and cranial regions. One would expect the location and quality of these strains to correlate with pain and altered balance mechanisms. The treatment principles of cranial osteopathy and balanced membranous techniques are often used in these children. These are gentle techniques aimed at rebalancing areas of dysfunction that may be interfering with normal function of the arousal-inhibition loop, altering sensory-motor processing, or in some way contributing to the child's inability to regulate his or her state of arousal.

Several studies have been published in the osteopathic literature concerning the role of osteopathic medicine in the treatment of children with ADHD. Unfortunately the findings in these studies are somewhat compromised by either a small enrollment or confounders. Nevertheless, they provide some intriguing data. Three studies have reported a prevalence of abnormal findings of the cranium and pelvis in children exhibiting behavioral problems, learning disabilities, and/or ADHD.[1-3] One study of 1250 children suggested that newborns with cranial strains and a history of difficult or prolonged labor and delivery are more likely to have symptoms of ADHD.[4] Another study reported improvement in neurological and behavioral parameters in children diagnosed with behavioral, developmental, and learning disabilities after osteopathic treatment.[4]

On osteopathic examination, there is a certain population of children with ADHD who have dysfunction involving the craniosacral and core-link mechanisms and only compensatory findings in the peripheral tissues.[2-6] Per their history, these children tend to have fewer repetitive stimulation behaviors. A significant finding in children with ADHD is altered brain wave activity in the frontal lobe as measured by EEG.[7] Children with ADHD have been reported to have increased slow wave (theta) activity and decreased fast β-activity in the frontal lobe. Theta wave activity is associated usually with revelry. Activity of β-waves, also called the *sensory-motor rhythms,* is associated with efficient processing of information. A published case study has demonstrated decreases in slow wave activity in one child with ADHD following osteopathic manipulation.[8]

Disrupted executive function and delay aversion force the child with ADHD to develop compensatory skills and strategies that are often of an undesirable character. Family, peer, and teacher response to these skills can be less than encouraging for the child. A dual pathway develops whereby the compensatory behaviors that develop in response to the ADHD in turn exacerbate or facilitate many of the symptoms of ADHD. In children with severe symptoms, osteopathic physicians often integrate manual techniques, dietary changes, parental training, and pharmacotherapeutics. Although there is no published literature assessing the efficacy of integrating osteopathic treatment into the care of the child with ADHD, the multifaceted nature of the disorder suggests that a multipronged attack would be most beneficial and would provide fertile ground for research.

Probiotics

Few studies have evaluated the use of probiotic therapy for patients with ADHD, and no definitive guidelines regarding dose or choice of specific microbes have been established. One published study employed probiotics combined with a variety of other supplements in a group of children with ADHD, whereas an equal number of children with the disorder received Ritalin.[1] The dietary supplements used were of significant number and included multivitamin and multimineral supplements and essential fatty acids, among others, as well as an unspecified dose of *Lactobacillus acidophilus* and *Bifidobacterium bifidus*. At the end of the study both groups of children experienced similar benefits from their respective therapies, suggesting that the supplements, and perhaps probiotic therapy, did provide a therapeutic effect.

Although benefit is possible, there is little to go on besides hypothetical considerations. However, probiotic therapy is quite safe and could conceivably be of help to a subset of patients with ADHD. Guidance with respect to choice of specific organisms and duration of therapy is sorely lacking. To further complicate matters, there seems little rationale behind the variety of dosages or combination of microbes employed in published studies. Often similar dosages have been utilized for distinct microbes, whereas widely disparate dosages have been employed by researchers studying the same probiotic. At this time, dosage recommendations are far from set in stone.

This author recommends using a 2- to 3-month trial of probiotic therapy for patients with ADHD, employing well-studied organisms shown to be safe, such as *Lactobacillus* GG (the microbe associated with the most supportive data), *Lactobacillus plantarum, Lactobacillus paracasei, Lactobacillus reuteri,* or *L. acidophilus.* Dosing guidelines to consider are 10 billion colony-forming units (CFU) for children <12 kg and 20 billion CFU for children weighing >12 kg. Treatment is extremely well tolerated, and palatability is an infrequent issue, as the capsules can be opened and mixed into drinks or soft foods. Sometimes the agents are available as a powder as well. If effective, treatment can continue indefinitely. Use with extreme caution, if at all, in those children at risk for infectious complications (e.g., immunosuppression or use of immunosuppressive agents, presence of central venous catheter, prematurity).

Psychology

Children with ADHD often experience significant impairment in academic, social, and family functioning in addition to the core symptoms of inattention, hyperactivity, and impulsivity. Psychological treatment aims to address all aspects of impairment. Many children utilize stimulant medication to manage their symptoms of ADHD. However, approximately 35% to 45% of patients diagnosed with inattentive type and 10% to 30% of those with combined type fail to respond to medication.[1] Other CAM psychological options are available to address concerns, and these treatments can be used in conjunction with traditional stimulant medication.

Treatments involve providing feedback (using biofeedback) for certain neuronal behaviors. For example, children may be trained in more appropriate levels of cortical arousal to improve attention. Some biofeedback protocols consist of enhancing β activity and suppressing theta activity, in addition to activating the frontal cortex.[2] One study found that children with ADHD demonstrated different learning curves on tests of continuous performance and intelligence following EEG biofeedback.[3] It has also been demonstrated that teaching self-control of slow cortical potentials led to a reduction by 25% in ADHD symptomology as reported by parents, as well as a significant decrease in impulsivity errors on a continuous performance test.[4] Some children with ADHD have significantly improved immediate recall of information and decreased levels of inattention and impulsivity with EEG biofeedback.[5]

Stimulant medication can be used in conjunction with biofeedback. A study that examined the role of biofeedback in changing cognitive functioning for children found that with stimulant medication and biofeedback, children showed significantly better attention and less hyperactive/impulsive behaviors as compared with those treated with medication alone.[6] After 1 year of medication treatment, the children then were taken off medication for 1 week. Those treated with biofeedback sustained their improvement, whereas those treated only with stimulant medication returned to baseline levels of functioning. Using an analysis of EEG recordings, significant differences in the degree of cortical arousal, as measured electrophysiologically over central and frontal brain locations, were found between the biofeedback and medication-alone groups once medication was discontinued. Essentially, the behavioral, neuropsychological, and electrophysiological improvements in the medication with biofeedback treatment group were maintained even after medication was stopped.

In addition to biofeedback, there are important psychosocial considerations for children with ADHD. Significant emotional concerns are associated with this condition. Many children feel demoralized and incompetent because of struggles with school, family and peers. It is important to explain to children that they have a neurological condition and their struggles are not their fault. Explaining the diagnosis to children and their parents can help them begin to understand their strengths and weaknesses. Within this context it is helpful to instill hope for the future and to explain that this is a highly treatable condition and families can take control of ADHD.

One way to gain control of the ADHD symptoms is through self-management skills training.[7] Often children with ADHD are highly disorganized and forgetful and have difficulty meeting goals. They may seem unable to create structure and routine in their lives. An important goal of treatment is to teach the skills necessary to be productive. Some basic steps include: practice proactive planning to prepare for the next day; keep "to do" lists and prominently display them; break down large tasks and assignments into smaller steps; use organizing systems (e.g., color-coded files, storage boxes, closet organizers); keep multiple sets of keys, glasses, gloves, and other easy-to-lose items; and use rewards when goals are met.[7]

Some treatments for ADHD are designed to specifically address the aggressiveness that can be associated with the disorder. Some components of these treatments can include problem solving skills, modeling, role playing, self-reinforcement and token systems, relaxation skills, and social skills development. To specifically address anger, it is important that the treatment teach the child how to identify angry feelings before becoming explosive and to be more aware of the cues for anger. Moreover, children with ADHD can misinterpret social situations such that they immediately respond in an aggressive or threatening manner. The theoretical model for these approaches is CBT. CBT aims to help the child understand the interaction between his or her thoughts, feelings, and actions. More specifically, how a child interprets or thinks about an event will affect how he or she feels and the subsequent behavioral response. Results suggest that this type of approach is effective in reducing hyperactivity, antisocial behavior, and social adjustment problems.[8]

Treatment Recommendations

Based on the literature discussed previously and the author's experience in working with hundreds of children and adults with ADHD, some steps can be easily incorporated into any treatment program without extensive training or the need for expensive biofeedback instruments.

During the first session it is essential to explain the neurophysiology of the condition in a way that is understandable to the parent and child. Children with ADHD tend to feel hopeless and inadequate because of the constant struggle in all areas of their lives (e.g., at home, academically, socially). Explaining that this is a highly treatable medical condition instills a feeling of hope for the future.

Self-management skills are typically underdeveloped in children with ADHD. It is possible, with specific instruction, to teach and improve this ability. Often completing things feels overwhelming to children with ADHD. Therefore teach the child to write a "to do" list and explain the types of tasks that go on such a list; break down tasks into small, manageable steps; outline when things needs to be completed; and plan ahead of time for the next day and, when possible, for the week.

Treatment should involve the parents so that they understand the changes that need to be made and help reinforce positive behavior. Immediate, specific, and consistent reinforcement is essential to effectively manage this condition. When a child begins to clean up or do homework, parents should use praise to reinforce the behavior. Often parents complain about what is not getting done, rather than focusing on strengths or accomplishments. Teaching parents to avoid lengthy dialogues with their children about why something should or should not happen is critical to increasing motivation.

Behavioral charts are easy to implement and are highly effective. Children tend to respond best to immediate consequences for their behavior. This is especially true when a child has ADHD. More specifically, have the parents and child list three behaviors that they would like to happen (e.g., feed pet, empty garbage can in kitchen to outside garbage can, set table for dinner), one of which the child is already successfully doing. These tasks should be as specific as possible. As soon as a task is completed, parents give lots of praise and then they or the child puts a sticker or check on the chart. At the end of the day a privilege that is previously agreed upon and desirable to the child can be earned (e.g., one check means 5 minutes of extra stay-up time, two checks mean 10 minutes,). As behavior improves, rewards can be accumulated to earn a bigger prize at the end of the week rather than every night (e.g., picking the family movie, choosing the restaurant).

With younger children it may be necessary to use pictures to guide behavior. For example, an easily distracted child may find it difficult to complete multiple tasks in the morning (e.g., brush teeth, wash face, comb hair). A picture of a toothbrush, soap, and a comb can be attached to the bathroom mirror as a visual cue.

A similar approach can help improve school performance. Often assignments seem daunting because a child with ADHD struggles with sequencing the steps necessary to complete something. A book report, for example, begins with choosing a book or, on a more basic level, going to the library. Depending on the needs of the child each step necessary should be identified and a time line for completion should be developed. Parents can provide valuable clues about a child's strengths and then build on those. For example, if a child is a visual learner, he can take notes on what is read on self-adhesive notes (e.g., Post-it notes) and then arrange them on a big board so that he can see the flow of the report. If he is more of an auditory learner, he can dictate ideas into a small recorder as he reads and then listen to them later.

The essential element to any treatment program is helping the child and family see that change is possible. Small successful steps instill hope and a new sense of confidence. Simple modifications often generalize to more profound change and greater success.

Qigong

Literature on behavior, learning, and ADHD has also been scant but promising. In one study at the University of Miami School of Medicine, 13 adolescents with ADHD participated in Tai Chi classes twice per week for 5 weeks. Teachers rated the adolescents' behaviors on the Conners Scale during the (1) baseline period, (2) after 5 weeks of Tai Chi twice per week, and (3) 2 weeks after treatment. After 10 Tai Chi lessons, the adolescents displayed less anxiety, daydreaming behaviors, inappropriate emotions, and hyperactivity and had improved conduct. These effects persisted during the 2-week follow-up period.[1]

From 2002 to 2003, an informal study revealed that, following a series of twelve 30-minute sessions of Tai Chi, elementary school teachers in St. George, Utah reported increased levels of attentiveness in their students. Therefore they concluded that Tai Chi may help children relax, regroup, and refocus, thus opening the door for teachers to be more successful. Tai Chi, as a commonly use form of Qigong, may give children the break they need in order to open their minds and more readily absorb the information imparted to them during the course of their school day.[2] Qigong is believed to enable the child and adolescent with ADHD to better utilize his or her inner resources.[3]

In TCM the heart is the primary responsible organ for intellectual and mental activities. However, because of the microcosm-macrocosm theory in TCM, it is never a single organ dysfunction but instead a multiplexed situation. Qigong assessment of a child with ADHD consists of passing the practitioner's hand over the body without touching the child to sense or "feel" the energy, which may manifest as energy excess in the Heart, Lung, and head, as well as a general Qi imbalance. The finding may vary at different occasions of assessment.

Qigong treatment may consist of Qigong exercises three or more times a day as needed to relax the child. The sessions can range from a few minutes to 30 minutes of Qigong exercise and meditation, including brushing energy gently away and outward from the center line of the body. Qipressure, which is adapted acupressure with intense breathing by both persons, can be applied on LI4 (between the thumbs and forefingers), LI11 (at the crook of the elbows), ST36 (4 inches down from the knee on the lateral side of the tibia), and SP6 (on the inner edge of the tibia, 4 inches up from the upper edge of the ankle bones). Positive mental attitude is also reinforced. (Therapy may vary at different occasions of assessment.)

The author has treated 12 cases and had excellent results, with improvements that included less disturbing behavior, more calmness, and better concentration.

References

Pediatric Diagnosis and Treatment

1. Shaywitz BA, Fletcher JM, Shaywitz SE: Attention-deficit/hyperactivity disorder, *Adv Pediatr* 44:331-367, 1997.
2. Kidd PM: Attention deficit/hyperactivity disorder (ADHD) in children: rationale for its integrative management, *Altern Med Rev* 5:402-428, 2000.
3. Schweitzer JB, Cummins TK, Kant CA: Attention-deficit/hyperactivity disorder, *Med Clin N Am* 85:757-777, 2001.
4. Worley KA, Wolraich ML: Attention-deficit hyperactivity disorder. In Wolraich ML, editor: *Disorders of development and learning*, ed 3, London, 2003, BC Decker.
5. American Academy of Pediatrics: Clinical practice guideline: diagnosis and evaluation of the child with attention-deficit/hyperactivity disorder, *Pediatrics* 105:1158-1170, 2000.
6. Richardson AJ, Ross MA: Fatty acid metabolism in neurodevelopmental disorder: a new perspective on associations between attention-deficit/hyperactivity disorder, dyslexia, dyspraxia and the autistic spectrum, *Prostaglandins Leukot Essent Fatty Acids* 63:1-9, 2000.
7. Schneider SC, Tan G: Attention-deficit hyperactivity disorder. In pursuit of diagnostic accuracy, *Postgrad Med* 101:231-232, 235-240, 1997.
8. Modigh K, Berggren U, Sehlin S: High risk for children with DAMP/ADHD to become addicts later in life [in Swedish], *Lakartidningen* 95:5316-5319, 1998.
9. Arnold LE: Sex differences in ADHD: conference summary, *J Abnormal Child Psychol* 24:555-69, 1996.
10. Shelley-Tremblay JF, Rosen LA: Attention deficit hyperactivity disorder: an evolutionary perspective, *J Genetic Psychol* 157:443-453, 1996.
11. Bradley JD, Golden CJ: Biological contributions to the presentation and understanding of attention-deficit/hyperactivity disorder: a review, *Clin Psychol Rev* 21:907-929, 2001.
12. Wolraich ML, Hannah JN, Pinnock TY et al: Comparison of diagnostic criteria for attention deficit/hyperactivity disorder in a county-wide sample, *J Am Acad Child Adolesc Psychiatry* 35:319-324, 1996.
13. Wolraich M, Hannah JN, Baumgaertel A et al: Examination of DSM-IV criteria for attention deficit/hyperactivity disorder in a county-wide sample, *J Dev Behav Pediatr* 19:162-168, 1998.
14. Taylor MA: Attention-deficit hyperactivity disorder on the frontlines: management in the primary care office, *Comprehensive Ther* 25:313-325, 1999.
15. Gibbs N: Latest on Ritalin, *Time* 152:86-96, 1998.
15a. Clayton V: *What's to blame for the rise in ADHD?* MSNBC, Sept. 8, 2004.
16. Ingram S, Hechtman L, Morgenstern G: Outcome issues in ADHD: adolescent and adult long-term outcome, *Ment Retard Dev Disabil Res Rev* 5:243-250, 1999.
17. Hechtman L: Assessment and diagnosis of attention-deficit/hyperactivity disorder, *Child Adolesc Psychiatr Clin North Am* 9:481-498, 2000.
18. Biederman J: Attention-deficit/hyperactivity disorder: a life-span perspective, *J Clin Psychiatr* 59(Suppl 7):4-16, 1998.
19. Faraone SV, Biederman J, Spencer T et al: Attention-deficit/hyperactivity disorder in adults: an overview, *Biol Psychiatry* 48:9-20, 2000.
20. Zuddas A, Ancilletta B, Muglia P et al: Attention-deficit/hyperactivity disorder: a neuropsychiatric disorder with childhood onset, *Europ J Paediatr Neurol* 4:53-62, 2000.
21. Wolraich ML, Wibblesman CJ, Brown TE et al: Attention deficit/hyperactivity disorder among adolescents: a review of the diagnosis, treatment, and clinical implications, *Pediatrics* 115:1734-1745, 2005.
22. Williams C, Wright B, Partridge I: Attention deficit hyperactivity disorder—a review, *Br J Gen Pract* 49:563-571, 1999.
23. Buitelaar JK, Kooij JJ: Attention deficit hyperactivity disorder (ADHD): etiology, diagnosis and treatment [in Dutch], *Ned Tijdschr Geneeskd* 144:1716-1723, 2000.
24. Denney CB: Stimulant effects in attention deficit hyperactivity disorder: theoretical and empirical issues, *J Clin Child Psychol* 30:98-109, 2001.
25. Eisenberg J, Zohar A, Mei-Tal G et al: A haplotype relative risk study of the dopamine D4 receptor (DRD4) exon III repeat polymorphism and attention deficit hyperactivity disorder (ADHD), *Am J Med Genetics* 96:258-261, 2000.
26. Faraone SV, Doyle AE: Genetic influences on attention deficit hyperactivity disorder, *Curr Psychiatry Rep* 2:143-146, 2000.
27. Levy F, Barr C, Sunohara G: Directions of aetiologic research on attention deficit hyperactivity disorder, *Austr N Z J Psychiatry* 32:97-103, 1998.
28. Lou HC: Etiology and pathogenesis of attention-deficit hyperactivity disorder (ADHD): significance of prematurity and perinatal hypoxic-haemodynamic encephalopathy, *Acta Pediatr* 85:1266-1271, 1996.
29. Mercugliano M: What is attention-deficit/hyperactivity disorder? *Pediatr Clin North Am* 46:831-843, 1999.
30. Faraone SV, Biederman J: Neurobiology of attention-deficit hyperactivity disorder, *Biol Psychiatry* 44:951-958, 1998.
31. Barkley RA: *Attention deficit hyperactivity disorder, a handbook for diagnosis and treatment*, New York, 1998, Guilford Press.
32. Baird J, Stevenson JC, Williams DC: The evolution of ADHD: a disorder of communication? *Rev Biol* 75:17-35, 2000.

33. Niedermeyer E, Naidu SB: Attention-deficit hyperactivity disorder (ADHD) and frontal-motor cortex disconnection, *Clin Electroencephalogr* 28:130-136, 1997.

34. Cameron J: Personal communication, April 2002.

35. Breakey J: The role of diet and behaviour in childhood, *J Pediatr Child Health* 33:190-194, 1997.

36. Boris M, Mandel FS: Foods and additives are common causes of the attention deficit hyperactive disorder in children, *Ann Allergy* 72:462-468, 1994.

37. Max JE, Lindgren SD, Knutson C et al: Child and adolescent traumatic brain injury: correlates of disruptive behaviour disorders, *Brain Injury* 12:41-52, 1998.

38. Accardo P: A rational approach to the medical assessment of the child with attention-deficit/hyperactivity disorder, *Pediatr Clin North Am* 46:845-856, 1999.

39. Blackman JA: Attention-deficit/hyperactivity disorder in preschoolers. Does it exist and should we treat it? *Pediatr Clin North Am* 46:1011-1025, 1999.

40. American Psychological Association: *Diagnostic and statistical manual of mental disorders*, ed 4, Washington, DC, 1994, American Psychiatric Press.

41. Pliszka SR: Patterns of psychiatric comorbidity with attention-deficit/hyperactivity disorder, *Child Adolesc Psychiatr Clin North Am* 9:525-540, vii, 2000.

42. Searight HR, Rottnek F, Abby SL: Conduct disorder: diagnosis and treatment in primary care, *Am Fam Physician* 63:1579-1588, 2001.

43. Faraone SV, Biederman J: Do attention deficit hyperactivity disorder and depression share familial risk factors? *J Nervous Mental Disord* 185:533-541, 1997.

44. Spencer T, Biederman J, Wilens T: Attention-deficit/hyperactivity disorder and comorbidity, *Pediatr Clin North Am* 46:915-927, vii, 1999.

45. Vance AL, Luk ES: Attention deficit hyperactivity disorder and anxiety: is there an association with neurodevelopmental deficits? *Austr N Z J Psychiatry* 32:650-657, 1998.

46. Brown R, Freeman WS, Perrin JM et al: Prevalence and assessment of attention deficit/hyperactivity disorder in primary care settings, *Pediatrics* 107:e43, 2001.

47. Lorch EP, Milich R, Sanchez RP: Story comprehension in children with ADHD, *Clin Child Fam Psychol Rev* 1:163-178, 1998.

48. Shaywitz BA, Fletcher JM, Shaywitz SE: Defining and classifying learning disabilities and attention-deficit/hyperactivity disorder, *J Child Neurol* 10(Suppl 1):S50-S57, 1995.

49. Chermak GD, Hall JW 3rd, Musiek FE: Differential diagnosis and management of central auditory processing disorder and attention deficit hyperactivity disorder, *J Am Acad Audiol* 10:289-303, 1999.

50. Damico JS, Damico SK, Armstrong MB: Attention-deficit hyperactivity disorder and communication disorders. Issues and clinical practices, *Child Adolesc Psychiatr Clin North Am* 8:37-60, vi, 1999.

51. Blondis TA: Motor disorders and attention-deficit/hyperactivity disorder, *Pediatr Clin North Am* 46:899-913, vi-vii, 1999.

52. Pineda D, Ardila A, Rosselli M et al: Executive dysfunctions in children with attention deficit hyperactivity disorder, *Int J Neurosci* 96:177-196, 1998. [Colombia.]

53. Janzen T, Graap K, Stephanson S et al: Differences in baseline EEG measures of ADD and normally achieving preadolescent males, *Biofeed Self Regulation* 20:65, 1995.

54. Comings DE: Serotonin and the biochemical genetics of alcoholism: lessons from studies of attention deficit hyperactivity disorder (ADHD) and Tourette syndrome, *Alcohol* (Suppl)2:237-241, 1993.

55. Stratton J, Gailfus D: A new approach to substance abuse treatment. Adolescents and adults with ADHD, *J Substance Abuse Treat* 15:89-94, 1998.

56. DiScala C, Lescohier I, Barthel M, Li G: Injuries to children with attention deficit hyperactivity disorder, *Pediatrics* 102:1415-1421, 1998.

57. American Academy of Pediatrics: Clinical practice guideline: treatment of the school-aged child with attention-deficit/hyperactivity disorder, *Pediatrics* 108:1033-1044, 2001.

58. Wilens TE, Spencer TJ: The stimulants revisited, *Child Adolesc Psychiatr Clin North Am* 9:573-603, viii, 2000.

59. Greenhill LL: Pharmacologic treatment of attention deficit hyperactivity disorder, pediatric psychopharmacology, *Psychiatr Clin North Am* 15:1, 1992.

60. Bennett FC, Brown RT, Craver J et al: Stimulant medication for the child with attention-deficit/hyperactivity disorder, *Pediatr Clin North Am* 46:929-944, vii, 1999.

61. Biederman J, Baldessarini RJ, Wright V et al: A double-blind placebo controlled study of desipramine in the treatment of ADD. I. Efficacy, *J Am Acad Child Adolesc Psychiatry* 8:777-784, 1989.

62. Casat CD, Pleasants DZ, Schroeder DH et al: Bupropion in children with attention deficit disorder, *Psychopharmacol Bull* 25:198, 1989.

63. Chen SW, Vidt DG: Patient acceptance of transdermal clonidine: a retrospective review of 25 patients, *Cleveland Clin J Med* 56:21, 1989.

64. Jensen PS, Hinshaw SP, Kraemer HC: ADHD comorbidity findings from the MTA study: comparing comorbid subgroups, *J Am Acad Child Adolesc Psychiatry* 40:147-158, 2001.

65. Dulcan MK: Using psychostimulants to treat behavioral disorders of children and adolescents, *J Child Adolesc Psychopharmacol* 1:7, 1990.

66. Ghuman JK, Ginsburg GS, Subramaniam G et al: Psychostimulants in preschool children with attention-deficit/hyperactivity disorder: clinical evidence from a developmental disorders institution, *J Am Acad Child Adolesc Psychiatry* 40:516-524, 2001.

67. Shevell M, Schreiber R: Pemoline-associated hepatic failure: a critical analysis of the literature, *Pediatr Neurol* 16:14-16, 1997.

68. Kappagoda C, Schell DN, Hanson RM et al: Clonidine overdose in childhood: implications of increased prescribing, *J Pediatr Child Health* 34:508-512, 1998.

69. Connor DF, Fletcher KE, Swanson JM: A meta-analysis of clonidine for symptoms of attention-deficit hyperactivity disorder, *J Am Acad Child Adolesc Psychiatry* 38:1551-1559, 1999.

70. Abikoff H: Cognitive training in ADHD children: less to it than meets the eye, *J Learn Disabil* 24:205, 1991.

71. Abikoff H, Gittleman R: Hyperactive children treated with stimulants: is cognitive training a useful adjunct? *Arch Gen Psychiatry* 42:953, 1985.

72. Brown RT, Wynne ME, Medenis R: Methylphenidate and cognitive therapy: a comparison of treatment approaches with hyperactive boys, *J Abnormal Child Pyschol* 13:69, 1985.

73. Ialongo NS, Horn WF, Pascoe JM et al. The effects of a multimodal intervention with attention deficit hyperactivity disorder children: a 9-month follow-up, *J Am Acad Child Adolesc Psychiatry* 32:182, 1993.

74. Lawrence JD, Lawrence DB, Carson BS: Optimizing ADHD therapy with sustained release methylphenidate, *Am Fam Physician* 55:1705, 1997.

75. Bennett DS, Power TJ, Rostain AL et al: Parent acceptability and feasibility of ADHD intervention, assessment, correlates, and predictive validity, *J Pediatr Psychiatry* 21:643, 1996.

76. Power TJ, Hess LE, Bennett DS: The acceptability of interventions for attention deficit hyperactivity disorder among elementary and middle school teachers, J Develop Behav Pediatr 16:238, 1995.

Acupuncture

1. Maciocia G: *The practice of Chinese medicine, the treatment of diseases with acupuncture and Chinese herbs*, London, 1994, Churchill Livingstone.
2. Loo M: *Pediatric acupuncture*, London, 2002, Elsevier.
3. Loo M, Naeser MA, Hinshaw S et al: Laser acupuncture treatment for ADHD. NIH grant #1 RO3 MH56009-01.
4. Gross-Tsur V, Lahad A, Shalev RS: Use of complementary medicine in children with attention deficit hyperactivity disorder and epilepsy, *Pediatr Neurol* 29:53-55, 2003.
5. Chan E, Rappaport LA, Kemper KJ: Complementary and alternative therapies in childhood attention and hyperactivity problems, *J Dev Behav Pediatr* 24:4-8, 2003.
6. Sinha D, Efron D: Complementary and alternative medicine use in children with attention deficit hyperactivity disorder, *J Paediatr Child Health* 41:23-26, 2005.
7. Stubberfield T, Parry T: Utilization of alternative therapies in attention-deficit hyperactivity disorder, *J Paediatr Child Health* 35:450-453, 1999.
8. Kim MR, Kim SJ, Lyu YS et al: Effect of acupuncture on behavioral hyperactivity and dopamine release in the nucleus accumbens in rats sensitized to morphine, *Neurosci Lett* 387:17-21, 2005.
9. Deadman P, Al-Khafaji M: *A manual of acupuncture*, Ann Arbor, Mich, 1998, Journal of Chinese Medicine Publications.
10. Maciocia G: *The foundations of Chinese medicine, a comprehensive text for acupuncturists and herbalists*, London, 1989, Churchill Livingstone.
11. O'Connor J, Bensky D, editors: *Acupuncture, a comprehensive text*, Seattle, 1981, Eastland Press.

Aromatherapy

1. Buckle J: *Clinical aromatherapy: essential oils in practice*, ed 2, Edinburgh, 2003, Churchill Livingstone.
2. Moss M, Cook J, Wesnes K et al: Aromas of rosemary and lavender essential oils differentially affect cognition and mood in healthy adults, *Int J Neurosci* 113:15-38, 2003.
3. Ilmberger J, Heuberger E, Mahrhofer C et al: The influence of essential oils on human attention. I: Alertness, *Chem Senses* 26:239-245, 2001.
4. Diego M, Aaron J, Field T et al: Aromatherapy positively affects mood, EEG patterns of alertness and math computations, *Int J Neurosci* 96:217-224, 1998.

Chiropractic

1. Giesen MF, Center DB, Leach RA: An evaluation of chiropractic manipulation as a treatment of hyperactivity in children, *J Manipulative Physiol Ther* 12:353-363, 1989.
2. Walton EV, Brozosowske: The effects of chiropractic treatment on students with learning and behavioral impairments due to neurological dysfunction, *Int Rev Chiropractic* 29:24-26, 1975.
3. Hospers LA, Zezula L, Sweat M: Life upper cervical adjustment in a hyperactive teenager, *Today's Chiropractic* 15:73-75, 1987.
4. Barnes TA: A multi-faceted chiropractic approach to attention deficit hyperactivity disorder: a case report, *ICA Int Rev Chiropractic* Jan/Feb:1-43, 1995.
5. Leisman NJ: A case study of ADHD, *ICA Int Rev Chiropractic* 54:54-61, 1998.
6. Arme J: Effects of biomechanical insult correction on attention deficit disorder, *J Chiropractic Case Rep* 1: 6-9, 1993.
7. Phillips CF: Case study: the effect of utilizing spinal manipulation and craniosacral therapy as the treatment approach for attention deficit hyperactivity disorder, *Proc Natl ICA Conf Chiropractic Pediatr* 57-74, 1991.

8. Langley C: Epileptic seizures, nocturnal enuresis, ADD, *Chiropractic Pediatr* 1:57-74, 1995.
9. Thomas MD, Wood J: Upper cervical adjustments may improve mental function, *J Man Med* 6:215, 1992.
10. Peet JB: Adjusting the hyperactive/ADD pediatric patient, *Chiropractic Pediatr* 2:12, 1997.
11. McClay R, Meleski ME: The role of chiropractic in the treatment of ADHD, *Dynamic Chiropractic* 21:60-64, 2003.
12. Anderson CD, Patridge JE: Seizures plus attention deficit hyperactivity disorder: a case report, *ICA Int Rev Chiropractic* Jul/Aug: 35-37, 1993.
13. Inselman PS: Is there any other way besides Ritalin? *Am Chiropractic* May/June:24, 1998.
14. Peet P: Child with chronic illness: respiratory infections, ADHD, and fatigue response to chiropractic care, *Chiropractic Pediatr* 3:12-13, 1997.
15. VandenBerg NL: The use of a weighted vest to increase on-task behavior in children with attention difficulties, *Am J Occup Ther* 55:621-628, 2001.
16. Khilnani S, Field T, Hernandez-Reif M et al: Massage therapy improves mood and behavior of students with attention deficit hyperactivity disorder, *Adolescence* 38:623-638, 2003.
17. Fritz S: Massage therapy and adjunctive soft tissue approaches, *J Bodywork Movement Ther* Jul:173, 2000.
18. Upledger JE: Relationship of craniosacral examination findings in grade school children with developmental problems, *J Am Osteopath Assoc* 77:760-776, 1978.
19. Davies NJ: *Chiropractic pediatrics*, London, 2000, Churchill Livingstone.
19a.Chan PA, Rabinowitz T: A cross-sectional analysis of video games and attention deficit hyperactivity disorder symptoms in adolescents, *Ann Gen Psychiatry*, 5:16-27, 2006.
20. Schetchikova NV: Children with ADHD: medical vs. chiropractic perspective and theory, *J Am Chiropractic Assoc* Jul:28-38, 2002.
21. O'Shea T: ADD/ADHD: the designer disease (part II), *Today's Chiropractic* 29:14-15, 2000.
22. Reichelt KL, Ekrem J, Scott H: Gluten, milk proteins and autism: dietary intervention effects on behavior and peptide secretion, *J Appl Nutr* 42:1-11, 1990.
23. Kidd PM: ADHD total health management, *Total Health* 22: 20-22, 2001.
24. US Food and Drug Administration: Food allergies: rare but risky, *FDA Consumer*, May 1994.
25. Sackett DL: Evidence based medicine, *Semin Perinatol* 21:3-5, 1997.
26. Kozielec T, Starobrat-Hermelin B: Assessment of magnesium levels in children with attention deficit hyperactivity disorder (ADHD): positive response to magnesium oral loading test, *Magnes Res* 10:149-156, 1997.
27. Murray MT, Pizzorno JT: *Encyclopedia of natural medicine*, Rocklin, Calif, 1998, Prima.
28. Sever Y, Ashkenazi A, Tyano S et al: Iron treatment in children with attention deficit hyperactivity disorder. A preliminary report, *Neuropsychobiology* 35:178-180, 1997.
29. Galland L: Nutritional supplementation for ADHD. In Bellanti JA, Crook WG, Layton RE, editors: *Attention deficit hyperactivity disorder: causes and possible solutions*, Jackson, TN, 1999, International Health Foundation Conference Proceedings.
30. Hagerman RJ, Falkenstein AR: An association between recurrent otitis media in infancy and later hyperactivity, *Clin Pediatr* 26:253-257, 1997.
31. Fallon JD: Otitis media and autism in childhood: is there a relationship? *ICA Rev* Fall:67-71, 2001.

32. Garvey F: Diet in autism and associated disorders, *J Fam Health Care* 12:34-38, 2002.

33. Willatts P, Forsyth JS: The role of long chain polyunsaturated fatty acids in infant cognitive developmen, *Prostaglandins Leukot Essent Fatty Acids* 63:95-100, 2000.

34. Makrides M, Neumann M Simmer K et al: Are long-chain polyunsaturated fatty acids essential nutrients in infancy? *Lancet* 345:1463-1468, 1995.

35. Bennett CN, Horrobin DF: Gene targets related phospholipid and fatty acid metabolism in schizophrenia and other psychiatric disorders: an update, *Prostaglandins Leukot Essent Fatty Acids* 63: 47-59, 2000.

36. Richardson AJ, Puri BK: The potential role of fatty acids in attention deficit/hyperactivity disorder, *Protaglandins Leukotr Essent Fatty Acids* 63:79-87, 2000.

37. Colquhon I, Bunday S: A lack of essential fatty acid as a possible cause of hyperactivity in children, *Med Hypothesis* 7:173, 1981.

38. Mitchell E, Lewis S, Cutler DR: Essential fatty acids and maladjusted behavior in children, *Protaglandins Leukotr Essent Fatty Acids* 12:281-287, 1983.

39. Stevens L, Zhang W, Peck L et al: EPA supplementation in children with inattention, hyperactivity and other disruptive behaviors. *Lipids* 38:1007-1021, 2003.

40. Stevens LJ, Zentall SS, Deck JL et al: Essential fatty acid metabolism in boys with attention deficit hyperactivity disorder, *Am J Clin Nut* 62:761-768, 1995.

41. Stevens LJ, Zentall SS, Abate ML et al: Omega-3 fatty acids in boys with behavior, learning and health problems, *Physiol Behav* 59:915-920, 1996.

42. Hamazaki T, Sawazaki S, Itomura M et al: The effect of docosahexaenoic acid on aggression in young adults, *J Clin Invest* 97:1129-1134, 1996.

43. DeMaria R: *Stop ADHD, ADD, ODD, hyperactivity: a drugless family guide to optimal health*, 2003, Drugless Healthcare Solutions.

44. Schetchikiva NV: Children with ADHD: medical vs. chiropractic perspective and theory. *J Am Chiro Assoc* p28-38, July 2002.

45. Shaffer RJ, Jacokes LE, Cassily JF et al: Effect of interactive metronome training on children with ADHD, *Am J Occup Ther* 55: 155-162, 2001.

46. Stein DB: *Unraveling the ADD/ADHD fiasco*, Kansas City, Mo, 2001, Andrews McMeel.

47. Stein DB: *Ritalin is not the answer*, San Francisco, Calif, 1999, Jossey Bass.

48. Stein DB: *Stop medicating, start parenting*, Lanham, Md, 2005, Taylor Trade.

Herbs—Chinese

1. Beinfield H, Korngold E: *Chinese medicine works clinical handbook,* San Francisco, 2007, www.chinesemedicineworks.com.

2. Natural Standard Research Collaboration. Available at www.naturalstandard.com. Accessed 2005.

3. Zhang H, Huang J. Preliminary Study of Traditional Chinese Medicine treatment of minimal brain dysfunction: analysis of 100 cases, *Chung Hsi I Chieh Ho Tsa Chih* 10:260, 278-279, 1990.

Herbs—Western

1. Chan E, Rappaport LA, Kemper KJ: Complementary and alternative therapies in childhood attention and hyperactivity problems, *J Dev Behav Pediatr* 24:4-8, 2003.

2. Lyon MR, Cline JC, Totosy de Zepetnek J et al: Effect of the herbal extract combination of *Panax quinquefolium* and *Gingko biloba* on attention deficit hyperactivity disorder: a pilot study, *J Psychiatry Neurosci* 26:221-228, 2001.

3. *Natural medicines in clinical management of ADHD*. Available at www.naturaldatabase.com. Accessed January 3, 2005.

4. Tenenbaum S, Paull JC, Sparrow EP et al: An experimental comparison of Pycnogenol and methylphenidate in adults with attention-deficit/hyperactivity disorder (ADHD), *J Atten Disord* 6:49-60, 2002.

5. Fetrow CW, Avila JR: *Professional's handbook of complementary & alternative medicines*, Springhouse, Pa, 1999, Springhouse.

6. Fewtrell MS, Abbott RA, Kennedy K et al: Randomized, double-blind trial of long-chain polyunsaturated fatty acid supplementation with fish oil and borage oil in preterm infants, *J Pediatr* 144:471-479, 2004.

7. Thomson MICROMEDEX: *MICROMEDEX Healthcare Series Vol. 123.* Available at www.micromedex.com. Accessed February 1, 2005.

8. Takwale A, Tan E, Agarwal S et al: Efficacy and tolerability of borage oil in adults and children with atopic eczema: randomised, double blind, placebo controlled, parallel group trial, *Br Med J* 327:1385, 2003.

9. Health Canada announces results of blue-green algal products testing—only Spirulina found Microcystin-free, Health Canada Sep:27, 1999. Available at www.hcsc.gc.ca/english/archives/releases/99_114e.htm. Accessed February 5, 2005.

Homeopathy

1. *ReferenceWorks Pro 4.2*, San Rafael, Calif, 2008, Kent Homeopathic Associates.

2. Reichenberg-Ullman J, Ullman R: *Ritalin-free kids*, ed 2, Roseville, Calif, 2000, Prima.

Massage Therapy

1. Field T, Quintino O, Hernandez-Reif M et al: Adolescents with attention deficit hyperactivity disorder benefit from massage therapy, *Adolescence* 33:129, 1998.

Mind/Body

1. Braud L: The effects of frontal EMG biofeedback and progressive relaxation upon hyperactivity and its behavioral concomitants, *Biofeed Self Regulation* 3:69-89, 1978.

2. Lee S: Biofeedback as a treatment for childhood hyperactivity: a critical review of the literature, *Psychol Rep* 68:163-192, 1991.

3. Denkowski K, Denkowski G: Is group progressive relaxation training as effective with hyperactive children as individual EMG biofeedback training? *Biofeed Self Regulation* 9:353-364, 1984.

4. Goldbeck L, Schmid K: Effectiveness of autogenic relaxation training on children and adolescents with behavioral and emotional problems, *J Am Acad Child Adolesc Psychiatry* 42:1046-1054, 2003.

5. Fuchs T, Birbaumer N, Lutzenberger W et al: Neurofeedback treatment for attention-deficit/hyperactivity disorder in children: a comparison with methylphenidate, *Appl Psychophysiol Biofeed* 28:1-12, 2003.

6. Linden M, Habib T, Radojevic V: A controlled study of the effects of EEG biofeedback on cognition and behavior of children with attention deficit disorder and learning disabilities, *Biofeed Self Regulation* 21:35-49, 1996.

7. Barkely R: Psychosocial treatments for attention-deficit/hyperactivity disorder in children, *J Clin Psychiatry* 12:36-43, 2002.

8. Arnold L: Alternative treatments for adults with attention-deficit hyperactivity disorder (ADHD), *Ann N Y Acad Sci* 931:310-341, 2001.

Nutrition

1. Swanson JM, Kinsbourne M: Food dyes impair performance of hyperactive children on a laboratory learning test, *Science* 207:1485-1487, 1980.
2. Carter CM, Urbanowicz M, Hemsley R et al: Effects of few food diet in attention deficit disorder, *Arch Dis Child* 69:564-568, 1993.
3. Pliszka SR, McCracken JT, Maas JW: Catecholamines in attention-deficit hyperactivity disorder: current perspectives, *J Am Acad Child Adolesc Psychiatry* 35:264-272, 1996.
4. Stevens LJ, Zentall SS Deck JL et al: Essential fatty acid metabolism in boys with attention-deficit disorder, *Am J Clin Nutrition* 62:761-768, 1995.
5. Mitchell EA, Aman MG, Turbott SH et al: Clinical characteristics and serum essential fatty acid levels in hyperactive children, *Clin Pediatr* 26:406-411, 1987.
6. Starobrat-Hermelin B: The effect of deficiency of selected bioelements on hyperactivity in children with certain metal disorders [in Polish], *Ann Acad Med Stetin* 44:297, 1998.
7. Pizzorno LU, Pizzorno JE, Murray MT: *Natural medicine instructions for patients*, London, 2002, Elsevier Science.
8. Egger J, Carter CM, Graham PJ et al: Controlled trial of oligoantigenic treatment in the hyperkinetic syndrome, *Lancet* 8355:865-869, 1985.
9. Boris M, Mandell FS: Foods and additives are common causes of the attention deficit hyperactive disorder in children, *Ann Allergy* 72:462-468, 1994.
10. Rapp D: Is this your child? Discovering and treating unrecognized allergies in children and adults, New York, 1991, William Morrow.
11. Bornstein RA, Baker GB, Carroll A et al: Plasma amino acids in attention deficit disorder, *Psychiatry Res* 33:301-306, 1990.
12. Kane P: Metabolic assessment and nutritional biochemistry. Clinical and research aspects. Symposium conducted at the Great Lakes College of Clinical Medicine, XXXI International Congress, Asheville, NC, 1999.
13. Harding KL, Judah RD, Gant C: Outcome-based comparison of Ritalin versus food supplement treated children with AD/HD, *Altern Med Rev* 8:319-330, 2003.
14. McDonough-Means SI, Cohen MW: Attention deficit disorder. In Rakel D, editor: *Integrative medicine*, St Louis, 2003, Saunders.

Osteopathy

1. Frymann VM: Relation of disturbances of craniosacral mechanism to symptomatology of the newborn, *J Am Osteopathic Assoc* 65:1059-1075, 1966.
2. Upledger JE: The relationship of craniosacral examination findings in grade school children with developmental problems, *J Am Osteopathic Assoc* 77:760-776, 1978.
3. Upledger JE: Craniosacral function in brain dysfunction, *Osteopath Ann* 11:318-324, 1983.
4. Frymann VM, Carney RE, Springall P: Effect of osteopathic medical management on neurological development in children, *J Am Osteopathic Assoc* 92:729-744, 1992.
5. Sutherland WG: *Teachings in the science of osteopathy*, Portland, Ore, 1990, Rudra Press.
6. Sutherland WG: *The cranial bowl*, ed 2, 1939, Sutherland.
7. Barry RJ, Clarke AR, Johnstone SJ: A review of electrophysiology in attention-deficit/hyperactivity disorder: I. Qualitative and quantitative electroencephalography, *Clin Neurophysiol* 114:171-183,2003.
8. Blood SD, Hurwitz BA: Brain wave pattern changes in children with ADD/ADHD following osteopathic manipulation: a pilot study, *Am Acad Osteopath J* 10:19-20, 2000.

Probiotics

1. Harding KL, Judah RD, Gant C: Outcome-based comparison of Ritalin versus food-supplement treated children with AD/HD, *Altern Med Rev* 8:319, 2003.

Psychology

1. Barkley RA: *Attention-deficit hyperactivity disorder: a handbook for diagnosis and treatment*, ed 2, New York, 1998, Guildford Press.
2. Kropotov JD, Grin-Yatsenko VA, Ponomarev VA et al: ERPs correlates of EEG relative beta training in ADHD children, *Int J Psychophysiol* 55:23-34, 2005.
3. deBeus R, Ball JD, deBeus ME et al: Attention training with ADHD children: preliminary findings in a double-blind placebo-controlled study, *J Neurother* 8:2, 2004.
4. Heinrich H, Gevensleben H, Freisleder FJ et al: Training of slow cortical potentials in attention-deficit/hyperactivity disorder: evidence for positive behavioral and neurophysiological effects, *Biol Psychiatr* 55:7, 2004.
5. Boyd WD, Campbell SE: EEG biofeedback in the schools: the use of EEG biofeedback to treat ADHD in a school setting, *J Neurother* 2:4 1998.
6. Monastra VJ, Monastra DM, George S: The effects of stimulant therapy EEG biofeedback and parenting style on the primary symptoms of attention-deficit/hyperactivity disorder, *Appl Psychophysiol Biofeed* 27:4, 2002.
7. Murphy K: Psychosocial treatments for ADHD in teens and adults: a practice-friendly review, *J Clin Psychol* 61:5, 2005.
8. Miranda A, Presentacion MJ: Efficacy of cognitive-behavioral therapy in the treatment of children with ADHD with and without aggressiveness, *Psychol Schools* 37:2, 2000.

Qigong

1. Field T: *Benefits from tai chi*. Available at www.dotaichi.com/Articles/ADHTBenefitsFromTaiChi.htm. Accessed July 2005.
2. *Ancient art of tai chi may enhance learning: exercises help calm children in a hyperactive world*. Available at www.prweb.com/releases/Nov%20/6/prweb182532.htm. Accessed July 2005.
3. Donahue K: *The treatment of ADHD*. Available at www.ofspirit.com/karendonahue1.htm. Accessed July 2005.

Autism

Pediatric Diagnosis and Treatment | Stephen Cowan

Acupuncture | May Loo

Chiropractic | Anne Spicer

Herbs—Western | Alan D. Woolf, Paula M. Gardiner,
Lana Dvorkin-Camiel, Jack Maypole

Homeopathy | Janet L. Levatin

Massage Therapy | Mary C. McLellan

Mind/Body | Timothy Culbert, Lynda Richtsmeier Cyr

Naturopathy | Matthew I. Baral

Nutrition | Joy A. Weydert

Osteopathy | Jane Carreiro

Probiotics | Russell H. Greenfield

✳ PEDIATRIC DIAGNOSIS AND TREATMENT

During the past 10 years we have seen a significant rise in the diagnosis of autism spectrum disorder (ASD) in North America and Europe. What was previously believed to be a rare genetic disorder with a prevalence of 1:2000 now is estimated to occur in as many as 1:165 children.[1,2] Initial denial by the medical community of a significant rise in prevalence has been refuted by studies that have shown this not to be due to improved diagnostics or shifts in the criteria for diagnosis.[3,4] The recognition that genetic syndromes do not rise epidemically has led researchers to search for possible alternative explanations for this devastating syndrome.

Terminology

The term *autism* was originally coined by Leo Kanner in 1943 and further described by Hans Asperger in 1944. They described a somewhat heterogeneous group of children with a "social-communication syndrome" who appeared detached and had a number of odd behaviors. In 1967 Dr. Bernard Rimland established the Autism Research Institute (ARI), a nonprofit organization devoted to conducting research on possible causes and treatment of autism. In 1994 the *Diagnostic and Statistical Manual of Mental Disorders*, fourth edition (DSM-IV), began referring to autism as a *spectrum* in order to stress the wide variation in signs and symptoms. This has been further refined to include other neurobehavioral disorders under the category of pervasive developmental disorder (PDD) (Box 14-1). The term "PDD–Not Otherwise Specified" (PDD-NOS) has been used to refer to children who do not meet the specific criteria for autism presented in the DSM IV-Revised but nevertheless have some social-communication dysfunction. Recently the term *autism spectrum disorder* has been used to describe this group of children.

Clinical Considerations

There is no doubt that the earlier a child is evaluated for possible autism spectrum, the better the prognosis. The American Academy of Pediatrics has recently highlighted the need for early diagnosis with its A.L.A.R.M. policy, which encourages early evaluation, diagnosis, referral, and parent education.[6]

The basic feature shared by children on the autistic spectrum and accounting for many of their symptoms is their difficulty with "relatedness." Although often subtle and frequently missed by parents and clinicians in very young children, the incapacity to "socially connect" may carry more predictive weight than delays in verbal expression. One aspect of relatedness is Receptive language skills. Parent and clinicians tend to concentrate more on the number of words a child can say rather than what he or she understands. Often parents do not realize that their child does not understand. Observing how a child uses a finger to point to specific objects will shed light on what he or she receptively understands. From this it is easy to understand why autistic children often have great difficulty following simple commands. In fact, some children will seem confused by simple facial expressions. Naturally, a child who confuses smiling for anger may appear to be responding quite bizarrely. This affects the ability to read social cues, a feature noted in higher-functioning disorders that lie on the spectrum, such as Asperger's syndrome. Relatedness also manifests as the inability to reciprocally interact. Typically, autistic children will have great difficulty taking turns. To assess this skill, ask a parent to roll a ball to a child and see whether and how many times the child will "get the game," rolling it back and forth.

How a child pretend plays also reflects his or her social-communication skills. An autistic child is unable to symbolically represent the world with language. This will limit a child's ability to mentally transform a pencil into a rocketship or fill a pretend bowel with pretend soup and feed it to the pretend person (doll). By extension, the clinician should observe the subtle signs of a child's sense of humor. Does he or she "get the joke"?

Finally, the clinician needs to observe the restrictions in the child's repertoire of activity. As a self-defense mechanism, many children with autism develop a rigid set of routines that protect them from the unpredictable world of human language and behavior. They often show intense resistance to change that can harden into obsessive compulsive behaviors. Many self-stimulatory behaviors develop as a way of blocking out the chaos of the world. An autistic child may choose sensory input that feels good and withdraw into it when overwhelmed. Some children with autism seem to get caught in the details of things, such as spinning shiny objects or studying the electrical

---

※ **Box 14-1**

DSM-IV-R Diagnostic Criteria for Diagnosis of Autism Spectrum Disorder

A. A total of six (or more) items from (1), (2), and (3), with at least two from (1), and one each from (2) and (3):
1. Qualitative impairment in social interaction, as manifested by at least two of the following:
   a. Marked impairment in the use of multiple nonverbal behaviors such as eye-to-eye gaze, facial expression, body postures, and gestures to regulate social interaction
   b. Failure to develop peer relationships appropriate to developmental level
   c. A lack of spontaneous seeking to share enjoyment, interests, or achievements with other people (e.g., by a lack of showing, bringing, or pointing out objects of interest)
   d. A lack of social or emotional reciprocity
2. Qualitative impairments in communication as manifested by at least one of the following:
   a. Delay in, or total lack of, the development of spoken language (not accompanied by an attempt to compensate through alternative modes of communication such as gesture or mime)
   b. In individuals with adequate speech, marked impairment in the ability to initiate or sustain a conversation with others
   c. Stereotyped and repetitive use of language or idiosyncratic language
   d. Lack of varied, spontaneous make-believe play or social imitative play appropriate to developmental level
3. Restricted repetitive and stereotyped patterns of behavior, interests, and activities, as manifested by at least one of the following:
   a. Encompassing preoccupation with one or more stereotyped and restricted patterns of interest that is abnormal either in intensity or focus
   b. Apparently inflexible adherence to specific, nonfunctional routines or rituals
   c. Stereotyped and repetitive motor mannerisms (e.g., hand or finger flapping or twisting, or complex whole-body movements)
   d. persistent preoccupation with parts of objects
B. Delays or abnormal functioning in at least one of the following areas, with onset prior to age 3 years: (1) social interaction, (2) language as used in social communication, or (3) symbolic or imaginative play.
C. The disturbance is not better accounted for by Rett's Disorder or "Childhood Disintegrative Disorder."

From *Diagnostic and Statistical Manual of Mental Disorders*, ed 4 [revised] (DSM-IVR), Arlington, Va, 2000, American Psychiatric Association.

---

circuitry of a room. It is as though they are attempting to understand the basic mechanisms of the universe. Self-stimulation (e.g., hand-flapping, spinning) is also related to the apparent heightened sensory awareness of children with autism. Many children will demonstrate extraordinary sensory abilities. These may result from the brain's compensation to limitations on the "social senses." This is analogous to the heightened visual acuity of a deaf child or the heightened sense of smell or touch of a visually impaired child.

Special Considerations

From a holistic perspective on child development, a number of important points should be considered before making a diagnosis of ASD. The first is to be mindful of the dynamic changes that take place as a child passes through various stages of development. The neurological system of a growing child is constantly being remodeled and refined, and research has described the process of apoptosis or "neurological pruning" that allows efficient neural pathways to be strengthened while inefficient pathways are destroyed.[7] This is the basis of all learning. In contrast to the conventional view of disease as a mechanical dysfunction, developmental dysfunction must be viewed as an organic process, influenced by a host of environmental factors. At best, a diagnosis of autism should be taken only as a snapshot of a moment in time in the constantly adapting child. Interestingly, there is recent radiological evidence that

a failure in the normal pruning process may occur, which leaves the autistic child with too many neurons and disordered white matter tracts.[8,9] This may account for the apparent sensory integration problems so common in children with autism.

A second important consideration in diagnosing children with autism is to remember the interdependency of all developmental skills. For example, an infant must learn to eat solid food before he or she can learn to speak. Likewise, difficulty with one particular developmental skill will exert an effect on other areas of development. This becomes very important when encountering young children with significant language dysfunction who exhibit odd behaviors such as self-stimulation and echolalia. These may be nonspecific signs of a child's attempt to comprehend the verbal world. Some children who initially appear to have characteristics of autism may in fact have a different developmental problem and will appear to outgrow their autism as they develop more receptive and expressive language. Careful evaluation and tracking is thus required to determine the nature and prognosis of each child. For examples of related syndromes to consider, see Box 14-2.

Etiology of ASD

At present, evidence indicates that this condition results from the cumulative effects of repeated exposures to causative agents in predisposed children, which ultimately results in the full-blown expression of autism. No single cause has been established.

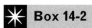

Box 14-2

Differential Diagnoses for Autism

Rett's disorder
Childhood disintegrative disorder
Asperger's disorder
Schizophrenia
Selective mutism
Expressive language disorder
Mixed receptive-expressive language disorder
Semantic pragmatic language disorder
Verbal apraxia
Nonverbal learning disability
Mental retardation
Stereotypic movement habit disorder

Genetic influences

Family studies in children with autism have noted an increased prevalence of autoimmune disease, inflammatory bowel disease, depression, obsessive-compulsive disorder, anxiety disorder, bipolar disorder, social phobia, and language disorders.[10-12] There is some evidence that relatives of autistic children show mild social, communicative, or repetitive behaviors that may place them on the normal end of the autistic spectrum. There is a 3:1 predilection for males over females in autism, indicating some degree of genetic influence. Additionally, in twin studies of autistic children, the incidence of autism in monozygotic twins is 60% to 90%. Investigation of specific genes for autism has been inconclusive, but there is evidence that multiple loci may be involved in the expression of autistic characteristics.[13] It must be remembered that the complexity of human neurodevelopment must not be oversimplified by the model of genetics. A more holistic way of understanding the role of our genes in the expression of disease is to recognize the organic nature of genes as reflected in their ability to be turned on and off by various environmental stressors. Important recent research has indicated that genetic variants (polymorphisms) are associated with the enzyme activity of methylenetetrahydrofolate reductase (MTHFR), which has been found in higher frequency in children with autism.[14] This enzyme is essential in the methionine synthase reaction, a major component of the detoxification process associated with production of glutathione, methyl B$_{12}$, and folate/folinic acid activation as well being involved in the activity of dopamine.

Prenatal influences

A number of factors have been retrospectively found to be associated with the etiology of autism. These include age of parents, exposure to epidural anesthesia, elective or emergency cesarean section, use of pitocin for labor induction, and threatened abortion.[15,16] Research is currently investigating the possible role of multiple prenatal ultrasounds, in vitro fertilization, fetal exposure to terbutaline during pregnancy, exposure to RhoGAM, use of selective serotonin reuptake inhibitor medications during pregnancy, and prenatal exposures to dietary heavy metals during pregnancy.

Postnatal influences

In order to explain the apparent exponential rise in prevalence of autism in recent years, researchers are looking at a number of potential environmental agents. Over the past decade, many articles have suggested the role of methylmercury exposure in autistic-like neurological disorders.[17-29] There appear to be remarkable similarities between mercury toxicity and autism. It has been proposed that the mechanism of action is complex and may result in both direct oxidative damage as well as indirect damage through the genetically predisposed MTHFR deficiency. A significant source of methylmercury has been found in thimerosal-containing vaccines. It has been suggested that the additive effect of multiple exposures to thimerosal-containing vaccines may result in dysregulation of the immune/detoxification systems, resulting in a generalized neuroinflammatory process. A significant aspect of this inflammatory process appears to be located in the digestive system and is known as *leaky gut syndrome.*

Leaky gut syndrome

A major component of the immune-regulatory system of an infant is located in the digestive tract. In genetically predisposed children, repeated exposures to toxins appear to result in chronic inflammatory processes in the intestinal wall with subsequent hyperpermeability that allows increased absorption ("leaking in") of macromolecules, diasaccharides, antigens, and toxins that result in neuroimmune dysfunction.[30-32] Both mercury exposure and recurrent antibiotic use result in the viscous cycle of gut mucosal damage, which leads to abnormal gut flora overgrowth or dysbiosis (e.g., yeast, pathogenic bacteria–like clostridia), which causes further gut mucosal damage. Evidence of dysbiosis, as reflected by the increased excretion of arabinose and analogs of Krebs cycle metabolites, has been found in children with autism.[33-36] Absorption of the toxic byproducts of abnormal gut flora (e.g., lactic acid, organic acids, arabinose, biologically active peptides) further aggravates brain function, leading to progressive neurological damage.[37-40]

A host of nonspecific symptoms can be early signs of leaky gut and include eczema, bloating, colic, hives, reflux, wheezing, diarrhea, and constipation. The presence of leaky gut in children does not necessarily lead to autism.

"The straw that breaks the camel's back"

It has been proposed that the current epidemic of autistic disorders may be a specific subtype of autism referred to as *regressive autism.*[41-43] It is suspected that some pivotal environmental exposure may occur that results in the full-blown regression seen in autism. The discovery of an apparent inflammatory enterocolitis in children with autism[44-47] has led some investigators to look at the possible role of live-virus vaccines in the development of this inflammatory process. It has been argued that because there is evidence of a relationship among measles infection, Crohn's disease, and other inflammatory bowel diseases,[48-50] live-virus vaccines such as the measles-mumps-rubella (MMR) vaccine may play a role in the immunological etiology of autism. This has been further supported by evidence of altered immunity in autism.[51-55] Although the connection of vaccinations with autism is controversial, further prospective studies are currently underway to clarify possible connections.

Thus we see that the etiology of autism results from progressive insults to the neuroimmunological system. It is possible that a child may develop minimal or no developmental symptoms if he or she is not exposed to repeated causative stages. This has importance in the preventive considerations when counseling siblings of children with autism. Early nonspecific symptoms such as eczema and chronic loose stools may be subtle signs of impending developmental dysfunction. Because no single insult may be responsible for the direct cause of autism, research must be aimed at considering the multiple variables at play. A careful history and tracking of symptoms is essential for diagnosis and has implications in determining management and prognosis.

Management

Early diagnosis is imperative in order to begin treatment as early as possible. As with other developmental disorders, prognosis is improved with early detection and treatment.[56,57] The first line of management is providing early intervention to support neurobehavioral development. Controversy over treatment has changed through the years. Ten years ago, conventional neurology/psychiatry denied the efficacy of treatments such as applied behavioral analysis (ABA) and sensory integration therapy, which have now become a standard of care in many areas. Certainly, referral to an early intervention program that offers a host of special education services including speech therapy, occupational therapy, physical therapy, and social interaction is the mainstay of any treatment plan. Determining a child's particular strengths and sensitivities is important in considering additional therapies, which may include the following:

- Auditory integration therapy
- Sensory integration therapy
- Visual training therapy
- Music therapy
- Craniosacral therapy

Conventional medical approaches to autism

Conventional medicine has relied primarily on the pharmacological management of aggressive or compulsive behaviors in autism. Medications such as risperidone, Abilify, Prozac, Paxil, Adderall, Depakote, propranolol, and other psychotropic medication are currently used in the psychiatric community.

Alternative medical management

For the past 10 years, the ARI has been developing a protocol to assess the efficacy of various alternative and nutritional interventions in autism. It is important to note here that many parents become desperate for a "cure" and will be easily led to try many treatments simultaneously. This can lead to exorbitant expense and little understanding of what is actually working. Parents should be advised to seek qualified, informed professionals. Clinicians who have been trained in the Defeat

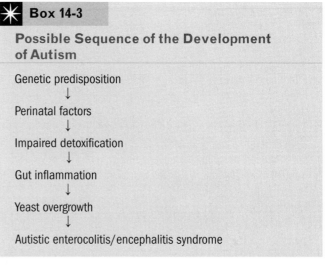

Box 14-3

Possible Sequence of the Development of Autism

Genetic predisposition
↓
Perinatal factors
↓
Impaired detoxification
↓
Gut inflammation
↓
Yeast overgrowth
↓
Autistic enterocolitis/encephalitis syndrome

Box 14-4

Alternative Medical Management of Autism

1. Treat dysbiosis
2. Heal the gut
3. Strengthen immunity and detoxification
4. Chelation of toxic elements
5. Neurometabolic fine-tuning

Autism Now (DAN) protocol are listed on the ARI website at www.autism.com.

Understanding the etiological sequence of events that leads to the full-blown expression of autism allow us to develop a specific treatment plan for each child (Box 14-3).

Thus treatment decisions are made based on specific aspects of physiological dysfunction, beginning with the digestive system (Box 14-4).

Treating dysbiosis

One of the first steps in managing a child with autism is to treat abnormal gut flora. Organic acid tests are available to determine the degree of dysbiosis. An immunoglobulin (Ig)-G food sensitivity test will reveal the degree of "leakiness" of the gut and serve as a guide to what foods to avoid. Often simply "lightening the load" of foods that are "toxic" to a leaky gut will have an immediate effect on behavior. Placing a child on a gluten-free, casein-free diet reduces the work that the digestive system must do. In some cases, the reduction of casomorphin absorption is enough to improve developmental progress. The treatment of *Candida* yeast overgrowth may require pharmaceutical antifungals such as nystatin or Diflucan. These can have powerful compromising effects on the liver's detoxification abilities and must be used with great care. Natural antifungals include garlic, grapefruit seed extract, and *Saccharomyces boulardii*. Parents should be counseled to watch for symptoms of die-off (the effects of absorption of toxins from dead yeast). These may include behavioral regressions, loose stools, increased self-stimulation, abdominal pain, and rashes. The addition of probiotics is essential to gut health, replacing pathogenic organisms with "good" bacteria. A trial of Elaine

Gottshall's Specific Carbohydrate Diet (SCD) has proven beneficial in treating dysbiosis.

Healing the gut

In addition to probiotics, the gut lining can be strengthened with some basic nutritional supplements that include zinc, calcium, magnesium, vitamin B_6, vitamin C, vitamin A, glutamine, licorice root, and aloe. Supplements that reduce inflammation of the gut include omega-3 essential fatty acids (EFAs), coenzyme Q10, grape seed extract, glutathione. Digestive enzymes improve absorption and should be given with meals. *It is important to remember to start ALL supplements at low doses. Often children will respond better to low doses than higher does of supplements because of their heightened level of sensitivity.*

Strengthening immunity and detoxification support

Reducing the oxidative stress on the body improves both gut and neurological function.[58] Reduced glutathione has antiinflammatory functions and supports the detoxification mechanism. In addition, high-dose vitamin C, carnosine, vitamin B_6, magnesium, zinc, selenium, and folinic acid work on various biochemical pathways involved in the protection against oxidative damage.

Chelation of Toxic Elements

It is important to strengthen the body's capacity to detoxify before trying to remove potentially toxic elements. The chelation process requires careful monitoring to avoid adverse reactions from both the chelating agents and the mobilization of toxic elements. Mineral supplementation is required during the process. A challenge of a chelator such as dimercaptosuccinic acid (DMSA) or topical DMPS followed by measurement of urinary metal excretion will determine the need for chelation. Natural chelators include garlic, cilantro, chlorella, chitosan, and hyaluronic acid. Allithiamine (TTFD) is an artificial garlic derivative that may potentiate removal of heavy metals.

Neurometabolic fine-tuning

Impaired function of methionine synthase affects the bioactivity of SAM, B_{12}, and glutathione, all of which are important chemical components in brain function. Supplementation with DMG (dimethylglycine), TMG (betaine), methyl B_{12}, amino acids, DMAE, L-theanine, acetyl-L-carnitine, coenzyme Q10, and specific neurotransmitter precursors such as tyrosine and 5-HTP can support proper brain function. Tests are available to indirectly assess relative imbalances in neurotransmitters.[59]

Homeopathy and Chinese medicine

Both homeopathy and Chinese medicine are complete "systems of medicine" that assess the child with autism, although careful consideration of each child's unique presentation is beyond the scope of this text. Homeopathy treats symptom complexes through the use of corresponding remedies. In traditional Chinese medicine (TCM) texts, children with mental disorders that bear similarities to autism are described as resulting from Phlegm misting the mind.[60] The origin of this Phlegm is thought to be internal trauma, excessive wetness, inappropriate diet, and food stagnation. This Phlegm corresponds to the inflammatory process described in recent research. Treatment is designed to address the Uprising Phlegm Fire with Chinese herbs and acupuncture. In TCM the digestive system is always considered of primary importance in the treatment of children. Treatment geared at supporting the spleen/stomach and liver is consistent with the recent research suggesting that autism be defined as an enterocolitis-encephalitis syndrome.

Summary

A careful history and an approach to management that respects the highly sensitive nature of children with autism can result in profound improvements in behavior and development. The ultimate goal of holistic pediatrics is to prevent problems from arising by considering the child within his or her context. An understanding of the complex factors involved in the development of autistic dysfunction requires a clinician to foster this holistic attitude, understanding the implications of diet, family, education, and toxins in the child's life.

✳ CAM THERAPY RECOMMENDATIONS

Acupuncture

TCM also regards autism as a complex disorder with multiple channel and organ imbalances and global effects on the child's emotional and even spiritual being. A thorough knowledge of TCM is needed for an understanding of the condition. A brief discussion is provided here for general reference.

In TCM, the Mind, Shen, resides in the Heart and is intimately related to the Liver Yin, which houses the Ethereal Soul, the Hun. Both are needed for thinking, consciousness, insight, memory, intelligence, and cognition. It is the Ethereal Soul that provides the Mind with the spiritual movement between self-recognition and introspection and the ability to project outward to relate to other people and the world.[1] The health of the Hun is reflected through the eyes, which can be corroborated by the Western idea that the eyes are windows to the soul. Autism therefore is primarily a disturbance of the Mind and the Spirit, due to Heart and Liver Yin deficiency. The Kidney Yin or Essence is also deficient, corresponding to genetic predisposition and decreased mental function in autism. Because children are constitutionally Spleen deficient,[2] the diminished SP function results in clouding or "Phlegm misting" the Mind.

There are no evidence-based data at this time on acupuncture treatment of autism. This author has treated autism by integrating conventional developmental pediatrics training with evaluation and treatment practices from acupuncture textbooks. The following are very basic and general treatment recommendations extracted from the clinic. Experienced practitioners who can assess and monitor the autistic child clinically should carry out more comprehensive treatments.

Global/General Points

GV20 and Sishenchong: raises clear Qi to the Mind

SP6 nourishes Yin, strengthens LR, SP, KI

For Liver Yin deficiency:
- LR8 nourishes LR Yin
- KI3, CV4 nourishes KI Yin
- BL18, BL47 root the Ethereal Soul

For Heart:
- HT7 nourishes Heart
- BL15, BL44 stimulates Mind's intellect, stimulates Shen

For KI Yin/Essence deficiency:
- CV4, CV7 nourish Essence
- KI3, KI6, SP6 nourish KI Yin
- CV4 nourishes KI Yin, calms Mind
- BL23, strengthens KI

For Spleen:
- ST40 resolves Phlegm
- CV12, ST36, SP6, BL20 to tonify Stomach and Spleen[1-5]

Chiropractic

An overview of the chiropractic role in management of autism looks at spinal integrity and its influence over neurobehavioral issues. Upon finding evidence of spinal subluxation, the chiropractor will correct this potential for neurological interference with a chiropractic adjustment. Many chiropractors also address the joints in the skull in the form of some method of cranial adjusting. Chiropractors also commonly address nutritional considerations, including the recommendation to utilize a trial of a gluten-free, casein-free diet and supplementation of omega-3 fats along with trace minerals when indicated.

Several case studies have demonstrated benefit to behavioral and other related symptoms in children with autism. One report was of a 5-year-old autistic girl born at 7.5 months' gestation; the pregnancy was complicated by maternal infection and maternal allergic reaction to magnesium sulfate. The parents reported that their daughter was allergic to cow's milk and apple juice and had a history of developmental delay, aggression, and chronic otitis media. The diagnosis of autism was confirmed at 3 years of age. The patient was assessed by infrared thermal scan and surface electromyography (EMG) as well as manual and motion palpation. Manual adjustments were provided to areas of concern (1 to 3 motion units or spinal segments) at a rate of four times per week. After 1 month, the patient was sleeping more soundly and had begun to verbalize, and her teachers noted a 30% improvement in social interaction. Her otitis media was cleared by this time and did not recur over the 2-year course in which this case was reported. Within 1 year, 80% improvement was noted in behavior, and communication skills and learning improved consistently.[1]

A 7-year-old boy was reportedly normal until the receipt of a DPT vaccine at 3 years of age. Regression was noted immediately and progressed until, by age 5, all vocabulary ceased and his bowel and kidney function were erratic and uncontrollable. After 2 months of chiropractic care, the child's vocabulary returned. After 1 year, the boy had infrequent bowel accidents and could communicate, and most of his autistic behaviors had diminished.[2]

A 5-year-old autistic girl presented with a complex symptom profile consisting of asthma, irritable bowel syndrome (IBS), strabismus, and illness susceptibility. Orthopedic, biomechanical, radiographic, and thermal scans were performed with noted irregularities at the upper cervical spine. Chiropractic adjustments were administered at the C0-C1 motion unit at a frequency of two times per week. By the end of week 1, the mother reported that the child had slept better than usual and that her violent tantrums had reduced by 40%, she was able to verbalize several emotions (hungry, tired, mad), and she was walking more flat-footed. By the end of week 2, the child's tantrums had reduced in frequency by 80% and had reduced significantly in intensity. The strabismus had improved in one eye and resolved in the other. The child spoke her first sentence, had a desire to be touched and hugged, and was sleeping through the night. By the end of week 4, tantrums, hyperactivity, and violent behaviors had ceased. There was no sign of strabismus, gait was normal, and the IBS continued to dramatically improve. The biomechanical, orthopedic, and thermal scans were normalized. She was reassessed in an autism center and declared to no longer have autism.[3] This was a very dramatic case indeed.

The Kentuckiana Children's Center (a nonprofit center providing chiropractic care to children with disabilities) reports that 75% of the 125 patient-cases per week are diagnosed with ASD.[4] One case involved a 16-year-old, high-functioning boy with autism who presented with encopresis. After 13 chiropractic adjustments and craniosacral therapy, the encopresis resolved and he also made improvement in his thought processes, as his mother indicated that he was able to carry on a conversation.[5] A 6-year-old boy was diagnosed with autism at age 2.5 years after a classic regression of language skills and eye contact as well as development of violent reactions to loud noises and persistent creation of guttural sounds or a long 'e' sound. He was delivered by emergency cesarean section and sustained a significant head injury at age 3. After approximately 9 sessions of spinal adjusting and cranial work, he stopped repeatedly standing on his head for long periods, began to make more eye contact, and started speaking. He was also being assessed according to the DAN protocols for nutritional deficiencies, toxicities, and metabolic abnormalities.[6]

Two more cases from Kentuckiana included a 5-year-old boy with autism and cerebral palsy who was managed with adjustive care for 17 months, during which time the child learned to walk independently and began to speak. The second case was that of a 3-year-old girl with classic autism symptoms and recurrent otitis media. Within 1 month, her ears cleared and her behavior began to improve. The addition of L-glutathione was associated with an advance in behavioral improvement, and another advance was noted with the addition of a gluten-free/casein-free diet. After 7 months of care, DMG was added to aid in detoxification; she again showed improvements. Within 18 months of the initial visit, the child was no longer throwing tantrums, injuring herself, isolated, or language delayed.[7]

A 5-year-old boy with autism was treated with chiropractic adjustments. After 2 weeks, he demonstrated 96% improvement as reported by "all involved parties." At a 3.5-year follow-up, the reported improvement by these same subjective and objective measures was 102%.[8]

A 7-year-old girl with autism was living in a state foster center. She had a history of sexual and physical abuse. She would not respond to verbal directions, would slowly turn in circles while singing an unintelligible song, and consistently maintained a glazed stare with blank expression. Spinal adjustments to the C1 vertebra were performed two times per week. By the end of 2 weeks, the girl stopped turning circles and singing. After 10 months, she was able to carry on a conversation, follow directions, and dress and groom herself. A setback occurred when the girl lost her home to a hurricane. She began spinning and singing again until she received a spinal adjustment 1 week later. This behavior immediately ceased. The chiropractor concluded that there was an emotional origin to the spinal subluxation complex associated with this girl's behavior.[9]

Although these case studies are provocative, clinical trials are sparse. One study evaluated 26 children with autism in a practice-based setting by supine leg check, infrared thermal scan, surface EMG, and plain film. All participants were adjusted in the upper cervical spine. Childhood Autism Rating Scales (CARS) scores were compiled before and after treatment. Although outcomes were variable and data collection was incomplete, the authors report improvement to some degree in all participants in both autistic behaviors and spinal balance.[10]

Chiropractic care was given over a 3- to 6-month period to six children with autism (aged 9 to 19 years) who attended a local school for children with autism. The teachers were aware that the children were receiving care but had no knowledge that data were being collected for study. Standard behavior charts were used to plot behaviors of interest including picking up toys, non-compliance, self-abuse, crying episodes, requests to use the bathroom, unprompted requests to play, use of correct verb tense, and appropriate response to a peer. These behaviors were plotted prior to chiropractic intervention, during intervention, and again after the termination of the chiropractic adjustments. Positive changes were noted in all observed areas.[11]

Autism may in part be due to abnormal sensory processing.[12-14] An elevated galvanic skin response is common among children with autism, and after deep skin pressure, the galvanic skin response is reduced and tension and anxiety are also reduced.[15] Chiropractic adjustments provide a similar reduction in galvanic skin response and reduction in abnormal behaviors.[16]

One theory posits that misalignment at the first cervical vertebra can cause distortion in the dentate ligament and therefore irritate the spinal cord directly, producing mechanically induced neurological symptomatology. Other theories include central nervous system (CNS) facilitation occurring as a result of a mechanical trauma, which results in abnormal hypomobility/hypermobility of spinal segments. It has also been suggested that brain cell hibernation may be a precursor to autistic behaviors and that the afferent stimulation of the chiropractic adjustment may influence normal brain function.

This author has noted some level of change in all patients with autism who were treated with chiropractic adjustments.

Changes range from notable reduction in self-stimulation behavior to reversal of autism diagnosis.

Examination of nutritional and GI factors related to autism is an ever-expanding field of study. There is clear evidence that people with autism have a high incidence of GI abnormalities in digestive physiology, mucosal biology, and immunoresponsiveness.[17]

Elimination of sugars, artificial coloring or flavoring agents, preservatives, and salicylates may offer some benefit through reduction of toxic load.[18]

The likelihood of toxic metabolites from gluten and casein ingestion is high in the autistic population, so elimination of dietary sources of both gluten and casein is recommended.[19] Care must be taken to maintain adequate nutrient intake in children on the restrictive diet.[20,21]

Addition of microflora may enhance gut function, which is found deficient in the majority of children with autism.[22,23] Microflora supplements from nondairy sources are available for children with dairy sensitivities.

Eicosapentaenoic acid/docosapentaenoic acid (EPA/DHA) enhances synaptic function in the brain and may result in more advanced cognitive and behavioral function.[24,26]

Vitamin A is consistently deficient in children with autism and is necessary to accommodate G-alpha protein defects to allow for normal language and sensory processing.[27] Selenium serves as a precursor to glutathione, which aids in oxidative stress and cellular toxicity management. Zinc is effective in managing damaging effects of mercury exposure.[28] The combination of B vitamins with magnesium improves neurological behavioral function.[29] Calcium is an important player in neuroplasticity. More than 50% of children with autism are also deficient in B vitamins, selenium, zinc, calcium, and magnesium.[30-32]

Copper should not be supplemented, as this nutrient is commonly seen in excess in children with autism and is inversely related to zinc levels.[33]

Heavy metal detoxification may be indicated through nutritional or pharmaceutical protocols.[34,35]

Assessment and intervention according to the DAN protocol (a 250-page manual of assessment tools, intervention protocols, and referral options based on scientific evidence) includes screening for trace mineral and vitamin deficiencies, toxic elements, gut permeability, and altered metabolism with specific and individualized management and monitoring. The basic organic assessment tools include blood chemistry with complete thyroid panel, complete blood count, urinalysis and urine amino acids, and serum ferritin and iron.

Although there are many forms of sensory therapy with varying degrees of success, participation in sensory integration and exercise programs may prove advantageous to those children with auditory sensitivities who seem to respond predictably to auditory integration therapies.[36]

Herbs—Western

In healthy adult individuals, gingko (*Ginkgo biloba L.*) has not been found to have clinically significant cognition-enhancing and memory-boosting effects. However, when used in adults with dementia, gingko was found to improve learning, cognitive function and recall (with 3- to 6-month treatment with 120 to 240 mg of *G. biloba* extract).[1] However, the use of this herb in children with cognitive impairment due to autism has not been studied. Gingko leaf is administered orally, but other plant parts are to be avoided owing to concern for potential severe allergic reactions.[2]

Doses of ginseng are prepared from the plant's roots and administered orally. These herbs may be found as a number of species, including American, *Panax ginseng*, and Asian ginseng has been studied variably for its impact on mental performance in healthy adults. Overall, in these adult studies, there is not a clear indication that it significantly boosts mental performance, memory, or cognitive ability.[3] There are no studies in children—neither in healthy, developmentally intact children nor in children with autism—regarding its effectiveness. The use of *P. ginseng* in infants and newborns is discouraged because of reports of intoxication.[2]

See Chapter 13, Attention-Deficit Hyperactivity Disorder, for information on the use of these herbs for attentiveness or impulsivity.

Homeopathy

Before using this section, please see Appendix A, Homeopathy, for definitions of practitioner expertise categories and general information on prescribing homeopathic medicines.

Practitioner Expertise Category 3

There are no controlled clinical trials of homeopathic treatment for autism, although the homeopathic literature contains evidence of its use in the form of accumulated clinical experience.[1] Most patients with autism need a comprehensive treatment plan including a variety of treatment modalities. Homeopathy can be used safely in combination with other treatment modalities, both alternative and conventional. Because autism is a complex and multifaceted developmental problem, successful homeopathic treatment usually requires extensive training in the art and science of homeopathy. Any one of many homeopathic medicines may be used to treat autism, depending on the characteristics of the patient being treated; sophisticated homeopathic analysis and long-term follow-up are required. For these reasons specific medicines for treating autism will not be presented here. Interested readers are referred to the homeopathic literature for further study.[1]

Massage Therapy

Often parents do not consider massage therapy for children with autism under their assumption that the autistic child would not tolerate the tactile stimulation. The contrary is true; massage provides a very predictable method of tactile communication for this population. Massage can also provide symmetrical tactile stimulation to both extremities together to promote recognition of the whole body for child with tactile and sensory difficulties.[1]

A study of autistic preschoolers reported that children in a touch therapy group had changes on the Autism Behavior Checklist, specifically decreases in sensory scale, relating scale, and total scale score compared with the touch control group. The touch therapy group also had improved ratings on the Early Social Communication Scale, which included joint attention, behavior regulation, and initiating behavior.[2] Parents who attended a touch therapy program for 8 weeks to massage their autistic child reported feeling that routine tasks were accomplished more easily, their child was more relaxed, and communication had improved between them and their child.[3]

The previous two studies suggest that massage therapy may be helpful for the child as well as the parents of the autistic child. If a parent or practitioner chooses to initiate massage therapy for an autistic child, it is incredibly helpful to keep the treatment structured as much as possible so the child may experience predictable touch. Swedish massage can be preformed in whichever position the child feels most secure. As some autistic children can have a component of tactile sensory integration disorders, massage can be done over the clothes if the provider feels the child would be more tactually comfortable. Light and/or fast massage strokes can be stimulating and should be avoided. Slow, rhythmic, moderate-pressure strokes helps the child predict where the provider's hands will be traveling and will facilitate the treatment. Performing the massage in the same position and/or at the same time of day will also help the child understand and prepare for the tactile stimulation he or she is about to receive. Often, after several sessions with the parent, it becomes evident that the child expects a comforting experience when placed into the massage position and begins to quiet his or her behavior even before the treatment is initiated.

For massage performed by the parent, having the child sit in the parent's lap may help the child integrate the touch better than if they were massaged "at" rather than "with." Parents and other practitioners can also sit close to the child, either on the floor or in an adjacent chair positioned perpendicular to the child. This allows the massage provider to be within the visual range of the child, whereas massaging from behind may be more difficult for the child to integrate. For some children, face-to-face massage may invade too much of their comfort zone.

For any autistic child, it is important to work within the child's comfort level and to be very conscious of disengagement behaviors. If a child begins to become agitated during the session, the massage provider should first try to stop the motion of the massaging hands and just let them lie on the child in a comforting position. The cessation of movement but persistence of contact allows the child the opportunity to regroup. If disengagement behaviors continue, it is best to end the session for the day.

Mind/Body

Anecdotally, mind/body approaches including hypnosis and biofeedback have been used to facilitate relaxation and self-control for children diagnosed with autism and PDD, but little has been published in this area. Mullins and Christian[1] provided a case report that progressive relaxation training was effective in reducing the disruptive behaviors of a young boy with autism. The authors have found that particularly in individuals with Asperger's syndrome and high-functioning autism, teaching the lowering of emotional (autonomic nervous system) arousal through surface EMG or skin conductance biofeedback can be helpful. Biophysical measures that include preferred sensory inputs can be calming and include massage, deep pressure, vibration, or rocking/swinging.

Naturopathy

The naturopathic approach to treating autism and other behavioral and developmental disorders in the autistic spectrum often utilizes therapies derived from DAN. DAN is a consensus group that consists of physicians and researchers who use integrative medicine to treat patients within the autism spectrum. The following is a very basic stepwise approach used by many DAN physicians:

1. Remove foods from the diet to which the child has intolerances.
    - The first step in improving digestion and behavior is avoidance of allergenic foods, in particular foods containing gluten and casein. Gluten-containing foods include barley, rye, oats, wheat, triticale, kamut, and spelt. Preexisting long-term constipation and/or diarrhea is common in the autistic population, and a restricted diet almost always improves these symptoms in patients. Avoidance of other allergenic foods such as corn, eggs, and soy may also prove beneficial.
    - Standard skin prick or IgE allergy tests may not detect delayed-type hypersensitivity reactions. There are several laboratories that can perform an IgG allergy test, which may be more helpful. An oligoantigenic diet, however, is the most effective way to determine a food intolerance or allergy. Improvements in behavior may be observed after a "washout" period of allergen avoidance. There are different opinions regarding what is the optimal time frame to avoid foods in order to see benefits in the patient. It seems that most physicians are suggesting a general range of at least 1 to 6 months.
    - It is thought that many autistic patients lack efficient levels of the digestive enzyme dipeptidyl peptidase IV (DPP-IV). DPP-IV is responsible for breaking down the opioid-like peptides gluteomorphin and caseomorphin, which are found in gluten-containing and casein-containing foods. Undigested peptides may pass through the digestive barrier and have an opiate effect on the brain of those with ASD. If families are traveling and they are not sure whether certain foods contain gluten or casein, an enzyme supplement with DPP-IV may be supplemented as a protective measure. Manufacturer's suggested dosages should be followed.
2. Evaluate nutritional status and supplement accordingly.
    - There are several reasons why autistic patients may have insufficient intake and absorption of vitamins and minerals. A recent study of more than 400 people with autism found that 48% reported chronic diarrhea or chronic constipation,[1] and these intestinal disorders are likely to affect the absorption of essential nutrients. Chronic intestinal inflammation has also been discovered in autistic patients,[2,3] which can affect absorption. A third reason is that autistic children typically have very restricted diets owing to their preferences, and these diets may be quite deficient in vitamins and minerals.

- A study of 500 children with autism revealed that more than 99% had an elevated ratio of serum copper:plasma zinc,[4] so patients with autism are advised to avoid copper-containing multivitamins and supplements with higher levels of zinc. A red blood cell elements test can provide information on vitamin status of the autistic patient.
- Elevated levels of methylmalonic acid in autistic patients led researchers to believe that a functional B_{12} deficiency may exist.[5] Dr. James Neubrander may be one of the most experienced physicians in the use of B_{12} supplementation in the form of methylcobalamin. His full evaluation and treatment protocol may be found on his website at www.drneubrander.com. A modified version of his treatment protocol includes preservative-free methylcobalamin, 25 mg/mL given at a dose of 64.5 mg/kg, every 3 days, with insulin syringes administered to the buttocks at a 30- to 45-degree angle.
- Calcium was also discovered to be deficient in autistic patients, and adequate intake should be ensured. Children 2 years and older may be given 800 mg of calcium per day. Calcium/magnesium supplements should be at a ratio of 1:1, as magnesium is also deficient in these patients and can aid in calcium absorption.
- Vitamin A supplementation may be beneficial, as Dr. Mary N. Megson discovered that a link may exist between a family history of nightblindness and endocrine abnormalities in family members and improvement in autistic children following supplementation of vitamin A. Megson prefers using cod liver oil as the method for providing vitamin A, as it is in the natural form. One teaspoon per 30 lb of body weight is a conservative dose. Vitamin D toxicity in cod liver oil is a concern during summer months or in those who live in particularly sunny climates. Fish oils other than cod liver oil will have much lower levels of vitamin D.
- Reductions in symptom severity with vitamin C supplementation have been reported, and these results were attributed to a hypothesized dopaminergic mechanism of action of ascorbic acid.[1] Doses used were approximately 100 mg/kg of body weight.
- A large body of literature shows the efficacy and safety of high doses of vitamin B6 and magnesium, including 11 double-blind placebo-controlled studies.[6-24] B6 is an essential cofactor in the synthesis of serotonin, γ-aminobutyric acid (GABA), dopamine, epinephrine, and norepinephrine. The combined treatment of B_6 and magnesium together can help decrease symptoms of autism. The addition of magnesium is important, as several physicians have reported that B_6 given alone can cause hyperactivity.

3. Evaluate gastrointestinal (GI) flora/dysbiosis and treat accordingly.
4. Evaluate heavy metal load in patients and chelate accordingly.
    - Consideration should be given to evaluating autistic patients for heavy metal toxicity. Autistic patients have been shown to have lower levels of mercury in hair when compared with controls, which signifies an impaired excretion ability.

- Check plasma cysteine levels (this author prefers Doctor's Data Laboratories). Cysteine is a precursor to glutathione, which is instrumental in protecting against exposure to environmental toxins, especially heavy metals. If levels are found to be low, supplementation with 500 to 600 mg/day of *n*-acetyl cysteine may help raise levels.
- Jill James discovered that supplementation with a combination of trimethylglycine, methylcobalamin, and folinic acid had a favorable effect on antioxidant and detoxification capacity. Doses used were 800 μg twice daily for folinic acid and 1000-mg trimethylglycine twice daily for 3 weeks. Levels of methylcobalamin may follow the dosing regimen by Dr. Neubrander as previously mentioned.
- It is essential that before considering chelation therapy, gut flora abnormalities must be corrected, cysteine levels should be adequate, and a chemistry panel should be performed and show adequate liver and kidney function.
- Perform a DMSA challenge. DMSA is traditionally used for treating patients with lead toxicity and is approved for use in patients as young as 1 year. DMSA can be administered orally at a dose of 25 mg/kg in one bolus, and urine is collected for 6 hours postadministration. If elevated levels are discovered, a conservative approach would be to give 10 mg/kg three times per day for 3 days, followed by 11 days of no therapy. This cycle may be repeated twice more, at which point urine may be collected for another 6 hours after the last dose of the last cycle and then sent for another toxic metal evaluation. A complete blood count and liver/kidney function evaluation, by way of a chemistry panel, should be performed at that time to ensure the safety of the patient. Zinc and cysteine (by way of *n*-acetyl cysteine) supplementation should always accompany chelation treatment, as DMSA tends to increase excretion of these nutrients.

Nutrition

Autism is a complex disorder thought to have multiple contributing factors: genetic, environmental, and metabolic. Current theories include dysregulation of neurotransmitters,[1] peptidase deficiency leading to the accumulation of opioid-like peptides,[2] food allergies and gut dysbiosis,[3] EFA imbalance or deficiency,[4] or disordered metal metabolism.[5]

Case reports using targeted amino acid therapy (TAAT) showed benefit in children with autism. The therapy, using dietary supplements, balances the level of inhibiting neurotransmitters with excitatory transmitters and is monitored by measuring urinary excretion of these neurotransmitters and observing behavioral changes.[6] Controlled studies have not been done with large groups to verify these results but would be of interest.

A randomized, controlled study to evaluate the effect of a gluten-free and casein-free diet in autistic children found that children on the diet were significantly better than controls after the 1-year period.[7] Other studies have found similar results.[8]

Because of the improvement in behavior seen in patients with other neuropsychiatric disorders treated with EFAs, it was theorized that children with autism would also show improvement. Parents reported improvement in general health, cognitive and motor skills concentration, eye contact and sociability, and other measures when their children with autism were supplemented with EPA-rich fish oils.[4] Large controlled trials have yet to be done in autistic children.

Treatment

- Recommend a gluten- and casein-free diet. To prevent withdrawal effects from the opioid-type metabolites from wheat or dairy, do this gradually—one meal at a time or one food at a time. Read labels carefully for "hidden" sources of wheat or diary such as "modified food starch," "hydrolyzed vegetable protein," or malted vinegars.
- Encourage organic, whole fresh foods to decrease exposure to toxins and to increase intake of natural sources of the essential nutrients.
- Identify and eliminate food allergens that may promote intestinal dysbiosis.
- Implement TAAT to rebalance the excitatory and inhibiting neurotransmitters.
- Restore and balance EFAs. A 1000-mg EFA supplement typically contains a mixture of 148-mg EPA, 99-mg DHA, and 40-mg γ-linolenic acid.

Osteopathy

The treatment of children with pervasive developmental disorders such as autism has been part of the osteopathic literature since its beginnings. The earliest writings by Andrew Taylor Still describe common osteopathic findings and approaches to treatment in children with a variety of developmental disorders. More recently several studies[1-5] and reports[6-9] have been published documenting the influence of osteopathic treatment on a number of associated symptoms. Unfortunately these were either small or not controlled. Within the osteopathic philosophy, the treatment of children with autism is viewed from several perspectives, depending upon which characteristics of the disorder the child predominantly manifests. Children with antisocial or high anxiety–type behaviors often have associated findings suggesting increased sympathetic nervous system activity and CNS irritability. The principles of osteopathy in the cranial field suggest that CNS irritability may be due to increased input from peripheral tissues or strain in the components of the cranial mechanism. Typical findings reported in these children include "strains" in the membranous and soft tissue components of the head, compression and restricted movement in the osseous mechanics of the head, and imbalances in the cerebral fluid systems.[1,8,10] Osteopathy in the cranial field is a gentle approach aimed at rebalancing strains and supporting optimal function of these areas.

From another perspective, some children with PDDs such as autism have the predominant appearance of being dissociated from their physical environment, including their own bodies. These children tend to have abnormally high thresholds for discomfort and pain and may even have self-mutilating tendencies. On osteopathic examination these children often have findings of tissue strain and mechanical compression throughout many areas that one would expect to be symptomatic but are not. The midline structures, such as the spine, ribcage, and the "core-link" as described by Sutherland[11,12] are often involved. Gentle, indirect osteopathic techniques can be used to relax tissue strains, improve function in these areas, and mechanically integrate the areas of dysfunction. Children with autism may also have GI and other visceral symptoms. One small study suggested that visceral osteopathic treatment may help with GI issues in children with autism.[2]

The child with autism can usually benefit from multiple therapeutic interventions. Osteopaths work in concert with other healthcare providers in the care of these children and those with other pervasive developmental problems. Tailoring therapeutic interventions to the needs and capacity of the child is very important. Overstimulation with too much well-intentioned therapy may result in an exacerbation of the child's behaviors. As such, good communication among all therapists and physicians and a well-informed parent are indispensable components of the child's healthcare plan.

Probiotics

One of the etiologies of ASD under consideration is exposure to environmental toxins or allergens. Because the GI tract is involved in detoxification of numerous environmental chemicals and microbes, some have proposed using probiotic therapy as part of a protocol to ameliorate potentially toxic CNS effects.[1] Data are essentially anecdotal in nature, but the theory is plausible. Probiotic therapy is generally regarded as safe and may prove beneficial for a subset of patients with autism.

Guidance with respect to choice of specific organisms and duration of therapy is sorely lacking. To further complicate matters, there seems little rationale behind the variety of dosages or combination of microbes employed in published studies. Oftentimes similar dosages have been utilized for distinct microbes, while widely disparate dosages have been employed by researchers studying the same probiotic. At this time, dosage recommendations are far from set in stone.

This author recommends using a 2- to 3-month trial of probiotic therapy for children with autism that includes well-studied organisms shown to be safe, such as *Lactobacillus GG* (the microbe associated with the most supportive data), *Lactobacillus plantarum*, *Lactobacillus paracasei*, *Lactobacillus reuteri*, or *Lactobacillus acidophilus*. Dosing guidelines to consider are 10 billion colony-forming units (CFU) for children weighing < 12 kg and 20 billion CFU for children > 12 kg. Treatment is extremely well tolerated, and palatability is an infrequent issue because the capsules can be opened and mixed into drinks or soft foods. Sometimes the agents are also available as a powder. If effective, treatment can be continued indefinitely. Use with extreme caution, if at all, for those children at risk for infectious complications (e.g., immunosuppression or use of immunosuppressive agents, presence of central venous catheter, prematurity).

References

Pediatric Diagnosis and Treatment

1. Bertrand J, Mars A, Boyle C et al: Prevalence of autism in a United States population: the Brick Township, New Jersey investigation, *Pediatrics* 108:1155-1161, 2001.
2. Newschaffer CJ, Falb MD, Gurney JG: National autism prevalence trends from United States special education data, *Pediatrics* 115:e277-e282, 2005.
3. Byrd RS: *Report to the legislature on the principal findings from the epidemiology of autism in California: a comprehensive pilot study*, San Diego, 2002, MIND Institute, University of California–Davis.
4. Yeargin-Allsopp M, Rice C, Karapurkar T et al: Prevalence of autism in a US metropolitan area, *J Am Med Assoc* 289:49-55, 2003.
5. American Psychiatric Association: *Diagnostic and statistical manual of mental disorders*, ed 4 [revised] (DSM-IVR), Washington, DC, 2000, American Psychiatric Association.
6. AAP Committee on Children with Disabilities: The pediatrician's role in the diagnosis and management of autistic spectrum disorder in children, *Pediatrics* 107:1221-1226, 2001.
7. Honig LS, Rosenberg RN: Apoptosis and neurologic disease, *Am J Med* 108:317-330, 2000.
8. Barnea-Goraly N, Kwon H, Menon V et al: White matter structure in autism: preliminary evidence from diffusion tensor imagery, *Biol Psychiatry* 55:323-326, 2004.
9. Coirchesne E, Karns CM, Davis HR et al: Unusual brain growth patterns in early life in patients with autistic disorder: an MRI study, *Neurology* 57:245-254, 2001.
10. Comi AM, Zimmerman A, Frye VH et al: Familial clustering of autoimmune disorders and evaluation of medical risk factors in autism, *J Child Neurol* 14:388-394, 1999.
11. Piven J, Palmer P, Jacobi D et al: Broader autism phenotype: evidence from a family history study of multiple-incidence autism families, *Am J Psychiatry* 154:185-190, 1997.
12. Micali N, Chakrabarti S, Fombonne E: The broad autism phenotype: findings from an epidemiological survey, *Autism* 8:21-37, 2004.
13. Muhle R, Trentacoste SV, Rapin I: The genetics of autism, *Pediatrics* 113:e472-486, 2004.
14. Boris M, Goldblatt PA, Galanko J et al: Association of MTHFR gene variants with autism, *J Am Phys Surg* 9:106-108, 2004.
15. Burd L, Severud R, Kerbeshian J et al: Prenatal and perinatal risk factors for autism, *J Perinat Med* 27:441-450, 1999.
16. Glasson EJ, Bower C, Petterson B et al: Perinatal factors and the development of autism: a population study, *Arch Gen Psychiatry* 61:618-627, 2004.
17. Alberti A, Pirrone P, Elia M et al: Sulphation deficit in "low-functioning" autistic children: a pilot study, *Biol Psychiatry* 46:420-424, 1999.
18. Impact of the 1999 AAP/USPHS joint statement on thimerosal in vaccines on infant Hepatitis B vaccination practices, JAMA 285:1568-1570, 2001.
19. American Psychiatric Association: *Diagnostic and statistical manual of mental disorders*, ed 4, Washington, DC, 1994, American Psychiatric Association.
20. Aronow R, Fleischmann L: Mercury poisoning in children, *Clin Pediatr* 15:936-945, 1976.
21. Aschner M, Aschner JL: Mercury neurotoxicity: mechanisms of blood-brain barrier transport, *Neurosci Behav Rev* 14:169-176, 1990.
22. Bagenstose LM, Salgame P, Monestier M: Mercury-induced autoimmunity in the absence of IL-4, *Clin Exp Immunol* 114:9-12, 1998.
23. Cagiano R, De Salvia MA, Renna G et al: Evidence that exposure to methyl mercury during gestation induces behavioral and neurochemical changes in offspring of rats, *Neurotoxicol Teratol* 12:23-28, 1990.
24. Centers for Disease Control and Prevention: Recommendations regarding the use of vaccines that contain thimerosal as a preservative, *MMWR Morbid Mortal Wkly Rep* 48:996-998, 1999.
25. Centers for Disease Control and Prevention: Thimerosal in vaccines: a joint statement of the American Academy of Pediatrics and the Public Health Service, *MMWR Morbid Mortal Wkly Rep* 48:563-565, 1999.

26. Clarkson TW: Mercury: major issues in environmental health, *Environ Health Perspect* 100:1-38, 1992.
27. Reference deleted in page proofs.
28. Deyab P, Gochfeldbc M, Reuhlabca K: Developmental methylmercury administration alters cerebellar PSA-NCAM expression and Golgi sialyltransferase activity, *Brain Res* 845:139-151, 1999.
29. Halsey NA: Limiting infant exposure to thimerosal in vaccines and other sources of mercury, *J Am Med Assoc* 282:18, 1999.
30. Manahan B: A brief evidence-based review of two gastrointestinal illnesses: irritable bowel and leaky gut syndrome, *Altern Ther Health Med* 10:14, 2004.
31. Kiefer D, Ali-Akbarian L: A brief evidence-based review of two gastrointestinal illnesses: irritable bowel and leaky gut syndromes, *Altern Ther Health Med* 10:22-30, 2004.
32. Verdu EF, Collins SM: Microbial-gut interactions in health and disease. Irritable bowel syndrome, *Best Pract Res Clin Gastroenterol* 18:315-321, 2004.
33. Kiehn T, Bernard E, Gold J et al: Candidiasis: detection by gas-liquid chromatography of D-arabitol, a fungal metabolite, in human serum, *Science* 206:577-580, 1979.
34. Shattock P, Savery D: Urinary profiles of people with autism: possible implications and relevance to other research. In *Proceedings of the Conference on Therapeutic Interventions for Autism: perspectives from research and practice*, 1996.
35. Shaw W: Role for certain yeast and bacteria byproducts discovered by organic acid testing in the etiology of a wide variety of human diseases, *Bull Great Plains Lab* 1999.
36. Shaw W, Kassen E, Chaves E: Increased excretion of analogs of Krebs cycle metabolites and arabinose in two brothers with autistic features, *Clin Chem* 41:1094-1104, 1995.
37. Shattock P, Lowdon G: Proteins, peptides and autism. Part 2: implications for the education and care of people with autism, *Brain Dysfunct* 4:323-334, 1991.
38. Reichelt K-L, Hole K, Hamberger A et al: Biologically active peptide containing fractions in schizophrenia and childhood autism, *Adv Biochem Psychopharmacol* 28:627-643, 1981.
39. Gupta S, Aggarwal S, Heads C: Dysregulated immune system in children with autism: beneficial effects of intravenous immune globulin on autistic characteristics, *J Autism Dev Disord* 26:439-452, 1996.
40. Gottschall EG: *Breaking the vicious cycle: intestinal health through diet* [revised edition], New York, 1994, Kirkton Press.
41. Rogers SJ, DiLalla DL: Age of symptom onset in young children with pervasive developmental disorders, *J Am Acad Child Adolesc Psychiatry* 29:863-872, 1990.
42. Tuchman R, Rapin I: Regression in pervasive developmental disorders: seizures and epileptiform electroencephalogram correlates, *Pediatrics* 99:560-566, 1997.
43. Schopler E, Reichler RJ, DeVellis RF et al: Toward objective classification of autism, *J Autism Dev Dis* 10:91, 1980.
44. D'Eufemia P, Celli M, Finocchiaro R et al: Abnormal intestinal permeability in children with autism, *Acta Pædiatr* 85:1076-1079, 1996.
45. Horvath K, Papadimitriou JC, Rabsztyn A et al: Gastrointestinal abnormalities in children with autistic disorder, *J Pediatr* 135:559-563, 1999.
46. Wakefield AJ, Anthony A, Murch SH et al: Enterocolitis in children with developmental disorders, *Am J Gastroenterol* 95:2285-2295, 2000.
47. Lewine JD, Andrews R, Chez M et al: Magnetoencephalographic patterns of epileptiform activity in children with regressive autism spectrum disorders, *Pediatrics* 104:405-418, 1999.
48. Ward B, Dewals P: Association between measles infection and the occurrence of chronic inflammatory bowel disease, *Can Commun Dis Rep* 23:1-5, 1997.
49. Pardi DS, Tremaine WJ, Sandborn WJ et al: Early measles virus infection is associated with the development of inflammatory bowel disease, *Am J Gastroenterol* 95:1480-1485, 2000.
50. Balzola FA, Khan K, Pera A et al: Measles IgM immunoreactivity in patients with inflammatory bowel disease, *Ital J Gastroenterol Hepatol* 30:378-382, 1998.
51. Vojdani A, Pangborn J: Binding of infectious agents, toxic chemicals, and dietary peptides to tissue enzymes and lymphocyte receptors are instigators of autoimmunity in autism, *Int J Immunopathol Pharmacol* 16:189-199, 2003.
52. Warren RP, Margaretten NC, Foster A: Reduced natural killer cell activity in autism, *J Am Acad Child Adolesc Psychiatry* 26:333-335, 1987.
53. Warren RP, Margaretten NC, Pace NC et al: Immune abnormalities in patients with autism, *J Autism Dev Disord* 16:189-197, 1986.
54. Singh V, Warren R, Odell J et al: Antibodies to myelin basic protein in children with autistic behavior, *Brain Behav Immun* 7:97-103, 1993.
55. Page T, Coleman M: Purine metabolism abnormalities in a hyperuricosuric subclass of autism, *Biochim Biophys Acta* 1500:291-296, 2000.
56. Osterling J, Dawson G: Early recognition of children with autism: a study of first birthday home videotapes, *J Autism Dev Disorders* 24:247-257, 1994.
57. Werner E, Dawson G, Osterling J et al: Brief report: recognition of autism spectrum disorder before one year of age: a retrospective study based on home videotapes, *J Autism Dev Disorders* 30:157-162, 2000.
58. McGinnis W: Oxidative stress in autism, *Altern Ther* 10:22-36, 2004.
59. *Neuroscience and autism*. Available at www.neurorelief.com. Accessed April 15, 2008.
60. Dharmananda S: *Autism* [lecture], Portland, Ore, 1997, Institute for Traditional Medicine.

Acupuncture

1. Maciocia G. *The practice of Chinese medicine: the treatment of diseases with acupuncture and Chinese herbs*, London, 1994, Churchill Livingstone.
2. Loo M: *Pediatric acupuncture*, London, 2002, Elsevier.
3. Deadman P, Al-Khafaji M: *A manual of acupuncture*, Ann Arbor, Mich, 1998, Journal of Chinese Medicine Publications.
4. Maciocia G: *The foundations of Chinese Medicine: a comprehensive text for acupuncturists and herbalists*, London, 1989, Churchill Livingstone.
5. O'Connor J, Bensky D, editors: *Acupuncture: a comprehensive text*, Seattle, 1981, Eastland Press.

Chiropractic

1. Warner SP, Warner TM: Case report: autism and chronic otitis media, *Today's Chiropractic* May/Jun:82-85, 1999.
2. Webster L: Chiropractic and autism, *Chiropractic J* Mar:36, 1995.
3. Amalu W: Autism, asthma, irritable bowel syndrome, strabismus and illness susceptibility: a case study in chiropractic management, *Today's Chiropractic* Sep/Oct:32-47, 1998.
4. Panter J: Kentuckiana: delivering special care for special needs, *Today's Chiropractic*, Sep/Oct:18-22, 2002.
5. Barnes T: Chiropractic management of the special needs child, *Top Clin Chiropractic* 4:9-18, 1997.
6. Barnes T: The story of John… a little boy with autism, *ICA Rev* Nov/Dec, 1996.
7. Khorshid K: Two special children and their parents are fighting autism and winning, *ICA Rev* Fall:59-64, 2001.

8. Potisk TJ: A case study of a five-year-old male with autism/pervasive development disorder who improved remarkably and quickly with chiropractic treatment, *Proceed World Fed Chiropractic Congress* May:320, 2001.

9. Rubenstein H: Case study—autism, *Chiropractic Pediatr* 1:23, 1994.

10. Aguilar AL, Grostic JD, Pfleger B: Chiropractic care and the behavior in autistic children, *J Clin Chirop Pediatr* 5:293-304, 2000.

11. Sandefur R, Adams E: The effect of chiropractic adjustments on the behavior of autistic children: a case review, *ICA J Chiropractic* Dec:21-25, 1987.

12. Delacato CH: *The ultimate stranger*, Novato, CA, 1974, Arena Press.

13. Grandin T: *Thinking in pictures*, New York, 1995, Doubleday.

14. Ornitz E: Neurophysiology of infantile autism, *J Am Acad Child Psychiatry* 24:251-262, 1985.

15. Edelson SM, Edelson MG, Kerr DCR et al: Behavioral and physiological effects of deep pressure on children with autism: a pilot study evaluating the efficacy of Grandin's hug machine, *Am J Occup Ther* 53:145-152, 1999.

16. Giesen MF, Center DB, Leach RA: An evaluation of chiropractic manipulation as a treatment of hyperactivity in children, *J Manipulative Physiol Ther* 12:353-363, 1989.

17. White JF: Intestinal pathophysiology in autism, *Exp Biol Med* 228:639-649, 2003.

18. Feingold Association of the United States: *Studies on diet, health and behavior*, Riverhead, NY, 2002, Feingold Association of the United States.

19. Reichelt KL, Ekrem J, Scott H: Gluten, milk proteins and autism: dietary intervention effects on behavior and peptide secretion, *J Appl Nutr* 42:1-11, 1990.

20. Cornish E: Gluten and casein free diets in autism: a study of the effect on food choice and nutrition, *J Hum Nutr Dietet* 15:261-269, 2002.

21. Kidd PM: Attention deficit/hyperactivity disorder (ADHD) in children: rationale for its integrative management, *Altern Med Rev* 5:402-428, 2001.

22. Fallon JD: Otitis media and autism in childhood: is there a relationship? *ICA Rev* Fall:67-71, 2001.

23. Garvey F: Diet in autism and associated disorders, *J Fam Health Care* 12:34-38, 2002.

24. Willatts P, Forsyth JS: The role of long chain polyunsaturated fatty acids in infant cognitive development, *Prostaglandins Leukot Essent Fatty Acids* 63:95-100, 2000.

25. Makrides M, Neumann M, Simmer K et al: Are long-chain polyunsaturated fatty acids essential nutrients in infancy? *Lancet* 345:1463-1468, 1995.

26. Bennett CN, Horrobin DF: Gene targets related phospholipid and fatty acid metabolism in schizophrenia and other psychiatric disorders: an update, *Prostaglandins Leukot Essent Fatty Acids* 63:47-59, 2000.

27. Megson M: Is autism a G-alpha protein defect reversible with natural vitamin A? *Med Hypotheses* 54:979-983, 2000.

28. Walker SJ, Segal J, Aschner M: Cultured lymphocytes from autistic children and non-autistic siblings up-regulate heat shock protein RNA in response to thimerosal challenge, *Neuro Toxicol* 27:685-692, 2006.

29. Mousain-Bosc M, Roche M, Polge A et al: Improvement of neurobehavioral disorders in children supplemented with magnesium-vitamin B6, *Magnes Res* 19:53-62, 2006.

30. Vogellar A: *Studying the effects of essential nutrients and environmental factors on autistic behavior*, San Diego, 2000, Autism Research Institute.

31. Shattock P, Whiteley P: *The Sunderland protocol: a logical sequencing of biomedical intervention for the treatment of autism and related disorders*, Sunderland, United Kingdom, 2000, University of Sunderland Autism Research Unit.

32. Bradstreet J, Kartzinel J: Biological interventions in the treatment of autism and PDD. In Rimland B, editor: *DAN! 2001 Fall Conference*, San Diego, Calif, 2001, Autism Research Institute.

33. Laidler JR: *Mercury detoxification consensus group position paper*, San Diego, Calif, 2001, DAN! Think Tank; Autism Research Institute.

34. Kidd PM: Freedom from toxins: reducing our total toxic load, *Total Health* 22:22-27, 2000.

35. Holmes A: Heavy metal toxicity in autistic spectrum disorders. In Rimland B, editor: *DAN! 2001 Fall Conference*, San Diego, Calif, 2001, Autism Research Institute.

36. Baranek GT: Efficacy of sensory and motor intervention for children with autism, *J Autism Dev Disord* 32:397-422, 2002.

Herbs—Western

1. Oken BS, Storzbach DM, Kaye JA: The efficacy of *Ginkgo biloba* on cognitive function in Alzheimer disease,. *Arch Neurol* 55:1409-1415, 1998.

2. Sorensen H, Sonne J: A double-masked study of the effects of ginseng on cognitive functions, *Curr Ther Res* 57:959-968, 1996.

3. McGuffin M, Hobbs C, Upton R et al, editors: *American Herbal Products Association's botanical safety handbook*, Boca Raton, Fla, 1997, CRC Press.

Homeopathy

1. *ReferenceWorks Pro 4.2*, San Rafael, Calif, 2008, Kent Homeopathic Associates.

Massage Therapy

1. Fleming-Drehobl K, Gengler-Fuhr M: *Pediatric massage for the child with special needs*, Tucson, Ariz, 1991, Therapy Skill Builders.

2. Field T, Lasko D, Mundy P et al: Brief report: autistic children's attentiveness and responsivity improve after touch therapy, *J Autism Dev Disord* 27:333-338, 1997.

3. Cullen L, Barlow J: Kiss, cuddle, squeeze: the experiences and meaning of touch among parents of children with autism attending a Touch Therapy Program, *J Child Health Care* 6:171-181, 2002.

Mind/Body

1. Mullins J, Christian L: The effects of progressive relaxation training on the disruptive behavior of a boy with autism, *Res Dev Disabil* 22:449-462, 2001.

Naturopathy

1. Schneider C, Melmed R: Presentation at Medical Basis of Autism Conference, Phoenix, Ariz, 2000.

2. Wakefield AJ, Anthony A, Murch SH et al: Enterocolitis in children with developmental disorders, *Am J Gastroenterol* 95:2285-2295, 2000.

3. Horvath K, Papadimitriou JC, Rabsztyn A et al: Gastrointestinal abnormalities in children with autistic disorder, *J Pediatr* 135:559-563, 1999.

4. Walsh W: Presentation at Defeat Autism Now! Conference, San Diego, Calif, 2001.

5. Wakefield AJ, Murch SH, Anthony A et al. Ileal-lymphoid-nodular hyperplasia, non-specific colitis, and pervasive developmental disorder in children, *Lancet* 351:637-641, 1998.

6. Dolske MC, Spollen J, McKay S et al. A preliminary trial of ascorbic acid as supplemental therapy for autism, *Prog Neuropsychopharmacol Biol Psychiatry* 17:765-774, 1993.

7. Barthelmey C, Garreau B, Leddet I et al: Behavioral and biological effect of oral magnesium, vitamin B6, and combined magnesium-B6 administration in autistic children, *Magnes Bull* 3:150-153, 1981.

8. Barthelmey C, Garreau B, Leddet I et al: Interet des eschelles de componement et des doages de l'acide homovanillque urinarie pour le controls des effets d'un traitement associant vitamin B6 et magnesium chez des enfants ayant un comportement autsigu. *Neuropsychiaurie de l'Enfance* 31:289-301, 1983.

9. Bonish VE: Erfahrungen mit pryithosin bei hirngeschadigten kinder mit autischem syndrom, *Proxis der Kinderpsychologie* 8:308-310, 1968.

10. Coleman M, Steinberg G, Tippell J et al: A preliminary study of the effect of pryidoxine administration in a subgroup of hyperkinetic children: a double blind crossover comparison with methylphenidate, *Biol Psychiatry* 4:741-751, 1979.

11. Ellman G: *Pyridoxine effectiveness on autistic patients at Sonoma State Hospital,* Paper presented at Research Conference on Autism, November 1, 1981, San Diego.

12. Garner C, Conroy E, Barthelemy C et al: Dopamine-beta hyroxylase (DBH) and homovanillic acid (HVA) in autistic children, *J Autism Dev Disord* 16:23-29, 1986.

13. Gaulterir CT, Von Bourgonndien ME, Hartx C et al: *Pilot study of pyridozine treatment in autistic children,* Paper presented at American Psychiatric Association meeting, New Orleans, May 1981.

14. Jonas C, Etienne T, Barthelemy C et al: Interetclinique et biochimque de l'associaton vitamine B6 + magnesium dans le traitement de l'autisme residuel à l'age adulte, *Therapie* 39:661-669, 1994.

15. LeLord G, Muh JP, Barthelemy C et al: Effects of pryidozine and magnesium on autistic symptoms: initial observations, *J Autism Dev Disord* 11:219-230, 1981.

16. LeLord G, Muh JP, Barthelemy C et al: Clinical and biological effects of vitamin B6 + magnesium in autistic subjects. In Leklem J, Reynolds R, editors: *Vitamin B6 responsive disorders in humans,* New York, 1988, Alan R. Liss.

17. Martineau J, Garreau B, Barthelemy C et al: Comparative effects of oral B6, B6-Mg, and Mg administration on evoked potentials conditioning in autistic children. In Rothenberger A, editor: *Proceedings: symposium on event-related potentials in children,* Amsterdam, 1982, Elsevier Biomedical Press.

18. Martineau J, Barthelemy C, Garreau B et al: Vitamin B6, magnesium and combined B6-Mg: therapeutic effects in childhood autism, *Biol Psychiatry* 20:467-468, 1985.

19. Martineau J, Barthelemy C, Lelord G: Long-term effects of combined vitamin B6-magnesium administration in an autistic child, *Biol Psychiatry* 21:511-518, 1986.

20. Rimland B: High dosage levels of certain vitamins in the treatment of children with severe mental disorders. In Hawkins D, Pauling L, editors: *Orthomolecular psychiatry,* New York, 1973, WH Freeman.

21. Rimland B: An orthomolecular study of psychotic children, *Orthomolec Psychiatry* 3:371-377, 1974.

22. Rimland B, Callaway E, Dreyfus P: The effects of high doses of vitamin B6 on autistic children: a double-blind crossover study, *Am J Psychiatry* 135:472-475, 1978.

23. Rimland B: Megavitamin B6 and magnesium in the treatment of autistic children and adolescents. In Schopler E, Mesibov GB, editors: *Neurobiological issues in autism,* New York, 1987, Plenum, pp 389-405.

24. Rossl P, Visconti P, Bergossi A et al: *Effects of vitamin B6 and magnesium therapy in autism,* Conference on the Neurobiology of Infantile Autism, Nov 10-11, 1990, Tokyo.

Nutrition

1. Eisenhofer G, Kopin IJ, Goldstein DS: Leaky catecholamine stores: undue waste or a stress response coping mechanism? *Ann N Y Acad Sci* 1018:224-230, 2004.

2. Reichelt KL, Knivsber AM: Can the pathophysiology of autism be explained by the nature of the discovered urine peptides? *Nutr Neurosci* 6:19-28, 2003.

3. D'Eufemia P, Celli M, Finocchiaro R et al: Abnormal intestinal permeability in children with autism, *Acta Paediatr* 85:1076-1079, 1996.

4. Bell JG, MacKinlay EE, Dick JR et al: Essential fatty acids and phospholipase A2 in autistic spectrum disorders, *Prostaglandin Leukot Essent Fatty Acids* 71:201-204, 2004.

5. Walsh WJ, Usman A, Tarpey J: *Disordered metal metabolism in a large autism population,* APA Annual Meeting, May 2001, New Orleans.

6. *Autism and Neurotoxins.* Available at www.neuroscienceinc.com.

7. Knivsber AM, Reichelt KL, Hoien T et al: A randomized, controlled study of dietary intervention in autistic syndromes, *Nutr Neurosci* 5:251-261, 2002.

8. Kidd P: Autism, an extreme challenge to integrative medicine, part II: medical management, *Alt Med Rev* 7:472-499, 2002.

Osteopathy

1. Upledger JE: Craniosacral function in brain dysfunction, *Osteopath Ann* 11:318-324, 1983.

2. Bramati-Castellarin I, Janossa M: Effect of visceral osteopathy on the gastrointestinal abnormalities in children with autistic disorders [see comments; meeting abstract], *J Osteopath Med (Austr)* 5:36-37, 2005.

3. Frymann VM, Carney RE, Springall P: Effect of osteopathic medical management on neurological development in children, *J Am Osteopathic Assoc* 92:729-744, 1992.

4. *The selected writings of Beryl E. Aurbuckle, D.O., F.A.C.O.P.,* Indianapolis, 1994, American Academy of Osteopathy.

5. Lassovetskaya L: Osteopathic treatment of schoolchildren with delayed psychic development of cerebral-organic origin, *J Osteopath Med (Austr)* 6:38, 2003.

6. Wales AL: *Osteopathic approach to the child with autism,* 2004.

7. Frymann VM: *Learning disabilities in childhood,* 1992 [unpublished work].

8. Infants and children. In Magoun HIS, editor: *Osteopathy in the cranial field,* Kirksville, Mo, 1951, CJ Krehbiel.

9. Magoun HIS: *Osteopathy in the cranial field,* ed 3, Kirksville, Mo, 1976, The Journal Printing.

10. Upledger JE: The relationship of craniosacral examination findings in grade school children with developmental problems, *J Am Osteopathic Assoc* 77:760-776, 1978.

11. Sutherland WG: *Contributions of thought,* ed 2, Portland, Ore, 1998, Rudra Press.

12. Sutherland WG: *Teachings in the science of osteopathy,* Portland, Ore, 1990, Rudra Press.

Probiotics

1. Brudnak MA: Probiotics as an adjuvant to detoxification protocols, *Med Hypotheses* 58:382, 2002.

CHAPTER 15

Bronchiolitis (Croup)

Acupuncture | May Loo

Chiropractic | Anne Spicer

Herbs—Chinese | Catherine Ulbricht, Jennifer Woods, Mark Wright

Homeopathy | Janet L. Levatin

Magnet Therapy | Agatha P. Colbert, Deborah Risotti

Massage Therapy | Mary C. McLellan

Osteopathy | Jane Carreiro

✳ PEDIATRIC DIAGNOSIS AND TREATMENT

Bronchiolitis is one of the most common acute, contagious, lower respiratory tract infections in infancy and early childhood.[1] By age 2 years nearly all children have been infected with respiratory syncytial virus (RSV).[2-4]

The disease is most severe among infants aged 1 to 3 months[5] and accounts for the largest number of hospital admissions for pediatric respiratory conditions. More than 100,000 U.S. infants—as many as 3% of all children in their first year of life[6]—are hospitalized with bronchiolitis annually, at an estimated cost of $700 million[1] and resulting in 3000 to 4000 deaths annually.[2] RSV is the major cause of bronchiolitis worldwide.[7-11] Other viral agents that cause bronchiolitis include human rhinoviruses (HRVs),[12] parainfluenza, and adenovirus.[13] Bacterial infection occurs only as a secondary superinfection.

Bronchiolitis is seasonal, with peak activity during winter and early spring.[8] The risk factors are babies less than 3 months old who are not being breastfed, crowded living conditions,[8] passive smoke exposure,[14] prematurity, cardiopulmonary disease, and immunodeficiency.[2,3,7,9,10]

RSV is a nonsegmented, single-stranded ribonucleic acid (RNA), negative-sense, enveloped virus.[2,10,15] The illness usually begins when the baby is exposed to an older sibling with mild upper respiratory tract symptoms—the RSV manifestation in older children.[3] An interplay of direct viral cytopathic effects and host inflammatory responses determines the severity of illness.[16,17]

RSV infection incites a complex and elaborate immune response involving eosinophils, immunoglobulin (Ig)-E antibodies, and a wide variety of cytokines and chemokines that trigger further inflammatory responses.[2,4,10] The vulnerable baby—such as one with a strong family history of asthma or other risk factors—develops respiratory distress and wheezing due to bronchiolar obstruction, which in turn lead to air trapping and overinflation. If obstruction is complete with resorption of trapped air, the child will then develop atelectasis. Normal pulmonary gas exchange is impaired, and the baby becomes hypoxic and even hypercapnic in severe cases. Chest radiography reveals hyperinflated lungs with patchy atelectasis. During the first 48 to 72 hours after onset of cough and dyspnea, the infant is at highest risk for further respiratory compromise.[8] Epidemiological and natural history studies have clearly demonstrated a link between bronchiolitis in infancy and asthma in later years.[4,11,14,18-20] One possible mechanism is that the RSV bronchiolitis enhances the development of "allergic" inflammatory responses when the child is later exposed to allergens.[21]

Treatment of RSV bronchiolitis is challenging and complicated because of the multifactorial nature of this infection.[17] Mild cases can be treated with supportive therapies such as fluids to prevent dehydration, nasal suctioning, and supplemental oxygen.[5] Infants younger than age 3 months, high-risk infants, and children in significant respiratory distress should be hospitalized. The mainstay of treatment is still supportive,[22] although medications are often used.[8,16] Overall, there is little evidence to support the usage of bronchodilators, corticosteroids, and the antiviral agent ribavirin.[6] Inhaled β2-agonist bronchodilators may produce modest short-term improvement in infants with mild or moderate bronchiolitis.[23] Usage of corticosteroids remains controversial when the antiinflammatory effects are weighed against the potent side effects in infants.[5,8,24] Antibiotics should not be used unless secondary bacterial pneumonia is present.

The best treatment is prevention. Parents and family members should be educated about hand washing, cleaning environmental surfaces, isolating infants and children with infection, and avoiding crowded places such as busy daycare centers.[17] Two immunoprophylaxis products, RSV intravenous immune globulin (RSV-IGIV) and palivizumab, a humanized murine monoclonal antibody, have been developed for clinical use in the prevention of serious RSV infection.[3,5] The American Academy of Pediatrics issued a policy statement in 2003 recommending prophylaxis for high-risk infants, and palivizumab is preferred over RSV-IGIV because of its ease of administration, safety, and effectiveness.[25] The Centers for Disease Control and Prevention have marked vaccine development for RSV as "a high priority."[26] Fortunately, the prognosis for the majority of normal infants who develop bronchiolitis is good.[7]

✳ CAM THERAPY RECOMMENDATIONS

Acupuncture

See Chapter 12, Asthma.

Chiropractic

Bronchiolitis

To date, there are no case studies or clinical trials by chiropractors in the management of bronchiolitis. However, this respiratory infection would be managed similarly to other respiratory conditions through elimination of physical, chemical, and emotional stressors. Evidence does exist that the chiropractic adjustment may be useful in minimizing respiratory conditions such as chronic obstructive pulmonary disease,[1] asthma,[2,3] and somatic dyspnea.[4] One study involving 55 patients showed improved lung function after the chiropractic adjustment to the upper cervical spine regardless of whether prior lung function was in the normal range or depressed.[5] In a study involving more than 4600 incidents of upper respiratory infections, only 5% of cases treated with spinal manipulative therapy developed secondary complications.[6] This is especially meaningful because bronchiolitis commonly begins with an upper respiratory tract infection.

After ruling out acute respiratory distress and dehydration, the chiropractor would assess the spinal column for evidence of the subluxation complex (SC), which interferes with optimal neurological function—thus diminishing immunological capacity. Any SC would be adjusted via a low-amplitude osseous maneuver with a velocity that is reflective of the child's age and condition. Evaluation for SC during this acute illness may be required daily owing to strong viscerosomatic reflexes secondary to the dense presence of chemoreceptors in the bronchial tree.[7] Commonly, an SC is identified in the upper cervical spine (relating to vagal or phrenic innervation), the upper thoracic spine (relating to primary respiratory musculature and sympathetics), and the cranium (relating to the primary respiratory mechanism).[8,9]

Maintenance of hydration is a must. Weight loss or clinical signs of dehydration are causes for medical referral. An urgent referral must also be made when the child shows signs of respiratory distress, such as dyspnea, retractions, diminished breath sounds, or cyanosis.

Percussion can be performed over the upper thoracic vertebrae (T1 to T4) by vigorously tapping over the spinous process with the fingertips. Intervals of 5 seconds of rapid percussion, followed by 15-second rests, repeated for 2 minutes, provides stimulation to the sympathetics.

Stimulation of the neurolymphatics is supportive. The points are located at the second intercostal space adjacent to the sternum and bilaterally on the posterior body wall, midway between the T2 spinous process and the tip of the transverse process.[10] Stimulation of these points is best achieved with firm focal massage.

Gentle hand-cupping percussion over the lung fields may improve drainage if administered with the child in a reverse incline position with the head lower than the thorax.[11]

Supplementation of immune-enhancing nutrients may prove beneficial. Vitamin C may be given to the young infant in the form of rose hip syrup or a buffered powder formula and should be dosed within gut tolerance.[7] An initial dose of 250 mg is a good starting place to aid in thinning of mucus. Zinc is available in liquid formulations for use in infants and toddlers and is vital to normal immune function. Other common recommendations include vitamin A/β-carotene and gut microflora to support the immune function, omega-3 fatty acids and eicospentaenoic acid/docosahexapentacnoic (EPA/DHA) for their antiinflammatory actions, vitamin E for its antioxidant and antiinflammatory properties,[12] and selenium for its potent

antioxidant capacity along with magnesium, because higher levels of both of these nutrients are associated with fewer respiratory abnormalities.[13-15]

The patient would be recommended to avoid consumption of dairy-based products during the course of the illness, as they have a tendency to increase mucous production.

Echinacea purpurea may be safely used as an immune stimulant.[16,17]

In the older child, blowing up balloons provides respiratory therapy in an enjoyable manner.

Croup

After ruling out acute respiratory distress and dehydration, the chiropractor would assess the spinal column for evidence of the SC, which interferes with optimal neurological function—thus diminishing immunological capacity. Any SC would be adjusted via a low-amplitude osseous maneuver with a velocity that is reflective of the child's age and condition. Commonly, an SC is identified in the upper cervical spine, the upper thoracic spine, and the cranium.[1,2]

Maintenance of hydration is a must.

Respiratory exposure to cool mist is often beneficial. If this is not sufficient to manage a mild episode of croup, then gradual exposure to steam, such as resting in an unventilated shower stall or bathroom with running hot water, may also prove useful. This can be followed by respiratory exposure to cool outdoor air, provided the child is bundled warmly.

Percussion can be performed over the upper thoracic vertebrae (T1 to T4) with the fingertips. An interval of 5 seconds of rapid percussion, followed by a 15-second rest, and then repeated for 2 minutes, provides stimulation to the sympathetics.

Stimulation of the neurolymphatics is also supportive to croup. The points are located at the first and second intercostal spaces adjacent to the sternum and bilaterally on the posterior body wall, midway between the T1 and T2 spinous processes and the tips of the corresponding transverse processes.[3]

Gentle hand-cupping percussion over the lung fields may discourage progression to the lungs if administered with the child in a reverse incline position with the head lower than the thorax.[4]

Supplementation of immune-enhancing nutrients may prove beneficial. Vitamin C may be given to the young infant in the form of rose hip syrup and should be dosed within gut tolerance.[5] An initial dose of 250 mg is a good starting place to aid in thinning of mucus. Zinc is available in liquid formulations for use in infants and toddlers and is vital to normal immune function. Other common recommendations include vitamin A/β-carotene and gut microflora to support the immune function, omega-3 fatty acids EPA/DHA for their antiinflammatory actions, vitamin E for its antioxidant and antiinflammatory properties,[6] and selenium for its potent antioxidant capacity along with magnesium because, higher levels of these nutrients are associated with fewer breathing abnormalities.[7-9]

The patient would be advised to avoid consumption of dairy-based products during the course of the illness, as they have a tendency to increase mucus production, thereby complicating the bronchiolar obstruction.

E. purpurea may be safely used as an immune stimulant.[10,11]

Emergency medical referral is necessary if the child with croup becomes cyanotic or shows signs of respiratory distress. An uncommon complication of croup is development of epiglottitis. The child will drool and have difficulty vocalizing. Observation of the oropharynx will reveal a visible, red epiglottis. Asphyxiation is possible from this condition and obviously makes this a critical medical emergency.

Herbs—Chinese

Preliminary research suggests that the Chinese herb Shuang Huang Lian may improve symptoms including cough, fever, wheezing, and chest signs as well as duration of stay in the hospital. Although Shuang Huang Lian may be safe and effective for treating bronchiolitis in children, more research is needed to verify efficacy of the herb.[1,2] Another study found that KingTo Nin Jiom Pei Pa Kao, a sweet Chinese cough syrup made from 15 different herbs—including bulb of *Fritillaria cirrhosa* D. Don (Chuan Bei Mu), leaf of *Eriobotrya japonica* (Thunb.) Lindl. (Pi Pa Ye), root of *Platycodon grandiflorum* (Jacq.) A. DC. (Jie Geng), mature pericarp of *Citrus reticulata* Blanco (Chen Pi), kernel of *Prunus armeniaca* L. (Xing Ren), root of *Glycyrrhiza uralensis* Fisch. (Gan Cao), fruit of *Schisandra chinensis* (Turcz.) Baill. (Wu Wei Zi), tuber of *Pinellia ternata* (Thunb.) Breitenb. (Ban Xia), root of *Adenophora tetraphylla* (Thunb.) Fisch. (Nan Sha Shen), stem and leaf of *Mentha haplocalyx* Briq. (Bo He), and honey—may have significant cough-relieving and sputum-removing effects.[2,3] The syrup is generally taken at 10 mL (2 tsp) for adults and 5 mL (1 tsp) for children, three times daily by mouth or stirred into hot water. Daily use is acceptable over a long period and is also regarded as being beneficial for tobacco smokers.[4] Further research is needed before a recommendation can be made.

According to TCM, the formula is also applicable for dry cough with little or no phlegm. The formula contains a number of herbs considered to "nourish the Yin" and "moisten dryness;" therefore, it would not be appropriate for a loose, productive cough. In the clinical experience of this author's associate, the formulation is best suited for low-grade, non-acute coughs that are not resolving and that can therefore be treated by a relatively gentle approach over a period of a week or more. In acute cases of cough, a more focused prescription would be preferable.

Homeopathy

Before using this section, please see Appendix A, Homeopathy, for definitions of practitioner expertise categories and general information on prescribing homeopathic medicines.

Practitioner Expertise Category 1

Category 1 includes bronchiolitis/croup with mild to moderate symptoms.

Practitioner Expertise Category 2

Category 2 includes bronchiolitis/croup with moderate to severe symptoms.

There are no controlled clinical trials of homeopathic treatment for bronchiolitis and croup, although the homeopathic literature contains much evidence for its use in the form of accumulated clinical experience.[1] Bronchiolitis and croup can often be treated very effectively with homeopathy. For bronchiolitis and croup unassociated with severe respiratory distress, respiratory compromise, or significant feeding difficulties, it is safe to try homeopathic treatment for 2 or 3 days prior to beginning conventional therapy or in combination with other therapies, either conventional or alternative. If more serious symptoms are present, conventional treatment should be sought for the patient without delay.

The goal in treating bronchiolitis and croup homeopathically is to determine the single homeopathic medicine whose description in the materia medica most closely matches the symptom picture of the patient. Often mental and emotional states, in addition to physical symptoms, are considered.

For croup, once the medicine has been selected, it can be given orally or sublingually in the 30C potency once every 15 to 60 minutes (use more frequent dosing when symptoms are more severe); for bronchiolitis, once the medicine has been selected, it can be given orally or sublingually three to four times daily. If the medicine has not helped in four to five doses, then another homeopathic medicine should be tried or some other form of therapy should be instituted, as needed. Once symptoms have begun to resolve, the medicine can be given less frequently or stopped. It can be repeated again for a relapse of symptoms.

The following is a list of homeopathic medicines commonly used to treat patients with bronchiolitis and croup. There are numerous homeopathic medicines for coughs caused by a variety of etiologies and with a variety of symptomatic expressions. It must be emphasized that this list is partial and represents only some of the probable choices from the homeopathic materia medica. If the symptoms of a given patient are not represented here, a search of the homeopathic literature would be needed to find the simillimum.

Bronchiolitis

Antimonium tartaricum

Antimonium tartaricum is one of the main homeopathic medicines to consider for bronchiolitis. The cough is loose and rattling, and the breathing may sound rattling. The chest sounds full of mucus, but the child may be too weak to expel it. Symptoms may be worse starting at 10 PM.

Ipecacuanha

Ipecacuanha should be considered when the patient has a dry, paroxysmal cough. The cough is accompanied by gagging, choking, retching, and/or vomiting. Symptoms are worse in the evening, from eating, or in a warm room and are better following cold drinks.

Kali sulphuricum

Kali sulphuricum is used for bronchiolitis accompanied by a rattling in the chest and a production of thick yellow mucus. There may also be nasal obstruction and postnasal drip. The patient is worse in the evening and at 2 AM or in a warm room and are better in cool, open air and from cold drinks.

Croup

Aconitum napellus

Aconitum napellus is the first homeopathic medicine to consider at the onset of acute croup. Usually the child who needs *Aconitum napellus* aconite awakens from sleep with the typical dry, barky cough of croup. The child is frightened, restless, and agitated. Croup responsive to *Aconitum napellus* often begins after exposure to a dry wind. If symptoms are severe, *Aconitum napellus* can be given and repeated every few minutes while the patient is en route to access emergency care.

Spongia tosta

Spongia tosta is also used for croup with the typical dry, barky cough, but it is usually given a little later in the course of the disease than is *Aconitum napellus*. The attack is worst around midnight. The cough is better when the child eats, drinks, or nurses; however, cold drinks may aggravate the condition. As for the child needing *Aconitum napellus,* he or she should be taken to an emergency care facility if symptoms are severe or the child is in respiratory distress.

Hepar sulphuris calcareum

Hepar sulphurus calcareum is used for croup with an onset at 2 to 4 AM or later in the morning. The cough is typically looser in character than the coughs seen in patients needing *Aconitum napellus* or *Spongia tosta*. The child is very sensitive to cold air, cold drinks, or becoming cold.

Magnet Therapy

Place an Accu-Band 800-G magnet on KD27, the tiny protrusion (bionorth) facing the skin bilaterally, and an 800-G Accu-Band magnet with the smooth side facing the skin on CV17.[1] Then palpate the upper back for tender points bilaterally near medial edge of each scapula. Place alternating north/south magnets (Accu-Band 800-G magnet) on tender points (maximum of two per side). Leave all magnets in place for 15 minutes. Treatment may be repeated two times per day. These magnets may be obtained from OMS (800-323-1839) or AHSM (800-635-7070).

Massage Therapy

In 1998, Children's Hospital Boston established the Center for Holistic Pediatric Education and Research (CHPER) to provide complementary and alternative medicine (CAM) consultations and education to inpatients at this hospital. Between 1999 and 2004, 762 consults were provided to patients on the pulmonary service; the chief complaints initiating the consultation were pain in the back, upper body, chest, and neck as well as anxiety. Chest, shoulder, neck, and back discomfort may develop from persistent cough during acute or chronic respiratory infections.[1-3] This pain or discomfort could lead to ineffective cough and deep breathing as a result of splinting.[1-3] To help decrease the musculoskeletal pain associated with coughing, children experiencing respiratory infections could benefit from back, shoulder, and anterior chest wall massage therapy with particular attention to the intercostals, scalenes, serratus, pectorals, and trapezius. Should cough-related pain or discomfort

extend to the abdomen, massage to the intercostals and external obliques may also be helpful. If children are splinting with cough or laughter or are indicating that it hurts too much to laugh, this would be a good indication of trying some massage to improve their comfort level. Children experiencing respiratory illness may feel more comfortable in an upright position during treatment rather than lying down. To treat the child in an upright position, they can be positioned in a chair with the head supported by a tabletop pillow or in the parent's lap. Infants and young children can readily be treated while cradled on their parent's shoulder or chest.

In addition to massage being helpful for cough-related pain, massage can also help relax or calm the child or infant who may be experiencing increased work of breathing or intermittent bronchospasms from their illness. Controlled studies have demonstrated decreased anxiety levels in children receiving parental Swedish massage who are diagnosed with asthma or cystic fibrosis.[4,5] These studies have also demonstrated increased peak flow readings and improved pulmonary function tests in the massage group compared with controls. Small studies in adult populations with pulmonary disease have also demonstrated improved peak flows[6,7] as well as decreased respiratory rate and increased chest wall expansion.[7]

Chest physiotherapy (CPT), which incorporates percussion and vibration, originated from use of massage in postoperative patients in the seventeenth century.[8] CPT has become a standard of care in hospital settings to prevent and treat atelectasis, ineffective cough, and respiratory secretion management.

Osteopathy

For osteopathic physicians, there are four important aspects to remember when dealing with children with respiratory disease. First, children have less elastic recoil in the lung parenchyma and more compliancy in the distal airways. This translates into an increased vulnerability for collapse and atelectasis. Second, the bronchial smooth muscle in children is thicker and more reactive, with a tendency for bronchospasm when irritated. Third, the musculoskeletal structures involved with breathing are mechanically and neurologically less effective than in adolescents. Fourth, the infant lung has more secretory glands such that when inflammation does occur, mucus production increases to a greater extent than in the adult.

The mechanics of breathing in toddlers and infants differ significantly from those used in older children. The compliancy of the thoracic cage limits the ventilatory pressures that the child can achieve. Too much pressure will cause the ribcage to retract, effectively inhibiting lung expansion. Efforts to increase oxygenation by increasing respiratory rate may also fail owing to the immaturity of the innervation patterns of respiratory muscles. Diseases that result in inflammation of the lung tissues are more likely to cause bronchospasm in children. Bronchial lymphatics play an important role in removing fluid and inflammatory products. Rhythmic fluctuations in intrathoracic pressure facilitate lymphatic drainage from the lungs and thoracic tissues via the low-pressure circulatory system. Children with restriction of respiratory mechanics may be unable to generate enough variation in pressures to facilitate this lymphatic pumping mechanism, thus prolonging tissue exposure to cellular waste and antigenic material. Biomechanical restrictions or strains in the muscles that stabilize the thoracic cage, such as the quadratus lumborum, scalene, trapezius, and serratus muscles, will alter respiratory volumes.

Osteopathic techniques focus on supporting respiratory mechanics to decrease the work of breathing. Addressing factors that might adversely affect pulmonary bronchial smooth muscle tone and pulmonary vascular tone is also important. These factors would include musculoskeletal findings indicative of vagus nerve irritation and the presence of somatic dysfunction that may influence autonomic tone via somatovisceral reflexes. An additional goal of osteopathic treatment would be supporting optimal function of the neuroendocrine-immune system through decreasing somatic nociception. Although there are no published data on the efficacy of osteopathic treatment in children with bronchiolitis, several published studies show improvements in respiratory function and decrease in illness parameters in adults.[1-9] Furthermore, specific osteopathic lymphatic techniques have been shown to be beneficial in stimulating immune responses[1,10-18] and decreasing symptoms of infection[2,5,9] in adults.

References

Pediatric Diagnosis and Treatment

1. Kuppermann N: Research network studying corticosteroid use for bronchiolitis, *Infect Dis Child* 39:12-13, 2005.
2. Ogra PL: Respiratory syncytial virus: the virus, the disease and the immune response, *Paediatr Respir Rev* 5(Suppl A):S119-S126, 2004.
3. Weisman LE: Current respiratory syncytial virus prevention strategies in high-risk infants, *Pediatr Int* 44:475-480, 2002.
4. Psarras S, Papadopoulos NG, Johnston SL: Pathogenesis of respiratory syncytial virus bronchiolitis-related wheezing, *Paediatr Respir Rev* 5(Suppl A):S179-S184, 2004.
5. Steiner RW: Treating acute bronchiolitis associated with RSV, *Am Fam Physician* 69:325-330, 2004.
6. King VJ, Viswanathan M, Bordley WC et al: Pharmacologic treatment of bronchiolitis in infants and children: a systematic review, *Arch Pediatr Adolesc Med* 158:127-137, 2004.
7. Jhawar S: Severe bronchiolitis in children, *Clin Rev Allergy Immunol* 25:249-257, 2003.
8. Behrman RE, Kliegman RM, Jenson HB, editors: *Nelson's textbook of pediatrics*, Philadelphia, 2004, Saunders.
9. Meissner HC: Selected populations at increased risk from respiratory syncytial virus infection, *Pediatr Infect Dis J* 22(2 Suppl): S40-S44. discussion S44-S45, 2003.
10. Welliver RC: Review of epidemiology and clinical risk factors for severe respiratory syncytial virus (RSV) infection, *J Pediatr* 143 (5 Suppl):S112-S117, 2003.
11. Openshaw PJ, Dean GS, Culley FJ: Links between respiratory syncytial virus bronchiolitis and childhood asthma: clinical and research approaches, *Pediatr Infect Dis J* 22(2 Suppl):S58-S64. discussion S64-S65, 2003.
12. Hayden FG: Rhinovirus and the lower respiratory tract, *Rev Med Virol* 14:17-31, 2004.
13. Rocholl C, Gerber K, Daly J et al: Adenoviral infections in children: the impact of rapid diagnosis, *Pediatrics* 113:e51-e56, 2004.
14. Gern JE: Viral respiratory infection and the link to asthma, *Pediatr Infect Dis J* 23(1 Suppl):S78-S86, 2004.
15. Rusk J: RSV presents same challenges, needs new approaches, *Infect Dis Child* 18:62-64, 2005.
16. Ovetchkine P: Antibiotic therapy for lower tract infections in children [in French], *Arch Pediatr* 11:1277-1281, 2004.
17. Jafri HS: Treatment of respiratory syncytial virus: antiviral therapies, *Pediatr Infect Dis J* 22(2 Suppl):S89-S92. discussion S92-S93, 2003.
18. Liu AH: Consider the child: how early should we treat? *J Allergy Clin Immunol* 113(1 Suppl):S19-S24, 2004.
19. Peebles RS Jr: Viral infections, atopy, and asthma: is there a causal relationship? *J Allergy Clin Immunol* 113(1 Suppl):S15-S18, 2004.
20. Martinez FD: Respiratory syncytial virus bronchiolitis and the pathogenesis of childhood asthma, *Pediatr Infect Dis J* 22 (2 Suppl):S76-S82, 2003.
21. Piedimonte G: Contribution of neuroimmune mechanisms to airway inflammation and remodeling during and after respiratory syncytial virus infection, *Pediatr Infect Dis J* 22(2 Suppl):S66-S74. discussion S74-S75, 2003.
22. Domachowske JB, Rosenberg HF: Advances in the treatment and prevention of severe viral bronchiolitis, *Pediatr Ann* 34:35-41, 2005.
23. Hartling L, Wiebe N, Russell K, et al: Epinephrine for bronchiolitis, *Cochrane Database Syst Rev* (1):CD003123, 2004.
24. Patel H, Platt R, Lozano JM, et al: Glucocorticoids for acute viral bronchiolitis in infants and young children, *Cochrane Database Syst Rev* (3):CD004878, 2004.
25. American Academy of Pediatrics Committee on Infectious Diseases and Committee on Fetus and Newborn Policy Statement: Revised indications for the use of palivizumab and respiratory syncytial virus immune globulin intravenous for the prevention of respiratory syncytial virus infections, *Pediatrics* 112:1442-1446, 2003.
26. Centers for Disease Control and Prevention: *Respiratory syncytial virus*. Available at www.cdc.gov/nicod/dvrd/revb/respiratory/rsvfeat.htm. Accessed August 2005.

Chiropractic

Bronchiolitis

1. Miller WD: Treatment of visceral disorder by manipulative therapy, In Goldstein M, editor: *The research status of spinal manipulative therapy*, Bethesda, Md, 1975, National Institiute of Neurological and Communicative Disorders and Stroke.
2. Nilsson N, Christiansen B: Prognostic factors in bronchial asthma in chiropractic practice, *Chiropractic J Austr* 18:85-87, 1988.
3. Nielsen N, Bronfort G, Bendix T et al: Chronic asthma and chiropractic spinal manipulation: a randomized clinical trial, *Clin Exp Allergy* 25:80-88, 1995.
4. Masarsky CS, Weber M: Somatic dyspnea and the orthopedics of respiration, *Chiropractic Technique* 3:26-29, 1991.
5. Kessinger R: Changes in pulmonary function associated with upper cervical specific chiropractic care, *J Vertebral Sublux Res* 1:43-49, 1997.
6. Purse FM: Manipulative therapy of upper respiratory infections in children, *J Am Osteopath Assoc* 65:964-972, 1966.
7. Davies N: *Chiropractic pediatrics*, London, 2000, Churchill Livingstone.
8. Homewood AE: *The neurodynamics of the vertebral subluxation*, St Petersburg, FL, 1977, Valkyrie Press.
9. Masarsky CS, Todres-Masarsky M: Breathing and the vertebral subluxation complex. In Masarsky CS, Todres-Masarsky M et al, editors: *The somatovisceral aspects of chiropractic*, Philadelphia, 2001, Churchill Livingstone.
10. Chaitow L: *Palpation skills: assessment and diagnosis through touch*, New York, 1977, Churchill Livingstone.

11. Bilgrai, Cohen K: *Clinical management of infants and children,* Santa Cruz, Calif, 1988, Extension Press.
12. Heffner JE, Repine JE: Pulmonary strategies of antioxidant defense, *Am Rev Resp Dis* 140:531-554, 1989.
13. Krueger A: Alternative remedies, *Altern Med* Jan/Feb:71, 2003.
14. Leviton R: Asthma—breathe easily again, *Altern Med* Sep:25:60, 1998.
15. Huntley A, White A, Ernst E: Complementary medicine for asthma, *Focus Altern Complement Ther* 5:11-116, 2000.
16. Bukovsky M, Vaverkova S, Kostalova D: Immunomodulating activity of *Echinacea glorios, Echinacea angustifolia* DC and *Rudbeckia speciosa Wenderoth* ethanol-water extracts, *Polish J Pharmacol* 47:175-177, 1995.
17. Melchart D, Linde K, Worku F et al: Results of five randomized studies on the immunomodulatory activity of preparations of Echinacea, *J Complement Altern Med* 1:145-160, 1995.

Croup

1. Homewood AE: *The neurodynamics of the vertebral subluxation,* St Petersburg, Fla, 1977, Valkyrie Press.
2. Masarsky CS, Todres-Masarsky M: Breathing and the vertebral subluxation complex. In Masarsky CS, Todres-Masarsky M, editors: *The somatovisceral aspects of chiropractic,* Philadelphia, 2001, Churchill Livingstone.
3. Chaitow L: *Palpation skills: assessment and diagnosis through touch,* New York, 1977, Churchill Livingstone.
4. Bilgrai Cohen K: *Clinical management of infants and children,* Santa Cruz, Calif, 1988, Extension Press.
5. Davies N: *Chiropractic pediatrics,* London, 2000, Churchill Livingstone.
6. Heffner JE, Repine JE: Pulmonary strategies of antioxidant defense, *Am Rev Resp Dis* 140:531-554, 1989.
7. Krueger A: Alternative remedies, *Altern Med* Jan/Feb:71, 2003.
8. Leviton R: Asthma—breathe easily again, *Altern Med* Sep:25:60, 1998.
9. Huntley A, White A, Ernst E: Complementary medicine for asthma, *Focus Altern Complement Ther* 5:11-116, 2000.
10. Bukovsky M, Vaverkova S, Kostalova D: Immunomodulating activity of *Ehinacea glorios, Echinacea angustifolia* DC and *Rudbeckia speciosa Wenderoth* ethanol-water extracts, *Polish J Pharmacol* 47:175-177, 1995.
11. Melchart D, Linde K, Worku F et al: Results of five randomized studies on the immunomodulatory activity of preparations of Echinacea, *J Complement Altern Med* 1:245-260, 1995.

Herbs—Chinese

1. Kong XT, Fang HT, Jiang GQ et al: Treatment of acute bronchiolitis with Chinese herbs, *Arch Dis Child* 68:468-471, 1993.
2. Natural Standard Research Collaboration. Available at www.naturalstandard.com. Accessed 2005.
3. Li ZL, Dai BQ, Liang AH et al: Pharmacological studies of nin jiom pei pa kao, *Zhongguo Zhong Yao Za Zhi* 19:362-384, 1994.
4. Zhu, Chun-han: *Clinical handbook of Chinese prepared medicines,* Brookline, Mass, 1989, Paradigm Publications.

Homeopathy

1. *ReferenceWorks Pro 4.2,* San Rafael, Calif, 2008, Kent Homeopathic Associates.

Magnet Therapy

1. Loo M: *Pediatric acupuncture,* London, 2002, Elsevier.

Massage Therapy

1. Boat TF: Cystic fibrosis, In Behrman RE, Kliegman R, Jenson HB, editors: *Nelson's textbook of pediatrics,* ed 17, Philadelphia, 2004, Saunders.
2. Shafer TH, Wolfson MR, Bhutani VK: Respiratory muscle function, assessment and training, *Phys Ther* 61:1711-1723, 1983.
3. Warren A: Mobilization of the chest wall, *Phys Ther* 48:582-585, 1968.
4. Field T, Henteleff T, Hernandez-Reif M et al: Children with asthma have improved pulmonary functions after massage therapy, *J Pediatr* 132:854-858, 1998.
5. Hernandez-Reif M, Field T, Krasnegor J et al: Children with cystic fibrosis benefit from massage therapy, *J Pediatr Psychol* 24: 175-181, 1999.
6. Beeken JE, Parks D, Cory J et al: The effectiveness of neuromuscular release massage therapy in five individuals with chronic obstructive lung disease, *Clin Nurs Res* 7:309-325, 1998.
7. Witt P, MacKinnon J: Psychological intergration: a method to improve chest mobility of patients with chronic lung disease, *Phys Ther* 66:214-217, 1986.
8. Fritz S: *Mosby's fundamentals of therapeutic massage,* St Louis, 1995, Mosby.

Osteopathy

1. Steele TF: Utilization of osteopathic lymphatic pump in the office and home for treatment of viral illnesses and after vaccine immunizations, *Fam Phys* 2:8-11, 1998.
2. Nelson KE: Osteopathic treatment of upper respiratory infections offers distinct therapeutic advantages, *Osteopath Fam Phys News* 2:10-12, 2002.
3. Paul FA, Buser BR: Osteopathic manipulative treatment applications for the emergency department patient, *J Am Osteopath Assoc* 96:403-409, 1996.
4. Schmidt IC: Osteopathic manipulative therapy as a primary factor in the management of upper, middle and pararespiratory infections, *J Am Osteopath Assoc* 81:382-388, 1982.
5. Stiles E: Manipulative management of chronic lung disease, *Osteopath Ann* 9:300-304, 1981.
6. Howell RK, Allen TW: The influence of osteopathic manipulative therapy in the management of patients with chronic lung disease, *J Am Osteopath Assoc* 75:757-760, 1974.
7. Mall R: An evaluation of routine pulmonary function tests as indicators of responsiveness of a patient with chronic obstructive lung disease to osteopathic health care, *J Am Osteopath Assoc* 73:327-333, 1973.
8. Noll DR, Shores J, Bryman PN et al: Adjunctive osteopathic manipulative treatment in the elderly hospitalized with pneumonia: a pilot study [see comments], *J Am Osteopath Assoc* 99:140, 1999.
9. Noll DR, Shores J, Bryman PN et al: Adjunctive osteopathic manipulative treatment in the elderly hospitalized with pneumonia: a pilot study, *J Am Osteopath Assoc* 99:143-152, 1999.
10. Degenhardt BF, Kuchera ML: Update on osteopathic medical concepts and the lymphatic system, *J Am Osteopath Assoc* 96: 97-100, 1996.
11. Mesina J, Hampton D, Evans R et al: Transient basophilia following the application of lymphatic pump techniques: a pilot study [see comments], *J Am Osteopath Assoc* 98:91-94, 1998.
12. Degenhardt BF, Werden SD, Noll DR et al: Quantitative analysis of elderly immune responses to influenza vaccination with osteopathic manipulation [meeting abstracts], *J Am Osteopath Assoc* 100:513, 2000.

13. Hampton D, Evans R, Banihashem M: Lymphatic pump techniques induce a transient basophilia [meeting abstract], *J Osteopath Med (Austr)* 6:41, 2003.

14. Paul RT, Stomel RJ, Broniak FF et al: Interferon levels in human subjects throughout a 24-hour period following thoracic lymphatic pump manipulation, *J Am Osteopath Assoc* 86:92-95, 1986.

15. Clymer DH, Levin FL, Sculthorpe RH: Effects of osteopathic manipulation on several different physiologic functions: part III. Measurement of changes in several different physiological parameters as a result of osteopathic manipulation, *J Am Osteopath Assoc* 72:204-207, 1972.

16. Kolman S, Getson P, Levin F et al: Effects of osteopathic manipulation on several different physiologic functions: part IV. Absence of crossover effect, *J Am Osteopath Assoc* 73:669-672, 1974.

17. Dugan EP, Lemley WW, Roberts CA et al: Effect of lymphatic pump techniques on the immune response to influenza vaccine, *J Am Osteopath Assoc* 101:472, 2001.

18. Jackson KM, Steele TF, Dugan EP et al: Effect of lymphatic and splenic pump techniques on the antibody response to hepatitis B vaccine: a pilot study, *J Am Osteopath Assoc* 98:155-160, 1998.

CHAPTER 16

Bruises

Acupuncture | May Loo
Aromatherapy | Maura A. Fitzgerald

Herbs—Western | Alan D. Woolf, Paula M. Gardiner, Lana Dvorkin-Camiel, Jack Maypole
Homeopathy | Janet L. Levatin

✳ PEDIATRIC DIAGNOSIS AND TREATMENT

Bruises or ecchymoses are skin lesions caused by capillary bleeding. They are large lesions that are flat and usually not palpable, whereas hematomas are accumulations of blood in the skin or deeper tissues. Hematomas in the skin are raised and palpable and often tender, whereas bruises are usually painless.[1,2]

It is not uncommon for normal children older than 9 months to have 20 or more bruises, especially during the summer time, in a region with temperate climate, or during team sports season. The bruises are predominantly on the lower extremities, most frequently on the shins and knees.[3]

The color of a bruise reflects its age and the depth of injury. A fresh bruise generally appears blue or reddish purple. If a bruise is older, then yellow, green, or brown is present.[2] A British review of 369 photographs of bruises from less than 6 hours to 21 days old concludes that a bruise with a yellow color was more than 18 hours old.[4] A German study used spectrophotometry to distinguish superficial from deep bruises. The results indicate that superficial bruises have a more reddish appearance, whereas deeper bruises have a more bluish color. The optical characteristics of the skin may be explained by the fact that blue wavelengths of the light are scattered (and thus reflected) to a greater extent than the red wavelengths.[5]

The location and uniformity of color are important factors to consider in distinguishing accidental bruising from child abuse.[6] Bruises that occur in nonmobile infants, those over soft tissue areas, and those that carry the imprint of the implement used or multiple bruises of uniform shape could be signs of physical abuse.[7] Bruises to the buttocks, genitals, back,[2] or numerous bruises in an infant younger than 9 months[3] are less likely to be due to an accident. Patterns of bruising in infants and children that do not match the injury scenario offered by caretakers also should raise the suspicion of abuse.[8]

Bruises with different colors on the same body surface generally are not compatible with a single event. Dark skin may mask bruises.[2] Wood lamp and digital photography can enhance visualization of faint bruises and bruises that are not readily visible.[8]

In the event of accidental bruising, it is important to make sure that there is no internal injury. Pain is usually associated with deeper trauma. Skin bruise corresponding to the site of the seat belt is known as the "seat belt mark" (SBM) sign and is associated with a high incidence of significant organ injuries, including thoracic trauma, myocardial contusion, and intraabdominal injuries, predominantly bowel and mesenteric lacerations that require laparotomy.[9]

The majority of bruises are self-limiting and do not require conventional treatment. However, the law requires that a child *suspected* of being abused or neglected should be reported immediately to Child Protective Services (CPS).[2]

✳ CAM THERAPY RECOMMENDATIONS

Acupuncture

There are no data on acupuncture treatment of bruises. This author has needled older children with large bruise lesions using the ancient "turtle technique" of surrounding the border of the bruised area with needles pointed toward the lesion. In younger children, massaging around the bruised area in a clockwise fashion, with the child as the clock, or applying magnets, alternating north and south polarities around the bruised area, would also be beneficial.

Aromatherapy

A number of essential oils are recommended for bruising, including caraway (*Carum carvi*), myrrh (*Commiphora myrrha*), German chamomile (*Matricaria recutita*), helichrysum (*Helichrysum angustifolium*), and hyssop (*Hyssopus officinalis*).[1,2] The oils are applied topically in a lotion. Additionally essential oils can be used for treatment of first-degree burns, including sunburn. Essential oils of German chamomile, lavender (*Lavandula angustifolia*), peppermint (*Mentha piperita*), and tea tree (*Melaleuca alternifolia*) are recommended and can be applied topically in a bath, by compress, or in a lotion.[1]

Herbs—Western

There are no specific herbal remedies that reduce bruising, although the vitamin C present in rose hips and other sources is an antioxidant known to promote wound healing.

Homeopathy

Before using this section, please see Appendix A, Homeopathy, for definitions of practitioner expertise categories and for general information on prescribing homeopathic medicines.

Practitioner Expertise Category 1 and 2

There are no recent controlled clinical trials to support the use of homeopathic treatment for the treatment of bruises, although the homeopathic literature contains much evidence for its use in the form of accumulated clinical experience.[1] Bruises can often be treated effectively with homeopathy. It is safe to use homeopathic treatment for bruises that are uncomplicated by other trauma, either alone or in combination with other therapies. Any bruise that is associated with more serious trauma, such as a fracture or an intracranial injury, will need to be evaluated at an emergency care facility, although homeopathic treatment can be provided as the patient is en route to such a facility.

The goal in treating bruises homeopathically is to determine the single homeopathic medicine whose description in the materia medica most closely matches the symptom picture of the patient. Sometimes mental and emotional states, in addition to physical symptoms, are considered. If the indicated homeopathic medicine is available, it is ideal to treat bruises as soon as possible; if the medicine is not available immediately, bruises can also be successfully treated after some time has elapsed. Once the medicine has been selected, it can be given orally or sublingually (except as noted later) in the 30C potency every 2 to 3 hours. For more serious or extensive bruises, a higher potency such as 200C may be helpful. If the medicine has not helped in four to five doses, then another homeopathic medicine should be tried, or some other form of therapy should be instituted, as needed. Once symptoms have begun to resolve, the medicine can be given less frequently or stopped. It can be repeated again for a relapse of symptoms.

Uncomplicated bruises are one of the few conditions that can be treated topically with homeopathic medicines. A topical preparation can be used instead of or in addition to an orally or sublingually administered homeopathic medicine. *Arnica montana* is available in cream, ointment, and gel forms and can be used to treat bruises with intact overlying skin. (*A. montana* may irritate the tissues under broken skin and therefore should not be used on areas where the skin integrity has been broken, on mucous membranes, or close to the eyes.) Creams containing a combination of homeopathic medicines for treating bruises are also available. One brand name is Topricin, and it contains *A. montana* 6X, *Rhus toxicodendron* 6X, *Ruta graveolens* 6X, *Lachesis muta* 8X, *Belladonna* 6X, *Echinacea* 6X, *Crotalus* 8X, *Aesculus* 6X, *Heloderma* 8X, *Naja* 8X, and *Graphites* 6X. Such creams should also be used only on intact skin. Application of the previously named substances in full strength should also be avoided, as many of them are irritating to the skin at full strength.

The following is a list of homeopathic medicines commonly used to treat patients with bruises. Except as noted for *A. montana*, the medicines are administered orally or sublingually. It must be emphasized that this list is partial and represents some of the probable choices from the homeopathic materia medica. If the symptoms of a given patient are not represented here, a search of the homeopathic literature would be needed to find the simillimum.

Arnica montana

Arnica montana is the most frequently used homeopathic medicine for bruises. *Arnica montana* can be topically applied in the form of an ointment or cream to acutely bruised area **with intact skin** (see previous section for restrictions to the topical use of *Arnica montana*). *Arnica montana* can be given orally or sublingually in the following situations: head trauma, including concussions; bruising to the periorbital tissues; post-surgical trauma with bruising and edema; bruising from labor and delivery (can be given to mother and/or baby); after dental procedures; bruising of extremities; and sore muscles after overexertion. *Arnica montana* can be tried in cases where a bruise sustained long ago never fully healed. (Any of the cases previously described may also need evaluation by conventional medical personnel, as indicated at the time.)

Bellis perennis

Bellis perennis is especially useful for bruising in the pelvic and abdominal regions after surgery or accidental trauma. Emergency care may also be required in the case of accidental trauma.

Ledum palustre

Ledum palustre should be considered when the bruised area is extremely painful. The bruised area is purplish, appears swollen or edematous, and feels cold to the touch. The bruised area feels better when it is kept warm. Cellulitis that develops after such a bruise may respond to *Ledum palustre*.

Conium maculatum

Conium maculatum is used for injuries of glands such as the testes. The bruised area may have a green discoloration and become indurated. These types of injuries will also need conventional medical evaluation. The medicine may also be given before or after a conventional medical evaluation has been completed; it is safe to use in concert with conventional care.

Hamamelis macrophylla

Hamamelis macrophylla is used for blunt trauma to the eye that results in bleeding inside the eye. If available, the medicine can be given orally or sublingually immediately after such a trauma is sustained. Evaluation at an emergency care facility or by an ophthalmologist must also be sought without delay. The medicine may also be given after a medical evaluation has been completed; it is safe to use in concert with conventional care.

Hypericum perforatum

Hypericum perforatum is used for injuries and bruises to nerve-rich areas such as the fingers or tongue. Shooting pains may be associated with the injury. Conventional medical evaluation may also be necessary.

Ruta graveolens

Ruta graveolens is used for bruises to the periosteum in areas where the bone is close to the surface of the body, such as the anterior tibia. It can also be used for bruises involving cartilage and tendons. Such injuries may also require emergency evaluation and conventional forms of treatment.

Symphytum officinale

Symphytym officinale is a medicine for blunt trauma sustained directly to the eyeball. If available, the medicine can be given orally or sublingually immediately after such a trauma is sustained. Evaluation at an emergency care facility or by an ophthalmologist must also be sought without delay. The medicine may also be given after a conventional medical evaluation has been completed; it is safe to use in concert with conventional care.

References

Pediatric Diagnosis and Treatment

1. Behrman RE, Kliegman RM, Jenson HB, editors: *Nelson textbook of pediatrics*, ed 17, Philadelphia, 2004, Saunders.
2. Kliegman RM, Greenbaum LA, Lye PS, editors: *Practical strategies in pediatric diagnosis and therapy*, ed 2, Philadelphia, 2004, Elsevier.
3. Labbe J, Caouette G: Recent skin injuries in normal children, *Pediatrics* 108:271-276, 2001.
4. Langlois NE, Gresham GA: The aging of bruises: a review and study of the colour changes with time, *Forensic Sci Int* 50:227-238, 1991.
5. Bohnert M, Baumgartner R, Pollak S: Spectrophotometric evaluation of the colour of intra- and subcutaneous bruises, *Int J Legal Med* 113:343-348, 2000.
6. Mudd SS, Findlay JS: The cutaneous manifestations and common mimickers of physical child abuse, *J Pediatr Health Care* 18:123-129, 2004.
7. Brunk D: Certain bruising patterns suggest abuse, *Pediatr News*, Mar 26, 2005.
8. Vogeley E, Pierce MC, Bertocci G: Experience with wood lamp illumination and digital photography in the documentation of bruises on human skin, *Arch Pediatr Adolesc Med* 156:265-268, 2002.
9. Velmahos GC, Tatevossian R, Demetriades D: The "seat belt mark" sign: a call for increased vigilance among physicians treating victims of motor vehicle accidents, *Am Surg* 65:181-185, 1999.

Aromatherapy

1. Battaglia S: *The complete guide to aromatherapy*, Virginia, Queensland, Australia, 1995, The Perfect Potion.
2. Keville K, Green M: *Aromatherapy: a complete guide to the healing art*, Berkeley, Calif, 1995, The Crossing Press.

Homeopathy

1. *ReferenceWorks Pro 4.2*, San Rafael, Calif, 2008, Kent Homeopathic Associates.

CHAPTER 17

Burns

Acupuncture | May Loo

Aromatherapy | Maura A. Fitzgerald

Chiropractic | Anne Spicer

Herbs—Western | Alan D. Woolf, Paula M. Gardiner, Lana Dvorkin-Camiel, Jack Maypole

Homeopathy | Janet L. Levatin

Massage Therapy | Mary C. McLellan

Mind/Body | Timothy Culbert, Lynda Richtsmeier Cyr

✳ PEDIATRIC DIAGNOSIS AND TREATMENT

Burns are a leading cause of unintentional death in children. Scald burns account for 85% of cases; flame burns, 13%; and the remainder are electrical and chemical burns.[1] Burn lesions are classified as first-, second-, or third-degree burns. First-degree burns involve only the epidermis and present as swelling, erythema, and pain, which usually resolves in 48 to 72 hours. Second-degree burns involve the entire epidermis and a variable portion of the dermal layer, characterized by vesicle and blister formation. Third-degree burns destroy the entire epidermis and dermis, leaving no residual epidermis cells to repopulate the damaged area.[1] This chapter will discuss treatment of only first- and second-degree dermal burns of less than 10% of body surface area.

Approximately 10% of cases of physical abuse in children involve burns,[2] but 18% of burns are due to abuse.[1] The shape or pattern of a burn may be diagnostic and reflect the pattern of an object or method of injury. Cigarette burns produce circular, punched-out lesions of uniform size. An immersion burn occurs when a child is placed in hot water intentionally or unintentionally. Immersion in 147° F (64° C) water for 1 second can result in a second-degree burn. Extremity immersions result in glove or stocking burn patterns. When a child's body is placed in hot water, the level of burn demarcation is uniform and distinct. Immersion burns are most common in infants.[2]

Conventional treatment consists of applying bacitracin ointment to small wounds, and dressing with bacitracin or silver sulfadiazine cream to larger wounds.[1] A major complication of superficial burns is secondary infection. Suspected child abuse should be reported immediately to Child Protective Services (CPS).

A Japanese clinical trial of 14 patients showed that when prostaglandin E1 (PGE1) ointment was applied to superficial second-degree to full-thickness dermal burns, more epithelialization occurred with less hypertrophic scarring compared to other therapies.[3] A Korean study found a pulsed laser to be effective in treating various types of scars, including scars from burns.[4]

✳ CAM THERAPY RECOMMENDATIONS

Acupuncture

There are no current data on acupuncture treatment of burns in children. A clinical trial from Mexico used acupuncture-like electrical stimulation on 10 adults with second-degree burn injuries who failed conventional medical treatment for wound healing. Lesions were covered with gauze soaked in a 10% (w/v) sterile saline solution; electrical stimulation was delivered via subcutaneously inserted needles surrounding the wound edges; a dose charge of 0.6 coulomb/cm²/day was delivered. Following electrostimulation, healing occurred in a thoroughly organized manner in all 10 patients regardless of the severity of the type of burn.[1]

Acupuncture can be used in pain management for severe burn cases. A U.S. controlled clinical trial of 11 inpatients administered bilateral acupuncture-like transcutaneous electrical nerve stimulation to six ear points after wound débridement, other wound care, and dressing changes. Pain was measured with the visual analog scale immediately before and after treatments and at 15, 30, and 60 minutes after treatment. Results revealed significant pain reduction.[2] Acupuncture anesthesia could also be used in severe burn cases.[3]

This author has needled older children with minor burn lesions using the ancient "turtle technique" of surrounding the border of the burn area with needles pointed toward the lesion. In younger children, massaging around the burned area in a clockwise fashion, with the child as the clock, or applying magnets, alternating north and south polarities around the burn area, would also be beneficial.

Aromatherapy

See Chapter 16, Bruises.

Chiropractic

Chiropractic management of the child with burns depends greatly on the location of the affected skin. Adjustments would be difficult, if not impossible, over burned areas in the inflammatory and proliferative phases. The exorbitant amount of afferent/efferent stimulation through the associated spinal area[1] is likely to predispose to focal spinal inflammatory changes and possibly resulting in a subluxation complex (SC) including kinesiopathology and myopathology along with neuropathology. Correction of the SC could theoretically enhance healing at the burn site via improved somatovisceral and somatosomatic function. Decreases in itching, anxiety, depression, and pain perception have been demonstrated with application of massage therapy[2] and may relate to the gate theory, which has also been cited as a theory in pain control through the chiropractic adjustment.

Nutritional considerations would take a priority in the chiropractic management for the duration of the collagen remodeling phase, with oral ingestion of adequate proteins (particularly those including arginine); vitamins A, C, and E; copper; and zinc.[3,4] Also beneficial to multiple systems repair, but of particular importance to the nervous system, are omega-3 fatty acids eicosapentaenoic acid and docosahexaenoic acid (EPA/DHA).

A singular case in the literature describing chiropractic participation in management of an adult burn victim may be extrapolated to children. A 61-year-old patient with steam burns developed spinal pain that resolved with chiropractic management. The chiropractors theorized that the pain symptoms were secondary to the inflammatory reaction and muscle splinting that occurs under acute trauma. The impaired tissue oxygenation triggers an immune reaction, which is manifest in the full body and resulted in the chiropractic SC. The correction of this spinal aberration was reported to have brought resolution of the spinal pain, but no discussion was offered regarding any direct benefit to the injured skin.[5]

Herbs—Western

Patients who have suffered burns that are severe, deep, extensive, or blistering should not rely on home remedies, but rather should be seen by a healthcare provider. Minor, superficial (first-degree) or partial thickness burns may benefit from the application of fresh aloe vera or an aloe vera–containing gel.[1,2]

In addition, calendula and chamomile extract are used for burns and radiation dermatitis; although calendula was promising (a calendula-based cream called *Pommade au Calendula par Digestion of Boiron* [Boiron, Sainte-Foy-lès-Lyon, France] was applied after each radiation session), the chamomile cream was not thought to be effective.[3,4]

Homeopathy

Before using this section, please see Appendix A, Homeopathy, for definitions of practitioner expertise categories and general information on prescribing homeopathic medicines.

Practitioner Expertise Category 1

Category 1 includes first-degree burns and second-degree burns with intact skin.

Practitioner Expertise Category 2

Category 2 involves second-degree burns with areas of open skin and third-degree burns in small areas.

Practitioner Expertise Category 3

Category 3 includes second-degree burns with area of open skin and third-degree burns in large areas.

There are no controlled clinical trials of homeopathy for treatment of burns, although the homeopathic literature contains much evidence for its use in the form of accumulated clinical experience.[1] Burns can often be treated effectively with homeopathy. It is safe to use homeopathic treatment for first-degree burns and second-degree burns with intact skin, either alone or in combination with other therapies. For more serious burns, such as third-degree burns and second-degree burns with areas of open skin, homeopathy can be used in conjunction with other forms of treatment; however, successful homeopathic treatment in such cases usually requires extensive training in the art and science of homeopathy. Therefore, in this chapter, only homeopathic treatment of less severe burns is included. Homeopathic treatment should help alleviate pain and encourage healing with less chance of scarring and infection.

When homeopathy is used for treatment of burns, there must be no delay in the patient's receiving any indicated conventional therapies. If the indicated homeopathic medicine is readily available, it is helpful if it is provided soon after a burn is sustained; however, it may also be given after a patient has received any necessary conventional treatment.

The goal in treating burns homeopathically is to determine the single homeopathic medicine whose description in the materia medica most closely matches the symptom picture of the patient. Sometimes mental and emotional states, in addition to physical symptoms, are considered. Once the medicine has been selected, it can be given orally or sublingually in the 30C potency once every 15 to 60 minutes. If the medicine has not helped in four to five doses, then another homeopathic medicine should be tried, or some other form of therapy should be instituted. Once symptoms have begun to resolve, the medicine can be given less frequently or stopped. It can be repeated again for a relapse of symptoms.

The following is a list of homeopathic medicines commonly used to treat patients with burns. It must be emphasized that this list is partial and represents some of the probable choices from the homeopathic materia medica. If the symptoms of a given patient are not represented here, a search of the homeopathic literature would be needed to find the simillimum.

Apis mellifica

Apis mellifica is used for minor burns with an excessive amount of erythema, swelling, and pain. The pain is relieved by the application of ice-cold compresses. If clinically indicated, the patient must seek care at an emergency care facility without delay.

Cantharis vesicatoria

Cantharis vesicatoria can be used for burns from scalds, chemicals, and acids. Burns to mucous membranes can be treated. The pain is severe but improves with cold applications. If clinically indicated, the patient must seek care at an emergency care facility without delay.

Urtica urens

Urtica urens is used for minor burns accompanied by itching. It is especially useful for scalds.

Hamamelis macrophylla

Hamamelis macrophylla is a medicine for burns of the mouth and tongue. If clinically indicated, the patient must seek care at an emergency care facility without delay.

Kali bichromicum

Kali bichromicum is a medicine for burns from steam. If clinically indicated, the patient must seek care at an emergency care facility without delay.

Massage Therapy

Massage should never be performed over areas where skin integrity may not be intact, such as over a burned or grafted area. Although massage may not benefit the recovery of the burned tissue, massage therapy could be helpful in managing burn patients' pain, anxiety, and emotional recovery from the burn trauma. Randomized controlled trials of adult and pediatric burn patients have demonstrated that patients receiving daily 20-minute massage prior to débridement had decreased pain scores, anxiety scores, anger, cortisol levels, and pruritus as well as improved behavior ratings compared with controls.[1-3] Nurses reported greater ease in completing dressing changes in the massage therapy group compared with controls.[3]

Massage may be an effective therapy to assist with pain management and emotional recovery for patients recovering from burn trauma. Massage can be done on unaffected areas and proximal to affected areas after post-trauma edema has resolved. Traditional Swedish massage techniques and/or trigger point therapy may be applied to these areas, with care taken to avoid the burned areas and donor graft sites. If inflammation is present from the burn trauma, massage distal to the burn site is not recommended, as it increases vasodilation of the massaged area and may increase the degree of inflammation present. Craniosacral therapy may be a very gentle, safe massage approach for a burn victim, especially if extensive burns are present. This modality may be applied over the patient's clothes, bed linens, or dressings as long as the integrity of the dressing is not impaired. Myofascial techniques would not be recommended until after tissue integrity has been achieved, as application of this technique may affect other body locations.

Mind/Body

Burn injuries often share characteristics of acute disorders as well as those of chronic illness. Mind/body approaches, as applied to the treatment of burn patients, require attention to the developmental and psychological principles underlying effective pediatric pain management more generally. Dise-Lewis provided an excellent overview of developmental considerations and psychological principles in pain management.[1] An effective approach to pain management needs to be multidisciplinary and culturally sensitive. Anticipatory anxiety and emotional distress are key components of the pain experience and, like pain itself, are amenable to modulation with a variety of mind/body approaches. Although not all the literature supporting mind/body therapies in chronic pain is specific to burn patients, many mind/body techniques, particularly self-hypnosis, generally apply to this population. In burn patients it is important to note that there is both the chronic, baseline pain component and the frequent acute pain exacerbations with procedures such as dressing changes.[2] Olness and Kohen[3] review applications of hypnosis in children with burns. Treatment protocols for hypnosis with burn patients include suggestions for pain control, symptom relief, general ego strengthening, adherence to treatment demands, improved body image, and ability to cope effectively following discharge from the hospital. Often problems for burn patients change quite quickly, and interventions need to be adapted for the situation.

Cognitive/behavioral techniques for managing pain and distress and improving coping skills are also very effective and should be considered for every pediatric pain patient.[4-6] In the authors' clinical experience, effective chronic pain treatment needs multimodality interventions that include both traditional and complementary approaches considering the patient's complex biological processes as well as developmental, socioemotional, psychological, and cultural factors.

References

Pediatric Diagnosis and Treatment

1. Antoon AY, Donovan MK: Burn injuries. In Behrman RE, Kliegman RM, Jenson HB, editors: *Nelson textbook of pediatrics*, ed 17, Philadelphia, 2004, Saunders.
2. Johnson CF: Abuse and neglect of children. In Kliegman RM, Greenbaum LA, Lye PS, editors: *Practical strategies in pediatric diagnosis and therapy*, ed 2, Philadelphia, 2004, Elsevier.
3. Gunji H, Ono I, Tateshita T et al: Clinical effectiveness of an ointment containing prostaglandin E1 for the treatment of burn wounds, *Burns* 22:399-405, 1996.
4. Kwon SD, Kye YC: Treatment of scars with a pulsed Er:YAG laser, *J Cutan Laser Ther* 2:27-31, 2000.

Acupuncture

1. Sumano H, Mateos G: The use of acupuncture-like electrical stimulation for wound healing of lesions unresponsive to conventional treatment, *Am J Acupunct* 27:5-14, 1999.
2. Lewis SM, Clelland JA, Knowles CJ et al: Effects of auricular acupuncture-like transcutaneous electric nerve stimulation on pain levels following wound care in patients with burns: a pilot study, *J Burn Care Rehabil* 11:322-329, 1990.
3. Extraordinary severe burn cases treated with integrated Chinese traditional and Western medicine, *Sci Sin* 20:125-134, 1977.

Chiropractic

1. Blaha J, Pondelicek I: Prevention and therapy of post burn scars, *Acta Chinergiae Plasticae* 39:17-21, 1997.
2. Vanderbilt S: Somatic research. Rising from the ashes: easing the healing path for burn patients, *Massage Bodywork* 16:118-120, 2001.
3. Dowsett J: Nutrition: the importance of nutrition in wound healing, *World Irish Nurs* 4:15-18, 1996.
4. Hildreth M: Nutrition therapy for the pediatric burn patient, *Topics Clin Nutr* 12:6-15, 1997.
5. Hendricks CL, Larkin-Thier SM: Thermal burns and chiropractic: a case study, *J Am Chiro Assoc* May:57-61, 1999.

Herbs—Western

1. Muller MJ, Hollyoak MA, Moaveni Z et al: Retardation of wound healing by silver sulfadiazine is reversed by aloe vera and nystatin, *Burns* 28:834-836, 2003.

2. Klein AD, Penneys NS: Aloe vera, *J Am Acad Dermatol* 18: 714-720, 1988.
3. Pommier P, Gomez F, Sunyach MP et al: Phase III randomized trial of *Calendula officinalis* compared with trolamine for the prevention of acute dermatitis during irradiation for breast cancer, *J Clin Oncol* 22:1447-1453, 2004.
4. Wickline MM: Prevention and treatment of acute radiation dermatitis: a literature review, *Oncol Nurs Forum* 31:237-247, 2004.

Homeopathy

1. *ReferenceWorks Pro 4.2,* San Rafael, Calif, 2008, Kent Homeopathic Associates.

Massage Therapy

1. Field T, Peck M, Krugman S et al: Burn injuries benefit from massage therapy, *J Burn Care Rehabil* 19:241-244, 1998.
2. Field T, Peck M, Scd et al: Postburn itching, pain, and psychological symptoms are reduced with massage therapy, *J Burn Care Rehabil*, 21:189-193, 2000.

3. Hernandez-Reif M, Field T, Largie S et al: Children's distress during burn treatment is reduced by massage therapy, *J Burn Care Rehabil* 22:191-195, 2001.

Mind/Body

1. Dise-Lewis JE: A developmental perspective on psychological principles of burn care, *J Burn Care Rehabil* 22:255-260, 2001.
2. Kazak A, Kunin-Batson A: Psychological and integrative interventions in pediatric procedure pain. In Finley A, McGrath P, editors: *Acute and procedure pain in infants and children,* Seattle, 2001, IASP Press.
3. Olness K, Kohen D: *Hypnosis and hypnotherapy with children,* New York, 1996, Guilford Press, pp 273-279.
4. Schechter NL: Pain and pain control in children, *Curr Prob Pediatr* 15:1-67, 1985.
5. Stoddard FJ, Sheridan RL, Saxe GN et al: Treatment of pain in acutely burned children, *J Burn Care Rehabil* 23:135-156, 2002.
6. Thurber CA, Martin-Hertz SP, Patterson DR: Psychosocial forum. Psychological principles of burn wound pain in children. I: theoretical framework, including commentary by Doctor M, *J Burn Care Rehabil* 21:376-387, 2000.

Cancer

Acupuncture | May Loo

Aromatherapy | Maura A. Fitzgerald

Homeopathy | Janet L. Levatin

Massage Therapy | Mary C. McLellan

Mind/Body | Timothy Culbert, Lynda Richtsmeier Cyr

Nutrition | Joy A. Weydert

Osteopathy | Jane Carreiro

✳ PEDIATRIC DIAGNOSIS AND TREATMENT

Approximately 12,000 new cases of cancer are diagnosed in children younger than 20 years annually in the United States.[1,2] Cancer remains the second most frequent cause of death, after injury, in children older than 3 months. Acute lymphoblastic leukemia, brain cancers, lymphomas, and sarcomas of soft tissue and bone predominate in children and adolescents.[2]

The mainstay of treatment consists of surgery, radiation, and chemotherapy. Many children are treated with two of the three modalities.[3] Pediatric oncologists face the unique challenges of treating a population that is still undergoing physical and emotional growth and development and must consider possible "late adverse effects"—serious long-term medical and psychosocial effects.[2,3]

The American Academy of Pediatrics recommends that children and adolescents with newly suspected and/or recurrent malignancy be referred to a pediatric cancer center for prompt and accurate diagnosis and management and should have their treatment coordinated by a board-certified pediatric hematologist/oncologist.[1]

Complementary and alternative medicine (CAM) therapies should not interfere with medical management but can be offered as complementary treatments for primary symptoms such as pain and for untoward side effects from medical treatments, such as nausea, vomiting, or fatigue with chemotherapy and pain and wound healing from procedures and surgery.

✳ CAM THERAPY RECOMMENDATIONS

Acupuncture

There are no good data on acupuncture treatment of childhood cancer. A few case reports from China indicate use of acupuncture for treatment of cancer in adults.[1-3] Although acupuncture is increasingly used by the general pediatric population, few children with cancer turn to acupuncture as part of the cancer treatment.[4]

Acupuncture has been shown to be effective for chemotherapy-induced nausea and vomiting.

In Canada, acupuncture is an option recommended for the prevention and management of acute chemotherapy-induced nausea and vomiting in children.[5] A multicenter, randomized crossover study from Germany found acupuncture reduced nausea and vomiting without the use of antiemetic medications in adolescent oncology patients. Acupuncture also enabled patients to experience higher levels of alertness during chemotherapy.[6]

Pain from cancer and treatment procedures continues to pose difficulties for oncology management.[7,8] Acupuncture as treatment of various pain syndromes is recognized by the National Institutes of Health.[9] Acupuncture can be used for pediatric oncology pain management. Acupuncture can also be used to treat the anxiety and depression often seen in oncology patients, young and old.

Acupuncture Treatment Recommendations

For nausea and vomiting: P6 (see Chapter 62, Vomiting).

For pain: The acupuncturist needs to individualize treatment according to organ, pain site, and specific procedure or surgery.

For depression: See Chapter 28, Depression.

Aromatherapy

Childhood Cancer

Although some references cite antitumoral effects of some essential oils,[1,2] primarily the study of aromatherapy for cancer has been in adults and for symptom management.[3-7] In most of these studies, aromatherapy is coupled with massage. In an analysis of eight randomized controlled trials (RCTs), a consistent finding was that use of aromatherapy led to a reduction of anxiety and that effects on other symptoms such as depression, pain, and nausea were mixed. The reviewer felt that more study was needed to determine the effect of aromatherapy on symptom management.[8] Although there are no large studies of children with cancer, the use of aromatherapy, either alone or with massage, in hospital and palliative care of children is considered to be safe and possibly useful for reduction of symptoms of pain and anxiety and for improvement of sleep.[9]

Given the lack of pediatric research, it is useful to consider studies that have been conducted with adults as a guideline. In a randomized controlled study of 46 adults with cancer in a day treatment unit, subjects were divided into standard care or standard care plus aromatherapy massage. There was no difference between groups on measures of mood, quality of life, and intensity of symptoms; however, all the patients in the aromatherapy massage group wished to continue the therapy.[10] In another RCT of 42 adult patients with advanced cancer, subjects were assigned to massage, aromatherapy massage, or no treatment. There was no change on pain intensity, anxiety, or quality of life indicators; sleep improved in both aromatherapy massage and massage groups, and depression decreased in the massage group.[11]

Finally, in a randomized study of 103 adult cancer palliative care patients, subjects were assigned to massage or aromatherapy massage groups. Reduction of anxiety after each treatment and overall improvement in psychological, quality of life, and physical indicators were observed for both groups with the aromatherapy massage group improving to a greater degree.[12]

In this author's experience, essential oils are useful for the treatment of cancer or chemotherapy-related side effects. Essential oils of peppermint *(Mentha piperita)*, ginger *(Zingiber officinalis)*, and spearmint *(Mentha spicata)* help relieve nausea (alone and in combination with antiemetic medications). Calming essential oils such as lavender *(Lavandula angustifolia)*, bergamot *(Citrus bergamia)*, and sweet orange *(Citrus sinensis)* will often help children and adolescents relax and improve their sleep. Alerting essential oils such as peppermint, basil *(Ocimum basilicum)*, and rosemary *(Rosmarinus officinalis)* can be helpful in combating fatigue. Additionally, using essential oils with massage therapy enhances the level of relaxation and increases pain reduction. Use of clinical aromatherapy offers children and adolescents some choice in their cancer care. They can choose the essential oil they want to use, how they want to use it (e.g., massage, inhalation), and when they want to use it.

Homeopathy

Before using this section, please see Appendix A, Homeopathy, for definitions of practitioner expertise categories and general information on prescribing homeopathic medicines.

Practitioner Expertise Category 3

There are no controlled clinical trials of homeopathy for childhood cancer, and the homeopathic literature contains virtually no anecdotal references to the use of homeopathy for this condition.[1] An experienced homeopathic practitioner could prescribe homeopathic medicines to be used in combination with other treatment modalities, conventional and/or alternative, in particular to alleviate the side effects of conventional treatment. Because childhood cancer and its treatment are complex and multifaceted problems, safe and effective homeopathic treatment requires extensive training in the art and science of homeopathy. For this reason professional treatment by an experienced practitioner is recommended if homeopathy is to be tried for childhood cancer or the side effects of its treatment. No specific treatment recommendations are included here.

Homeopathy has been used successfully for treatment of a variety of adult cancers. For more information on this subject, interested readers are referred to Ramakrishnan and Coulter's *A Homoeopathic Approach to Cancer.*[2]

Massage Therapy

Massage therapy for cancer patients can be very beneficial; however, many precautions and considerations need to be addressed in providing massage to this patient population. Massage therapy is included as a possible nonpharmacological tool for treating cancer pain as part of a multimodality approach, according to the National Comprehensive Cancer Network Clinical Practice Guidelines in Oncology and the American College of Chest Physicians Evidence-Based Clinical Practice Guidelines.[1-4] Pilot studies and RCTs have reported cancer patients who received massage therapy experienced increased relaxation,[5-8] decreased pain,[5,7-14] decreased anxiety and stress,[5,11-16,18-20] improved mood,[6,11,12,15,19] decreased depression,[13,15,16,19] improved quality of life indicators,[7] decreased fatigue, and decreased cancer and chemotherapy-related physical symptoms.[6-8,11,17,21,22] Massage therapy has been shown to be an effective adjunct therapy for pain management in patients with acute and chronic pain (see Chapter 21).

A literature review of potential therapies to decrease stress behaviors for children undergoing bone marrow transplantation suggests that massage may be one of the therapies to be most beneficial.[18] Research specific to pediatric cancer patients receiving chemotherapy reported massage therapy and healing touch decreased pain ratings, nonsteroidal antiinflammatory drug (NSAID) use, anxiety, and lowered mood disturbance compared to controls.[12]

A 3-year study of 1290 adult cancer patients receiving either inpatient or outpatient Swedish massage, light touch massage, or foot massage reported a 60% reduction in anxiety scores, a 45% reduction in pain scores, and a 43% reduction in fatigue. The outpatients in this study reported greater improvements in symptoms than did inpatients. The cancer patients reported that they had more benefit from Swedish massage or light touch compared with the foot massage treatments.[13] An RCT examining the use of massage therapy and acupuncture for cancer patients postoperatively had 25.5% reduction in pain from baseline and a brief improvement in tension, anxiety, and nausea compared to the control group.[14]

One study reported acupressure to be an effective adjunct in the treatment of chemotherapy-induced nausea and vomiting when used in conjunction with antiemetics compared with antiemetic therapy only.[22] A similar study reported that massage treatment during chemotherapy infusions decreased nausea in women with breast cancer compared to the control treatment.[17]

Physical measures from a pilot RCT reported, in addition to improved psychological indicators as previously mentioned, that the adult cancer patients had increased dopamine and serotonin levels, as well as increased natural killer cell and lymphocyte numbers.[19] A subsequent RCT evaluated the same indicators comparing effects of massage therapy, progressive muscle relaxation, and a standard of care control. The study reported improvement in depressed mood, reduced anxiety scores, and decreased pain in both the massage and muscle relaxation group compared to the controls. The massage group had decreased anger scores, improved vigor scores, increased dopamine and serotonin levels, and significant increase in NK cells and lymphocytes compared to the other two groups, with the progressive relaxation group experiencing a significant increase in NK cytotoxicity.[15]

Patient reports of improved symptom management with aromatherapy massage have prompted some small pilot studies. One study did not find any statistically significant difference between cancer patients who received aromatherapy massage with lavender oil compared with massage with unscented oil,[23] whereas another study reported improvement when Roman chamomile oil was used compared with unscented oil.[24]

Caregivers of oncology patients often experience stress, depression, and fatigue caring for their patient or loved one. Massage therapy can be utilized to help provide the caregivers with support through the process of caring for a cancer patient. A study of massage therapy provided to oncology caregivers reported decreased anxiety scores, depression, and motivational and emotional fatigue.[20] Teaching these caregivers some massage techniques that they may use for the patient can help empower the caregiver to contribute to the comfort and disposition of the patient. Care must be taken in assessing whether a parent would like to participate in such a role. Many parents are eager for any opportunity to make their child more comfortable, but some parents may perceive this as another burden or task they must perform. Many parents are very dedicated to remaining at their child's bedside throughout the hospitalization process. Often parents will seize the opportunity while a massage therapist is present to take a much-needed break for themselves with the confidence and reassurance that their child is receiving a treatment that provides comfort and a person is present with their child during their brief absence. A massage provider should always ask the parents whether they would like to remain during the treatment; many times after observing the first massage treatment and the child's response, the parent readily leaves during subsequent sessions.

Before any massage session begins with an oncology patient, the provider should always assess whether there are any contraindications for massage (see Chapter 3). Contraindications common within this patient population include thrombocytopenia (platelets <50,000), areas of disrupted skin integrity from radiation or prolonged bed rest, presence of indwelling lines or feeding tubes, and presence of a tumor. Assessment for contraindications should take place for each massage visit, even if the patient is treated regularly, as an oncology patient's health status may change drastically in a short time period.

If contraindications are present, the modality and/or approach to the massage session may be adapted to provide comfort to the patient. The American Massage Therapy Association recommends using caution when a patient is thrombocytopenic, as bruising can occur from the massage treatment. Avoiding deep pressure modalities, such as trigger point therapy, would be advised in this setting. Many of the energy-related modalities and those that require very light touch could be effective adaptations, such as craniosacral therapy, polarity therapy, Reiki, healing touch, therapeutic touch, and somatoemotional release.[25] Areas of impaired skin integrity, presence of a tumor, or presence of indwelling medical device can be avoided while the rest of the body is treated.

A recent study reported increased bacterial counts present on massage therapists' palms following a massage session, even after hand washing has been performed, with simultaneously decreased counts on the patient's skin suggesting bacterial transfer from patient to therapist.[26] If a massage provider is treating other patients as well as an oncology patient, extra care must be taken to thoroughly wash the hands before treating a potentially neutropenic patient to protect the immunocompromised patient from risk. Ideally, treating these patients before other patients may help decrease their exposure to pathogens. Many massage providers will use well-fitting disposable nonlatex gloves in conjunction with vegetable-based massage oils to provide massage to this patient population to further protect the patient from disease. If a massage provider (e.g., a parent) wears artificial nails, the use of gloves should strongly be considered because artificial nails may have high bacteria counts present. Removing all jewelry prior to treatment is also recommended, as bacteria may be present beneath rings and stones.

If thrombocytopenia is not present, Swedish massage, myofascial release, trigger point therapy, and neuromuscular therapy may be used in addition to energy modalities during the acute phase of cancer treatment. The location and nature of the massage treatment will depend on the patient's need at the time of treatment. During the acute treatment period, a cancer patient may not tolerate a session longer than 10 to 20 minutes, so it is best to ask the patient how they can best be helped for that session. Often the answer may vary—one day it could be to treat leg cramps, another day to just help the patient rest better.

From a musculoskeletal consideration, hospitalized cancer patients often have muscular tension, congestion, and trigger points in the legs due to decreased activity. Contractures may begin to form, so particular attention to the Achilles tendon may be helpful to prevent leg pain when the patient is resuming ambulation. Muscles in the neck (especially sternocleidomastoid and suboccipital muscles) and the upper shoulders (especially levator scapulae and upper trapezius) may also be affected following episodes of retching. These areas would be excellent areas of focus using any of the previously mentioned massage modalities. If the patient has esophagitis or mucositis present, massage in the neck region may be uncomfortable and should be avoided until the conditions resolve.

There has been much discussion regarding the use of lymphatic manual drainage (LMD) massage for cancer patients. It had been theorized several decades ago that this technique would increase the spread of cancer. In 1995, the International Society of Lymphology Executive Committee concluded LMD's ability to spread cancer was "speculative and thus far unconvincing and unfounded."[25,27] Furthermore, this group indicated LMD may be helpful in the palliative treatment of pain related to lymphedema in cancer patients.[25] A massage therapist may still wish to consult with the patient's physician prior to providing this therapy in order to avoid any miscommunication regarding the patient's treatment plan.

Myofascial release therapy may be helpful when contractures are present or beginning to form. This relatively gentle technique is tolerated by most patients. A pilot study of myofascial release in women 2 months post-lumpectomy and radiation therapy reported reduction of chest wall pain, and more than half of the women reported complete resolution of the pain.[28]

If the patient is currently being treated for palliative care, some of the more aggressive massage modalities may not be indicated or tolerated. The patient may not have the energy to change position or the stamina for sustained massage treatment. Providing relaxation massage with gentle effleurage of the extremities in conjunction with hand and/or foot massage may be the relaxing relief the patient needs at that moment. Effleurage to these areas are very easy to teach to parents.

Mind/Body

Although mind/body approaches are increasingly being used with pediatric cancer patients to promote comfort and decrease pain and anxiety, there are few RCTs in the literature. Cognitive-behavioral approaches and relaxation training have been effectively used to reduce procedure-related pain.[1] Cotanch and colleagues[2] report in a pilot study that patients who received imagery-based interventions with suggestion experienced decreased intensity and duration of nausea and vomiting compared with patients who received active cognitive distraction combined with relaxation. In a similar comparison study, Zeltzer et al.[3] report that nausea and vomiting severity was reduced by imagery with suggestion and active cognitive distraction with relaxation. Subjects in this study met with the therapist once for 30 minutes during a routine clinic visit prior to chemotherapy administration. Distraction techniques included helping the child focus on objects in the treatment room, taking deep breaths, enjoying laughter and jokes, and playing guessing games. The hypnotic intervention involved using "favorite place" imagery, and posthypnotic suggestions were given to use imagery at home and to have a good appetite and a restful sleep following the session. In an RCT, Zeltzer et al.[4] found that both interventions (imagery with suggestion versus active cognitive distraction with relaxation) resulted in shorter duration of nausea compared with an attention-control group, but that only the imagery treatment group had shorter duration of vomiting. In the adult literature, pilot studies are currently being conducted with breast cancer patients to determine the benefits of mindfulness-based, stress-reduction meditation[5] and autogenic training[6] on immune status, psychological functioning, and general stress management.

In the authors' clinical experience, self-regulation skills training (e.g., biofeedback, hypnosis, guided imagery, meditation, cognitive-behavioral interventions) is helpful in reducing stress associated with cancer treatment, as well as reducing symptoms of nausea and pain. A primary focus is on enhancing the child's sense of self-control of his or her own behavior, feelings, and thoughts. Mind/body approaches provide tools for self-care by improving stress management skills, balancing the autonomic nervous system, and establishing a sense of mastery and control for the pediatric patient. Children are taught a variety of mind/body skills so that they will have a toolbox of skills at hand. This often begins by teaching them diaphragmatic breathing, progressive muscle relaxation, and "safe place" imagery. Mental imagery with cancer patients can also focus on modification of the disease process (e.g., "black knight" cancer cells being attacked by "white

knight" healthy blood cells).[7] The authors also blend mind/body strategies with other CAM approaches, including massage, healing touch, clinical aromatherapy, and acupuncture, for optimal benefits.

Nutrition

Strong links have been made between dietary habits and the incidence of various adult cancers. Excess calorie intake, high-fat diets, and low fiber intakes have been implicated in breast, colon, and prostate cancers. These correlations have been investigated in the etiology of childhood cancers. A recent study obtained dietary histories from a diverse population of children. It found that regular consumption of oranges, bananas, and orange juice during the first 2 years of life was associated with a reduced risk of leukemia diagnosed between ages 2 and 14 years.[1] No association between eating hot dogs or lunch meat and the increased risk of leukemia was found.

Another study assessed the maternal dietary intake in the 12 months prior to pregnancy. Consumption of the vegetable, protein, and fruit food groups was inversely associated with acute lymphocytic leukemia (ALL). Among nutrients, consumption of pro-vitamin A carotenoids and the antioxidant glutathione were inversely associated with ALL.[2]

A third study found that childhood fruit consumption may have a long-term protective effect on cancer risk in adults.[3] It is believed that the antioxidants found in fruits and vegetables stimulate the production of anti-cancer enzymes, thus increasing the immune system response. It is also believed that these same antioxidants can be helpful for those undergoing chemotherapy, as they may increase the effectiveness of the chemotherapeutic agents and decrease the adverse effects from the chemotherapy. Organically grown foods have been found to be higher in antioxidants than foods grown conventionally.[4]

Rodent studies suggested that antioxidants may decrease the effectiveness of chemotherapy, which often are oxidizing agents, but this has not been observed consistently in the human studies.

Other theories suggest that modulating the effects of inflammation with omega-3 fatty acids has effects on overall immune cell function and tumor cell division. The essential fatty acids also activate kinase C, which retards tumor growth and metastasis.[5] This and other studies have been conducted in laboratory animals and need to be validated in humans.

Because elevated fasting serum glucose levels and a diagnosis of diabetes are independent risk factors for several major cancers, and because the risk tends to increase with an increased level of fasting serum glucose,[6] early childhood efforts to prevent obesity and type 2 diabetes would reduce cancer risks. Following a low-glycemic-load diet would not only provide the essential nutrients and antioxidants that can be cancer protective, but would also prevent glucose intolerance.

Treatment

The following strategies can be implemented not only as a means to prevent cancers, but also to help cancer therapy patients:

- Encourage intake of organically grown fruits and vegetables starting in early childhood.

- Increase daily intake of omega-3 fatty acids in the diet.
- Reduce sugar intake and encourage a low-glycemic-load diet.

Osteopathy

Within the osteopathic philosophy, the child with cancer is treated from the perspectives of optimizing function of the immune and neuroendocrine systems and, when possible, facilitating the healing processes of the body. The primary role of the neuroendocrine-immune system is to maintain a dynamic homeostasis among the various cells, fluids, and tissues of the body. Although science has traditionally viewed them as three separate systems, the extent of interdependence between the endocrine, immune, and nervous systems makes the boundaries almost nonexistent. Various factors can affect function of the neuroendocrine and immune systems, undermining the child's ability to respond to the therapeutic regimens being employed. One such factor is nociceptive input from primary afferent fibers in muscles and fascia.[1] Nociception, along with emotional, psychological, and other stressors, can affect overall health by altering function of the immune, endocrine, and nervous systems.[2-10] Chemotherapy, radiation therapy, and surgery all address the cancer, but the child's capacity for healing is what determines the ultimate therapeutic outcome.

Osteopathy does not destroy the cancer; osteopathy supports the child's capacity for healing. As such, osteopathic manipulation is always used in conjunction with and as an adjunct to the oncological regimen. The goal of an osteopathic treatment is to promote an exchange among all the fluid systems in all the tissues of the body.[11,12] This allows the self-healing, self-correcting forces within the child to take full advantage of the chemotherapeutic agents and other cancer therapies the child is receiving. Osteopathic manipulation may be used in conjunction with homeopathy, acupuncture, naturopathy, Chinese medicine, and herbal remedies. There are no published studies on the efficacy of osteopathic manipulation in the treatment of cancer. However, several studies have demonstrated improvement in immune function[13-20] and changes in autonomic tone[19,21-25] with osteopathic manipulation.

Techniques are chosen based on the type of cancer, the presence and extent of metastasis, and the overall bioenergetic capacity of the child. Techniques that promote localized drainage of lymphatic tissue are contraindicated in cases of lymphatic involvement or metastasis.[26,27] Instead, balancing techniques addressing autonomic nervous system function via the sympathetic chain ganglia and cranial techniques such as compression of the fourth ventricle (CV-4) may be used. Children undergoing aggressive polypharmacy protocols have low levels of energy. In these cases, less is often more, with only short treatments aimed at supporting the child's inner resources during the chemotherapy cycle. In the period between chemotherapy sessions, the child may be treated with gentle balancing techniques directed at promoting relaxation and restfulness, thereby supporting the bioenergetic capacity of the child. A child who is receiving radiation therapy would be approached from the perspective of preventing fascial and tissue scarring. Gentle techniques that promote fluid exchange and maintenance of normal tissue relationships would be used in these children. Once the child has completed a cycle of therapy, whether it be radiation or chemotherapy, osteopathic manipulative techniques would be directed at relieving any compensatory tissue strains and dysfunctions, balancing autonomic tone, and addressing findings that may amplify the child's level of stress and discomfort. Throughout the child's treatment, the overreaching goals of osteopathic manipulative treatment is to facilitate normal function of the fluid and cellular components of the body, promote an inner sense of well-being and peace, and support the child's inherent capacity for health.

References

Pediatric Diagnosis and Treatment

1. AAP Policy Statement: Guidelines for pediatric cancer centers, *Pediatrics* 113:1833-1835, 2004.
2. Gurney JG, Bondy ML: Epidemiology of childhood and adolescent cancer. In Behrman RE, Kliegman RM, Jenson HB, editors: *Nelson textbook of pediatrics,* ed 17 Philadelphia, 2004, Saunders.
3. Childhood cancer survivors may face late effects of the disease, *UCLA Pediatr Update* 11:1-3, 2004.

Acupuncture

1. Guo XZ, Li CJ, Gao BH et al: Acupuncture treatment of benign thyroid nodules. Clinical observation of 65 cases, *J Tradit Chin Med* 4:261-264, 1984.
2. Wu XJ, Wang LQ, Huang BY et al: Treatment of 35 cases of leukoplakia vulvae with helium-neon laser radiation at acupuncture points, *J Tradit Chin Med* 3:62, 1983.
3. Yin X, Yin D, Liu X et al: Treatment of 104 cases of chemotherapy-induced leukopenia by injection of drugs into Zusanli, *J Tradit Chin Med* 21:27-28, 2001.
4. Friedman T, Slayton WB, Allen LS et al: Use of alternative therapies for children with cancer, *Pediatrics* 100:E1, 1997.
5. Dupuis LL, Nathan PC: Options for the prevention and management of acute chemotherapy-induced nausea and vomiting in children, *Paediatr Drugs* 5:597-613, 2003.
6. Reindl TK, Geilen W, Hartmann R et al: Acupuncture against chemotherapy-induced nausea and vomiting in pediatric oncology: interim results of a multicenter crossover study, *Support Care Cancer* 14:172-176, 2006.
7. Zernikow B, Bauer AB, Andler W: Pain control in German pediatric oncology: an inventory [in German], *Schmerz* 16:140-149, 2002 (abstract).
8. Stevens MM, Dalla Pozza L, Cavalletto B et al: Pain and symptom control in paediatric palliative care, *Cancer Surv* 21:211-231, 1994.
9. The National Institutes of Health (NIH) Consensus Development Program: *Acupuncture.* NIH Consensus Development Conference Statement, November 1997.

Aromatherapy

1. Gould MN: Cancer chemoprevention and therapy by monoterpenes, *Environ Health Perspect* 105(Suppl 6):977-979, 1997.
2. Dwivedi C, Abu-Ghazaleh A: Chemopreventive effects of sandalwood oil on skin papillomas in mice, *Eur J Cancer Prev* 6:399-401, 1997.
3. Zappa SB, Cassileth BR: Complementary approaches to palliative oncological care, *J Nurs Care Quality* 18:22-26, 2003.
4. Evans B: An audit into the effects aromatherapy massage and the cancer patient in palliative and terminal care, *Complement Ther Med* 3:239-241, 1995.

5. Kite SM, Maher EJ, Anderson K, Young T et al: Development of an aromatherapy service at a cancer centre, *Palliat Med* 12:171-180, 1998.
6. Buckley J: Massage and aromatherapy massage: nursing art and science, *Int J Palliat Nurs* 8:276-280, 2002.
7. Ernst E: A primer of complementary and alternative medicine commonly used by cancer patients, *Med J Austr* 174:88-92, 2001.
8. Fellowes D, Barnes K, Wilkinson S: Aromatherapy and massage for symptom relief in patients with cancer, *Cochrane Database Syst Rev* 2:CD002287, 2004.
9. Styles J: The use of aromatherapy in hospitalized children with HIV disease, *Complement Ther Nurs Midwifery* 3:16-20, 1997.
10. Wilcock A, Manderson C, Weller R et al: Does aromatherapy benefit patients with cancer attending a specialist palliative care day centre? *Palliat Med* 18:287-290, 2004.
11. Soden K, Vincent K, Craske S et al: A randomized controlled trial of aromatherapy massage in a hospice setting, *Palliat Med* 18:87-92, 2004.
12. Wilkinson S, Aldridge J, Salmon I et al: An evaluations of aromatherapy massage in palliative care, *Palliat Med* 13:409-417, 1999.

Homeopathy

1. *ReferenceWorks Pro 4.2*, San Rafael, Calif, 2008, Kent Homeopathic Associates.
2. Ramakrishnan AU, Coulter CR: *A homoeopathic approach to cancer*, St Louis, 2001, Quality Medical.

Massage Therapy

1. National Comprehensive Cancer Network: *Clinical practice guidelines in oncology: adult cancer pain v1*, 2007. Available at www.nccn.org. Accessed: February 2008.
2. National Comprehensive Cancer Network: *Clinical practice guidelines in oncology: pediatric cancer pain v1*, 2007. Available at www.nccn.org. Accessed: February 2008.
3. National Comprehensive Cancer Network: *Clinical practice guidelines in oncology: cancer related fatigue v4*, 2007. Available at www.nccn.org. Accessed: February 2008.
4. Cassileth BR, Deng GE, Gomez JE et al: Complementary therapies and integrative oncology in lung cancer: ACCP evidence-based clinical practice guidelines (2nd edition), *Chest*, 132:340S-354S, 2007.
5. Ferrell-Tory AT, Glick OJ: The use of therapeutic massage as a nursing intervention to modify anxiety and the perception of cancer pain, *Cancer Nurs* 16:93-101, 1993.
6. Tope DM, Hann DM, Pinkson B: Massage therapy: an old intervention comes of age, *Quality Life A Nurs Challenge* 3:14-18, 1994.
7. Wilkinson S: Get the massage, *Nurs Times* 92:61-64, 1996.
8. Grealish L, Lomasney A, Whiteman B: Foot massage: a nursing intervention to modify the distressing symptoms of pain and nausea in patients hospitalized with cancer, *Cancer Nurs* 23:237-243, 2000.
9. Weinrich SP, Wienrich MC: The effect of massage on pain in cancer patients, *Appl Nurs Res*, 3:140-145, 1990.
10. Smith MC, Kemp J, Hemphill L et al: Outcomes of therapeutic massage for hospitalized cancer patients, *J Nurs Scholar* 34:257-262, 2002.
11. Smith MC, Reeder F, Daniel L et al: Outcomes of touch therapies during bone marrow transplantation, *Altern Ther Med* 9:40-49, 2003.
12. Post-White J, Kinney ME, Savik K et al: Therapeutic massage and healing touch improve symptoms in cancer, *Integr Cancer Ther* 2:332-344, 2003.

13. Cassileth BR, Vickers AJ: Massage therapy for symptom control: outcome study at a major cancer center, *J Pain Symptom Manage* 28:3, 2004.
14. Mehling WE, Jacobs B, Acree M et al: Symptom management with massage and acupuncture in postoperative cancer patients: a randomized controlled trial, *J Pain Symptom Manage* 33:258-266, 2007.
15. Hernandez-Reif M, Field T, Ironson G, et al: Natural killer cells and lymphocytes increase in women with breast cancer following massage therapy, *Intern J Neuroscience*, 115:495-510, 2005.
16. Wilkinson SM, Love SB, Westcombe AM et al: Effectiveness of aromatherapy massage in the management of anxiety and depression in patients with cancer: a multi-center randomized controlled trial, *J Clin Oncol* 25:532-538, 2007.
17. Billhult A, Bergbom I, Stener-Victorin E: Massage relieves nausea in women with breast cancer who are undergoing chemotherapy, *J Altern Complement Med* 13:53-57, 2007.
18. Phipps S: Reduction of distress associated with pediatric bone marrow transplant: complementary health promotion interventions, *Pediatr Rehabil* 5:223-234, 2003.
19. Hernandez-Reif M, Ironson G, Field T et al: Breast cancer patients have improved immune and neuroendocrine functions following massage therapy, *J Psychosom Res* 57:45-52, 2004.
20. Rexilius SJ, Mundt C, Erickson Megel M et al: Therapeutic effects of massage therapy and handling touch on caregivers of patients undergoing autologous hematopoietic stem cells, *Oncol Nurs Forum* 29:E35-E44, 2002.
21. Sims S: Slow stroke back massage for cancer patients, *Nurs Times* 82:47-50, 1986.
22. Collins KB, Thomas DJ: Acupuncture and acupressure for the management of chemotherapy-induced nausea and vomiting, *J Am Acad Nurse Pract* 16:76-80, 2004.
23. Wilkinson S: Aromatherapy and massage in palliative care, *Int J Palliat Nurs* 1:21-30, 1995.
24. Soden K, Vincent K, Craske S et al: A randomized control trial of aromatherapy massage in a hospice setting, *Palliat Med* 18:87-92, 2004.
25. MacDonald G: *Medicine hands: massage therapy for people with cancer*, Tallahassee, Fla, 1999, Findhorn Press.
26. Donoyama N, Wakuda T, Tanitsu T et al: Washing hands before and after performing massages? Changes in bacterial survival count on skin of a massage therapist and a client during massage therapy, *J Altern Complement Med* 10:684-686, 2004.
27. The Diagnosis and Treatment of Peripheral Lymphedema: Consensus Document of the International Society of Lymphology Executive Committee, *Lymphology* 28:113-117, 1995.
28. Crawford J: Myofascial release provides symptomatic relief from chest wall tenderness occasionally seen following lumpectomy and radiation in breast cancer patients, *Int J Oncol Biol Physics* 34:1188-1189, 1996.

Mind/Body

1. Powers S: Empirically supported treatment in pediatric psychology: procedure-related pain, *J Pediatr Psychol* 24:131-145, 1999.
2. Cotanch P, Hockenberry M, Herman S: Self-hypnosis as antiemetic therapy in children receiving chemotherapy, *Oncol Nurs Forum* 12:41-46, 1985.
3. Zeltzer L, LeBaron S, Zeltzer P: The effectiveness of behavioral intervention for reduction of nausea and vomiting in children and adolescents receiving chemotherapy, *J Clin Oncol* 2:684-690, 1984.
4. Zeltzer L, Dolgin M, LeBaron S et al: A randomized, controlled study of behavioral intervention for chemotherapy distress in children with cancer, *Pediatrics* 88:34-42, 1991.

5. Shapiro SL, Bootzin RR, Figueredo AJ et al: The efficacy of mindfulness-based stress reduction in the treatment of sleep disturbance in women with breast cancer: an exploratory study, *J Psychosom Res* 54:85-91, 2003.

6. Hidderley M, Holt M: A pilot randomized trial assessing the effects of autogenic training in early stage cancer patients in relation to psychological status and immune system responses, *Eur J Oncol Nurs* 8:61-65, 2004.

7. Olness K: Hypnosis in pediatric practice, *Curr Probl Pediatr* 12: 1-47, 1981.

Nutrition

1. Kwan ML, Block G, Selvin S et al: Food consumption by children and the risk of childhood acute leukemia, *Am J Epidemiol* 160:1098-1107, 2004.

2. Jensen CD, Block G, Buffler P et al: Maternal dietary risk factors in childhood acute lymphoblastic leukemia (United States), *Cancer Causes Control* 15:559-570, 2004.

3. Maynard M, Gunnell D, Emmett P et al: Fruit, vegetables, and antioxidants in childhood and risk of adult cancer: the Boyd Orr cohort, *J Epidemiol Community Health* 57:218-225, 2003.

4. Asami DK, Hong YJ, Barrett DM et al: Comparison of the total phenolic and ascorbic acid content of freeze-dried and air-dried marionberry, strawberry, and corn grown using conventional, organic, and sustainable agricultural practices. *Agric Food Chem* 51:1237-1241, 2003.

5. Chen J, Stavro PM, Thompson LU: Dietary flaxseed inhibits human breast cancer growth and metastasis and downregulates expression of insulin-like growth factor and epidermal growth factor receptor, *Nutr Cancer* 43:187-192, 2002.

6. Jee SH, Ohrr H, Sull JW et al: Fasting serum glucose level and cancer risk in Korean men and women, *J Am Med Assoc* 293:194-202, 2005.

Osteopathy

1. Willard FH, Mokler DJ, Morgane PJ: Neuroendocrine-immune system and homeostasis. In Ward RC, editor: *Foundations for osteopathic medicine*, Baltimore, 1997, Williams and Wilkins.

2. McEwen BS: Allostasis, allostatic load, and the aging nervous system: role of excitatory amino acids and excitotoxicity, *Neurochem Res* 25:1219-1231, 2000.

3. McEwen BS: Allostasis and allostatic load: implications for neuropsychopharmacology, *Neuropsychopharmacol* 22:108-124, 2000.

4. Seeman TE, McEwen BS, Rowe JW et al: Allostatic load as a marker of cumulative biological risk: MacArthur studies of successful aging, *Proc Natl Acad Sci U S A* 98:4770-4775, 2001.

5. McEwen BS: The neurobiology of stress: from serendipity to clinical relevance, *Brain Res* 886:172-189, 2000.

6. McEwen BS, Seeman T: Protective and damaging effects of mediators of stress. Elaborating and testing the concepts of allostasis and allostatic load, *Ann N Y Acad Sci* 896:30-47, 1999.

7. McEwen BS: Stress, adaptation, and disease. Allostasis and allostatic load. *Ann N Y Acad Sci* 840:33-44, 1998.

8. McEwen BS, Stellar E: Stress and the individual. Mechanisms leading to disease, *Arch Intern Med* 153:2093-2101, 1993.

9. Esterling BA, Kiecolt-Glaser JK, Glaser R: Psychosocial modulation of cytokine-induced natural killer cell activity in older adults, *Psychosom Med* 58:264-272, 1996.

10. Kiecolt-Glaser JK, Glaser R. Stress and immune function in humans. In Ader R, Felton DL, Cohen N, editors: *Psychoneuroimmunology*, ed 2, San Diego, 1991, Academic Press.

11. Sutherland WG: *Teachings in the science of osteopathy*, Portland, Ore, 1990, Rudra Press.

12. Sutherland WG: *Contributions of thought*, ed 2, Portland, Ore, 1998, Rudra Press.

13. Dugan EP, Lemley WW, Roberts CA et al: Effect of lymphatic pump techniques on the immune response to influenza vaccine, *J Am Osteopath Assoc* 101:472, 2001.

14. Hampton D, Evans R, Banihashem M: Lymphatic pump techniques induce a transient basophilia [meeting abstract], *J Am Osteopath Assoc (Austr)* 6:41, 2003.

15. Van Buskirk RL: Nociceptive reflexes and the somatic dysfunction: a model, *J Am Osteopath Assoc* 90:792-809, 1990.

16. Degenhardt BF, Werden SD, Noll DR et al: Quantitative analysis of elderly immune responses to influenza vaccination with osteopathic manipulation [meeting abstracts], *J Am Osteopath Assoc* 100:513, 2000.

17. Steele TF: Utilization of osteopathic lymphatic pump in the office and home for treatment of viral illnesses and after vaccine immunizations, *Fam Phys* 2:8-11, 1998.

18. Jackson KM, Steele TF, Dugan EP et al: Effect of lymphatic and splenic pump techniques on the antibody response to hepatitis B vaccine: a pilot study, *J Am Osteopath Assoc* 98:155-160, 1998.

19. Celander E, Koenig AJ, Celander DR: Effect of osteopathic manipulative therapy on autonomic tone as evidenced by blood pressure changes and activity of the fibrolytic system, *J Am Osteopath Assoc* 67:1037-1038, 1968.

20. Degenhardt BF, Kuchera ML: Update on osteopathic medical concepts and the lymphatic system, *J Am Osteopath Assoc* 96: 97-100, 1996.

21. Kolman S, Getson P, Levin F et al: Effects of osteopathic manipulation on several diferent physiologic functions: Part IV. Absence of crossover effect, *J Am Osteopath Assoc* 73:669-672, 1974.

22. Clymer DH, Levin FL, Sculthorpe RH: Effects of osteopathic manipulation on several different physiologic functions: Part III. Measurement of changes in several different physiological parameters as a result of osteopathic manipulation, *J Am Osteopath Assoc* 72:204-207, 1972.

23. Walko EJ, Janouschek C: Effects of osteopathic manipulative treatment in patients with cervicothoracic pain: pilot study using thermography, *J Am Osteopath Assoc* 94:135-141, 1994.

24. Rogers F, Glassman J, Kavieff R: Effects of osteopathic manipulative treatment on autonomic nervous system function in patients with congestive heart failure, *J Am Osteopath Assoc* 86:605, 1986.

25. Paul RT, Stomel RJ, Broniak FF et al: Interferon levels in human subjects throughout a 24-hour period following thoracic lymphatic pump manipulation, *J Am Osteopath Assoc* 86:92-95, 1986.

26. Kuchera ML, Kuchera WA: *Osteopathic considerations in systemic disease*, Columbus, OH, 1994, Greydon Press.

27. Ward RC, Hruby RJ, Jerome JA et al: *Foundations for osteopathic medicine*, ed 2, St Louis, 2003, Lippincott Williams and Wilkins.

CHAPTER 19

Cerebral Palsy

Acupuncture | May Loo

Chiropractic | Anne Spicer

Herbs—Western | Alan D. Woolf, Paula M. Gardiner, Lana Dvorkin-Camiel, Jack Maypole

Homeopathy | Janet L. Levatin

Magnet Therapy | Agatha P. Colbert, Deborah Risotti

Mind/Body | Timothy Culbert, Lynda Richstmeier Cyr

Osteopathy | Jane Carreiro

✳ PEDIATRIC DIAGNOSIS AND TREATMENT

Cerebral palsy (CP) is a descriptive term for a group of disorders of movement, muscle tone, or other features that reflect abnormal control over motor function by the central nervous system (CNS).[1] It is the most common chronic motor disability that begins in childhood, with a prevalence of 2 per 1000 live births in term infants but as many as 50 to 80 per 1000 preterm, low–birth-weight infants.[1-3]

Possible etiology appears to be multiple but the precise cause remains unknown, although it is most often related to prenatal insults and prematurity, when the immature brain is vulnerable to hypoxia and hemorrhage. CP in term infants is found in postnatal infections or in various metabolic conditions, such as Reye syndrome.[4]

CP is classified primarily as (1) spastic (or pyramidal), which includes subtypes of quadriplegia (motor involvement of all four extremities), diplegia (primarily the lower extremities), and hemiplegia (involvement of one side of the body); or (2) dyskinetic (extrapyramidal) with choreoathetoid and ataxic subtypes.[1] Children can often exhibit more than one type of CP.

Evaluation often involves a multidisciplinary team approach with a pediatric developmentalist, physical therapist, psychologist, and speech therapist. Neurological findings include abnormal resting muscle tone, increased deep tendon reflexes, pathological reflexes (such as the Babinski or plantar reflex), abnormal primitive reflexes, and delayed protective postural responses.[1] Various pediatric outcome instruments, such as the Gross Motor Function Classification System (GMFCS), can be used to assess levels of severity of ambulatory CP.[5]

Physical therapy is a major component of treatment. A nonrandomized cohort study with 62 months' (mean) follow-up of 10 premature infants with CNS insults at risk for developing spastic diplegic CP revealed a consistently applied physiotherapy program resulted in better motor outcomes.[6] Botulinum toxin A (Btx-A) is now widely used in CP[7-9] to provide temporary reduction of spasticity and delay the shortening of spastic muscle. Btx-A blocks the release of acetylcholine from the axon terminal into the synaptic cleft of the motor endplate, resulting in paresis of the injected musculature. Such localized, temporary chemodenervation of affected muscles can lead to functional gains and may improve the child's daily routine and rehabilitative care.[10,11]

Intrathecal baclofen therapy has also been administered for children with more severe spastic CP.[12-14]

Various surgical procedures include lengthening of the medial and lateral hamstring,[15] tenomuscular lengthening of the Achilles tendon,[16] multilevel surgery,[17] or selective dorsal rhizotomy.[1,15,18,19]

✳ CAM THERAPY RECOMMENDATIONS

Acupuncture

Acupuncture treatment for CP is usually incorporated as part of an integrative, multidisciplinary regimen consisting of various forms of acupuncture such as body acupuncture or scalp acupuncture, physical therapy, occupational therapy, massage, and other therapies including hydrotherapy, osteopathic manipulation, social adaptation, electroneurostimulation, biofeedback, or conductive training.[1-4] The children in China are often hospitalized and given intensive therapies 5 days per week for several months.[1-3] One particular form of acupuncture is sometimes used in isolation, such as tongue acupuncture. At this time, there is an ongoing collaborative study between Beijing Children's Hospital and the University of Arizona to incorporate acupuncture as part of an five-treatment protocol.

Chiropractic

The efforts of the chiropractor in the management of a child with CP are to remove interference to optimal function. The doctor of chiropractic is also concerned with preventing deformities that may arise secondary to postural variations, joint immobilization, falls, and spasticity.[1]

The most common spinal finding by the chiropractor is at the C0 to C1 level, and the most common cranial finding is at the occipital base and sphenobasilar junction.[2] It is interesting to note that suboccipital stretching techniques have been found to improve range of motion at the hip.[3] Addressing upper cervical spinal function is therefore foundational to enhanced gait maintenance, which is related to the abundant mechanoreceptors at the upper cervical spine that serve to direct postural control.[4,5]

Also noted is that with chiropractic adjustments to the lower cervical spine, significant changes occurred in the muscle tone at the lumbar pelvis.[6] Maintenance of improved postural control and muscle tone gives rise to higher function in activities of daily living and will decrease further muscular and spinal asymmetries. This in turn decreases pain levels and reduces incidence of injury.

Chiropractic management of the child with CP should include an assessment of the temporomandibular joint and corresponding musculature to aid in control of drooling and minimize influence into the cervical spine.

Also included in the care regimen should be trigger point therapy at the lateral thigh, which aids in bladder control and decreases scissor-gait patterning. This can be performed in the office by the chiropractor as well as at home by the child or the child's caregivers.

Parents of infants are encouraged to breastfeed or, if bottle-feeding, alternate the baby's position from the left arm to the right arm holding position in an effort to alternately stimulate the hemispheres of the brain. Development of binocular vision and binaural hearing may be stimulated passively by engaging all ranges of visual and auditory fields. Physical therapy is recommended especially when homolateral patterning is seen before 6 months of age and cross-crawl patterning begins by 10 months of age.

Passive stretches directed at reaching a maximal range of joint motion can minimize joint immobilization sequelae. These stretches are best tolerated when initiated slowly to not stimulate spastic reactions from the activated muscle. In a child with hemiparesis, full range of motion, mirror-image exercises at the higher functioning side of the body will increase the ranges of motion at the same joint on the opposite side of the body.

Nutritional considerations relate primarily to muscle contracture. A calcium/magnesium/vitamin D combination supplement supports the muscle under contracture. Trace mineral supplements strengthen the bone mineral against the contractile pressure.

A pilot study involving adults and children was conducted to evaluate the upper cervical adjustment on neurological dysfunction secondary to CP. Measures included surface electromyography (SEMG), brainstem evoked potentials (BSEP), balance platform, and grip strength. Ten participants were studied and received upper cervical adjustments. After the adjustments, the SEMG showed decreased muscle tone and increased symmetry between the right and left side of the body. The BSEP showed observable improvements in all evaluated subjects. The balance was conducted on a computer-evaluated platform, and all patients assessed showed improved balance. Grip strength was difficult to evaluate in the children but appeared to be improving as well. Subjective reports of improvement in other areas of life were also reported. These reports included improved sleep, decreased irritability, decreased pain, decreased incidence of respiratory infections, and (in one case) a correction of strabismus.[7]

One reported case involved a 5-year-old boy with CP who was treated with an upper cervical adjustment. SEMG recordings were taken before and after the adjustment. The recordings clearly indicate a reduction in muscle activity after the chiropractic adjustment.[8]

Four children with CP were studied for changes related to chiropractic intervention. All four children demonstrated improvements in muscle tone as well as in independent mobility, feeding, and postural control.[9]

Kentuckiana Children's Center in Louisville, Kentucky, is an integrative chiropractic clinic for children with special challenges. Children with CP are commonly treated there, with case studies reporting complete resolution of mild CP symptoms and improvement in hundreds more.[10]

Electrode stimulation at the C2 to C4 cord level has the ability to decrease spasticity and improve motor control in individuals with CP.[11]

Several chiropractic case studies exist that demonstrate an improvement in manifestations of CP after chiropractic adjustments, particularly at the cervical spine.[12-15]

Herbs—Western

Cerebral palsy is a disability caused by brain damage before or during birth that may result in a loss of voluntary muscular control and coordination. By definition, CP is a permanent condition that affects neuromuscular development. Consequently, treatment for this condition primarily seeks to maximize function and minimize symptoms such as spasticity, weakness, or contractures. In some cases, CP is associated with children who have developmental delay or mental retardation.

In healthy adult individuals, ginkgo (*Ginkgo biloba L.*) has been found to have clinically significant cognition-enhancing and memory-boosting effects. Furthermore, when used in adults with dementia, ginkgo was found to improve learning, cognitive function, and recall.[1] (See Chapter 14, Autism.) However, the use of this herb in children with cognitive impairment or mental retardation associated with CP has not been studied. Ginkgo leaf is administered orally; ginkgo's fruit and pulp are to be avoided because of concern for potential severe allergic reactions. In addition, consumption of raw or roasted ginkgo plant seeds may lower seizure thresholds, causing seizures or death in children,[2-4] making this of particular concern for children with CP who have a higher incidence of seizures.

Doses of ginseng are prepared from the plant's roots and are administered orally. These herbs may be found as a number of species. Asian ginseng has been studied variably for its impact on mental performance in healthy adults. Overall, in these adult studies there is not a clear indication that it significantly boosts mental performance, memory, or cognitive ability.[5] There are no studies in children of the effectiveness of any ginseng species—neither in healthy, developmentally intact children nor in children with cognitive deficits associated with CP. The use of *Panax ginseng* in infants and newborns is discouraged because of reports of intoxication.[3,4]

See Chapter 13, Attention-Deficit Hyperactivity Disorder, for information on the use of these herbs for attentiveness or impulsivity.

Homeopathy

Before using this section, please see Appendix A, Homeopathy, for definitions of practitioner expertise categories and general information on prescribing homeopathic medicines.

Practitioner Expertise Category 3

There are no controlled clinical trials of homeopathic treatment for CP, although the homeopathic literature contains a few references regarding its use.[1] Homeopathic treatment can be used safely and in combination with other treatment modalities, both alternative and conventional. Because CP is a complex and multifaceted problem with protean manifestations, successful homeopathic treatment usually requires extensive training in the art and science of homeopathy. Any one of many homeopathic medicines may be used to treat CP, depending on the characteristics of the patient being treated; sophisticated homeopathic analysis and long-term follow-up are required. For these reasons, specific medicines for treating CP will not be presented here. Interested readers are referred to the homeopathic literature for further study.[1]

Magnet Therapy

The Magnessage (Painfree Lifestyles, Bracey, Va.) can be used to gently massage all sides of the arms and legs that have spasticity of muscles. Perform massage therapy daily for 10 to 15 minutes to obtain maximum relaxation of muscles. The Magnessage may be obtained from Painfree Lifestyles (800-480-8601).

Mind/Body

Biofeedback training as an adjunctive therapy has assisted children with CP in improving ambulation and decreasing muscle spasticity. Dursun et al.[1] demonstrated in a randomized controlled trial that 21 children with spastic CP who received EMG biofeedback training in addition to their conventional exercise program obtained statistically significant improvements in gait function compared with the 15 children in the control group who received only the conventional exercise program. Research by Colborne et al.[2] suggested that EMG biofeedback may be an effective adjunctive therapy for children with spastic hemiplegia secondary to CP. In this study of seven children (ages 8 to 15 years), EMG biofeedback training for muscle relaxation and activation was compared with physical therapy in two 8-week periods in a crossover design. The biofeedback training, compared with physical therapy, had a positive impact on stride length, velocity, and gait symmetry.[3]

Individuals with CP often experience chronic pain secondary to their musculoskeletal problems. EMG biofeedback and relaxation/mental imagery may provide treatment options to decrease pain in this population, and future research is warranted.

Mauersberger et al.,[4] in a pilot study of children with spastic quadriplegic CP, were able to demonstrate that training in self-hypnosis reduced muscle tension readings as measured by surface EMG in three of four subjects and that two of the subjects were better able to control involuntary movements.

Osteopathy

Ultimately the goal of osteopathic treatment is to facilitate and nurture health within the child and within the family. In general, the physical goals of osteopathic treatment of the child with CP are to improve function, decrease pain, and limit or prevent contractures, hip dislocations, and scoliosis. Osteopathic techniques are used to facilitate normal function of the different tissues of the child's body that may be interfering with the child's ability to reach his or her full potential. Although no conclusive study has yet been done, many osteopaths have written of the relationship between osteopathic findings, particularly cranial somatic dysfunction, and CP.[1-11]

An important goal of osteopathic treatment in children with CP is to decrease pain. Chronically elevated muscle tone can cause pain and discomfort that disrupt normal activities such as sleep. Osteopathic techniques aimed at passive or isometric muscle stretch, such as muscle energy techniques, are effective in the older child who can follow directions. Counterstrain techniques, especially in the shoulder and hip girdle, can also provide relief and be taught to parents and other caregivers. Depending on the skill of the practitioner, counterstrain techniques can be used in the toddler and young child. Balanced ligamentous and other "indirect" techniques are appropriate, well tolerated, and useful in all age groups, especially very young children or children unable to follow commands.

Another goal of osteopathic manipulative treatment in a child with CP is to influence changes in proprioceptive input from joints, connective tissues, and muscle, which may be compromising posture, balance, and movement. Joint contractures, scoliosis, and hip dislocation may all be complications of chronic muscle spasm, abnormal postural forces, and altered joint mechanics. In addition, children with CP are creating, refining, and incorporating movement strategies to interact with their environment. Often this involves the development of compensatory movement patterns that create or exacerbate abnormal postural mechanisms. Osteopathic treatment would be directed toward alleviating some of these abnormal or stressful inputs resulting from the compensatory changes. This will help the child create motor strategies that are minimally encumbered by these compensatory changes. Although the baseline hypertonia remains, appropriate osteopathic treatment is directed at alleviating muscle spasm and articular strain that has developed secondarily and is now contributing to the overall level of tone in the child. This should facilitate the child's ability to perform motor planning and execute movement.

A third goal of osteopathic treatment is to maintain muscle tone at a baseline level. For the child with spastic CP, every movement made with the affected limb has the potential to increase the resting muscle tone through the unmodulated spinal reflex.[3,12] Altered use of the affected limb leads to compensatory biomechanical changes in the limb stabilizers and postural muscles. These compensatory changes will often exacerbate or summate with the baseline muscle tone resulting from the neurological insult. Consequently the level of spasticity due to the neurological insult may be lower than the tone the child is functioning with on a daily basis. Thus even a child with a mild spasticity is at risk for developing further muscle contraction and deleterious impact on function of a limb if appropriate therapies are started too late or discontinued too early.

When a child has increased tone in a muscle group, development of postural and cortical function is affected. Biomechanical strains have been shown to influence cortical mapping of somatosensory input.[13,14] Increased muscle tone alters joint mechanics and proprioception. Thus spasticity can influence primary somatosensory mapping, muscle coupling, and movement strategies. It has been suggested that the abnormal postural control in children with some forms of spasticity is due to biomechanical rather than neurological factors.[15] Although definitive studies are lacking, empirical evidence suggests that the addition of osteopathic treatment to more traditional early intervention protocols may aid in the child's overall development.

In a child with CP, somatic dysfunction in the neck and torso may alter the proprioceptive input from these areas and further compromise stability and posture. Alleviating biomechanical stresses with osteopathic manipulation may help the child by normalizing input from joint afferents and balancing agonist/antagonist muscle tone. In older children, well-developed compensatory mechanisms for stability may be compromised by changes in environmental demands or biomechanical stresses.[3] Frequent postural adjustments can be misinterpreted as inattentiveness and distractability. Yet in the child with CP, this movement may be necessary to maintain stability or relieve muscle ache and fatigue.

Many children with CP will have associated problems in other systems. These need to be diagnosed and addressed as early as possible to avoid further compromising the child's development. Approximately 40% of children with CP have visual perception problems, most of which are visual processing problems that may be related to altered somatosensory mapping. Complicating this is the fact that children with CP are more reliant on visual input for balance control than most children. Overcorrection of visual acuity may alter postural mechanics and adversely affect the child's balance. Osteopathic physicians often work closely with functional optometrists and pediatric neuroophthalmologists who manage vision correction from a whole-body, whole-system perspective.

Children with CP seem to respond best to osteopathic approaches that influence proprioception and joint position. Slow, gentle techniques that rely on activating forces within the patient appear to be most effective. Counterstrain, Sutherland's approach, and facilitated positional release tend to be very helpful in younger children. In older children who can follow directions, muscle energy techniques using isotonic eccentric contraction and reciprocal inhibition can be quite effective and may be taught to parents as part of an at-home program. Anecdotally, the addition of osteopathic manipulative procedures that influence joint position and proprioceptive function appear to enhance the child's response to physical therapy and rehabilitation programs.

Children with CP need consistent osteopathic treatment to maintain minimal baseline levels of spasticity. Most children will need to be treated fairly regularly, at least as often as every growth spurt, provided that they also receive appropriate therapies at home or school. Osteopathic physicians typically work as part of a team approach, coordinating with the child's orthotist, orthopedic surgeon, and speech, occupational, and physical therapists. Good communication with an orthotist, who can sculpt orthotic devices that support the body's inherent capabilities, and therapists, who can springboard from the changes created through osteopathic treatment, is very beneficial for the child.

CP is a very complicated disorder to manage because the issues change as the child matures and develops. The health of the child's family needs to be supported and nurtured as well. Good communication among all healthcare providers and well-informed parents is essential. Family resources are often stretched financially, physically, and emotionally. Parents and siblings may be struggling with feelings of guilt and apprehension for the future. Some families may find fortification in counseling or group support meetings. Other families will work it out by themselves. Ultimately, the family needs to be a family, not a household of people focusing on this one child with a cerebral injury. As with each individual, each family is different. A good clinician must be able to step back and see the whole picture, not just the child's neurological condition.

References

Pediatric Diagnosis and Treatment

1. Petersen MC, Whitaker TM: *Cerebral palsy in disorders of development and learning*, ed 3, London, 2003, BC Decker.
2. Surveillance of Cerebral Palsy in Europe: Surveillance of cerebral palsy: a collaboration of cerebral palsy surveys and registers, *Dev Med Child Neurol* 42:816-824, 2000.
3. Behrman RE, Kliegman RM, Jenson HB, editors: *Nelson's textbook of pediatrics*, Philadelphia, 2004, Saunders.
4. Cans C, McManus V, Crowley M et al; Surveillance of Cerebral Palsy in Europe Collaborative Group: Cerebral palsy of postneonatal origin: characteristics and risk factors, *Paediatr Perinat Epidemiol* 18:214-220, 2004.
5. Oeffinger DJ, Tylkowski CM, Rayens MK et al: Gross Motor Function Classification System and outcome tools for assessing ambulatory cerebral palsy: a multicenter study, *Dev Med Child Neurol* 46:311-319, 2004.
6. Kanda T, Pidcock FS, Hayakawa K et al: Motor outcome differences between two groups of children with spastic diplegia who received different intensities of early onset physiotherapy followed for 5 years, *Brain Dev* 26:118-126, 2004.
7. Wallen MA, O'Flaherty SJ, Waugh MC: Functional outcomes of intramuscular botulinum toxin type A in the upper limbs of children with cerebral palsy: a phase II trial, *Arch Phys Med Rehabil* 85:192-200, 2004. Erratum in: *Arch Phys Med Rehabil* 85:862, 2004.
8. O'Brien CF: Treatment of spasticity with botulinum toxin, *Clin J Pain* 18(6 Suppl):S182-S190, 2002.
9. Yang TF, Fu CP, Kao NT et al: Effect of botulinum toxin type A on cerebral palsy with upper limb spasticity, *Am J Phys Med Rehabil* 82:284-289, 2003.
10. Berweck S, Heinen F: Use of botulinum toxin in pediatric spasticity (cerebral palsy), *Mov Disord* 19(Suppl 8):S162-S167, 2004 [review].
11. Hurvitz EA, Conti GE, Brown SH: Changes in movement characteristics of the spastic upper extremity after botulinum toxin injection, *Arch Phys Med Rehabil* 84:444-454, 2003.
12. Awaad Y, Tayem H, Munoz S et al: Functional assessment following intrathecal baclofen therapy in children with spastic cerebral palsy, *J Child Neurol* 18:26-34, 2003.
13. Murphy NA, Irwin MC, Hoff C: Intrathecal baclofen therapy in children with cerebral palsy: efficacy and complications, *Arch Phys Med Rehabil* 83:1721-1725, 2002.
14. Campbell WM, Ferrel A, McLaughlin JF et al: Long-term safety and efficacy of continuous intrathecal baclofen, *Dev Med Child Neurol* 44:660-665, 2002.
15. Kay RM, Rethlefsen SA, Hale JM et al: Comparison of proximal and distal rotational femoral osteotomy in children with cerebral palsy, *J Pediatr Orthop* 23:150-154, 2003.
16. Weigl D, Copeliovitch L, Itzchak Y et al: Sonographic healing stages of Achilles tendon after tenomuscular lengthening in children with cerebral palsy, *J Pediatr Orthop* 21:778-783, 2001.

17. Saraph V, Zwick EB, Zwick G et al: Multilevel surgery in spastic diplegia: evaluation by physical examination and gait analysis in 25 children, *J Pediatr Orthop* 22:150-157, 2002.
18. Steinbok P, McLeod K: Comparison of motor outcomes after selective dorsal rhizotomy with and without preoperative intensified physiotherapy in children with spastic diplegic cerebral palsy, *Pediatr Neurosurg* 36:142-147, 2002.
19. Tsirikos AI, Chang WN, Shah SA et al: Preserving ambulatory potential in pediatric patients with cerebral palsy who undergo spinal fusion using unit rod instrumentation, *Spine* 28:480-483, 2003.

Acupuncture

1. Loo M: Personal observations, Shanghai Xinhua Hospital, Beijing Children's Hospital, May 2004.
2. Zhou XJ, Zheng K: Treatment of 140 cerebral palsied children with a combined method based on traditional Chinese medicine (TCM) and western medicine, *J Zhejiang Univ Sci B* 6:57-60, 2005.
3. Zhou XJ, Chen T, Chen JT: 75 infantile palsy children treated with acupuncture, acupressure and functional training [in Chinese], *Zhongguo Zhong Xi Yi Jie He Za Zhi* 13:197, 220-222, 1993.
4. Shaitor IN, Bogdanov OV, Shaitor VM: The combined use of functional biocontrol and acupuncture reflexotherapy in children with the spastic forms of infantile cerebral palsy [in Russian], *Vopr Kurortol Fizioter Lech Fiz Kult* Nov/Dec:38-42, 1990.

Chiropractic

1. Mikawa Y, Watanabe R, Shikata J: Cervical myelo-radiculopathy in athetoid cerebral palsy, *Arch Orthop Trauma Surg* 116:116-118, 1997.
2. Waltz JM: Spinal chord stimulation for palsies, *Patient Care* 13:18-206, 1997.
3. Amalu WC: Cortical blindness, cerebral palsy, epilepsy, and recurring otitis media: a case study in chiropractic management, *Today's Chiropractic* May/Jun:16-25, 1998.
4. Sweat R, Ammons D: Case study: treatment of a cerebral palsy patient, *Today's Chiropractic* Nov/Dec:51-52, 1988.
5. Webster LL: Case study—mental retardation/cerebral palsy, *Chiropractic Pediatr* 1:15-16, 1994.
6. Golden L, VanEgmond C: Longitudinal clinical case study: multidisciplinary care of child with multiple functional and developmental disorders, *J Manipulative Physiol Ther* 17:279, 1994.
7. McMullen M: Chiropractic and the handicapped child/cerebral palsy, *ICA Int Rev Chiropractic* Sep/Oct:39-45, 1990.
8. Pollard H, Ward G: A study of two stretching techniques for improving hip flexion range of motion, *J Manipulative Physiol Ther* 20:443-447, 1997.
9. Fitz-Ritzon D: Therapeutic traction: a review of neurological principles and clinical applications, *J Manipulative Physiol Ther* 7:39-49, 1984.
10. Richmond F, Abrahams V: Morphology and distribution of muscle spindles in dorsal muscles of the cat neck, *J Neurophysiol* 38:1322-1339, 1975.
11. Nansel DD, Waldorf T, Cooperstein R: Effect of cervical spinal adjustments on lumbar paraspinal muscle tone: evidence for facilitation of intersegmental tonic neck reflexes, *J Manipulative Physiol Ther* 16:91-95, 1993.
12. Feeley Collins K: The efficacy of upper cervical chiropractic care on children and adults with cerebral palsy: a preliminary report, *Chiropractic Pediatr* 1:13-15, 1994.
13. Hospers LA, Daso JA, Steinie LV: Electromyographic patterns of mentally retarded cerebral palsy patient after upper cervical adjustment, *Today's Chiropractic* Sep/Oct:13-14, 1986.

14. McCoy M, Malakhova E, Safronov Y: Improvement in paraspinal muscle tone, autonomic function and quality of life in four children with cerebral palsy undergoing subluxation based chiropractic care: four retrospective case studies, *J Vertebral Subluxation Res* 4:19-21, 2000.
15. Like a flower unfolding: chiropractic offers hope for cerebral palsy, *J Am Chiropractic Assoc* Aug:46-50, 2002.

Herbs—Western

1. Oken BS, Storzbach DM, Kaye JA: The efficacy of *Ginkgo biloba* on cognitive function in Alzheimer disease, *Arch Neurol* 55:1409-1415, 1998.
2. Kajiyama Y, Fujii K, Takeuchi H et al: Ginkgo seed poisoning, *Pediatrics* 109:325-327, 2002.
3. McGuffin M, Hobbs C, Upton R et al, editors: *American Herbal Products Association's botanical safety handbook*, Boca Raton, Fla, 1997, CRC Press.
4. *Panax ginseng*. Available at www.naturaldatabase.com. Accessed Jan 25, 2005.
5. Sorensen H, Sonne J: A double-masked study of the effects of ginseng on cognitive functions, *Curr Ther Res* 57:959-968, 1996.
6. Arenz A, Kelin M, Flehe K et al: Occurrence of neurotoxic 4'-o-methylpyridoxine in *Ginkgo biloba* leaves, ginkgo medications and Japanese ginkgo food, *Planta Med* 62:548-551, 1996.

Homeopathy

1. *ReferenceWorks Pro 4.2*, San Rafael, Calif, 2008, Kent Homeopathic Associates.

Mind/Body

1. Dursun E, Dursun N, Alican D: Effects of biofeedback treatment on gait in children with cerebral palsy, *Disabil Rehabil* 26:116-120, 2004.
2. Colborne G, Wright F, Naumann S: Feedback of triceps surae EMG in gait of children with cerebral palsy: a controlled study, *Arch Phys Med Rehabil* 75:40-45, 1994.
3. Engel J, Jensen M, Schwartz L: Outcome of biofeedback-assisted relaxation for pain in adults with cerebral palsy: preliminary findings, *Appl Psychophysiol Biofeedback* 29:135-140, 2004.
4. Mauersberger K, Artz K, Duncan B et al: Can children with spastic cerebral palsy use self-hypnosis to reduce muscle tone? A preliminary study, *Integr Med* 2:93-96, 2000.

Osteopathy

1. Infants and children. In Magoun HIS, editor: *Osteopathy in the cranial field*, Kirksville, Mo, 1951, CJ Krehbiel.
2. Arbuckle B: The value of occupational and osteopathic therapy in the rehabilitation of the cerebral palsy victim. In Patriquin DA, editor: *The selected writings of Beryl E. Arbuckle, DO, FAAO*, ed 2, Indianapolis, 1994, American Academy of Osteopathy.
3. Carreiro JE: *Cerebral palsy: an osteopathic approach to children*, London, 2003, Churchill Livingstone.
4. Sutherland WG: *Teachings in the science of osteopathy*, Portland, Ore, 1990, Rudra Press.
5. Arbuckle B: Subclinical signs of trauma, *J Am Osteopath Assoc* 58:227-237, 1958.
6. Arbuckle B: The infant—an entity, *J Am Osteopath Assoc* 49:474-477, 1950.
7. Arbuckle B: Guidance for necessary environment for the cerebral palsied child, *Osteopath Prof* 19:18-19, 1952.
8. Arbuckle B: Cranial technic: reactions in infant brain resulting from pressure at or prior to birth, *Osteopath Prof* 15:11-38, 1948.

9. Arbuckle B: The CP patient: II. Rehabilitation through osteopathic manipulation and occupational therapy, *J Osteopath* 69:28-38, 1962.

10. Arbuckle B: The CP Patient: I. Rehabilitation through occupational and manipulative therapy, *J Osteopath* 69:24-39, 1962.

11. Wilson P: Cerebral palsy: a study of 92 cases, *Osteopath Prof* 21:11-15, 1954.

12. Carreiro JE: *Neurology: an osteopathic approach to children*, London, 2003, Churchill Livingstone.

13. Merzenich MM, Schreiner C, Jenkins W et al: Neural mechanisms underlying temporal integration, segmentation, and input sequence representation: some implications for the origin of learning disabilities, *Ann N Y Acad Sci* 682:1-22, 1993.

14. Merzenich MM, Recanzone GH, Jenkins WM et al: Adaptive mechanisms in cortical networks underlying cortical contributions to learning and nondeclarative memory, *Cold Spring Harb Symp Quant Biol* 55:873-887, 1990.

15. Woollacott MH, Burtner P, Jensen J et al: Development of postural responses during standing in healthy children and children with spastic diplegia, *Neurosci Biobehav Rev* 22:583-589, 1998.

CHAPTER 20

Childhood Illnesses: General Overview

Acupuncture | May Loo

Herbs—Chinese | Catherine Ulbricht, Jennifer Woods, Mark Wright

Homeopathy | Janet L. Levatin

Massage Therapy | Mary C. McLellan

✳ PEDIATRIC DIAGNOSIS AND TREATMENT

The conditions in this chapter are grouped together because they share similar characteristics:

1. They are often endemic and are controlled by vaccination in developed countries.
2. They affect infants and young children.
3. The time and severity of clinical presentation may be influenced by maternal antibodies transmitted through the placenta.
4. They have characteristic, readily recognizable rashes or clinical presentations.

This chapter will focus on measles, mumps, rubella, roseola, varicella (chickenpox), and fifth disease. The pros and cons of vaccination is a controversial topic among general pediatricians and CAM practitioners and will not be discussed here.

Measles (Rubeola)

Measles is highly contagious and was endemic before the measles vaccine was developed. Before the vaccine, there were approximately 500,000 cases and 500 deaths reported annually with epidemic cycles every 2 to 3 years. After measles vaccination began in 1963, the incidence of measles decreased by more than 98%, and 2- to 3-year epidemic cycles no longer occurred. However, measles still causes childhood morbidity and mortality in developing countries.[1,2]

Measles appears as an acute viral infection characterized by an eruption of a maculopapular rash that progresses from the neck and face to the trunk, arms, and legs. Toward the end of the illness, a high fever accompanies the rash. Infants can acquire immunity transplacentally from mothers who had measles or received the vaccine. Immunity may persist and interfere with the infant's vaccination before 12 months of age.[2] Treatment is supportive with no specific antiviral therapy.

Rubella (German Measles)

Rubella was widespread in the past but now occurs infrequently. The primary purpose for vaccination against rubella is the prevention of congenital rubella syndrome (CRS), which may affect all of the internal organs and cause multiple birth defects such as microcephaly, deafness, and mental retardation, as well as heart, liver and spleen damage. Infants with CRS can shed large quantities of the virus from body secretions for up to 1 year and can therefore transmit the disease to anyone caring for them who is susceptible, especially pregnant women.[1]

The most characteristic clinical sign is tender lymphadenopathy followed by a rapidly spreading discrete maculopapular rash from the face throughout the body. Treatment is supportive with no specific antiviral therapy.[2]

Mumps

Before 1967, when the mumps vaccine was licensed, the disease was widespread and occurred primarily in 5- to 9-year–old children. In the 1980s there was a shift towards older children. Since 1989 there has been a steady decline after institution of the second mumps vaccine.[1] Mumps is characterized by painful enlargement of the salivary glands. Treatment is supportive with no specific antiviral therapy.[2]

Varicella (Chickenpox)

Chickenpox occurs in almost all children, with the majority of cases being mild and self-limiting. Because of complications that include secondary bacterial infection, pneumonia (rare in children), and central nervous system manifestations ranging from aseptic meningitis to encephalitis,[1] vaccination was initially given to immune-compromised children in 1995 and was added to routine pediatric immunization in 2001.[3] The characteristic rash begins as intensely pruritic erythematous macules that evolve quickly from papules to clear, fluid-filled vesicles. Treatment with antiviral acyclovir is not recommended for healthy children with uncomplicated varicella.

Roseola

Roseola is a mild, febrile, exanthematous illness occurring almost exclusively during infancy. More than 95% of roseola cases occur in children younger than 3 years, with a peak at 6 to 15 months of age. Transplacental antibodies likely protect most infants until 6 months of age. The illness is generally characterized by high body temperature (101° to 101° F), although the child appears healthy. The fever may resolve abruptly, followed by the eruption of a pink, generalized, nonpruritic rash. Treatment is supportive in uncomplicated cases.[2]

Fifth Disease (Erythema Infectiosum)

Fifth disease is a benign, self-limiting illness that appears with prodromal, low-grade fever and URI symptoms followed by the appearance of the hallmark "slapped cheek" erythematous rash that quickly spreads to the trunk and extremities. Treatment of uncomplicated cases is supportive.[2]

✳ CAM THERAPY RECOMMENDATIONS

Acupuncture

Chinese medicine posits that most childhood diseases are due to "womb toxin," or residual effects of infections the mother contracted and passed along to the child in utero. The energy or Qi of the maternal illness still lingers even when the serum antibody is no longer present. It is a natural process for the child to "expel" these toxins through childhood illnesses. If this normal outlet for accumulated toxins is blocked, the toxins can remain in the body and give rise to problems or diseases at a later age.[1-5]

Recommendations

These recommendations for symptomatic care can be applied after vaccination:

- Fever: GV14, LI11
- Cough: CV22, LU7, P6
- Boost immunity: ST36
- Itching/pruritus: ST15, GB31[6,7]

Herbs—Chinese

The Chinese herb *Clinacanthus nutans* (Burm. f.) Lindau (Qing Jian), which is not a classically documented herb but a relatively recent addition to the Chinese herbal materia medica, is able to kill varicella zoster virus (VZV) and other herpes viruses in test tubes. Small studies have compared an extract of the herb with a placebo in the treatment of shingles. Research suggests that a topical application of *C. nutans* extract may shorten the length of time that skin lesions are present. More research is needed before any recommendations can be made.[1,2]

Chinese herbal prescription can be divided into two discrete phases. In the first phase, the Wind-Heat is considered to be relatively superficial and would be treated by the prescription Yin Qiao San, which includes flower of *Lonicera japonica* Thunb. (Jin Yin Hua), fruit of *Forsythia suspensa* (Thunb.) Vahl (Lian Qiao), fruit of *Arctium lappa* L. (Niu Bang Zi), and stem and leaf of *Mentha haplocalyx* Briq. (Bo He). It is a classically established prescription and is available in prepared form. These herbs are all considered to clear Heat from the superficial layers of the body. If the "heat pathogen" is not expelled in time and "sinks into the body," then it would be more appropriate to use Qing Li Jie Du Tang, which comprises an entirely different group of herbs, including root of *Scutellaria baicalensis* Georgi (Huang Qin), rhizome of *Coptis chinensis* Franch. (Huang Lian), root-bark of *Paeonia suffruticosa* Andrews (Mu Dan Pi), and fresh root of *Rehmannia glutinosa* (Gaertn.) Libosch. (Sheng Di Huang). Scientific evidence for these prescriptions is lacking.

Homeopathy

This section contains clinical information on measles and other self-limited viral infections of childhood that are included in this book, fifth disease (parvovirus B$_{19}$ infection), mumps, rubella, and roseola.*

Before using this section, please see Appendix A, Homeopathy, for definitions of practitioner expertise categories and general information on prescribing homeopathic medicines.

Practitioner Expertise Category 1

Category 1 includes uncomplicated measles and other childhood diseases.

There are no controlled clinical trials of homeopathy for treatment of measles and the other self-limited viral illness of childhood, although the homeopathic literature contains evidence for its use in the form of accumulated clinical experience.[1] Although these viral illnesses are usually relatively minor and resolve on their own (with the exception of measles, which can be more serious, especially in malnourished individuals, and mumps when it affects the testes), homeopathy can be used to lessen the symptoms and help patients resolve the illnesses more quickly than they would without treatment. For uncomplicated measles and other viral illnesses, it is safe to try homeopathic treatment alone or in combination with other therapies such as herbs, hydrotherapy, and conventional antipyretics.

The goal in treating a viral illness homeopathically is to determine the single homeopathic medicine whose description in the materia medica most closely matches the symptom picture of the patient. Study of a homeopathic repertory in cases of viral illness would focus on one or more of the following organs or symptom expressions: skin (eruption section), face (eruption and discoloration [redness] sections), fever, cough, external throat (cervical glands), eyes (discharge), nose (coryza, catarrh, and discharge sections), chest, and others, as needed, for the case being analyzed.[2] Often mental and emotional states in addition to physical symptoms are considered.

Once the medicine has been selected, it can be given orally or sublingually in the 30C potency three to four times daily. If it has not helped after 1 to 2 days, then another homeopathic medicine should be tried or some other form of therapy should be instituted as needed. Once symptoms have begun to resolve, the medicine can be given less frequently or stopped. It can be repeated again for a relapse of symptoms. If a child's condition worsens at any time during the course of a viral illness, conventional medical care must be sought without delay if clinically indicated.

Following is a list of homeopathic medicines commonly used to treat patients with measles, mumps, roseola, and fifth disease (rubella is such a mild illness in children that it usually does not require treatment). It must be emphasized that this list is partial and represents only some of the probable choices

---

*The incidence of measles, mumps, and rubella is very low in children in the developed areas of the world, where most children are vaccinated for these diseases. In less developed areas, the incidence of these diseases is higher; therefore this section of homeopathic recommendations might be useful for practitioners in these areas.

from the homeopathic materia medica. If the symptoms of a given patient are not represented here, a search of the homeopathic literature would be needed to find the simillimum.

Measles

Aconitum napellus

Aconitum napellus can be given at the onset of measles when the patient experiences fever, a dry cough, conjunctivitis, and coryza. *Aconitum napellus* is most useful before the eyes and nose develop the purulent discharges that occur in the later stages of measles. The patient who needs *Aconitum napellus* is restless and may be agitated and fearful with the fever.

Euphrasia officinalis

Euphrasia officinalis is useful for measles when there are profuse, thin discharges from the nose and eyes. Typically, the nasal discharge is bland and the eye discharge is irritating. The eyes feel hot, irritated, and are sensitive to light.

Gelsemium sempervirens

Patients who need *Gelsemium sempervirens* are listless, lethargic, apathetic, and fatigued. (They feel dull and heavy, both physically and mentally.) The muscles (especially those of the back, neck, and periorbital area) feel achy and heavy. There may be a dull headache. The face is hot and flushed. The patient is usually thirstless and experiences chills, especially in the back. (*Gelsemium sempervirens* is also an excellent medicine for influenza, when indicated.)

Pulsatilla nigricans

Pulsatilla nigricans is a commonly used medicine for measles. The patient has copious purulent discharges from the nose and eyes and has a low thirst, feels warm, and has changeable moods. *Pulsatilla nigricans* should also be considered in cases in which the patient never fully returns to his or her normal state of health after having measles.

Sulphur

The patient needing *Sulphur* is usually warm, sweaty, and thirsty with a rash that is particularly itchy and is aggravated by heat, at night, and from bathing. The patient's sweat and stools may have an offensive smell.

Mumps

Abrotanum

Abrotanum is a medicine for cases of mumps that begin in the parotid glands and move to the testes.

Belladonna

Belladonna can be given at the beginning of mumps, or any other viral illness, when the symptoms match those of the belladonna picture. The patient has the sudden onset of a high fever with a flushed, red face and dilated pupils. There may be throbbing pains in the inflamed area. The face is hot to the touch, whereas the hands and feet may feel cold. Usually the thirst is low, although the patient may be thirsty for lemonade. The patient may become delirious and experience hallucinations.

Phytolacca decandra

Phytolacca decandra is an excellent medicine for mumps, as it treats hard, painful swellings of glands, including the parotid gland, which is affected in mumps. Pain may radiate to the ear when the patient swallows. Symptoms are relieved when the patient drinks cold liquids.

Roseola

See the previous recommendations for *Aconitum napellus*, *Belladonna*, *Gelsemium sempervirens*, *Pulsatilla nigricans*, and *Sulphur*.

Fifth Disease

Ferrum phosphoricum

Ferrum phosphoricum can be considered for use in the early stages of fifth disease (or other viral illnesses) when the patient has a fever and a flushed face. There are usually not many localizing symptoms, although the patient may have tonsillitis or a headache. The patient who needs this medicine usually prefers cold drinks.

See also the previous recommendations for *Aconitum napellus*, *Belladonna*, *Gelsemium sempervirens*, *Pulsatilla nigricans*, and *Sulphur*.

Massage Therapy

Chickenpox

As a general rule, massage should not be applied to any areas of the body where skin integrity is compromised.[1,2] As a result, standards of massage therapy practice consider chickenpox a contraindication for massage treatment, as it may increase the risk of spreading bacterial infection to open skin areas of draining vesicles. A recent study demonstrated increased bacterial counts on massage therapists' hands during and after massage treatments, although lower on the clients' skin.[3] In addition, children may have a lower touch threshold during the presence of an acute infection.[4]

Energy massage modalities (e.g., Reiki, Therapeutic Touch, polarity therapy) that may be performed over the patient's clothes or even without touching the patient could be considered as an alternative.

Measles, Rubella, Roseola, Fifth Disease

Cautious use of massage therapy is advised because it may stimulate pruritus while rash is present. Massage may be applied to unaffected areas of the body to help comfort and soothe the child. Children may have a lower threshold to touch during an acute illness,[4] and the therapist should carefully monitor the child's response to massage. If a rash is present and the child would like massage treatment, but the affected areas cannot be avoided, broad, flat effleurage strokes using a moderate pressure would be less stimulating to the skin than light strokes. Although massage strokes are typically recommended as working distal to proximal, using a slow, steady pressure working proximal to distal would have less stimulation to the hair follicles, which in turn may have less pruritic effect.

The following limitation applies to conjunctivitis, ringworm, and yeast infections: massage should be avoided over skin conditions considered contagious through contact to avoid further spread of the disease to the child or the massage practitioner.[1,2] A recent study demonstrated increased bacterial counts on massage therapists' hands during and after massage treatments, although counts were lower on the client's skin.[3]

References

Pediatric Diagnosis and Treatment

1. *Epidemiology and prevention of vaccine-preventable diseases: the pink book,* ed 6, Waldorf, Md, 2001, Public Health Foundation.
2. Nelson WE, Kliegman RM, Jenson HB, editors: *Nelson textbook of pediatrics,* ed 17, Philadelphia, WB Saunders, 2004.
3. Centers for Disease Control and Prevention: *Vaccine information statement: varicella,* Washington, DC, 2001, U.S. Department of Health and Human Services

Acupuncture

1. Loo M: *Pediatric acupuncture,* London, 2002, Elsevier.
2. Cao J: *Essentials of traditional Chinese pediatrics,* Beijing, 1990, Foreign Language Press.
3. Diagnosis and treatment of gynecology and pediatrics. In *Chinese Zhenjiuology, a series of teaching videotapes,* Beijing, 1990, Chinese Medical Audio-Video Organization and Meditalent Enterprises.
4. Flaws B: *A handbook of TCM pediatrics, a practitioner's guide to the care and treatment of common childhood diseases,* Boulder, Colo, 1997, Blue Poppy Press.
5. Scott J: *Acupuncture in the treatment of children,* London, 1991, Eastland Press.

6. Deadman P, Al-Khafaji M: *A manual of acupuncture,* Ann Arbor, Mich, 1998, Journal of Chinese Medicine Publications.
7. O'Connor J, Bensky D, editors: *Acupuncture, a comprehensive text,* Seattle, 1981, Eastland Press.

Herbs—Chinese

1. Sangkitporn S, Chaiwat S, Balachandra K et al: Treatment of herpes zoster with *Clinicanthus nutans* (bi phaya yaw) extract, *J Med Assoc Thai* 78:624-627, 1995.
2. Natural Standard Research Collaboration. Available at www.naturalstandard.com. Accessed October 2005.

Homeopathy

1. *ReferenceWorks Pro 4.2,* San Rafael, Calif, 2008, Kent Homeopathic Associates.
2. *MacRepertory Pro 7.5,* San Rafael, Calif, 2008, Kent Homeopathic Associates.

Massage Therapy

1. Tappan F: *Healing massage techniques: holistic, classic, and emerging methods,* Norwalk, Conn, 1988, Appleton and Lange.
2. Fritz S: *Mosby's fundamentals of therapeutic massage,* St Louis, 1995, Mosby.
3. Donoyama N, Wakuda T, Tanitsu T et al: Washing hands before and after performing massages? Changes in bacterial survival count on skin of a massage therapist and client during massage therapy, *J Altern Complement Med* 10:684-686, 2004.
4. Fleming-Drehobl K, Gengler-Fuhr M: *Pediatric massage for the child with special needs,* Tucson, Ariz, 1991, Therapy Skill Builders.

CHAPTER 21

Chronic Pain

Acupuncture | May Loo

Aromatherapy | Maura A. Fitzgerald

Homeopathy | Janet L. Levatin

Magnet Therapy | Agatha P. Colbert, Deborah Risotti

Massage Therapy | Mary C. McLellan

Mind/Body | Timothy Culbert, Lynda Richtsmeier Cyr

Nutrition | Joy A. Weydert

Osteopathy | Jane Carreiro

✳ PEDIATRIC DIAGNOSIS AND TREATMENT

Children, even newborns, experience pain.[1] Severe or repetitive pain in infants can result in immediate and long-lasting harmful consequences to the nervous system.[2]

Pain is usually described in physical terms: location, quality, duration, frequency, and intensity. However, pain has sensory, emotional, cognitive, and behavioral ramifications that interrelate with environmental, developmental, sociocultural, and contextual factors. The American Academy of Pediatrics (AAP) and the American Pain Society (APS) jointly issued a statement emphasizing that pain is an inherently subjective multifactorial experience and that pediatricians need to ensure humane and competent treatment of pain and suffering in all infants, children, and adolescents.[3]

Although many children with chronic pain have specific organic conditions, such as arthritis, chronic pain without a definite cause—often referred to as *functional* or *idiopathic*—is also common among children.[4] Even neuropathic pain occurs more often in the pediatric population than previously believed. Experience of pain in early life can often lead to long-term consequences.[5]

The mainstay of conventional management consists of nonopioid and opioid medications.[6] No potent analgesics have received approval from the Food and Drug Administration for use in children.[3] Because of difficulties in treating pediatric chronic pain, physicians have accepted and integrated various complementary and alternative medicine (CAM) therapies as part of pain management in children. These therapies include but are not limited to acupuncture, hypnosis, relaxation, biofeedback, and massage.[6] Readers should refer to the chapters on specific pain syndromes, such as headache (Chapter 40) or abdominal pain (Chapter 8), for more detailed and precise CAM approaches.

✳ CAM THERAPY RECOMMENDATIONS

Acupuncture

Acupuncture has been most widely used for treatment of both chronic and acute pain. Chronic pain in traditional Chinese medicine (TCM) can have numerous underlying etiologies that include: obstruction of Qi and Blood flow, Qi deficiency or stagnation; Yin organ deficiency, such as Kidney deficiency; or blood stasis, especially with history of trauma. Acupuncture approach would first decipher the underlying causes of chronic pain, some of which may have conventional correlations, such as migraine headache and arthritis. Pain clinics throughout the world have incorporated acupuncture into their multidisciplinary approach to chronic pain.[1-10] Neurophysiologically, acupuncture efficacy in pain can be explained by its numerous analgesic and antiinflammatory mechanisms, discussed in detail in Chapter 6.

Evidence-Based Information in Children

Despite its increasing use to treat pain, acupuncture is rarely considered by pediatricians. This may in part be due to perceptions that it will not be acceptable to children. A retrospective case study of 47 adolescents with various chronic pain syndromes rated the therapy as pleasant and helpful.[11] A Phase I investigation examined the effect of combining acupuncture and hypnosis for chronic pediatric pain in 33 children aged 6 to 18 years and revealed significant improvements in symptoms of various chronic pain syndromes.[12]

Acupuncture Treatment Recommendations

For any child with pain, especially chronic pain, it is important to evaluate the etiology so that acupuncture treatment does not mask the symptoms and delay diagnosis. Once the etiology is known, treatment should be directed toward relieving pain, improving lifestyle, and healing the underlying condition.

For specific treatments, see the chapters on individual conditions such as headache (Chapter 40), inflammatory bowel disease (Chapter 46), or arthritis (Chapter 11).

General Points That Can Be Used for Nonspecific Pain

- ST36 and LI4 for general pain relief: A word of caution in applying LI4 in children: because LI4 is a very strong dispersing (sedating) point, it would not be advisable to use it alone, especially in children who are Qi deficient.
- Zusanli (ST36) can be used to treat any abdominal pain.[13]
- Chu-Chih (LI11) + Ho-Ku (LI4) + Zusanli (ST36) can treat painful syndromes with fever.[14]

Aromatherapy

Chronic pain can be caused by injury, disease process, stress, or a combination of all three. Aromatherapy can be a useful addition to a plan that blends a number of approaches including analgesic medication, physical therapy, stress management techniques, and manual and energy therapies.[1] A number of essential oils are purported to have analgesic effects, including lavender (*Lavandula angustifolia*), peppermint (*Mentha piperita*), rosemary (*Rosmarinus officinalis*), lemongrass (*Cymbopogon citratus*), and Roman chamomile (*Chamaemelum nobile*).[2,3]

The choice of essential oil depends on the properties of specific oils and patient preference. Some essential oils, such as peppermint, feel cool when placed on the skin, whereas others, such as rosemary, feel warm. Others, such as lavender, have a neutral effect. Children often have an idea whether cooling or warming feels better to them when they are in pain. When used for pain management, essential oils are most effective when applied topically during therapeutic massage, applied in a compress, or lightly rubbed on the skin. In the author's experience, aromatherapy for chronic pain is particularly useful to help reduce pain sensation when the child is trying to rest or sleep. Lavender, which has both analgesic and calming properties, is ideal for bedtime. Other essential oils that are more alerting, such as rosemary or peppermint, can be applied to the skin while a more relaxing essential oil, such as lavender or sweet orange, is diffused in the room.

Homeopathy

Before using this section, please see Appendix A, Homeopathy, for definitions of practitioner expertise categories and general information on prescribing homeopathic medicines.

Practitioner Expertise Category 3

There are no controlled clinical trials of homeopathy for chronic pain, although the homeopathic literature contains evidence for its use in the form of accumulated clinical experience.[1] Homeopathic treatment can be used safely in combination with other treatment modalities, both alternative and conventional. Because chronic pain is a complex and multifaceted problem with many causes, successful homeopathic treatment usually requires extensive training in the art and science of homeopathy. Any one of many homeopathic medicines may be used to treat chronic pain, depending on the characteristics of the patient being treated; sophisticated homeopathic analysis and long-term follow-up are required. For these reasons, specific medicines for treating chronic pain will not be presented here. Interested readers are referred to the homeopathic literature for further study.[1]

Magnet Therapy

Chronic pain syndrome may involve any of a number of different sites on the body. When using magnets to treat children with chronic pain conditions, it is best to work with a physical therapist or a massage therapist who is able to identify relevant tender points or active trigger points. The practitioner should be aware that these points may be found at some distance from where the child actually feels the pain. An example of finding the relevant tender point was reported by Holcomb.[1] A 15-year-old boy complained of aching in his right thoracolumbar region, right groin, and right lower abdominal quadrant with intermittent radiation into the testes. Careful palpation and pressure applied to the spinous processes in the thoracolumbar region elicited the same symptoms of pain radiating to the right testis. In this situation the magnets were applied over points on the thoracolumbar spine that were tender and/or reproduced the painful sensations of which the boy complained. Relief occurred within 10 minutes of placing the magnets on these points, using the diagram for pediatric acupuncture at A10. The north side of Neodymium Spot magnets, which may be obtained from Painfree Lifestyles (800-480-8601), can be taped into place over the identified tender points.

Massage Therapy

Massage therapy has long been used as an adjunct to traditional pain management methods: people intuitively massage areas of pain to make the area feel better. Research has shown elevated plasma β-endorphin levels following massage therapy,[1] which may explain some of its pain-reducing properties. Theorists have postulated that massage therapy may decrease substance P levels during massage treatment, but controlled studies have not yet been performed. A systematic review of 22 articles on the effects of massage therapy on relaxation and comfort indicated significantly decreased anxiety or perception of tension in 8 of 10 articles; physiological relaxation was indicated in 7 of 10 articles; and 3 studies demonstrated it was effective at reducing pain.[2]

It is not unusual for some chronic pain to be related to musculoskeletal restrictions and/or immobility. In cases where mobility restrictions are a source of chronic pain, massage can be beneficial as an adjunct to a person's management (see Chapter 3 for details on muscle rehabilitation and pain), especially to facilitate passive and active ranges of motion during physical therapy. Controlled studies have found massage to be more effective than relaxation techniques for musculoskeletal pain reduction.[3-6] Studies comparing effectiveness of massage therapy versus traditional therapies (traditional Chinese acupuncture, self-care measures, progressive muscle relaxation, soft tissue manipulation, exercise, or placebo) for chronic low back pain demonstrated massage to be more effective for reducing symptoms and improving function.[5-8] In addition, massage therapy had beneficial effects for almost a year after active treatment when used in conjunction with exercise and education.[7] A recent systematic Cochrane review of massage for low back pain concluded from the eight studies reviewed that massage therapy may be beneficial for patients with subacute and chronic low back pain, especially when combined with exercise and education.[9] A randomized controlled trial demonstrated massage therapy to be effective in improving range of motion and reducing pain in patients with chronic shoulder pain.[10] Massage was as effective as transcutaneous electrical nerve stimulation (TENS) in decreasing pain in fibromyalgia patients, but was more effective in overall pain reduction, improved sleep patterns, and decreased fatigue and stiffness.[11] Another systematic review of 23 articles suggested that there is evidence for massage therapy to be a useful approach for pain relief in numerous chronic, nonmalignant pain conditions, specifically musculoskeletal pain complaints.[12]

The efficacy of massage therapy to decrease pain scores during acute postoperative pain has been demonstrated.[10,13-16] Numerous randomized controlled trials reported decreased pain in patients with cancer who received massage therapy[17-25] and the Clinical Practice Guidelines of both the National Comprehensive Cancer Network and the American College of Chest Physicians include massage therapy as part of a multimodality approach in treating cancer pain.[26-29]

Mind/Body

Pain is a multifactorial phenomenon and is often associated with chronic disease in children. Pain in chronic disease is less predictable than acute pain and thus has been more difficult to treat. Teaching children techniques that cultivate deep relaxation, facilitate a sense of control, and access altered states of awareness can be very helpful for decreasing anticipatory anxiety. This also teaches children to modulate the pain experience so that it is less distressing. Biofeedback-based relaxation training, meditation, autogenics, and diaphragmatic breathing all represent reasonable ways to assist an individual in achieving a lowered state of arousal, which in turn may mediate the pain experience.[1]

Clinical experience suggests that meditation results in changes in brain wave activity, increased parasympathetic activity, increased heart rate variability, and changes in neurotransmitter levels. Mindfulness meditation also has an excellent track record in adults with chronic pain and would be a reasonable consideration with children and adolescents as well.[2,3] In the author's clinical experience, children and adolescents benefit from a variety of meditation skills including mindfulness meditation, concentrative mediations (e.g., belly breathing, visualization, Qigong, yoga), and expressive meditations (e.g., shaking and dancing). When working with children, it is important to explain that any activity can be a meditation. When teaching meditation to children, it is often helpful to first do an active meditation (e.g., yoga, shaking and dancing) followed by a quiet meditation (e.g., a focus on belly breathing). It is important for children and adolescents to choose a practice that feels right for them and practice it daily for a period of time. As with any mind/body therapy, it is important to coordinate medication needs with the appropriate medical provider. Often patients need less medication once they have established a mind/body practice.

For many children with chronic conditions, recurrent procedures such as lumbar punctures (LPs), venipuncture, and radiological procedures are a major source of anxiety and discomfort. In a recent review, Wild and Espie[4] concluded that there is not enough robust research evidence at present to recommend that hypnosis be a part of the best practice guidelines for the management of procedure-related pain in pediatric oncology. However, the authors used a description of the process of hypnosis in children, which includes six phases similar to the usual process for adults. One of their criteria for assessing the nine studies is whether these six phases are mentioned. For example, authors state that the hypnotic treatment in a study reported by Zeltzer and LeBaron[5] should be more "accurately labeled as guided imagery as there was no hypnotic induction phase." Inasmuch as there is no way to prove that guided imagery does not induce a hypnotic state, the criteria demanded by Wild and Espie[4] seem contrived.

Medical procedures can be a cause of recurrent pain for many children. A recent study examining the use of hypnosis for children undergoing voiding cystourethrography (VCUG) is noteworthy in that it studied children who had previous uncomfortable experiences with VCU and demonstrated a robust, positive result.[6] The study involved 44 children (mean age 7.6 years) scheduled for VCU who were randomized to receive either hypnosis or routine care while undergoing the procedure.

Results indicate benefits for the hypnosis group relative to the control group in four areas:

1. Parents of subjects in the hypnosis group rated their child's experience as significantly less traumatic than those in the control group.
2. Observational ratings of distress for children in the hypnosis group were significantly less than those for subjects in the control group.
3. Medical staff reported significantly less difficulty in conducting the procedure for children in the hypnosis group.
4. Total procedural time was significantly shorter in the hypnosis group by almost 14 minutes.

In a recent study, Huth et al.[7] reported that imagery in combination with routine analgesics reduced children's anxiety and pain 1 to 4 hours after tonsillectomy and/or adenoidectomy surgery, but there was no significant improvement for the experimental imagery group 22 to 27 hours after discharge.

Common techniques for hypnotic pain control include dissociation, direct suggestion for analgesia/anesthesia, distancing from pain, suggestions for feelings antithetical to pain, distraction, and directing attention to pain itself. For all pediatric interventions, it is important to consider the developmental stage of the patient and adjust the mind/body skills techniques accordingly. Hypnotic techniques for very young children could include rocking and motion, singing, visual and auditory distractions, and playing with puppets. Techniques for preschool-aged children could include storytelling, animal metaphors, and pretend play. School-aged children may benefit from hypnotic interventions that use favorite place imagery, biofeedback-based inductions, and control metaphors (e.g., pain switches). In working with preadolescents and adolescents, hypnotic techniques could include favorite place imagery, progressive muscle relaxation, and mastery imagery.

Nutrition

Symptom management with pharmaceuticals has been the mainstay in treating pain in children. This is undoubtedly helpful in the short term, but when pain becomes a chronic problem, nutrition can be an avenue for long-term treatment. Specific recommendations are discussed under various pediatric conditions in this text.

Neurotransmitters and hormones, which are derived from the foods we eat, play a role in pain transmission and perception. A greater understanding of how the manipulation of these neurotransmitters through diet can affect pain has occurred over the past decade, opening new modalities of therapy.

γ-Aminobutyric acid (GABA) is the major inhibitory neurotransmitter in the brain and plays an important role in memory, depressed moods, and pain. It also helps in relaxation and maintenance of focus and control. GABA is derived from glutamine, which is found in fish, meat, beans, dairy, and spinach. In one study, germinated barley foodstuff (GBF), which mainly consists of dietary fiber and glutamine-rich protein, was able to attenuate the symptoms of ulcerative colitis in a relatively short time.[1]

Serotonin, another inhibitory neurotransmitter that controls mood, sleep, appetite, and the pain threshold, is derived from L-tryptophan. Serotonin-releasing brain neurons are unique in that the amount of neurotransmitter they release is normally controlled by food intake: Carbohydrate consumption, acting via insulin secretion and the "plasma tryptophan ratio," increases serotonin release. Many people overeat carbohydrates (particularly snack foods, which are rich in carbohydrates and fats) to make themselves feel better, which indicates how food is often used as a therapeutic agent.[2]

More research is being conducted in the use of targeted amino acid therapy for treating a variety of chronic pain syndromes, as these amino acids are the precursors to the neurotransmitters necessary for normal neurological balance.[3]

Two comorbid states often arise in children experiencing chronic pain that only increase that experience—dehydration and constipation. These may occur as side effects of medications, altered appetite, or lack of activity/mobility, but they often augment the pain experience. Headaches, back pain, arthritis, or ulcers may be prevented in some cases with the normalization of fluid levels. The brain is more than 75% water, and when it detects a shortage of available fluids, it implements a water-rationing process by producing histamines, which direct certain subordinate water regulators to redistribute the amount of water in circulation. This system helps move water to areas where it is needed for basic metabolic activity and survival. When histamine and its subordinate regulators for water intake and distribution come across pain-sensing nerves in the body, they cause strong and continual pain. Constipation not only causes localized discomfort in the abdomen, but can contribute to general malaise, which worsens the pain experience. Correcting these two problems can be helpful in alleviating chronic pain.

Magnesium is being increasingly recognized as a significant pain reliever. Magnesium is vital for muscle contraction and nerve conduction. Without sufficient amounts of magnesium, the cellular energy and electrical stability of the cells falter. Chronic pain often has associated myalgias and a sensitized nervous system. Case reports of patients with persistent pain were found to have magnesium deficiency; correction relieved the pain.[4] Many studies have shown the effectiveness of supplemental magnesium for preventing and treating migraine and tension-type headaches.[5,6] Magnesium appears to affect the N-methyl-D-aspartate (NMDA) receptors that play a crucial role in pain perception. In deficient states, NMDA receptors develop a hypersensitivity to pain. Magnesium acts as an NMDA receptor antagonist, much in the same way that ketamine does, to reduce pain.

Treatment

Nutritional management of chronic pain might include the following recommendations:

- A diet rich in whole foods (not processed), to include whole grains, fresh fruits and vegetables, and a healthy source of protein including the plant sources, will provide the necessary amino acids and nutrients to support normal neurotransmitter function. These foods also provide fiber for healthy elimination.
- Encourage proper hydration with water.
- Avoid sources of aspartame and monosodium glutamate, as these stimulate the excitatory neurotransmitters, specifically glutamate, and the NMDA receptors.
- Magnesium supplementation in the form of glycinate, gluconate, aspartate, or oxide in a dose of 500 mg twice per day works as a natural muscle relaxant and pain reliever. Good sources of dietary magnesium include avocados, pork, milk, clams, mushrooms, spinach, barley, quinoa, sunflower and pumpkin seeds, and chocolate.
- Provide daily sources of omega-3 fatty acids, either through supplementation with fish oil, flaxseed oil, or hemp oil at 1000 mg per day, or with dietary sources including salmon, mackerel, herring, flaxseed, hemp seeds, or walnuts. Omega-3 fatty acids have natural antiinflammatory qualities to help reduce pain. Make sure the fish sources are free of heavy metal (mercury) and pesticide contamination.

Osteopathy

We do not feel pain with our bodies; we feel it with our brains. As such, the influences of somatic, emotional, hormonal, psychological, and immune factors on the perception of pain in adults is an accepted aspect of neuroscience. Unfortunately, modern medicine has only recently accepted that these same mechanisms are operating in our youngest patients. The osteopathic approach views the interrelationship of these factors as paramount in helping the child with chronic pain. Somatic dysfunction and altered biomechanics will exacerbate a child's threshold for pain and alter normal function of other areas of the body. This in turn creates compensatory tissue stresses and coping mechanisms, which influence the way the child perceives and interacts with the world.

Children with chronic pain can benefit from the therapeutic aspect of gentle tissue manipulation as well as the therapeutic aspect of physical contact. Decreasing nociceptive drive from compensatory tissue strains is one of the primary goals of osteopathic treatment in the child with chronic pain. Another goal is promoting relaxation and homeostasis through supporting the inherent forces within the child's body.

Chronic pain is associated with imbalances in the neuroendocrine-immune network. This occurs via the hypothalamic-pituitary-adrenal axis and via sympathetic stimulation through the hypothalamus. Chronic pain has been associated with sleep disorder, cardiovascular disease, and melancholic depression.[1,2] One cranial technique, CV4, is thought to promote relaxation, fluid balance, and equilibrium of the autonomic nervous system.[3-5] This and other cranial techniques have been described as useful in the treatment of sleep disorders and depression. Other gentle techniques such as myofascial, functional, and balancing techniques are typically used to promote normal tissue function, facilitate the removal of cellular waste products, encourage oxygen delivery to tissues, and enhance autonomic "tone" (i.e., balance in the autonomic nervous system). Viscerosomatic reflexes, Chapman's points, tender points, and trigger points all have additive effects on the child's overall level of nociception. Consequently, these and other findings of somatic dysfunction need to be addressed. Although there are no published random controlled studies investigating the efficacy of osteopathic manipulation in the treatment of children with chronic pain, several studies have shown some benefit in adults with various chronic pain conditions.[6-9]

Osteopathic treatment of the child with chronic pain must occur as part of a team effort. Homeopathy, naturopathy, biofeedback, and acupuncture all support and are supported by the osteopathic approach. Likewise diet, lifestyle changes, and counseling can also benefit the child. Activities that reinforce the idea of wholeness and motion as life help to build the child's self-confidence and coping strategies.

References

Pediatric Diagnosis and Treatment

1. Mathew PJ, Mathew JL: Assessment and management of pain in infants, *Postgrad Med J* 79:438-443, 2003.
2. Mitchell A, Boss BJ: Adverse effects of pain on the nervous systems of newborns and young children: a review of the literature, *J Neurosci Nurs* 34:228-236, 2002.
3. Committee on Psychosocial Aspects of Child and Family Health, Task Force on Pain in Infants, Children, and Adolescents. American Academy of Pediatrics Policy: The assessment and management of acute pain in infants, children, and adolescents, *Pediatrics* 108:793-797, 2001.
4. Malleson P, Clinch J: Pain syndromes in children, *Curr Opin Rheumatol* 15:572-580, 2003.
5. Howard RF: Current status of pain management in children, *J Am Med Assoc* 290:2464-2469, 2003.
6. Behrman RE, Kliegman RM, Jenson HB, editors: *Nelson's textbook of pediatrics*, Philadelphia, 2004, Saunders, pp 357-366.

Acupuncture

1. Buenaventura RM, McSweeney TD, Benedetti C et al: The qualifications of pain physicians in Ohio, *Anesth Analg* 100:1746-1752, 2005.
2. Blossfeldt P: Acupuncture for chronic neck pain—a cohort study in an NHS pain clinic, *Acupunct Med* 22:146-151, 2004.
3. Orpen M, Harvey G, Millard J: A survey of the use of self-acupuncture in pain clinics—a safe way to meet increasing demand? *Acupunct Med* 22:137-140, 2004.
4. Eshkevari L: Acupuncture and pain: a review of the literature, *AANA J* 71:361-370, 2003.
5. Giles LG, Muller R, Winter GJ: Patient satisfaction, characteristics, radiology, and complications associated with attending a specialized government-funded multidisciplinary spinal pain unit, *J Manipulative Physiol Ther* 26:293-299, 2003.
6. Israel HA, Ward JD, Horrell B et al: Oral and maxillofacial surgery in patients with chronic orofacial pain, *J Oral Maxillofac Surg* 61:662-667, 2003.

7. Meng A: Acupuncture therapy with TENS in chronic pain at the Neurologic Pain-Acupuncture Ambulatory Care Clinic of the Vienna Lainz Hospital [in German], *Wien Med Wochenschr* 148:443-446, 1998 (abstract).
8. Tsibuliak VN, Zagorul'ko OI, Kartavenko SS: Our general chronic pain (centers for treatment chronic pain: therapeutic and organizational work principles) [in Russian], *Anesteziol Reanimatol* Sep/Oct:54-59, 1998.
9. Woollam CH, Jackson AO: Acupuncture in the management of chronic pain, *Anaesthesia* 53:593-595, 1998.
10. Elkayam O, Ben Itzhak S, Avrahami E et al: Multidisciplinary approach to chronic back pain: prognostic elements of the outcome, *Clin Exp Rheumatol* 14:281-288, 1996.
11. Kemper KJ, Sarah R, Silver-Highfield E et al: On pins and needles? Pediatric pain patients' experience with acupuncture, *Pediatrics* 105:941-947, 2000.
12. Zeltzer LK, Tsao JC, Stelling C et al: A Phase I study on the feasibility and acceptability of an acupuncture/hypnosis intervention for chronic pediatric pain, *J Pain Symptom Management* 24:437-446, 2002.
13. Xu S, Liu Z, Xu M: Treatment of cancerous abdominal pain by acupuncture on zusanli (ST 36)—a report of 92 cases, *J Tradit Chin Med* 15:189-191, 1995.
14. Lin MT, Chandra A, Chen-Yen SM et al: Needle stimulation of acupuncture loci Chu-Chih (LI-11) and Ho-Ku (LI-4) induces hypothermia effects and analgesia in normal adults, *Am J Chin Med* 9:74-83, 1981.

Aromatherapy

1. Chambliss CR, Heggen J, Copelan DN et al: The assessment and management of chronic pain in children, *Paediatric Drugs* 4:737-746, 2002.
2. Buckle J: Use of aromatherapy as a complementary treatment for chronic pain, *Altern Ther Health Med* 5:42-51, 1999.
3. Battaglia S: *The complete guide to aromatherapy*, Virginia, Queensland, Australia, 1995, The Perfect Potion.

Homeopathy

1. *ReferenceWorks Pro 4.2*, San Rafael, Calif, 2008, Kent Homeopathic Associates.

Magnet Therapy

1. Holcomb RR, Worthington WB, McCullough BA et al: Static magnetic therapy for pain in the abdomen and genitals, *Pediatr Neurol* 23:261-264, 2000.

Massage Therapy

1. Kaada B, Torsteinbo O: Increase of plasma endorphins in connective tissue massage, *Gen Pharmacol* 20:487-489, 1989.
2. Richards KC, Gibson R, Overton-McCoy AL: Effects of massage in acute and critical care, *AACN Clin Issues* 11:77-96, 2000.
3. Quinn C, Chandler C, Moraska A: Massage therapy and frequency of chronic tension headaches, *Am J Public Health* 92:1657-1661, 2002.
4. Hasson D, Arnetz B, Jelveus L et al: A randomized clinical trial of the treatment effects of massage compared to relaxation tape recordings on diffuse long-term pain, *Psychotherapy Psychosom* 73:17-24, 2004.
5. Hernandez-Reif M, Field T, Krasnegor J et al: Lower back pain is reduced and range of motion increased after massage therapy, *Int J Neurosci* 106:131-145, 2001.
6. Cherkin DC, Sherman KJ, Deyo RA et al: A review of the evidence for the effectiveness, safety, and cost of acupuncture, massage therapy, and spinal manipulation for back pain, *Ann Intern Med* 138:898-906, 2003.

7. Cherkin DC, Eisenberg DM, Sherman KJ et al: Randomized trial comparing traditional Chinese medical acupuncture, therapeutic massage, and self-care education for chronic low back pain, *Arch Intern Med* 161:1081-1088, 2001.

8. Preyde M: Effectiveness of massage therapy for subacute low-back pain: a randomized controlled trial, *CMAJ* 162:1815-1820, 2000.

9. Furlan AD, Brosseau L, Imamura I et al: Massage for low back pain: a systematic review within the framework of the Cochrane Collaboration Back Review Group, *Spine* 27: 1896-1910, 2002.

10. van der Dolder PA, Roberts DL: A trial into the effectiveness of soft tissue massage in the treatment of shoulder pain, *Austr J Physiother* 49:183-188, 2003.

11. Sunshine W, Field T, Quintino O et al: Fibromyalgia benefits from massage therapy and transcutaneous electrical stimulation, *J Clin Rheumatol* 2:18-22, 1996.

12. Tsao JC: Effectiveness of massage therapy for chronic, non-malignant pain: a review, *Evid Based Complement Alternat Med* 4:165-179, 2007.

13. Piotrowski MM, Paterson C, Mitchinson A et al: Massage as adjuvant therapy in the management of acute postoperative pain: a preliminary study in men, *J Am Coll Surg* 197:1037-1046, 2003.

14. Taylor AG, Galpner DI, Taylor P et al: Effects of adjunctive Swedish massage and vibration therapy on short-term postoperative outcomes: a randomized, controlled trial, *J Altern Complement Med* 9:77-89, 2003.

15. LeBlanc-Louvry I, Costaglioli B, Boulon C et al: Does mechanical massage of the abdominal wall after colectomy reduce postoperative pain and shorten the duration of ileus? Results of a randomized study, *J Gastrointest Surg* 6:43-49, 2002.

16. Mitchinson AR, Kim HM, Rosenberg JM et al: Acute postoperative pain management using massage as an adjuvant therapy: a randomized trial, *Arch Surg* 142:1158-1167, 2007.

17. Ferrell-Tory AT, Glick OJ: The use of therapeutic massage as a nursing intervention to modify anxiety and the perception of cancer pain, *Cancer Nurs* 16:93-101, 1993.

18. Wilkinson S: Get the massage, *Nurs Times* 92:61-64, 1996.

19. Grealish L, Lomasney A, Whiteman B: Foot massage: a nursing intervention to modify the distressing symptoms of pain and nausea in patients hospitalized with cancer, *Cancer Nurs* 23:237-243, 2000.

20. Weinrich SP, Wienrich MC: The effect of massage on pain in cancer patients, *Appl Nurs Res* 3:140-145, 1990.

21. Smith MC, Kemp J, Hemphill L et al: Outcomes of therapeutic massage for hospitalized cancer patients, *J Nurs Scholar* 34:257-262, 2002.

22. Smith MC, Reeder F, Daniel L et al: Outcomes of touch therapies during bone marrow transplantation, *Altern Ther Med* 9:40-49, 2003.

23. Post-White J, Kinney ME, Savik K et al: Therapeutic massage and healing touch improve symptoms in cancer, *Integr Cancer Ther* 2:332-344, 2003.

24. Cassileth BR, Vickers AJ: Massage therapy for symptom control: outcome study at a major cancer center, *J Pain Symptom Manage* 28:3, 2004.

25. Mehling WE, Jacobs B, Acree M et al: Symptom management with massage and acupuncture in postoperative cancer patients: a randomized controlled trial, *J Pain Symptom Manage* 33:258-266, 2007.

26. National Comprehensive Cancer Network: *Clinical practice guidelines in oncology: adult cancer pain v1,* 2007. Available at www.nccn.org. Accessed February 2008.

27. National Comprehensive Cancer Network: *Clinical practice guidelines in oncology. pediatric cancer pain v1,* 2007 Available at www.nccn.org. Accessed: February 2008.

28. National Comprehensive Cancer Network: *Clinical practice guidelines in oncology. cancer related fatigue v4,* 2007. Available at www.nccn.org. Accessed: February 2008.

29. Cassileth BR, Deng GE, Gomez JE et al: Complementary therapies and integrative oncology in lung cancer: ACCP Evidence-Based Clinical Practice Guidelines (2nd edition), *Chest* 132:340-354, 2007.

Mind/Body

1. Andrasik F: The essence of biofeedback, relaxation, and hypnosis. In Dworkin R, Breitbart W, editors: *Psychosocial aspects of pain: a handbook for health care providers,* Seattle, 2004, IASP Press.

2. Kabat-Zinn J, Lipworth L, Burney R: Four-year follow-up of a meditation-based program for the self-regulation of chronic pain: treatment outcomes and compliance, *Clin J Pain* 12:159-173, 1987.

3. Kabat-Zinn J, Lipworth L, Burney R: The clinical use of mindfulness meditation for the self-regulation of chronic pain, *J Behav Med* 8:163-190, 1985.

4. Wild MR, Espie CA: The efficacy of hypnosis in the reduction of procedural pain and distress in pediatric oncology, *Devel Behav Pediatr* 25:207-213, 2004.

5. Zeltzer L, LeBaron S: Hypnotic and nonhypnotic techniques for reduction of pain and anxiety during painful procedures in children and adolescents with cancer, *J Pediatr* 101:1032-1035.

6. Butler LD, Symons BK, Henderson SL et al: Hypnosis reduces distress and duration of an invasive medical procedure for children, *Pediatrics* 115:e77-e85, 2005.

7. Huth M, Broome M, Good M: Imagery reduces children's postoperative pain, *Pain* 110:439-448, 2004.

Nutrition

1. Kanauchi O, Mitsuyama K, Homma T et al: Treatment of ulcerative colitis patients by long-term administration of germinated barley foodstuff: multi-center open trial, *Int J Mol Med* 12:701-704, 2003.

2. Wurtman RJ, Wurtman JJ: Brain serotonin, carbohydrate-craving, obesity and depression, *Obes Res* 3(Suppl 4):477S-480S, 1995.

3. Purvis K, Kellermann G, Cross D et al: An experimental evaluation of targeted amino acid therapy with at-risk children, *J Alt Complement Med* (in press). Available at www.neuroscienceinc.com.

4. Bilbey DL, Prabhakaran VM: Muscle cramps and magnesium deficiency—case reports, *Can Fam Physician* 42:1348-1351, 1996.

5. Wang F, Van Den Eeden SK, Acherson LM et al: Oral magnesium oxide prophylaxis of frequent migrainous headache in children: a randomized, double-blind, placebo-controlled trial, *Headache* 32:601-610, 2003.

6. Altura BM, Altura BT: Tension headaches and muscle tension: is there a role for magnesium? *Med Hypothesis* 57:705-713, 2001.

Osteopathy

1. Gold P, Goodwin F: Clinical and biochemical manifestations of depression: part II, *N Engl J Med* 319:413-420, 1988.

2. Gold P, Goodwin F: Clinical and biochemical manifestations of stress: part I, *N Engl J Med* 319:348-353, 1988.

3. Magoun HIS: *Osteopathy in the cranial field,* Kirksville, Mo, 1951, The Journal Printing Company.

4. Kuchera ML, Kuchera WA: *Osteopathic considerations in systemic disease,* Columbus, OH, 1994, Greydon Press.

5. Sutherland WG: *Teachings in the science of osteopathy*, Portland, Ore 1990, Rudra Press.

6. Andersson GB, Lucente T, Davis AM et al: A comparison of osteopathic spinal manipulation with standard care for patients with low back pain, *N Engl J Med* 341:1426-1431, 1999.

7. Walko EJ, Janouschek C: Effects of osteopathic manipulative treatment in patients with cervicothoracic pain: pilot study using thermography, *J Am Osteopath Assoc* 94:135-141, 1994.

8. Gamber RG, Shores JH, Russo DP et al: Osteopathic manipulative treatment in conjunction with medication relieves pain associated with fibromyalgia syndrome: results of a randomized clinical pilot project, *J Am Osteopath Assoc* 102:321-325, 2002.

9. Wright HOL: Rheumatoid arthritis: the incurable disease, *J Am Osteopath Assoc* 2:11-12, 1992.

CHAPTER 22

Chronic Urticaria

Acupuncture | May Loo

Chiropractic | Anne Spicer

Homeopathy | Janet L. Levatin

Probiotics | Russell H. Greenfield

✳ PEDIATRIC DIAGNOSIS AND TREATMENT

Although urticaria is commonly encountered in children,[1] chronic idiopathic urticaria (CIU), a disabling condition[2] lasting more than 6 weeks, is rare in childhood.[3] Initial diagnosis is made by careful history and physical examination, as routine laboratory studies tend to be normal. CIU has an increased association with Hashimoto thyroiditis[4] but is usually not associated with any other systemic disease or malignancy.[2]

Establishing a cause for CIU can be challenging. Although infection, allergies to drugs and foods, and physical factors are the most common causes of acute urticaria,[4] when these factors are entered into the differential for CIU,[3] an exogenous cause of chronic urticaria is rarely identified. A significant portion of chronic urticarial cases are now considered to have an autoimmune etiology.[1,5] About one third of patients with CIU have circulating functional autoantibodies against the high-affinity immunoglobulin (Ig)-E receptor or against IgE.[2] Approximately 35% to 40% of patients with chronic urticaria have a positive autologous skin test: when serum from the patient is intradermally injected into their skin, a significant wheal and flare reaction is observed, which supports the autoimmune theory of pathogenesis.[4,6] Biopsy of the typical lesion consists of a non-necrotizing perivascular mononuclear cell infiltrate.[4]

Although a primary role for infection is controversial, concurrent infections seem to exacerbate chronic urticaria.[7] Food is rarely a cause of chronic urticaria.[8]

Chronic urticaria resolves spontaneously in 30% to 55% of patients within 5 years, but it can persist for many years.[2]

Management of chronic urticaria in children is difficult because the pathogenesis can be unclear and multifactorial such that a specific treatment is not feasible.[7,9] Treatment is aimed first at avoiding any known underlying causative or exacerbating factors. Histamine H1 receptor antagonists remain the mainstay of oral treatment for all forms of urticaria. Sedating antihistamines have more adverse effects but are useful if symptoms are causing sleep disturbance.[2] Combination of H$_1$- and H$_2$-type antihistamines, steroids, leukotriene antagonist, intravenous immunoglobulins, and plasmapheresis have all been used to treat CIU.[2,4,10] In severe cases, immunosuppressive therapy may even be required.[5]

✳ CAM THERAPY RECOMMENDATIONS

Acupuncture

Acupuncture has long been used to treat urticaria in the Asian world.[1] A clinical study from China comparing acupuncture with desensitization therapies in 143 subjects including children showed a higher curative effect in the acupuncture group for chronic urticaria.[2] No controlled studies on acupuncture for urticaria in children are available.

Clinical reports from experienced practitioners in China indicate that needle acupuncture has been beneficial for the treatment of urticaria in adults.[3] Clinical reports from Taiwan indicate that the four acupuncture points most commonly used to treat acute urticaria (hives) are LI11 (Quchi), SP10 (Xuehai), SP6 (Sanyinjiao), and S36 (Zusanli). Treatment of chronic urticaria needs to combine stimulation of body points with other modalities, such as concomitantly treating the auricular microsystem or injecting acupuncture points with thiamine (vitamin B$_1$).[1] Some U.S. clinicians recognize that acupuncture may be helpful for urticaria.[4]

Chiropractic

The chiropractor views chronic urticaria as an immunosensitivity reaction and would approach this child with a goal of restoring normal neuroimmune function after removal of suspected provocative agents (See Chapter 10, Allergies). Another possibility is a chronic infective state, which can typically be established through a blood workup. The chiropractor evaluates the child for subluxation complex and corrects this condition with the manual osseous adjustment, keeping in mind that facilitation of the sympathetics is associated with an increased inflammatory response and increased vagal activity would reduce this response.[1] Recommendation is made to specifically assess C6 to T3 for thyroid involvement and T7 to T12 for adrenal involvement, L4 to L5, and the second sacral segment.[2] The chiropractic adjustment has modulatory neuroimmune influence over natural killer cell production and autonomic balance,[3] immunoglobulin (IgA, G, and M) levels and B-cell lymphocyte count,[4] polymorphonuclear neutrophils, monocytes,[5] and even CD4 counts.[6] This potent influence on the immune system directly regulates immunocompetence and may provide a benefit in the child with immunological dysfunction.

A specialized and controversial technique used by a small percentage of chiropractors, called *applied kinesiology muscle testing,* correlates with more than 90% of items found on radioallergosorbent testing (RAST) for IgE and IgG and may also find items unidentified by conventional allergy testing.[7] This chiropractic technique is particularly useful when conventional laboratory testing is inadequate or unobtainable.

Another possibility is a chronic infective state, which can be established typically with laboratory profiling.

Nutrients supportive of the immune system would be useful and include omega-3 fatty acids, zinc, and vitamins A and C.

Homeopathy

Before using this section, please see Appendix A, Homeopathy, for definitions of practitioner expertise categories and general information on prescribing homeopathic medicines.

Practitioner Expertise Category 1

Category 1 includes chronic urticaria uncomplicated by other conditions.

Practitioner Expertise Category 2

Category 2 includes chronic urticaria associated with other mild to moderate allergic symptoms or coexisting conditions.

Practitioner Expertise Category 3

Category 3 includes chronic urticaria associated with anaphylaxis or other severe allergic reactions.

There have been no controlled clinical trials of homeopathy for chronic urticaria, although the homeopathic literature contains evidence for its use in the form of accumulated clinical experience.[1] Chronic urticaria, as well acute urticaria, can frequently be treated effectively with homeopathy. For urticaria unassociated with other severe reactions, homeopathic treatment is safe to try alone or in combination with other therapies, either conventional or alternative. If urticaria is associated with allergic symptoms that compromise respiration or circulation, emergency care must be sought for the patient without delay.

The goal in treating urticaria homeopathically is to determine the single homeopathic medicine whose description in the materia medica most closely matches the symptom picture of the patient. Often mental and emotional states, in addition to physical symptoms, are considered. Once the medicine has been selected, it can be given orally or sublingually in the 30C potency two to four times daily (more frequently in acute cases, less frequently in chronic cases). Some patients with chronic urticaria may benefit from use of a 200C potency. If the medicine has not helped after a few days, then another homeopathic medicine should be tried or some other form of therapy should be instituted as needed. Once symptoms have begun to resolve, the medicine can be given less frequently or stopped. It can be repeated again for a relapse of symptoms.

The following is a list of homeopathic medicines commonly used to treat patients with urticaria. It must be emphasized that this list is partial and represents some of the probable choices from the homeopathic materia medica. If the symptoms of a given patient are not represented here, a search of the homeopathic literature would be needed to find the simillimum.

Apis mellifica

Apis mellifica will successfully treat a significant percentage of patients with urticaria. The hives are hot, red, swollen, and experienced by the patient as very itchy or burning. They are worse from heat and exercise and better from the application of cold compresses or ice. Swelling of the lips, the conjunctiva, and the tissue around the eyes may occur. The patient is quite irritable. In some patients who need *Apis mellifica*, the symptoms can progress to anaphylaxis. Such patients should seek emergency care without delay.

Chloralum hydratum

Chloralum hydratum is a medicine to consider for the patient with urticaria and insomnia. The hives occur mostly on the face, around the eyes, and on the extremities. The patient is worse from becoming slightly chilled and better from warmth. Symptoms are better during the day.

Natrum muriaticum

Natrum muriaticum is a good medicine for patients whose hives are aggravated by emotional stress. They are also worse from exercise or becoming overheated. The eruptions occur primarily at the joints and on the hands and may be pale in color before they are rubbed or scratched.

Rhus toxicodendron

Rhus toxicodendron is a medicine for large hives that are very red and located primarily on the hands and arms. The hives are worse from cold air and better from very hot water.

Urtica urens

The hives that will be successfully treated by *Urtica urens* are very itchy, burning, and stinging. The desire to scratch or rub is constant. The patient feels worse from exercise and becoming overheated and better from lying down.

Probiotics

A trial of probiotic therapy may prove beneficial for a subset of patients experiencing chronic urticaria, although little or no data exist in this regard. Because the pathophysiology of this malady is inflammatory in nature, the reported antiinflammatory actions of probiotic therapy may help ameliorate processes that drive symptoms. That stated, few studies have evaluated the use of probiotic therapy in this situation, and there are no definitive guidelines regarding dose or choice of specific microbe.

Support for probiotic therapy in the setting of chronic urticaria is largely extrapolated from data pertaining to eczema, food allergies, and immune system function. In theory, specific microbial strains may affect the modification/degradation of antigens, optimize mucosal barrier function, regulate secretion of inflammatory mediators, and promote proper immune system function.[1,2] Research also suggests that probiotic therapy may help lessen activation of cells important to an inflammatory response. A study of 14 consecutive subjects, ages 6 to 48 years, with clinical symptoms of asthma and/or conjunctivitis, rhinitis, urticaria, atopic dermatitis, food allergy, and irritable bowel syndrome was published in 2004. The subjects were given a daily mixture of *Lactobacillus acidophilus*, *Lactobacillus delbrueckii*, and *Streptococcus thermophilus* (a total of 1 billion live bacteria) for 30 days. Circulating CD34+ cell values decreased significantly after the treatment.[3]

Guidance with respect to choice of specific organisms and duration of therapy is sorely lacking. To further complicate matters, there seems little rationale behind the variety of dosages or combination of microbes employed in published studies. Similar dosages have often been used for distinct microbes, whereas widely disparate dosages have been employed by researchers studying the same probiotic. At this time, dosage recommendations are far from set in stone.

Clinical experience suggests only moderate success, but this author recommends a 2- to 3-month trial of probiotic therapy for chronic urticaria employing well-studied organisms shown to be safe, such as *Lactobacillus* GG (the microbe associated with the most supportive data), *Lactobacillus plantarum*, *Lactobacillus paracasei*, *Lactobacillus reuteri*, or *L. acidophilus*. Dosing guidelines to consider are 10 billion colony-forming units (CFU) for children weighing less than 12 kg and 20 billion CFU for children weighing more than 12 kg. Treatment is extremely well tolerated, and palatability is an infrequent issue, as the capsules can be opened and mixed into drinks or soft foods. Sometimes the agents are also available as a powder. If effective, treatment can continue indefinitely. Use with extreme caution, if at all, for those children at risk for infectious complications (e.g., immunosuppression or use of immunosuppressive agents, presence of central venous catheter, prematurity).

References

Pediatric Diagnosis and Treatment

1. Baxi S, Dinakar C: Urticaria and angioedema, *Immunol Allergy Clin North Am* 25:353-367, 2005.
2. Kozel MM, Sabroe RA: Chronic urticaria: aetiology, management and current and future treatment options, *Drugs* 64:2515-2536, 2004.
3. Hamel-Teillac D: Chronic urticaria in children [in French], *Ann Dermatol Venereol* 130:S69-S72, 2003.
4. Behrman RE, Kliegman RM, Jenson HB, editors: *Nelson's textbook of pediatrics*, Philadelphia, 2004, Saunders, pp 778–781.
5. Clarke P: Urticaria, *Austr Fam Physician* 33:501-503, 2004.
6. Amsler E: Allergy in chronic urticaria [in French], *Ann Dermatol Venereol* 130:S105-S120, 2003.
7. Wedi B, Raap U, Kapp A: Chronic urticaria and infections, *Curr Opin Allergy Clin Immunol* 4:387-396, 2004.
8. Burks W: Skin manifestations of food allergy, *Pediatrics* 111:1617-1624, 2003.
9. Stone KD: Advances in pediatric allergy, *Curr Opin Pediatr* 16:571-578, 2004.
10. Pescollderungg L: Role of leukotriene antagonists in non-asthmatic disorders [in Italian], *Minerva Pediatr* 56:151-155, 2004.

Acupuncture

1. Chen CJ, Yu HS: Acupuncture treatment of urticaria, *Arch Dermatol* 134:1397-1399, 1998.
2. Lai X: Observation on the curative effect of acupuncture on type I allergic diseases, *J Tradit Chin Med* 13:243-248, 1993.
3. Chen CJ, Yu HS: Acupuncture, electrostimulation, and reflex therapy in dermatology, *Dermatol Ther* 16:87-92, 2003.
4. Charlesworth EN, Beltrani VS: Pruritic dermatoses: overview of etiology and therapy, *Am J Med* 113(Suppl 9A):25S-33S, 2002.

Chiropractic

1. Zeichner A, Boczkowski JA: Clinical application of biofeedback techniques for the elderly, *Clinical Gerontology* 5:457-473, 1996.
2. Buerger MA: History and physical assessment. In Anrig C, Plaugher G, editors: *Chiropractic pediatrics*, Baltimore, 1998, Williams and Wilkins.
3. Leach RA, Burgess SC: Neuroimmune hypothesis. In Leach RA, editor: *The chiropractic theories*, Baltimore, 2004, Lippincott Williams and Wilkins.
4. Brennan PC, Kokjohn K, Triano JJ et al: Immunologic correlates of reduced spinal mobility: preliminary observations in a dog model. In Wold S, editor: *Proceedings of the 1991 international conference on spinal manipulation*, Arlington Va, 1991, Foundation for Chiropractic Education and Research.
5. Brennan PC, Kokjohn K, Kaltinger CJ et al: Enhanced phagocytic cell respiratory burst induced by spinal manipulation: potential role of substance P, *J Manipulative Physiol Ther* 14:399-408, 1991.
6. Hightower BC, Pfleger B, Selano JL et al: The effects of specific upper cervical adjustments on the CD4 counts of HIV positive patients, *Chiro Res J* 3:32-39, 1994.
7. Schmitt WH Jr, Leisman G: Correlation of applied kinesiology muscle testing findings with serum immunoglobulin levels for food allergies, *Int J Neurosci* 96:237-244, 1998.

Homeopathy

1. *ReferenceWorks Pro 4.2*, San Rafael, Calif, 2008, Kent Homeopathic Associates.

Probiotics

1. Isolauri E: Dietary modification of atopic disease: use of probiotics in the prevention of atopic dermatitis, *Curr Allergy Asthma Rep* 4:270-275, 2004.
2. Isolauri E: Probiotics in the prevention and treatment of allergic disease, *Pediatr Allergy Immunol* 2001;12(Suppl):56-59, 2001.
3. Mastrandrea F, Coradduzza G, Serio G et al: Probiotics reduce the CD34+ hemopoietic precursor cell increased traffic in allergic subjects, *Allerg Immunol (Paris)* 36:118-122, 2004.

Colic

Acupuncture | May Loo

Aromatherapy | Maura A. Fitzgerald

Chiropractic | Anne Spicer

Herbs—Western | Alan D. Woolf, Paula M. Gardiner, Lana Dvorkin-Camiel, Jack Maypole

Homeopathy | Janet L. Levatin

Massage Therapy | Mary C. McLellan

Naturopathy | Matthew I. Baral

Nutrition | Joy A. Weydert

Osteopathy | Jane Carreiro

Probiotics | Russell H. Greenfield

✳ PEDIATRIC DIAGNOSIS AND TREATMENT

Colic is a common condition of infants, affecting approximately one of five infants, or more than 700,000 infants in the United States each year.[1] In spite of its prevalence, colic remains mysterious and puzzling to pediatric healthcare professionals.[2]

A review of pediatric medical literature indicates that infantile colic is difficult to define, both in terms of its etiology and symptomatology.[3]

Colic usually begins between the second and sixth week of life and is rare after the fourth month of life.[4] The most common description of colic is intense, "paroxysmal" crying that is markedly different from normal fussing and crying. It can also occur as prolonged, unpredictable crying,[5] and the infant is restless and unconsolable.[6] The crying episode can last for minutes or even hours. Crying may occur any time of the day without obvious cause but is most common after the evening feeding.[4] The colicky episode is often accompanied by distention of the abdomen and cold feet. Often the baby seems to feel better after passing gas or a stool.

Various etiologies of colic have been proposed, including variation in infant behavior and development, temperament, gastrointestinal (GI) and feeding abnormalities, and dysfunction in the mother-infant relationship.

Infant Behavior and Development/Temperament

Early infancy is a developmental stage that represents a complex interaction between the baby and their environment. One conception of colic can be an expression of developmental stress,[7] possibly from unmet biological needs. A study on early infant behavior revealed a progressive drop in colicky symptoms by the eighth week of life, which can be interpreted as a maturation process.[8] Some infants may have a temperamental predisposition to colic. A study of 40 infants and their mothers revealed that the irritable infants demonstrated an increase in the amount and intensity of crying, more disruption in sleep-wake states,[6] and increased settled and awake periods.[8] Follow-up at 4 years of age revealed that formerly colicky children displayed more negative emotions, more negative moods, and more reported stomachaches.[9]

Gastrointestinal

Colicky babies manifest various feeding difficulties and GI variants. Hypermotility, an overagitated colon, may explain the symptoms.[10]

One survey of 2773 infants revealed colicky babies tend to have slow or gluttonous feeding with various digestive symptoms.[11] Although no difference was found in the intestinal microflora of the colicky infants at the time of colic compared with controls, a difference in bacterial cellular fatty acid profiles at the age of 3 months was found to correlate with severe infantile colic.[12]

Colic has been attributed to feeding, both the timing and the content. Early introduction of bottles may account for less effective suckling with more air swallowing that results in colic.[13] Cow's milk allergy has been repeatedly found in breastfed babies with colic. When mothers were put on a diet free of cow's milk protein, colicky symptoms disappeared in many infants.[14-18]

Dysfunction in Mother-Infant Relationship

The lack of synchrony in mother-infant interaction has received a great deal of attention as the cause of colic. Studies are supportive of finding difficulty in mother-infant interaction.[6] Several possible factors contribute to the dysfunction: maternal perception of infant behavior, maternal age, inadequate parenting skills, and mother's poor self-image. Colic may in fact begin during a woman's pregnancy or at birth.

A retrospective study of 25 4- to 8-month-old infants revealed that mothers of infants with colic were more bothered by the infants' mood than mothers of infants without colic.[19] This was not attributed to the possible difficult temperament of the baby but to maternal perception. A prospective study of colicky infants with age-matched controls indicate that although there is no significant difference in temperament between the colicky and noncolicky babies, the mothers of colicky babies perceive them as more intense in their reactions, more distractible, and negative.[20] Postpartum depression in the mother has also been found to correlate with development of colic in the infant.[21] A question survey of 76,747 infants in London revealed that the mother's young age, parity, and socioeconomic status remain the most important risk factors for infantile colic.[22]

Parenting skills play a significant role in colic. In a survey of 2773 infants, the parents of colicky babies needed more advice on diet and hygiene and tended to give their babies more medications.[11] Some parents who put forth a great deal of effort to console crying babies may actually be stimulating them excessively, resulting in the characteristic behavior of colic.[23] Mothers' own feelings of inadequacy may also play a role in colic. Compared with mothers with normal infants, mothers of colicky infants feel less competent as mothers and tend to have more separation anxiety.[24] Unable to calm her infant's distress, a mother may experience doubts as to her own mothering ability[25] or even feel rejected.[26] This may be associated with abuse or thoughts of abuse, as 70% of mothers revealed explicit aggressive thoughts and fantasies and 26% admitted thoughts of infanticide during their babies' colic episodes.[27]

Colic may begin in the womb and at birth. A study from Finland looked at associations between characteristics of families during pregnancy and development of colic. Results indicate that when women experience emotional stress, physical symptoms, dissatisfaction with the sexual relationship during pregnancy, and negative experiences during childbirth, the incidence of colic in their babies increases.[28]

However, it is comforting to know that although colic causes added anxiety and conflict to a family, one study revealed that 3 years after the colicky period, families with moderate and severe colicky infants did not differ significantly from control families with respect to psychological family characteristics.[29]

Treatment is advisable not so much because of the condition itself, but more because of the negative effect it can have on the parent-infant relationship. Because the precise etiology is not understood, the therapeutic goal of Western medicine is not aimed at "curing" colic, but at containment of the crying.[1] Prevention of attacks may consist of improving feeding techniques, including "burping," providing a stable emotional environment, identifying possibly allergenic foods in the infant's or nursing mother's diet, and avoiding underfeeding or overfeeding. During the attack, holding the infant upright or prone across the lap or on a hot water bottle or heating pad occasionally helps. Prolonged attacks may require sedation of the baby or both the mother and baby. Temporary hospitalization of the infant offers respite for the mother and may help in extreme cases.[10]

✳ CAM THERAPY RECOMMENDATIONS

Acupuncture

Currently there are no data on acupuncture treatment of infantile colic. The traditional Chinese medicine explanation of colic is a digestive problem due to an inherently weak Spleen. Food accumulation and Qi stagnation result in abdominal distention, gaseousness, and transformation into heat, causing colicky symptoms. Because the infant is in the Water phase of development, the Kidney is vulnerable and fear is the underlying emotion that motivates many behaviors.

These explanations correlate well with the proposed Western etiologies:

GI symptoms: Spleen is the digestive Yin organ that is responsible for formation of nutritive Qi and for transformation and transportation of food, Qi, and fluid.

Milk allergy: Cow's milk causes phlegm accumulation and further weakens the Spleen.

Dysfunctional relationship with mother: Chinese medicine posits that maternal physical and emotional health during pregnancy influences the physical and emotional health of the fetus. If the mother experiences stress and worry during pregnancy, the fetus may be predisposed to developing various weaknesses, including Spleen deficiency. Western clinicians have become concerned that colic may in fact begin during pregnancy.

The mother's own weaknesses after pregnancy—Spleen, Kidney, and Liver—predispose her to emotional states of excess worry, fear, or anger, which can manifest as various maternal issues such as poor self-image and a more disturbed perception of the baby. The mother's mental state would in turn affect the mental state of the baby, who becomes more irritable.

Infant temperament and development: The infant is in the Water phase of development, when the Kidney, which influences the marrow, the Western brain, is the dominant and the most vulnerable organ. The emotion associated with the Kidney is fear. The various irritating behaviors of the baby—increase in intensity and amount of crying, disruption in sleep-wake states—which Western medicine explains as based on unmet biological needs, may be explained as motivated by Fear, such as the instinctual fear of abandonment, especially when the mother is aloof because of depression or feelings of inadequacy.

Types of Colic

Colic can be classified in Chinese medicine as two basic types[2-5]:

1. Excess colic: Signs of Heat and excess Yang due to Spleen Yin deficiency: red face, warm extremities, intense cry, abdominal distention, agitation
2. Deficient colic: Signs of Spleen Qi deficiency and Kidney deficiency: pale face, cold extremities, abdominal distention, cry prolonged but not intense, possible loose stools

Management

The management is the same for both types of colic and needs to be directed toward both the infant and the mother.

Infant

Avoid overfeeding the baby: Excess milk or formula result in food and Qi accumulation in the Stomach and Intestines. Parents are more likely to overfeed a bottle-fed baby, as parents usually want to "finish the bottle" even when the baby is full, compared with the more natural self-limiting in breastfeeding.

Tonify abdominal Qi: Daily abdominal massage should be performed clockwise in the direction of the large intestine flow: up the right side (ascending colon), across the top (transverse colon), down the left side (descending colon), and back across the bottom to the right side again.

Keep CV8 warm. Babies should wear clothing that does not expose the umbilicus.

Tonify spleen: The mother can be taught to massage SP6, ST36. Although the infant's bony structures are not well formed, the mother can perform massage in the general area.

Tonify the kidney: Massage KI3.

Calm the baby: Massage Yintang to calm the baby.

For infants with signs of Heat: Massage LI11.

Mother

Diet: Breastfeeding mothers need to avoid phlegm- and gas-producing foods such as milk, milk products, cabbage, broccoli, cauliflower, Brussels sprouts, tomatoes, citrus, garlic, onions, chocolate, coffee, beans, rhubarb, peaches, and melons. They should also avoid excess energetically Hot or Cold foods.

Treat mother's deficiencies: Find the underlying weakness/deficiency in the mother, and treat her with acupuncture, herbs, and/or diet.

Calm the mother: Teach the mother to massage her own Yintang point and perform calming exercises, such as simple breathing or Qigong exercises that take only seconds or 1-2 minutes, which she can practice throughout the day for calming effects.

Aromatherapy

Essential oils recommended for colic include bergamot (*Citrus bergamia*), Roman chamomile (*Chamaemelum nobilis*), ginger (*Zingiber officinalis*), and mandarin (*Citrus reticulata*).[1] The most effective method of administration for colic is to mix a 0.5% to 1% solution, applied to the infant's stomach in an abdominal massage. Abdominal massage should be firm and strokes should follow the normal passage of stool through the large bowel. Circular strokes should go from the child's right to left side, and scooping strokes should go from top to bottom.[2] Abdominal massage can be completed in a few minutes and can be done two or three times per day.

Chiropractic

The success of chiropractic management of colic is substantial enough to suggest that colic may be a neurologically based condition of spinal origin. The chiropractic approach to the infant with colic is to look carefully at any historical indication of spinal/neural injury including abnormal positioning or constraint in utero, as well as difficult labor, delivery, and postpartum.[1] Rotational and/or distractive forces into the newborn cervical spine, which are common during delivery, have been demonstrated to be associated with injury to the upper cervical structures.[2-7] The chiropractor would observe for postural indications of spinal injury, such as a preference for trunk or head positions at rest, preference for unilateral breastfeeding, torticollis, scoliosis, or a need to be held in a specified posture. Increased irritability and feeding difficulties are known to be associated with such injuries.[8,9] The chiropractic regimen in the case of an infant with colic centers primarily upon assessing and correcting the spinal subluxation.

The most common areas adjusted by the chiropractor are found in the upper cervical spine (C0 to C2) and the middle thoracic spine (T4 to T9).[10-17] The most common subluxation patterns are extension of the occiput on C1, extension of C2 on C3 without rotation or laterality, and laterality of C2 on C3, in that order.[18]

The chiropractic adjustment at the C1 to C2 region has been recorded through electrogastrogram as normalizing gastric tone.[19] This result is likely due to the fact that parasympathetic regulation of the GI tract is vagal in both efferent and afferent innervation. The vagus exits the skull through the jugular foramen adjacent to the occipital condyle and traverses the anterolateral cervical spine, just deep to the sternocleidomastoid (SCM) muscle.[20]

The sympathetic influence is found in the thoracic sympathetic trunk from T4 to T6 as well as the superior thoracic splanchnic from T6 to T9.[21] Overstimulation of the sympathetic system or suppression of the parasympathetic system may cause contraction of the sphincter tone while inhibiting gastric secretions and peristalsis. A functional assessment of the nervous system through motion and position of the vertebrae, especially at the primary nerve pathways, is therefore central to the chiropractic management of colic.

A retrospective uncontrolled parental questionnaire of 132 infants with colic reported that 91% responded favorably with an average of three chiropractic adjustments.[22] As a follow-up to this questionnaire, a prospective study was undertaken with 316 infants diagnosed with colic. In this study, parents recorded daily colic symptoms prior to and during a course of chiropractic adjustments. After 2 weeks of chiropractic care (average of three adjustments) colic stopped in 60%, 34% showed improvement, 4% had no change, and 2% worsened.[23] A 94% improvement rate is a success indeed.

In a randomized clinical control trial, the chiropractic adjustment was compared with dimethicone in the management of infant colic. Both groups showed some improvement in the first 5 days of the study (daily crying reduced by 1 hour in the dimethicone group and by 2.5 hrs in the chiropractic group), but thereafter only the chiropractic group demonstrated continued improvement.[24]

A study done in South Africa compared the chiropractic adjustment with a nonfunctional ultrasound application (placebo). After a maximum of six adjustments over a 2-week course, 93% of the infants had a complete recovery from colic symptoms.[25]

Another study was conducted as a double-blind randomized control trial. This study found a 70% rate of improvement with adjustments but no difference between the group receiving adjustments and the control group.[26] However, the *maximum* number of adjustments was three, which was the *average* number in the three previous studies.

Multiple case studies also support reduction or resolution of colic symptoms with administration of chiropractic intervention.[27-32]

Secondary assessments by chiropractors involve identifying abnormal muscular tone, which may influence vertebral position and motion. If the SCM is hypertonic owing to injury or as a secondary manifestation of a vertebral subluxation, irritation may be placed on the vagus as it traverses the cervical spine, causing autonomic imbalance into the GI tract.

Decompression of the occiput with cranial techniques may provide some relief.[33]

Pressure points over the abdomen and the soles of the feet are also sometimes used supplementally to regulate peristalsis. The abdominal points are treated by finger-pad pressure (just at the point of tissue resistance) with vibration sustained for approximately 10 seconds each. The points are treated in order 1 to 5 and are stimulated approximately four times per day (Figure 23-1).

The pressure on the soles of the feet is applied with the thumb pad stroking first along the lateral arch from heel to the fifth digit and then circling back across at the level of the metatarsal-phalangeal joint (Figure 23-2).

In cases in which the adjustment does not provide the anticipated reduction in symptoms, specific food eliminations may be recommended to the breastfeeding mother, with dairy being the most common.[34] Other foods passing into breast milk that may be caustic or irritating to the newborn gut include coffee, black teas, black pepper, chocolate, and alcohol. It has been found that formula-fed infants who are lactose intolerant may have fewer symptoms on a lactose-free formula. Cross reactivity with soy is common in infants who have milk protein intolerance, and a hydrolyzed formula may be best tolerated in these cases.

Microflora is recommended to enhance digestion.

In breastfed infants, feeding from only one breast per feeding may be beneficial because of increased consumption of higher-calorie hindmilk.[35]

A tea made of fennel seed, vervain, chamomile, licorice, and/or balm mint may be given to the infant to calm the stomach.[36]

Herbs—Western

Gripe water has historically been promoted for colicky infants and labeled for gripes, acidity, and flatulency as a quick and gentle way of relieving the baby's hiccups, minor stomach upsets, and teething.[1,2] To date there have been no clinical studies on gripe water, but in recent years it has gained popularity though anecdotal evidence. The original formula included combinations of alcohol, sodium bicarbonate, or dill seed oil. However, many modern formulations do not include alcohol or sucrose and substitute fennel and ginger in place of dill.

Chinese star anise (*Illicium verum*) is used as an herbal tea for the treatment of colic and is popular among Caribbean and Latino populations.[3] Chinese star anise has been commonly regarded as being safe and nontoxic because of its long traditional use. Although Chinese star anise is considered safe for consumption, this species also contains toxic compounds named veranisatins A, B, and C. Of note, neurological symptoms are observed at higher doses.[4] Recent case reports noted that veranisatins in sufficient quantities may produce adverse reactions in susceptible infants.[3,4] A larger concern has been the adulteration of Chinese star anise (*I. verum*) with a closely related species, Japanese star anise (*Illicium anisatum*), which has been well documented as causing both neurological and GO toxicities.[5-9] There are no clinical trials on the use of star anise for colic.

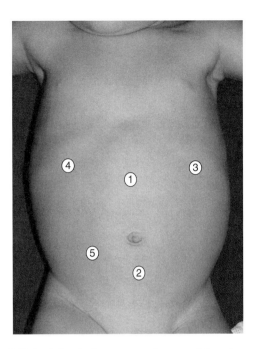

FIGURE 23-1 Abdominal pressure points. *1,* Midway between the umbilicus and the xiphoid; *2,* midway between the umbilicus and the superior rim of the symphysis pubis; *3,* inferior to the rib margin at the nipple line on the left side; *4,* inferior to the rib margin at the nipple line on the right side; *5,* over the location of the ileocecal valve.

Chamomile (*Matricaria chamomilla*) has long been used to treat colic in infants. In a prospective randomized double-blind, placebo-controlled study, 68 healthy, full-term, colicky infants (2 to 8 weeks old) received either herbal tea (Calma Bebi from Italy) or placebo with each colic episode no more than three times per day for 7 days. Calma Bebi contains extracts of German chamomile (*M. chamomilla*), vervain (*Verbena officinalis*), licorice (*Glycyrrhiza glabra*), fennel (*Foeniculum vulgare*), and balm mint (*Melissa officinalis*) with natural flavors and glucose. There was a statistically significant difference in colic in 57% of the infants, whereas placebo was helpful in only 26% ($p < 0.01$). No adverse effects were noted in either group.[10]

Fennel (*F. vulgare*) is another traditional herb used for the treatment of infant colic. Fennel seed oil for the treatment of infantile colic was examined in a double-blind, randomized, placebo-controlled trial in two large multi-specialty clinics in Russia. One hundred and twenty five infants, 2 to 12 weeks of age, who met definition of having colic (according to the Wessel criteria) were randomized to either a water emulsion of 0.1% fennel seed oil and 0.4% polysorbate-80 or placebo (4% polysorbate-80). The use of fennel oil emulsion eliminated colic in 65% of infants in the treatment group, which was significantly better than 23.7% of infants in the control group. No side effects were reported for infants in either group during the trial.[11]

Homeopathy

Before using this section, please see Appendix A, Homeopathy, for definitions of practitioner expertise categories and general information on prescribing homeopathic medicines.

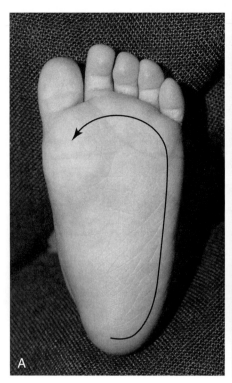 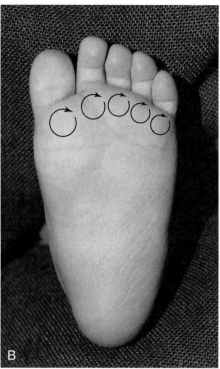

FIGURE 23-2 Pressure on the soles of the feet is applied with the thumb pad, stroking first along the lateral arch from the heel to fifth digit (**A**) and then circling back across at the level of the metatarsal-phalangeal joint (**B**).

Practitioner Expertise Category 1

Category 1 includes colic unassociated with other pathology requiring treatment.

There are no controlled clinical trials of homeopathy for treatment of colic, although the homeopathic literature contains much evidence for its use in the form of accumulated clinical experience.[1] After other treatable causes of distress in an infant have been ruled out and a diagnosis of colic has been made, it is safe to try homeopathic treatment for colic. Homeopathy can be used in conjunction with dietary changes and other treatment modalities, either conventional or alternative.

The goal in treating colic homeopathically is to determine the single homeopathic medicine whose description in the materia medica most closely matches the symptom picture of the patient. Often mental and emotional states as well as physical symptoms are considered. Once the medicine has been selected, it can be given orally or sublingually in the 30C potency two to four times daily. If it has not helped within four or five doses, then another homeopathic medicine should be tried or some other form of therapy should be instituted as needed. Once symptoms have begun to resolve, the medicine can be given less frequently or stopped. It can be repeated again for a relapse of symptoms.

The following is a list of homeopathic medicines commonly used to treat patients with colic. It must be emphasized that this list is partial and represents some of the probable choices from the homeopathic materia medica. If the symptoms of a given patient are not represented here,

a search of the homeopathic literature would be needed to find the simillimum. For more homeopathic medicines that might be useful in treating colic, please also see Chapter 8, Abdominal Pain; Chapter 30, Diarrhea; and Chapter 62, Vomiting.

Aethusa cynapium

The infant needing *Aethusa cynapium* cannot digest milk well and vomits curds of milk shortly after feeding. The abdomen is bloated, tense, and sensitive to touch. The infant may have severe vomiting and diarrhea, with thin green stools, and may become weak and dehydrated. If clinically indicated, an infant who is beginning to become dehydrated should be taken for emergency care without delay.

Chamomilla vulgaris

The infant needing *Chamomilla vulgaris* is very irritable, even inconsolable, and consoling efforts are usually rejected. The infant is generally hot, red, sweaty, and thirsty. He or she arches the back with the pains. Symptoms improve when the infant is carried. The stools are green and mucoid and appear like chopped spinach.

Colocynthinum

The infant needing *Colocynthenum* is angry and impatient. Crampy pains cause the infant to double over. He or she may vomit and have diarrhea, especially after ingesting fruit. The pain is relieved with firm pressure on the abdomen and by warmth. The colic may be worse during teething.

Dioscorea villosa

For patients who need *Dioscorea villosa*, the key symptom is abdominal pain that is relieved by bending backward such that the infant arches the back. The infant feels better after belching. Diarrhea may be present.

Magnesia phosphorica

Magnesia phosphorica treats colic that is better from the application of hot compresses, pressure, bending forward, and massage. The infant is bloated and gassy.

Nux vomica

The infant with colic needing *Nux vomica* is angry and arches the back. The infant may be constipated or have diarrhea alternating with constipation. The pain is worse from tight clothes and cold and better from warmth and after passing a stool.

Massage Therapy

Abdominal massage for infants and children has long been used by parents to help treat colic or constipation. Massage can help restore communication and improve bonding between the infant and parent, which can be very helpful in the case of a colicky infant.

Infant abdominal massage ideally should not be done immediately following a feeding; waiting at least 30 minutes may help prevent vomiting or spitting up that could occur from pressure applied to a full stomach.[1] If the child is distressed at the time of the massage, it is best to try to soothe the infant before beginning the massage, as crying engages and uses the abdominal muscles. Resting the distressed infant against the parent's chest with the knees pulled up similar to a fetal position can help to decrease tension on the abdomen and comfort the infant. If the colicky infant has not received massage before, it is best to introduce the infant to massage when not in a distressed state.

Placing the infant in a seated position in the parent's lap facing the parent, with the infant's feet resting on the parent's chest, will relax the abdominal muscles and facilitate the massage.[1] An infant with a history of reflux could be placed more upright in the lap either using pillows or having the parent's knees flexed. Abdominal massage should be in the direction of the large intestines at all times.[1,2] For the massage, slow, rhythmic strokes applied with the firm pressure of a relaxed hand will be relaxing and prevent tickling the infant.[1,2] A light amount of oil or lotion may be used to facilitate the hand gliding along the infant's abdomen.[1,2] The massage strokes should each be repeated approximately 5 to 10 times each. (If the infant has an abdominal feeding tube in place or a stoma, avoid the area and continue the rest of the massage as instructed.)

The first stroke is a hand-over-hand motion starting below the rib cage, stroking down the middle of the abdomen with one hand, to the pelvic bone. This is then repeated with the alternate hand, thereby always keeping contact with the infant.[1,2] For the second step, strokes are applied in a clockwise, circular motion (with the child as the clock) along the entire abdomen, avoiding the navel area.[1,2] Firmer pressure should be added from the 9 o'clock to the 5 o'clock positions.[1] Repeat in a continuous motion.[1,2]

The last step has three separate strokes.[1,2] The first stroke starts on the child's left side below the rib cage, moving the hand downward to the hip, following the descending colon. Repeat several times before proceeding to the next stroke. The second stroke follows the transverse and descending colon. Begin the stroke on the infant's right side under the rib cage, gliding the hand below the ribs toward the left and then downward, in the figure of an upside-down L. Repeat several times. The final stroke begins at the infant's right hip, then upward below the ribs and along to the left and then down in the figure of an upside-down U. This last stroke follows the ascending, transverse, and descending colon and completes the massage.[1,2]

A recent study compared the effectiveness of massage to a crib vibrator for colicky infants less than 7 weeks of age. A control was not present in this study. Parents were instructed to keep a structured cry journal and provide the assigned treatments three times per day for 3 weeks. Parents reported total cry time decreased by almost 50% and colicky crying decreased by slightly more than 50% for both groups. In both groups, 93% of the parents thought that the colic symptoms had decreased with the interventions.[3]

Naturopathy

Colic is a common complaint among families with newborns, and treating this problem should be relatively simple.

Address Baby's Diet

Reviews on colic research reveal that cow's milk and soy allergies may play a major role in colic.[1] Rather than giving medications that attempt to decrease the symptoms, such as simethicone, addressing the root of the cause by removing the offending food from the diet or switching to a predigested protein formula[2] may be more effective. Introduction of solid foods at too early an age may also cause colic and predispose the child to development of atopy. It is recommended that solid food introduction be started at 6 months of age at the earliest.

Address Mother's Diet

There is some supporting evidence that the diet of the breastfeeding mother can affect colic,[3] and removal of these foods can be a very helpful treatment.[4] Foods such as wheat, dairy, eggs, spicy food, caffeinated beverages, or any foods that seem to cause intestinal gas in the mother may be eliminated for several days to verify whether the diet changes have a beneficial effect.

Botanical Medicine

Several herbal species are reported to be quite successful and safe when used appropriately for colic. A common recipe called "gripe water" is available at most health food stores, and most formulations contain herbs such as ginger, fennel, chamomile, catnip, dill, lemon balm, and anise. Research is limited on botanical treatment for colic, but one study in infants showed improvement in colic symptoms when given an herbal tea preparation that contained several of these ingredients.[5] These products are safe and useful if the manufacturer's recommendations are followed.

In her book *Encyclopedia of Natural Healing for Children and Infants*, naturopathic physician Mary Bove gives two helpful recipes for colic. Catnip, considered to have antispasmodic properties, may be used in alcohol tincture form by adding 40 drops to 1 ounce of water, sweetened with rice syrup and given by the dropper every 15 minutes. Seeds that contain volatile oils, such as fennel, dill, caraway, and anise, can be used to make a tea at home. Add 1 teaspoon of seeds from one of these sources to 8 ounces of hot water, steep for 10 minutes, add 3 ounces of vegetable glycerine, and store in a bottle. The recommended dose is ¼ to ½ teaspoon every half hour in acute colic situations or 15 minutes before feeding. Chamomile tea may be made from teabags and given 1 teaspoon at a time throughout the day for babies with colic. It may be sweetened with maple syrup or brown rice syrup for taste.

Chinese star anise is another plant that has been traditionally used for colic, but recent products were discovered to be contaminated with the neurotoxic species of Japanese star anise and caused significant neurological problems in a group of infants.[6]

Address Functional Issues

Feeding position and overfeeding should always be considered as possible aggravating factors in colic. The baby should feed with the head above the stomach in order to avoid reflux. Overfeeding can also lead to reflux and inadequate digestion.

Physical Medicine

A common folk remedy of abdominal massage has been passed down for many generations, which helps facilitate movement of trapped abdominal gas. Gently massage from the right lower quadrant in the direction of the colon, moving clockwise. This may be done at any time the baby is having a bout of colic.

Another effective remedy is the castor oil pack. Some health food stores actually sell premade packs. To make the pack at home, saturate a flannel cloth with castor oil and place on the child's abdomen and cover with a hot water bottle for approximately 1 hour, as needed throughout the day. The pack may be reused for several weeks.

Nutrition

Various nutritional strategies have been implicated for the infant with colic. For exclusively breastfed infants, fully emptying the first breast before starting on the second breast provides more of the hindmilk that is richer in fat content and therefore more satisfying, causing the babies to be more content. The mother's diet also needs to be assessed for foods that may contribute to colic symptoms in infants. One survey of more than 270 breastfeeding women and their infants found an increased relative risk of colic symptoms when the women ingested cruciferous vegetables such as cauliflower, broccoli, or cabbage; onion; chocolate; and cow's milk.[1] Cow's milk protein can affect formula-fed infants as well. Changing to a soy or hydrolyzed casein or whey formula may be helpful to some.

Another study found the relationship of colic symptoms with the infant's intake of fruit juices containing sorbitol and high fructose:glucose ratio (apple juice).[2] Breath hydrogen gas analysis found carbohydrate malabsorption in the infants who received this juice but not in those who received white grape juice.

Probiotics may help colic by improving digestion and reducing carbohydrate malabsorption, especially if there is

a history of prenatal/perinatal use of antibiotics. Probiotics restore the natural intestinal flora that may have been disrupted by antibiotics or stress. Chamomile, fennel, peppermint, and ginger are foods and herbs that can easily be made into a tea and safely used to treat infants with colic.[3]

Treatment

- Evaluate the mother's diet and eliminate any offending foods such as dairy products, cruciferous vegetables, onions, or chocolate.
- Observe breastfeeding techniques to ensure that the infant is feeding fully.
- Eliminate fruit juices that contain high fructose or sorbitol from the infant's diet.
- If there is evidence of cow's milk protein intolerance, consider changing to soy or hydrolyzed formula.
- Herbal teas containing chamomile, fennel, peppermint, or lemon balm can be used safely if the herbs are derived from reputable sources. Cool the tea to room temperature before giving it to the infant.

Osteopathy

Theories concerning the etiology and pathophysiology of colic are broad and varied, ranging from food sensitivities to gut and nervous system immaturity to poor caregiving techniques. From an osteopathic perspective, all but the latter of these has some merit and in fact the clinical presentation of colic may represent different pathology manifesting with a similar sign/symptom complex. Based upon osteopathic structural findings, most children presenting with colic fall into one of three groups: functional GI disturbance, persistent nociceptive or painful stimuli, or some combination of the two. This hypothesis is based on the observation that the osteopathic structural examination findings present in the baby with colic are similar to findings in patients who are able to communicate their complaints. It is probable that the somatic dysfunction produces a similar symptom in the infant who has limited means of communication.

In traditional osteopathic teaching, colic has been described as resulting from vagal nerve irritation associated with tissue strain patterns in the cranial base, petrobasilar, and occipitomastoid areas.[1-4] These strains may contribute to vagal irritation by compressing the nerve's vasa nervosum or nervi nervosum. Gut motility and function are immature in newborns, resulting in increased transit times and immature hormone and enzyme function.[5] These factors promote the production of intestinal gases. Vagal or parasympathetic influences on the gut act to increase tonic contractions. The lack of mature innervation patterns in the gut wall results in an uncoordinated contraction rather than the peristaltic wave seen in adults. It is thought that vagal irritation may exacerbate this process.[2] The symptoms of colic usually arise sometime between the second and fourth week of life in the term infant. This period of time coincides with the initial development of voluntary control of the posterior cervical muscles. The head and neck extensor muscles attach to the areas of the cranium commonly found to have biomechanical strain in infants with colic. One hypothesis suggests that the engagement of the posterior cervical muscles exacerbates minor tissue strains in this area.[3] Other common findings on osteopathic examination include tissue strains in the thorax, abdomen, or pelvis similar to those found in adults with functional bowel complaints.[4] Viscerosomatic reflexes in the mid to lower thoracic area may also be present in infants with severe symptoms.

Another group of infants diagnosed with colic presents with a preponderance of signs of anxiety and irritability rather than GI dysfunction. Their symptoms are often not related to feeding. Parents often report that symptoms began immediately after birth rather than into the second or third week. Palpatory findings in these children often suggest nociceptive or painful stimuli usually involving somatic dysfunction in the thoracic, cervical, or cranial areas, particularly compressive and nonphysiological strains as described by Sutherland's model.[2] These findings are similar to those of adults with chronic headache or neck pain.[2,6-8] Coincidently the medical literature also recognizes a subgroup of colicky infants whose symptom complex suggests immaturity or irritability of the central nervous system. Normal adults have the ability to screen out stimulus through gating mechanisms in the spinal cord and cortex. The immature infant nervous system does not have this ability. Consequently, areas of nociception or tissue stress may be perceived as more irritating than would be expected in an adult. Furthermore, sensory input summations onto areas of the spinal cord and brain effectively decrease the threshold for activation of the arousal systems. Areas of constriction, irritation, and dysfunction in the body will contribute to this summation.[9-17] Osteopathic cranial techniques, balancing techniques, and functional techniques are used to treat the findings in the head and neck. These techniques, in addition to inhibition techniques, may also be used to address the viscerosomatic reflexes.

Many of the aforementioned GI and neurological factors begin to mature by age 4 to 5 months, which coincides with the time at which untreated colic usually resolves. Nevertheless, osteopathic treatment of associated findings may help the infant compensate until these systems mature and give the parents a much-needed break.

Probiotics

Research into the use of probiotic therapy for the prevention or treatment of colic is in its earliest stages. One study evaluating the long-term safety of probiotic therapy in healthy infants aged 3 to 24 months receiving >10 million colony-forming units (CFU) of *Bifidobacterium lactis* and *Streptococcus thermophilus* did, however, report a lower incidence of colic and irritability in children who received probiotic-supplemented formula compared with standard formula.[1]

A trial of probiotic therapy should be safe in infants and could prove beneficial for a subset of patients with colic. Guidance with respect to use of specific organisms, dose, and duration of therapy is not yet firmly established. This author recommends using a 2- to 3-month trial of therapy for infants with colic employing well-studied organisms shown to be safe, such as *Lactobacillus* GG, *Lactobacillus reuteri*, *Lactobacillus plantarum*, *Lactobacillus acidophilus*, or *Bifidobacterium* species. Dosing guidelines to consider are 10 billion CFU for children < 12 kg. Treatment is extremely well tolerated, and palatability

is an infrequent issue, as the capsules can be opened and mixed into drinks or soft foods. Some agents are also available as a powder. If effective, treatment can continue indefinitely. Use with extreme caution, if at all, for those children at risk for infectious complications (e.g., immunosuppression or use of immunosuppressive agents, presence of central venous catheter, prematurity).

References

Pediatric Diagnosis and Treatment

1. Pinyerd BJ: Strategies for consoling the infant with colic: fact or fiction? *J Pediatr Nurs* 7:403-411, 1992.
2. Barr RG: Crying in the first year of life: good news in the midst of distress, *Child Care Health Dev* 24:425-439, 1998.
3. Gupta SK: Is colic a gastrointestinal disorder? *Curr Opin Pediatr* 14:588-592, 2002.
4. Colon AR, DiPalma JS: Colic, *Am Fam Physician* 40:122-124, 1989.
5. James-Roberts IS, Conroy S, Wilsher K: Bases for maternal perceptions of infant crying and colic behavior, *Arch Dis Child* 75:375-384, 1996.
6. Keefe MR, Kotzer AM, Froese-Fretz A et al: A longitudinal comparison of irritable and nonirritable infants, *Nurs Res* 45:4-9, 1996.
7. Hewson P, Oberklaid F, Menahem S: Infant colic, distress, and crying, *Clin Pediatr* Feb:69-76, 1987.
8. Walker AM, Menahem S: Normal early infant behavior patterns, *J Pediatr Child Health* 30:260-262, 1994.
9. Canivet C, Jakobsson I, Hagander B: Infantile colic. Follow-up at four years of age: still more "emotional," *Acta Paediatr* 89:13-17, 2000.
10. Behrman RE, Kliegman RM, Jenson HB, editors: *Nelson textbook of pediatrics*, ed 17, Philadelphia, 2004, Saunders.
11. Stagnara J, Blanc JP, Danjou G et al: Clinical data on the diagnosis of colic in infants. Survey in 2,773 infants aged 15-119 days, *Arch Pediatr* 4:959-966, 1997.
12. Lehtonen L, Korvenranta H, Eerola E: Intestinal microflora in colicky and noncolicky infants: bacterial cultures and gas-liquid chromatography, *J Pediatr Gastroenterol Nutrition* 19:310-314, 1994.
13. Newman J: Breastfeeding problems associated with the early introduction of bottles and pacifiers, *J Human Lact* 6:59-63, 1990.
14. Jakobsson I, Lindberg T: Cow's milk as a cause of infantile colic in breast-fed infants, *Lancet* 2:437-439, 1978.
15. Jakobsson I, Lindberg T: Cow's milk proteins cause infantile colic in breast-fed infants: a double-blind crossover study, *Pediatrics* 71:268-271, 1983.
16. Jenkins GH: Milk-drinking mothers with colicky babies, *Lancet* 2:261, 1981.
17. Gerrard JW: Allergies in breastfed babies to foods ingested by the mother, *Clin Rev Allergy* 2:143-149, 1984.
18. Colon AR, DiPalma JS: Colic. Removal of cow's milk protein from the diet eliminates colic in 30% of infants, *Am Fam Physician* 40:122-124, 1989.
19. Jacobson D, Melvin N: A comparison of temperament and maternal bother in infants with and without colic, *J Pediatr Nurs* 10:181-188, 1995.
20. Lehtonen L, Korhonen T, Korvenranta H: Temperament and sleeping patterns in colicky infants during the first year of life, *J Dev Behav Pediatr* 15:416-420, 1994.
21. Miller AR, Barr RG, Eaton WO: Crying and motor behavior of six-week-old infants and postpartum maternal mood, *Pediatrics* 92:551-558, 1993.

22. Crowcroft NS, Strachan DP: The social origins of infantile colic: questionnaire study covering 76,747 infants, *Br Med J* 314: 1325-1328, 1997.
23. McKenzie S: Troublesome crying in infants: effect of advice to reduce stimulation, *Arch Dis Child* 66:1416-1420, 1991.
24. Stifter CA, Bono MA: The effect of infant colic on maternal self-perceptions and mother-infant attachment, *Child Care Health Dev* 24:339-351, 1998.
25. Menahem S: The crying baby—why colic? *Austr FamPhysician* 7:1262-1266, 1978.
26. Pauli-Pott U, Becker K, Mertesacker T et al: Infants with "colic"—mothers' perspectives on the crying problem, *J Psychosom Res* 48:125-132, 2000.
27. Levitzky S, Cooper R: Infant colic syndrome—maternal fantasies of aggression and infanticide, *Clin Pediatr* 39:395-400, 2000.
28. Rautava P, Helenius H, Lehtonen L: Psychosocial predisposing factors for infantile colic, *Br Med J* 307:600-604, 1993.
29. Raiha H, Lehtonen L, Korhonen T et al: Family functioning 3 years after infantile colic, *J Dev Behav Pediatr* 18:290-294, 1997.

Acupuncture

1. Loo M: *Pediatric acupuncture*, London, 2002, Elsevier.
2. Cao J: *Essentials of traditional Chinese pediatrics*, Beijing, 1990, Foreign Language Press.
3. Diagnosis and treatment of gynecology and pediatrics. In *Chinese Zhenjiuology, a series of teaching videotapes*, Beijing, 1990, Chinese Medical Audio-Video Organization and Meditalent Enterprises.
4. Flaws B: *A handbook of TCM pediatrics, a practitioner's guide to the care and treatment of common childhood diseases*, Boulder, Colo, 1997, Blue Poppy Press.
5. Scott J: *Acupuncture in the treatment of children*, London, 1991, Eastland Press.

Aromatherapy

1. Price S, Parr PP: *Aromatherapy for babies and children*, San Francisco, 1996, Thorsons.
2. McClure V: *Infant massage*, New York, 2000, Bantam.

Chiropractic

1. Hogdall CK, Vestermark V, Birsch M et al: The significance of pregnancy, delivery and postpartum factors for the development of infant colic, *J Perinat Med* 19:251-257, 1991.
2. Giles FH, Bina M, Sotrel A: Infantile atlanto-occipital instability: the potential danger of extreme extension, *Am J Dis Child* 133: 30-37, 1979.
3. Biedermann H: Kinematic imbalance due to suboccipital stain in newborns, *Manuelle Medizin* 6:151-156, 1992.
4. Menticogluou SM, Perlman M, Manning FA: High cervical spinal cord injury in neonates delivered with forceps: report of 15 cases, *Obstet Gynecol* 86:589-594, 1995.
5. Towbin A: Latent spinal cord and brainstem injury in newborn infants, *Dev Med Child Neurol* 11:54-68, 1969.
6. Byers RK: Spinal cord injuries during birth, *Dev Med Child Neurol* 17:103-110, 1975.
7. Davies N: *Chiropractic pediatrics*, London, 2000, Churchill Livingstone.
8. Gutmann G: The atlas fixation in the baby and infant. *Manuelle Medizin* 25:5-10, 1987.
9. Gottlieb MS: Neglected spinal cord, brain stem and musculoskeletal injuries stemming from birth trauma, *J Manipulative Physiol Ther* 16:537-543, 1993.
10. Nillson N: Infant colic and chiropractic, *Eur J Chiropractic* 33: 264-265, 1985.
11. Klougart N, Nilsson N, Jacobsen J: Infantile colic treated by chiropractors: a prospective study of 316 cases, *J Manipulative Physiol Ther* 12:281-288, 1989.
12. Wiberg JM, Nordsteen J, Nilsson N: The short-term effect of spinal manipulation in the treatment of infantile colic: a randomized controlled clinical trial with a blinded observer, *J Manipulative Physiol Ther* 22:517-522, 1999.
13. Mercer C, Nook BC: The efficacy of chiropractic spinal adjustment as a treatment protocol in the management of infantile colic, *WFC's 5th Congress: symposium presentation*, May 1999, World Federation of Chiropractors.
14. Olafsdottir E, Forshei S, Fluge G et al: Randomised controlled trial of infantile colic treated with chiropractic spinal manipulation, *Arch Dis Child* 84:138-141, 2001.
15. Leach RA: Differential compliance instrument in the treatment of infantile colic: a report of two cases, *J Manipulative Physiol Ther* 25:58-62, 2002.
16. Van Loon M: Colic with projectile vomiting: a case study, *J Clin Chiropractic Pediatr* 3:207-210, 1998.
17. Killinger LZ, Azad A: Chiropractic care of infantile colic: a case study, *J Clin Chiropractic Pediatr* 3:203-206, 1998.
18. Pluhar GR, Schobert PD: Vertebral subluxation and colic: a case study, *J Chiropractic Res Clin Invest* 7:75-76, 1991.
19. Krauss LL: Case study: birth trauma results in colic, *Chiropractic Pediatr* 2:10-11, 1995.
20. Cuhel JM, Powel M: Chiropractic management of an infant patient experiencing colic and difficulty breastfeeding: a case report, *J Clin Chiropractic Pediatr* 2:150-154, 1997.
21. Munck LK, Hoffmann H, Nielsen AA: treatment of infants in the first year of life by chiropractors. Incidence and reasons for seeking treatments, *Ugeskr Laeger* 150:1841-1844, 1988.
22. Sheader WE: Chiropractic management of an infant experiencing breastfeeding difficulties and colic: a case study, *J Clin Chiropractic Pediatr* 4:245-247, 1999.
23. Leach RA: Differential compliance instrument in the treatment of infantile colic: a report of two cases, *J Manipulative Physiol Ther* 25:58-62, 2002.
24. Klougart N, Nilsson N, Jacobsen J: Infantile colic treated by chiropractors: a prospective study of 316 cases, *J Manipulative Physiol Ther* 12:281-288, 1989.
25. Wiberg JM, Nordsteen J, Nilsson N: The short-term effect of spinal manipulation in the treatment of infantile colic: a randomized controlled clinical trial with a blinded observer, *J Manipulative Physiol Ther* 22:517-522, 1999.
26. Van Loon M: Colic with projectile vomiting: a case study, *J Clin Chiropractic Pediatr* 3:207-210, 1998.
27. Killinger LZ, Azad A: Chiropractic care of infantile colic: a case study, *J Clin Chiropractic Pediatr* 3:203-206, 1998.
28. Pluhar GR, Schobert PD: Vertebral subluxation and colic: a case study, *J Chiropractic Res Clin Invest* 7:75-76, 1991.
29. Krauss LL: Case study: birth trauma results in colic, *Chiropractic Pediatr* 2:10-11, 1995.
30. Davies N: *Chiropractic pediatrics*, London, 2000, Churchill Livingstone.
31. Wiles MR: Observations on the effects of upper cervical manipulations on the electrogastrogram: a preliminary report, *J Manipulative Physiol Ther* 3:226-228, 1980.

32. Gray H: *Gray's anatomy*, Philadelphia, 1973, Lea and Febiger.
33. Bilgrai Cohen K: *Clinical management of infants and children: a hand book for chiropractors*, Santa Cruz, Calif, 1988, Extension Press.
34. Iacono G, Carroccio A, Montalto G et al: Severe infantile colic and food intolerance: a long-term prospective study, *J Pediatr Gastroenterol Nutr* 12:332-335, 1991.
35. Kerner JA: Formula allergy and intolerance, *Gastroenterol Clin North Am* 24:1-25, 1995.
36. Weizman Z, Alkrinawi S, Goldfarb D et al: Efficacy of herbal tea preparations in infantile colic, *J Pediatr* 122:650-652, 1993.

Herbs—Western

1. Wisniowski L: *FDA detention of Woodword's Gripe Water.* Available at www.fda.gov/ora/fiars/ora-import-ia6609.html.
2. Blumenthal I: The gripe water story, *J R Soc Med* 93:172-174, 2000.
3. Ize-Ludlow D: Neurotoxicities in infants seen with the consumption of star anise tea, *Pediatrics* 114:653-656, 2004.
4. Okuyama E, Nakamura T, Yamazaki M: Convulsants from star anise (*Illicium verum* Hook. F.), *Chem Pharma Bull* 41:1670-1671.
5. Biessels GJ, Vermeij FH, Leijten FS: Epileptic seizure after a cup of tea: intoxication with Japanese star anise [in Dutch], *Nederlands Tijdschrift voor Geneeskunde* 146:808-811, 2002.
6. Garzo Fernandez C, Gomez Pintado P, Barrasa Blanco A et al: Cases of neurological symptoms associated with star anise consumption used as a carminative [in Spanish], *Anales Españoles de Pediatria Asociacion Espanola de Pediatria (Madrid)* 4:290-294, 2002.
7. Johanns ES, van der Kolk LE, van Gemert HM et al: An epidemic of epileptic seizures after consumption of herbal tea [see comment] [in Dutch], *Nederlands Tijdschrift voor Geneeskunde* 146:813-816, 2002.
8. Vandenberghe N, Pittion-Vouyovitch S, Flesch F et al: Generalized tonic-clonic convulsions beginning after consumption of Japanese star anise [in French], *Presse Medicale Editions Masson (Paris)* 1:27-28, 2003.
9. Ize-Ludlow D, Ragone S, Bernstein JN et al: Chemical composition of Chinese star anise (*Illicium verum*) and neurotoxicity in infants, *J Am Med Assoc* 291:562-563, 2004.
10. Weizman Z, Alkrinawi S, Goldfarb D et al: Efficacy of herbal tea preparation in infantile colic, *J Pediatr* 122:650-652, 1993.
11. Alexandrovich I, Rakovitskaya O, Kolmo E et al: The effect of fennel (*Foeniculum vulgare*) seed oil emulsion in infantile colic: a randomized, placebo-controlled study, *Altern Ther Health Med* 9:58-61, 2003.

Homeopathy

1. *ReferenceWorks Pro 4.2*, San Rafael, Calif, 2008, Kent Homeopathic Associates.

Massage Therapy

1. Fleming-Drehobl K, Gengler-Fuhr M: *Pediatric massage for the child with special needs*, Tucson, Ariz, 1991, Therapy Skill Builders.
2. McClure VS: *Infant massage, a handbook for loving parents*, New York, 1989, Bantam.
3. Huhtala V, Lehtonen L, Heinonen R et al: Infant massage compared with crib vibrator in the treatment of colicky infants, *Pediatrics* 105:E84, 2000.

Naturopathy

1. Cirgin Ellett ML: What is known about infant colic? *Gastroenterol Nurs* 26:60-65, 2003.
2. Swadling C, Griffiths P: Is modified cow's milk formula effective in reducing symptoms of infant colic? *Br J Community Nurs* 8: 24-27, 2003.
3. Hill DJ, Hudson IL, Sheffield LJ et al: A low allergen diet is a significant intervention in infantile colic: results of a community-based study, *J Allergy Clin Immunol* 96:886-892, 1995.
4. Heine RG, Elsayed S, Hosking CS et al: Cow's milk allergy in infancy, *Curr Opin Allergy Clin Immunol* 2:217-225, 2002.
5. Weizman Z, Alkrinawi S, Goldfarb D et al: Efficacy of herbal tea preparation in infantile colic, *J Pediatr* 122:650-652, 1993.
6. Ize-Ludlow D, Ragone S, Bruck IS et al: Neurotoxicities in infants seen with the consumption of star anise tea, *Pediatrics* 114: e653-e656, 2004.

Nutrition

1. Lust KD, Brown JE, Thomas W: Maternal intake of cruciferous vegetables and other foods and colic symptoms in exclusively breast-fed infants, *J Am Diet Assoc* 96:46-48, 1996.
2. Duro D, Rising R, Cedillo M et al: Association between infantile colic and carbohydrate malabsorption from fruit juices in infancy, *Pediatrics* 109:797-805, 2002.
3. Weizman Z, Alkrinawi S, Goldfarb D et al: Efficacy of herbal tea preparation in infantile colic, *J Pediatr* 122:650-652, 1993.

Osteopathy

1. Sutherland WG: *Teachings in the science of osteopathy*, Portland, Ore, 1990, Rudra Press.
2. Magoun HIS: *Osteopathy in the cranial field*, Kirksville, Mo, 1951, The Journal Printing Company.
3. Carreiro JE: *An osteopathic approach to children*, London, 2003, Churchill Livingstone.
4. Kuchera ML, Kuchera WA: *Osteopathic considerations in systemic disease*, Columbus, Ohio, 1994, Greydon Press.
5. Milla PJ: The ontogeny of intestinal motor acti. In Walker WA, Durie PR, Hamilton JR et al, editors: *Pediatric gastrointestinal disease*, St Louis, 1996, Mosby.
6. FitzGerald R.T.D.: Observations on trigger points, fibromyalgia, recurrent headache and cervical syndrome, *J Man Med* 6:124-129, 1991.
7. Ward RC, editor: *Foundations for osteopathic medicine*, Philadelphia, 2003, Lippincott.
8. Bogduk N: The anatomical basis for cervicogenic headache, *J Manipulative Physiol Ther* 15:67-70, 1992.
9. Wallace KG: The pathophysiology of pain, *Crit Care Nurs Q* 15: 1-13, 1992.
10. Yaksh TL: The spinal pharmacology of facilitation of afferent processing evoked by high-threshold afferent input of the postinjury pain state, *Curr Opin Neurol Neurosurg* 6:250-256, 1993.
11. Randich A, Gebhart GF: Vagal afferent modulation of nociception, *Brain Res Brain Res Rev* 17:77-99, 1992.
12. Scarinci IC, McDonald-Haile J, Bradley LA et al: Altered pain perception and psychosocial features among women with gastrointestinal disorders and history of abuse: a preliminary model [see comments], *Am J Med* 97:108-118, 1994.
13. Gold P, Goodwin F: Clinical and biochemical manifestations of depression: part II, *N Engl J Med* 319:413-420, 1988.
14. Gold P, Goodwin F: Clinical and biochemical manifestations of stress: part I, *N Engl J Med* 319:348-353, 1988.

15. Ganong W: The stress response—a dynamic overveiw, *Hosp Prac* 23:155-171, 1988.
16. Willard FH, Mokler DJ, Morgane PJ: Neuroendocrine-immune system and homeostasis. In Ward RC, editor: *Foundations for osteopathic medicine*, Baltimore, 1997, Williams and Wilkins, pp 107-135.
17. Donnerer J: Nociception and the neuroendocrine-immune system. In Willard FH, Patterson M, editors: *Nociception and the neuroendocrine-immune connection*, Indianapolis, 1992, American Academy of Osteopathy.

Probiotics

1. Saavedra JM, Abi-Hanna A, Moore N et al: Long-term consumption of infant formulas containing live probiotic bacteria: tolerance and safety, *Am J Clin Nutr* 79:261, 2004.

CHAPTER 24

Concussion

Acupuncture | May Loo
Chiropractic | Anne Spicer

Homeopathy | Janet L. Levatin
Osteopathy | Jane Carreiro

✳ PEDIATRIC DIAGNOSIS AND TREATMENT

Concussion is the most common sequela of mild head injury.[1] It is an alteration of mental status ranging from a brief period of neural dysfunction to a prolonged period of unconsciousness.[2]

The constellation of complaints includes disturbance of vision and equilibrium, retrograde amnesia and other cognitive dysfunction, and headache. Multiple concussions can cause cognitive impairment, including impaired memory, attention, and activity planning, as well as emotional lability and fatigue.[1]

The predominant causes are accidental: motor vehicle crashes, falls, play activity, and sports injuries. Concussion is the most common head injury occurring in sports participation and is occurring at epidemic proportions in high schools and universities as sports become increasingly violent and aggressive.[3] Approximately 300,000 sport-related concussions occur annually in the United States.[4]

Improved equipment standards for helmets and the enforcement of rules to prohibit the use of the head as the point of initial contact when tackling have resulted in some decrease in the incidence of sports-related catastrophic head injuries.[1]

Sixty-three percent of mild traumatic head injuries in high school sports occur in football. The other sports in descending frequency of head injuries include wrestling, soccer, basketball, softball, field hockey, and volleyball.

A prospective U.K. review of 4258 children (3341 boys and 917 girls) aged 6 to 16 years who participated in national and international tae kwon do tournaments revealed the head as the most often injured body part, with cerebral concussion the second most common accident. Boys were injured at a higher rate than girls. The unblocked attack was the major cause of injury.[5]

Despite a paucity of research on female athletes and youth athletes, there is evidence that female athletes are at higher risk for injury than males and that concussions may affect children and young adolescents differently than older adolescents and adults.[6]

Physical abuse should be suspected in head injuries in children younger than 6 years.[7]

In addition to a complete neurological examination, the Colorado Medical Society Guidelines can be used to evaluate severity of concussion according to the level of confusion, amnesia, and loss of consciousness. The Glasgow Coma Scale (GCS) is commonly used to assess children with an altered level of consciousness and provides very rapid assessment of cerebral cortical function. Patients with a GCS score of 8 or less may require aggressive management, including mechanical ventilation and intracranial pressure monitoring.[1]

The care and management of children with concussions is challenging because each patient has different symptoms.[8] Understanding of the sequelae of cerebral concussion, education on proper sport techniques, body conditioning, and equipment upkeep are the mainstay of vigilant sport injury treatment and prevention.[9] It is important to recognize that emotional disturbances such as anxiety are sometimes associated with mild traumatic brain injury.[10]

Baseline neuropsychological or balance evaluation of athletes would be helpful for assessment of recovery after injury, as the absence of symptoms at rest and with increasing intensity of exercise are often the criteria for allowing an athlete to return to play.[8] Children with concussion with brief loss of consciousness are often admitted for observation, even with a normal central nervous system (CNS) finding, negative computed tomography (CT) scan, and a low GCS score.[11] A National Collegiate Athletic Association (NCAA) prospective cohort study of 1631 collegiate football players revealed that these athletes may require several days for recovery of symptoms, cognitive dysfunction, and postural instability after concussion.[12]

Postconcussional syndrome may develop 2 weeks to 2 months after a minimal brain trauma,[13,14] which may consist of symptoms such as attention deficits, hyperactivity, or conduct disorder that may interfere with other aspects of the child's life.[14]

The complementary and alternative medicine (CAM) therapist needs to be able to recognize concussion symptoms and promptly refer the child to the physician for evaluation, management, and possible hospitalization. The CAM therapist can function in a complementary role in providing CAM treatment for symptoms such as headache, fatigue, or attention issues.

✳ CAM THERAPY RECOMMENDATIONS

Acupuncture

At this time there is no evidence-based information on acupuncture treatment of concussion in children.

Chinese medicine considers a blow to the head as the cause of Blood stasis in the area of the trauma. Acupuncture treatment can be instituted to treat Blood stasis and headaches if neurological examination and laboratory evaluations are negative for skull fracture or CNS bleed. There are four major stasis points:

1. BL17, the Hui-meeting point of Blood, invigorates Blood and dispels stasis.
2. SP10 for general treatment for Blood stasis.
3. Taiyang acupoint for Blood stasis in the temple region.
4. TB18 for Blood stasis in the occiput.

Treatment of headache depends on the location of the headaches, which is usually at the site of trauma. Treatment can begin with Ah Shi tender points as local points, followed by a distal point along the channel that connects to the Ah Shi point. For example, if the tender point is on the forehead along the ST line, treat the tender Ah Shi point and then choose a distal point on the ST channel; if the tender point is a GB point on the side of the head, treat the Ah Shi point as a local point and then treat a distal GB point.

Chiropractic

Although chiropractors do not directly treat concussions, the traumatic physical effects are managed quite well by chiropractic care. The subluxation complex (SC) and all its ramifications are often a direct result of trauma, as with concussion.

Careful examination, including radiographs, is indicated in the case of trauma before care begins. Presence of fracture and dislocation must be identified. In the absence of gross pathology, the SC is identified and corrected. Specific locations of postconcussive headaches may give the chiropractor clues to the dysfunctional spinal level.[1]

- Pain in the frontal region is often associated with the C0-C1 or C2-C3.
- Pain in the retroorbital region is often associated with C2-C3.
- Pain in the temporosphenoidal or occiput region is often associated with C1-C2.
- Pain in the suboccipital region or into the neck is often associated with the lower cervical spine, thoracolumbar junction, or lumbosacral junction.

Cranial therapies may be employed with the understanding that intracranial bleeding can occur in any postconcussive child. The peak bleed typically occurs within 72 hours of onset. It is therefore advisable to wait until such time as confirmed stabilization occurs, prior to commencing with cranial therapies.

A case study was reported of a postconcussive 2-year old with persistent vomiting, lethargy, and "strange behavior." Chiropractic examination revealed an SC at the atlantooccipital junction. After one adjustment to the occiput, the vomiting ceased and the child's energy returned. The child was adjusted three more times for a complete recovery of all symptoms.[2]

Although not exclusively a concussion case, there was a remarkable case report of a 21-year-old man in a coma following a motor vehicle accident.[3] After being comatose for 1 year, the man was adjusted in the upper cervical spine. He awakened after the third adjustment; with further care he was able to walk with the aid of crutches.

A study of 11 children with head injuries found immune system suppression following these injuries.[4] However, there is evidence that the chiropractic adjustment has influence over natural killer cell production,[5] immunoglobulin (IgA, IgG, and IgM) levels, B-cell lymphocyte count,[6] polymorphonuclear neutrophils and monoctyes,[7] and even CD4 counts.[8]

Individuals may be allowed to return to participation in physical activities after an observation period of 24 to 72 hours (depending on severity) following resolution of symptoms and when they have cleared agility and mental acuity tests. If symptoms persist, return to physical activity is postponed until such time as all symptoms have abated at rest and do not return with exertion.

Homeopathy

Before using this section, please see Appendix A, Homeopathy, for definitions of practitioner expertise categories and general information on prescribing homeopathic medicines.

Practitioner Expertise Category 1

Category 1 includes minor concussions without significant coexisting trauma.

Practitioner Expertise Category 2

Category 2 includes minor concussions with minor coexisting trauma, or slightly more severe concussions.

Practitioner Expertise Category 3

Category 3 includes patients with more serious concussions, patients with coexisting trauma, and patients who are suffering from the chronic aftereffects of a concussion.

There is a small amount of research evidence to support the use of homeopathy for treatment of the aftereffects of head injuries (mild traumatic brain injury). A randomized, double-blind, placebo-controlled trial published in 1999 showed that patients with chronic problems (including speech and language problems, disorders of memory and affect, and difficulties with day-to-day situations) after head injuries benefited from receiving individualized homeopathic medicines.[1] Additionally, the homeopathic literature contains much evidence for the homeopathic treatment of concussions in the form of accumulated clinical experience.[2]

For acute head injuries that appear serious, it is appropriate to administer a homeopathic medicine, if available, while the patient is in the process of seeking evaluation and treatment at an emergency care facility; the indicated homeopathic medicine can also be administered after such an evaluation has been completed. Because patients with chronic sequelae after a head injury present with more complex and multifaceted problems, successful homeopathic treatment usually requires extensive training in the art and science of homeopathy (such patients might be under the care of a neurologist and other specialists as well as a homeopathic doctor). For this reason, most of the recommendations in this section are for acute situations. When clinically indicated, any patient with a head injury or concussion should seek emergency evaluation and treatment without delay.

The goal in treating concussions homeopathically is to determine the single homeopathic medicine whose description in the materia medica most closely matches the patient's symptom picture. Mental and emotional states, in addition to physical symptoms, are considered. Once the medicine has been selected, it can be given orally or sublingually in the 30C potency every 15 to 60 minutes. (As alternatives in a poorly responsive patient, one granule of the medicine can be placed between the cheek and the gums on the buccal mucosa; or the medicine can be diluted in purified water, and 2 to 4 drops can be placed on the patient's lips with a dropper. If some of the liquid reaches the oral mucosa, the correct medicine is able produce an effect when administered this way.) In more serious situations, higher potencies such as 200C or 1M (1000C) may be required. If the medicine has not helped in four to five doses, then another homeopathic medicine should be tried or some other form of therapy should be instituted as indicated. Once symptoms have begun to resolve, the medicine can be given less frequently or stopped. It can be repeated again for a relapse of symptoms.

The following is a list of homeopathic medicines commonly used to treat patients with concussions. It must be emphasized that this list is partial and represents some of the probable choices from the homeopathic materia medica. If the symptoms of a given patient are not represented here, further research in the homeopathic literature would be needed to find the simillimum.

Arnica montana

Arnica montana is the most frequently used homeopathic medicine for concussions. The medicine can be given for any head trauma with bruising, swelling, or pain. The patient may seem shocked or dazed, denying that anything is wrong and asking to be left alone. There may be frank loss of consciousness for periods of time. The patient may feel that the bed or pillow is too hard, and he or she will be aggravated from being moved or jarred. This patient should also be taken for emergency treatment if clinically indicated.

Hypericum perforatum

Hypericum perforatum is the medicine to try for the patient who experiences sharp, shooting pains after a head injury or with an injury involving the spinal cord. Consider *H. perforatum* when convulsions occur very soon after a head injury. This patient would also require emergency treatment without delay.

Hyoscyamus niger

The patient needing *Hyoscyamus niger* experiences excitation of the nervous system after a concussion. The patient may be delirious, agitated, and restless. He or she may be cursing and/or exhibiting other inappropriate behavior. This patient would also require emergency care without delay.

Opium

Consider *Opium* when the patient is in a stupor or a coma after a concussion. The face appears red, bloated, and sweaty, and the pupils are constricted. The patient may be snoring (this patient can be given the remedy in liquid form with a dropper, as described earlier). If not comatose, the patient needing opium will be confused, slow, or sleepy and seem to not be experiencing pain commensurate with the severity of the injury. This patient should also receive conventional medical care.

Osteopathy

The osteopathic approach to the treatment of the child with concussion or postconcussional syndrome is twofold: (1) alleviate any musculoskeletal tissue strains produced by the injury, and (2) improve any secondary somatic or biomechanical dysfunction that may be compounding or exacerbating the child's symptoms. The most common symptom of concussion and postconcussional syndrome is headache. The membranous, osseous and cartilaginous structures of the head and neck absorb the forces of the impact. The principles of osteopathy in the cranial field deal specifically with tissue strains and altered fluid mechanics in the head. Several techniques described by Sutherland have been reported to be useful in treating patients with closed head trauma and postconcussion symptoms.[1,2] These are very gentle techniques used often by therapists in various clinical scenarios. However, side effects requiring medical intervention have been reported in patients with closed head injury treated with craniosacral manipulation.[3] Consequently, it is important that these techniques be used judiciously by trained physicians capable of handling the potential side effects.

It goes without saying that an appropriate workup including CT scan must be done to rule out intracranial bleed if postconcussion symptoms persist. Although there are no supportive studies, children with abnormal positron emission tomography (PET) scan secondary to closed brain injury may benefit from osteopathic treatment. The specific osteopathic treatment in the postconcussion phase will vary depending upon the child's predominant symptoms. Within the concept of the structure-function relationship, the child's predominant symptoms are a manifestation of restrictions in functional anatomy. Patients with postconcussional syndrome generally display one of four clusters of symptoms: predominantly somatic, predominantly sensory, predominantly affective, or predominantly cognitive.[4] Somatic symptoms include feelings of lightheadedness, coordination problems, nausea, and increased motion sickness. These children usually have strains involving the tissues at the craniocervical junction, cranial base, occipitomastoid area, and temporal bones. Altered fluid mechanics, typically described as "lateral fluctuations,"[5] are also common in these children. Secondary strains may be found in the pelvis and sacrum. Indirect, cranial, and balancing techniques can be used to address these findings. Children with sensory symptoms may have hyperacusis, photophobia, and complaints of "funny feelings" in the extremities or body. Osteopathic findings in these cases may include somatic dysfunction in the cranial vault, cranial base, and core-link mechanics as described by Sutherland. Tissue texture changes suggestive of autonomic imbalance or increased tone of the sympathetic nervous system are also found. Children with primarily cognitive symptoms typically present with loss of energy, slowed thinking, poor concentration, and forgetfulness. These children often have findings of compression in the cranial base and vault, disturbance in the core-link and reciprocal tension mechanisms, and disruption of intracranial fluid mechanics. Finally, children with primarily affective symptoms will be irritable, depressed, easily frustrated, and anxious. Within the model of osteopathy in the cranial field and biodynamics, in addition to somatic strains in the cranium, these children also exhibit irritability of the nervous system or strains at the potency-fluid interface. Cranial, biodynamic, balancing, and indirect techniques may all be used depending upon the age of the child and mechanism of injury. Although classically cases and reports of osteopathic treatment deal with the postconcussion symptoms, treating the child in the acute phase following the injury may prevent the development of compensatory tissue strains. For example, dysfunction of the musculoskeletal tissues of the cervical spine is common in patients with postconcussion cephalgia[6,7]; from an osteopathic perspective these findings may be from the acute injury or a secondary compensation[7] that is avoidable.

References

Pediatric Diagnosis and Treatment

1. Behrman, RE, Kliegman RM, Jenson HB, editors: *Nelson's textbook of pediatrics*, Philadelphia, 2004, Saunders, pp 2313-2314.
2. Poirier MP, Wadsworth MR: Sports-related concussions, *Pediatr Emerg Care* 16:278-283; quiz 284-286, 2000.
3. Proctor MR, Cantu RC: Head and neck injuries in young athletes, *Clin Sports Med* 19:693-715, 2000.
4. Guskiewicz KM, McCrea M, Marshall SW et al: Cumulative effects associated with recurrent concussion in collegiate football players: the NCAA Concussion Study, *J Am Med Assoc* 290:2549-2555, 2003.
5. Pieter W, Zemper ED: Head and neck injuries in young tae kwon do athletes, *J Sports Med Phys Fitness* 39:147-153, 1999.
6. McKeever CK, Schatz P: Current issues in the identification, assessment, and management of concussions in sports-related injuries, *Appl Neuropsychol* 10:4-11, 2003.
7. Reece RM, Sege R: Childhood head injuries: accidental or inflicted? *Arch Pediatr Adolesc Med* 154:11-15, 2000.
8. Landry GL: Central nervous system trauma management of concussions in athletes, *Pediatr Clin North Am* 49:723-741, 2002.
9. Faillace WJ: Management of childhood neurotrauma, *Surg Clin North Am* 82:349-363, vii, 2002.
10. Putukian M, Echemendia RJ: Psychological aspects of serious head injury in the competitive athlete, *Clin Sports Med* 22:617-630, xi, 2003.
11. Adams J, Frumiento C, Shatney-Leach L et al: Mandatory admission after isolated mild closed head injury in children: is it necessary? *J Pediatr Surg* 36:119-121, 2001.
12. McCrea M, Guskiewicz KM, Marshall SW et al: Acute effects and recovery time following concussion in collegiate football players: the NCAA Concussion Study, *J Am Med Assoc* 290:2556-2563, 2003.
13. Mittenberg W, Wittner MS, Miller LJ: Postconcussion syndrome occurs in children, *Neuropsychology* 11:447-452, 1997.
14. Davidhizar R, Bartlett D: Management of the patient with minor traumatic brain injury, *Br J Nurs* 6:498-503, 1997.

Acupuncture

1. Loo M: *Pediatric acupuncture*, London, 2002, Elsevier.

Chiropractic

1. Davies N: *Chiropractic pediatrics*, London, 2000, Churchill Livingstone.
2. Araghi JH: Post-traumatic evaluation and treatment of the pediatric patient with head injury: a case report, *ICA Int Rev Chiropractic* Jan/Feb:29-31, 1995.
3. Plaugher G, Alcantasa J, Doble RW, et al: Chiropractic management of spinal fractures and dislocations with closed reduction methods: a report of nine cases. In Wolk S, editor: *Proceedings of the 1992 International Conference on Spinal Manipulation*, Arlington, Va, 1992, Foundation for Chiropractic Education and Research.
4. Meert KL, Long M, Kaplan J et al: Alterations in immune function following head injury in children, *Crit Care Med* 23:822-828, 1995.
5. Leach RA, Burgess SC: Neuroimmune hypothesis. In Leach RA, editor: *The chiropractic theories*, Baltimore, 2004, Lippincott Williams and Wilkins.
6. Brennan PC, Kokjohn K, Triano JJ et al: Immunologic correlates of reduced spinal mobility: preliminary observations in a dog model. In Wold S, editor: *Proceedings of the 1991 International Conference on Spinal Manipulation*, Arlington, Va, 1991, Foundation for Chiropractic Education and Research.
7. Brennan PC, Kokjohn K, Kaltinger CJ et al: Enhanced phagocytic cell respiratory burst induced by spinal manipulation: potential role of substance P, *J Manipulative Physiol Ther* 14:399-408, 1991.
8. Selano JL, Hightower BC, Pfleger B et al: The effects of specific upper cervical adjustments on the CD4 counts of HIV positive patients, *Chiropractic Res J* 3:32, 1994.

Homeopathy

1. Chapman EH, Weintraub RJ, Milburn MA et al: Homeopathic treatment of mild traumatic brain injury: a randomized, double-blind, placebo-controlled clinical trial, *J Head Trauma Rehabil* 14:521-542, 1999.
2. *ReferenceWorks Pro 4.2*, San Rafael, Calif, 2008, Kent Homeopathic Associates.

Osteopathy

1. Sutherland WG: *The cranial bowl*, ed 2, 1939, Sutherland.
2. Sutherland WG: *Teachings in the science of osteopathy*, Portland, Ore, 1990, Rudra Press.
3. Greenman PE, McPartland JM: Cranial findings and iatrogenesis from craniosacral manipulation in patients with traumatic brain syndrome, *J Am Osteopathic Assoc* 95:182-191, 1995.
4. Cicerone KD, Kalmer K: Persistent post-concussion syndrome: the structure of subjective complaints after mild traumatic brain injury, *J Head Trauma Rehabil* 10:1-17, 1995.
5. Magoun HIS: *Osteopathy in the cranial field*, ed 3, Kirksville, Mo, 1976, The Journal Printing Company.
6. Treleaven J, Jull G, Atkinson L: Cervical musculoskeletal dysfunction in post-concussional headache [see comments], *Cephalalgia* 14:273-279; discussion 257, 1994.
7. Stoll ST, Mitra M: Post-traumatic headache of cervical origin, *AAOJ* 12:38-41, 2002.

Conjunctivitis

Acupuncture | May Loo

Chiropractic | Anne Spicer

Herbs—Chinese | Catherine Ulbricht, Jennifer Woods, Mark Wright

Herbs—Western | Alan D. Woolf, Paula M. Gardiner, Lana Dvorkin-Camiel, Jack Maypole

Homeopathy | Janet L. Levatin

Massage Therapy | Mary C. McLellan

Naturopathy | Matthew I. Baral

Osteopathy | Jane Carreiro

✳ PEDIATRIC DIAGNOSIS AND TREATMENT

Conjunctivitis, or pink eye, is very common in childhood. It can be caused by a wide range of both infectious and noninfectious agents. The infections are usually viral and bacterial, and noninfections are due to a variety of allergens, irritants, and toxins. The cardinal sign is redness in the eyes, accompanied by different types of discharges and possibly other symptoms.

Infectious Conjunctivitis

Viral conjunctivitis

Viral conjunctivitis, generally characterized by a watery discharge, is commonly due to adenovirus infection and may be associated with systemic viral infections such as upper respiratory tract infection and measles.[1]

Bacterial conjunctivitis

Bacterial conjunctivitis is characterized by purulent discharge, often accompanied by edema or swelling of the eyes and some discomfort, but usually does not have any vision change or ocular pain. Sometimes children have a history of morning crusting and difficulty opening the eyelids.[2] The majority of cases in children are caused by nontypable *Haemophilus influenzae, Streptococcus pneumoniae, Moraxella catarrhalis,* and less commonly by staphylococci.[1-3] Although there are no data currently to support a direct infection of the conjunctivae from acute otitis media (AOM), given the similarities among upper respiratory infection, it is possible that there is retrograde spread of the organisms through nasal lacrimal ducts, such that suspicion of concomitant AOM in bacterial conjunctivitis is reasonable.[3] Although conjunctival smear and culture are helpful in differentiating specific types,[4] they are rarely done in a pediatric outpatient clinic. The standard treatment is with broad-spectrum antibiotic eye drops and local measures such as warm compresses. Complications of infectious conjunctivitis, such as keratitis, cellulitis, or abscess formation, should be referred for ophthalmological evaluation and treatment.[4]

The newborn is given silver nitrate instillation immediately after birth to prevent gonorrheal conjunctivitis. Inclusion blennorrhea, a common form of ophthalmia neonatorum, is caused by *Chlamydia trachomitis.* The infection is contracted from the maternal genital tract during birth. The incubation period is usually 1 week or longer. The newborn develops an acute purulent conjunctivitis, but the discharge and scrapings are negative for bacteria and positive for the diagnostic intracytoplasmic inclusion bodies.[1]

Noninfectious Conjunctivitis

Allergic conjunctivitis

Allergic conjunctivitis is the most common noninfectious conjunctivitis in children and shares pathophysiology similar to other allergic conditions.[5]

Allergic conjunctivitis presents with red, itchy eyes with profuse watery discharge and conjunctival edema. Children often rub the eyes, which aggravates the condition. History can often reveal the source of the allergen, with the onset of symptoms associated with being around cats or seasonal pollen allergens. Treatment consists of avoiding the offending allergen if possible. Using saline eyedrops is simple, nontoxic, and effective in up to 30% to 35% of cases.[6] Local treatment with cold compresses and topical antihistamine eye drops resolves the majority of cases. Corticosteroid eye drops are rarely indicated and should be used only with the close supervision of an ophthalmologist.[4] Allergic conjunctivitis frequently accompanies allergic rhinitis in children[7] and responds to oral antihistamines.

Chemical conjunctivitis

Chemical conjunctivitis is caused by an irritant to the conjunctivae. Silver nitrate can cause a chemical conjunctivitis in the newborn. Other common offenders are smoke, smog, industrial pollutants, and household cleaning substances and sprays.

✳ CAM THERAPY RECOMMENDATIONS

Acupuncture

Chinese medicine[1] correlates both viral and allergic conjunctivitis to Wind-Cold invasion and bacterial conjunctivitis to Wind-Heat invasion. There is no current study on acupuncture treatment of conjunctivitis in children. A report from Russia indicates that acupuncture increased the resistance to allergens by 100-fold and significantly reduced the content of immuno-globulin (Ig) E,[2] the immune globulin that increases with allergic reactions. A clinical report from China used acupuncture and bloodletting to treat acute, fulminant red eyes in adults.[3]

Treatment

Traditional treatment consists of expelling Wind invasions when systemic symptoms are present and treating local and distal points for conjunctival symptoms of the eyes.

For Wind-Cold and Wind-Heat treatments, please see Appendix B for general protocols.

Local treatments of eyes

Apply saline eye drops.

Local points: Because it is difficult to insert needles or even apply noninvasive modalities such as electrical stimulation or magnets to points near or around the eyes in children, the best way to treat local points for conjunctivitis is with acupressure:
- Massage BL1, BL2, GB1, ST1
- Distal points: GB42, GB43[4-8]

In children with recurrent Wind invasions, tonify them with the immune tonification protocol. (See Chapter 43, Immune System)

Chiropractic

Although the chiropractic literature does not cite any cases of conjunctivitis, the chiropractor would identify any interference to normal function in the child presenting with conjunctivitis. Adjustment of the subluxation complex would enhance the immune function and allow for optimal neuroimmune function. There is evidence that the chiropractic adjustment has influence over natural killer cell production and autonomic balance,[1] immunoglobulin (IgA, IgG, and IgM) levels and B-cell lymphocyte count,[2] polymorphonuclear neutrophils and monocytes,[3] and even CD4 counts.[4]

Deep focal pressure at the anterior head of the humerus and along the suboccipital ridge may stimulate healing of eye conditions.[5]

In the breastfed infant, topical application of freshly expressed breast milk may hasten the resolution of conjunctivitis owing due to its antibacterial properties.

In the infant and older child, an application of a warm compress made with eyebright tincture or tea serves to reduce inflammation and improve healing time.

Oral administration of a vitamin A/β-carotene and omega-3 fatty acids/fish oil provide support to the immune system and are particularly useful in visual conditions.

Oral administration of zinc and vitamin C is also highly beneficial.

Echinacea has an immunosupportive effect when used with viral conditions.

Herbs—Chinese

According to TCM, allergic conjunctivitis may be thought of as a condition with deficiency of Yin, which correlates to "cool and moist." An infectious conjunctivitis is caused by an attack by Wind-Heatpathogens.

The infectious type may be treated by topical application of flowers of *Chrysanthemum morifolium* Ramat. (Ju Hua) and *Lonicera japonica* Thunb. (Jin Yin Hua). Topical treatment works fast, although sometimes an oral prescription may also be given and often includes Ju Hua, Jin Yin Hua and fruit of *Forsythia suspensa* (Thunb.) Vahl (Lian Qiao). Extracts of these three herbs have been shown to be inhibitive to various bacteria. For example, in vitro aqueous extract of Jin Yin Hua dramatically inhibits *Shigella dysenteriae, Salmonella typhi, Escherichia coli, Staphylococcus aureus, Streptococcus hemolyticus,* and *Hemophilus pertussis,*[1] as well as *Bacillus typhi, Bacillus paratyphi, Proteus* spp., *Pseudomonas aeruginosa, Streptococcus* spp., *Staphylococcus* spp., and *Meningococcus* spp.[2] Similar data are available for Ju Hua and Lian Qiao.

Method of Application

A small handful of the dried flowers of each of Jin Yin Hua and Ju Hua is taken and placed in the bottom of a standard drinking mug. Boiling water is poured onto the blossom to cover it. It is left to steep for 10 minutes or so, with occasional mixing. When it is of a suitable temperature, a lightly squeezed pad of wet flower heads is placed over the closed, affected eye and the patient lies for 10 to 15 minutes with the pad in place. The process is repeated several times a day.

Results are usually rapid, with the condition clearing in 24 to 48 hours. No details of a scientific study of patients under treatment are available, but the broad-spectrum antibacterial effects of the phytochemical constituents of the herbs would tend to support the traditional claim. Data from actual case trials would be useful.

The recurrent, allergic type of conjunctivitis would require follow-up treatment with Yin tonics. A proprietary formulation such as Liu Wei Di Huang Wan (the ingredients of this are listed in full in Chapter 12, Asthma) or its derivative Qi Ju Di Huang Wan would traditionally be indicated. Qi Ju Di Huang Wan comprises Liu Wei Di Huang Wan with Ju Hua and fruit of *Lycium chinense* Mill. (Gou Qi Zi). No data are available to substantiate the outcome of long-term use of these prescriptions as a remedy to recurrent allergic conjunctivitis.[3]

Herbs—Western

Eyebright, or *Euphrasia rostkoviana* and *Euphrasia officinalis,* belongs to the Scrophulariaceae family. Eyebright has been used traditionally in ophthalmic solutions in the management of multiple eye conditions. One controlled study in children and one open-label trial in adults have investigated eyebright for conjunctivitis. Safety data are insufficient, with concerns regarding potential contamination of products and risk of infection and insufficient scientific evidence to recommend this herb for the treatment of conjunctivitis.

Orally or topically, 10 to 60 drops of eyebright tincture may induce mental confusion, headache, increased eye pressure with lacrimation, itching, redness, swelling of eyelid margins, dim vision, photophobia, weakness, sneezing, nausea, toothache, constipation, cough, dyspnea, insomnia, polyuria, and sweating.[1]

Allergic Conjunctivitis

Any drops applied to the eyes directly should be sterile to prevent infection. Note also that nonprescription eyedrops may actually worsen the redness and irritation of conjunctivitis when used chronically. See the previous discussion of eyebright.

Chamomile *(Matricaria chamomilla)*, which is found in many foodstuffs and cosmetic products, may be applied topically for conjunctivitis. A case series found that chamomile applications may actually provoke allergic conjunctivitis in adults attempting to treat their eye problems. Eye washing with chamomile tea can induce allergic conjunctivitis and therefore should not be done in children.[2]

Homeopathy

Before using this section, please see Appendix A, Homeopathy, for definitions of practitioner expertise categories and general information on prescribing homeopathic medicines.

Practitioner Expertise Category 1

Category 1 includes nonallergic conjunctivitis unassociated with other pathology, such as periorbital cellulitis, uveitis, or otitis media.

Practitioner Expertise Category 2

Category 2 includes conjunctivitis associated with allergies.

Conjunctivitis has many etiologies including bacterial, viral, allergic, and chemical. The recommendations in this section can be used to treat conjunctivitis of any etiology. It may also be useful to refer to Chapter 10, Allergies, as it contains information on hay fever and allergic rhinitis, which are often accompanied by conjunctivitis.

There are no controlled clinical trials of homeopathic treatment of bacterial or viral (nonallergic) conjunctivitis, although the homeopathic literature contains evidence for its use in the form of accumulated clinical experience.[1] Usually conjunctivitis is treated topically with antimicrobial drops or ointment. It is safe to use orally or sublingually administered homeopathic medicines in combination with conventional topical therapy. Alternative topical treatments are also available, and can be used in conjunction with homeopathy and/or alternated with conventional topical therapy. Herbal tinctures can be diluted and used to flush the eyes three to four times daily (2 drops of *Euphrasia* or *Calendula* tincture diluted in 1 oz (30 mL) purified water). Commercially available homeopathic eye drops can also be an effective form of therapy. One brand of homeopathic eye drops is Similasan Pink Eye Relief, which contains *Euphrasia* 6X, *Hepar sulphuris calcareum* 12X, and *Belladonna* 6X.

The goal in treating conjunctivitis homeopathically with a systemic medicine is to determine the single homeopathic medicine whose description in the materia medica most closely matches the symptom picture of the patient. Sometimes mental and emotional states, in addition to physical symptoms, are considered. As mentioned previously, other symptoms such as those of hay fever or rhinitis might also be considered. Once the medicine has been selected, it can be given in the 30C potency three times daily for 3 days. If the medicine has not helped after four to five doses, then another homeopathic medicine should be tried or some other form of therapy should be instituted as needed. Once symptoms have begun to resolve, the medicine can be given less frequently or stopped. It can be repeated again for a relapse of symptoms. If any eye pathology beyond simple conjunctivitis is present, treatment from an ophthalmologist should be sought without delay.

The following is a list of homeopathic medicines commonly used to treat patients with conjunctivitis. It must be emphasized that this list is partial and represents some of the probable choices from the homeopathic materia medica. If the symptoms of a given patient are not represented here, a search of the homeopathic literature would be needed to find the simillimum.

Pulsatilla nigricans

Pulsatilla nigricans is the most commonly used homeopathic medicine for conjunctivitis and can be used for infectious or allergic conjunctivitis. In the case of infection, the conjunctivae are red and the eyes produce thick yellow or green discharge. Often there is an accompanying upper respiratory infection, otitis media, or measles. The child may be warm and have a low level of thirst. *P. nigricans* can be used to treat some infants with blocked and infected nasolacrimal ducts.

Aconitum napellus

Conjunctivitis responsive to aconite *(Aconitum napellus)* usually develops after exposure to a cold wind or after a trauma to the eye, including acquiring a foreign body. The eye is red and intensely painful. If clinically indicated, the child should also be seen at an emergency care facility or by an ophthalmologist.

Argentum nitricum

The patient needing *Argentum nitricum* has conjunctivae that are acutely or chronically enflamed. The inner canthi in particular are red, and a purulent discharge is present. The symptoms are worse in a warm room.

Belladonna

Try *Belladonna* when the eye is acutely inflamed and painful, but a discharge has not yet occurred. The eye may feel as though it is throbbing.

Euphrasia officinalis

Euphrasia officinalis can be used for infectious or allergic conjunctivitis. The eye feels hot and itchy, and the lids are red and swollen. The eye discharge is watery and irritating to the surrounding skin.

Graphites naturalis

The hallmark of *Graphites naturalis* conjunctivitis is dryness and cracking around the eyes, especially at the inner canthi. The eyelids may be stuck together with dried discharged matter.

Mercurius solubilis hahnemanni

The patient with mercurius conjunctivitis who needs *Mercurins solubilis hahnemanni* will have green or possibly bloody discharge from the eye. The whole eyelid is inflamed and painful. The symptoms are worse from heat. The patient may have an accompanying upper respiratory tract or other infection and be suffering from fever with chills and sweats. If clinically indicated, the child should also be seen at an emergency care facility or by an ophthalmologist.

Silica terra

Silica terra is a medicine for conjunctivitis, blepharitis, and infections of the tear ducts. It can treat chronic or recurrent infections that result from injuries to or foreign bodies of the cornea. The discharge is thick, yellow, and crusty. The symptoms are worse in the Cold and Wind. If clinically indicated, this type of patient should also be under the care of an ophthalmologist.

Sulphur

Sulphur is a medicine for conjunctivitis or blepharitis with yellow, burning discharge. The eyes are red, as are the lids. There may be seborrhea of the lash area with itching and scaling.

Massage Therapy

Massage should be avoided over skin conditions considered contagious thorough contact to avoid further spread of the disease to the child or the massage practitioner.[1,2] A recent study demonstrated increased bacterial counts on massage therapists' hands during and after massage treatments, although lower on the client's skin.[3]

Naturopathy

Treating conjunctivitis should include both topical and systemic measures.

Topical Treatments

Botanical eyewashes are a safe way to treat most cases of conjunctivitis. To date, there is a lack of scientific literature on the use of the treatments listed here. These treatments have been found by the author and his colleagues to be very effective with little or no adverse reactions. A body of research from India and China has reported the success of formulations frequently used in those countries,[1-5] but these formulations are difficult to find in the United States and therefore not commonly used in this country.

- Herbal eye drops: A popular botanical combination by Herbpharm, called *Rue Fennel,* combines several different herbs that have a soothing effect as well as astringent and antibacterial properties. The ingredients include rue (*Ruta graveolens*), fennel (*Foeniculum*), eyebright (*E. officinalis*), goldenseal (*Hydrastis canadensis*), mullein (*Verbascum thapsus*), and boric acid. Dosage: 5 to 15 drops in 1 oz distilled/sterile water. **NOTE: Never apply undiluted drops to the eyes.** The amount of drops used in the mixture should be in a stepwise fashion. Parents should start conservatively and test the solution first in their own eyes before applying the drops to the child. If the concentration does not sting, the drops may be applied to the child. It is normal for the drops to make the eye feel slightly dry because of its astringent properties, but this is a temporary effect. In children 1 year and older, 2 to 4 drops should be applied to the affected eye, four to six times per day.
- Another combination may include *E. officinalis,* yarrow (*Achillea millefolium*), and Oregon grape root (*Berberis aquifolium*).

White and Mavor[6] give the following directions to create a useful solution at home:

4 tsp *E. officinalis*
2 tsp *A. millifolium* flowers and leaves
¼ tsp *B. aquifolium*
Pinch of salt
2 cups distilled water
Add *B. aquifolium* to water and boil for 10 minutes.
Add *E. officinalis, A. millefolium,* and salt, and allow to steep and cool.
Strain the mixture through a damp cloth and then through two different coffee filters. It should be noted that children who are allergic to flowers in the daisy family should not be exposed to *A. millefolium.*

- Pot marigold (*Calendula officinalis*) is another useful herb that has antibacterial, antiinflammatory, and analgesic actions. It may be added to any of the above combinations.
- Breastmilk applied to the eye may also be beneficial. The high amount of IgA in breastmilk helps protect against further infection. It also contains lactoferrin, which will deprive bacteria and virus of iron, thereby slowing microbial growth. Lysozymes and other bacteriolytic enzymes destroy bacteria cell membranes. Ascorbic acid and zinc are antioxidant nutrients that are found in breastmilk and can provide additional antimicrobial action.

Systemic Treatments

It is important to address the whole patient when treating any condition. It is easy to get into the habit of treating symptoms, but internal immune system support is essential when treating infections of any kind.

- Euphrasia tea is available in most health food stores, and several cups per day is safe in children older that one year. One tablespoon of the loose herb may be added to a cup of hot water and steeped for 10 minutes. Eyebright tea also comes in individual tea bags, and one bag may be used for 8 ounces of water. In younger children who may not be able to drink more than a cup can sip on the 8 ounces of tea throughout the day, by cooling and adding to juice. Diluting the juice with the tea will help reduce the amount of sugar in the mixture, which is advised during infections.
- Antioxidant vitamins and minerals can be supplemented during the infection, again in children older than 1 year old:
  - Vitamin C: 1 to 4 g daily, to bowel tolerance
  - Vitamin A: Large doses of vitamin A (not β-carotene) is well tolerated and safe for a limited time during the infection. The author uses <50,000 IU per day in the form of liquid drops in children. Studies show that this dose is well tolerated in the short term[7] and does not have adverse side effects.[8]
  - Zinc: 15 to 60 mg per day with food
  - Vitamin E: 400 IU per day
  - Selenium: 100 to 200 μg per day

Osteopathy

The goal of osteopathic treatment in children with conjunctivitis is to improve vascular and lymphatic flow to the eye, thus facilitating the body's ability to heal itself. Infections and disorders of the eye may be treated with specific osteopathic techniques described by T.J. Ruddy, an osteopathic ophthalmologist.[1] Ruddy's techniques require some cooperation from the patient, so they are used in older children capable of following instructions. Young children and infants can be treated with cranial techniques that address the structure-function relationship of the orbital bones, extraocular muscles, and fascias. Techniques addressing facial strains may also be employed to facilitate drainage through the nasolacrimal duct. Myofascial tender points in the upper neck, occipitalis, and orbicularis oculi muscles may exacerbate the discomfort of conjunctivitis and are treated with functional or Jones counterstrain techniques. The primary goals of these techniques are to improve arterial, venous, and lymphatic drainage of the eye; to balance the tissue stresses of the extraocular muscles and fascias; and to remove any tissue strains acting as pain generators. Most reports in the osteopathic literature refer to the usefulness of these techniques in the treatment of strabismus,[2] amblyobia,[2,3] and glaucoma.[1,2] Although there have been no specific studies evaluating their usefulness in the treatment of conjunctivitis, the principles of facilitating vascular flow and tissue function are applicable in cases of eye infections as well.

References

Pediatric Diagnosis and Treatment

1. In Behrman RE, Kliegman RM, Jenson HB, editors: *Nelson's textbook of pediatrics*, Philadelphia, 2004, Saunders, pp 2099-2102.
2. Friedlaender MH: A review of the causes and treatment of bacterial and allergic conjunctivitis, *Clin Ther* 17:800-810; discussion 779, 1995.
3. Gigliotti F: *A pediatric view of conjunctivitis*. Presented at the 17th Annual Infectious Diseases in Children Symposium, New York, November 2004.
4. Howes DS: The red eye, *Emerg Med Clin North Am* 6:43-56, 1988.
5. Aprile A, Lucarelli S, Vagnucci B et al: The use of antileukotrienes in paediatrics, *Eur Rev Med Pharmacol Sci* 5:53-57, 2001.
6. Joss JD, Craig TJ: Seasonal allergic conjunctivitis: overview and treatment update, *J Am Osteopath Assoc* 99(7 Suppl):S13-S18, 1999.
7. Perdomo de Ponce D, Uribe M et al: Allergic and nonallergic rhinitis: their characterization in a tropical environment [in Italian], *Investig Clin* 31:129-138, 1990.

Acupuncture

1. Loo M: *Pediatric acupuncture*, London, 2002, Elsevier.
2. Nezabudkin SN, Kachan AT, Fedoseev GB et al: The reflexotherapy of patients with respiratory allergoses [in Russian], *Ter Arkh* 64:64-67, 1992.
3. Deng SF: Treatment and prevention of fulminant red-eye by acupuncture and bloodletting, *J Tradit Chin Med* 5:263-264, 1985.
4. Deadman P, Al-Khafaji M: *A manual of acupuncture*, East Sussex, United Kingdom, 1998, Journal of Chinese Medicine Publications.
5. Diagnosis and treatment of gynecology and pediatrics. In *Chinese Zhenjiuology, a series of teaching videotapes*, Beijing, 1990, Chinese Medical Audio-Video Organization and Meditalent Enterprises Ltd.
6. Ellis E, Wiseman N, Boss K: *Fundamentals of Chinese acupuncture, revised edition*, Brookline, Mass, 1991, Paradigm Publications.
7. Flaws B: *A handbook of TCM pediatrics, a practitioner's guide to the care and treatment of common childhood diseases*, Boulder, Colo, 1997, Blue Poppy Press.
8. Maciocia G: *The foundations of Chinese medicine, a comprehensive text for acupuncturists and herbalists*, London, 1989, Churchill Livingstone.

Chiropractic

1. Leach RA, Burgess SC: Neuroimmune hypothesis. In Leach RA, editor: *The chiropractic theories*, Baltimore, 2004, Lippincott Williams and Wilkins.
2. Brennan PC, Kokjohn K, Triano JJ et al: Immunologic correlates of reduced spinal mobility: preliminary observations in a dog model. In Wold S, editor: *Proceedings of the 1991 International Conference on Spinal Manipulation*, Arlington, Va, 1991, Foundation for Chiropractic Education and Research.
3. Brennan PC, Kokjohn K, Kaltinger CJ, et al: Enhanced phagocytic cell respiratory burst induced by spinal manipulation: potential role of substance P, *J Manipulative Physiol Ther* 14:399-408, 1991.
4. Selano JL, Hightower BC, Pfleger B et al: The effects of specific upper cervical adjustments on the CD4 counts of HIV positive patients, *Chiropractic Res J* 3:32, 1994.
5. Chaitow L: *Palpation skills: assessment and diagnosis through touch*, New York, 1977, Churchill Livingstone.

Herbs—Chinese

1. Hsu H, Chen Y, Shen S et al: *Oriental materia medica: a concise guide*, Long Beach, Calif, 1986, Oriental Healing Arts Institute.
2. Anonymous: *Newly compiled Chinese officinal dictionary* [in Chinese]. Taipei, Taiwan, 1984, Xin Wen Feng Chu Ban Gong Si.
3. Natural Standard Research Collaboration. Available at www.naturalstandard.com. Accessed 2005.

Herbs—Western

1. Newall CA, Anderson LA, Philpson JD: *Herbal medicine: a guide for healthcare professionals*, London, 1996, Pharmaceutical Press.
2. Subiza J, Subiza JL, Alonso M et al: Allergic conjunctivitis to chamomile tea, *Ann Allergy* 65:127-132, 1990.

Homeopathy

1. *ReferenceWorks Pro 4.2*, San Rafael, Calif, 2008, Kent Homeopathic Associates.

Massage Therapy

1. Tappan F: *Healing massage techniques: holistic, classic, and emerging methods*, Norwalk, Conn, 1988, Appleton and Lange.
2. Fritz S: *Mosby's fundamentals of therapeutic massage*, ed 3, St Louis, 1995, Mosby.
3. Donoyama N, Wakuda T, Tanitsu T et al: Washing hands before and after performing massages? Changes in bacterial survival count on skin of a massage therapist and client during massage therapy, *J Altern Complement Med* 10:684-686, 2004.

Naturopathy

1. Siddiqui TA, Zafar S, Iqbal N: Comparative double-blind randomized placebo-controlled clinical trial of a herbal eye drop formulation (Qatoor Ramad) of Unani medicine in conjunctivitis, *J Ethnopharmacol* 83:13-17, 2002.
2. Wei H, Zeng F, Lu M et al: Studies on chemical constituents from the root of *Coriaria nepalensis* Wall (*Coriaria sinica* Maxim), *Yao Xue Xue Bao* 33:688-692, 1998.

3. Sharma P, Singh G: A review of plant species used to treat conjunctivitis, *Phytother Res* 16:1-22, 2002.
4. Biswas NR, Gupta SK, Das GK et al: Evaluation of Ophthacare eye drops—a herbal formulation in the management of various ophthalmic disorders, *Phytother Res* 15:618-620, 2001.
5. Biswas NR, Beri S, Das GK et al: Comparative double blind multicentric randomised placebo controlled clinical trial of a herbal preparation of eye drops in some ocular ailments, *J Indian Med Assoc* 94:101-102, 1996.
6. White L, Mavor S: *Kids, herbs, and health,* Loveland, Colo, 1998, Interweave Press.
7. Humphrey JH, Agoestina T, Wu L et al: Impact of neonatal vitamin A supplementation on infant morbidity and mortality, *J Pediatr* 128:489-496, 1996.
8. Humphrey JH, Agoestina T, Juliana A et al: Neonatal vitamin A supplementation: effect on development and growth at 3 y of age, *Am J Clin Nutr* 68:109-117, 1998.

Osteopathy

1. Ruddy TJ: Osteopathic manipulation in eye, ear, nose and throat disease, *AOA Yearbook* 133-140, 1962.
2. Magoun HIS: *Osteopathy in the cranial field,* ed 3, Kirksville, Mo, 1976, The Journal Printing Company.
3. Kuchera ML, Kuchera WA: *Osteopathic considerations in systemic disease,* Columbus, Ohio, 1994, Greydon Press.

CHAPTER 26

Constipation

Acupuncture | May Loo

Aromatherapy | Maura A. Fitzgerald

Chiropractic | Anne Spicer

Herbs—Chinese | May Loo, Harriet Beinfield, Efrem Korngold

Herbs—Western | Alan D. Woolf, Paula M. Gardiner, Lana Dvorkin-Camiel, Jack Maypole

Homeopathy | Janet L. Levatin

Magnet Therapy | Agatha P. Colbert, Deborah Risotti

Massage Therapy | Mary C. McLellan

Mind/Body | Timothy Culbert, Lynda Richtsmeier Cyr

Naturopathy | Matthew I. Baral

Nutrition | Joy A. Weydert

Osteopathy | Jane Carreiro

Psychology | Anna Tobia

✴ PEDIATRIC DIAGNOSIS AND TREATMENT

Constipation is common in children. It is estimated that between 5% and 10% of pediatric patients have constipation and/or encopresis. Constipation is the second most referred condition in pediatric gastroenterology practices, accounting for as many as 25% of all visits.[1]

Constipation in children is defined by the Constipation Subcommittee of the Clinical Guidelines Committee of the North American Society for Pediatric Gastroenterology and Nutrition as a delay or difficulty in defecation that is present for 2 or more weeks.[2]

Constipation should refer to the character rather than frequency of the stool and to associated symptoms such as abdominal discomfort, as constipation may represent the regular passage of firm or hard stools.[3]

The list of differential diagnoses for constipation is long: functional constipation; improper diet, such as excessive intake of cow's milk or lack of fiber; drug induced, such as antihistamines and antidepressants; anatomical malformations such as anal stenosis; association gastrointestinal (GI) disorders such as celiac disease; with endocrine disorders such as hypothyroidism; with metabolic disorders such as renal tubular acidosis; and with genetic disorders such as Down syndrome.[3-5]

A careful history taking and interpretation is necessary so that diagnostic tests are reserved only for severe constipation or for those suspected of having a primary disorder.[1] Diagnosis can also be complicated by familial, cultural, and social factors and normal childhood development. Psychogenic factors, various methods involved in toilet training, diet, and misuse or abuse of laxatives and enemas may influence the advent of constipation. Natural childhood motor and social development can also contribute to constipation: as infants become more ambulatory, they are distracted by many new and exciting activities such that they would pass just enough stool to relieve the pressure while continuing to play, and gradually they can develop the capacity to ignore the rectal fullness. In older children, school, games, social events, and the hurried pace of life may all interfere with any pattern of regularity. Many teenage girls, for example, may become constipated because of reluctance to use toilet facilities other than at home.[3] Diagnostic evaluation ranges from a simple history and physical examination[3] to the use of sophisticated technical instrumentation such as anorectal manometry.[6]

The exact pathophysiology of constipation in children is not known[7] but most likely involves interaction of several factors, such as low-fiber diet, early weaning, painful bowel movement, fecal retention, disturbance of intestinal motility, and genetic predisposition.[8] The end result is either defect in filling or emptying the rectum.[5]

Infants and toddlers often manifest hard and painful bowel movements by screaming and stool-holding maneuvers. Constipation is practically unknown in breastfed infants receiving an adequate amount of milk. A nursing infant may have very infrequent stools of normal consistency. True constipation in the neonatal period is most likely secondary to Hirschsprung disease, intestinal pseudo-obstruction, or hypothyroidism.[5]

The clinical presentation of older children with constipation can be variable, as the daily bowel habits of children are extremely susceptible to any changes in routine environment.[1] Some children are not diagnosed until they develop complications such as soiling, abdominal pain, and urinary abnormalities.[8]

Childhood constipation can be difficult to treat.[1] There is no single treatment protocol for constipation, and many children do not respond to multiple therapeutic trials and continue to have chronic problems.[7]

A prospective examination of primary care physicians' treatment of 119 children between 2 and 7 years of age revealed nearly 40% of children remain symptomatic after 2 months of treatment, the majority of which treatment consisted of laxative or stool softener, and dietary intervention was prescribed in half the cases.[9]

Most treatment consists of fecal disimpaction, laxatives to prevent future impaction, promotion of regular bowel habits, and retraining of the child in toilet habits. New treatments consist of various prokinetic agents.[7] Behavioral and psychological interventions are not recommended for routine managmnet[10] but would be beneficial in functional constipation. Children who are resistant to standard care may benefit from a combination of intensive medical management and behavioral therapy.[11]

The long-term control of chronic constipation depends on the acquisition of dietary habits that provide an adequate intake of dietary fiber. It is possible that a high-fiber diet is important not only to the control of constipation, but may also reduce the risk for diet-related chronic diseases during adulthood.[8]

Young infants with constipation or older children with longstanding stool impaction should be referred to a specialist for further diagnostic and therapeutic management.[12]

Children with constipation also need a great deal of understanding and emotional support. A case-controlled evaluation using a health-related quality of life tool during initial outpatient consultation of 224 children aged 10.6 ± 2.9 years indicated that constipated children had lower quality of life scores than did those with inflammatory bowel disease, gastroesophageal reflux disease, and healthy children.[13] Therefore successful management requires prolonged support by physicians and parents, frequent explanations, and most importantly the child's cooperation.[1] Parents should be reassured that although this disorder is not life-threatening, several months to years of intervention may be required for effective treatment.[14]

✳ CAM THERAPY RECOMMENDATIONS

Acupuncture

Currently there is only one study from Israel on acupuncture treatment of chronic constipation in children. Seventeen children who experienced constipation for at least 6 months were treated with five weekly placebo acupuncture sessions, followed by 10 weekly true acupuncture sessions. Frequency of bowel movements increased after the true acupuncture sessions.[1] Acupuncture has also been found to be effective in the treatment of postoperative rehabilitation in children who underwent surgery for Hirschsprung disease, suggesting its potential for treatment of postoperative complications.[2] In a randomized controlled trial from Germany on adults with constipation, electroacupuncture (10 Hz) performed on LI4, ST25, LR3, and BL25 did not change stool frequency.[3] Case reports from China of 21 adult patients with diabetes mellitus treated with daily acupuncture at BL32, TE6, and ST36 for 5 days showed improvement. Only 4 patients needed a second course at 6-month follow-up.[4] A Canadian review of studies from both the Chinese and Western literature found that acupuncture was effective in regulating GI motor activity and secretion through opioid and other neural pathways.[5]

From the traditional Chinese medicine (TCM) perspective, physiological bowel movements require sufficient Qi in multiple organs and an adequate supply of Fluids, a Yin constituent. Digestion of Fluids begins in the Stomach, where Fluid is propelled downward. The Intestines rely on the Spleen to transform and transport Fluids. The Liver directs smooth flow of Qi in the organs, including the Intestines. The Kidney is very important in being the foundation of Yin and Yang of all the organs, therefore influencing the Fluids and Yang Qi in the Lower Energizer, and also in controlling both the urethra and the anus, thus influencing defecation.

TCM posits several factors that can interfere with normal physiological function, producing constipation, and that may offer explanations for pathophysiology that is puzzling to Western medicine:

Diet: The major cause of constipation relates to improper food intake: excess Phlegm-producing foods or energetically Hot and Cold foods in the modern children's diet. Constipation associated with cow's milk is due to excess Phlegm production.

Energetically Cold foods and ice-cold drinks diminish the Spleen's function of transportation, resulting in colonic inability to move the stool downward. Energetically Hot foods dry up the fluids in the Stomach and Intestines, resulting in dry and hard stools that are difficult to propel through the Intestines.

Excess internal Cold: Excess internal Cold occurs frequently in children, secondary to recurrent invasions by Cold pathogens, from consumption of excess energetically Cold foods or drinks, medications that deplete Qi and Yang, and any chronic conditions. Excess Cold in the Intestines slows the normal peristalsis movement of the Intestines.

Stress: A stressful lifestyle, worry, frustration, and anger can all cause Qi stagnation, specifically in the Liver and also in the Spleen. This type of constipation is usually accompanied by abdominal distention and sometimes pain as well.

Excess mental activity, such as studying long hours without adequate rest, can deplete Spleen Qi and Kidney Yin and Yang. All can lead to Coldness in the Lower Energizer, in the intestines, and can result in slower peristalsis and constipation.

Excess or lack of physical activity: An appropriate amount of exercise stimulates all metabolic activities, including peristalsis of the Large Intestine. Excess physical activity can often deplete Qi, whereas lack of exercise would slow the movement of stool down the Large Intestine.

Repeated illness-related fevers: Repeat occurrences of fever results in interior Heat and dries up Fluids, which can manifest as constipation.

Medications: Antibiotics are antiinflammatory and therefore are considered as energetically "Cold." Excess antibiotics can lead to constipation due to Coldness in the Lower Energizer. Western literature lists antihistamine as a potential cause of constipation without an explanation for pathophysiology. TCM can explain the role of antihistamine as a drying agent that depletes the child's Yin, resulting in constipation.

Constitutional weaknesses: Children are constitutionally Spleen deficient. Some children also have familial predisposition for Spleen deficiency and therefore are more prone to developing Spleen deficiency conditions, including constipation.

TCM Evaluation of the Constipated Child

TCM evaluation includes the following steps:

Taking a detailed history: The age of onset, diet, previous illnesses, frequency of fever, maximum body temperature, mental and physical activities, emotional stress, medications (especially frequency of antibiotics and antihistamines), and any associated symptoms such as abdominal distention or pain.

Determining the possible constitutional weakness: A detailed family history to reveal GI disorders and constipation, physical and emotional health and well-being of the parents at conception, and mother's health during pregnancy—specifically if dietary factors or emotional stress such as excess worry could have contributed to Spleen deficiency in the parents and been transmitted to the child in pre-Heaven Qi and Essence. A family history of Kidney deficiencies would predispose the child to Kidney Yin and Yang deficiencies.

Using the Developmental theory to help determine the origin. For children younger than age 6, consider Kidney deficiency as a contributing factor to constipation. For children older than age 6, consider Liver Qi stagnation as a component of constipation.

Determining the type of constipation:
- Constipation with excess Cold: Facial pallor, general feeling of coldness, cold hands and feet, and abdominal pain that improves with pressure.
- Constipation with excess Heat: Dry, hard, infrequent stools; thirst; dry mouth; red face; and occasionally abdominal pain that worsens with pressure.
- Constipation with Qi stagnation: Firm stools every 3 to 4 days, and abdominal distention with belching.

TCM Diagnosis

There are three major diagnostic categories for childhood constipation, and many children may have a combination of two or all three types:
1. Spleen Qi deficiency
2. Liver Qi stagnation
3. Yin deficiency

Spleen Qi deficiency

Constipation can be accompanied by other Spleen Qi deficiency signs, such as facial pallor, fatigue, and muscle weakness. This type of constipation can explain the majority of Western diagnoses: functional constipation, improper diet, drug-induced constipation (causing internal Cold), and constipation secondary to chronic illnesses. Encopresis may be the concomitant occurrence of Spleen-deficient constipation and Spleen Cold diarrhea, when loose stools seep around impacted dry stools.

Liver Qi stagnation

Liver Qi stagnation constipation is accompanied by excess signs, such as abdominal distention and pain.

Yin deficiency

Yin-deficiency constipation can be accompanied by other signs of Yin deficiency, such as dry skin, dry mouth, and Heat signs owing to Yin deficiency, such as red skin rashes. Kidney Yin deficiency signs may be present, such as concentrated, scanty urine.

General Treatment
Expel stool

The first goal is to propel the stool through the colon. Anatomically, the large intestine begins on the right with the ascending colon, then goes across the upper abdomen as the transverse colon and down on the left side as the descending colon to the rectum. The mother can massage the child's abdomen in a clockwise direction (with the child as the clock), beginning at the child's right lower abdomen, massaging upward to below the ribs, then across the top of the abdomen to the child's left, and then down the left side. Massage 50 times at least once per day.

Modify diet

Decrease or eliminate Phlegm-producing foods, artificially sweet foods, greasy or fried foods, and excess energetically Cold or Hot foods.

Modify lifestyle

Balance rest, study, and physical activities.

Acupuncture Treatment
Spleen Qi deficiency

Tonify the Spleen:
    ST36
    SP3, SP6, BL20
Or use the Four-Point Protocol:
    Tonify SP2, HT8; sedate SP1, LR1
ST40 to expel Damp.
If there are signs of Coldness, expel Cold from the Spleen:
    SP2, SP9
Or use the Four-Point protocol:
    Tonify SP2, HT8; sedate SP9, KI10.
    Moxa CV8 to warm the Middle Energizer; avoid exposing the umbilicus (CV8) to Cold.
    Tonify the Kidney in children younger than age 6 in the Water phase of Development: KI3, KI6, KI7, BL23.

Liver Qi stagnation

LR13, LR14 to promote the smooth flow of Liver Qi and relieve Qi stagnation.
ST40 to expel Damp.
Tonify the Spleen:
    ST36
    SP3, SP6, BL20
Or use the Four-Point protocol:
    Tonify SP2, HT8; sedate SP1, LR1.

Yin deficiency

Eliminate or decrease energetically Hot foods.
KI3, KI6, SP6 to globally tonify Yin.
LI11 to disperse Heat.
LI2 to tonify Large Intestine Yin.
Use the Two-Point or Four-Point protocol to disperse Heat from the large intestine:
    Tonify LI2, sedate LI5.
    Tonify LI2, BL66; sedate LI5, SI5.
Tonify the Spleen:
    ST36
    SP3, SP6, BL20
Or use the Four-Point protocol:
    Tonify SP2, HT8; sedate SP1, LR1.[6-18]

Aromatherapy

Aromatherapy was coupled with massage in an observational study conducted on 15 adult subjects with constipation related to cancer.[1] All subjects were taught abdominal massage techniques; the massage was provided by the subjects' caretakers, or the subjects performed it on themselves. Massage lotion with essential oils of black pepper *(Piper nigrum)* and Roman chamomile *(Chamaemelum nobile)* were provided. All patients reported a decline in distention and flatulence after the first week. After 6 weeks, bowel function normalized (by patient definition) for 3 subjects improved but was not considered normal by 3 subjects, and 4 subjects were lost to follow-up.

In this author's experience, aromatherapy treatment of constipation should be done in conjunction with abdominal massage as well as dietary management. Price and Parr recommend an abdominal massage oil of a combination of 3 drops ginger *(Zingiber officinalis)*, 3 drops rosemary *(Rosmarinus officinalis)*, and 2 drops of mandarin *(Citrus reticulata)* in 50 mL of oil.[2]

Chiropractic

The goal of the chiropractor in managing the child with constipation is to eliminate any interference to normal intestinal function. Physical, chemical, and emotional stressors commonly disrupt normal gut function. First and foremost in the chiropractic evaluation is an assessment of the physical interference to nerve function at the spinal level: the subluxation complex (SC).

The sympathetic regulation of the GI tract is vagal in both efferent and afferent innervation. The efferent and afferent parasympathetic influence is found in the cervical and thoracic sympathetic trunks at T4 to T6 as well as in the the superior thoracic splanchnic nerves at T6 to T9.[1] Overstimulation of the sympathetic system or suppression of the parasympathetic system may inhibit gastric secretions and peristalsis.

The SC that affects nerves to the intestinal region correlates strongly with individuals with digestive organ disease.[2] Furthermore, the chiropractic adjustment at the C1-C2 region has been recorded through electrogastrogram as normalizing peristaltic wave patterns and increasing gastric tone as compared with a control group.[3] In a study of 316 infants with colic, spinal adjustments (primarily to the upper cervical and middle thoracic regions) resulted in improvement in 94% of the participants.[4]

Common recommendations include utilizing a Logan Basic contact at the sacrotuberous ligament, specific upper cervical adjustments, occipital decompression, and cranial adjusting.[5] Parasympathetic stimulation can be accomplished by percussion over the sacrum, which is done by fingertip percussion for a period of 5 seconds followed by a 15-second rest and then repeated percussion/rest intervals for a 2-minute period.[6]

A case report was documented of a 5-year-old girl with progressively worsening constipation during the past 3 years. At the initial visit, the girl was experiencing only one bowel movement per week induced by medication. After two adjustments to the cervical spine, she experienced 4 to 6 bowel movements per week without pharmaceutical induction.[7]

A 7-month-old girl had a bowel movement frequency of once every 1 to 3 days since birth. Each bowel movement was precipitated by hours of crying and resulted in "rabbit pellet" stools. Her spine and cranium were adjusted on two occasions in 2 days. Following the second visit, she began to have daily soft bowel movements. Two follow-up visits occurred in the following 6 weeks. At a 1-year follow-up, the bowel movements continued to be daily and soft.[8]

Another case of a 10-month-old girl with a 4-month history of constipation is reported in chiropractic literature. This child was having painful bowel movements at a frequency of once every 7 to 10 days, generally manually stimulated. After her second chiropractic visit, she began to have bowel movements on her own and within 2 weeks of care the frequency reached 3 to 4 times per week, unassisted and apparently pain free. With continued care, the frequency became daily.[9]

In support of the chiropractic adjustment, nutritional modifications are commonly recommended. Adequate fluid intake is essential. A quality diet high in fresh fruit and vegetable fiber is always recommended. Avoidance of constipating foods such as carrots, bananas, white rice, processed flour, and cheese with the addition of loosening foods such as apricots, pears, plums, prunes, and white grapes may be enough to manage milder challenges. Severe chronic constipation may be secondary to allergy.[10,11] Common foods associated with constipation include dairy, wheat, and eggs. A trial of elimination of these foods in such cases may prove corrective up to 70% of the time.

A therapeutic supplementation of magnesium may be utilized in the initial stages of healing. A magnesium load of 5 mg per pound of body weight may cause relaxation of the intestine and produce stool.

In cases of chronic constipation secondary to brain injury, buffered vitamin C may be used safely on a daily basis to gut tolerance.

Psyllium seed may be used in children older than 2 years.[12]

Pressure points over the abdomen and the soles of the feet are also sometimes used supplementally to regulate peristalsis. The abdominal points are located as follows: (1) midway between the umbilicus and the xiphoid, (2) midway between the umbilicus and the superior rim of the symphysis pubis, (3) inferior to the rib margin at the nipple line on the left, (4) inferior to the rib margin at the nipple line on the right, and (5) over the location of the ileocecal valve. The abdominal points are treated by finger pad pressure (just at the point of tissue resistance) with vibration sustained for approximately 10 seconds each. The points are treated in order 1 to 5 and are stimulated approximately four times per day. This technique is commonly followed by light massage in a clockwise direction over the entire abdomen (Figure 26-1).

Foot reflexology is used for various GI disturbances and has been found to be productive in the management of constipation.[13] Pressure on the soles of the feet is applied with the thumb pad stroking first along the lateral arch from the heel to fifth digit and then circling back across at the level of the proximal interphalangeal joint (Figure 26-2).

Deep muscle massage over the quadratus lumborum bilaterally and also along the tensor fasciae latae bilaterally may relax a spastic constipation.[14]

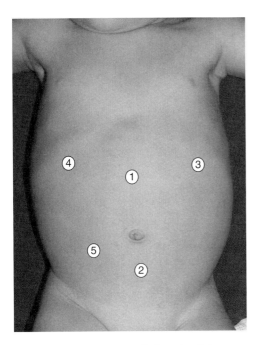

FIGURE 26-1 Points marked on the abdomen.

Herbs—Chinese

TCM herbal treatment of constipation is to quickly relieve the stagnation of food and stool without excessive moistening and overstimulation of the bowel that can result in diarrhea.[1]

Easy Going is a variation of Tummy Tamer (Gentle Warrior Pediatric Formula, Kan Herb Company, Scotts Valley, Calif.)

with the addition of flax (hu ma ren) and rhubarb (da huang) to lubricate the colon and activate intestinal peristalsis. Although rhubarb rhizome (da huang) is a moderately strong laxative, its influence is tempered by the other ingredients in the formula including pogostemon (huo xiang), aucklandia (mu xiang), citrus (chen pi), poria (fu ling), atractylodes (bai zhu), cardamon (sha ren), and licorice (gan cao).[1]

Dosage: 1 to 2 droppersful of Easy Going as needed every 4 to 6 hours.[1]

Caution: Acute gastroenteritis (stomach or intestinal flu); high fever (temperature of 102° F or higher); thirst, dehydration, sweating, weakness or lethargy; or suspected appendicitis or bowel obstruction.[1]

Herbs—Western

Bulk Laxatives

Blond psyllium husk consists of the ground husk of the psyllium seed *(Plantago ovata)*, a mixture of polysaccharides composed of pentoses, hexoses, and uronic acids. Psyllium is a predominantly soluble fiber, and numerous adult clinical studies have evaluated the effect of psyllium in subjects with constipation.[1-3] We were unable to identify any trials of children in the treatment of constipation; however, some studies show its efficacy for the treatment of high cholesterol in children. Patients should be warned that consuming large amounts of fiber can cause abdominal bloating or flatulence; this can be modulated by starting with small amounts and slowly increasing according to tolerance and efficacy. Psyllium is safe for children and may typically be given as ¼ to ½ teaspoon mixed in water or juice up to three times daily. However, psyllium is contraindicated in cases of allergic

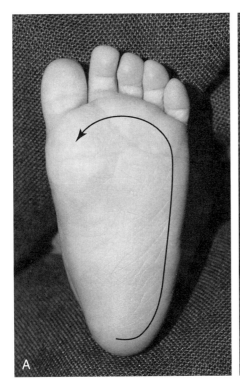 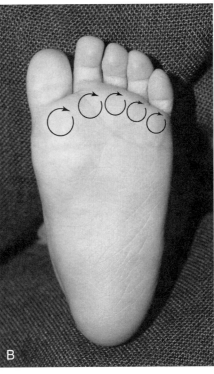

FIGURE 26-2 Pressure on the soles of the feet is applied with the thumb pad stroking first along the lateral arch from the heel to fifth digit (**A**) and then circling back across at the level of the metatarsal-phalangeal joint (**B**).

reaction to psyllium, intestinal obstruction, fecal impaction, difficulty in swallowing, and esophageal narrowing.[4-6]

Anthraquinone Laxatives

Extracts of aloe *(Aloe vera)*, barbaloin, or aloin are derived from the inner sheath cells of the leaves; it is a very powerful laxative and can cause stomach cramps. Although there are clinical trials of efficacy in adults, aloe latex is too strong for most childhood cases of constipation and should be avoided in children younger than 12 years and used with caution (keeping in mind its propensity for rebound constipation) for children older than 12 years.[4,7] In addition, anthraquinone glycoside constituents of the leaf juice may be secreted into breast milk; therefore aloe and aloin should be avoided during lactation.[4]

Cascara sagrada *(Rhamni purshiani)* and senna *(Sennae folum)* both have clinical and historical evidence for use in the treatment of constipation in adults and children. Cascara sagrada and senna have been approved by the U.S. Food and Drug Administration for adults and children older than 2 years for bowel preparation and constipation. Irritant/stimulant laxatives such as senna and cascara sagrada should be used sparingly and only for the treatment of acute constipation unable to be treated with fiber. They are not recommended for long-term use. They both have a high potential for dependence and abdominal discomfort side effects.[8] The use of senna preparations in young children and infants has been associated with severe diaper rash, blisters, and skin sloughing.[9]

Homeopathy

Before using this section, please see Appendix A, Homeopathy, for definitions of practitioner expertise categories and general information on prescribing homeopathic medicines.

Practitioner Expertise Category 1

Category 1 includes constipation that is of relatively recent onset and is unassociated with other serious pathology.

Practitioner Expertise Category 2

Category 2 includes constipation that is longstanding or associated with other conditions.

There are no controlled clinical trials of homeopathy for treatment of constipation, although the homeopathic literature contains much evidence for its use in the form of accumulated clinical experience.[1] After causes of constipation in an infant requiring early surgical intervention (such as Hirschsprung disease) have been ruled out, it is safe to try homeopathic treatment for constipation. Homeopathy can be used in conjunction with dietary changes and other treatment modalities, either conventional or alternative.

The goal in treating constipation homeopathically is to determine the single homeopathic medicine whose description in the materia medica most closely matches the symptom picture of the patient. Often mental and emotional states in addition to physical symptoms are considered. Once the medicine has been selected, it can be given in the 30C potency two to three times daily. If it has not helped in 3 to 4 days, then another homeopathic medicine should be tried or some other form of therapy should be instituted as needed. Once symptoms have begun to resolve, the medicine can be given less frequently or stopped. It can be repeated again for a relapse of symptoms.

The following is a list of homeopathic medicines commonly used to treat patients with constipation. It must be emphasized that this list is partial and represents some of the probable choices from the homeopathic materia medica. If the symptoms of a given patient are not represented here, a search of the homeopathic literature would be needed to find the simillimum.

Aluminum oxydatum

Aluminum oxydatum can be given for constipation where the rectum is dry and the stools are hard and dry, although there may be constipation with soft stools as well. Very little urging is felt by the patient, and the stools may need to be mechanically evacuated.

Calcarea carbonica hahnemanni

The child needing *Calcarea carbonica* has constipation that tends to be chubby and may be slow in developing (e.g., late teething or walking). The child may be prone to sweating. There may be little urging felt by the patient, and a passed stool may be claylike.

Lycopodium clavatum

The child needing *Lycopodium clavatum* is bloated and gassy with audible intestinal rumbling. This child is sensitive to tight clothing around the abdomen. The child is hungry immediately on waking and may fill up quickly while eating or have a voracious appetite. Some stools are hard and small. Other stools may start hard and then be followed by soft or liquid stool. The child's features may be fine, and the head may appear too large for the body.

Nux vomica

The child needing *Nux vomica* is very irritable and sensitive to stimuli such as light and noise. He or she is colicky and has frequent, ineffectual urging to pass stools but passes only small amounts.

Opium

The child needing *Opium* has serious constipation with no urge to defecate. This may lead to fecal impaction and bowel obstruction. In some cases colicky pains may occur. The patient may be a heavy sleeper with snoring respirations.

Silica terra

The child needing *Silica terra* has constipation with no urge to defecate. Hard stools may also be produced with straining. One characteristic described in the homeopathic literature is "bashful stools," which recede back into the rectum after almost being expelled. Anal fissures may be present.

Magnet Therapy

Apply the ½- or ¾-inch Neodymium nylon–coated magnets in a pattern of alternating north/south polarities on the lower abdomen at CV6, bilateral KD15, and LR13. Magnets may be left in place up to 24 hours and treatment repeated three times per week. These magnets may be obtained from Painfree Lifestyles (800-480-8601).

Massage Therapy

Historically massage has been used to help treat infants, children, and adults with constipation.[1] Stimulation of the parasympathetic nervous system from massage therapy increases intestinal peristalsis and circulation to the GI tract. Direct application of massage to the abdomen assists with the mechanical action of peristalsis. Prior to the use of current medical therapies, parents of children with cystic fibrosis massaged their child's abdomen to help prevent blockage.

Use of abdominal massage to prevent constipation in hospice patients during palliative care is beginning to be reinvestigated as a potential therapy.[2] A recent systematic review of four controlled clinical trials suggests that massage therapy could be a potential treatment for chronic constipation.[1] Another recent study evaluated the efficacy of six 30-minute sessions of foot reflexology (a massage modality in which pressure is applied to reflex areas on the feet, hands, and ears that correspond to other body parts and organs[3]) weekly for children diagnosed with encopresis and chronic constipation.[4] The parents reported that their children had more bowel movements and fewer episodes of soiling.[4]

Ideally, abdominal massage should not be done immediately after a feeding or meal; waiting at least 30 minutes may help prevent vomiting or spitting up that could occur from pressure applied to a full stomach.[5] If an infant is being treated, placing the infant in a seated position in the parent's lap, facing the parent, with the infant's feet resting on the parent's chest, will relax the abdominal muscles and facilitate massage.[5] An infant with a history of reflux could be placed more upright in the lap either by using pillows or having the parent flex the knees. For a child, abdominal massage can easily be done with the child lying on the back with the knees bent. If the child is old enough, the child could learn the abdominal massage routine to perform alone when needed.

Abdominal massage should be in the direction of the large intestines at all times.[5,6] For the massage, slow, rhythmic strokes applied with firm pressure of a relaxed hand will be relaxing and prevent tickling the infant or child.[5,6] A small amount of oil or lotion may be used to facilitate the hand gliding along the infant's abdomen.[5,6] The massage strokes should be repeated approximately 5 to 10 times each. (If the infant or child has an abdominal feeding tube in place or a stoma, avoid the area and continue the rest of the massage as instructed.)

The first stroke is a hand-over-hand motion starting below the ribcage and stroking down the middle of the abdomen with one hand to the pelvic bone. This is then repeated with the alternate hand, thereby always maintaining contact with the child.[5,6] For the second step, strokes are applied in a clockwise, circular motion (with the child as the clock) along the entire abdomen with the exception of over the navel.[5,6] Firmer pressure should be added from the 9 o'clock to 5 o'clock regions.[5] Repeat in a continuous motion.[5,6]

The last step has three separate strokes.[5,6] The first stroke starts on the child's left side below the ribcage, moving the hand downward to the hip, following the descending colon. Repeat several times before proceeding to the next stroke. The second stroke follows the transverse and descending colon. Begin the stroke on the child's right side under the ribcage, gliding the hand below the ribs toward the left and then downward, in the figure of an upside-down L. Repeat several times. The final stroke begins at the child's right hip, then upward below the ribs and along to the left and then down, in the figure of an upside-down U. This last stroke follows the ascending, transverse, and descending colon and completes the massage.[5,6]

Mind/Body

Simple constipation in childhood can be complicated by stress and at times by withholding behavior. In children who experience constipation with high stress levels, mind/body strategies directed at stress management would make sense as an adjunctive approach. Children who actively withhold stool secondary to fear of painful elimination (defecation anxiety) often benefit from basic relaxation training such as diaphragmatic breathing, progressive muscle relaxation, and cognitive-behavioral techniques combined with appropriate medical management (stool softeners and laxatives). In one author's experience (Culbert), pelvic floor surface electromyographic (EMG) biofeedback training has also proven useful.

Some children with constipation evolve into a more significant picture that includes fecal soiling, or encopresis, which includes rectal stretching, some loss of sensitivity, and overflow soiling. For some of these children, disordered defecation dynamics can play a role. Biofeedback training using surface EMG, anorectal EMG, and manometric (pressure) feedback can assist in rehabilitation of the muscles involved and a return to normal defecation dynamics.[1-4] Relaxation training to ensure complete release of the external anal sphincter and more complete evacuation of the rectosigmoid is also well supported.[5] A review of 23 studies reported a 72% mean success rate for biofeedback for fecal incontinence in a pediatric population with diverse etiology.[6]

In certain yoga traditions (Iyengar and others), specific poses have been developed for certain medical conditions, including constipation, although to our knowledge no randomized study of this has been published. In general, physical activity promotes more regular bowel movements and thus yoga is a reasonable adjunctive choice on that basis alone.

The author's usual protocol includes combining a high-fiber, dairy restricted diet with a behavioral bowel training program, a symptom diary (in the form of a sticker chart), and the use of an osmotic laxative such as polyethylene glycol 3350 powder. Relaxation exercises for children who have defecation anxiety can be added at toileting practice times as indicated. Children who are still struggling after an 8 to 12 week trial of this protocol are then offered the option of either pelvic floor surface EMG biofeedback or anorectal EMG biofeedback to increase body awareness, retrain dysfunctional defecation dynamics, and reduce overactive pelvic activity when indicated. Self-hypnosis to improve body awareness and sense of control can be included, with suggestions such as "imagine telephone lines between the brain and the poop muscles, and make sure the volume is turned up so they can hear each other."

Naturopathy

Constipation in the pediatric population is a common complaint of parents and is often undertreated by physicians.[1] Constipation should always be treated as a symptom rather than a condition. If the underlying cause of the constipation is addressed, normal function of the bowels should follow. Healthy bowel frequency should be 1 to 5 bowel movements per day in infants and children. It is not uncommon for individuals in industrialized countries to have a very infrequent stooling pattern owing to our consumption of a low-fiber diet, sedentary activity levels, stressful lifestyle, and lack of adequate fluid intake. Many patients consider days without a bowel movement to be normal and expected. However, it is important to note that the body's process of elimination exists to remove waste products that contain absorbable toxins. As bowel frequency increases, the chance of exposure to these toxins that can predispose patients to cancer of the colon in later life[2] or development of diverticulosis decreases.

Breastfeeding is without question the best choice for babies, and breastfed babies are protected from development of constipation in the first few months of life.[3] In addition, breastfed babies can often follow the mother's bowel patterns, such that treatment of the mother will have beneficial effects on the child. Beets are a well-tolerated food that the breastfeeding mother can consume to alleviate constipation in her child. When solids are introduced into a baby's diet, stool frequency may decrease as a result of relative dehydration. It is therefore essential to stay aware of breast milk and/or fluid intake at the onset of solid food consumption. A child should be drinking one third of his or her body weight in ounces, and the first liquid introduced to a baby should be water or diluted juice instead of straight juice to avoid high consumption of sugars.

Elimination of foods from the diet has been effective in relieving chronic constipation, and cow's milk intolerance is commonly implicated,[4-6] resulting in gut lymphoid nodular hyperplasia.[7] Erosions and inflammation of the GI mucosa have been discovered in patients who have intolerance to certain foods, especially cow's milk. This inflammation can lead to a chronic proctitis directly related to the constipation these patients experience when consuming these foods, especially cow's milk.[8]

Treatment

Treatment recommendations include the following:

- Remove commonly allergenic foods from the diet of the breastfeeding mother or the child who is consuming solid foods. Consider elimination trial of dairy, wheat, eggs, corn, or soy.
- Increase exercise and/or activity of the child.
- Flax seeds: ½ to 1 tsp of fresh seeds ground in a coffee grinder and mixed in food two to three times per day.
- Increase consumption of fruits and vegetables. In particular, oats, beets, prunes, and apricots are high in fiber and can increase the number of bowel movements.
- Osmotic agents such as vitamin C and magnesium citrate can be used for temporary normalization of bowel movement frequency. Children older than 1 year can consume 250 mg vitamin C several times per day until stools soften.

The dose acquired may be maintained as other treatments are utilized. Magnesium may be administered at 50 to 100 mg two to three times per day, again until stools soften. (Magnesium is only for spastic constipation; do not use magnesium in atonic constipation but instead use plateau dose of senna.)

- Home formula: 2 dried prunes, 2 dried apricots, 1 cinnamon stick in 1 cup of water. Bring to a boil and let sit overnight. Add to breakfast or drink throughout the day.[9]
- Cascara sagrada/buckthorn (*R. purshiana*) is most indicated in chronic constipation and is safe for the pediatric population. A dosage regimen should start with gradual increase from once-daily dosages for 1 week and increase weekly to three times daily dosage. When bowels normalize, a gradual weaning in the opposite fashion may follow. Powdered bark: 1 to 2.5 g per dose; liquid extract: 2 to 5 mL per dose; decoction of root: 1 to 2 tsp/cup water/dose; 1:5 tincture: 0.5 to 1 mL per dose.[9]
- Probiotics in the treatment of constipation have shown mixed results. *Lactobacillus* species *Lactobacillus casei Shirota*,[10] *Lactobacillus rhamnosus*,[11] and others have shown promising effects,[12] whereas *Lactobacillus* GG was not shown to be helpful in the treatment of constipation in children.[13] Because supplementation with probiotics will not be detrimental, a multi-month trial of several different species may reveal benefits.
- Senna (*Cassia acutifolia*) is a strong laxative but may be habit forming, as the bowels tend to depend on it if used long term. It may be too harsh a remedy for the pediatric population, and the other options mentioned previously should be considered for these patients before using senna.

Nutrition

After all the ominous causes of constipation have been ruled out, the most common findings of functional constipation are lack of water and lack of fiber. A goal would be one or two soft bowel movements per day passed without pain, mucus, or blood. If this is not the norm, use nutritional strategies to correct the problem, starting with increased intakes of water (not juice, fruit drinks, soda, or tea). Next, increase the intake of dietary fiber. A general rule of thumb for the recommended amount of fiber is *age + 5 = total grams of fiber per day*. Sources of fiber and fiber grams are listed in Table 26-1.[1] Various recipes and home remedies can be used safely to treat common constipation.

1. Power Pudding: Equal portions (⅓ cup) of bran cereal, prune juice, and applesauce mixed together and sweetened if desired. Give 1 tablespoon with meals three times per day.
2. Prune juice cocktail: 4 oz prune juice plus 2 oz lemon-lime soda served over ice.
3. Chocolate fiber cookies: 1 large chocolate candy bar plus just enough Fiber One cereal (General Mills, Golden Valley, Minn.) to be well coated with chocolate (more chocolate than cereal). Melt chocolate in microwave for 2 minutes. Stir in cereal. Drop clusters of mixture on wax paper and sprinkle with cake decorations or candy if desired. Refrigerate until clusters are firm. Makes 6 to 12 cookies. Do not exceed intake of more than 1 to 2 cookies per day.

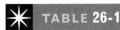

TABLE 26-1

Sources of Fiber

	PORTION	FIBER (GRAMS)
High-fiber Foods		
Whole wheat bread	2 slices	6
All-bran cereal	½ cup	10
Wheaties cereal	1 oz	2.5
Whole wheat spaghetti	1 cup	3.5
Lentils	½ cup cooked	3.5
Kidney beans	½ cup cooked	9
Broccoli	¾ cup cooked	7
Baked potato with skin	1 medium	5
Spinach	½ cup cooked	7
Yam baked in skin	1 medium	7
Apple with skin	1 medium	3.5
Raspberries	½ cup	3.5
Blackberries	½ cup	5
Figs, dried	3	10
Baked beans	½ cup cooked	8
Low-fiber Foods		
Bagel	1	<1
Cornflakes	1 oz	<1
Grapes	20	<1
Watermelon	1 cup	<1
Lettuce	1 cup	<1

4. Flax seed: Grind 1 tablespoon in a coffee grinder and blend in apple juice, fruit smoothies, or oatmeal, or sprinkle on a salad. This has a natural laxative effect and also provides omega-3 fatty acids that are released when seeds are crushed.
5. Laxative tea: 2 tablespoons honey plus 2 tablespoons raw vinegar added to 1 cup hot tea.[2]

Osteopathy

Constipation is a common concern for parents of infants and toddlers and reportedly accounts for one fourth of visits to pediatric gastroenterologists, yet the clinical syndrome of constipation is not well defined or understood. Within the osteopathic concept, several factors are thought to contribute to this condition. Fascial strains in the pelvis and abdomen may impede the low-pressure circulatory system, leading to venous and lymphatic congestion. This in turn alters the milieu of the neural components of the mesenteric and submucosal plexus in the distal colon. These cells are immature at birth and remain so throughout the first 2 years of life and thus may be more susceptible to alterations in tissue pH and exposure to cellular waste products. Gut transit time is significantly delayed in children with constipation, with most prolonged clearance times occurring in the distal colon or rectum.[1,2] Children with constipation may present with signs of tissue congestion in the pelvic diaphragm, altered mechanics at the sacroiliac joints, and increased tone and tender points in the muscles of the lower back and pelvis. Depending upon the age and disposition of the child, these findings may be addressed with direct or indirect techniques.[3-6]

Altered parasympathetic and sympathetic tone in the gut is another factor to be considered in the child with constipation. Various osteopaths and others have written on the association between signs of altered autonomic tone and abnormal bowel function.[3,4,7-9] In children with constipation this often presents as viscerosomatic reflexes in the paraspinal muscles of the lower thoracic and upper lumbar areas[9,10] or Chapman's reflexes,[8,11] areas of tissue texture changes thought to be associated with neurolymphatic changes. Anterior visceral techniques aimed at addressing the fascias surrounding the mesenteric ganglia are often indicated in these patients.[3,7] These and other visceral techniques are well tolerated. Modified rib raining, myofascial, and indirect techniques can be used to address the sympathetics in the lower thoracic area. Patients can also be taught some myofascial and soft tissue techniques to apply to their child at home.[12]

Psychology

Throughout the psychology literature, constipation and encopresis tend to be seen as synonymous, and children with constipation, incontinence, and constipation plus incontinence tend to be grouped together. Some key features of each disorder are the possible significant impact of encopresis on a child's social and emotional functioning. Children can experience low self-esteem related to teasing and a sense of their own incompetence at handling this basic skill. The significant effects of constipation are abdominal pain and pain during defecation. For all groups, the normal physiological process of defecation and the appropriate behavioral response needed for socially acceptable toileting can be negatively affected when children experience pain and fear about defecation. Children must have the opportunity to toilet without tension or anxiety because it is very important to be able to relax during the process. If children are unable to relax, toileting can become an aversive experience that results in an avoidance response. Children may also become habituated to the sensation of fullness in the rectal area, which leaves them unaware of the need to defecate.

Most psychological treatments include a comprehensive medical intervention (e.g., cleanout with laxative and dietary recommendations) in conjunction with psychological interventions. Biofeedback for constipated children typically focuses on external anal sphincter (EAS) contraction and correcting paradoxical contraction. Overall, biofeedback plus medical management is more effective than medical management alone and has met efficacy criteria for children with constipation and encopresis.[1] Adding a behavioral intervention may help further improve outcome. When a behavioral program of positive reinforcement, skills training, and toileting schedule was added to a biofeedback and medical management treatment program, improvement was significantly higher (85% improved) than for biofeedback and medical management (61%) and medical management alone (45%).[2] In this study, biofeedback training included EAS contraction, correction of paradoxical contraction, and home practice of EAS tightening and relaxation.

Even behavioral approaches without biofeedback can be effective for children with encopresis and constipation. A comprehensive behavioral program that focuses on fiber education, bowel activity records, goal setting, sitting schedule, reinforcement, and skills-building techniques such as how to relax while on the toilet teach children the necessary skills to manage their bowels. In a study examining this protocol, 89% of children had no soiling at the end of treatment.[3]

Treatment Recommendations

During the first session with a CAM psychologist, a comprehensive interview would be conducted that covers the history of the problem, any approaches the family has already tried, how accidents are managed, and the current diet. Understanding the baseline level of functioning, including frequency of accidents, willingness to toilet, and pain with defecation, will provide a valuable reference for progress. Food choices that will facilitate bowel movements and the importance of adequate water intake must be discussed. It may be necessary to begin with a laxative clean-out if the child has not had any bowel movement for several days.

Treatment should focus on developing a regular sitting on the toilet schedule. Approximately 30 minutes after each meal, the patient should attempt to defecate. It may be necessary to develop a reinforcement program if the child has had a painful or negative experience with toileting. Rewards should be easy to administer and motivating for the child (e.g., 5 minutes of a video game, music, a special coloring book). Parents should record successful bowel movements on a chart so that the child can monitor progress. This is important because children need to be invested in the process. If they struggle or resist toileting, it can create stress and tension and become a power struggle with parents. The tension can then lead to tighter muscles and more difficulty defecating.

Another important component of treatment is for children to learn to relax for defecation. This is necessary because children tense up or constrict their anal muscles to hold in their feces. Often showing a picture of their anatomy facilitates awareness of the muscles that should be relaxed. It is important to teach basic diaphragmatic breathing. For example, teach the child to breathe in slowly, allowing the belly and diaphragm area to fill up with air. Have him imagine he is filling up a balloon inside of him and then breathe out slowly as though the balloon were deflating. The child can be instructed to feel his body becoming loose and relaxed as he breathes in and out slowly. A child can practice alternatively squeezing his gluteal muscles together and then relaxing them and then doing this while sitting on the toilet.

The following is a more specific example of a script that could be used:

> Imagine you have to squeeze through a tight hole to get to the magic land where everyone is relaxed and happy. Make yourself as skinny as you can—pull in your stomach and butt muscles. Pull in everything tight. Hold it in. Make yourself as skinny as possible to squeeze through the fence. And now that you are through, let your body relax. Let your body become loose and relaxed as you pop through the other side of the fence. Let out your breath. Feel every muscle in your butt relax. Take a deep breath, and let it go slowly.

This exercise can be repeated several times. The contrasting tensing and relaxing of muscles will increase the child's awareness of the different ways muscles can feel.

Children with constipation and encopresis can learn to have healthy defecation habits, and these psychological treatments do not pose a safety risk. Overall, a combined approach that incorporates medical interventions of dietary changes and initial laxative use with behavioral and/or biofeedback may help improve outcome.

References

Pediatric Diagnosis and Treatment

1. Youssef NN, Di Lorenzo C: Childhood constipation: evaluation and treatment, *J Clin Gastroenterol* 33:199-205, 2001.
2. Baker SS, Liptak GS, Colletti RB et al: Constipation in infants and children: evaluation and treatment. A medical position statement of the North American Society for Pediatric Gastroenterology and Nutrition, *J Pediatr Gastroenterol Nutr* 29:612-626, 1991.
3. Roy CC, Silverman A, Alagille D: *Pediatric clinical gastroenterology*, ed 4, New York, 1995, Mosby.
4. Loening-Baucke V: Management of chronic constipation in infants and toddlers, *Am Fam Physician* 49:397-400, 403-406, 411-413, 1994.
5. Behrman RE, Kliegman RM, Jenson HB, editors: *Nelson's textbook of pediatrics*, Philadelphia, 2004, Saunders.
6. Messina M, Meucci D, Di Maggio G et al: Idiopathic constipation in children: 10-year experience [in Italian], *Pediatr Med Chir* 21:187-191, 2000.
7. Nurko S: Advances in the management of pediatric constipation, *Curr Gastroenterol Rep* 2:234-240, 2000.
8. Morais MB, Maffei HV: Constipation [in Portuguese], *J Pediatr (Rio J)* 76(Suppl 1):S147-S156, 2000.
9. Borowitz SM, Cox DJ, Kovatchev B et al: Treatment of childhood constipation by primary care physicians: efficacy and predictors of outcome, *Pediatrics* 115:873-877, 2005.
10. Brooks RC, Copen RM, Cox DJ et al: Review of the treatment literature for encopresis, functional constipation, and stool-toileting refusal, *Ann Behav Med* 22:260-267, 2000.
11. Splete H: Behavioral therapy effective with constipation when other care fails, *Pediatr News* May:46, 2005.
12. Koletzko S: Constipation in childhood—from the pediatric viewpoint [in German], *Kinderarztl Prax* 61:245-249, 1993.
13. Youssef NN, Langseder AL, Verga BJ et al: Chronic childhood constipation is associated with impaired quality of life: a case-controlled study, *J Pediatr Gastroenterol Nutr* 41:56-60, 2005.
14. Loening-Baucke V: Functional constipation, *Semin Pediatr Surg* 4:26-34, 1995.

Acupuncture

1. Broide E, Pintov S, Portnoy S et al: Effectiveness of acupuncture for treatment of childhood constipation, *Dig Dis Sci* 46:1270-1275, 2001.
2. Khasaev KM, Svarich VG, Kopylov SM: A rehabilitative method for children operated on for Hirschsprung's disease [in Russian], *Vestn Khir Im I I Grek* 150:71-73, 1993.
3. Klauser AG, Rubach A, Bertsche O et al: Body acupuncture: effect on colonic function in chronic constipation, *Z Gastroenterol* 31:605-608, 1993.
4. Xiong XH, Deng DM: Acupuncture treatment of constipation due to diabetes mellitus: an observation of 21 cases, *Int J Clin Acupunct* 6:19-21, 1995.

5. Li Y, Tougas G, Chiverton SG et al: The effect of acupuncture on gastrointestinal function and disorders, *Am J Gastroenterol* 87:1372-1381, 1992.
6. Loo M: *Pediatric acupuncture*, London, 2002, Elsevier.
7. Diehl DL: Acupuncture for gastrointestinal and hepatobiliary disorders, *J Altern Complement Med* 5:27-45, 1999.
8. Cao J: *Essentials of traditional Chinese pediatrics*, Beijing, 1990, Foreign Language Press.
9. *China Zhenjiuology, a series of teaching videotapes*, Beijing, China, 1990, Chinese Medical Audio-Video Organization and Meditalent Enterprises Ltd.
10. Deadman P, Al-Khafaji M: *A manual of acupuncture*, East Sussex, UK, 1998, Journal of Chinese Medicine Publications.
11. Diagnosis and treatment of gynecology and pediatrics. In *Chinese Zhenjiuology, a series of teaching videotapes*, Beijing, China, 1990, Chinese Medical Audio-Video Organization and Meditalent Enterprises.
12. Ellis E, Wiseman N, Boss K: *Fundamentals of Chinese acupuncture, revised edition*, Brookline, Mass, 1991, Paradigm Publications.
13. *English-Chinese encyclopedia of practical traditional Chinese medicine*, vols 1-14, Beijing, 1990, Higher Education Press.
14. Helms J: *Acupuncture energetics, a clinical approach for physicians*, Berkeley, Calif, 1995, Medical Acupuncture Publishers.
15. Maciocia G: *The foundations of Chinese medicine, a comprehensive text for acupuncturists and herbalists*, London, 1989, Churchill Livingstone.
16. Maciocia G: *The practice of Chinese medicine, the treatment of diseases with acupuncture and Chinese herbs*, London, 1994, Churchill Livingstone.
17. *Nei Ching. the Yellow Emperor's classic of internal medicine*, Berkeley, Calif, 1949, University of California Press (translated by I Veith).
18. O'Connor J, Bensky D, editors: *Acupuncture, a comprehensive text*, Seattle, 1981, Eastland Press.

Aromatherapy

1. Preece J: Introducing abdominal massage in palliative care for the relief of constipation, *Complement Ther Nurs Midwifery* 8:101-105, 2002.
2. Price S, Parr PP: *Aromatherapy for babies and children*, San Francisco, 1996, Thorsons.

Chiropractic

1. Gray H: *Gray's anatomy*, Philadelphia, 1973, Lea and Febiger.
2. Jorgensen LS, Fossgreen J: Back pain and spinal pathology in patients with functional upper abdominal pain, *Scand J Gastroenterol* 25:1235-1241, 1990.
3. Wiles MR: Observations on the effects of upper cervical manipulations on the electrogastrogram: a preliminary report, *J Manipulative Physiol Ther* 3:226-228, 1980.
4. Klougart N, Nilsson N, Jacobsen J: Infantile colic treated by chiropractors: a prospective study of 316 cases, *J Manipulative Physiol Ther* 12:281-288, 1989.
5. Davies N: *Chiropractic pediatrics*, London, 2000, Churchill Livingstone.
6. Swenson R: Pediatric disorders. In Lawrence DJ, editor: *Fundamentals of chiropractic diagnosis and management*, Baltimore, 1991, Williams and Wilkins.
7. Eriksen K: Effects of upper cervical correction on chronic constipation, *Chiropractic Res J* 3:19-22, 1994.
8. Hewitt EG: Chiropractic treatment of a 7-month-old with chronic constipation: a case report, *Chiropractic Tech* 5:101-103, 1993.
9. Marko SK: Case study—the effect of chiropractic care on an infant with problems of constipation, *Chiropractic Pediatr* 1:23-24, 1994.
10. Iacono G, Cavataio F, Montacto G: Intolerance of cow's milk and chronic constipation in children, *N Engl J Med* 339:1100-1104, 1998.
11. Shaf N, Lindley K, Milla P: Cow's milk and chronic constipation in children, *N Engl J Med* 340:891-892, 1999.
12. Bilgrai Cohen K: *Clinical management of infants and children*, Santa Cruz, Calif, 1988, Extension Press.
13. Bishop E, McKinnon E, Weir E et al: Reflexology in the management of encopresis and chronic constipation, *Pediatr Nurs* 15:20-21, 2003.
14. Chaitow L: *Palpation skills: assessment and diagnosis through touch*, New York, 1977, Churchill Livingstone.

Herbs—Chinese

1. Beinfield H, Korngold E: *Chinese medicine works clinical handbook*, San Francisco, 2007, www.chinesemedicineworks.com.

Herbs—Western

1. McRorie JW, Daggy BP, Morel JG et al: Psyllium is superior to docusate sodium for treatment of chronic constipation, *Aliment Pharmacol Ther* 12:491-497, 1998.
2. Dettmar PW, Sykes J: A multi-centre, general practice comparison of ispaghula husk with lactulose and other laxatives in the treatment of simple constipation, *Curr Med Res Opin* 14:227-233, 1998.
3. Cheskin LJ, Kamal N, Crowell MD et al: Mechanisms of constipation in older persons and effects of fiber compared with placebo, *J Am Geriatr Soc* 43:666-669, 1995.
4. Blumenthal M, editor: *The complete German Commission E monographs: therapeutic guide to herbal medicines*, Austin, Tex, 1998, American Botanical Council.
5. Schneider RP: Perdiem causes esophageal impaction and bezoars, *South Med J* 82:1449-1450, 1989.
6. Newall CA, Anderson LA, Phillipson JD: *Herbal medicines: a guide for health-care professionals*, London, 1996, Pharmaceutical Press.
7. McGuffin M, Hobbs C, Upton R et al: *American Herbal Products Association's botanical safety handbook*, Boca Raton, Fla, 1997, CRC Press.
8. Gardiner P, Kemper KJ: For GI complaints: which herbs and supplements spell relief? *Contemp Ped*, May 2005. Available at http://mommd.mediwire.com/main/Default.aspx?P=Content&ArticleID=174258. Accessed February 2, 2008.
9. Spiller HA, Winter ML, Weber JA et al: Skin breakdown and blisters from senna-containing laxatives in young children, *Ann Pharmacother* 37:636-639, 2003.

Homeopathy

1. *ReferenceWorks Pro 4.2*, San Rafael, Calif, 2008, Kent Homeopathic Associates.
2. Morrison R: *Desktop guide to keynotes and confirmatory symptoms*, Albany, Calif, 1996, Hahnemann Clinic.

Massage Therapy

1. Ernst E: Abdominal massage therapy for chronic constipation: a systematic review of controlled clinical trials, *Forsch Komplementarmed* 6:149-151, 1999.
2. Preece J: Introducing abdominal massage in palliative care for the relief of constipation, *Complement Ther Nurs Midwifery* 8:101-105, 2002.
3. Association of Reflexologists. Available at www.reflexology.org/index.html. Accessed August 2005.

4. Bishop E, McKinnon E, Weir E et al: Reflexology in the management of encopresis and chronic constipation, *Paediatr Nurs* 15: 20-21, 2003.
5. Fleming-Drehobl K, Gengler-Fuhr M: *Pediatric massage for the child with special needs*, Tucson, 1991, Therapy Skill Builders.
6. McClure VS: *Infant massage, a handbook for loving parents*, New York, 1989, Bantam Books.

Mind/Body

1. Loening-Baucke V: Modulation of abnormal defecation dynamics by biofeedback treatment in chronically constipated children with encopresis, *J Pediatr* 116:214-222, 1990.
2. Olness K, McParland F, Piper J: Biofeedback: a new modality in the management of children with fecal soiling, *J Pediatr* 96: 505-509, 1980.
3. Cox D, Sutphen J, Borowitz S et al: Simple electromyographic biofeedback treatment for chronic pediatric constipation/encopresis: preliminary report, *Biofeed Self-Regulat* 19:41-50, 1994.
4. Wang J, Luo M, Qi Q et al: Prospective study of biofeedback retraining in patients with chronic idiopathic functional constipation, *World J Gastroenterol* 9:2109-2113, 2003.
5. McGrath J, Mellon M, Murphy L: Empirically supported treatments in pediatric psychology: constipation and encopresis, *J Pediatr Psychol* 24:225-254, 2000.
6. Jorge J, Harb-Gama A, Wexner S: Biofeedback therapy in the colon and rectal practice, *Appl Psychophysiol Biofeed* 28:47-61, 2003.

Naturopathy

1. Borowitz SM, Cox DJ, Kovatchev B et al: Treatment of childhood constipation by primary care physicians: efficacy and predictors of outcome, *Pediatrics* 115:873-877, 2005.
2. Watanabe T, Nakaya N, Kurashima K et al: Constipation, laxative use and risk of colorectal cancer: the Miyagi Cohort Study, *Eur J Cancer* 40:2109-2115, 2004.
3. Aguirre AN, Vitolo MR, Puccini RF et al: Constipation in infants: influence of type of feeding and dietary fiber intake, *J Pediatr (Rio J)* 78:202-208, 2002.
4. Heine RG, Elsayed S, Hosking CS et al: Cow's milk allergy in infancy, *Curr Opin Allergy Clin Immunol* 2:217-225, 2002.
5. Daher S, Tahan S, Sole D et al: Cow's milk protein intolerance and chronic constipation in children, *Pediatr Allergy Immunol* 12: 339-342, 2001.
6. Iacono G, Cavataio F, Montalto G et al: Intolerance of cow's milk and chronic constipation in children, *N Engl J Med* 339: 1100-1104, 1998.
7. Turunen S, Karttunen TJ, Kokkonen J: Lymphoid nodular hyperplasia and cow's milk hypersensitivity in children with chronic constipation, *J Pediatr* 145:606-611, 2004.
8. Carroccio A, Scalici C, Maresi E et al: Chronic constipation and food intolerance: a model of proctitis causing constipation, *Scand J Gastroenterol* 40:33-42, 2005.
9. Alschuler L: Personal communication, 2000.
10. Koebnick C, Wagner I, Leitzmann P et al: Probiotic beverage containing *Lactobacillus casei Shirota* improves gastrointestinal symptoms in patients with chronic constipation, *Can J Gastroenterol* 17:655-659, 2003.
11. Ouwehand AC, Lagstrom H, Suomalainen T et al: Effect of probiotics on constipation, fecal azoreductase activity and fecal mucin content in the elderly, *Ann Nutr Metab* 46:159-162, 2002.
12. Marteau P, Boutron-Ruault MC: Nutritional advantages of probiotics and prebiotics, *Br J Nutr* 87(Suppl 2):S153-S157, 2002.
13. Banaszkiewicz A, Szajewska H: Ineffectiveness of *Lactobacillus* GG as an adjunct to lactulose for the treatment of constipation in children: a double-blind, placebo-controlled randomized trial, *J Pediatr* 146:364-369, 2005.

Nutrition

1. Mahan LK, Escott-Stump S, editors: *Krause's food, nutrition, and diet therapy*, ed 10, Philadelphia, 2000, Saunders.
2. Beard LM: Constipation, *Pediatr News* Nov:27, 2004. Available at www.epediatricnews.com.

Osteopathy

1. Arhan P, Devroede G, Jehannin B et al: Idiopathic disorders of fecal continence in children, *Pediatrics* 71:774-779, 1983.
2. Arhan P, Devroede G, Jehannin B et al: Segmental colonic transit time, *Pediatrics* 24:625-629, 1981.
3. Kuchera ML, Kuchera WA: *Osteopathic considerations in systemic disease*, Columbus, Ohio, 1994, Greydon Press.
4. Herrmann E: Postoperative adynamic ileus: its prevention and treatment by osteopathic medicine, *D O*:163-164, 1965.
5. Goodridge JP, Kuchera WA: Muscle energy techniques for specific areas, In Ward R, editor: *Foundations of osteopathic medicine*, Baltimore, 1997, Williams & Wilkins.
6. Douglas J: *OMT in postoperative ileus* residency research presentation, 2000, Maine Osteopathic Association.
7. Barral JP, Mercier P. *Visceral manipulation*, Seattle, 1988, Eastland Press.
8. Owen C: *An endocrine interpretation of Chapman's reflexes*, ed 2, Boulder, Colo, 1963, American Academy of Osteopathy.
9. Strong WB: Disorders of the digestive system, In Hoag JM, editor: *Osteopathic medicine*, New York, 1969, McGraw-Hill.
10. Beal MC: Viscerosomatic reflexes: a review, *J Am Osteopath Assoc* 85:786-801, 1985.
11. Mitchell FL Jr: The influence of Chapman's reflexes and the immune reactions, *Osteopath Ann* 2:12, 1974.
12. Carreiro JE: *An osteopathic approach to children*, London, 2003, Churchill Livingstone.

Psychology

1. McGrath ML, Mellon MW, Murphy L: Empirically supported treatments in pediatric psychology: constipation and encopresis, *J Pediatr Psychol* 25:225-254, 2000.
2. Cox DJ, Sutphen J, Borowitz S et al: Contribution of behavior therapy and biofeedback to laxative therapy in the treatment of pediatric encopresis, *Ann Behav Med* 20:70-76, 1998.
3. Stark LJ, Owens-Stively J, Spirito A et al: Group treatment of retentive encopresis, *J Pediatr Psychol* 15:659-671, 1990.

Cough

Acupuncture | May Loo

Aromatherapy | Maura A. Fitzgerald

Herbs—Chinese | May Loo

Herbs—Western | Alan D. Woolf, Paula M. Gardiner, Lana Dvorkin-Camiel, Jack Maypole

Homeopathy | Janet L. Levatin

Magnet Therapy | Agatha P. Colbert, Deborah Risotti

Massage Therapy | Mary C. McLellan

Mind/Body | Timothy Culbert, Lynda Richtsmeier Cyr

✳ PEDIATRIC DIAGNOSIS AND TREATMENT

Cough is a healthy reflex response of the lower respiratory tract to stimulation of irritant or cough receptors in the airway's mucosa.[1,2] Cough receptors also reside in the pharynx, paranasal sinuses, stomach, and external auditory canal; therefore the source of a persistent cough may be outside of the lungs.[2] Chronic cough, defined as coughing for more than 3 or 4 weeks, is a common childhood complaint.[3-6]

The majority of children with isolated cough are normal.[7] However, it is important to rule out more serious causes.

A systematic approach to the diagnosis and treatment of chronic cough in children begins with a comprehensive history to assess possible atopic conditions such as asthma, eczema, urticaria, allergic rhinitis, or a strong family history of atopic conditions; gastrointestinal symptoms such as reflux or malabsorption symptoms; or a family history of cystic fibrosis. There is worldwide consensus that exposure to tobacco smoke causes persistent cough or other chronic respiratory symptoms in children.[8-11] Foreign body aspiration should be suspected in a child between 9 and 36 months of age.[10-13]

Symptoms suggestive of serious etiologies that warrant evaluation include persistent fever, ongoing limitation of activity, failure to grow, cyanosis, respiratory distress, and productive cough with sputum or blood.[2,6] Physical examination may reveal an overinflated chest, wheezing, rales, rhonchi, diminished intensity of breath sounds, coarse crackles, or clubbing of the digits. Chest radiograph is often abnormal.

The most common causes of chronic cough in children are reactive airways (asthma), chronic allergic rhinosinusitis causing postnasal drip, and gastroesophageal reflux disease.[3,4,14] Asthma is the most frequent diagnosis given to children with lingering cough. However, it is important to point out that cough as the sole symptom of asthma is unusual.[13,15,16] The diagnosis of asthma must have other findings such as wheezing, shortness of breath, cough during sleep or exercise, or a family or personal history of atopic symptoms.[10,13] Treatment of cough with underlying pathology is directed toward the specific condition.

In a child with isolated cough, a detailed history and examination should allow the practitioner to distinguish between "benign" cough and cough with pathology.[7] Although some practitioners adopt a prudent "'wait and see'" approach, with reassurance to the parents that the cough is not serious,[15] many practitioners, however, often recommend nonprescription, nonspecific, over-the-counter (OTC) medicines, which in general have not been found to be helpful.[7,17]

Habit cough, sometimes called *psychogenic cough*, is characterized by a cough that occurs as often as several times per minute with regularity, that has lasted for weeks or months, that has been refractory to treatment, that disappears with sleep, and that typically has a harsh, "barking" quality. It typically begins with an upper respiratory infection but then lingers. The child misses many days of school because the cough disrupts the classroom. This cough occurs more frequently in teenagers, who are often referred for psychological and speech therapy.[2,9]

✳ CAM THERAPY RECOMMENDATIONS

Acupuncture

The precise etiology of cough in children, especially chronic cough, needs to be thoroughly evaluated. The following acupuncture recommendations are for *symptomatic* treatment of cough (see also Appendix B).

- For cough with watery phlegm, disperse LU Cold:
  - Four-point protocol: Tonify LU10, HT 8; sedate LU5, KI10.
  - Two-point protocol: Tonify LU10, sedate LU5.
- For cough with yellow, thick phlegm, disperse LU Heat:
  - Four-point protocol: Tonify LU5, KI10; sedate LU10, HT8.
  - Two-point protocol: Tonify LU5, sedate LU10
- Magnets with ion pumping cords and laser can be used.[1]
- General treatment of cough:
  - CV22, LU7
- Treatment of persistent or chronic cough:
  - BL13
  - BL10+LI11[2]
  - BL13+ST40 for cough with abundant phlegm

In Chinese medicine, LU and SP are closely related, especially in children,[1] and because LU is the Yin couple organ to the large intestine (LI), cough may be accompanied by gastrointestinal symptoms such as diarrhea. Diarrhea can be treated separately (see Chapter 30, Diarrhea). SP5 can be used to treat cough and diarrhea with no desire to eat.[3]

Aromatherapy

Essential oils recommended for cough include frankincense (*Boswellia carteri*), spike lavender (*Lavandula spica*), cedarwood (*Cedrus atlantica*), and eucalyptus (*Myrtaceae globulus*).[1,2] Both inhalation and topical application work well. Topically a 0.5% to 2% solution in lotion or oil is rubbed on the chest. The child will inhale the essential oil as it vaporizes, and it will be absorbed through the skin. For inhalation the essential oils can be steamed or diffused in the room. Diffusion is particularly good for a nighttime cough.

Herbs—Chinese

An acute cough proceeds from a common cold through seven distinct stages, each requiring a different herbal prescription, in order to regulate various pathological presentations as heat, cold, dryness, wetness, microbial toxins and phlegm. Bronchiolitis/Croup is considered to be in the lung fire stage. Herbs can be given every 3 or 4 hours for acute cough, and 3 times a day for chronic cough.[1] See Appendix C for manufacturers and dosage administration, as well as Chapter 12, Asthma, and Chapter 15, Bronchiolitis.

Wind-Cold Cough

Wind-Cold cough can be present as an early upper respiratory tract infection or asthma.

Prescription

- Xiao Qing Long Tang (Minor Blue Dragon Decoction) to warm the lungs and dispel pathogenic wind cold.
- Folk-remedy: Grate 1 teaspoon of fresh ginger, steep in boiling water, strain and administer dosage as listed in Appendix C.[1]
- Lung Qi Jr. (Blue Poppy Herb, Boulder, Colo.) is used to treat asthmatic and bronchiolitic coughing and wheezing. It is a formula of 15 herbs that clears heat and transforms phlegm. Dosage is 1 to 2 droppersful for younger children and 3 to 4 droppersful for older children. During an acute asthmatic episode, doses can be given every hour or more frequently, and three times per day during remission.[2]

Wind-Heat Cough

Wind-Heat cough a as a sudden onset of a mild dry cough that often follows a sore throat. It may be considered as the first stage of a common cold.

Prescription

- Sang Ju Yin (Morus, Chrysanthemum Decoction) is used for clearing Wind-Heat and stopping coughing. It is not appropriate for treating a cough with phlegm.[1]
- Chest Relief (Kan Herb Company, Scotts Valley, Calif.) is a formulation of 20 herbs and is designed to soothe the throat and chest, dispel phlegm, aid expectoration, replenish moisture, rectify the Qi of the Lung, and purge Wind and Heat. The formula comes as a liquid alcohol extract. The alcohol can be removed by placing the drops in a little hot water and allowing it to cool before administration. Dosage is

1 dropperful every 3 hours in babies, and 2 to 3 droppersful for children 2 years and older.[2]

Lung-Fire Cough

Lung-Fire cough is an acute, harsh, hacking cough that is often painful to the chest and may be accompanied by sore throat, headache, but without phlegm. Western diagnoses may include croup, bronchiolitis, asthma, and early stages of pertussis. The cough may begin without phlegm and progress to producing thick phlegm.

Prescription

- Qing Fei Yi Huo Pian (Clear Lungs Restrain Fire Tablet) is a strong formula that is used to clear Lung Fire. *Caution:* this formula contains a large amount of Rhubarb Da Huang (Radix et Rhizoma Rhei). If loose stools develop, reduce the dose accordingly.
- Yang Yin Qing Fei Tang Jiang (Support Yin, Clear Lung Decoction Thick-Syrup) is a patent medicine that comes as a syrup and is easily administered to infants every three hours or three times per day.
- Hsiao Keh Chuan: Special Medicine For Bronchitis (Xiao Ke Chuan Zhuan Zhi Qi Guan Yan, "Disperse Cough, Asthma Specific Treat Bronchitis"). This syrup contains a single herb, Rhododendron Man Shan Hong (Radix Rhododendri Daurici), which has strong antibacterial and antiviral effects. Use is limited to three days, administered three times per day.[1]

Pipe Cleaner (Kan-Chinese Modular Solution, Kan Herb Company, Scotts Valley, Calif.) is a formula of 12 herbs designed to treat bronchitis with the accumulation of Phlegm, Heat, and toxins that block the downward movement of Lung Qi, dry up the Yin, and deplete the Qi of the Lung and Kidney. It is indicated when phlegm and expectoration are thick and yellow-green with a slight to moderate fever (temperature <102° F). Dose is 1 dropperful every 3 hours in infants, and 2 to 3 droppersful for children 2 years and older.[2]

Profuse Phlegm-Heat

Profuse Phlegm-Heat apears as a persistent, rattling cough throughout the day and often at night. Older children may expectorate a bright yellow or yellow-phlegm. Younger children tend to swallow their phlegm, but manifest this symptom as a thick nasal discharge. This discharge may correlate to bronchitis and pertussis. Untreated Phlegm-Heat cough can last from seven days to three weeks. Although Chinese herbs are very effective, it can still take three to ten days to completely resolve the symptoms, with progressive lessening of cough and phlegm production.

Prescription

- Qing Qi Hua Tan Wan (Clear Qi, Transform Phlegm Pills) This formula is readily available from many manufacturers. It includes herbs that clear heat, transform phlegm, and stop cough. Administered three times per day, it is often combined with:
- Loquat and Fritillary Extract (Chuan Bei Pi Pa Lu, [Fritillaria, Eriobotrya Liquid]) is a pleasant tasting syrup that helps to relieve cough throughout the day and especially at night.

Sticky Phlegm-Heat Cough

Sticky Phlegm-Heat cough is a chronic, persistent cough that often follows the Phlegm-Heat stage, although it may also be seen after Lung-Fire. The phlegm is scanty, sticky, and difficult to expectorate because of the presence of chronic Heat in the Lungs. The child will cough in an attempt to expectorate.

Prescription

- Ning Sou Wan (Peaceful Cough Pills) The herbs in this formula stop cough, moisten the lung, and clear phlegm.

Profuse Phlegm-Damp Cough

The profuse Phlegm-Damp chronic cough following Phlegm-Heat is uncommon in children and appears with expectoration of white or clear frothy phlegm.

Prescription

- Er Chen Wan (Two-Aged Pill) transforms Phlegm-Damp to stop coughing.

Yin Deficiency Cough

Yin deficiency cough is a chronic, dry, weak cough accompanied by a general lethargy. There may also be hoarse voice and dry throat. The treatment strategy is to moisten the Lung and tonify Lung Qi.

Prescription

- Sha Shen Mai Dong Tang (Glehnia, Ophiopogon Decoction)
- Bai He Gu Jin Wan (Lilium Secure Metal Pills)

Herbs—Western

Eucalyptus oil is widely found in OTC cold remedies and may be applied directly as a decongestant and/or expectorant. However, there is a lack of evidence to establish its effectiveness. Furthermore, direct application of eucalyptus oil in children poses a risk of toxicity, especially in terms of aspiration when ingested, or for central nervous system depression or seizures in children. Camphor may be applied topically as an antitussive; the U.S. Food and Drug Administration (FDA) has approved its use in concentrations less than 11%. However, its use in children has not been proven effective. Furthermore, young children, especially those younger than 12 months, may be vulnerable to its side effects and toxicity, which may be potentially deadly.[1]

White horehound, or *Marrubium vulgare* of the Lamiaceae/Labiatae family, has been used in many medical traditions (Ayurvedic, Native American, and Australian Aboriginal medicines, and even in ancient Egypt) for its expectorant qualities and ingredients assisting in respiratory conditions. The FDA banned horehound from cough drops in 1989 owing to insufficient evidence supporting its effectiveness. However, this herb is used widely in Europe and is found in European-made herbal cough remedies sold in the United States (e.g., Ricola; Ricola, Ltd., Laufen, Switzerland)). Reliable information available about the effectiveness of white horehound is insufficient. Orally, large amounts of white horehound can cause purgative effects.[2,3]

A suggested adult dose is 1 to 2 g dried above-ground parts or 1 cup of tea three times daily before meals as an expectorant.[4] By contrast, there are no specific evidence-based dosage recommendations for children.

Homeopathy

Before using this section, please see Appendix A, Homeopathy, for definitions of practitioner expertise categories and general information on prescribing homeopathic medicines.

Practitioner Expertise Category 1

Category 1 includes acute coughs with no accompanying respiratory distress or coexisting serious conditions.

Practitioner Expertise Categories 2 and 3

Categories 2 and 3 include serious acute coughs, chronic coughs, and coughs associated with other conditions such as asthma.

There are no controlled clinical trials of homeopathic treatment of cough, although the homeopathic literature contains much evidence for its use in the form of accumulated clinical experience.[1] Both acute and chronic coughs can often be treated effectively with homeopathy; however, because cough is a very common symptom with many variations in its symptomatic expression and many associated illnesses and conditions, there are many homeopathic medicines that can treat coughs. This makes accurate homeopathic prescribing a challenging undertaking.

For acute coughs that are not associated with respiratory distress or coexisting serious conditions, it is safe to try homeopathic treatment for a few days prior to beginning conventional therapy. Homeopathy can also be used in conjunction with other treatments for cough, both conventional and alternative. Successful homeopathic treatment of chronic coughs or more serious acute coughs usually requires extensive training in the science and art of homeopathy; therefore the following discussion will focus primarily on relatively minor acute coughs.

The goal in treating cough homeopathically is to determine the single homeopathic medicine whose description in the materia medica most closely matches the symptom picture of the patient. Often mental and emotional states in addition to physical symptoms are considered. Once the medicine has been selected, it can be given orally or sublingually in the 30C potency every 2 to 3 hours, or two to three times daily, depending on the frequency and severity of the cough. If the medicine has not helped in five to six doses, then another homeopathic medicine should be tried or some other form of therapy should be instituted as needed. Once symptoms have begun to resolve, the medicine can be given less frequently or stopped. It can be repeated again for a relapse of symptoms.

The following is a list of homeopathic medicines commonly used to treat patients with cough. It must be emphasized that this list is partial and represents some of the probable choices from the homeopathic materia medica. If the symptoms of a given patient are not represented here, further research in the homeopathic literature would be needed to find the simillimum. For more homeopathic medicines that might be useful in treating cough, see Chapter 15, Bronchiolitis (Croup).

Bryonia alba

The cough requiring *Bryonia alba* is painful; the jarring caused by the cough causes pain in the chest and/or head. The patient may hold the head or chest while coughing. The cough is dry and is worse from deep breathing and eating. The patient may be constipated and thirsty for large amounts of fluid.

Coccus cacti

Coccus cacti is used for a tickling, paroxysmal cough. The cough is worse from 6 to 7 AM or after 11:30 PM. The patient is worse in warm air and better in cold air. The cough may be productive of large amounts of thick mucus that is difficult to expel.

Kali carbonincum

Kali carbonicum covers a dry, tickling cough that is worse from 2 to 4 AM or when first going to sleep. There may be stitching pains in the chest with the cough.

Pulsatilla nigricans

The cough treated with *Pulsatilla nigricans* is loose and rattling. The patient may expel green phlegm. The cough is worse in bed in the evening or night and better from a slow walk in the open air. This medicine covers coughs in children who have otitis media or other upper respiratory tract infection symptoms particularly those accompanied by mucus production.

Rumex crispus

The cough treated with *Rumex crispus* is due to tickling in the anterior throat (larynx and trachea). The cough is worse at 11 PM, from cold air, and when the patient goes from cold air to warm air or warm air to cold air.

Magnet Therapy

Ask the child to point to the area of the neck where he or she feels the cough is starting, and place a ½- or ¾-inch Neodymium spot magnet with the designated north side facing the skin. Next, gently massage the Immune point near the child's elbow. The Immune point near LI11 is located as the child is lying supine with arms placed along the side of the body, dorsal side up and slightly bent at the elbow.[1] The point in this area that is most tender should have the side of the magnet designated as biosouth facing the skin over the Immune point. Magnets on the neck and Immune point may be left in place as long as 30 minutes. These magnets may be obtained from Painfree Lifestyles (800-480-8601).

Massage Therapy

In 1998 Children's Hospital Boston established the Center for Holistic Pediatric Education and Research (CHPER) to provide complementary and alternative medicine consultations and education to inpatients at this hospital. Between 1999 and 2004, 762 consults were provided to patients on the pulmonary service; the chief complaints that initiated the consultation were pain in the back, upper body, chest, and neck as well as anxiety. During acute or chronic respiratory infections, chest, shoulder, neck, and back discomfort may develop from persistent cough.[1-3] This pain or discomfort could lead to ineffective cough and deep breathing as a result of splinting.[1-3] To help decrease the musculoskeletal pain associated with coughing, children experiencing respiratory infections could benefit from back, shoulder, and anterior chest wall massage therapy with particular attention to the intercostals, scalenes, serratus, pectorals, and trapezius. Should cough-related pain or discomfort extend to the abdomen, massage to the intercostals and external obliques may also be helpful. If children are splinting with cough or laughter or indicating that it hurts too much to laugh, this would be a good indication to try some massage to improve their comfort level. Children experiencing respiratory illness may feel more comfortable in an upright position during treatment rather than lying down. To treat the child in an upright position, the child can be positioned in a chair with the head supported by a tabletop pillow or in the parent's lap. Infants and young children can readily be treated while cradled on the parent's shoulder or chest.

In addition to massage being helpful for cough-related pain, massage can also help relax or calm the child or infant who may be experiencing increased work of breathing or intermittent bronchospasms due to illness. Controlled studies have demonstrated decreased anxiety levels in children receiving parental Swedish massage who are diagnosed with asthma or cystic fibrosis.[4,5] These studies have also demonstrated increased peak flow readings and improved pulmonary function tests in the massaged children compared with controls. Small studies in adult populations with pulmonary disease have also demonstrated improved peak flows[6,7] as well as decreased respiratory rate and increased chest wall expansion.[7]

Chest physiotherapy (CPT), which incorporates percussion and vibration, originated from use of massage in postoperative patients in the seventeenth century.[8] CPT has become a standard of care in hospital settings to prevent and treat atelectasis, ineffective cough, and respiratory secretion management.

Mind/Body

Habit Cough

A retrospective chart review study reported 51 children and adolescents who were taught self-hypnosis for habit cough.[1] The habit cough resolved during or immediately after the initial hypnosis instruction session in 78% of subjects, within 1 week in an additional 8%, and within 1 month in an additional 4%. Authors correctly called for controlled prospective clinical studies.

The authors find that working clinically with patients to increasingly lengthen the interval between coughing episodes by using a variety of mind/body techniques, positive self-talk, and physical means (drinking water) to be quite useful. Imagery about reducing the "tickle spot" in the throat and directed therapeutic suggestion about the cough urge not "needing to bother so much" offer effective options within the context of self-hypnosis practice.

References

Pediatric Diagnosis and Treatment

1. Padman R: The child with persistent cough, *Del Med J* 73:149-156, 2001.
2. Behrman RE, Kliegman RM, Jenson HB, editors: *Nelson textbook of pediatrics,* ed 17, Philadelphia, 2004, Saunders.

3. Chow PY, Ng DK: Chronic cough in children, *Singapore Med J* 45:462-468, 2004.

4. Pradal M, Retornaz K, Poisson A: Chronic cough in childhood, *Rev Mal Respir* 21:743-762, 2004. [Article in French.]

5. Chang AB, Lasserson TJ, Gaffney J et al: Gastro-oesophageal reflux treatment for prolonged non-specific cough in children and adults, *Cochrane Database Syst Rev* (2):CD004823, 2005.

6. de Jongste JC, Shields MD: Cough. 2: Chronic cough in children, *Thorax* 58:998-1003, 2003.

7. Bush A: Paediatric problems of cough, *Pulm Pharmacol Ther* 15:309-315, 2002.

8. Jaakkola JJ, Jaakkola MS: Effects of environmental tobacco smoke on the respiratory health of children, *Scand J Work Environ Health* 28(Suppl 2):71-83, 2002.

9. Schwartz J: Air pollution and children's health, *Pediatrics* 113 (4 Suppl):1037-1043, 2004.

10. Donato L, Gaugler C, Weiss L et al: Chronic cough in children: signs of serious disease and investigations, *Arch Pediatr* 8(Suppl 3): 638-644, 2001.

11. Rushton L: Health impact of environmental tobacco smoke in the home, *Rev Environ Health* 19:291-309, 2004.

12. Swanson KL, Edell ES: Tracheobronchial foreign bodies, *Chest Surg Clin N Am* 11:861-872, 2001.

13. Fardy HJ: A coughing child: could it be asthma? *Austr Fam Physician* 33:312-315, 2004.

14. Lack G: Pediatric allergic rhinitis and comorbid disorders, *J Allergy Clin Immunol* 108(1 Suppl):S9-S15, 2001.

15. de Benedictis FM, Selvaggio D, de Benedictis D: Cough, wheezing and asthma in children: lesson from the past, *Pediatr Allergy Immunol* 15:386-393, 2004.

16. Marguet C, Couderc L, Bocquel N et al: Chronic cough, asthma and allergy [in French], *Arch Pediatr* 8(Suppl 3):623-628, 2001.

17. Schroeder K, Fahey T: Over-the-counter medications for acute cough in children and adults in ambulatory settings, *Cochrane Database Syst Rev* (4):CD001831, 2004.

Acupuncture

1. Loo M: *Pediatric acupuncture*, London, 2002, Elsevier.

2. O'Connor J, Bensky D, editors: *Acupuncture, a comprehensive text*, Seattle, 1981, Eastland Press.

3. Deadman P, Al-Khafaji M: *A manual of acupuncture*, Ann Arbor, Mich, 1998, Journal of Chinese Medicine Publications.

Aromatherapy

1. Battaglia S: *The complete guide to aromatherapy*, Virginia, Queensland, Australia, 1995, The Perfect Potion.

2. Price S, Parr PP: *Aromatherapy for babies and children*, San Francisco, 1996, Thorsons.

Herbs—Chinese

1. Fratkin JP: Personal communication, 2005.

2. Neustaedter R: Personal communication, 2005.

Herbs—Western

1. American Academy of Pediatrics Policy Statement: Camphor revisited: focus on toxicity (RE9422), Pediatrics 94:127-128, 1994. Available at: http://www.aap.org/policy/00300.html.

2. Newall CA, Anderson LA, Philpson JD: *Herbal medicine: a guide for healthcare professionals*, London, 1996, Pharmaceutical Press.

3. McGuffin M, Hobbs C, Upton R et al, editors: *American Herbal Products Association's botanical safety handbook*, Boca Raton, Fla, 1997, CRC Press.

4. Wichtl MW: *Herbal drugs and phytopharmaceuticals*, Stuttgart, 1994, Medpharm Scientific (translated by NM Bisset).

Homeopathy

1. *ReferenceWorks Pro 4.2*, San Rafael, Calif, 2008, Kent Homeopathic Associates.

Magnet Therapy

1. Loo M: *Pediatric acupuncture*, London, 2002, Elsevier.

Massage Therapy

1. Boat TF: Cystic fibrosis. In Behrman RE, Kliegman R, Jenson HB, editors: *Nelson's textbook of pediatrics*, ed 17, Philadelphia, 2004, Saunders.

2. Shafer TH, Wolfson MR, Bhutani VK: Respiratory muscle function, assessment and training, *Phys Ther* 61:1711-1723, 1983.

3. Warren A: Mobilization of the chest wall, *Phys Ther* 48:582-585, 1968.

4. Field T, Henteleff T, Hernandez-Reif M et al: Children with asthma have improved pulmonary functions after massage therapy, *J Pediatr* 132:854-858, 1998.

5. Hernandez-Reif M, Field T, Krasnegor J et al: Children with cystic fibrosis benefit from massage therapy, *J Pediatr Psychol* 24: 175-181, 1999.

6. Beeken JE, Parks D, Cory J et al: The effectiveness of neuromuscular release massage therapy in five individuals with chronic obstructive lung disease, *Clin Nurs Res* 7:309-325, 1998.

7. Witt P, MacKinnon J: Psychological integration: a method to improve chest mobility of patients with chronic lung disease, *Phys Ther* 66:214-217, 1986.

8. Fritz S: *Mosby's fundamentals of therapeutic massage*, ed 3, St Louis, 2005, Mosby.

Mind/Body

1. Anbar RD, Hall HR: Childhood habit cough treated with self-hypnosis, *J Pediatr* 144:213-217, 2004.

CHAPTER 28

Depression

Acupuncture | May Loo

Aromatherapy | Maura A. Fitzgerald

Chiropractic | Anne Spicer

Herbs—Western | Alan D. Woolf, Paula M. Gardiner, Lana Dvorkin-Camiel, Jack Maypole

Homeopathy | Janet Levatin

Magnet Therapy | Agatha P. Colbert, Deborah Risotti

Massage Therapy | Mary C. McLellan

Nutrition | Joy A. Weydert

Psychology | Anna Tobia

Spirituality | Tobin Hart

✴ PEDIATRIC DIAGNOSIS AND TREATMENT

Depression among children and adolescents is common but often unrecognized. It affects approximately 2% of prepubertal children and 5% to 8% of adolescents.[1] Childhood depression appears to be the effect of an interaction between genetics and environment. The child with a high genetic risk—a strong family history of depression, especially in parents—may be more vulnerable to adverse environmental stressors such as family disruption, certain chronic or debilitating illnesses, or poor school performance.[1-3] More than one fifth of adolescents with major depression reported suicide attempt.[2] The National Youth Risk Behavior Survey conducted by the Centers for Disease Control and Prevention in 2003 indicated 16.9% of normal adolescents in grades 9 to 12 had seriously considered attempting suicide in the previous 12 months and 8.5% had attempted suicide at least once in that time period.[4] Suicide is the third leading cause of death for adolescents 15 to 19 years old.[3]

The high risk of school failure and suicide necessitate prompt referral or close collaboration with a mental health professional. Evaluation should first include a complete medical assessment to rule out underlying medical causes. A structured clinical interview and various rating scales such as the Pediatric Symptom Checklist are helpful in determining whether a child or adolescent is depressed.[1] The *Diagnostic and Statistical Manual for Primary Care, Child and Adolescent Version*, describes a clinical spectrum of "sadness" symptoms, from sadness problem to a full-blown major depression.[5]

Because childhood depression is frequently comorbid with other psychiatric disorders, it is imperative to rule out other conditions such as anxiety disorder, attention-deficit hyperactivity disorder (ADHD), and conduct disorder.[6] An untreated major depressive episode can last as long as 7 to 9 months, with about 40% recurrence within 2 years and 70% within 5 years. The earlier the onset of depression, the more severe and recurrent the course. Untreated major depression persists into adulthood, resulting in impaired psychological, social, and academic functioning.[2]

Treatment with antidepressants has been controversial. A recent review of studies suggests that the benefit of antidepressants may have been exaggerated and that they may have little clinical significance. Adverse effects of these drugs may have also been downplayed, and pharmaceutical companies often funded clinical trials advocating the use of these drugs.[7] A systematic review of 82 charts revealed that 22% of children treated with selective serotonin reuptake inhibitors (SSRIs) manifested treatment emergent psychiatric adverse events (PAEs), the most common being mood disturbances. PAEs were not associated with psychiatric diagnosis(es), age, sex, concurrent medications, doses, or specific serotonin reuptake inhibitors. The onset of PAE was observed typically 3 months after SSRI exposure (median 91 days).[8] Furthermore, 2 out of 100 patients on SSRI either attempted suicide or exhibited suicidal ideation.[4] On March 22, 2004, the U.S. Food and Drug Administration (FDA) announced that "Prozac (fluoxetine) is [the only SSRI] approved for use in children and adolescents for the treatment of major depressive disorder"; and on September 16, 2004, the FDA released a statement requiring pharmaceutical companies to add a "black box" warning about the increased risk of suicidal behavior with antidepressants in pediatric patients.[9,10] A metaanalysis conducted in Italy investigated the frequency of side effects induced by fluoxetine. The authors concluded that activating side effects (insomnia, agitation, tremor, and anxiety) and gastrointestinal (GI) adverse events (nausea, vomiting, diarrhea, weight loss, and anorexia) were significantly more frequent in fluoxetine-treated patients, whereas cholinergic side effects were significantly less frequent. The side effects often necessitate additional pharmacotherapy or other management strategies, leading to discontinuation, noncompliance, and increasing costs.[11]

Pharmacotherapy appears to be more effective than psychotherapy alone, and combining an SSRI with cognitive-behavioral therapy (CBT) might be more effective in treating depression. The clinician must balance the increased short-term risk of SSRIs versus the potentially decreased long-term risk of suicidal thoughts and behavior due to depression, must follow the FDA's monitoring suggestions, and must inform the family of the potential risks and benefits.[4] A report in 2005 indicates a 10% drop in the number of children taking antidepressants.[12]

The complementary and alternative medicine (CAM) therapist should be informed of the risks, medical treatments, and prognosis of childhood depression and should work closely with the conventional pediatric practitioner. The role of the CAM therapist can be in recommending safe management of untoward physical side effects (e.g., nausea, diarrhea) if the medication needs to be maintained. See the respective sections that correspond to the side effects of Prozac for CAM recommendations such as allergic rash, constipation, headache, nausea, and diarrhea.

✳ CAM THERAPY RECOMMENDATIONS

Acupuncture

Whereas conventional medicine uses depression as a broad diagnosis that encompasses a wide spectrum of symptoms, traditional Chinese medicine (TCM) evaluates the symptoms for specific organ and channel imbalances. The assessment and management is further complicated by the TCM belief that all emotional conditions have a spiritual component.

At the center of depression of any mental-emotional disorder is a disturbance of the Heart, which houses the Mind.[1] The Mind is intimately related to the Ethereal Soul, the Hun, which resides in the Liver. Both Shen and Hun are needed for thinking, consciousness, insight, memory, intelligence, and cognition. The Ethereal Soul provides the Mind with the spiritual "movement" between self-recognition and introspection and the ability to relate to other people and the world.[1]

It is important to tease out the root of the symptoms, as outward manifestation of depression or withdrawal may have originated from an emotion other than sadness; for example, from fear or obsessive thoughts. Because each Yin organ is associated with a major emotion, and all organs have their own Yin-Yang balance within as well as interrelatedness with all the other organs, the diagnosis is a complex interplay of excesses and deficiencies of Qi, Yang, Blood, and Yin.

An experienced acupuncturist would take a detailed history that includes any physical or emotional stress, family history of depression to assess possible genetic (Kidney) predisposition, current and past diet and medications, lifestyle such as excess studying or sports, and a thorough examination with observation, palpation, and listening. A specialized treatment plan needs to be formulated to address the child's specific mental-spiritual symptoms.[1,2] It is also important to recognize that the condition is an ever-evolving one, as the symptom complex undergoes constant changes not only with treatment but also with all internal and external influences. For example, a child who catches a cold can develop lung deficiency that can aggravate his sadness.

The most common causes of childhood depression are Liver Yin deficiency that leads to Heart Yin deficiency, Kidney Yin deficiency, and Spleen deficiency.

Current Evidence-Based Information

There are no current data on acupuncture treatment of depression in children. Although many of the studies in adults seem inadequate[3] and insufficient,[4] a few emerging studies have promising results. A small clinical study from China in which 12 patients were treated with scalp acupuncture revealed increased glucose metabolism in various brain regions with improvement of symptoms in depressed patients.[5] Another small clinical study from China using electroacupuncture (EA) treatments showed acupuncture to have results comparable to medication, with less side effects and better symptomatic improvement.[6] The results from a randomized controlled U.S. study indicates that acupuncture holds promise for the treatment of depression during pregnancy.[7]

A clinical trial demonstrated symptomatic improvement with stimulation of ST36 and GB20, which has been demonstrated in the laboratory to increase intracephalic blood flow and may indirectly increase the quantity of serotonin released.[8] Animal studies demonstrated that EA accelerates the synthesis and release of serotonin (5-HT) and norepinephrine in the central nervous system. Clinical data from China have demonstrated that EA has efficacy similar to that of antidepressants.[9] A Russian clinical study demonstrated that acupuncture normalized blood serotonin levels.[10] A great deal of research is needed.

Treatment Recommendations

A depressed child should be under the care of an experienced acupuncturist who can assess and monitor progress and changes and adjust treatments accordingly. The treatment regimen should also include dietary and lifestyle management, as all children are Spleen deficient, and the modern child tends to have a poor diet and either participates in excess sports and activities or is sedentary, spending hours in front of the television.

A few general points can be used for depression due to any imbalance:

- GV20, Sichenchong, brings clear Qi to the Mind.
- Tonify KI Yin (Chinese medicine posits that one can never overtonify the Kidney): KI3, KI6, BL23.
- Tonify LR Yin (children are constitutionally Yin deficient and liver vulnerable):
  - LR3, LR8, BL18
  - BL47 to root the Ethereal Soul
- Tonify HT Yin: HT7 calms the Mind and nourishes the Heart.
- Tonify Spleen, expel Damp: SP9, UB20, ST40.

Aromatherapy

Aromatherapy in the treatment of depression in children has not been studied. In a non-blinded, randomized study, 32 adults undergoing inpatient or (predominantly) day treatment for depression or anxiety were assigned to receive massage with aromatherapy or massage alone. Treatment was done every 14 days during a 12-week period. Both groups improved in measures of depression and anxiety, but the aromatherapy massage group improvement was significantly greater than the massage-alone group. Patients also reported improvement in other symptoms, including sleep and headaches.[1]

In this author's experience, some adolescents with depression are interested in exploring options to assist their own management of mood. Essential oils can be useful adjuncts to primary therapy. Relaxation essential oils such as lavender (*Lavandula angustifolia*), sweet orange (*Citrus sinensis*), and bergamot (*Citrus bergamia*) are useful if the individual is struggling with insomnia. Alternatively, alerting essential oils can help relieve mental fatigue; these would include peppermint

(*Mentha piperita*), lemon (*Citrus limon*), and rosemary (*Rosmarinus officinalis*). Aromatherapy coupled with massage is a way to offer a pleasurable touch therapy and aid the reduction of any anxiety. Because of the serious effects of depression, it is always important to emphasize that clinical aromatherapy is an adjunctive option and does not replace antidepressant medication or CBT. Because no clear guidelines exist, it is important to work closely with the child or adolescent to develop an aromatherapy plan that is acceptable to the patient.

Chiropractic

There is no specific chiropractic literature pertaining to outcomes of adjustments on depressive states. However, in a text written in 1906 about the works of the founder of chiropractic, D.D. Palmer describes a man with depression and presumably schizophrenia.[1] This man was reported to have found some symptomatic relief when receiving chiropractic adjustments on a regular basis. More recent studies have provided possible explanations for this occurrence. Researchers have demonstrated an increase in endorphin levels within minutes of an upper cervical adjustment.[2,3] Substance P has been used as a treatment for anxiety and depression and has been found to increase following adjustments to the thoracic spine.[4] Corticoid levels are also often increased in depression,[5] and spinal manipulation reduces cortisol, reflecting a decreased stress response.[6] Some evidence exists that depression is associated with a reduced cerebral blood flow.[7,8] The chiropractic adjustment has the ability to increase cerebral circulation.[9,10] Although not a depressive condition, a study involving phobic college students found that the intensity of emotional arousal was diminished after spinal manipulation.[11] Influence over other behavioral conditions is reported by chiropractors in the areas of autism and ADHD. (See Chapter 13, Attention-Deficit Hyperactivity Disorder, and Chapter 14, Autism.) Because anxiety and depression are closely associated with ADHD,[12] the implied relationship is apparent.

Cerebral conditions involving intracranial neurological and neurovascular disorders are commonly associated with subluxation complex at C0 to C4 and T1 to T3.[13]

Aerobic exercise is an important therapeutic approach in reduction of depression.[14,15]

Several nutritional therapies have shown benefit, including omega-3 fatty acids,[16] 5-hydroxytryptophan (5-HTP) with pyridoxal 5 phosphate,[17] L-phenylalanine,[18,19] magnesium with calcium,[17] and S-adenosylmethionine.[20]

Herbal remedies that may also be of benefit are St. John's wort,[21] valerian, and kava kava.[22]

Herbs—Western

All adults and children who suffer from severe depression require the support and involvement of a healthcare provider. St. John's wort is the most extensively studied herbal therapy. Taken orally, most studies have evaluated St. John's wort in mild to moderately depressed adults. However, there is also some evidence that it might be effective for mild to moderate depression in children 6-16 years old.[1,2] Taken orally, St. John's wort is usually well tolerated. Side effects can include insomnia, vivid dreams, restlessness, anxiety, agitation, irritability, GI discomfort, fatigue, dry mouth, dizziness, and headache. Furthermore, it should be used cautiously owing to the potential side effects and interactions. St. John's wort users may suffer from photosensitivity. Caution is advised for multiple potential drug interactions, including reduced therapeutic effect of digitalis and antiretroviral medication, oral contraceptives, cyclosporine, and others.[1,3,4]

5-HTP is often produced commercially from the seeds of the African plant *Griffonia simplicifolia* and may be effective against treatment-resistant depression in adults. Evidence of its effectiveness in children is insufficient Notably, impurities exist in 5-HTP that have been implicated in causing potentially fatal eosinophilia-myalgia syndrome.[5,6] Thus 5-HTP use in children should be avoided.

There are no evidence and/or clinical trials to assess the effectiveness of *Ginkgo biloba* for the treatment of depression in children. It has been assessed in adults for seasonal affective disorder but was not found to be an effective treatment.[5,7]

Homeopathy

Before using this section, please see Appendix A, Homeopathy, for definitions of practitioner expertise categories and general information on prescribing homeopathic medicines.

Practitioner Expertise Category 3

There are no controlled clinical trials of homeopathy for childhood depression, although the homeopathic literature contains evidence for its use in the form of accumulated clinical experience.[1] Homeopathic treatment can be used safely and effectively for childhood depression, either alone or in combination with other treatment modalities, both alternative and conventional. Because childhood depression is a complex and multifaceted problem, successful homeopathic treatment usually requires extensive training in the art and science of homeopathy. Any one of many homeopathic medicines may be used to treat childhood depression, depending on the characteristics of the patient being treated; sophisticated homeopathic analysis and long-term follow-up are required. For these reasons specific medicines for treating childhood depression will not be presented here. Interested readers are referred to Reichenberg-Ullman and Ullman's *Prozac-Free*,[2] the most comprehensive discussion of the use of homeopathy for depression in adults and children.

Magnet Therapy

For children 12 years of age and older, apply alternating bionorth/biosouth magnets (9000 G Accuband 9000 REC magnets) to Nagano's toe points for 20 minutes daily for 2 weeks. This treatment can be repeated when needed. Nagano's toe points are the traditional TCM Ba Fen points. They are located on the dorsal aspect of the foot at the four web spaces. These magnets may be obtained from OMS (800-323-1839) or AHSM (800-635-7070).

Massage Therapy

In addition to promoting opportunities for relaxation, receiving massage therapy on a regular basis decreased anxiety[1-12] and depression scores in a large number of randomized controlled trials.[3,6-7,10-12] Consistently controlled trials of children with psychiatric disorders have reported decreased symptoms of psychiatric disturbances, decreased anxiety, decreased depression, and improved behavior ratings.[13-17]

Because depression is not a musculoskeletal disorder, no particular type of massage modality has been identified as more beneficial than another for treating patients with depression. Many patients report that they feel improved after massage treatments that have a component of energy work integrated into the session. Many of the massage modalities incorporated with the structural integration realm may be difficult for a patient suffering from depression, as the patient is expected to take an active role in his or her own therapy (i.e., homework exercises between sessions). This active expectation may be overwhelming for some depressed patients.

If the depression has been induced from a chronic disease process, the massage modality may need to vary based upon the patient's physical needs and restrictions.

Nutrition

The etiology of depression in children cannot be explained by one mechanism, as it is likely a combination of biology, personality traits, and life events. Other etiological theories include neurotransmitter imbalance or change in neurotransmitter receptor function,[1,2] hypothalamic-pituitary-adrenal (HPA) axis activation,[3] imbalance of essential fatty acids,[4] vitamin and mineral depletion, food/chemical/environmental allergies,[5] or low albumin levels.[6]

The essential amino acids are precursors to the neurotransmitters associated with depressions: serotonin, norepinephrine, phenylethylamine, and histamine. Hypoalbuminemia and tryptophan-depleted diets have been associated with increased symptoms of depression, which are reversible when the essential amino acids are supplied.[7,8] Amino acids are converted to the active neurotransmitters in the presence of the B vitamins, Vitamin C, zinc, copper, and magnesium. Deficiencies in these essential nutrients prevent the production of neurotransmitters, leading to symptoms of depression.[9] Increased stress and the production of cortisol downregulates the serotonin receptors and increases the catabolism of tryptophan, further causing a decrease in serotonin.[10]

The essential fatty acids help maintain normal function of all cell membranes and improve the function of serotonin receptors. The addition of omega-3 fatty acid was found to have benefits when added to standard treatment of unipolar depression.[4] Essential fatty acids are natural antiinflammatory agents and therefore decrease the production of cytokines and histamine, which can contribute to neurotransmitter imbalance.

Food/chemical/environmental sensitivities can cause an imbalance of histamine, norepinephrine, and acetylcholine via an inflammatory response, triggering symptoms of depression.[5] Excess glutamate or aspartame is neurotoxic for most humans. Any exogenous intake of these in the diet, such as through MSG or artificial sweeteners, may be enough to disrupt the neurotransmitter balance. Hypoglycemia has been associated with mood disorders and may be a reaction to sugar, caffeine, or alcohol.

Treatment

- Balance and restore normal neurotransmitter levels through a diet complete in the essential amino acids, vitamins, and minerals. Symptoms of irritability, anxiety, and sleeplessness indicate a relative lack of serotonin; therefore increasing tryptophan in the presence of vitamins B and C may be of benefit. Tryptophan is abundant in turkey, nuts, soybeans, and cooked beans and peas. If symptoms of lethargy, fatigue, hypersomnolence, and immobility predominate, more tyrosine may be needed to boost norepinephrine levels. Tyrosine is found in eggs, aged cheese, tofu, and seafood. Key vitamins and minerals are found naturally in a variety of fruits, vegetables, whole grains, seeds, and nuts.
- Replace and balance the essential fatty acids, particularly omega-3 fatty acids. These are found in cold-water fish and fish oils, flax seeds and oil, hemp seeds and oil, walnuts, and algae.
- Correct or prevent hypoglycemia by limiting or completely eliminating intakes of refined sugar products, caffeine, and alcohol. Following a low glycemic load diet will promote a better range of blood sugar levels.
- Assess for food and environmental sensitivities by measuring immunoglobulin (Ig)-E and IgG antibodies for acute and delayed sensitivity reactions, respectively. Eliminate those foods that are most problematic.

Psychology

The etiological pathway to the development of depression in children is complex and differs for each child. The prevailing conceptual model that underlies most CAM psychological interventions is a diathesis-stress model. In this framework, stress interacts with vulnerability within the child and results in a depressive disorder. The onset of stress can be chronic or acute and can include things such as a chronic medical condition, daily hassles, major life events, and family stress such as insecure attachment, conflict, or separation. The diathesis may involve neurohormonal dysregulation, family history of depression, or negative and hopeless attribution styles.[1]

Cognitive behavioral therapy (CBT) is a widely used approach to treating depression that focuses on both the diathesis and stress aspects of the disorder.[2] From this perspective, depression is characterized by a disturbance in cognitions that is activated by vulnerability to stressful events. The cognitive disturbance produces a negative distortion in the way the child sees himself (e.g., "I am stupid"), his world (e.g., "All the teachers hate me"), and his future (e.g., "I'll never be good in school).[3]

CBT focuses on the development of healthier ways of interpreting and responding to situations and people. By teaching effective ways to stop negative thoughts and counter them with positive thoughts, CBT seeks to alter the core psychological mechanism believed to underlie depression and, in so doing, it is effective at reducing the severity of depression and producing remission of symptoms.[4] A form of CBT known as the *Coping with Depression Intervention* emphasizes identifying and changing depressive cognitions, developing healthier coping strategies, and seeking out pleasurable activities and positive social interactions.[5] Another effective component to CBT may include relaxation training to enhance coping with stress.[6]

Family members can also be included in CBT with a depressed child. Family education about depression and the impact of pervasive negative thinking can promote a more supportive family environment. Parents can also be instrumental in transferring the skills learned in therapy into the home environment. For example, therapy may include discussion of emotional spirals such as how people's responses to stress (their behavior and cognitions) can create downward spirals in which they feel worse or upward spirals in which they feel better.[7] Parents can help support upward spirals. Similarly, an important component of CBT is increasing pleasurable activities. Parents can help arrange fun events for their children and can encourage participation. Finally, parents may be unaware of ways that they contribute to their child's depression. For example, statements such as "You are a failure" or "You will never amount to anything" support and contribute to the cognitive disturbances that underlie the depressive symptoms.

Treatment Recommendations

Once a child has experienced a depressive episode, it is more likely that they will experience depression again in the future. Therefore effective treatment must teach skills to manage the symptoms of depression and cope with future stress.[4] A CAM psychologist would begin treatment by teaching children to identify and manage feelings more effectively. Most depressed children are unaware of the connection among their thoughts, feelings, and behavior.

One activity that can be helpful is a version of the game Pictionary, in which different emotions are written on index cards and the player guesses the emotion based on the drawing. The child and therapist alternate choosing cards and then drawing a picture of a person experiencing that feeling (i.e., what the person might be doing), and then identifying the negative thoughts that accompany the scene. For example, if the emotion is "sad," the drawing could be of a child sitting alone in his bedroom. The thought might be, "All of the kids hate me—I'll never have any friends." The therapist and child could then discuss what could be done to feel better (e.g., play with siblings, find neighbors to play with, arrange a play date). Another version of this is to act out the emotions, rather than draw them, and then provide a solution using more adaptive coping.

Children tend to draw or act themes from their own life, which can be discussed as well. Children can write down their negative, depressive cognitions (e.g., "it will never work," "I'm a loser," "I can't pass this class," "the teacher hates me") and then write down counter-positive thoughts (e.g., "I can try to make it work," "I have good qualities," "if I get extra help and finish my assignment I will pass," "my teacher was probably just upset that I haven't done my work"). By countering every negative thought with a more positive one, life will not seem so gloomy and hopeless.

Depressed children tend to dwell on the negative aspects of life. A sticker chart that keeps track of fun activities and good things can help increase awareness of the positive. Sometimes depressed children do not anticipate pleasure from activities, so they tend not to look forward to things and are more resistant to participating. It can be helpful to have them rate how much fun they think something will be on a scale of 1 to 10 and then rate how much fun it actually was. This will increase awareness of the impact of depressive distortions.

In being able to more realistically appraise life events and problem solve, and also by being more aware of their emotional state, children will be more likely to have a positive mood and maintain their improvements over time.

Spirituality

There is little literature on spiritual or religious intervention of childhood depression.[1,2]

Symptoms can emerge from different roots, and childhood depression is no exception. What appears as depression may have roots ranging from nutritional deficiency (e.g., anemia) to parental conflict to existential crises to alleged past life memory. As a result, accurate assessment is particularly important if treatment is to extend beneath the surface of the symptom and offer fundamental and enduring healing. In cases such as depression, simply ameliorating the symptom may mask the more serious, underlying conditions—the root that has generated the symptom. The symptom may temporarily go underground only to return, perhaps in a more entrenched and dangerous manifestation. Beyond basic psychological, psychosocial, and even cultural and religious assessment, a "spiritual" assessment may be revealing. This assessment invites questions about meaning and hope, boundaries and connections, multidimensional perceptions, and sources of comfort and counsel,[3,4] which may reveal sources of pathology and healing. For example, recognizing a source of inner wisdom or developing capacity for awareness may provide a life-long healing resource. Because of the different etiological paths, it is impossible to provide a generic intervention method. Accurate and ongoing interactive assessment is essential. A sample case presentation can illustrate the spiritual approach.

"Jane," aged 10, had previously been diagnosed with mood, eating, and sleep disorders. Physical examinations revealed no unusual findings; psychosocial assessment did not reveal family conflict, abuse history, residual grief, or other contributing factors. Prepubescent hormones may have amplified emotional responses but did not seem to be a primary cause. No learning difficulties appeared present. Although she had a history of friendships, she increasingly seemed to withdraw from others. She would sleep long hours, was described as very withdrawn, experienced suicidal ideation at times, and sometimes had intense emotional outbursts. In a spirituality-oriented assessment, it was discovered that that she was extremely sensitive to others' emotional states. She recognized that she often picked up others' feelings but was not sure what to do with this sensitivity and was sometimes overwhelmed both with others' feelings and also her own sense of hopelessness at wanting to help others. In treatment, her deep or transpersonal experience of empathy was acknowledged and explained, giving her a possible map for understanding the liabilities and value of her empathic capacity.[5] She then was coached in discerning between her own feelings and those feelings that might belong to another. Through some simple questioning and practice she developed an awareness of the qualitative difference in her thinking or feeling, and especially her bodily sensations, between responses that seemed to come from within her and those that seemed to come from someone else. In addition, explicit questions such as "What color is this? Where is it in your body? What shape (e.g., movement, density, texture, sound, taste) does it have? What comes to mind when you pay attention to this? What does it have to say?" may be helpful to bring awareness to these sensations. Through this simple process of enhancing her awareness of what is "hers" and what is "not hers," the depression started "moving" or "breaking up," and its impact on Jane's emotional well-being began to decrease.

A home regimen could also help Jane clear unwanted energy. She often seemed overwhelmed and either agitated or exhausted upon returning home from a school day. She and her mother would sit in front of each other in silence for a few minutes, touch hands, set an intention or prayer to release safely into the universe any accumulated energy that was not helpful, and then take some deep breaths together. Sometimes they imagined this energy draining out of their bodies. This provided a very simple clearing that seemed to work remarkably well. (The notion of picking up "airs" or "wind" or energy from a place or a person is recognized in Native American tradition and is traditionally cleared through ritual smudging with a plant such as sage.)

In the heat of a difficult or sensitive day, an empathically sensitive child (or adult) may just need to form a temporary boundary. A simple technique of imaging a bubble around oneself, perhaps in a favorite color that may turn opaque as needed, can sometimes provide a sense of protection and modulation from the day's energy.

In addition to simple awareness, imagery, and clearing practices, helping the child to develop the capacity to witness the contents of consciousness (e.g., feelings) rather than just being reactive to them is an important centering skill found in many traditions. William James referred to this distinction as the difference between being awash in the "me"—the content of our consciousness, such as thoughts, feelings, and sensations—and witnessing from the "I".[6] To do so, Jane was invited to notice how a situation seemed when she concentrated on her solar plexus, above the diaphragm, a region typically more emotionally reactive, and then in turn notice the scene when her attention was moved to her "third eye," a point in the center of the forehead between the eyebrows. With the latter, one typically notices a less reactive, clearer, more spacious view of a situation, which provides a kind of centered, nonattached, witness position rather than an emotionally reactive or overwhelmed one. Children are surprisingly adept at developing this kind of awareness.

Empathic capacity often leads to compassion. Empathy has been described as the root of moral development and even the quality that makes people most human.[7,8] When an individual connects so directly with the experience of another, compassion may be a natural outcome. Sometimes natural compassion extends beyond people to entire nations, nature, or perhaps the whole planet. The result is that an overwhelming sense of responsibility, frustration for not being able to help, and ultimately demoralization and hopelessness at one's impotence in the face of the world's needs may emerge. In such a situation it can be helpful for a young person to find the means and power of compassionate service. All expressions of love are maximal. Like a drop of water, which has the same composition as a whole ocean, an expression of compassion, whatever the scale, contains the same nourishing spiritual power. Thus although children might not be able to solve all the world's

problems, they can express the energy of compassion by offering what they can. Perhaps they may walk by a homeless person and offer a glance, the next day say a prayer or a hello, another day give a sandwich, and one distant day perhaps they serve in some new way. The challenge is just to get the compassionate energy moving in some way; the result to the giver is nourishment and movement; without it, they may feel discouragement or harden their hearts as a form of protection.

This difficulty represents one small consideration of a type of spiritual-oriented treatment. In this instance, appropriate assessment was especially important to direct treatment.

References

Pediatric Diagnosis and Treatment

1. Son SE, Kirchner JT: Depression in children and adolescents, *Am Fam Physician* 62:2297-2308, 2311-2312, 2000.
2. Jenkins RR: Depression. In Behrman RE, Kliegman RM, Jenson HB, editors: *Nelson's textbook of pediatrics*, ed 17, Philadelphia, 2004, Saunders.
3. AAP Policy Statement, Committee on Adolescence: Suicide and suicide attempts in adolescents, *Pediatrics* 105:871-874, 2000.
4. Wachter K: Balance SSRI benefits with risks for children, *Pediatric News* 39:23, 2005.
5. American Psychological Association: *Diagnostic and statistical manual of mental disorders, fourth edition (DSM-IV)*, Washington, DC, 1994, American Psychiatric Press.
6. Ryan ND: Diagnosing pediatric depression, *Biol Psychiatry* 49:1050-1054, 2001.
7. Jureidini JN, Doecke CJ, Mansfield PR et al: Efficacy and safety of antidepressants for children and adolescents, *Br Med J* 328: 879-883, 2004.
8. Wilens TE, Biederman J, Kwon A et al: A systematic chart review of the nature of psychiatric adverse events in children and adolescents treated with selective serotonin reuptake inhibitors, *J Child Adolesc Psychopharmacol* 13:143-152, 2003.
9. U.S. Food and Drug Administration: *Antidepressant use in children, adolescents, and adults*, 2004. Available at www.fda.gov/cder/drug/antidepressants/default.htm. Accessed February 12, 2008.
10. AAP Priority Drugs and Pediatric Labeling Education Project Advisory Committee: Prozac labeled as safe, effective for depression in children, *AAP News* Jun:26-28, 2005.
11. Brambilla P, Cipriani A, Hotopf M et al: Side-effect profile of fluoxetine in comparison with other SSRIs, tricyclic and newer antidepressants: a meta-analysis of clinical trial data, *Pharmacopsychiatry* 38:69-77, 2005.
12. Kilgore C: Antidepressant prescriptions for youth drop 10%, *Pediatric News* 39:1, 24, 2005.

Acupuncture

1. Maciocia G: *The foundations of Chinese medicine, a comprehensive text for acupuncturists and herbalists*, London, 1989, Churchill Livingstone.
2. Schnyer RN: Personal communications, 2005.
3. Smith CA, Hay PP: Acupuncture for depression, *Cochrane Database Syst Rev* (2):CD004046, 2005.
4. Mukaino Y, Park J, White A et al: The effectiveness of acupuncture for depression—a systematic review of randomised controlled trials, *Acupunct Med* 23:70-76, 2005.
5. Huang Y, Li DJ, Tang AW et al: Effect of scalp acupuncture on glucose metabolism in brain of patients with depression [in Chinese], *Zhongguo Zhong Xi Yi Jie He Za Zhi* 25:119-122, 2005 (abstract).

6. Han C, Li X, Luo H et al: Clinical study on electro-acupuncture treatment for 30 cases of mental depression, *J Tradit Chin Med* 24:172-176, 2004.

7. Manber R, Schnyer RN, Allen JJ et al: Acupuncture: a promising treatment for depression during pregnancy, *J Affect Disord* 83:89-95, 2004.

8. Chen A: An introduction to sequential electric acupuncture (SEA) in the treatment of stress related physical and mental disorders, *Acupunct Electrother Res* 17:273-283, 1992.

9. Han JS: Electroacupuncture: an alternative to antidepressants for treating affective diseases? *Int J Neurosci* 29:79-92, 1986.

10. Markelova VF, Belitskaia RA, Mikhailova AA et al: Serotoninergic and catecholaminergic indices in patients with neurotic and depressive disorders and changes in them as a result of reflexotherapy [in Russian], *Zh Nevropatol Psikhiatr Im S S Korsakova* 86:1708-1712, 1986 (abstract).

Aromatherapy

1. Lemon K: An assessment of treating depression and anxiety with aromatherapy, *Int J Aromatherapy* 14:63-69, 2004.

Chiropractic

1. Palmer BJ: *The science of chiropractic*, Davenport, Iowa, 1906, The Palmer School of Chiropractic.

2. Vernon HT, Dhami MS, Howley TP et al: Spinal manipulation and beta-endorphin: a controlled study of the effect of a spinal manipulation on plasma beta-endorphin levels in normal males, *J Manipulative Physiol Ther* 9:115-123, 1986.

3. Christian GF, Stanton GJ, Sissons D et al: Immunoreactive ACTH, beta-endorphin, and cortisol levels in plasma following spinal manipulative therapy, *Spine* 13:1411-1317, 1988.

4. Brennan PC, Triano JJ, McGregor M et al: Enhanced neutrophil respiratory burst as a biological marker for manipulation forces: duration of the effect and association with substance P and tumor necrosis factor, *J Manipulative Physiol Ther* 15:83-89, 1992.

5. Leach RA, Burgess SC: Neuroimmune hypothesis. In Leach RA, editor: *The chiropractic theories: a textbook of scientific research*, Baltimore, 2004, Lippincott Williams and Wilkins.

6. Rosner A: Endocrine disorders. In Masarsky CS, Todres-Masarsky M, editors: *The somatovisceral aspects of chiropractic*, Philadelphia, 2001, Churchill Livingstone.

7. Mathew RJ, Unwin DH: Cerebral blood flow in depression, *Am J Psychiatry* 137:1449-1450, 1980.

8. Mathew RJ, Weinman ML, Barr DL: Personality and regional cerebral blood flow, *Br J Psychiatry* 144:529-532, 1984.

9. Risley W: Impaired arterial blood flow to the brain as a result of a cervical subluxation: a clinical report, *J Am Chiropractic Assoc* 32:61, 1995.

10. Haldeman S: The influence of the autonomic nervous system on cerebral blood flow, *J Can Chiropractic Assoc* 18:6, 1974.

11. Peterson DB: The effects of spinal manipulation on the intensity of emotional arousal in phobic subjects exposed to a threat stimulus: a randomized, controlled double-blind clinical trial, *J Manipulative Physiol Ther* 20:602-606, 1997.

12. Power TJ, Costigan TE, Eiraldi RB et al: Variations in anxiety and depression as a function of ADHD subtypes defined by DSM-IV: do subtype differences exist or not? *J Abnorm Child Psychol* 32:27-37, 2004.

13. Lawrence DJ, editor: *Fundamentals of chiropractic diagnosis and management*, Baltimore, 1991, Williams and Wilkins.

14. Martinsen EW: Benefits of exercise for the treatment of depression, *Sports Med* 9:380-390, 1990.

15. Martinsen EW, Medhus A, Sandivik L: Effects of aerobic exercise on depression: a controlled study, *Br Med J* 291:109-111, 1985.

16. Stoll AL, Severus WE, Freeman MP et al: Omega-3 fatty acids in bipolar disorder: a preliminary double-blind placebo-controlled trial, *Arch Gen Psychiatry* 56:407-412, 1999.

17. Souza TA: *Differential diagnosis and management for the chiropractor: protocols and algorithms*, ed 3, Sudbury, Mass, 2005, Jones and Bartlett.

18. Von Prang HM, Lemus C: Monoamine precursors in the treatment of psychiatric disorders. In Wurtman RJ, Wurtman JJ, editors: *Nutrition and the brain*, New York, 1986, Raven Press.

19. Sabelli HC, Fawcett J, Gusovsky F et al: Clinical studies on the phenylethylamine hypothesis of affective disorder: urine and blood phenylacetic acid and phenylalanine dietary supplements, *J Clin Psychiatry* 47:66-70, 1986.

20. Bressa GM: S-Adenosyl-1-methionine (SAMe) as antidepressant: meta-analysis of clinical studies, *Acta Neurol Scand* 154:S7-S14, 1994.

21. Linde D, Ramirez G, Mulrow CD et al: St. John's wort for depression—an overview and meta-analysis of randomized clinical trials, *Br Med J* 313:253-258, 1996.

22. DeSmet P: Herbal remedies, *N Engl J Med* 347:2046-2056, 2002.

Herbs—Western

1. Hubner WD, Kirste T: Experience with St. John's wort *(Hypericum perforatum)* in children under 12 years with symptoms of depression and psychovegetative disturbances, *Phytother Res* 15:367-370, 2001.

2. Walter G, Rey JM: Use of St. John's wort by adolescents with a psychiatric disorder, *J Child Adolesc Psychopharmacol* 9:301-311, 1999.

3. Hennessy M, Kelleher D, Spiers JP et al: St. John's wort increases expression of P-glycoprotein: implications for drug interactions, *Br J Clin Pharmacol* 53:75-82, 2002.

4. Findling RL, McNamara NK, O'Riordan MA et al: An open-label pilot study of St. John's wort in juvenile depression, *J Am Acad Child Adolesc Psychiatry* 42:908-914, 2003.

5. *Natural medicines in clinical management of depression*. Available at www.naturaldatabase.com. Accessed Jan 4, 2005.

6. U.S. Food and Drug Administration: *Information paper on L-tryptophan and 5-hydroxy-L-tryptophan*, Office of Nutritional Products, Labeling, Dietary Supplements; Center for Food Safety and Applied Nutrition, Feb 2001.

7. Lingaerde O, Foreland AR, Magnusson A: Can winter depression be prevented by *Ginkgo biloba* extract? A placebo-controlled trial, *Acta Psychiatr Scand* 100:62-66, 1999.

Homeopathy

1. *ReferenceWorks Pro 4.2*, San Rafael, Calif, 2008, Kent Homeopathic Associates.

2. Reichenberg-Ullman J, Ullman R: *Prozac-free*, ed 2, Berkeley, Calif, 2002, North Atlantic Books.

Massage Therapy

1. Hernandez-Reif M, Field T, Krasnegor J et al: Lower back pain is reduced and range of motion increased after massage therapy, *Int J Neurosci* 106:131-145, 2001.

2. Fraser J, Kerr JR: Psycho-physiological effects of back massage on elderly institutionalized patients, *J Adv Nurs* 18:238-245, 1993.

3. Field T, Ironson G, Scafidi F et al: Massage therapy reduces anxiety and enhances EEG patterns of alertness and math computations, *Int J Neurosci* 3:197-205, 1996.

4. Field T, Peck M, Krugman S et al: Burn injuries benefit from massage therapy, *J Burn Care Rehabil* 19:241-244, 1998.

5. Moyer CA, Rounds J, Hannum JW: A meta-analysis of massage therapy research, *Psychol Bull* 130:3-18, 2004.

6. Field T, Morrno C, Valdeon C et al: Massage reduces anxiety in child and adolescent psychiatric patients, *J Am Acad Adolesc Psychiatry* 31:125-131, 1992.

7. Field T, Sunshine W, Hernandez-Reif M et al: Chronic fatigue syndrome: massage therapy effects of depression and somatic symptoms in chronic fatigue, *J Chronic Fatigue Syndr* 3:43-51, 1997.

8. Post-White J, Kinney ME, Savik K et al: Therapeutic massage and healing touch improve symptoms in cancer, *Integr Cancer Ther* 2:332-344, 2003.

9. Schachner L, Field T, Hernandez-Reif M et al: Atopic dermatitis decreased in children following massage therapy, *Pediatr Dermatol* 15:390-395, 1998.

10. Field T, Peck M, Scd et al: Post-burn itching, pain, and psychological symptoms are reduced with massage therapy, *J Burn Care Rehabil* 21:189-193, 2000.

11. Rexilius SJ, Mundt C, Erikson Megel M et al: Therapeutic effects of massage therapy and handling touch on caregivers of patients undergoing autologous hematopoietic stem cells, *Oncol Nurs Forum* 29:E35-E44, 2002.

12. Sunshine W, Field T, Quintino O et al: Fibromyalgia benefits from massage therapy and transcutaneous electrical stimulation, *J Clin Rheumatol* 2:18-22, 1996.

13. Cullen L, Barlow J: 'Kiss, cuddle, squeeze': the experiences and meaning of touch among parents of children with autism attending a Touch Therapy Programme, *J Child Health Care* 6:171-181, 2002.

14. Field T, Lasko D, Mundy P et al: Brief report: autistic children's attentiveness and responsivity improve after touch therapy, *J Autism Devel Disord* 27:333-338, 1997.

15. Field T, Quintino O, Hernandez-Reif M et al: Adolescents with attention deficit hyperactivity disorder benefit from massage therapy, *Adolescence* 33:105-108, 1998.

16. Field T, Schanberg S, Kuhn C et al: Bulimic adolescents benefit from massage therapy, *Adolescence* 33:557-563, 1998.

17. Jones NA, Field T: Massage and music therapies attenuate frontal EEG asymmetry in depressed adolescents, *Adolescence* 34:529-534, 1999.

Nutrition

1. Melzter H: Serotonergic dysfunction in depression, *Br J Psychiatry* 155:25-31, 1989.

2. Delgado PL, Moreno FA: Role of norepinephrine in depression, *J Clin Psychiatry* 61(Suppl 1):5-12, 2000.

3. Pichot W, Herrera C, Ansseau M: HPA axis dysfunction in major depression: relationship to 5-HT$_{1A}$ receptor activity. *Neuropsychobiology* 44:74-77, 2001.

4. Nemets B, Stahl Z, Belmaker RH et al: Addition of omega-3 fatty acids to maintenance medication treatment for recurrent unipolar depressive disorder, *Am J Psychiatry* 159:477-479, 2002.

5. Rapp DJ: *Is this your child's world? How you can fix the schools and homes that are making your child sick*, New York, 1997, Bantam.

6. Huang SY, Chiu CC, Shen WW et al: Hypoalbuminemia in drug-free patients with major depressive disorder compared with a dietary matched control group: a clinical meaning beyond malnutrition, *Eur Neuropsychopharmacol* 15:227-230, 2005.

7. Spillman MK, Van der Does AJ, Rankin MA et al: Tryptophan depletion in SSRI-recovered depressed patients, *Psychopharmacology* 155:123-127, 2001.

8. Van Praag HM: : Serotonin precursors in the treatment of depression, *Adv Biochem Psychopharmacol* 34:259-286, 1982.

9. Young SN: The use of diet and dietary components in the study of factors controlling affect in humans: a review, *J Psychiatry Neurosci* 18:235-244, 1993.

10. De Souza E: Corticotropin-releasing factor receptors: physiology, pharmacology, biochemistry and role in central nervous system and immune disorders, *Psychoneuroendocrinology* 20:789-819, 1995.

Psychology

1. Burke P, Elliott M: Depression in pediatric chronic illness, *Psychosomatics* 40:5-17, 1999.

2. Southham-Gerow MA, Kendall PC: Cognitive-behaviour therapy with youth: Advances, challenges, and future directions, *Clin Psychol Psychother* 7:5, 2000.

3. Kendall PC, Strak KD, Adam T: Cogntive deficit or cognitive distortion in childhood depression, *J Abnorm Child Psychol* 18:255-270, 1990.

4. Stark K, Sander JB, Yancy MG et al: Treatment of depression in childhood and adolescence. In Kendall PC, editor: *Child and adolescent therapy*, New York, 2000, Guilford Press.

5. Lewinsohn PM, Clarke GN, Hops H et al: Cognitive-behavioral treatment for depressed adolescents, *Behav Ther* 21, 1990.

6. Roberts MC, Lazicki-Puddy TA, Puddy RW et al: The outcomes of psychotherapy with adolescents: a practitioner-friendly research review, *J Clin Psychol* 59:1177-1191, 2003.

7. Asarnow JR, Scott CV, Mintz J: A combined cognitive-behavioral family education intervention for depression in children: a treatment development study, *Cognitive Ther Res* 26:2, 2002.

Spirituality

1. Houskamp BM, Fisher LA, Stuber ML: Spirituality in children and adolescents: research findings and implications for clinicians and researchers, *Child Adolesc Psychiatr Clin N Am* 13:221-230, 2004.

2. Little TD, Perez JE: 2003 religiousness and depressive symptoms among adolescents, *J Clin Child Adolesc Psychol* 32:267, 2003.

3. Hart T: *The secret spiritual world of children*, Makawao, Hawaii, 2003, Inner Ocean.

4. Hart T, Waddell A: *Spiritual issues in counseling and psychotherapy: toward assessment and treatment*, 2003. Available at www.childspirit.net/hart%20and%20waddell.pdf. Accessed August 26, 2004.

5. Hart T: Deep empathy. In Hart T, Nelson PL, Puhakka K, editors: *Transpersonal knowing: exploring the horizon of consciousness*, Albany, NY, 2000, State University of New York Press, pp 253-270.

6. James W: *The varieties of religious experience*, New York, 1936, Modern Library.

7. Azar B: Defining the trait that makes us most human, *APA Monitor* 28:1-15, 1997.

8. Hoffman ML: Empathy and justice motivation, *Motivation Emotion* 14:151-172, 1990.

CHAPTER 29

Diaper Rash (Yeast Infection)

Acupuncture | May Loo

Aromatherapy | Maura A. Fitzgerald

Herbs—Chinese | Catherine Ulbricht, Jennifer Woods, Mark Wright

Herbs—Western | Alan D. Woolf, Paula M. Gardiner, Lana Dvorkin-Camiel, Jack Maypole

Homeopathy | Janet L. Levatin

Massage Therapy | Mary C. McLellan

✴ PEDIATRIC DIAGNOSIS AND TREATMENT

Irritant diaper dermatitis (IDD) occurs when there is disruption of the barrier function of the skin through prolonged contact with feces and urine in a non–toilet trained or an incontinent child.[1] It usually peaks between 7 and 12 months of age.[2] The inflammation of the skin covered by the diaper is caused by an interaction of multiple factors: increased wetness, elevated pH due to urine, fecal enzymes, and microorganisms.[3]

In addition, children are more vulnerable because the adult sex hormones that enhance the health of genital skin are deficient.[4]

Diaper rash begins as an erythematous rash occurring on the convex surfaces of skin under the diaper.[3] *Candida* spp. dermatitis commonly develops because infants usually carry *Candida albicans* in their intestinal tract and the warm, moist, occluded skin of the diaper area provides an optimal environment for its growth. Both diarrhea and oral antibiotics also lead to candidal diaper rash: diarrhea provides increased wetness, while antibiotics alter normal bacterial flora, allowing yeast overgrowth. The characteristic appearance is an intensely erythematous plaque with satellite lesions.[5] Excoriated skin can lead to secondary bacterial infection or impetigo.

Diaper rash not only causes discomfort to babies but is also distressing to parents and caregivers, who often feel guilty and ill prepared for this problem.[2]

The most effective prevention and treatment is keeping the diaper area clean and dry.[2,6] More absorbent diapers have reduced incidence and severity of diaper rash.[3,7] Barrier preparations can be used to protect the skin by coating the surface of the skin and/or supplying lipids that can penetrate the intercellular spaces of the stratum corneum.[1]

Topical antimonilial ointments such as nystatin are usually prescribed. Although topical corticosteroids are in general contraindicated,[8] they are often used for their antiinflammatory effects. Secondary bacterial impetiginous lesions are treated with antibiotic creams. Education of and support for the caregivers are also necessary components of diaper care.[9-11]

✴ CAM THERAPY RECOMMENDATIONS

Acupuncture

Diaper rash, like eczema, represents generalized accumulation of internal Damp-Heat in the skin. There are no data at this time on acupuncture or herbal treatment of diaper rash. Traditional Chinese medicine recommendations would be to disperse Heat and Dampness.

- Keep the diaper area dry.
- ST40 disperses generalized Dampness.
- LI11 disperses Heat.
- LR8 Water point of the Liver channel to sedate Heat in the Blood and also Heat to the genital area.
- KI6 tonifies Yin.
- Decrease energetically Hot or phlegm-producing foods in the child's diet.
- In children with recurrent diaper rash, overall tonification of Spleen can decrease internal dampness and minimize recurrence.
- Single point: SP3 or SP6
- Four-Point protocol: tonify SP2, HT8; sedate SP1, LR1.[1-6]

Aromatherapy

Essential oils recommended for diaper rash include bergamot (*Citrus bergamia*), roman chamomile (*Chamaemelum nobile*), frankincense (*Boswellia carteri*), geranium (*Pelargonium graveolens*), lavender (*Lavandula angustifolia*), and sandalwood (*Santalum album*).[1] The oils are mixed in a carrier oil or soothing lotion in a 0.5% to 1% solution and applied to reddened areas once or twice per day. The oils also can be added to the baby's bath.

Herbs—Chinese

Chinese herbal therapy may help relieve discomfort with redness and itchiness.[1,2]

Talcum, which is usually in the form of powder, is administered topically to the affected area. Qing Dai is the leaf of *Baphicacanthus cusia* (Nees) and *Isatis tinctoria* L. The activite component indirubin helps relieve the discomfort of diaper rash. Flower of *Lonicera Japonica* Thunb. (Jin Yin Hua), rhizome of *Coptis chinensis* Franch. (Huang Lian), root-bark of *Dictamnus dasycarpus* Turcz. (Bai Xian Pi), bark of *Phellodendron amurense* Rupr. (Huang Bai), root of *Sophora japonica* L. (Ku Shen Gen), rhizome of *Anemarrhena asphodeloides* Bunge (Zhi Mu), and root of *Glycyrrhiza uralensis* Fisch. (Gan Cao) have also been used to treat children with diaper rash. However, scientific evidence is lacking on their safety and efficacy.[1,2]

Herbs—Western

Minor chafing of the diaper area can be treated with fresh aloe vera or an aloe vera–containing gel to promote healing and hydrate the skin. Teas made from calendula are used as diaper rashes, eye washes, gargles, or compresses to treat conjunctivitis, pharyngitis, aphthous stomatitis and gingivostomatitis, and other inflammatory conditions of the skin and mucous membranes.[1,2]

Homeopathy

Please see Chapter 58, Thrush.

Massage Therapy

To avoid further spread of the disease to the child or the massage practitioner,[1,2] massage should be avoided over skin conditions considered contagious through contact. A recent study demonstrated increased bacterial counts on massage therapists' hands during and after massage treatments, although counts were lower on the client's skin.[3]

References

Pediatric Diagnosis and Treatment

1. Atherton DJ: A review of the pathophysiology, prevention and treatment of irritant diaper dermatitis, *Curr Med Res Opin* 20: 645-649, 2004.
2. Scowen P: Nappy rash: let's give mothers more help, *Prof Care Mother Child* 10:26-28, 30, 2000.
3. Prasad HR, Srivastava P, Verma KK: Diaper dermatitis—an overview, *Indian J Pediatr* 70:635-637, 2003.
4. Fiorillo L: Therapy of pediatric genital diseases, *Dermatol Ther* 17:117-128, 2004.
5. Behrman RE, Kliegman RM, Jenson HB, editors: *Nelson's textbook of pediatrics*, Philadelphia, 2004, Saunders.
6. Boiko S: Treatment of diaper dermatitis, *Dermatol Clinic* 17: 235-240, 1999.
7. Odio M, Friedlander SF: Dermatitis and advances in diaper technology, *Curr Opin Pediatr* 12:342-346, 2000.
8. Chosidow O, Lebrun-Vignes B, Bourgault-Villada I: Local corticosteroid therapy in dermatology [in French], *Presse Med* 28:2050-2056, 1999 (abstract).
9. Singleton JK: Pediatric dermatoses: three common skin disruptions in infancy, *Nurse Practitioner* 22:32-33, 37, 43-44, 1997.
10. Caputo RV: Fungal infections in children, *Dermatol Clin* 4: 137-149, 1986.
11. Neville EA, Finn OA: Psoriasiform napkin dermatitis—a follow-up study, *Br J Dermatol* 92:279-285, 1975.

Acupuncture

1. Loo M: *Pediatric acupuncture*, London, 2002, Elsevier.
2. Cao J: *Essentials of traditional Chinese pediatrics*, Beijing, 1990, Foreign Language Press.
3. Flaws B: *A handbook of TCM pediatrics, a practitioner's guide to the care and treatment of common childhood diseases*, Boulder, Colo, 1997, Blue Poppy Press.
4. Maciocia G: *The foundations of Chinese medicine, a comprehensive text for acupuncturists and herbalists*, London, 1989, Churchill Livingstone.
5. O'Connor J, Bensky D, editors: *Acupuncture, a comprehensive text*, Seattle, 1981, Eastland Press.
6. Scott J: *Acupuncture in the treatment of children*, London, 1991, Eastland Press.

Aromatherapy

1. Price S, Parr PP: *Aromatherapy for babies and children*, San Francisco, 1996, Thorsons.

Herbs—Chinese

1. *Dermatitis, diaper*, 2005. Available at www.herbchina2000.com/therapies/LDD.shtml. Accessed April 2005.
2. Natural Standard Research Collaboration. Available at www. naturalstandard.com. Accessed 2005.

Herbs—Western

1. *Calendula*. Available at www.naturaldatabase.com. Accessed Mar 21, 2005.
2. Newall CA, Anderson LA, Philpson JD: *Herbal medicine: a guide for healthcare professionals*, London, 1996, The Pharmaceutical Press.

Massage Therapy

1. Tappan F: *Healing massage techniques: holistic, classic, and emerging methods*, Norwalk, Conn, 1988, Appleton and Lange.
2. Fritz S: *Mosby's fundamentals of therapeutic massage*, ed 3, St Louis, 2005, Mosby.
3. Donoyama N, Wakuda T, Tanitsu T et al: Washing hands before and after performing massages? Changes in bacterial survival count on skin of a massage therapist and client during massage therapy, *J Altern Complement Med* 10:684-686, 2004.

Diarrhea

Acupuncture | May Loo

Chiropractic | Anne Spicer

Herbs—Chinese | May Loo, Harriet Beinfield, Efrem Korngold

Herbs—Western | Alan D. Woolf, Paula M. Gardiner, Lana Dvorkin-Camiel, Jack Maypole

Homeopathy | Janet L. Levatin

Naturopathy | Matthew I. Baral

Osteopathy | Jane Carreiro

Probiotics | Russell H. Greenfield

✳ PEDIATRIC DIAGNOSIS AND TREATMENT

Diarrhea is a significant cause of pediatric morbidity and mortality in both developed and underdeveloped countries,[1,2] especially in children younger than 5 years. *Diarrhea* is defined as an alteration in normal bowel movement characterized by increases in the water content (decrease in consistency), volume, and frequency to > 3 stools/day. Acute diarrhea is an episode of diarrhea ≤14 days in duration. The majority of pediatric acute diarrhea is "infectious diarrhea," an episode due to an infectious etiology. Persistent diarrhea is diarrhea of more than 14 days' duration, whereas chronic diarrhea lasts more than 30 days.[3]

Acute Infectious Diarrhea

In the United States, acute gastroenteritis accounts for more than 1.5 million pediatric outpatient visits, 200,000 hospitalizations, and approximately 300 deaths per year.[4] Children younger than 3 years have an average of approximately 2.5 episodes of gastroenteritis per year.[3] Preschoolers placed in childcare centers are at increased risk for diarrhea because of greater potential for person-to-person transmission.[5] Internationally, it is estimated that 1.5 billion episodes and 1.5-2.5 million deaths from diarrhea occur annually in children younger than 5 years.[6-8]

The infectious pathogens that cause acute diarrheal episodes in children include viruses, bacteria, and parasites.[9] Transmission is most likely via the fecal-oral route, from ingesting contaminated food or water,[10] or in infants and toddlers, by mouthing contaminated toys. The nature of foodborne diseases is changing as more mass-produced, minimally processed, and widely distributed foods result in nationwide and international outbreaks of diarrheal disease instead of just a few individuals who shared a meal.[3] The majority of cases are due to viral infections. Rotavirus is the most prevalent, causing approximately one third of all hospitalizations for diarrhea among U.S. children aged < 5 years, incurring $250 million/year of direct medical cost and an estimated $1 billion per year in total costs to society.[4] Human astrovirus (HAstV) is a significant cause of diarrheal outbreaks.[10] Other viruses include enteric adenoviruses, cytomegalovirus (CMV), norovirus, caliciviruses, and herpes simplex viruses.[11] Frequently, children are coinfected by several viruses.[10]

Viral diarrhea tends to involve the small bowel, producing large, watery, but relatively infrequent stools. These illnesses usually have short, self-limiting courses, typically lasting between 3 and 7 days.[12] However, they can be devastating to children with compromised immune systems or structural abnormalities of the gastrointestinal (GI) tract.[3]

The most common bacterial agents are enteropathogenic *Escherichia coli*, *Shigella* spp., *Salmonella* spp., *Campylobacter* spp., *Clostridium difficile*, *Clostridium perfringens*, *Staphylococcus aureus*, *Yersinia* spp., *Cryptosporidium* spp., and *Vibrio* spp.[11] These are much more virulent pathogens than viruses and usually cause mucosal injury in the small and large intestines, producing frequent, often bloody stools containing leukocytes. *E. coli* has become an important public health problem in recent years, causing more than 20,000 cases of infection and up to 250 deaths per year in the United States.[13] Transmission of infection is most commonly linked to consumption of contaminated meat, water, unpasteurized milk, leafy lettuce, alfalfa sprouts, goat's milk, and exposure to contaminated water in recreational swimming sites.[1,11,14] The different strains of enteropathogenic *E. coli* produce an inflammatory diarrhea by attaching to the intestinal mucosa and releasing toxins that injure cells and cause hemorrhage and necrosis.[15] The acute diarrhea, accompanied by abdominal cramping, progresses to bloody stools and often leads to serious complications such as hemolytic-uremic syndrome and thrombotic thrombocytopenic purpura.[14] *Shigella* spp. and *Salmonella* spp. cause similar inflammatory injuries that result in bloody stools and fecal leukocytes.[12] The Foodborne Diseases Active Surveillance Network (FoodNet) of the Centers for Disease Control and Prevention (CDC) Emerging Infections Program collects data from 10 U.S. sites on diseases caused by enteric pathogens transmitted commonly through food. The 2004 data indicate declines in the incidence of infections caused by *Campylobacter* spp., *Cryptosporidium* spp., Shiga toxin–producing *E. coli* (STEC) O157, *Listeria* spp., *Salmonella* spp., and *Yersinia* spp. Declines in *Campylobacter* spp. and *Listeria* spp. incidence are approaching national health objectives; for the first time, the incidence of STEC O157 infections in FoodNet is below the 2010 target.[16]

The most common parasitic infection is *Giardia lamblia*, which often causes secretory diarrhea without blood[12] and often leads to chronic diarrhea.[17] Other parasitic pathogens include *Entamoeba histolytica, Strongyloides stercoralis, Balantidium coli*, and spore-forming protozoa, which include *Cryptosporidium parvum, Cyclospora cayetanensis, Isospora belli, Enterocytozoon bieneusi*, and *Encephalitozoon intestinalis*. The latter three agents have been found most often in persons with acquired immune deficiency syndrome (AIDS). *B. coli, Trichuris trichiura*, and *E. histolytica* infections can produce bloody diarrhea in humans.[11] Diagnosis and treatment are still inconsistent. Because most acute diarrhea cases are self-limited, physicians often do not obtain stool cultures or examination for ova and parasites, as the results are sometimes not available for several days. Stool culture can identify different types of bacteria, but detection of specific enteropathogenic strains of *E. coli* requires specific serotyping that is not performed in routine stool cultures.[13] Serotyping is expensive, time consuming, and often not sufficiently specific or sensitive, so it is not recommended for routine diagnosis.[15]

The primary treatment focus is on correction of dehydration, which is the most important cause of morbidity and mortality in acute diarrhea. Oral rehydration treatment (ORT) with solutions containing appropriate concentrations of electrolytes and carbohydrates has been recommended by the World Health Organization (WHO) and has significantly reduced mortality.[18] On April 29, 2004, the American Academy of Pediatrics endorsed and accepted as its policy the guidelines issued by the CDC.[19] The rationale for ORT is that the intestinal sodium transport is enhanced by glucose, and this mechanism remains intact despite entertoxin injury to the small intestine epithelium.[16] ORT encompasses two phases of treatment: (1) a rehydration phase, in which water and electrolytes are administered as oral rehydration solution (ORS) to replace existing losses, and (2) a maintenance phase, which includes both replacement of ongoing fluid and electrolyte losses and adequate dietary intake.[20] Zinc with ORT reduces stool output and duration of diarrhea.[21]

Early refeeding is important for reducing diarrheal duration, severity, and nutritional impact.[22] Breastfed infants should continue nursing. Formula-fed infants should continue their usual formula[20] (not with lactose-free formulas as previously recommended)[23] and with age-appropriate, non-restricted diet.[20] Probiotics, live microorganisms in fermented foods that promote optimal health by establishing an improved balance in intestinal microflora, have been found to be safe and effective as treatment for infectious diarrhea.[24,25] ORT is contraindicated in children who are in hemodynamic shock or have abdominal ileus or intussusception.[20] Because the majority of acute infectious diarrhea cases are viral, antimicrobial therapy is not necessary. The rotavirus vaccine was first marketed in the United States in October 1998. This vaccine, as the natural infection, decreases the risk of acute rotavirus diarrhea by 50% and the risk of severe diarrhea with dehydration by more than 70%.[26] Breastfeeding is one of the most important preventive measures. Continuation of breastfeeding has also been found to control acute diarrheal episodes.[22] Improved hygiene such as hand washing is also important, especially in daycare centers.

Treatment with antimicrobial therapy must be instituted carefully only upon specific identification of pathogen and of drug sensitivity. Antibiotic resistance is increasing such that commonly used antibiotics are ineffective in acute diarrhea. Treatment of salmonellosis with antibiotics can prolong the carrier state and lead to a higher clinical relapse rate.[3] Injudicious antimicrobial therapy can also lead to susceptibility to other infections, enhance colonization of resistant organisms, and disrupt the normal intestinal flora, the body's natural defense against infection.[27] A recent CDC report indicates that a new epidemic strain of *C. difficile* has emerged, resulting in an increase in the rates of *C. difficile*–associated diseases from 2001 to 2004.[28]

Persistent Diarrhea

After acute gastroenteritis, delayed recovery and protracted diarrhea may occur, leading to postenteritis enteropathy. The diarrhea persists for more than 14 days, with continual small intestinal mucosal damage.[1,29] It occurs most frequently in very young infants, especially those living in poor, crowded conditions;[1] in bottlefed, malnourished infants, and after rotavirus infection.[1]

Clinically, the infant is listless, irritable, often has a "worried look," and begins to show weight loss and wasting with persistent diarrhea. If the watery stool is profuse, the abdomen may become distended and tympanitic. The precise pathogenesis for ongoing diarrhea following a bout of infectious gastroenteritis remains undetermined but is most likely multifactorial: (1) persistence of the intestinal pathogen; (2) malnutrition from the acute episode exerts an adverse effect on the repair of the intestinal mucosa and on the recovery of normal motility; (3) dysmotility-engendered bacterial contamination and overgrowth; and (4) young age with immature immune response to antigenic stimuli.[1] Secondary lactose and sucrose malabsorption and small bowel bacterial overgrowth have been detected. The finding of lymphocytic infiltration of intestinal mucosa suggests a cell-mediated immune response to environmental antigens, such as dietary, microbial, or both.[1,30]

Whereas the major complication due to acute diarrhea is dehydration, persistent diarrhea even at 2- to 3-week duration can result in malnutrition and failure to thrive. Despite intensive field-based and laboratory studies spanning 3 decades, many questions remain unanswered about prevention and the best approaches to management.[1] Children with secondary lactose intolerance would have more watery diarrhea, accompanied by bloating, flatulence, and crampy abdominal pain after ingestion of lactose.[12]

Chronic Diarrhea

Chronic diarrhea, defined as diarrhea lasting more than 30 days,[3] seems to be increasing globally in the pediatric population.[31] A long list of differentials includes congenital anomalies, such as disaccharidase deficiencies, inborn errors of metabolism, cystic fibrosis, enteric infections such as giardiasis, extraintestinal infection such as urinary tract infection, acquired sugar and protein intolerance, inflammatory bowel disease, immune defects, and endocrinopathies.[1,11] Malnutrition due to chronic diarrhea affects hundreds of millions of young children and annually causes more than 3 million deaths in children younger than 5 years.[1] Infections remain the most common cause of chronic diarrhea in children of all ages,[32] with an expanding number of potential viral, bacterial, and parasitic pathogens.[33] Just as in acute diarrhea, identification of specific pathogen and drug sensitivity is important for management of infectious chronic diarrhea. Treatment of noninfectious conditions such as inflammatory bowel disease needs to be directed toward the primary disorder. In all cases of chronic diarrhea, fluid intake needs to be closely monitored and malnutrition needs to be treated vigorously to prevent growth failure and mortality. Micronutrients such as zinc[34] and vitamins need to be supplemented.[31] Probiotics and vaccinations are assuming increasingly more important roles in the management of chronic diarrhea.[33]

Chronic diarrhea without malnutrition is considered toddler's diarrhea, or chronic nonspecific diarrhea (CNSD). It is the most frequent cause of chronic diarrhea in children between 6 months and 3 years of age.[1,11] The typical clinical presentation is a young child who was a colicky baby and gradually begins to have three to six loose stools per day. Most of the stools are passed early during the waking hours and contain undigested foods and mucus.[35] The child is otherwise active and healthy looking, with normal growth.[11] Stress and infection can precipitate bouts of diarrhea, which are made worse by a low-residue, low-fat, and high-carbohydrate diet.[1]

The precise etiology is still undetermined. There is often a strong family history of functional bowel disorders such that it may be an early manifestation of irritable bowel syndrome. From an infectious standpoint, bacterial invasion of the small intestine by the upper respiratory tract microflora is a possibility.[1] Current evidence also suggests that CNSD is primarily a gut motility disorder, modulated by dietary factors.[1,36] Diminished upper small intestinal motility may be a physiological, developmental phenomenon.[37] Some children demonstrate intestinal mucosal injury[38] with villous atrophy. The mechanisms that lead to mucosal injury are elusive.[31]

Dietary factors include low dietary fat, high carbohydrate, and high fluid consumption, especially apple juice.[39] The overconsumption of apple juice has received the most attention as the causative agent. Previously, children were given orange juice to prevent scurvy. In recent years, apple juice has become the juice of choice for children younger than age 5.[40] In many children with CNSD, apple juice constitutes 25% to 60% of daily dietary intake.[41] Apple juice is high in sorbitol and has a high fructose:glucose ratio,[42] thus contributing to a carbohydrate imbalance. In addition, compared with the freshly pressed and unprocessed ("cloudy") apple juice, enzymatically processed ("clear") apple juice significantly promotes diarrhea. This suggests that the increased amount of nonabsorbable monosaccharides and oligosaccharides as a result of the enzymatic processing of apple pulp is an important etiological factor in apple juice–induced CNSD.[39]

Normally, 95% to 98% of the intestinal fluid is reabsorbed. Disordered intestinal motility combined with excessive fluid and carbohydrate intake contribute to development of diarrhea.[1] Other proposed theories of pathogenesis include food allergy and intolerance,[35,43] behavioral problems,[43]

hypogammaglobulinemia,[44] congenital sucrase-isomaltase deficiency,[25] and iatrogenic causes of excess ORT and elimination diet.[45] CNSD seems to be self-limiting, resolving spontaneously in a mean time of 1.7 years.[45] However, symptoms may resurface later in childhood,[1] such as in teenagers who have diarrhea while on a fruit and juice diet.[42] Treatment generally consists of normalization of the child's diet, especially with regard to fat, fiber, fluids, and fruit juices,[1,11] and alleviating parental anxiety.[1]

✳ CAM THERAPY RECOMMENDATIONS

Acupuncture

Acupuncture has long been used for various GI conditions.[1] Research data on adults—albeit often considered of substandard quality—support the beneficial effects of acupuncture in diarrhea. The treatment protocols in point selections generally depend on traditional Chinese medicine (TCM) diagnoses, with the majority of points located on Stomach and Spleen channels such as SP3, SP4, SP6, ST25, and ST36.[2-6]

Chinese physicians have reported success in treating diarrhea using back-Shu points.[7] Shallow needling, the mere puncturing of the skin, is well tolerated by children and has been shown to enhance both humoral and cellular immunity and regulate intestinal peristaltic function. One study from China demonstrated that such needling was successful in treating diarrhea in children, using either back BL points or abdominal and leg points CV6, CV9, ST25, ST36, SP3, and SP4.[8]

Recent studies attempt to elucidate the physiological effects of acupuncture on the GI tract.[1] A Japanese animal study showed gastric motility was inhibited by acupuncture-like stimulation applied to the abdomen and lower chest region but was often excited when the limbs were stimulated. The researchers demonstrated that the gastric responses were reflexes mediated via neural pathways. In addition, because the responses were not influenced by naloxone, the endogenous opioids did not appear to be involved.[9] A Canadian review of studies, however, reveals that acupuncture regulates GI motility and secretion through both opioid and neural pathways.[10] A recent Japanese animal study demonstrated that by just treating GV1—an acupoint historically used successfully to treat diarrhea—the colonic motility and inflammation in colitic rats were significantly reduced. Naloxone pretreatment blocked these effects, which suggests that the therapeutic effects of acupuncture at GV1 in colitis may involve endogenous opioid pathways.[11] An animal study from Korea also demonstrated antiinflammatory effects of GV1. The researchers induced enteropathogenic *E. coli* diarrhea in 32 young pigs, then compared acupuncture treatment at GV1 with intramuscular antibiotics and no-treatment controls. The acupuncture- and antibiotic-treated pigs had normal GI linings compared with severe inflammation found in the control pigs.[12] A U.S. study of nine healthy adults demonstrated that electrical stimulation of acupuncture points may enhance the regularity of gastric myoelectrical activity and may be an option for treatment of gastric dysrhythmia.[13] A Chinese study revealed that electroacupuncture at Zusanli (ST36) regulates pylorus peristaltic function.[14]

Treatment

TCM explains acute diarrhea as external Cold and Damp-Heat pathogenic invasions, which correlate to viral and bacterial infections.[15] Chronic diarrhea is primarily due to internal imbalances of Spleen and Stomach deficiency and Kidney Yang deficiency. Improper diet can cause both acute and chronic diarrhea. In addition to acupuncture treatment, parents can be taught a home treatment program of acupuncture and massage to help alleviate symptoms and shorten the course of diarrhea. TCM food recommendations can add another perspective to the dietary management of diarrhea.

Treatment of all diarrhea

GV1: shallow needling without retention can be applied in infants and young children.

Parents can be instructed to do acupressure for all children.

For acute diarrhea, prevent dehydration with ORT.

Acute diarrhea

Acute diarrhea is best managed with an integrative approach. It is important to obtain the appropriate laboratory studies; namely, stool cultures for bacteria and examinations for ova and parasites, especially in bloody diarrhea or in water stools of more than 7 days' duration. Antibiotic sensitivity should be determined to avoid giving medications indiscriminately. Fluid management with ORT should be part of the immediate treatment regimen. Acupuncture can be used to alleviate pain, shorten the course by expelling the pathogens, and strengthen the child's immune system.

Viral gastroenteritis. Viral gastroenteritis correlates with external Cold pathogenic invasion into the gastrointestinal channels.

Avoid raw and Cold foods; avoid Phlegm-producing foods that injure the Spleen.

Moxa or warm CV8, the umbilicus.

KI7 to expel Cold.

Initial treatment to stop diarrhea: ST39, ST25, CV12, CV6, CV10.

Four-Point, Five-Element protocol for expelling Cold from the Small Intestine: Tonify SI5, TB6, sedate SI2, BL66.

If the course of diarrhea is > 4 to 5 days: Four-Point, Five-Element protocol to expel ST and LI Cold:
  Stomach: Tonify ST41, SI5; sedate ST44, BL66.
  Large Intestine: Tonify LI5, SI5; sedate LI2, BL66.

In young children, use only the two meridian points:
  Stomach: Tonify ST41; sedate ST44.
  Large Intestine: Tonify LI5; Sedate LI2.
  Tonify Spleen: Two points or four points.
  Continue ST25, CV12, CV6, CV10, and warm CV8; ST37.

If diarrhea is >1 week duration:
  Vigorously tonify Spleen and expel Cold from the Intestines.
  ST37, ST39 to regulate the Intestines.

After diarrhea has resolved, vigorously strengthen the immune system.

Home treatment:

Abdominal massage: With warm palms, parents can massage the child's abdomen in a counter-clockwise direction around the umbilicus 50 to 100 times.

Warming CV 8

Bacterial infection. Bacteria infection correlates with External Damp-Heat pathogenic invasions.

Prevent dehydration as soon as possible with ORT.

Avoid energetically Hot foods; avoid Phlegm-producing foods.

BL25, BL22, SP9, SP6.

GV14 to treat fever.

LI11 to resolve Heat.

ST40 to resolve Damp.

BL20 to tonify Spleen, resolve Dampness.

For the first 1 to 2 days:
  ST25 to stop diarrhea.
  CV12, CV6, CV10.
  Begin tonification of the Spleen and the immune system.
  ST39 to regulate the Small Intestine.
  Disperse Small Intestine Heat: Tonify SI2, SI5; sedate SI5, TB6.
  In small children, use the two SI points: Tonify SI2; sedate SI5.

When there is high fever and sweating and the child is very thirsty:
  Disperse ST and LI Heat:
    Stomach: Tonify ST44, BL66; sedate ST41, SI5.
    Large Intestine: Tonify LI2, BL66; sedate LI5, SI5.
  In small children, use only the channel points:
    Stomach: Tonify ST44; sedate ST41.
    Large Intestine: Tonify LI2; sedate LI5.
  Tonify Spleen: Two points or Four-Point protocol.
  ST39 to regulate the Large Intestine.

After diarrhea has resolved, vigorously strengthen the immune system.

Home treatment: Perform abdominal massage as in Cold diarrhea, but do not apply warmth to CV8.[15]

Chronic diarrhea

Chronic diarrhea can be due to SP deficiency (which can explain CNSD of infancy and early childhood), Kidney Yang deficiency, or improper diet.

For SP deficiency

Vigorously tonify Spleen with the Five-Element, Four-Point protocol:
  Tonify SP2, HT8; sedate SP1, LR1.

Add BL20, BL21, SP6, ST36, CV12 to tonify the Stomach and Spleen.

Moxa or warm CV8.

ST25, ST37 to stop chronic diarrhea.

Avoid Cold, greasy, Phlegm-producing foods, such as dairy products.

Avoid excess apple juice.

Modify the child's lifestyle: decrease school workload or extracurricular activities to allow more rest; decrease any stress that can precipitate worry and frustration.

Teach parents the same home treatment regimen as for acute Cold diarrhea.[15]

Kidney Yang deficiency. Kidney Yang deficiency usually manifests as early morning diarrhea with abdominal pain, borborygmi during the bowel movement with a feeling of cold.

Chinese case reports indicate that Kidney deficiency diarrhea responds to treatment of combining GV4 (Mingmen) with CV4 (Guanyuan.)[16]

Tonify Kidney Yang: KI3, KI7, CV4, CV6, BL23.

Overall tonification of Kidney with Five-Element, Four-Point protocol:

Tonify KI7, LU8; sedate KI3, SP3.

Tonify Spleen: Tonify SP2, HT8; sedate SP1, LR11.

ST25, ST37.

Avoid Cold, raw foods; avoid greasy, Phlegm-producing foods such as dairy products.

Modify the child's lifestyle to minimize Fear.

Teach parents the home treatment regimen.

Improper diet. Diet with excess of foods that are artificially sweetened, greasy, Phlegm-producing, salty, or energetically too Hot or too Cold can result in Spleen deficiency that can then lead to Kidney deficiency and Liver Qi stagnation.

Eliminate excess inappropriate foods.

ST21, ST44, SP4, CV12, BL20, BL21, ST36, SP6, ST25, ST37.

Five-Element, Four-Point protocol (see Appendix B) to treat specific deficiencies:

Tonify Spleen.

Tonify Kidney.

LR3, LR13 to move Liver Qi.[15]

Chiropractic

No case studies or clinical trials are available in the chiropractic literature on management of diarrhea. However, after organic disease states have been ruled out, the chiropractic approach, as always, is to normalize body function through removal of physical, chemical, and emotional influences.

GI disturbances are highly irritating to the nervous system and therefore commonly cause recurrent subluxation via the viscerosomatic reflex pathways.[1]

The chiropractor would stimulate the sympathetic system at the area of T1 to T4 with an adjustment, if indicated, or with percussive stimulation at the same location.[2] Parasympathetic suppression may be accomplished with sustained firm pressure over the sacrum for more than 30 seconds. If an adjustment at the lumbars or sacrum is required, a stretch-type technique is recommended to avoid overstimulation of the parasympathetics.[3]

Persistent diarrhea may be secondary to allergy and intolerance. The most common agent is dairy. Therefore a dairy elimination trial is an appropriate step in management. A digestive stool analysis may prove instructive in the course of management.

Breastfeeding must be encouraged.

Microflora supplementation is advisable in many GI conditions and especially in the case of diarrhea, which may effectively reduce the colonization and lead to other complications.[4-8]

Intake of foods that have a tendency to bind the stool may be useful. These foods include cooked carrots, white rice, applesauce, and bananas. A mixture of rice and lentils has been successfully used in children malnourished by diarrhea with a good measure of success in decreasing diarrheal duration as well as enhancing weight gain.[9]

Signs of dehydration are an indication to involve medical comanagement.

Herbs—Chinese

TCM posits that diarrhea in children may result from a number of causes including food stagnation, excessive intake of raw or cold food, food poisoning or food intolerance (starch, dairy, or gluten sensitivity), side effects of medication (antibiotics, laxatives, carbohydrate sweeteners), emotional upset, infections of the GI tract (gastroenteritis, candidiasis, parasites), or any combination of these factors. Chinese herbal treatment of diarrhea emphasizes a gradual lessening of intestinal activity and mucous secretion without producing constipation from excessive astringency and inhibition of peristalsis.[1]

Acute Diarrhea

The Belly Binder (Gentle Warrior Pediatric Formula, Kan Herb Company, Scotts Valley, Calif.) emphasizes astringing secretions and dispelling of external and internal pathogens (Wind, Cold, Summer Heat, Dampness, Damp Heat, and Toxins) as well as elimination of food stagnation. In the case of diarrhea associated with indigestion, food poisoning, acute gastroenteritis, or emotional or physical distress, this remedy can quickly and gently restore normal intestinal function.

Herbal formulation: Hawthorn fruit (shan zha), citrus peel (chen pi), and perilla fruit (zi su ye) aid digestion and eliminate food stagnation. White atractylodes rhizome (bai zhu), dioscorea rhizome (shan yao), poria fungus (fu ling), dolichoris seed (bai bian dou), lotus seed (lian zi), eupatorium herb (pei lan), pogostemon herb (huo xiang), and alisma rhizome (ze xie) dispel exterior Wind Damp, disperse internal Dampness, strengthen the Spleen, and consolidate Moisture and Qi, thus checking excessive secretions, toning the membranes of the bowel, and normalizing peristalsis. In addition, pulsatilla root (bai tou weng) dispels the interior Damp Heat that often accompanies acute diarrhea, while cardamon seed (sha ren) warms the Spleen and Stomach and soothes the intestines and reduces abdominal distention. Finally, licorice root (gan cao) not only harmonizes the formula but also aids pulsatilla (bai tou weng) and perilla fruit (zi su ye) in dispelling Heat and Toxins.

Dosage: 1 to 2 droppersful as needed every 2 to 4 hours.

Caution: Alternating constipation and diarrhea; acute gastroenteritis (intestinal flu); food poisoning; weakness or lethargy, thirst, dehydration, and high fever (102° F or above).

Chronic or Recurring Diarrhea

Chronic or recurring diarrhea can lead to weight loss and a failure to thrive due to depletion of Qi and Blood, Yin and Yang, particularly of the Spleen and Stomach. In these conditions, it is better to use tonifying formulas such as *Grow and Thrive* or *Strengthen Spleen* (Gentle Warrior Pediatric Formula, Kan Herb Company, Scotts Valley, Calif.).

Herbs—Western

Although rehydration is the gold standard in the treatment for diarrhea, certain herbs have been traditionally used in the treatment of diarrhea. For example, as a soothing agent the demulcent herbs marshmallow and slippery elm taken as a tea are popular. Other traditional herbs include green tea *(Camellia sinensis)*, bilberry *(Vaccinium myrtillus)*, blackberry *(Rubus fruticosus)*, and raspberry *(Rubus idaeus)*.

Chamomile *(Matricaria recutita)* has also been used for diarrhea. In a double-blind, randomized, multicenter study that included 79 children between ages 6 months and 5.5 years with acute, non-complicated diarrhea, patients randomly received both an apple pectin and chamomile extract (Diarrhoesan) or placebo for 3 days. The apple/pectin preparation decreased the duration of diarrhea when compared with placebo.[1]

Berberine is a constituent from the roots of goldenseal *(Hydrastis canadensis)* and Oregon grape root *(Berberis aquifolium)*. Berberine is active against many parasites and bacteria that cause diarrhea. Berberine has shown mixed results in the treatment of diarrhea in clinical trials in children.[2-6] In terms of safety, some practitioners consider berberine to cause severe acute hemolytic and neonatal jaundice in babies with glucose-6 phosphate deficiency; therefore treatment of newborns with neonatal jaundice is contraindicated.[7,8]

Homeopathy

Before using this section, please see Appendix A, Homeopathy, for definitions of practitioner expertise categories and general information on prescribing homeopathic medicines.

Practitioner Expertise Category 1

Category 1 includes acute childhood diarrhea.

Practitioner Expertise Categories 2 and 3

Categories 2 and 3 include chronic diarrhea.

There is a small body of research on homeopathic treatment of acute childhood diarrhea that shows a significant decrease in the length of diarrhea with homeopathic treatment. Jacobs et al. conducted three double-blind trials on homeopathic treatment of diarrhea in children aged 6 months to 5 years, with two trials in Nicaragua and one trial in Nepal.[1-3]

Because the methodology was similar in these three studies, the data were pooled and analyzed together to gain greater statistical power.[4] It was found that with individualized homeopathic treatment, the mean duration of diarrhea was 4.1 days in the placebo group compared with 3.3 days in the active group ($p = 0.008$). The five most commonly used medicines in this study were *Podophyllum peltatum, Arsenicum album,* sulphur, *Chamomilla vulgaris,* and *Calcarea carbonica;* these medicines were used to treat 85% and 78% of cases in Nepal and Nicaragua, respectively. In addition to the aforementioned research evidence, the homeopathic literature contains much evidence in the form of accumulated clinical experience to support the use of homeopathic treatment for diarrhea.[5]

Homeopathic treatment of childhood diarrhea, when used in conjunction with ORT, could make a significant impact on childhood mortality in developing countries. Further study of homeopathic treatment for diarrhea is indicated.

Homeopathic treatment is safe to try for acute diarrhea not associated with other serious conditions and before a child becomes significantly dehydrated owing to fluid loss. If the patient does not respond quickly to homeopathic treatment, then conventional care may be necessary. Homeopathic treatment should be used in combination with dietary modifications (withholding of dairy products and other foods that prolong diarrhea). Probiotics are also often helpful and can be used in conjunctions with homeopathy.

The goal in treating diarrhea homeopathically is to determine the single homeopathic medicine whose description in the materia medica most closely matches the symptom picture of the patient. Often mental and emotional states in addition to physical symptoms are considered. Once the medicine has been selected, it can be given orally or sublingually in the 30C potency after each episode of diarrhea, up to six times per day. If the patient is also vomiting, a few (4 to 6) granules of the medicine can be diluted in 3 oz (90 mL) of water, and a few drops can be placed in the patient's mouth whenever a dose of the medicine is needed. The medicine does not need to be swallowed to be effective; the simillimum will work even if it remains in the mouth for only a brief period of time. If the medicine has not helped after six doses, another homeopathic medicine should be tried and/or some other form of therapy should be instituted. Once symptoms have begun to resolve, the medicine can be given less frequently or stopped. It can be repeated again for a relapse of symptoms.

The following is a list of homeopathic medicines commonly used to treat patients with acute diarrhea. It must be emphasized that this list is partial and represents some of the probable choices from the homeopathic materia medica. If the symptoms of a given patient are not represented here, further research in the homeopathic literature would be needed to find the simillimum. The section on homeopathic treatment of colic (see Chapter 23) also contains some information on treating diarrhea.

Podophyllum peltatum

Podophyllum peltatum is one of the main medicines for acute diarrhea in children. The child has profuse, gushing diarrhea that is watery, green or yellow, and offensive. There is gurgling in the abdomen with passage of gas. Often the diarrhea is painless, although some cramping may occur prior to passing a stool. Despite having diarrhea, the child does not seem too ill, although he or she may begin to seem tired if the diarrhea persists for a few days. This medicine is sometimes also needed in cases in which diarrhea and constipation alternate.

Arsenicum album

Arsenicum album is another medicine commonly used for acute diarrhea. This medicine covers diarrhea caused by food poisoning as well as other etiologies. The stool is watery and feels hot to the patient. The patient is anxious, restless, and weak, and feels chilly. The diarrhea may be worse from midnight to 2 AM. The abdomen feels better with the application of warm cloths. The patient may be thirsty, but only for sips of water.

Chamomilla vulgaris

Chamomilla vulgaris is one of the main medicines for diarrhea during teething. The stool is green and slimy and possibly mucous. The diarrhea may be worst at 9 AM. The child is hot and very irritable.

Sulphur

Sulphur is used to treat diarrhea that causes the patient to awaken in the morning near 5 AM. The stool is foul smelling and painful and may cause redness and burning around the anus. The patient is generally warmblooded.

Veratrum album

Diarrhea that responds to *Veratrum album* is profuse, watery, and odorless. The stool may occur simultaneously with vomiting. The patient may break into a cold sweat on the forehead.

Naturopathy

It is important to know the cause of diarrhea in order to apply the appropriate treatment. In some cases physicians and parents are tempted to alleviate the symptoms without addressing the cause or allowing the body to clear itself from organisms that may be causing the diarrhea. There seem to be three main causes of diarrhea: infectious agents, antibiotics, and foods. The conventional categories include infectious, persistent, and chronic. However, the causes of persistent and chronic diarrhea are often overlooked and, as a result, treatment is frequently unsuccessful.

Dietary

Dietary instruction should always accompany diarrhea symptoms regardless of the cause. Avoid sorbitol, a sugar alcohol found in cookie mixes, brownie mixes, imitation maple syrup, dietetic foods, candies, gums, apples, pears, peaches, and prunes, because it can exacerbate diarrhea. Because of this effect, the previously mentioned fruits are commonly used to treat constipation. Foods with mannitol, high-sugar foods, and fruit juices should also be avoided. The diet should consist of well-cooked foods, non-spicy foods, and low fiber. In some cases a dairy-free diet can often improve chronic diarrhea that is unrelated to lactose intolerance.

Antibiotic-Induced Diarrhea

It is common knowledge that when a patient receives antibiotics, beneficial bacteria in the gut are eliminated, giving way to pathogenic bacteria. A simple way to combat this issue is to replenish the gut with the necessary flora. A growing body of research demonstrates that this therapy, often referred to as *probiotics*, is quite effective in the prevention and treatment of diarrhea caused by antibiotics.

- *Lactobacillus* GG supplementation has been shown to reduce the risk of diarrhea caused by antibiotics[1] and to be somewhat effective for treatment of *C. difficile* infection.[2] Both *Lactobacillus* GG and *Bifidobacterium* have shown effectiveness in antibiotic-associated diarrhea.[3] They may be provided at a dose of 1 to 10 billion colony forming units (CFU) per day.[4]
- *Saccharomyces boulardii* is moderately successful in treating antibiotic-induced diarrhea[5] and effective in treating acute diarrhea in hospitalized children.[6] The dose range is 250 mg once to three times per day, or approximately 3 billion units per day.
- Antibiotic-induced diarrhea was also prevented with *Bifidobacterium lactis* and *Streptococcus thermophilus*.[7]

Acute Infectious Diarrhea

Several botanicals and certain food supplements can be helpful in treating infections of the GI tract.

- Botanicals that contain high levels of antimicrobial berberines, such as goldenseal *(Hydrastis)*, Oregon grape *(Berberis aquifolium)*, or barberry *(Berberis vulgaris)*, may be helpful for infectious diarrhea.[8,9] Berberines were also found to be more effective for treating the symptoms of *Giardia* spp. infection than metronidazole, but less effective in treating *Giardia*-positive stools.[10] A common dose of 5 mg/kg/day may be used.
- Wheat germ can be effective in treating *Giardia* spp. infections, as it contains a lectin that binds to the N-acetyl glucosamine residues of *Giardia* spp.[11] One teaspoon three times per day is an appropriate dose.
- Grapefuit seed extract, which has antimicrobial properties, can be provided at 10 drops, three times per day. It has a bitter taste, so compliance may be difficult in smaller children.
- Garlic and garlic extracts have antimicrobial properties. Two to four grams per day in children older than 1 year old is an appropriate dose.

Other Diarrheal Conditions

It is interesting to note that the common age range of CNSD is during the period that solid foods are introduced to the child. Chronic and persistent diarrhea may indeed be due to either the early introduction of solid foods, introduction of foods that the child is having difficulty digesting, or introduction of foods to which the child is having a delayed-type hypersensitivity reaction. The latter case seems more feasible when considering that family history will often show other irritable bowel diseases or syndromes. This should remind the clinician that dietary factors should always be considered. Removal of commonly allergenic foods such as wheat, dairy, eggs, soy, or corn can show excellent results in these cases. Probiotics may also prove helpful in patients with unexplained diarrhea, even in children who have not been exposed to antibiotics.

The following treatments may be used in both infectious and chronic diarrheal states, as they can serve to soothe the GI mucosa:

- Robert's formula is a botanical combination frequently used by naturopathic physicians to treat intestinal inflammation from either an infectious cause or inflammatory bowel diseases such as Crohn's or ulcerative colitis. It consists of mucilage-containing herbs such as marshmallow *(Althea officinalis)* and slippery elm *(Ulmus fulva)*; antibacterial herbs such as wild indigo *(Baptisia tinctoria)*, echinacea, and goldenseal *(Hydrastis canadensis)*; cranesbill (geranium) as an astringent; and cabbage powder and pokeroot *(Phytolacca* spp.) as ulcer-healing constituents. Patients who can swallow capsules may take two capsules three to four times per day. The capsules may also be opened and mixed with diluted juice.

- Slippery elm powder may be given by itself if Robert's formula is rejected for its taste. An appropriate regimen is 1 to 6 teaspoons per day in divided doses mixed in water or diluted juice.
- Rosemary is an astringent herb and can be used as an infusion: 1 teaspoon of herb per cup of water, with ¼-½ cup three times per day, or 2 tablespoons every 2 hours.
- One tablespoon of tomato juice plus 1 tablespoon of sauerkraut juice taken throughout the day may reduce diarrhea.
- Bentonite clay, rye flour, and unsweetened carob powder can all produce a beneficial binding effect. Any of these ingredients mixed in applesauce, yogurt, or diluted juice will help decrease diarrheal episodes. One to six teaspoons per day mixed in food may be given depending on the severity of the stools. It is important to provide these powders in a graded fashion, as too much can result in constipation.
- Carob powder may be used by itself and needs to be mixed with water or milk or added to applesauce. Use ½ to 1 teaspoon per dose up to six times per day. Slippery elm *(Ulmus fulva)* powder may also be mixed with carob in a 1:1 ratio.
- Infusions of either raspberry or blackberry leaves are very astringent. They may be given in ¼-cup doses every 2 to 3 hours in cases of acute diarrhea.
- Geranium (cranesbill root) tincture can be helpful in most cases of diarrhea, as it is astringent to the GI tract. It may be given as a tea or tincture. To make the tea, add 1 to 2 teaspoons of the root to 2 cups of water, simmer 10 to 15 minutes, and drink 1 cup three times per day. The tincture may be taken as a 1:5 concentration, 2 to 4 mL three times per day.

Osteopathy

Within osteopathic teaching, idiopathic diarrhea may be due to overactivity of the parasympathetic innervation to the colon.[1] Both the vagus nerve and pelvic splanchnic nerves may be involved. Parasympathetic activity causes increased motility and glandular secretion.[1,2] Viscerosomatic reflexes in the lower thoracic area may play a role in maintaining irritability of the lower gut[3,4] by altering secretory cell activity that responds to autonomic influences and stimulating tonic contractions of visceral smooth muscle. Visceral strains that interfere with the inherent motility of the gut, as described by Barral, may also play a role in chronic diarrhea[5] by altering hemodynamics and normal peristalsis. Furthermore, congestion within the mesenteric lymphatic system may alter the cellular milieu, adversely affecting electrochemical gradients responsible for slow wave activity in the colon.[1,2] Osteopathic techniques including balancing, inhibition, and visceral and functional techniques can be used to address these issues. Chapman's reflexes have been associated with recurrent and chronic diarrhea; improvement in symptoms has been reported when these reflexes are treated.[1,6] Visceral techniques also appear to be beneficial in decreasing cramping, pain, and frequency of bowel movements in functional or idiopathic diarrhea.[5] Likewise, inhibition and lymphatic techniques are thought to facilitate normal function of the colon. No published studies have been performed on children with chronic diarrhea, but several reports and small studies in the adult population exist in the osteopathic literature.[3,5,7-9]

Probiotics

Perhaps the clearest indication for probiotic therapy, and that associated with the strongest supportive research, is for the prevention and treatment of diarrheal disease. This is especially true with respect to acute infectious viral diarrhea (notably rotavirus).[1-5]

One study used *Lactobacillus* GG in a dose of 100 billion CFU in 71 well-nourished children with acute diarrhea between 4 and 45 months of age. The groups receiving either *Lactobacillus* GG in a fermented milk product or in a freeze-dried powder had a significantly shorter duration of illness when compared with the placebo group.[6] Another trial focused on children aged 6 to 36 months who were hospitalized with acute diarrhea. Those receiving 10 billion CFU of *Lactobacillus reuteri* daily experienced a shorter duration of watery diarrhea as compared with those receiving placebo.[7] In a trial of 100 children with diarrhea, 61 of whom had rotavirus diarrhea, who received either oral rehydration alone or oral rehydration plus *Lactobacillus* GG, those in the experimental arm experienced an almost 50% shorter duration of illness than those who received rehydration alone. In addition, therapy with *Lactobacillus* GG shortened the duration of rotavirus excretion and risk to other children.[8] In a study of infants aged 5 to 24 months who were admitted to a chronic care hospital, children were randomized to receive a standard infant formula or the same formula supplemented with *B. bifidum* (900 million CFU) and *S. thermophilus* (1.4 billion CFU). Supplementation reduced the incidence of acute diarrhea and rotavirus shedding.[9] A trial of 49 children aged 6 to 35 months with rotavirus gastroenteritis randomly assigned participants to either *Lactobacillus* GG, *Lactobacillus rhamnosus*, or a combination of *S. thermophilus* and *Lactobacillus bulgaricus* twice daily for 5 days. The mean duration of diarrhea was shortest for those receiving *Lactobacillus* GG, followed by *L. rhamnosus* and then the combination therapy. Evaluation also showed a rotavirus-specific immune augmentation with *Lactobacillus* GG.[10]

Data are also quite strong with respect to those prone to antibiotic-associated diarrhea. A capsule form of *S. boulardii*, a nonpathogenic yeast, was given concurrently to 180 hospitalized patients who were receiving antibiotics. Only 9.5% of those receiving *S. boulardii* 250 mg twice daily developed diarrhea as compared with 22% of those receiving placebo.[11] The efficacy of *Lactobacillus* GG yogurt in preventing antibiotic-associated diarrhea was studied in 16 healthy volunteers who were given erythromycin acistrate 400 mg three times daily for 1 week. The volunteers were randomly assigned to take twice daily 125 mL of either *Lactobacillus* GG–fermented yogurt or pasteurized regular yogurt as placebo during the drug treatment. Those receiving *Lactobacillus* GG yogurt with erythromycin had less diarrhea and fewer side effects, such as abdominal distress, than those taking pasteurized yogurt.[12] Probiotic therapy may also be of benefit in the setting of recurrent *C. difficile* infection because, in theory, antibiotics damage the protective colonic microflora, thereby permitting colonization by and then infection with *C. difficile*.[13-17]

Data are less convincing with respect to bacterial enteritis or traveler's diarrhea. In one placebo-controlled, double-blind study, however, *Lactobacillus* GG was effective in preventing traveler's diarrhea in one group of people traveling to one of two destinations in southern Turkey, especially in older age groups. No side effects were noted.[18]

Many experts believe that any child with likely viral diarrhea, antibiotic-associated diarrhea, or recurrent *C. difficile* infection should receive a course of probiotic therapy of at least 3 to 4 weeks' duration. Although controversial, a growing number of experts also contend that any child offered antibiotic therapy should be offered simultaneous probiotic therapy that extends at least 1 week beyond the full course of antibiotics. Although some practitioners have recommended a delay between the time of administration of antibiotic and that of probiotic in order to enhance viability of the probiotic organisms, this author believes the two can be administered at the same time with minimal, if any, impact on therapeutic efficacy and with clear benefit regarding compliance.

Prevention and treatment of diarrhea is one of the few clinical arenas where adequate information exists to guide choice of organism, dose, and duration of therapy. These recommendations are far from set in stone, but they provide much-needed guidelines for therapy (many of which have been applied to other clinical settings).

Although duration of use employed in studies has varied widely, this author recommends using a 1- to 2-month trial of probiotic therapy for treatment of diarrhea employing well-studied organisms shown to be safe and typically effective in specific circumstances. When trying to prevent an episode of acute diarrhea, good data exist for *Lactobacillus GG, L. reuteri, B. bifidum,* and perhaps *S. thermophilus.* When treating acute diarrhea, the data appear to support benefits from the use of *Lactobacillus GG, L. reuteri, S. boulardii, S. thermophilus,* and *L. bulgaricus,* with some support as well for the use of *Lactobacillus acidophilus.* This author chooses not to use *S. boulardii,* in part due to lack of experience with the agent, but also because of case reports documenting rare infectious complications with the microbe in non-immunocompromised patients who were nonetheless ill.[19,20] Although the risk appears to be minimal, eradication of the rare bacterial complication from lactobacilli or *Bifidobacteria* spp. seems more amenable to treatment than fungal infection, albeit rare as well. *Lactobacillus GG* remains the organism best studied for the prevention and treatment of diarrheal disease.

Dosing guidelines to consider for non-yeast probiotic therapy are 10 billion CFU for children <12 kg and 20 billion CFU for children >12 kg. Treatment is extremely well tolerated, and palatability is an infrequent issue, as the capsules can be opened and mixed into drinks or soft foods. Sometimes the agents are available as a powder as well. If effective, treatment can continue indefinitely. Use with extreme caution, if at all, for those children at risk for infectious complications (e.g., immunosuppression or use of immunosuppressive agents, presence of central venous catheter, prematurity).

References

Pediatric Diagnosis and Treatment

1. Roy CC, Silverman A, Alagille D: *Pediatric clinical gastroenterology,* ed 4, St Louis, 1995, Mosby.
2. Northrup RS, Flanigan TP: Gastroenteritis, *Pediatr Rev* 15:461-472, 1994.
3. Guerrant RL, Van Gilder T, Steiner TS et al: Practice guidelines for the management of infectious diarrhea. Infectious Diseases Society of America, *Clin Infect Dis* 32:331-350, 2001.
4. Tucker AW, Haddix AC, Bresee JS et al: Cost-effectiveness analysis of a rotavirus immunization program for the United States, *J Am Med Assoc* 279:1371-1376, 1998.
5. Thompson SC: Infectious diarrhoea in children: controlling transmission in the child care setting, *J Pediatr Child Health* 30:210-219, 1994.
6. Kosek M, Bern C, Guerrant RL: The global burden of diarrhoeal disease, as estimated from studies published between 1992 and 2000, *Bull World Health Organ* 81:197-204, 2003.
7. Black RE, Morris SS, Bryce J: Where and why are 10 million children dying every year? *Lancet* 361:2226-2234, 2003.
8. Parashar U, Hummelman E, Bresee J et al: Global illness and deaths caused by rotavirus disease in children, *Emerg Infect Dis* 9:565-572, 2003.
9. Laney DW Jr, Cohen MB: Approach to the pediatric patient with diarrhea, *Gastroenterol Clin North Am* 22:499-516, 1993.
10. Walter JE, Mitchell DK: Role of astroviruses in childhood diarrhea, *Curr Opin Pediatr* 12:275-279, 2000.
11. Behrman RE, Kliegman RM, Jenson HB, editors: *Nelson's textbook of pediatrics,* Philadelphia, 2004, Saunders.
12. Mason JD. The evaluation of acute abdominal pain in children. Gastrointestinal emergencies, part I, *Emerg Med Clin North Am* 14:629-643, 1996.
13. Koutkia P, Mylonakis E, Flanigan T: Enterohemorrhagic *Escherichia coli* O157:H7—an emerging pathogen, *Am Fam Physician* 56:853-856, 859–861, 1997.
14. Trachtman H, Christen E: Pathogenesis, treatment, and therapeutic trials in hemolytic uremic syndrome, *Curr Opin Pediatr* 11:162-168, 1999.
15. Hart CA, Batt RM, Saunders JR: Diarrhoea caused by *Escherichia coli, Ann Trop Pediatr* 13:121-131, 1993.
16. Preliminary FoodNet Data on the incidence of infection with pathogens transmitted commonly through food—10 sites, United States, 2004, *MMWR Morbid Mortal Wkly Rep* 54:352-356, 2005.
17. Hjelt K, Paerregaard A, Krasilnikoff PA: Giardiasis in children with chronic diarrhea. Incidence, growth, clinical symptoms and changes in the small intestine [in Danish], *Ugeskr Laeger* 155:4083-4086, 1993 (abstract).
18. Shahani R: *Sustaining health with innovative R&D and health infrastructure,* 2004. Available at www.who.int/intellectualproperty/events/en/shahani2.pdf. Accessed August 2005.
19. American Academy of Pediatrics, statement of endorsement: Managing acute gastroenteritis among children: oral rehydration, maintenance, and nutritional therapy, *Pediatrics* 114:507, 2004.
20. King CK, Glass R, Bresee JS et al; Centers for Disease Control and Prevention: Managing acute gastroenteritis among children: oral rehydration, maintenance, and nutritional therapy, *MMWR Recomm Rep* 52(RR-16):1-16, 2003.
21. Bhatnagar S, Bahl R, Sharma PK et al: Zinc with oral rehydration therapy reduces stool output and duration of diarrhea in hospitalized children: a randomized controlled trial, *J Pediatr Gastroenterol Nutr* 38:34-40, 2004.
22. Gracey M: Nutritional effects and management of diarrhoea in infancy, *Acta Pediatria Suppl* 88:110-126, 1999.
23. DeWitt TG: Acute diarrhea in children, *Pediatr Rev* 11:6-13, 1989.
24. D'Souza AL, Rajkumar C, Cooke J et al: Probiotics in prevention of antibiotic associated diarrhoea: meta-analysis, *Br Med J* 324:1361-1366, 2002.

25. Szajewska H, Kotowska M, Mrukowicz JZ et al: Efficacy of *Lactobacillus* GG in prevention of nosocomial diarrhea in infants, *J Pediatr* 138:361-365, 2001.

26. Schmitz J: Anti-rotavirus vaccinations [in French], *Arch Pediatr* 6:979-984, 1999 (abstract).

27. McFarland LV: Microecologic approaches for traveler's diarrhea, antibiotic-associated diarrhea, and acute pediatric diarrhea, *Curr Gastroenterol Rep* 1:301-307, 1999.

28. McDonald LC: Emergence of an epidemic strain of *Clostridium difficile* in the United States, 2001-2004: potential role for virulence factors and antimicrobial resistance traits, LB-2. Presented at the 42nd Annual Meeting of the Infectious Diseases Society of America, Boston 2004.

29. Paerregaard A, Hjelt K, Krasilnikoff PA: Vitamin B12 and folic acid absorption and hematological status in children with postenteritis enteropathy, *J Pediatr Gastroenterol Nutr* 11:351-355, 1990.

30. Hugot JP, Cezard JP: Diarrhea in children [in French], *Rev Prat* 48:382-388, 1998.

31. Mehta DI, Blecker U: Chronic diarrhea in infancy and childhood, *J LA State Med Soc* 150:419-429, 1998.

32. Leung AK, Robson WL: Evaluating the child with chronic diarrhea, *Am Fam Physician* 53:635-643, 1996.

33. Rudolph JA, Cohen MB: New causes and treatments for infectious diarrhea in children, *Curr Gastroenterol Rep* 1:238-244, 1999.

34. Hambidge KM: Zinc and diarrhea, *Acta Paediatr Suppl* 381:82-86, 1992.

35. Bonamico M, Culasso F, Colombo C et al: Irritable bowel syndrome in children: an Italian multicentre study—collaborating centres [in Italian], *Ital J Gastroenterol* 27:13-20, 1995 (abstract).

36. Kneepkens CM, Hoekstra JH: Chronic nonspecific diarrhea of childhood: pathophysiology and management, *Pediatr Clin North Am* 43:375-390, 1996.

37. Rasquin-Weber A, Hyman PE, Cucchiara S et al: Childhood functional gastrointestinal disorders, *Gut* 45(Suppl 2). II60-II8, 1992.

38. Montes RG, Perman JA: Lactose intolerance: pinpointing the source of nonspecific gastrointestinal symptoms, *Postgrad Med* 89:175-184, 1991.

39. Hoekstra JH, van den Aker JH, Ghoos YF et al: Fluid intake and industrial processing in apple juice induced chronic non-specific diarrhoea, *Arch Dis Child* 73:126-130, 1995.

40. Dennison BA: Fruit juice consumption by infants and children: a review, *J Am Coll Nutr* 15(5 Suppl):4S-11S, 1996.

41. Smith MM, Lifshitz F: Excess fruit juice consumption as a contributing factor in nonorganic failure to thrive, *Pediatrics* 93:438-443, 1994.

42. Ament ME: Malabsorption of apple juice and pear nectar in infants and children: clinical implications, *J Am Coll Nutr* 15 (5 Suppl):26S-29S, 1996.

43. Panizon F: Food allergy and psychosomatic medicine: new frontiers [in Italian], *Pediatr Med Chir* 9:671-677, 1987 (abstract).

44. Perlmutter DH, Leichtner AM, Goldman H et al: Chronic diarrhea associated with hypogammaglobulinemia and enteropathy in infants and children, *Dig Dis Sci* 30:1149-1155, 1985.

45. Boehm P, Nassimbeni G, Ventura A: Chronic non-specific diarrhoea in childhood: how often is it iatrogenic? *Acta Pediatria* 87:268-271, 1998.

Acupuncture

1. Diehl DL: Acupuncture for gastrointestinal and hepatobiliary disorders, *J Altern Complement Med* 5:27-45, 1999.

2. Lin YC: Observation of the therapeutic effects of acupuncture treatment in 170 cases of infantile diarrhea, *J Tradit Chin Med* 7:203-204, 1987.

3. Feng WL: Acupuncture treatment for 30 cases of infantile chronic diarrhea, *J Tradit Chin Med* 9:106-107, 1989.

4. Jiang R: Analgesic effect of acupuncture on acute intestinal colic in 190 cases, *J Tradit Chin Med* 10:20-21, 1990.

5. Su Z: Acupuncture treatment of infantile diarrhea: a report of 1050 cases, *J Tradit Chin Med* 12:120-121, 1992.

6. Xu JH, Lin LH, Zhang PY: Treatment of infantile diarrhea with anisodamine by the injection method of Zu San Li acupuncture points [in Chinese], *Zhonghua Hu Li Za Zhi* 31:345, 1996.

7. Wang M, Zhu Y: Clinical experience of Dr. Shao Jingming in treatment of diseases by puncturing back-shu points, *J Tradit Chin Med* 16:23-26, 1996.

8. Lin Y, Zhou Z, Shen W et al: Clinical and experimental studies on shallow needling technique for treating childhood diarrhea, *J Tradit Chin Med* 13:107-114, 1993.

9. Sato A, Sato Y, Suzuki A et al: Neural mechanisms of the reflex inhibition and excitation of gastric motility elicited by acupuncture-like stimulation in anesthetized rats, *Neurosci Res* 18:53-62, 1993.

10. Li Y, Tougas G, Chiverton SG et al: The effect of acupuncture on gastrointestinal function and disorders, *Am J Gastroenterol* 87:1372-1381, 1992.

11. Kim HY, Hahm DH, Pyun KH et al: Effects of acupuncture at GV01 on experimentally induced colitis in rats: possible involvement of opioid system, *Jpn J Physiol* 55:205-210, 2005.

12. Park ES, Jo S, Seong JK et al: Effect of acupuncture in the treatment of young pigs with induced *Escherichia coli* diarrhea, *J Vet Sci* 4:125-128, 2003.

13. Lin X, Liang J, Ren J et al: Electrical stimulation of acupuncture points enhances gastric myoelectrical activity in humans, *Am J Gastroenterol* 92:1527-1530, 1997.

14. Qian LW, Lin YP: Effect of electroacupuncture at zusanli (ST36) point in regulating the pylorus peristaltic function [in Chinese], *Zhongguo Zhong Xi Yi Jie He Za Zhi* 13:336-339, 324, 1993 (abstract).

15. Loo M: *Pediatric acupuncture*, London, 2002, Elsevier.

16. Shen X: Acupuncture treatment for kidney deficiency with combined application of points mingmen and guanyuan, *J Trad Chin Med* 16:275-277, 1996.

Chiropractic

1. Davies N: *Chiropractic pediatrics*, London, 2000, Churchill Livingstone.

2. Bilgrai Cohen K: *Clinical management of infants and children*, Santa Cruz, Calif, 1988, Extension Press.

3. Swenson R: Pediatric disorders. In Lawrence DJ, editor: *Fundamentals of chiropractic diagnosis and management*, Baltimore, 1991, Williams and Wilkins.

4. Van Niel CW, Feudtner C, Garrison MM et al: *Lactobacillus* therapy for acute infectious diarrhea in children: a meta-analysis, *Pediatrics* 109:678-684, 2002.

5. Isolauri E, Kaila M, Mykkänen H et al: Oral bacteriotherapy for viral gastroenteritis, *Dig Dis Science* 39:2595-2600, 1994

6. Perdigon G, Nader de Macias ME, Alvarez S et al: Prevention of gastrointestinal infection using immunobiological methods with milk fermented with *Lactobacillus casei* and *Lactobacillus acidophilus*, *J Dairy Res* 57:255-264, 1990.

7. Boudraa G, Touhami M, Pochart P et al: Effect of feeding yogurt versus milk in children with persistent diarrhea, *J Pediatr Gastoenterol Nutr* 11:509-512, 1990.

8. Saavedra JM, Bauman NA, Oung I et al: Feeding of *Bifidobacterium bifidum* and *Streptococcus thermophilus* to infants in hospital for prevention of diarrhea and shedding of rotavirus, *Lancet* 334:1046-1049, 1994.

9. Bhutta ZA, Nizami SQ, Isani Z: Lactose intolerance in persistent diarrhoea during childhood: the role of a traditional rice-lentil (khitchri) and yogurt diet in nutritional management, *J Pak Med Assoc* 47:20-24, 1997.

Herbs—Chinese

1. Beinfield H, Korngold E: *Chinese medicine works clinical handbook,* San Francisco, 2007, www.chinesemedicineworks.com.

Herbs—Western

1. De La Motte S, Boese O'Reilly S, Heinisch M et al: Double-blind comparison of a preparation of pectin/chamomile extract and placebo in children with diarrhea [in German], *Arzneimittel Forschung* 47:1247-1249, 1997.

2. Choudhry VP, Sabir M, Bhide VN: Berberine in giardiasis, *Indian Pediatr* 9:143-146, 1972.

3. Desai AB, Shah KM, Shah DM: Berberine in treatment of diarrhoea, *Indian Pediatr* 8:462-465, 1971.

4. Chauhan RK, Jain AM, Bhandari B: Berberine in the treatment of childhood diarrhoea, *Indian J Pediatr* 37:577-579, 1970.

5. Chauhan RK, Jain AM, Dube MK et al: A combination of sulfadimidine, neomycin and berberine in the treatment of infectious diarrhoea, *Indian J Pediatr* 36:242-244, 1969.

6. Lahiri SC, Dutta NK: Berberine and chloramphenicol in the treatment of cholera and severe diarrhoea, *J Indian Med Assoc* 48:1-11, 1967.

7. Mills S, Bone K, editors: *The essential guide to herbal safety,* St Louis, 2005, Elsevier.

8. Ho NK: Traditional Chinese medicine and treatment of neonatal jaundice, *Singapore Med J* 37:645-651, 1996.

Homeopathy

1. Jacobs J, Jiménez LM, Gloyd S et al: Homeopathic treatment of acute childhood diarrhoea, *Br Homeopath J* 82:83-86, 1993.

2. Jacob J, Jiménez LM, Gloyd S et al: Treatment of acute childhood diarrhea with homeopathic medicine: a randomized clinical trial in Nicaragua, *Pediatrics* 93:719-735, 1994.

3. Jacobs J, Jiménez LM, Malthouse S et al: Homeopathic treatment of acute childhood diarrhea: results from a clinical trial in Nepal, *J Altern Complement Med* 6:131-139, 2000.

4. Jacobs J, Jonas WB, Jiménez-Perez M et al: Homeopathy for childhood diarrhea: combined results and metaanalysis from three randomized, controlled clinical trials, *Pediatr Infect Dis J* 22:229-234, 2003.

5. *ReferenceWorks Pro 4.2,* San Rafael, Calif, 2008, Kent Homeopathic Associates.

Naturopathy

1. Hawrelak JA, Whitten DL, Myers SP: Is *Lactobacillus rhamnosus* GG effective in preventing the onset of antibiotic-associated diarrhoea: a systematic review, *Digestion* 72:51-56, 2005.

2. Surawicz CM: Probiotics, antibiotic-associated diarrhoea and *Clostridium difficile* diarrhoea in humans, *Best Pract Res Clin Gastroenterol* 17:775-783, 2003.

3. Cremonini F, Di Caro S, Santarelli L et al: Probiotics in antibiotic-associated diarrhoea, *Dig Liver Dis* 34(Suppl 2):S78-S80, 2002.

4. Murray M: Lactobacilli abstracts and commentary, *Am J Nat Med* April 1997.

5. Szajewska H, Mrukowicz J: Meta-analysis: non-pathogenic yeast *Saccharomyces boulardii* in the prevention of antibiotic-associated diarrhoea, *Aliment Pharmacol Ther* 22:365-372, 2005.

6. Kurugol Z, Koturoglu G: Effects of *Saccharomyces boulardii* in children with acute diarrhoea, *Acta Paediatr* 94:44-47, 2005.

7. Correa NB, Peret Filho LA, Penna FJ et al: A randomized formula controlled trial of *Bifidobacterium lactis* and *Streptococcus thermophilus* for prevention of antibiotic-associated diarrhea in infants, *J Clin Gastroenterol* 39:385-389, 2005.

8. Subbaiah TV, Amin AH: Effect of berberine sulphate on *Entamoeba histolytica*, *Nature* 215:527-528, 1967.

9. Amin AH, Subbaiah TV, Abbasi KM: Berberine sulfate: antimicrobial activity, bioassay, and mode of action, *Can J Microbiol* 15:1067-1076, 1969.

10. Choudhry VP, Sabir M, Bhide VN: Berberine in giardiasis, *Indian Pediatr* 9:143-146, 1972.

11. Ortega-Barria E, Ward HD, Evans JE et al: N-acetyl-D-glucosamine is present in cysts and trophozoites of *Giardia lamblia* and serves as receptor for wheatgerm agglutinin, *Mol Biochem Parasitol* 43:151-165, 1990.

Osteopathy

1. Kuchera ML, Kuchera WA: *Osteopathic considerations in systemic disease*, Columbus, Ohio, 1994, Greydon Press.

2. Carreiro JE: *An osteopathic approach to children*, London, 2003, Churchill Livingstone.

3. Strong WB: Disorders of the digestive system. In Hoag JM, editor: *Osteopathic medicine*, New York, 1969, McGraw-Hill.

4. Denslow J: Functional colitis: etiology, *AAO Yearbook* 1:192-197, 1965.

5. Barral JP, Mercier P: *Visceral manipulation*, Seattle, 1988, Eastland Press.

6. Owen C: *An endocrine interpretation of Chapman's reflexes,* ed 2, Boulder, Colo, 1963, American Academy of Osteopathy.

7. Masterson EV: Irritable bowel syndrome: an osteopathic approach, *Osteopath Ann* 12:12-18, 1984.

8. Bramati-Castellarin I, Janossa M: Effect of visceral osteopathy on the gastrointestinal abnormalities in children with autistic disorders [see comments; meeting abstract], *J Osteopath Med (Austr)* 5:36-37, 2002.

9. Fitzgerald M, Stiles E: Osteopathic hospital's solution to DRG's may be OMT, *D O* 97-101, 1984.

Probiotics

1. Gorbach SL: Efficacy of *Lactobacillus* in treatment of acute diarrhea, *Nutr Today* 31:19S, 1996.

2. Marteau PR, de Vrese M, Cellier CJ et al: Protection from gastrointestinal diseases with the use of probiotics, *Am J Clin Nutr* 73(Suppl):430S, 2001.

3. Saavedra J: Probiotics and infectious diarrhea, *Am J Gastroenterol* 95(Suppl):S16, 2000.

4. Van Niel CW, Feudtner C, Garrison MM et al: *Lactobacillus* therapy for acute infectious diarrhea in children: a meta-analysis, *Pediatrics* 109:678-684, 2002.

5. Allen SJ, Okoko B, Martinez E et al: Probiotics for treating infectious diarrhoea (Cochrane Review), *Cochrane Library* 3, 2004.

6. Isolauri E, Juntunen M, Routanen T et al: A human *Lactobacillus* strain (*Lactobacillus casei* sp. strain GG) promotes recovery from acute diarrhea in children, *Pediatrics* 88:90, 1991.

7. Shornikova A-V, Casas IA, Isolauri E et al: *Lactobacillus reuteri* as a therapeutic agent in acute diarrhea in young children, *J Pediatr Gastroenterol* 24:399, 1997.

8. Guarino A, Canani RB, Spagnuolo MI et al: Oral bacterial therapy reduces the duration of symptoms and of viral excretion in children with mild diarrhea, *J Pediatr Gastroenterol Nutr* 25:516-519, 1997.

9. Saavedra J, Bauman NA, Oung I et al: Feeding of *Bifidobacterium bifidum* and *Streptococcus thermophilus* to infants in hospital for prevention of diarrhea, and shedding of rotavirus, *Lancet* 344:1046-1049, 1994.

10. Majamaa H, Isolauri E, Saxelin M et al: Lactic acid bacteria in treatment of acute rotavirus gastroenteritis, *J Pediatr Gastroenterol Nutr* 20:333-338, 1995.

11. Surawicz CM, Elmer G, Speelman P et al: Prevention of antibiotic-associated diarrhea by *Saccharomyces boulardii*: a prospective study, *Gastroenterology* 96:981-988, 1989.

12. Siitonen S, Vapaatalo H, Salminen S et al: Effect of *Lactobacillus GG* yoghurt in prevention of antibiotic associated diarrhoea, *Ann Med* 22:57-59, 1990.

13. Pochapin M: The effect of probiotics on *Clostridium difficile* diarrhea, *Am J Gastroenterol* 95(Suppl):S11-S13, 2000.

14. Gorbach SL, Chang TW, Goldin B: Successful treatment of relapsing *Clostridium difficile* colitis with *Lactobacillus* GG [letter], *Lancet* 2:1519, 1987.

15. McFarland LV: Biotherapeutic agents for *Clostridium difficile*-associated disease. In Elmer GW, McFarland LV, Surawicz CM, editors: *Biotherapeutic agents and infectious diseases*, Totowa, NJ, 1999, Humana Press.

16. Biller JA, Katz AJ, Flores AF et al: Treatment of recurrent *Clostridium difficile* colitis with *Lactobacillus* GG, *J Pediatr Gastroenterol Nutr* 21:224-226, 1995.

17. Colombel JF, Cortot A, Neut C et al: Yoghurt with *Bifidobacterium longum* reduces erythromycin-induced gastrointerstinal effects [letter], *Lancet* 2:43, 1987.

18. Oksanen PJ, Salminen S, Saxelin M et al: Prevention of diarrhea by *Lactobacillus* GG, *Ann Med* 22:53-56, 1990.

19. Pletincx M, Legein J, Vandenplas Y: Fungemia with *Saccharomyces boulardii* in a 1-year-old girl with protracted diarrhea, *J Pediatr Gastroenterol Nutr* 21:113-115, 1995.

20. Rijnders BJ, Van Wijngaerden E, Verwaest C et al: *Saccharomyces fungemia* complication *Saccharomyces boulardii* treatment in a non-immunocompromised host, *Intens Care Med* 26:825, 2000.

CHAPTER 31

Drooling

Acupuncture | May Loo

Chiropractic | Anne Spicer

Homeopathy | Janet L. Levatin

✳ PEDIATRIC DIAGNOSIS AND TREATMENT

Drooling, or sialorrhea, occurs in normal infants until approximately 6 months of age, when muscular reflexes that initiate swallowing and lip closure are more developed. Later, the irritation of teething may lead to temporary drooling.[1] Drooling frequently occurs in children with multiple handicaps,[2] especially neurological dysfunction. An estimated 10% of children with neurological impairment such as cerebral palsy have excessive drooling that interferes with everyday living.[3,4] Contrary to common belief, this condition is not due to hypersalivation. The primary pathophysiology is the inefficient swallowing of saliva because of oromotor incoordination, resulting in excessive pooling of saliva in the anterior part of the mouth and consequent overspill.[5,6]

Although it is not a serious health problem, drooling is an unpleasant physical affliction and can have a significant negative social impact on children, especially the handicapped children who may feel further social isolation with drooling added to their other disabilities.[7-9] Drooling is also difficult for parents and caregivers who need to constantly change bibs or clothing.[10]

Mild cases are usually not treated. More severe cases are managed by various treatment modalities that include behavioral therapy, medication, biofeedback, physiotherapy, biofunctional oral appliances, and surgery.[5,11]

A British review of 78 children ages 3-17 years who were treated in a multidisciplinary oral-motor clinic revealed that 18% responded to oral skills training alone, 30% had good results with a palatal training appliance, 8% needed medication, and 47% underwent some form of surgery to control their drooling.[9]

Anticholinergic drugs such as benztropine, glycopyrrolate, and scopolamine can offer some symptom relief.[2,8] Recently, botulinum toxin (BTX) was introduced for the treatment of hypersialorrhea. A 2003 German review indicated that hypersialorrhea was reduced in almost all affected children for up to 6 months by using ultrasound-guided intraglandular BTX injections.[12] The first controlled clinical trial demonstrated a reduction in drooling in children with cerebral palsy, achieving maximum effect 2 to 8 weeks after injection, with fewer side-effects than transdermal scopolamine.[2]

Patients with intractable drooling are referred for surgical procedures, such as submandibular duct relocation and submandibular gland excision.[1] One of the newest procedures is the four-duct ligation: combined ligation of the submandibular and parotid ducts. A U.S. report of 21 patients who underwent this procedure and were followed up to 14 months after surgery indicated improvement of symptoms in 17 patients. No patient's sialorrhea was worse after surgery.[7]

Parents fear side effects of drugs and often do not wish to subject their children to irreversible surgery. Various complementary and alternative medicine (CAM) therapies offer safe and more effective treatment modalities for a condition that has physical and social consequences.

✳ CAM THERAPY RECOMMENDATIONS

Acupuncture

There is little information on acupuncture treatment of drooling.[1]

The best point appears to be the local point, ST4,[2] which has recently been demonstrated to be effective in treating children with cerebral palsy, with the application of a biosouth (+) magnet facing downward on the point.[3]

Treatment of excess Stomach water: Sedate ST44.

Tonification of Spleen can promote better movement and circulation of fluid:

Four-Point protocol: Tonify SP2, HT8; sedate SP1, LR1.

Two points: Tonify SP2; sedate SP1.

Or use meridian tonification: Connect with ion pumping cord: black on lower SP point (e.g., SP3 or SP6); red on SP9. If using magnets, place bionorth (−) pole facing down on SP3 or SP6 and biosouth (+) pole facing down on SP9, and connect with ion pumping cord as above.

Because the majority of drooling occurs in children with neurological impairment, which correlates to Kidney deficiency, tonification of Kidney would help improve neurological function:

Tonify KI7, LU8; sedate KI3, SP3.

A clinical trial in Hong Kong treated 10 children with neurological disability and severe drooling using five tongue acupoints. The children received daily treatments for a total of 30 sessions. Statistically significant improvement in drooling was observed. Although this is a painful form of acupuncture, it may be tried prior to considering invasive surgical procedures.[4]

Chiropractic

Chiropractic literature makes one reference to control of drooling in its relationship to brain injury.[1] This report recommends that the chiropractor address the function of the temporomandibular joint (TMJ) and its supportive musculature, particularly the masseter and the pterygoids. Adjustments to the TMJ would be provided as necessary, along with manual stimulation and stretch of the associated musculature. Muscle work in this area may be painful, and care should be taken to remain within the tolerance of the child.

The chiropractic adjustment at the C0 to C1 region is also helpful in tongue retraction and therefore drooling.

Homeopathy

Before using this section, please see Appendix A, Homeopathy, for definitions of practitioner expertise categories and general information on prescribing homeopathic medicines.

Drooling is a symptom associated with a number of medical conditions including teething, gingivostomatitis, developmental disorders, pharyngitis, and neurological disorders, among others. Drooling, or excessive salivation, is mentioned frequently as a symptom in the homeopathic literature[1]; however, from a homeopathic perspective drooling is not considered a condition to be treated in and of itself, but rather part of the whole symptom picture that a patient presents. When drooling is a prominent symptom in a case, it should be included in the analysis that is done to determine the simillimum. Homeopathic treatment may be effective for drooling when the simillimum is given to the patient for the overall condition. For the reason cited previously, however, it is not practical to provide specific medicines for treatment of drooling in this chapter. Interested readers are referred to the homeopathic literature for further study of the medical conditions that may include drooling as a symptom.[1]

References

Pediatric Diagnosis and Management

1. Behrman RE, Kliegman RM, Jenson HB, editors: *Nelson's textbook of pediatrics*, Philadelphia, 2004, Saunders.
2. Jongerius PH, van Tiel P, van Limbeek J et al: A systematic review for evidence of efficacy of anticholinergic drugs to treat drooling, *Arch Dis Child* 88:911-914, 2003.
3. Wolraich ML: *Disorders of development and learning*, ed 3, London, 2003, BC Becker.
4. O'Dwyer TP, Conlon BJ: The surgical management of drooling—a 15 year follow-up, *Clin Otolaryngol* 22:284-287, 1997.
5. Shapira J, Becker A, Moskovitz M: The management of drooling problems in children with neurological dysfunction: a review and case report, *Spec Care Dentist* 19:181-185, 1999.
6. Lespargot A, Langevin MF, Muller S et al: Swallowing disturbances associated with drooling in cerebral-palsied children, *Devel Med Child Neurol* 35:298-304, 1993.
7. Shirley WP, Hill JS, Woolley AL et al: Success and complications of four-duct ligation for sialorrhea, *Int J Pediatr Otorhinolaryngol* 67:1-6, 2003.
8. Tscheng DZ: Sialorrhea—therapeutic drug options, *Ann Pharmacother* 36:1785-1790, 2002.
9. Lloyd Faulconbridge RV, Tranter RM, Moffat V et al: Review of management of drooling problems in neurologically impaired children: a review of methods and results over 6 years at Chailey Heritage Clinical Services, *Clin Otolaryngol* 26:76-81, 2001.
10. Shott SR, Myer CM 3rd, Cotton RT: Surgical management of sialorrhea, *Otolaryngol Head Neck Surg* 101:47-50, 1989.
11. Hussein I, Kershaw AE, Tahmassebi JF et al: The management of drooling in children and patients with mental and physical disabilities: a literature review, *Int J Paediatr Dent* 8:3-11, 1998.
12. Guntinas-Lichius O: Management of Frey's syndrome and hypersialorrhea with botulinum toxin, *Facial Plast Surg Clin North Am* 11:503-513, 2003.

Acupuncture

1. Loo M: *Pediatric acupuncture*, London, 2002, Elsevier.
2. Deadman P, Al-Khafaji M: *A manual of acupuncture*, East Sussex, United Kingdom, 1998, Journal of Chinese Medicine Publications.
3. Colbert A: Lecture and personal communication, 1999.
4. Wong V, Sun JG, Wong W: Traditional Chinese medicine (tongue acupuncture) in children with drooling problems, *Pediatr Neurol* 25:47-54, 2001.

Chiropractic

1. McMullen M: Chiropractic and the handicapped child/cerebral palsy, *ICA Int Rev Chiropractic* Sep/Oct:39-45, 1990.

Homeopathy

1. *ReferenceWorks Pro 4.2*, San Rafael, Calif, 2008, Kent Homeopathic Associates.

Eczema

Acupuncture | May Loo

Aromatherapy | Maura A. Fitzgerald

Chiropractic | Anne Spicer

Herbs—Chinese | May Loo, Harriet Beinfield, Efrem Korngold

Herbs—Western | Alan D. Woolf, Paula M. Gardiner, Lana Dvorkin-Camiel, Jack Maypole

Massage Therapy | Mary C. McLellan

Mind/Body | Timothy Culbert, Lynda Richtsmeier Cyr

Naturopathy | Matthew I. Baral

Nutrition | Joy A. Weydert

Probiotics | Russell H. Greenfield

✳ PEDIATRIC DIAGNOSIS AND TREATMENT

Atopic dermatitis (AD), or atopic eczema, is the most common chronic skin condition in children in industrialized countries.[1] It affects between 5% and 20% of all children from birth to 11 years at one time or another[2] and accounts for 20% of all dermatologic referrals. Recent data indicate that its prevalence is increasing,[2,3] and many cases persist into adulthood.[1]

The precise etiology and pathophysiology is still unknown.[1] There appear to be two forms of this disorder: an allergic (extrinsic) form and a nonallergic (intrinsic) form, each with clear genetic, humoral, and cellular distinctions.[4] The allergic variant is an exaggerated response of the immune system to external substances,[5] engendering both immunoglobulin (Ig)-E production and T cell–mediated responses.[6] Various environmental allergens have been implicated, the most common being grass, tree pollens, the house dust mite, products from pets and other animals, agents encountered in industry, wasp and bee venom, drugs, and certain foods.[2,5] *Food intolerance* is a better term than *food allergy*, as many individuals with eczema do not demonstrate an alteration in the immune system with food challenges.[5]

Recent research has demonstrated that maternal atopy during pregnancy may have an important effect on the developing immune response of the fetus and may predispose the child to developing allergies. Maternal IgE, IgG, and amniotic fluid cytokines, combined with the presence of allergen in the fetomaternal environment, are all possible factors that influence infant responses to common environmental antigens. Immune modulation at this stage of development may, in the future, be a way forward in the prevention of allergy.[7]

The Canadian Cochrane Database examined preventive studies that prescribed an antigen avoidance diet to high-risk mothers during pregnancy and lactation. A high-risk woman is one with the atopic disease, and a high-risk fetus or infant is one with eczema in the mother, father, or a sibling. Current data seem to suggest that when lactating mothers with high-risk infants are given the diet, the incidence of eczema is decreased during the child's first 12 to 18 months of life,[8] whereas in a small clinical trial in which the diet was prescribed to lactating mothers of infants who already have atopic eczema, the severity of the baby's eczema was not significantly affected.[9] When a high-risk mother was placed on the restrictive diet during pregnancy, the incidence of giving birth to an atopic child was not reduced, and the diet may have had an adverse effect on maternal and/or fetal nutrition.[10]

Eczema is a chronic condition with a wide spectrum of clinical presentations, ranging from a few patches of dry, pruritic, thickened skin to fulminant, severe, generalized dermatitis that fluctuates between acute flare-up of red, intensely pruritic, inflammatory skin and periods of relative quiescence.[1,4,11] Eczema often occurs in patients with a family history of the atopic triad (asthma, allergic rhinitis, and atopic dermatitis).[11]

Treatment

Although eczema is not life threatening, the discomfort from the symptoms, the unsightly rash, and the chronic nature of the condition are distressing to both the child and the parents[1] and have an effect on the child's and family's quality of life.[12] The excoriated skin from scratching is susceptible to developing secondary bacterial infection as purulent, weepy, impetiginous lesions. Treatment is therefore challenging and complicated and needs to address not only the physical symptoms, but also the psychosocial impact on the lives of the child and the caregivers. As a result, eczema engenders significant cost for the family and healthcare systems.[2,13]

The physical manifestations are treated symptomatically, often by elimination of allergenic foods or avoidance of environmental allergens.[6,14] Topical steroids have been the treatment of choice for eczema.[11,15,16] Steroid-free treatments with a more favorable safety profile have become available recently. Tacrolimus ointment, a topical immunomodulator, became available in early 2001 and is indicated for moderate to severe AD. A similar but highly skin-selective cytokine inhibitor, pimecrolimus cream 1%, became available in March 2002.[11] Although many studies and reviews expound on the efficacy of tacrolimus and pimecrolimus,[11,16,17] evidence from randomized controlled trials is still limited.[15] In February 2005, after reviewing various safety and efficacy reports of possible adverse events associated with tacrolimus (Protopic) and pimecrolimus (Elidel) the U.S. Food and Drug Administration (FDA) pediatric advisory committee recommended that these two drugs carry a black-box warning for possible risk of malignancy and other adverse side effects.[18,19]

✳ CAM THERAPY RECOMMENDATIONS

Acupuncture

Acupuncture[1] has been found to be successful in treating both the pruritic symptoms[2] and the skin lesions in eczema.[3-5] The possible mechanisms include an antiinflammatory mechanism that minimizes IgE and eosinophils.[5]

From the traditional Chinese medicine (TCM) standpoint, the pathophysiology of eczema is manifold: accumulation of Heat and Damp combined with Blood and Yin deficiency.[4] Multiple organ and channel dysfunction can be involved: Lung, Spleen, Kidney, or Liver. Lingering Heat and Damp from previous illnesses and a diet rich in Damp and energetically Hot foods would predispose children to accumulate Heat and Damp in the skin and in the Blood. In TCM the skin is part of the Lung, which explains the frequent manifestation of eczema in patients with asthma. Spleen deficiency can manifest as accumulation of Damp. A child may have a prenatal predisposition to Dampness and eczema when there is a strong familial tendency toward Spleen deficiency; when parents engage in excess mental work, have excess worry, or have digestive weakness due to poor diet or alcohol abuse during conception; and when the mother has these experiences during pregnancy. Living in a Damp environment, such as in the basement, close to the ocean, or in a rainy climate; eating Damp-producing foods, such as milk products, greasy fried foods, peanuts, sweets, and white sugar; and engaging in excess mental activities can subject the child to Spleen deficiency and the development of eczema. Although Dampness usually affects the lower part of the body, it can easily enter the Middle Burner; from there it rises upward to affect the Upper Burner, the Lung and its corresponding organ, the skin. The Lung houses the Corporeal Soul, which gives us the capacity for physical sensations. When the Lung is not in balance, the Corporeal Soul is responsible for manifestation of excess physical sensations, such as itching in eczema. Kidney and Liver Yin deficiencies can predispose the child to Blood and Yin deficiencies and Heat accumulation, which manifest as red, dry skin.

Treatment for eczema is directed toward dispersing Heat and Damp in acute flare-ups and tonifying chronic deficiencies.

Acute Eczema

ST40 to disperse Damp and Heat.
SP10, BL17, LI11 to remove Blood Heat.
Avoid energetically Hot foods and Phlegm-producing foods.
Minimize application of dermocorticosteroids. From the TCM
standpoint, these ointments tend to keep Dampness and
Heat in the skin, which may predispose the child to develop
Damp and Heat conditions elsewhere.

Treat lesions according to specific location:
Local points and Ah Shi points: for example, BL40 for popliteal fossa; GV14, GB20, BL12 for head and neck.
Combine proximal and distal points of the corresponding channels to the area:
Head, neck, upper back: GV and BL channels
Face: Yangming ST channel
Upper extremities:
Flexor surface—LU, HT, P
Extensor surface—SI, LI, TB
Lower extremities:
Flexor surface—KI, BL, LR
Extensor surface—ST, SP, GB

Chronic Eczema

The recommended treatment for specific channels and organs is to select the Yuan (source) point, He (Sea) point, and Back Shu points of each organ[12]:

SOURCE	HE (SEA)	BACK SHU
SP: SP3	SP9	BL20
KI: KI3	KI10	BL23
LU: LU9	LU5	BL13
LR: LR3	L48	BL18

BL17 to tonify Blood.
ST40 to disperse Damp and Heat.
SP10, BL17, LI11 to remove Blood Heat.
Avoid energetically Hot foods and phlegm-producing foods.
Tonify Spleen to minimize Dampness:
Tonify SP2, HT8; sedate SP1, LR1.

Itching/Pruritis

ST15, GB31 for generalized itching.[6]

Tonification of the Immune System

Because eczema has immune components, use the immune protocol to strengthen the child.[1]

Aromatherapy

Aromtherapy with massage was tested in a small pilot study of eight children, 3-7 years of age, with atopic eczema. Subjects were randomly assigned to either massage alone or aromatherapy massage. In each group, massage was performed one time per week by a massage therapist, and mothers provided daily massage after instruction. This was done for a total of 8 weeks. Mothers selected three essentials oils from a group of eight oils. These oils were mixed in equal parts and added to the massage lotion and to the child's bath. The essential oils used for this study were sweet marjoram (*Origanum majorana)*, frankincense (*Boswellia carteri)*, German chamomile (*Matricaria recutita)*, myrrh (*Commiphora myrrha)*, benzoin (*Styrax benzoin)*, May chang (*Litsea cubeba)*, spike lavender (*Lavandula spica)*, and thyme (*Thymus vulgaris)*. Mothers rated change in daytime irritation and nighttime disturbance. Both mothers and medical practitioners rated change in general improvement. Nighttime and daytime disturbance scores dropped for both groups with no difference between groups. General improvement scores also showed no difference between groups. However, after a subsequent 8 weeks of therapy, nighttime disturbance scores increased for the aromatherapy group. The authors express concern that contact dermatitis was provoked by the essential oil.[1]

Recognizing that there is little research on essential oils for skin conditions, one author recommends essential oils that are antiinflammatory, such as German chamomile (*M. recutita*) and yarrow (*Achillea millefolium*) for treatment of psoriasis.[2] However, given the results of the previous study, although allergic reactions are infrequent, essential oils should be used with care in children with demonstrated sensitivities.[3]

Chiropractic

Eczema classically results from hyperreactivity to a chemical exposure, particularly foods. The section on chiropractic management of allergies (see Chapter 10 Allergies) is reflective of the management of eczema as well.

Prevention of atopy may occur with exposure to endotoxins and infectious diseases early in life, whereas exposure to antibiotics in utero and in early life increases the risk of development of eczema.[1] Therefore the chiropractor is not generally an advocate of universal use of antimicrobial and disinfectant products in the child's environment. Integrated therapies are also recommended in infancy and childhood in an effort to avoid the use of antibiotics unless and until vitally necessary. Maintenance of healthy gut microflora from infancy supports normal immune function and may reduce even intrinsic forms of eczema.

Control of the itching associated with eczema is advantageous. This can be done with application of a hypoallergenic moisturizing lotion, use of oatmeal baths, and avoidance of products that dry the skin.

Natural-fabric clothing is preferable and should be washed in nonallergenic laundry products.

Daily brief to moderate sun exposure and fresh air may help reduce inflammation, whereas long periods of sun exposure can worsen eczema.

Herbs—Chinese

One Chinese herbal approach may aim toward helping the child neutralize and eliminate phlegm, as well as normal byproducts of metabolism and toxins absorbed from the environment, such as food or environmental allergens.

Fire Fighter (Gentle Warrior Pediatric Formula, Kan Herb Company, Scotts Valley Calif.) is a broadly focused remedy for assisting the body in getting rid of internally and externally accumulated toxins.

Herbal formula: The leading ingredient, *Oldenlandia* herb (bai hua she she cao), is assisted by *Scrophularia* root (xuan shen), dandelion root (pu gong ying), honeysuckle flower (jin yin hua), *Forsythia* bud (lian qiao), and *Arctium* fruit (niu bang zi) in the action of clearing Heat, neutralizing Toxins, softening and dispersing Phlegm nodules, and eliminating pus. *Platycodon* root (jie geng) enhances the action of dissolving Phlegm and eliminating pus as well as facilitating—directing—the formula into the channels and collaterals (jing-luo) that, in modern terms, correspond to

peripheral circulation of blood and lymph including the small capillaries, venules, lymphatic vessels, and lymph nodes. Peppermint herb (bo he), jujube fruit (da zao), cloves (ding xiang), and licorice root (gan cao) tone the Stomach and aid digestion, moderating the strong cooling and detoxifying properties of the primary ingredients.[1]

Dosage: 1 to 2 droppersful as needed 2 to 4 times per day.[1]
Caution: Suspected bacterial infection with high fever; while nursing; diarrhea.[1]

Herbs—Western

See also Dermatitis, Allergic or Atopic.

Eczema (also known as AD) is a chronic skin rash that affects the flexor surfaces of the arms and legs, although it may also commonly involve the face, neck, and abdomen. Steroid-containing creams are viewed as the mainstay of therapy. However, both flaxseed oil (given as 15 to 30 mL in adults)[1] and evening primrose oil (doses of 3 g/day for 16 weeks have been used in children with apparent safety)[2] taken orally contain EFAs that can enhance the skin's healing from eczema and help relieve itching and inflammation. Children with AD are thought to have a reduced rate of conversion from linoleic acid to GLA, dihomo-γ-linolenic acid, or arachidonic acid as compared with healthy subjects.[3-5] Replacement of GLA, in the form of primrose oil or borage oil, may therefore benefit the treatment of these patients. In fact, more than 20 randomized controlled studies assessing the effects of GLA have been performed, with most studies indicating an improved epidermal barrier on GLA application. In one recent study, topical application of 20% evening primrose oil caused a statistically significant stabilizing effect on the epidermal barrier in patients with AD as evaluated by transepidermal water loss and stratum corneum hydration. When compared with placebo, the water-in-oil emulsion of primrose oil proved effective, whereas the amphiphilic emulsion did not, which emphasizes the importance of the vehicle. In addition, borage oil (40 drops twice daily for 12 weeks), which contains a large quantity of GLA, improved pruritus, erythema, vesiculation, and oozing in atopic adult patients when compared with placebo-treated patients.

Some other investigations of herbs used for eczema are mentioned here briefly. AD did not improve in children and adults following 12 weeks of treatment with borage oil in a randomized, double-blind, placebo-controlled trial.[6] The use of evening primrose oil applied orally to children with eczema showed little to no difference to comparison groups receiving placebo therapy.[3,5,7-10] Chamomile has been used in the treatment of eczema and has been found in adult studies to be as effective as 0.25% hydrocortisone and superior to topical glucocorticoid preparations.[11]

Massage Therapy

In a small study of children with AD who were being treated with standard topical care and received parental massage for 20 minutes per day for 1 month, lower anxiety scores and improvement in clinical measures were reported, including redness, scaling, lichenification, excoriation, and pruritus when compared with controls.[1] A small pilot study (without controls) evaluated use of daily parental massage with or without essential oils, plus weekly massage by a therapist, in children with AD while receiving their traditional management over an 8-week period. The parents reported improvement in irritation scores and nighttime disturbance scores, but a deterioration in the eczematic condition occurred with continued use of essential oils after the 8-week study period.[2]

Patients have reported the use of aromatherapy and aromatherapy massage to treat the symptoms of AD.[3] In recent case reports, aromatherapists[4-6] and people[7,8] who use aromatherapy products have developed contact dermatitis from exposure to essential oils used in aromatherapy. A recent survey of 350 massage therapists assessed self-reported incidence of AD during a 12-month period. Hand dermatitis occurred in almost one fourth of the therapists; use of aromatherapy products in the massage oils, creams, and lotions and a history of AD were identified as significant risk factors.[9]

Small studies suggest that massage may be helpful in the management of AD symptoms.[1,2] Publications have demonstrated that occupational exposure of essential oils could contribute to development of dermatitis.[4-6,9] Products containing essential oils and/or aromatherapy products should be avoided in patients with a history of AD until further safety and efficacy studies have been performed.

Vegetable-based massage oils or lotions are preferred to mineral oil–based massage products, as they prevent clogged pores. Many unscented massage products are available, which avoids the potential risk of aggravating the eczema with essential oils. If the child is prone to allergies, especially nut allergies, nut-based oils such as almond oil would best be avoided. Jojoba oil, which is considered a wax ester and not an oil, is considered hypoallergenic and may be preferred for children with allergies.

Massage should not be performed over areas where there is a loss of tissue integrity, as it increases the risk of bacterial infection[10]; care should be taken to examine the eczematic areas to ensure that there is no skin breakdown from scratching and inflammation. A massage practitioner should inquire whether topical treatments have been applied to the affected skin; if so, the practitioner may consider avoiding the area to prevent their own exposure to the pharmaceuticals present or prevent an unknown interaction between the topical ointment and the massage lotion. This can best be accomplished by massaging over clothes rather than direct skin-to-skin contact if large surface areas of eczema are present.

Mind/Body

The important role of psychological factors in the development of, maintenance of, and recovery from certain skin conditions such as eczema (AD) via the neuroimmune axis is generally accepted. The psychological issue most consistently associated with eczema is stress.[1]

Several studies in adults have supported the beneficial effects of biofeedback-based relaxation training (usually bifrontal surface electromyography or thermal biofeedback) and other relaxation strategies (including autogenics) in improving eczema and associated symptoms such as itching.[2,3] Clinical experience suggests that these same techniques are equally applicable to childhood eczema, and other mind/body

techniques, including yoga, meditation, progressive relaxation, and diaphragmatic breathing are also likely to be beneficial as one component of therapy aimed at mediating the negative effects of stress. Self-hypnosis can be added with specific suggestions for reducing inflammatory activity in the body; imagining soft, healthy skin, and giving one's own immune system ("control center") various positive messages about functioning properly and reducing eczema. Sokel et al.[4] have provided a comparison of hypnotherapy and biofeedback in the treatment of childhood atopic eczema.

Naturopathy

With skin conditions in particular, the naturopathic belief is that they are a manifestation of an imbalance within the body. Creating an optimal diet changes the internal environment and therefore decreases inflammation and reactions to allergens. Essential nutrients are also provided so that common deficiencies that may lead to AD development are eliminated.

Diet of Child

Diet plays a role in many pediatric conditions. Removing the offending foods from the diet can result in vast improvements in those that are related to the "atopic march,"[1,2] a group of conditions that usually present first as eczema and then progress to asthma and allergic rhinitis later in life. Avoidance of that food should occur for at least 4 to 6 weeks, with a challenge of the food followed by an observation period of 2 to 3 days,[3] as some cases will not show immediate reactions to foods.[4] It should be noted that skin tests for food allergens are often unreliable in determining delayed hypersensitivity responses. Food additives such as coloring agents, preservatives, citric acid, and flavoring agents can also have a detrimental effect on patients with eczema,[5-9] so convenience or fast foods should be avoided. This is also supported by the fact that patients with AD were found to consume more refined sugar and saturated fats.[10,11]

Essential fatty acids

Consideration of essential fatty acids (EFAs) is crucial when creating a treatment plan for any child who has a condition characterized by inflammation. Because patients with AD have been shown to have a lower omega-3:omega-6 ratio,[12] consumption of animal fats should be limited, with the exception of some fish and their oils. Administration of γ-linolenic acid (GLA) in the form of evening primrose oil has been shown to improve AD.[13,14] The dosing and safety of evening primrose oil are not well studied in children; however, limited research data indicate that 1.5 g twice per day is a reasonable dosage in patients 1 year or older. δ-6-desaturase, the enzyme required for the conversion of dietary fats to GLA, may be either defective or inhibited in patients with eczema.[15] It is thought by some physicians that positive and negative "modulators" of this enzyme exist, and supplementing or ensuring a diet high in these nutrient modulators may improve symptoms. Positive modulators may include zinc, B_6, B_3, magnesium, and vitamin C, whereas negative modulators may include trans-fatty acids and insulin. Interestingly, atopic patients have been shown to have higher serum levels of copper[16] and lower levels of zinc,[17,18] and patients with severe zinc deficiency develop acrodermatitis enteropathica, a condition reminiscent of atopic eczema. The recommended dietary allowance for zinc, 10 mg, should at least be supplemented in patients 1 to 10 years old. In younger patients, a dose of at least 5 mg per day should be provided.

Because convenience foods contain high levels of trans-fatty acids in the form of hydrogenated oils as well as dramatically raised insulin levels due to high refined sugar intake, it is again stressed that atopic patients should limit their intake of these foods. Other sources of long-chain polyunsaturated fatty acids (FAs) that have been found to be helpful in treating AD are hemp seed oil[19] and fish oils that provide eicosapentaenoic acid (EPA) and docosahexaenoic acid (DHA).[20-22] α-Linolenic acid, a precursor to EPA and DHA, can be supplied by flax oil, hemp seed oil, or fish oils; current recommendations are 500 mg total per day for the first year of life.[23] Regarding doses for older children, there is no standardized dosing schedule. Many practitioners suggest 1 to 3 teaspoons per day of flax, hemp, or fish oil to children older than 1 year without any adverse effects.

Diet of Mother

The diet of mothers who are breastfeeding can affect their children, as discussed in Chapter 23, Colic. Mothers of infants with AD have been found to have abnormal FA composition of their breast milk,[24] in particular low levels of long-chain polyunsaturated FAs.[25] Therefore it would be wise to have those mothers on a healthy essential FA supplement during breastfeeding. Borage or evening primrose oil can be given to the mother at a dose of 3 to 6 g per day. It should also be noted that supplementation of the mother with omega-3 polyunsaturated FAs in the form of fish oil during pregnancy resulted in decreased rates of atopy in their children who were at an increased risk.[26] Pregnant women may take 3 to 4 g of fish oil per day. Purity of fish oil should always be considered, and reputable companies should give detailed descriptions of purification processes.

Topical Treatments

Ointment with chamomile as its main ingredient has been shown to be more effective than hydrocortisone and placebo.[27]

Intestinal Flora and Permeability

It is thought that atopic patients have an abnormal intestinal milieu, which can lead to increased gut permeability. Probiotic supplementation can prevent the development of this permeability[28-30] and therefore prevent AD.[31] Indeed there is evidence that these patients will benefit from probiotic treatment, in particular *Lactobacillus GG*,[32] *Lactobacillus rhamnosus,* and *Lactobacillus reuteri*.[33] Another justification for the use of probiotics is that patients with eczema often have a history of frequent antibiotic use due to otitis media and sinusitis. See the discussion of naturopathy in Chapter 12, Asthma, for specific information on probiotic supplementation and elimination of intestinal overgrowth with antifungals such as nystatin and fluconazole as well as treatment for intestinal permeability. In one study, the use of a low-salt water decreased intestinal permeability in patients with AD.[34] A lactulose-mannitol test may provide useful information that can help in determining how to prioritize treatments.

Environment

Conventional medicine concurs that certain materials or detergents should be evaluated as a possible cause or compounding factor in eczema. Synthetic clothing has been known to aggravate this condition, as well as deodorant soaps with certain chemical fragrances added. A wide array of hypoallergenic soaps and detergents are available in most stores.

Other Therapies

It is interesting to note that patients suffering from eczema have been found to sweat less than control subjects.[35] Some alternative medicine providers believe that eczema is a result of accumulated toxins in the body. Encouraging perspiration may be beneficial in some patients by way of sauna treatments or increased physical exercise. However, this should be done with caution, as the increased perspiration may aggravate AD.

In a study intended to reveal the benefit of essential oils in the treatment of eczema, it was found that infants who received massage (either with or without essential oils) improved.[36] This poses an interesting discovery that massage may in fact help alleviate symptoms.

Some patients with AD worsen when they are exposed to stressful situations or experience stress. Improvement in symptomology was seen when patients were provided with relaxation therapy and cognitive-behavioral treatment,[37] which thus may be another beneficial treatment option.

Nutrition

Discussion

Children with eczema, similar to those with asthma, are more likely to have symptoms when exposed to foods or food additives that trigger sensitivities, which indicates the role of dieting factors in this disease process.[1] These children may have immune system abnormalities that cause histamine responses to various triggers.[2] Identifying these food triggers via IgE and IgG antibody testing to immediate and delayed sensitivities is imperative. Children suffering from eczema also have low levels of omega-3 FAs and altered FA and prostaglandin metabolism, causing a relative inflammatory state.[3]

In one study, 40 drops twice daily of high-EPA borage oil improved pruritus, erythema, vesiculation, and oozing in atopic patients compared with patients treated with placebo.[4]

Studies have found that probiotic-supplemented yogurt resulted in trends in reduced inflammation and reduced allergic symptoms. Pregnant women who had at least one first-degree relative or partner with eczema, allergies, or asthma (related diseases) were given the probiotic *Lactobacillus* GG until 6 months postpartum. In the group of women who took probiotics, the incidence of infant eczema was half that of the women who took a placebo.[5]

A prospective investigation of the influence of maternal antioxidant intake during pregnancy on the development of asthma and eczema in children was undertaken. The results of this study suggested that maternal dietary antioxidant intakes during pregnancy may modify the risks of developing wheeze and eczema during early childhood.[6]

Treatment

- Increase consumption of foods high in omega-3 FAs, such as cold-water fish, flax seeds and oil, hemp seeds and oil, walnuts, and algae.
- Foods high in quercetin inhibit the release of histamine, thereby reducing eczema symptoms.[7] Leading food sources include onions, spinach, apples, cabbage, white grapefruit, pears, and grapes.
- Vitamin C is necessary for skin formation and can also act as an antioxidant and antihistamine. Good sources of vitamin C include strawberries, red cabbage, red bell peppers, oranges, tangerines, and kiwi fruit. If the patient is allergic to citrus fruits, vitamin C can be obtained from other food sources.
- Zinc is necessary for skin and collagen formation but is also important to support the immune system and to process EFAs. Leading sources of zinc include wheat, chicken, barley, oysters, and turkey.
- Use probiotics if there is a history of antibiotic use and possible dysbiosis.

Probiotics

Probiotic therapy for the treatment of eczema and other atopic disorders is an area of intense investigation. Some trials suggest that probiotic therapy may help to lessen the activation of cells important to an inflammatory response. A study of 14 consecutive subjects, aged 6 to 48 years, with clinical symptoms of asthma and/or conjunctivitis, rhinitis, urticaria, AD, food allergy, or irritable bowel syndrome was published in 2004. The subjects were given a daily mixture of *L. acidophilus, Lactobacillus delbrueckii,* and *Streptococcus thermophilus* (a total of 1 billion live bacteria) for 30 days. Circulating CD34$^+$ cell values decreased significantly after the treatment.[1] Many investigators have reported that probiotic therapy can ameliorate symptoms associated with eczema. In one such trial, 27 exclusively breastfed infants (mean age 4.6 months) with atopic eczema were weaned to probiotic-supplemented, extensively hydrolyzed whey formulas (containing *Bifidobacterium lactis* Bb-12 or *Lactobacillus* GG) or to the same formula without probiotics. After 2 months, a significant improvement in skin condition occurred in patients given probiotic-supplemented formulas as compared with the unsupplemented group. The authors remarked that the data suggest that probiotics may counteract inflammatory responses beyond the intestinal milieu.[2] One trial employed *L. rhamnosus* and *L. reuteri* (10 billion colony-forming units [CFU] of each microbe) given to 41 children with moderate and severe AD for 6 weeks. Gastrointestinal symptoms were determined before and during treatment, and small intestinal permeability was measured. Gastrointestinal symptoms decreased significantly during probiotic therapy, as did eczema. The authors suggest that impairment of the intestinal mucosal barrier is an integral part of the pathogenesis of AD and that probiotic supplementation may stabilize the intestinal barrier function.[3] Even more exciting, data suggest that exposure to probiotics in the perinatal period and during infancy may help *prevent* eczema and that the effect extends beyond infancy.[4-6]

The majority of research supporting the use of probiotic therapy for the prevention or treatment of eczema has employed *Lactobacillus* GG. This author recommends using a 2- to 3-month course of therapy employing organisms such as *Lactobacillus* GG for children with established eczema. Strong consideration should also be given to providing probiotic therapy to expectant mothers during the latter half of the third trimester if they have a significant family history of atopic disease. Dosing guidelines to consider are 10 billion CFU for children <12 kg and 20 billion CFU for children >12 kg and adults. Treatment is extremely well tolerated, and palatability is an infrequent issue, as the capsules can be opened and mixed into formula, drinks, or soft foods. Sometimes the agents are available as a powder as well. If effective, treatment can continue indefinitely. Use with extreme caution, if at all, for those at risk for infectious complications (e.g., immunosuppression or use of immunosuppressive agents, presence of central venous catheter, prematurity).

References

Pediatric Diagnosis and Treatment

1. Thestrup-Pedersen K: Clinical aspects of atopic dermatitis, *Clin Exp Dermatol* 25:535-543, 2000.
2. Fennessy M, Coupland S, Popay J et al: The epidemiology and experience of atopic eczema during childhood: a discussion paper on the implications of current knowledge for health care, public health policy and research, *J Epidemiol Comm Health* 54:581-589, 2000.
3. O'Connell EJ: The burden of atopy and asthma in children, *Allergy* 59(Suppl 78):7-11, 2004.
4. Bardana EJ Jr.: Immunoglobulin E-(IgE) and non-IgE-mediated reactions in the pathogenesis of atopic eczema/dermatitis syndrome (AEDS), *Allergy* 59(Suppl 78):25-29, 2004.
5. Kay AB, Lessof MH: Allergy: conventional and alternative concepts—a report of the Royal College of Physicians Committee on Clinical Immunology and Allergy, *Clin Exp Allergy* 22(Suppl 3):1-44, 1992.
6. Werfel T, Breuer K: Role of food allergy in atopic dermatitis, *Curr Opin Allergy Clin Immunol* 4:379-385, 2004.
7. Warner JA, Warner JO: Early life events in allergic sensitisation, *Br Med Bull* 56:883-893, 2000.
8. Kramer MS: Maternal antigen avoidance during lactation for preventing atopic disease in infants of women at high risk, *Cochrane Database Syst Rev* (2):CD000132, 2000.
9. Kramer MS: Maternal antigen avoidance during lactation for preventing atopic eczema in infants, *Cochrane Database Syst Rev* (2):CD000131, 2000.
10. Kramer MS: Maternal antigen avoidance during pregnancy for preventing atopic disease in infants of women at high risk, *Cochrane Database Syst Rev* (2):CD000133, 2000.
11. Weinberg JM: Formulary review of therapeutic alternatives for atopic dermatitis: focus on pimecrolimus, *J Manag Care Pharm* 11:56-64, 2005.
12 Ben-Gashir MA: Relationship between quality of life and disease severity in atopic dermatitis/eczema syndrome during childhood, Curr Opin Allergy Clin Immunol 3:369-373, 2003.
13. Jones Lewis-Jones S: Atopic dermatitis in childhood, *Hosp Med* 62:136-143, 2001.
14. Fiocchi A, Bouygue GR, Martelli A et al: Dietary treatment of childhood atopic eczema/dermatitis syndrome (AEDS), *Allergy* 59(Suppl 78):78-85, 2004.
15. Ross T, Ross G, Varigos G: Eczema—practical management issues, *Austr Fam Physician* 34:319-324, 2005.
16. Thestrup-Pedersen K: Tacrolimus treatment of atopic eczema/dermatitis syndrome, *Curr Opin Allergy Clin Immunol* 3:359-362, 2003.

17. Garside R, Stein K, Castelnuovo E et al: The effectiveness and cost-effectiveness of pimecrolimus and tacrolimus for atopic eczema: a systematic review and economic evaluation, *Health Technol Assess* 9:1-230, 2005.

18. *FDA issues health adivisory informing health care providers of safety concerns associated with the use of two eczema drugs, Elidel and Protopic,* 2005. Available at www.fda.gov/bbs/topics/ANSWERS/2005/ANS01343.html.

19. Grassia T: Black box recommended for atopic dermatitis creams, *Infect Dis Child* Mar:14-15, 2005.

Acupuncture

1. Loo M: *Pediatric acupuncture*, London, 2002, Elsevier.

2. Lun X, Rong L: Twenty-five cases of intractable cutaneous pruritus treated by auricular acupuncture, *J Tradit Chin Med* 20:287-288, 2000.

3. Sun Y, Wang D: Acupuncture treatment of dermopathies and pediatric diseases, *J Tradit Chin Med* 16:214-217, 1996.

4. Lu S: Acupuncture and moxibustion in the treatment of dermatoses, *J Tradit Chin Med* 13:69-75, 1993.

5. Liao SJ: Acupuncture for poison ivy contact dermatitis. A clinical case report, *Acupunct Electrother Res* 13:31-39, 1988.

6. Deadman P, Al-Khafaji M: *A manual of acupuncture*, Ann Arbor, Mich, 1998, Journal of Chinese Medicine Publications.

Aromatherapy

1. Anderson C, Lis-Balchin M, Kirk-Smith M: Evaluation of massage with essential oils on childhood atopic eczema, *Phytother Res* 14:452-456, 2000.

2. Bensouliah J: Psoriasis and aromatherapy, *Int J Aromatherapy* 13:2-8, 2003.

3. Maddocks-Jennings W: Critical incident: idiosyncratic allergic reactions to essential oils, *Complement Ther Nurs Midwifery* 10:58-60, 2004.

Chiropractic

1. Zutavern A, von Klot S, Gehring U et al: Pre-natal and post-natal exposure to respiratory infection and atopic diseases development: a historical cohort study, *Respir Res* 7:81, 2006.

Herbs—Chinese

1. Beinfield H, Korngold E: *Chinese medicine works clinical handbook,* San Francisco, 2007, www.chinesemedicineworks.com.

Herbs—Western

1. *Flaxseed oil.* Available at www.naturaldatabase.com. Accessed Mar 25, 2005.

2. Aman MG, Mitchell EA, Turbott SH: The effects of essential fatty acid supplementation by Efamol in hyperactive children, *J Abnorm Child Psychol* 15:75-90, 1987.

3. Biagi PL, Bordoni A, Hrelia S et al: The effect of gamma-linolenic acid on clinical status, red cell fatty acid composition and membrane microviscosity in infants with atopic dermatitis, *Drugs Exp Clin Res* 20:77-84, 1994.

4. Don M, Melli P, Braida F et al: Efficacy of essential fatty acids in the treatment of atopic dermatitis and correlations of their changes with clinical response, *Ital J Pediatr* 29:427-432, 2003.

5. Hederos CA, Berg A: Epogam evening primrose oil treatment in atopic dermatitis and asthma, *Arch Dis Child* 75:492-497, 1996.

6. Takwale A, Tan E, Agarwal S et al: Efficacy and tolerability of borage oil in adults and children with atopic eczema: randomised, double blind, placebo controlled, parallel group trial, *Br Med J* 327:1385, 2003.

7. Berth-Jones J, Graham-Brown R: Placebo-controlled trial of essential fatty acid supplementation in atopic dermatitis, *Lancet* 341:1557-1560, 1993.

8. Biagi PL, Bordoni A, Hrelia S et al: The effect of gamma-linolenic acid on clinical status, red cell fatty acid composition and membrane microviscosity in infants with atopic dermatitis, *Drugs Exp Clin Res* 20:77-84, 1994.

9. Bamford J, Gibson R, Reiner C: Atopic eczema unresponsive to evening primrose oil (linoleic and [gamma]-linolenic acids), *J Am Acad Dermatol* 13:959-965, 1985.

10. Wright S, Burton JL: Oral evening-primrose-seed oil improves atopic eczema, *Lancet* 2:1120-1122, 1982.

11. Aertgeerts P, Albring M, Klaschka F et al: Comparative testing of Kamillosan cream and steroidal (0.25% hydrocortisone, 0.75% fluocortin butyl ester) and non-steroidal (5% bufexamac) dermatologic agents in maintenance therapy of eczematous diseases, *Z Hautkr* 60:270-277, 1985.

Massage Therapy

1. Schachner L, Field T, Hernandez-Reif M et al: Atopic dermatitis decreased in children following massage therapy, *Pediatr Dermatol* 15:390-395, 1998.

2. Anderson C, Lis-Balchin M, Kirk-Smith M: Evaluation of massage with essential oils on childhood atopic eczema, *Phytother Res* 14:452-456, 2000.

3. Nicolaou N, Johnston GA: The use of complementary medicine by patients referred to a contact dermatitis clinic, *Contact Dermatitis* 51:30-31, 2004.

4. Cockayne SE, Gawkrodger DJ: Occupational contact dermatitis in an aromatherapist, *Contact Dermatitis* 37:306-307, 1997.

5. Keane FM, Smith HR, White IR et al: Occupational allergic contact dermatitis in two aromatherapists, *Contact Dermatitis* 43:49-51, 2000.

6. Bleasel N, Tate B, Rademaker M: Allergic contact dermatitis following exposure to essential oils. *Australas J Dermatol* 43:211-213, 2002.

7. Weiss RR, James WD: Allergic contact dermatitis from aromatherapy, *Am J Contact Dermat* 8:250-251, 1997.

8. Schaller M, Korting HC: Allergic airborne contact dermatitis from essential oils used in aromatherapy, *Clin Exp Dermatol* 20:2, 143-145, 1995.

9. Crawford GH, Katz KA, Ellis E et al: Use of aromatherapy products and increased risk of hand dermatitis in massage therapists, *Arch Dermatol* 140:991-996, 2004.

10. Donoyama N, Wakuda T, Tanitsu T et al: Washing hands before and after performing massages? Changes in bacterial survival count on skin of a massage therapist and a client during massage therapy, *J Altern Complement Med* 10:684-686, 2004.

Mind/Body

1. Koo J, Lebwohl A: Psycho dermatology: the mind and skin connection, *Am Fam Physician* 64:1873-1878, 2001.

2. Ehlers A, Stangier U, Gieler U: Treatment of atopic dermatitis: a comparison of psychological and dermatological approaches to relapse prevention, *J Consult Clin Psychol* 63:624-635, 1995.

3. McMenamy CJ, Katz RC, Gipson M: Treatment of eczema by EMG biofeedback and relaxation training: multiple baseline analysis, *J Behav Ther Exp Psychiatry* 19:221-227, 1988.

4. Sokel B, Kent CA, Lansdown R et al: A comparison of hypnotherapy and biofeedback in the treatment of childhood atopic eczema, *Contemp Hypnosis* 10:145-154, 1993.

Naturopathy

1. Kanny G: Atopic dermatitis in children and food allergy: combination or causality? Should avoidance diets be initiated? *Ann Dermatol Venereol* 132:S190-S103, 2005.
2. Resano A, Crespo E, Fernandez Benitez M et al: Atopic dermatitis and food allergy, *J Investig Allergol Clin Immunol* 8:271-276, 1998.
3. Niggemann B: Role of oral food challenges in the diagnostic workup of food allergy in atopic eczema dermatitis syndrome, *Allergy* 59(Suppl 78):32-34, 2004.
4. Broberg A, Engstrom I, Kalimo K et al: Elimination diet in young children with atopic dermatitis, *Acta Derm Venereol* 72:365-369, 1992.
5. Worm M, Ehlers I, Sterry W et al: Clinical relevance of food additives in adult patients with atopic dermatitis, *Clin Exp Allergy* 30:407-414, 2000.
6. Kanny G, Hatahet R, Moneret-Vautrin DA et al: Allergy and intolerance to flavouring agents in atopic dermatitis in young children, *Allerg Immunol (Paris)* 26:204-206, 209–210, 1994.
7. Fuglsang G, Madsen G, Halken S et al: Adverse reactions to food additives in children with atopic symptoms, *Allergy* 49:31-37, 1994.
8. Fuglsang G, Madsen C, Saval P et al: Prevalence of intolerance to food additives among Danish school children, *Pediatr Allergy Immunol* 4:123-129, 1993.
9. Van Bever HP, Docx M, Stevens WJ: Food and food additives in severe atopic dermatitis, *Allergy* 44:588-594, 1989.
10. Soyland E, Funk J, Rajka G et al: Dietary supplementation with very long-chain n-3 fatty acids in patients with atopic dermatitis. A double-blind, multicentre study, *Br J Dermatol* 130:757-764, 1994.
11. Solvoll K, Soyland E, Sandstad B et al: Dietary habits among patients with atopic dermatitis, *Eur J Clin Nutr* 54:93-97, 2000.
12. Sakai K, Okuyama H, Shimazaki H et al: Fatty acid compositions of plasma lipids in atopic dermatitis/asthma patients, *Arerugi* 43:37-43, 1994.
13. Biagi PL, Bordoni A, Hrelia S et al: The effect of gamma-linolenic acid on clinical status, red cell fatty acid composition and membrane microviscosity in infants with atopic dermatitis, *Drugs Exp Clin Res* 20:77-84, 1994.
14. Morse PF, Horrobin DF, Manku MS et al: Meta-analysis of placebo-controlled studies of the efficacy of Epogam in the treatment of atopic eczema. Relationship between plasma essential fatty acid changes and clinical response, *Br J Dermatol* 121:75-90, 1989.
15. Manku MS, Horrobin DF, Morse NL et al: Essential fatty acids in the plasma phospholipids of patients with atopic eczema, *Br J Dermatol* 110:643-648, 1984.
16. David TJ, Wells FE, Sharpe TC et al: Serum levels of trace metals in children with atopic eczema, *Br J Dermatol* 122:485-489, 1990.
17. De Luca L, Vacca C, Pace E et al: Immunological and trace element study in 50 children with various diseases caused by food allergens and aeroallergens, *Pediatr Med Chir* 9:589-591, 1987.
18. David TJ, Wells FE, Sharpe TC et al: Low serum zinc in children with atopic eczema, *Br J Dermatol* 111:597-601, 1984.
19. Callaway J, Schwab U, Harvima I et al: Efficacy of dietary hempseed oil in patients with atopic dermatitis, *J Dermatolog Treat* 16:87-94, 2005.
20. Bjorneboe A, Soyland E, Bjorneboe GE et al: Effect of n-3 fatty acid supplement to patients with atopic dermatitis, *J Intern Med Suppl* 731:233-236, 1989.
21. Mayser P, Mayer K, Mahloudjian M et al: A double-blind, randomized, placebo-controlled trial of n-3 versus n-6 fatty acid-based lipid infusion in atopic dermatitis, *J Parenter Enteral Nutr* 26:151-158, 2002.
22. Bjorneboe A, Soyland E, Bjorneboe GE et al: Effect of dietary supplementation with eicosapentaenoic acid in the treatment of atopic dermatitis, *Br J Dermatol* 17:463-469, 1987.
23. Mahan LK, Escott-Stump S, editors: *Krause's food, nutrition, and diet therapy*, ed 11, Philadelphia, 2003, Saunders.
24. Wright S, Bolton C: Breast milk fatty acids in mothers of children with atopic eczema, *Br J Nutr* 62:693-697, 1989.
25. Businco L, Ioppi M, Morse NL et al: Breast milk from mothers of children with newly developed atopic eczema has low levels of long chain polyunsaturated fatty acids, *Allergy Clin Immunol* 91:1134-1139, 1993.
26. Dunstan JA, Mori TA, Barden A et al: Fish oil supplementation in pregnancy modifies neonatal allergen-specific immune responses and clinical outcomes in infants at high risk of atopy: a randomized, controlled trial, *J Allergy Clin Immunol* 112:1178-1184, 2003.
27. Patzelt-Wenczler R, Ponce-Poschl E: Proof of efficacy of Kamillosan cream in atopic eczema, *Eur J Med Res* 5:171-175, 2000.
28. Bongaerts GP, Severijnen RS: Preventive and curative effects of probiotics in atopic patients, *Med Hypotheses* 64:1089-1092, 2005.
29. Probiotics for atopic diseases, *Drug Ther Bull* 43:6-8, 2005.
30. Rosenfeldt V, Benfeldt E, Valerius NH et al: Effect of probiotics on gastrointestinal symptoms and small intestinal permeability in children with atopic dermatitis, *J Pediatr* 145:612-616, 2004.
31. Kalliomaki M, Salminen S, Poussa T et al: Probiotics and prevention of atopic disease: 4-year follow-up of a randomised placebo-controlled trial, *Lancet* 361:1869-1871, 2003.
32. Viljanen M, Savilahti E, Haahtela T et al: Probiotics in the treatment of atopic eczema/dermatitis syndrome in infants: a double-blind placebo-controlled trial, *Allergy* 60:494-500, 2005.
33. Rosenfeldt V, Benfeldt E, Nielsen SD et al: Effect of probiotic *Lactobacillus* strains in children with atopic dermatitis, *J Allergy Clin Immunol* 111:389-395, 2003.
34. Dupuy P, Casse M, Andre F et al: Low-salt water reduces intestinal permeability in atopic patients, *Dermatology* 198:153-155, 1999.
35. Stern UM, Salzer B, Schuch S et al: Sex-dependent differences in sweating of normal probands and atopic patients in cardiovascular stress, *Hautarzt* 49:209-215, 1998.
36. Anderson C, Lis-Balchin M, Kirk-Smith M: Evaluation of massage with essential oils on childhood atopic eczema, *Phytother Res* 14:452-456, 2000.
37. Ehlers A, Stangier U, Gieler U: Treatment of atopic dermatitis: a comparison of psychological and dermatological approaches to relapse prevention, *J Consult Clin Psychol* 63:624-635, 1995.

Nutrition

1. Fuglsang G, Madsen G, Jalken S et al: Adverse reactions to food additives in children with atopic symptoms, *Allergy* 49:31-37, 1994.
2. Chandra RK: Nutrition and immunity, *Contemp Nutr* 11:1-4, 1986.
3. Gil A: Polyunsaturated fatty acids and inflammatory diseases, *Biomed Pharmacother* 56:388-396, 2002.
4. Andreassis M, Forleo P, Lorio AD et al: Efficacy of γ-linolenic acid in the treatment of patients with atopic dermatitis, *J Int Med Res* 25:266-274, 1997.
5. Kalliomaki M, Salminen S, Arvilommi H et al: Probiotics in primary prevention of atopic disease: a randomised placebo-controlled trial, *Lancet* 357:1076-1079, 2001.
6. Martindale S, McNeill G, Devereux G et al: Antioxidant intake in pregnancy in relation to wheeze and eczema in the first two years of life, *Am J Respir Crit Care Med* 171:121-128, 2005.
7. Pizzorno LU, Pizzorno JE, Murray MT: *Natural medicine: instructions for patients*, London, 2002, Churchill Livingstone.

Probiotics

1. Mastrandrea F, Coradduzza G, Serio G et al: Probiotics reduce the CD34+ hemopoietic precursor cell increased traffic in allergic subjects, *Allerg Immunol (Paris)* 36:118-122, 2004.
2. Isolauri E, Arvola T, Sutas Y et al: Probiotics in the management of atopic eczema, *Clin Exp Allergy* 30:1605-1610, 2000.
3. Rosenfeldt V, Benfeldt E, Valerius NH et al: Effect of probiotics on gastrointestinal symptoms and small intestinal permeability in children with atopic dermatitis, *J Pediatr* 145:612-616, 2004.
4. Kalliomaki M, Salminen S, Arvilommi H et al: Probiotics in primary prevention of atopic disease: a randomized placebo-controlled trial, *Lancet* 57:1076-1079, 2001.
5. Rautava S, Kalliomäki M, Isolauri E: Probiotics during pregnancy and breastfeeding might confer immunomodulatory protection against atopic disease in the infant, *J Allergy Clin Immunol* 109:119-121, 2002.
6. Isolauri E: Probiotics in the prevention and treatment of allergic disease, *Pediatr Allergy Immunol* 12(Suppl):56-59, 2001.

CHAPTER 33

Enuresis

Acupuncture | May Loo

Chiropractic | Anne Spicer

Homeopathy | Janet L. Levatin

Mind/Body | Timothy Culbert, Lynda Richtsmeier Cyr

Osteopathy | Jane Carreiro

Psychology | Anna Tobia

✳ PEDIATRIC DIAGNOSIS AND TREATMENT

Nocturnal enuresis, or bed-wetting, is a complex disorder with poorly understood pathogenicity and pathophysiology. It affects children all over the world[1-4]: approximately 5-7 million children in the United States[5] and as many as 30% of school-age children in Italy.[2]

The prevalence is highest at age 5 years: 7% for males and 3% for females. At age 10 years, the prevalence is 3% for males and 2% for females, and at age 18 years, 1% for males and extremely rare in females.[1] *Enuresis* is defined as inappropriate or involuntary voiding during the night at an age when urinary control should be achieved, occurring twice per week for at least 3 consecutive months, or when wetting causes clinically significant distress in the child's life.[1]

Enuresis is classified as primary nocturnal enuresis (PNE) when the child has never been dry at night or as secondary nocturnal enuresis (SNE) when wetting follows a dry 6-month period and usually occurs after an identifiable stress.[1] The majority (as many as 85%) of PNE cases are monosymptomatic in that the enuresis is not accompanied by other voiding disorders or daytime incontinence.[1,2,6] Most children with primary monosymptomatic bed-wetting have either a large nighttime urine production and a normal bladder capacity or a small bladder capacity with normal urine production.[7] Further classification involves nocturnal enuresis (voiding urine at night) and diurnal enuresis (voiding urine while awake). Primary nocturnal enuresis represents approximately 90% of all cases.[1] By age 8 years, 87% to 90% of children should have nighttime dryness. Enuresis improves with maturity, with a natural, spontaneous remission rate of 15% per year of age.[1] It is possible that different factors may be predominant in different age groups.[8]

Etiology and Pathophysiology

Both the etiology and pathophysiology of enuresis are still not well understood. There appears to be a wide spectrum of possible pathogenic factors for enuresis: functional/psychological causes, delayed maturation of the central nervous system (CNS), genetic predisposition, and infrequently, organic/anatomical dysfunction.

Functional/psychological

Many investigators consider PNE to be a disorder with a strong functional component.[9-11] Psychological factors may affect as many as 95% of children with enuresis.[11] It is interesting to note that fear reactions have been reported to be significantly higher in enuretic children.[4,12] Enuresis has been linked to night terror, nightmares, and sleepwalking.[13,14]

Secondary enuresis is often associated with life stress and/or traumatic experiences.[1] Marital separation or birth of a sibling were also found to be precipitating factors, especially for nightwetters.[15] Evidence indicates clear connections between childhood enuresis and mental well-being.[16] Most likely, this disorder is a highly complex interaction between somatic and psychiatric factors.[10]

Central nervous system

Nocturnal enuresis may be due to a maturational lag in the development of the CNS.[1,17] A popular theory posits that low nocturnal vasopressin secretion results in high nocturnal urine output, which explains why enuretic patients respond to 1-deamino-8-D-argininge casopressin (DDAVP), an exogenous vasopressin. However, there may be a more complex, dual CNS developmental delay in both the afferent and efferent limbs: the CNS fails to recognize and respond to bladder fullness or contraction during sleep and also fails to suppress the micturition reflex arc during sleep. The child may manifest other signs of developmental delay, such as slower growth, poorer visual-motor and spatial perception, or signs of neurological dysfunction.[15] The pathology does not appear to relate to sleep physiology, as the sleep cycle appears normal and enuretic episodes have been found to occur in every sleep stage.[10] There may in fact be a close correlation between biological and psychological factors, in that extreme CNS disorganization may result in psychological symptoms.[18]

For instance, children with nocturnal enuresis may both hyposecrete arginine vasopressin (AVP) generally and be less responsive to the lower urine osmolality associated with fluid loading. Independent evidence suggests that tubular sodium-potassium exchange in the kidney, partly influenced by AVP secretion, is associated with nocturnal enuresis. Evidence also suggests that AVP receptor function in the tubule may be a key factor in the pathophysiology of the disorder. On the other hand, associations between sleep and enuresis may also exist. Although enuresis may occur at any stage of sleep, there is some support for a relationship among sleep architecture, diminished capacity to be aroused from sleep, and abnormal bladder function in enuretic patients.[1]

Genetic predisposition

PNE has a strong hereditary component.[3,8,15,18] Twin studies show a marked familial pattern: A 68% concordance rate in monozygotic twins and a 36% concordance rate in dizygotic twins have been documented.[1] Many families seem to manifest an autosomal dominant mode of inheritance.[10] At this time, molecular genetics have identified numerous loci on more than 10 chromosomes.[10,19]

Organic/anatomical dysfunction

Organic factors include infectious, most often urinary tract infection, and anatomical anomalies such as epispadias, ectopic ureter, spinal coral lesion, or urethral obstacle.[20] Organic/anatomical dysfunction can also be a feature of many conditions, including renal,[21] neurological, and organic disease states.[22]

Secondary Enuresis

SNE accounts for about one fourth of patients with bed-wetting.[23] There is significant association of psychiatric problems with SNE,[10,23] both causally and reactively following the enuresis.[10] The organic conditions that feature primary enuresis can also be the cause of secondary enuresis.[22,23] Enuresis has been associated with behavioral disorders such as attention-deficit hyperactivity disorder.[24-28] SNE has also been reported with trauma, such as car and motorcycle accidents, and in such cases may be due to psychological trauma or organic head trauma.[29] SNE has been reported to be associated with upper airway obstruction[30] and constipation.[17] It is important to consider micturition deferral (e.g., when the normal preschool child waits until the last minute to void urine).[1]

Treatment

Although enuresis is considered benign and mostly self-limiting, treatment is warranted because of the adverse personal, family, and psychosocial effects of the disorder.[5,8,31] Nocturnal enuresis delays early autonomy and socialization owing to decreased self-esteem and self-confidence[6] and fear of detection by peers.[31] The child may be at increased risk for emotional or even physical abuse from family members.[31] The conventional treatment modalities are still controversial. Because the vast majority of PNE resolves spontaneously with time, treatment should carry minimal or no risk. Conservative measures should be tried first, such as decreasing fluid intake before bedtime; making sure that the child voids before going to bed; giving positive reinforcement or rewarding the child for dry nights; and using an alarm clock to wake the child once 2 to 3 hours after falling asleep. The moisture alarm is safe, inexpensive,[8] and effective.[32] Medical treatment should be placed in a biopsychosocial framework, with medication prescribed in conjunction with psychosocial interventions.[11,33] Imipramine is now seldom used[34] because it is associated with cardiac conduction disturbances and is deadly in overdose.[1] DDAVP is frequently prescribed.[1,35] Its fast action makes it convenient

for special occasions (such as overnight stays) when rapid control of enuresis is desired. Unfortunately, it is expensive and the relapse rate upon discontinuation of DDAVP is very high. DDAVP is also associated with rare side effects of hyponatremia[36] and water intoxication, with resulting seizures.[37]

✸ CAM THERAPY RECOMMENDATIONS

Acupuncture

Worldwide literature is supportive of acupuncture as a valid treatment modality for the enuretic child.[1-22] Although the reported success rate can be as high as 98.2%,[21] positive support for acupuncture treatment of enuresis is often rejected because of small sample size[2] or poor methodology.[23]

Clinical trials have found acupuncture to be successful both in decreasing occurrence of enuresis during treatment and in exerting persistent, long-term effect after treatment.[7-9] Parents also report a decrease in sleep arousal threshold.[8] The therapeutic efficacy improves with combined treatment of DDAVP and acupuncture.[17] Although the precise mechanism of acupuncture is still unknown, a multidisciplinary approach including acupuncture demonstrated on electroencephalography that treatment normalized activities of the cerebral cortex,[18] whereas an Italian study and a Russian report showed that acupuncture treatment was effective in suppressing uninhibited bladder contractions and decreasing bladder instability.[19,20] A preliminary study in which only BL33 (Zhongliao) was needled for treatment of monosymptomatic nocturnal enuresis found the treatment to significantly increase nocturnal bladder capacity.[5]

For those children who are fearful of needles, laser and acupressure have also been found to be effective. A randomized controlled trial (RCT) from Austria found laser acupuncture treatment to be just as effective as desmopressin.[6] A German clinical trial used laser acupuncture for weekly treatment of 5 to 12 year olds with classic monosymptomatic nocturnal enuresis. The points chosen were CV3, bilateral ST36, bilateral P6, bilateral BL33, and CV6. Preliminary data on 24 children showed improvement in 87.5% of subjects. After 12 treatments, 25% were completely dry. The authors recommend laser as a painless, noninvasive, and cost-effective treatment for children with therapy-resistant, monosymptomatic nocturnal enuresis.[3] Since the early 1980s, simple acumassage has been demonstrated to be beneficial to the enuretic child.[22] A more recent RCT from Turkey compared the efficacy of acupressure versus oxybutinin. Acupressure was taught to the parents to apply to the children at home. The points chosen were GV4, GV15, GV20, BL23, BL28, BL32, HT7, HT9, ST36, SP4, SP6, SP12, CV2, CV3, CV6, KI3, and KI5. Results indicate that the noninvasive, painless, and cost-effective acupressure was more effective than medication for treating nocturnal enuresis.[4]

Although it is not possible to precisely correlate the Western diagnosis of enuresis with Chinese medicine impressions, PNE can be explained in the acupuncture paradigm as Kidney Yang and Kidney Essence deficiency, and SNE as Spleen and Lung Qi deficiency and Yin deficiency.

Treatment for Kidney Yang and Kidney Essence Deficiency

Restrict fluid at and after dinner to decrease urine production.

Diet: Avoid energetically Cold foods; avoid excess salt; increase Warming foods.

Keep warm; especially keep the abdomen warm; advise mothers not to dress young children with the abdomen partially exposed.

KI3 tonifies both Kidney Yin and Kidney Yang.

KI6, CV4, SP6 tonifies KI Yin/Essence.

KI7, BL23 tonifies KI Yang.

Use the Five-Element, Four-Point protocol to disperse Cold from the Kidney and tonify both the Kidney Yin and Yang:

Disperse Kidney Cold: Tonify KI2, HT8; sedate KI10.

Tonify Kidney: Tonify KI7, LU8; sedate KI3, SP3.

CV6 to tonify Lower Energizer.

Acupuncture Treatment for Spleen and Lung Qi Deficiency

Avoid excessive sweet or spicy foods. Also avoid Phlegm-producing and Cold foods.

Change lifestyle to provide plenty of rest and diversification of activities.

Perform calming exercises.

Tonify Spleen:

Two points: Tonify SP2; sedate SP1.

Four points: Tonify SP2, HT8; sedate SP1, LR1.

Tonify Lung:

Two points: Tonify LU9; sedate LU10.

Four points: Tonify LU9, SP3; sedate LU10, HT8.

Moxa CV 8 to tonify Middle Burner.

CV17 to tonify Upper Energizer.

Treatment for Yin Deficiency Enuresis

Avoid excessive intake of sour or bitter foods. Avoid taking medication unnecessarily, especially over-the-counter pills.

Parents can massage Yintang point for calming.

KI6, SP6, CV4 to tonify Yin.

BL18 to tonify LR Yin.

BL47, Hunmen, "Gate of the Ethereal Soul," to calm the Hun.

LR3 to subdue Liver Yang and nourish Liver Yin.

LR13 to regulate LR Qi and harmonize LR and SP.[24-34]

Chiropractic

As with all conditions, the chiropractic approach is not determined exclusively by the condition, but rather by the presence of the subluxation complex (SC) and its effect on the body. Organic pathologies and life-threatening conditions are ruled out, and chiropractic adjustments are applied as indicated to remove barriers to optimal function. According to Davies, author of *Chiropractic Pediatrics,* "any child who wets consistently beyond the (age of 3) should be considered for chiropractic management."[1]

Neurological input to the detrusor muscle of the bladder and external sphincter arises via the second, third, and fourth sacral segments (pudendal and pelvic splanchnic).[2] Sympathetic fibers to the bladder arise from the T11 to T12 levels.[3]

The most common area adjusted in cases of enuresis is the sacrum, with S2 gaining primary attention. Sacral segments remain unfused until the early second decade of life and therefore can be individually adjusted in children. Secondary areas related to the sacral segments include the sacroiliac joints, low lumbar vertebrae, and coccyx. Success has also been reported with adjustments to the upper cervical spine and thoracolumbar junction. Correction of the SC commonly identified in these areas improves the efferent-afferent neurological controls to the genitourinary system.

Urinalysis may reveal the presence of infective agents or diabetes underlying the enuresis. Psychological contributors should also be historically investigated.

Plain film radiographs may reveal evidence of other neurological causes such as spina bifida occulta. It should be noted that the presence of this abnormality does not prohibit chiropractic correction of the condition, but may warrant modifications in technique application.

Multiple case studies document benefit from chiropractic adjustment in cases of enuresis.[4-15]

Although individual cases suggest a benefit from chiropractic adjustments, the largest chiropractic clinical trial, which involved 171 children with enuresis, produced results that suggest the chiropractic adjustment may be only marginally better, if at all, than the natural course of the condition.[16] The study's use of chiropractic student interns to provide the adjustments may be a significant reason for the rather neutral results.

Another smaller study (46 subjects) comparing a sham protocol versus the chiropractic adjustment determined a 17.9% decrease overall in frequency of wet nights, with 25% of the subjects showing a 50% reduction.[17]

Chiropractic is most likely to be successful when the child has non-enuretic parents or grandparents.[18]

Cranial evaluation and indicated corrections may prove beneficial,[18] particularly occipital decompression and sacrooccipital synchronization.[19]

In some cases, allergic/sensitivity reactions may increase symptoms. Classic allergens (dairy, wheat, corn, berries, yeast) may be excluded from the diet on a 1-month trial basis.[19] Elimination of refined sugars will help stabilize glucose utilization.

Deep focal muscle stimulation at the umbilicus and the symphysis pubis as well as at the superior aspect of the transverse processes of L2 may provide some relief.[20]

Some chiropractors recommend a two-step process founded in TCM: the first step is focal stimulation at the inferior medial aspect of the clavicles while contacting the umbilicus, and then the second step is to stimulate the tip of the coccyx while maintaining an umbilical contact.

If a trial of chiropractic management is unproductive in altering the course of the enuresis, a referral to a behavioral therapist for a modified dry bed training program or bell-and-pad system is in order.

Limitation of stimulating behaviors (e.g., television, video games, physical play) before bedtime may also be useful.

Because of many side effects, recommendation to use pharmaceuticals would remain a last resort to the chiropractor.

Homeopathy

Before using this section, please see Appendix A, Homeopathy, for definitions of practitioner expertise categories and general information on prescribing homeopathic medicines.

Clinical Expertise Categories 2 and 3

There are no controlled clinical trials of homeopathy for enuresis or nocturnal enuresis, although the homeopathic literature contains evidence for its use in the form of accumulated clinical experience.[1] Homeopathic treatment can be used safely either alone or in combination with other treatment modalities, both alternative and conventional. Because enuresis and nocturnal enuresis are problems relating to general child development, urinary tract pathology, and/or sleep problems, successful homeopathic treatment usually requires extensive training in the art and science of homeopathy. Any one of many homeopathic medicines may be used to treat enuresis, depending on the characteristics of the patient being treated; sophisticated homeopathic analysis and close follow-up are required. For these reasons, specific medicines for treating enuresis will not be presented here. Interested readers are referred to the homeopathic literature for further study.[1]

Mind/Body

Enuresis can be divided into different domains including nocturnal enuresis (bed-wetting), diurnal enuresis (daytime wetting), and children who experience both. In terms of mind/body approaches, biofeedback has a particularly strong track record in the treatment of children with dysfunctional voiding.

Nocturnal Enuresis

The best researched mind/body approach for nighttime wetting is the urine alarm conditioning device. Considered a form of biofeedback, these devices are connected to the child's underwear or pajamas at bedtime and the moisture sensor picks any urine flow, which in turns triggers an alarm to awaken the child. In a systemic review from 2000, Mellon and McGrath[1] support the use of an alarm device as first-line, sufficient treatment for most children with nocturnal enuresis. As many as 70% of children who use this approach will achieve dryness, with a low relapse rate. Schulman and colleagues[2] did a retrospective cohort review of patients with nocturnal enuresis 1 year following assessment and found that 56% of patients who used the urine alarm were completely dry compared with 18% who used desmopressin acetate.

Cognitive-behavioral techniques that promote positive expectations may also play a role in a comprehensive approach to this problem.

Hypnosis can also be a very effective nonpharmacological approach for children with nocturnal enuresis. The advantage of offering hypnosis as treatment for enuresis in children is that it provides them with a sense of personal participation in treatment and enhances their sense of mastery and competency. Numerous clinical reports demonstrate successes in teaching children self-hypnosis for treatment of enuresis. As is true with all symptoms, it is important that careful diagnostic evaluation precede the recommendation for any type of treatment for enuresis. Although PNE is common until age 6 years and is usually not associated with anatomical or metabolic disorders, the development of enuresis may reflect an acquired condition such as diabetes, hyperthyroidism, constipation, or urinary tract infection.

Two studies[3,4] concluded that hypnotherapy is not likely to help children with enuresis if marked improvement does not occur after the first three or four visits. A number of clinical case reports in which children learned self-hypnosis for control of enuresis found complete resolution in 70% within a few weeks.[4-6] In general, the children who did not succeed were those who did not continue daily self-hypnosis practice. Banerjee et al.[7] compared treatment with hypnotherapy to treatment with imipramine in two groups of 25 children, ages 5 to 16 years. Comparable results were found between groups after 3 months of treatment, with 75% of the imipramine group and 72% of the hypnosis group achieving positive responses (defined as all dry beds or substantial decreases in the frequency of wet beds). After 3 months of treatment and reinforcement, imipramine was discontinued and active follow-up visits were discontinued for both groups. Six months later, only 24% of the imipramine group had maintained a positive response, whereas 68% of the hypnosis group had maintained a positive response without clinical reinforcement.

One key treatment approach, as is the case with most mind/body problems but particularly with this condition, is setting positive expectancy. Children are asked to establish a dryness "ruler" with which they rate their gradation of dryness each night from 0 to 10 or 0 to 5 on a visual analog scale. Various techniques such as conditioning alarms, mental imagery, and behavioral reinforcement can all be combined concurrently as needed. In the author's experience, imagery is particularly helpful for children with enuresis and can be utilized with great creativity and imagination. Visualizations about "keeping the muscle gate on the bladder closed all night" or "closing the dam on the river all night" are quite useful. Children can also incorporate therapeutic suggestions about the "pride and comfort they will feel waking up in a dry bed each morning," about how their "brain and bladder can learn to talk to each other every night to help control things," and how their kidneys can also help by "decreasing the production of pee while they are sleeping."

Diurnal Enuresis

Children with dysfunctional voiding that includes detrusor-sphincter dyssynergia and pelvic floor muscle coordination problems often can benefit from pelvic floor surface electromyography (SEMG) biofeedback training and bladder manometric feedback.[8,9] A subset of children with behavioral urinary urgency and frequency symptoms (termed *pollakiuria*) can benefit from SEMG biofeedback, relaxation, and diaphragmatic breathing training, especially to address the anxiety component that commonly accompanies this disorder. Many of these children have anxiety when they have even a mild urge to urinate, such as worry that they will not make it the bathroom in time. The authors typically teach positive coping statements together with easy, abdominal breathing, which usually reduces any excess pelvic floor activity that might be squeezing the bladder as well as stops the unhelpful thoughts associated with the urinary urge. Self-hypnosis, including images of the child urinating at longer intervals throughout the day and feeling confident and in control, can also be added to the practice regimen.

Osteopathy

From an osteopathic perspective, one factor that must be considered in children with enuresis is the mechanism by which children are awakened when their bladder is full. The conscious sensation of bladder fullness and the capacity to control urination develop together as the child matures. This sensation of fullness must reach a conscious level in the sleeping child in order for him to awaken. The sleeping child may not be sensitized to the discomfort of bladder expansion in the presence of nociceptive input from the tissues of the low back or pelvis. Low-grade chronic nociception may alter the child's sensitivity to visceral discomfort from that same area. According to the older osteopathic literature, musculoskeletal strains in the back and pelvis are a typical finding in children with enuresis.[1-4] Furthermore, when these findings are treated with osteopathic manipulation, the child's enuresis improves.

In most people, musculoskeletal strains produce symptoms of pain. However, children younger than 8 or 9 years are not always able to localize pain or discomfort and may not be able to articulate their symptoms when awake. Once asleep, the child becomes "acclimated" to the level of nociception coming from the pelvis and is not awakened by signals of bladder distention. Another theory is that some children with enuresis have a higher threshold for nociception and are not conscious of the discomfort associated with bladder distention. These children typically do not complain when hurt and tend to be more stoic than their siblings.

In children with enuresis, osteopathic findings typically include altered involuntary mechanics of the sacrum and somatic dysfunction involving the pelvis, sacrum, lower lumbar spine, and/or pelvic diaphragm. Although no studies are available, one would expect children to respond well to osteopathic treatment in conjunction with an alarm system that can be used to reinforce the child's alertness to signals of bladder distention.

Psychology

Nocturnal enuresis without daytime wetting or other medical problems can be conceptualized as a biobehavioral problem. It is a physical problem that can be managed with learning-based treatments that rely on conditioning. A careful medical screening to rule out diseases of the urinary tract is essential. The behavioral treatment program, although effective, requires high motivation by both the parent and child, and parents are not recommended to attempt this treatment unless they are fully committed to the process.

The most effective behavioral program, known as *dry bed training*, requires the family to utilize a urine alarm that activates if a child urinates while sleeping, verbal praise for the child, positive practice, and cleanliness training. It has an average success rate of 75%.[1] The urine alarm can be sewn into a child's underpants or can be a mat on which the child sleeps. The alarm sounds when any wetness occurs. When the urine alarm is activated, the child must fully wake up, finish urinating in the toilet,

and help change the sheets before returning to sleep. A parent typically wakes up with the child to facilitate this process. In the initial stages of treatment, this can involve frequent wakings during the night, which can be difficult for many families. Children who are not motivated may turn off the alarm and return to sleep. However, if the family follows the behavioral program, the likely outcome is positive.[2,3] The dry bed training can be used in combination with pharmacological treatment.

Treatment Recommendations

The first complementary and alternative medicine (CAM) psychology treatment session would typically begin with an interview of the parents and child to review the nighttime routine and strategies parents are currently using to manage the problem. Some parents may resort to punishment for nighttime wetting because of their own frustration. It is important to emphasize that the child does not have conscious control over this condition.

The urine alarm works by increasing awareness of the physiological cues for the need to urinate. In order for this conditioning to effectively occur, the child needs to have multiple learning trials. What this means for the family is that for treatment to be effective over the long-term, in the beginning, the more times the child wets during the night, the better. This will provide the most chances for the alarm to go off and hence for the child to change. Therefore parents should not restrict fluids before bedtime.

It must be explained to the parents that they will be waking up with the child multiple times per night. The child must be fully awakened and finish urinating in the bathroom as necessary. The sheets can be quickly changed, the urine alarm reset, and everyone returns to sleep until the next awakening. It is helpful to emphasize that this is a highly effective treatment, although difficult to implement in the beginning.

As a means of tracking progress and reinforcing the family's efforts, this author recommend charting the progress with a simple bar graph of number of accidents per night for each night that the family is in treatment. Reinforcement for dry nights is not encouraged because this is not within the child's control. Instead it is preferable to reinforce effort; for example, helping change sheets or waking up independently.

Subsequent sessions are designed to ensure that the parents are following the protocol and the child is having several wet nights to provide the opportunity for learning to occur. Parents and children may need ongoing reinforcement, especially during the first few weeks of treatment. At this time it is helpful to show parents the bar graph that marks their progress. One possible explanation for treatment failure is when parents do not reset the alarm after the first awakening. It would then be helpful to review the program step by step to make sure that the protocol is being followed correctly.

References

Pediatric Diagnosis and Treatment

1. Behrman RE, Kliegman RM, Jenson HB, editors: *Nelson textbook of pediatrics*, ed 17, Philadelphia, 2004, Saunders.
2. Caione P, Nappo S, Capozza N et al: Primary enuresis in children: which treatment today [in French], *Minerva Pediatr* 46:437-443, 1994 (abstract).

3. Chao SM, Yap HK, Tan A et al: Primary monosymptomatic nocturnal enuresis in Singapore—parental perspectives in an Asian community, *Ann Acad Med Singapore* 26:179-183, 1997.

4. Bhatia MS, Dhar NK, Rai S et al: Enuresis: an analysis of 82 cases, *Indian J Med Sci* 44:337-342, 1990.

5. Miller K: Concomitant nonpharmacologic therapy in the treatment of primary nocturnal enuresis, *Clin Pediatr (Phila)* Jul: 32-37, 1993.

6. Chiozza ML: An update on clinical and therapeutic aspects of nocturnal enuresis [in Italian], *Pediatr Med Chir* 19:385-390, 1997 (abstract).

7. Djurhuus JC, Rittig S: Current trends, diagnosis, and treatment of enuresis, *Europ Urol* 33(Suppl 3):30-33, 1998.

8. Alon US: Nocturnal enuresis, *Pediatr Nephrol* 9:94-103, 1995.

9. Schwobel M, Bodmer C: Urodynamic studies in the child with urinary incontinence [in German], *Wien Med Wochenschr* 148: 508-510, 1998 (abstract).

10. Von Gontard A, Lehmkuhl G: Enuresis nocturna—new studies of genetic, pathophysiologic and psychiatric correlations [in German], *Prax Kinderpsychol Kinderpsychiatr* 46:709-726, 1997 (abstract).

11. Kelleher RE: Daytime and nighttime wetting in children: a review of management, *J Soc Pediatr Nursing* 2:73-82, 1997.

12. MacKeith R: A frequent factor in the etiology of enuresis: fear in the third year of life [in Czech], *Cas Lek Cesk* 108:36-37, 1969 (abstract).

13. Guilleminault C, Anders TF: The pathophysiology of sleep disorders in pediatrics. Part II. Sleep disorders in children, *Adv Pediatr* 22:151-174, 1976.

14. Kales A, Soldatos CR, Kales JD: Sleep disorders: insomnia, sleepwalking, night terrors, nightmares, and enuresis, *Ann Intern Med* 106:582-592, 1987.

15. Jarvelin MR, Moilanen I, Kangas P et al: Aetiological and precipitating factors for childhood enuresis, *Acta Paediatr Scand* 80: 361-369, 1991.

16. Moilanen I, Tirkkonen T, Jarvelin MR et al: A follow-up of enuresis from childhood to adolescence, *Br J Urol* 81(Suppl 3):94-97, 1998.

17. Robson WL, Leung AK, Van Howe R: Primary and secondary nocturnal enuresis: similarities in presentation, *Pediatrics* 115: 956-959, 2005.

18. Maizels M, Gandhi K, Keating B et al: Diagnosis and treatment for children who cannot control urination, *Curr Probl Pediatr* 23: 402-450, 1993.

19. Djurhuus JC: Definitions of subtypes of enuresis, *Scand J Urol Nephrol* 202:5-7, 1999.

20. Brueziere J: Enuresis [in French], *Ann Urol (Paris)* 26:218-224, 1992 (abstract).

21. Heiliczer JD, Canonigo BB, Bishof NA et al: Noncalculi urinary tract disorders secondary to idiopathic hypercalciuria in children, *Pediatr Clin North Am* 34:711-718, 1987.

22. Lettgen B: Differential enuresis nocturna diagnosis [in German], *Wien Med Wochenschr* 148:515-516, 1998.

23. Robson WL, Leung AK: Secondary nocturnal enuresis, *Clin Pediatr (Phila)* 39:379-385, 2000.

24. Diamond JM, Stein JM: Enuresis: a new look at stimulant therapy, *Can J Psychiatry* 28:395-397, 1983.

25. Hjalmas K: Desmopressin treatment: current status, *Scand J Urol Nephrol Suppl* 202:70-72, 1999.

26. Kong DS: Psychiatric disorders in pre-schoolers, *Singapore Med J* 36:318-321, 1995.

27. Hara H: Diagnosis and drug treatment in hyperactive children [in Japanese], *No To Hattatsu* 26:169-174, 1994 (abstract).

28. Robson WL, Jackson HP, Blackhurst D et al: Enuresis in children with attention-deficit hyperactivity disorder, *South Med J* 90: 503-505, 1997.

29. Eidlitz-Markus T, Shuper A, Amir J: Secondary enuresis: posttraumatic stress disorder children after car accidents, *Israel Med Assoc J* 2:135-137, 2000.

30. Nowak KC, Weider DJ: Pediatric nocturnal enuresis secondary to airway obstruction from cleft palate repair, *Clin Pediatr (Phila)* 37:653-657, 1998.

31. Warzak WJ: Psychosocial implications of nocturnal enuresis, *Clin Pediatr (Phila)* Jul:38-40, 1993.

32. Neveus T: Alarm defends its position. Comments to meta-analysis of alarm treatment of nocturnal enuresis [in Swedish], *Lakartidningen* 98:3212-3215, 2001 (abstract).

33. Wiener JM: Psychopharmacology in childhood disorders, *Psychiatr Clin North Am* 7:831-843, 1984.

34. Gepertz S, Neveus T: Imipramine for therapy resistant enuresis: a retrospective evaluation, *J Urol* 171:2607-2610, 2004; discussion 2609-2610.

35. Neveus T, Lackgren G, Tuvemo T et al: Enuresis—background and treatment, *Scand J Urol Nephrol* Suppl(206):1-44, 2000.

36. Robson WL, Norgaard JP, Leung AK: Hyponatremia in patients with nocturnal enuresis treated with DDAVP, *Eur J Pediatr* 155:959-962, 1996.

37. Robson WL, Leung AK: Side effects and complications of treatment with desmopressin for enuresis, *J Natl Med Assoc* 86: 775-778, 1994.

Acupuncture

1. Loo M: *Pediatric acupuncture*, London, 2002, Elsevier.

2. Glazener CM, Evans JH, Cheuk DK: Complementary and miscellaneous interventions for nocturnal enuresis in children, *Cochrane Database Syst Rev* (2):CD005230, 2005.

3. Heller G, Langen PH, Steffens J: Laser acupuncture as third-line therapy for primary nocturnal enuresis: first results of a prospective study [in German], *Urologe A* 43:803-806, 2004 (abstract).

4. Yuksek MS, Erdem AF, Atalay C et al: Acupressure versus oxybutinin in the treatment of enuresis, *J Int Med Res* 31:552-556, 2003.

5. Honjo H, Kawauchi A, Ukimura O et al: Treatment of monosymptomatic nocturnal enuresis by acupuncture: a preliminary study, *Int J Urol* 9:672-676, 2002.

6. Radmayr C, Schlager A, Studen M et al: Prospective randomized trial using laser acupuncture versus desmopressin in the treatment of nocturnal enuresis, *Eur Urol* 40:201-205, 2001.

7. Serel TA, Perk H, Koyuncuoglu HR et al: Acupuncture therapy in the management of persistent primary nocturnal enuresis—preliminary results, *Scand J Urol Nephrol* 35:40-43, 2001.

8. Bjorkstrom G, Hellstrom AL, Andersson S: Electro-acupuncture in the treatment of children with monosymptomatic nocturnal enuresis, *Scand J Urol Nephrol* 34:21-26, 2000.

9. Caione P, Nappo S, Capozza N et al: Primary enuresis in children: which treatment today [in Italian], *Minerva Pediatr* 46:437-443, 1994 (abstract).

10. Roje-Starcevic M: The treatment of nocturnal enuresis by acupuncture [in Romanian], *Neurologija* 39:179-184, 1990 (abstract).

11. Huo JS: Treatment of 11 cases of chronic enuresis by acupuncture and massage, *J Tradit Chin Med* 8:195-196, 1988.

12. Yang CP: Acupuncture of guanyuan (Ren 4) and Baihui (Du 20) in the treatment of 500 cases of enuresis, *J Tradit Chin Med* 8:197, 1988.

13. Chen Z, Chen L: The treatment of enuresis with scalp acupuncture, *J Tradit Chin Med* 11:29-30, 1991.

14. Xu B: 302 cases of enuresis treated with acupuncture, *J Tradit Chin Med* 11:121-122, 1991.
15. Hu J: Acupuncture treatment of enuresis, *J Tradit Chin Med* 20:158-160, 2000.
16. Bjorkstrom G, Hellstrom AL, Andersson S: Electro-acupuncture in the treatment of children with monosymptomatic nocturnal enuresis, *Scand J Urol Nephrol* 34:21-26, 2000.
17. Capozza N, Creti G, De Gennaro M et al: The treatment of nocturnal enuresis: a comparative study between desmopressin and acupuncture used alone or in combination [in Italian], *Minerva Pediatr* 43:577-582, 1991 (abstract).
18. Tret'iakova EE, Komissarov VI: Characteristics of the electric activity of the projection areas of the large hemispheres in children with enuresis [in Russian], *Zh Nevropatol Psikhiatr Im S S Korsakova* 90:41-44, 1990 (abstract).
19. Minni B, Capozza N, Creti G et al: Bladder instability and enuresis treated by acupuncture and electro-therapeutics: early urodynamic observations [in Italian], *Acupunct Electrother Res* 15:19-25, 1990 (abstract).
20. Kachan AT, Trubin MI, Skoromets AA et al: Acupuncture reflexotherapy of neurogenic bladder dysfunction in children with enuresis [in Russian], *Zh Nevropatol Psikhiatr Im S S Korsakova* 93:40-42, 1993 (abstract).
21. Tuzuner F, Kecik Y, Ozdemir S et al: Electro-acupuncture in the treatment of enuresis nocturna, *Acupunct Electrother Res* 14:211-215, 1989 (abstract).
22. Bartocci C, Lucentini M: Acupuncture and micro-massage in the treatment of idiopathic nocturnal enuresis [in Italian], *Minerva Med* 72:2237, 1981 (abstract).
23. Bower WF, Diao M, Tang JL et al: Acupuncture for nocturnal enuresis in children: a systematic review and exploration of rationale, *Neurourol Urodyn* 24:267-272, 2005.
24. Cao J, Xu X, Cao J et al: *Essentials of traditional Chinese pediatrics*, Beijing, 1990, Foreign Language Press.
25. Deadman P, Al-Khafaji M: *A manual of acupuncture*, East Sussex, United Kingdom, 1998, Journal of Chinese Medicine Publications.
26. Diagnosis and treatment of gynecology and pediatrics. In *Chinese Zhenjiuology, a series of teaching videotapes,* Bejing, 1990, Medical Audio-Video Organization and Meditalent Enterprises.
27. Ellis E, Wiseman N, Boss K: *Fundamentals of Chinese acupuncture*, revised edition, Brookline, Mass, 1991, Paradigm Publications.
28. *English-Chinese encyclopedia of practical traditional Chinese medicine*, vol 1-14, Beijing, 1990, Higher Education Press.
29. Helms J: *Acupuncture energetics, a clinical approach for physicians*, Berkeley, Calif, 1995, Medical Acupuncture Publishers.
30. Maciocia G: *The foundations of Chinese medicine, a comprehensive text for acupuncturists and herbalists*, London, 1989, Churchill Livingstone.
31. Maciocia G: *The practice of Chinese medicine, the treatment of diseases with acupuncture and Chinese herbs*, London, 1994, Churchill Livingstone.
32. *Nei Ching, The Yellow Emperor's classic of internal medicine*, Berkeley, Calif, 1949, University of California Press (Translated by I Vieth).
33. O'Connor J, Bensky D, editors: *Acupuncture, a comprehensive text*, Seattle, 1981, Eastland Press.
34. Shanghai Xin-Hua Hospital, personal observations, March 1999.

Chiropractic

1. Davies N: *Chiropractic pediatrics*, London, 2000, Churchill Livingstone.
2. Guyton AC: *Textbook of medical physiology*, ed 11, Philadelphia, 2006, Saunders.
3. Moore KL: *Clinically oriented anatomy*, ed 5, Baltimore, 2006, Lippincott Williams and Wilkins.
4. Sweeney A: Resolution of enuresis with chiropractic adjustments in Romania, *ICA Rev* 53:69-72, 1997.
5. Stude D, Bergmann T, Finer B: A conservative approach for a patient with traumatically induced urinary incontinence, *J Manipulative Physiol Ther* 21:363-367, 1998.
6. Molina N: Chiropractic vertebral subluxation and enuresis, *Dynamic Chiropractic*, 2000. Available at http://www.chiroweb.com/archives/18/21/08.html. Accessed April 8, 2008.
7. Anrig C: Nocturnal enuresis, *Dynamic Chiropractic*, 1999. Available at http://www.chiroweb.com/archives/17/03/34.html. Accessed April 8, 2008.
8. Marko RB: Bed-wetting; two case studies, *Chiropractic Pediatr* 1:21-22, 1994.
9. Langley C: Epileptic seizures, nocturnal enuresis, ADD, *Chiropractic Pediatr* 1:22, 1994.
10. Bachman TR, Lantz CA: Management of pediatric asthma and enuresis with probable traumatic etiology, *JCA Rev* 51:37-40, 1995.
11. Fysh PN: Chiropractic management of enuresis, *Dynamic Chiropractic* 11:12-13, 1993.
12. Borregard PE: Neurogenic bladder and spina bifida occulta: a case report, *J Manipulative Physiol Ther* 10:122, 1987.
13. Vallone SA: Chiropractic management of a 7-year-old female with recurrent urinary tract infections, *Chiropractic Technique* 10:113-117, 1998.
14. Blomerth PR: Functional nocturnal enuresis, *J Manipulative Physiol Ther* 17:335-338, 1994.
15. Gemmel HA, Jacobson BH: Chiropractic management of enuresis: time-series descriptive design, *J Manipulative Physiol Ther* 12:386-389, 1989.
16. Leboeuf C, Brown P, Herman A et al: Chiropractic care of children with nocturnal enuresis: a prospective outcome study, *J Manipulative Physiol Ther* 14:110-115, 1991.
17. Reed WR, Beavers S, Reddy SK et al: Chiropractic management of primary nocturnal enuresis, *J Manipulative Physiol Ther* 17:156-185, 1994.
18. Davies N: *Chiropractic pediatrics*, London, 2000, Churchill Livingstone.
19. Bilgrai Cohen K: *Clinical management of infants and children*, Santa Cruz, Calif, 1988, Extension Press.
20. Chaitow L: *Palpation skills: assessment and diagnosis through touch*, New York, 1977, Churchill Livingstone.

Homeopathy

1. *ReferenceWorks Pro 4.2*, San Rafael, Calif, 2008, Kent Homeopathic Associates.

Mind/Body

1. Mellon M, McGrath M: Empirically supported treatments in pediatric psychology: nocturnal enuresis, *J Pediatr Psychol* 25:193-214, 2000.
2. Schulman S, Colish Y, von Zuben F et al: Effectiveness of treatments for nocturnal enuresis in a heterogeneous population, *Clin Pediatr* 29:359-364, 2000.
3. Kohen DP, Colwell SO, Heimel A et al: The use of relaxation/mental imagery (self hypnosis) in the management of 505 pediatric behavioral encounters, *J Devel Behav Pediatr* 5:21-25, 1984.
4. Stanton HE: Short term treatment of enuresis, *Am J Clin Hypnosis* 22:103-107, 1979.
5. Olness K: Treatment of enuresis with self hypnosis, an evaluation of 40 cases, *Clin Pediatr* 14:273-279, 1975.

6. Edwards SD, van der Spuy HI: Hypnotherapy as a treatment for enuresis, *J Child Psychol Psychiatry* 26:161-170, 1985.
7. Banerjee S, Srivastav A, Palan BM: Hypnosis and self hypnosis in the management of nocturnal enuresis: a comparative study with imipramine therapy, *Am J Clin Hypnosis* 36:113-119, 1993.
8. Porena M, Costantini E, Rociola W et al: Biofeedback successfully cures detrusor-sphincter dyssynergia in pediatric patients, *J Urol* 163:1927-1931, 2000.
9. Combs A, Glassberg A, Gerdes D et al: Biofeedback therapy for children with dysfunctional voiding, *Urology* 52:312-315, 1998.

Osteopathy

1. Gamble H: Defects corrected by osteopathic treatment, *Osteopath Prof* 13:8, 1946.
2. Bowman ER: Diagnosis: problems common to office practice exemplified in these case records of general practitioner, *Osteopath Prof* 15:22-54, 1948.
3. Priest T: Enuresis, *Osteopath Prof* 12:46-54, 1945.
4. Holt WL: Osteopathic notes: a wholly manipulative approach to osteopathic disorders, *Osteopath Prof* 7:6, 1940.

Psychology

1. Mellon M, McGrath M: Empirically supported treatments in pediatric psychology: nocturnal enuresis, *J Pediatr Psychol* 25: 193-214, 2000.
2. Bollard J, Nettlebeck T: A component analysis of dry-bed training for treatment of bedwetting, *Behav Res Ther* 20:383-390, 1982.
3. Butler R, Brewing C, Forsythe W: A comparison of two approaches to the treatment of nocturnal enuresis and the prediction of effectiveness using pretreatment variables, *J Child Psychol Psychiatry* 29:501-509, 1988.

Epilepsy

Acupuncture | May Loo
Aromatherapy | Maura A. Fitzgerald

Magnet Therapy | Agatha P. Colbert, Deborah Risotti
Osteopathy | Jane Carreiro

✳ PEDIATRIC DIAGNOSIS AND TREATMENT

Epilepsy is among the most common serious neurological disorders in childhood.[1] It occurs in approximately 10% of children[2] and has a variety of etiologies and manifestations.[4] By definition, a *seizure* is a paroxysmal disturbance of consciousness, motor function, sensation, perception, behavior, or emotion resulting from a cortical neuronal discharge. The symptoms can occur singly or in any combination.[4] The immature and developing brain of children, especially infants, has a lower seizure threshold and therefore is vulnerable toward developing seizures.[5] Epilepsy is present when two or more unprovoked seizures occur at an interval greater than 24 hours apart.[2]

More than two thirds of all seizures begin in childhood.[6] It is an important disorder because it can significantly affect not only the health but also the quality of life of the child and the family.[6] Childhood seizure represents a broad and complex range of disorders that vary from benign to severely disabling diseases.[7] The spectrum of causes encompasses genetic predisposition, birth and perinatal complications, congenital anomalies, metabolic disorders, infections, head trauma, and brain tumor. A significant number of seizures are considered idiopathic (without known cause).[8] Various non-neurological disorders, such as breath-holding spells, can mimic seizures.[9] Epileptic children have higher incidence of psychiatric disorders.[1]

Less than one third of seizures in children are actually caused by recurrent triggers from within the brain.[2] Neuronal hyperexcitability is the common pathophysiology in the various epileptic syndromes.[10] Neurochemical mechanisms include neurotransmitters γ-aminobutyric acid (GABA) and catecholamines and opioid peptides.[10]

Seizures in children are frequently misdiagnosed and inappropriately managed.[11] The International Classification of Seizures Disorders broadly categorizes seizures into generalized, partial (focal, local), and unclassified seizures. Each class has a long list of differentials with complex dimensions.[8] This section briefly focuses on the major seizures of childhood: generalized seizures: febrile, grand mal, and absence seizures; and partial, focal seizures.

Generalized Seizures

The generalized seizures have clinical presentations that indicate involvement of both cerebral hemispheres. Consciousness may be impaired and may in fact be the initial manifestation. Motor manifestations are bilateral. Electroencephalogram (EEG) reflects widespread neuronal discharges in both hemispheres.[8]

Febrile convulsions

Febrile seizures are the most common seizure disorder in childhood, occurring in 2% to 5% of children.[12] Most often febrile seizures are generalized tonic-clonic convulsions. They usually occur hours after onset of a febrile illness and are usually self-limiting and brief, lasting only a few seconds to a few minutes. They occur in children between 3 months and 5 years of age, with predominant presentation between 18 and 22 months.[13] There is no precise temperature elevation for seizure to occur, as the temperature threshold varies among children and even within the same child during different illnesses.[13]

Although children with preexisting neurological or developmental abnormalities may be more vulnerable to febrile seizures, they usually occur in normal children and are considered benign.[7,14] The recurrence rate is 30% to 40%.[15] A specific genetic defect is associated with a child's vulnerability to febrile seizures.[10] About 10% of parents of children with febrile seizures have had seizures themselves, chiefly the febrile type. Maternal illness and smoking during pregnancy also contribute to increased risk.[8] Treatment of most simple febrile seizures consists of fever control and counseling parents,[16] who understandably become very upset on seeing their young child convulse. The American Academy of Pediatrics (AAP) has determined that simple febrile convulsions are not associated with long-term adverse effects, and the risk of developing epilepsy is extremely low. Furthermore, even in those children who do become epileptic, there is no evidence that recurrent simple febrile seizures produce structural central nervous system (CNS) damage. Therefore long-term treatment of simple febrile convulsions is not recommended because the potential toxicities associated with antiepileptic therapy outweigh the relatively minor risks associated with simple febrile seizures.[12] In these cases, EEG changes tend to resolve even within hours or days after the acute episode, and EEG is of limited diagnostic and prognostic value.[8] Neuroimaging is not recommended.[13] Antipyretic treatment does not reduce the recurrence rate.[15] Intermittent diazepam prophylaxis at times of fever may or may not reduce the recurrence rate significantly. There are no data to suggest that it improves the long-term outcome, as compared with short-term seizure control, in terms of intelligence quotient, cognition, academic progress, motor control, and subsequent epilepsy.[15]

Grand mal seizures

Grand mal seizures are the most common type of convulsive disorders in children.[17] The seizures are characterized by generalized tonic-clonic movements that reflect involvement of both hemispheres. There is usually impairment of consciousness and a postictal period of drowsiness or confusion. EEG reveals higher amplitude of waves during tonic phase and slower waves during clonic phase.[8]

Grand mal seizures have numerous causes. Convulsions are often associated with CNS infections such as viral encephalitis or bacterial meningitis. Generalized seizure may be the first presentation of bacterial sepsis and meningitis in infants and young children. Mechanisms of seizure production in infection include venous thrombosis, cerebritis, abscess formation, and subdural effusions. In neonates and infants, grand mal seizures may be due to congenital anomalies, prenatal and perinatal complications, or metabolic dysfunctions. The majority of primary grand mal seizures in older children are idiopathic, often with a strong genetic predisposition.[17] Vascular lesions and even brain tumors usually present with focal seizures. Head trauma seizures tend to be focal when the onset is within 24 hours and generalized when the onset is delayed, usually within 3 years after the injury.[8]

Evaluation begins with a thorough history and neurological examination. The AAP endorses and accepts as its policy the Practice Parameter developed by the Quality Standards Subcommittee of the American Academy of Neurology for evaluating a first nonfebrile seizure in children and recommends a routine EEG to "predict the risk of recurrence and to classify the seizure type and epilepsy syndrome."[12] Other studies, such as laboratory evaluations and neuroimaging studies, are recommended based on specific clinical circumstances.[18]

Treatment with long-term anticonvulsants is important because hypoxemia during an acute episode of seizures can have serious CNS sequelae. Overall, epileptic children have diminished mental processing abilities, have poorer concentration, and are less alert than age-matched controls.[10] Because seizure medications have significant side effects, physicians are often confronted with the difficult decision of maintaining a child on long-term treatment or discontinuing drugs and risking the relapse of seizures.[20] Medically intractable, disabling seizures maybe treated with surgery.[7,21,22]

Benign epilepsy of childhood

This form of partial or generalized seizure is associated with genetic predisposition and maturational process. Some cases have transient worsening, including cognitive troubles.[23]

Absence Seizures

Absence, or petit mal epilepsy, remains one of the most enigmatic neurological disorders. In a typical simple absence attack, the child abruptly loses consciousness and ceases ongoing activity without even change in posture. The child's eyes stare vacantly straight ahead or may roll upward. There is no movement except possibly some subtle fluttering of the eyelids and twitching of the perioral muscles. The episode lasts for a brief moment, usually a few seconds, and the child suddenly resumes previous activity as though nothing had happened. No postical confusion or drowsiness occurs. Dozens to hundreds of seizures may occur in a single day. Intellectual and school performance may deteriorate because of the frequent interruptions of concentration. The child may be labeled as a daydreamer, lazy, or dull. These attacks tend to abate by adolescence.[7] although many children continue to suffer absence seizures well into adulthood.[24]

EEG exhibits a typical pattern of bilaterally synchronous, frontally predominant 3 Hz spike-and-slow-wave activity. These are thought to be abnormal oscillations between the thalamus and cerebral cortex.[25] Research has demonstrated a neurochemical basis involving GABA, catecholamines, and "endogenous" epileptogens[24] that activate burst firing of thalamic neurons, initiating an absence seizure.[26] These seizures are usually managed with medication.[7] There is no widely accepted theory of a precise etiology,[24] except for well-established evidence of genetic predisposition.[26,27]

Partial, Focal Seizures

Partial, focal seizures have clinical and EEG changes that indicate initial activation of neurons limited to part of one cerebral hemisphere. The seizures may or may not have impaired consciousness and often progress to generalized motor convulsions.[8] Some may become generalized so quickly that the initial focal nature of the seizures is masked. Others become generalized after an appreciable time has elapsed. EEG tracing may indicate initial activation of neurons limited to a localized area in one cerebral hemisphere.[8] The mechanisms that initiate, promulgate, and terminate seizures remain unknown.

In children, approximately 30% to 50% of focal seizures have no known etiological cause. A genetic factor may determine whether a focal lesion becomes epileptogenic. Cerebral damage during or near the time of birth may result in seizures in early infancy or later in childhood. CNS tumor is rare in children. Head trauma is the most common cause of focal seizures. Closed head injuries, which constitute most of pediatric injuries, are associated with only a 5% incidence of epilepsy. The best results (of head trauma) were associated with normal computed tomography scans.[28] Linear or depressed skull fractures have an approximately 50% incidence of posttraumatic seizures. Fifty percent of seizures have their onset within 24 hours of injury and tend to be focal in nature. Seizures occurring within 3 years of injury are more frequently generalized tonic-clonic grand mal seizures.[28] The pathogenesis of seizure due to head injury may be extravasation of blood that stimulates epileptogenic processes. Management may require neurosurgical evacuation of subdural hematomas, followed by long-term use of anticonvulsant medications.

A recent, unreported, randomized survey of 350 children with chronic neurological disorders, 60% with epilepsy, revealed 37% of surveyed caregivers reported current or past use of complementary and alternative medicine (CAM), consisting of massage, herbal therapies, acupuncture, chiropractic, and vitamin therapy; 81% reported that CAM therapy was efficacious.[29]

❋ CAM THERAPY RECOMMENDATIONS

Acupuncture

The first description of grand mal seizures appeared in *The Yellow Emperor's Classic of Internal Medicine, Huang Di Nei Ching* (770-221 BCE).[1] Pediatric textbooks have indicated successful treatment with acupuncture. Current acupuncture data have demonstrated varying degrees of success in treatment of adult epilepsy—mostly the chronic, medically intractable seizures.[2-5] A retrospective study from Israel indicated that one third of epileptic children in their lifetime used CAM therapy, including acupuncture.[6] Scalp acupuncture has been shown to improve cerebral blood flow in children, which would increase the delivery of oxygen and nutrients to the cortical tissues. This can theoretically be beneficial in childhood epilepsy.[7]

Several animal studies from China have elucidated the possible biochemical mechanisms of acupuncture in epilepsy. One study, in which corresponding GV26 and GV24 points were treated on rats, revealed an increase in brain GABA levels.[8] Two studies demonstrated acupuncture's effect on nitric oxide (NO), a diffusible neurotransmitter that is neurotoxic when overproduced, which is found in ischemia and in epilepsy. Electroacupuncture may exert anticonvulsant effect by antagonizing the ischemia-elicited rise of NO[9] and by decreasing the neuronal NO synthase.[10] One study demonstrated that electrical stimulation of ear acupoints diminished convulsive behaviors and significantly decreased hippocampal amino acid neurotransmitters.[11]

An integrative approach to pediatric seizure disorder can combine Western neurological examination and laboratory evaluations for diagnosis. Because acupuncture has minimal or no side effects, it can be administered concomitantly with seizure medications. Tapering of medications, however, should be carried out carefully with close coordination with the neurologist.

Acupuncture Differentiation and Treatment Recommendations

According to Chinese medicine, epileptic convulsions are Internal Wind disturbances that can be due to both external and internal causes.[12]

Generalized seizures

Grand mal generalized seizures can be caused by external pathogenic invasion or internal imbalances.

External pathogenic invasion: Wind-Cold and Wind-Heat. Seizures are acute manifestations of severe-stage Wind-Cold (viral) and Wind-Heat (bacterial) invasions (infections), correlating to the sepsis and meningitis of Western diagnoses.

Acupuncture can be used as complement treatment to dissipate Heat, subdue internal Wind, and tonify the child:

GV14 to dissipate Heat and subdue Wind.
GV16, GB20 to subdue Wind.
LR2 to clear Jue Yin Liver Heat.
LR3 to subdue Liver Wind and nourish Liver Yin and Blood.
SI3 to expel Wind from GV channel.
GV20 to increase Qi to the CNS.

Kidney Yin deficiency/Liver Yin deficiency. Kidney Yin and Liver Yin deficiencies correspond to the idiopathic seizures with strong genetic predisposition, CNS congenital anomalies or lesions, perinatal complications, or metabolic dysfunctions. Benign epilepsy of children and febrile convulsions may be milder forms of this imbalance, whereas infantile spasm is on the other end of the spectrum, being the most severe manifestation.

Treatment for acute seizure: GV26, KI1.
Prophylactic treatment to prevent recurrence:
    GV14, LI11 to clear Heat from the system.
    GV16, GB20 to subdue Wind,
Tonify Kidney Yin and Liver Yin:
    KI6 tonifies KI Yin, an important point for seizures.
    LR8 tonifies LR Yin.
    LR3 subdues LR Yang and LR Wind; tonifies Liver Yin.
    SP6, KI6 tonify Yin.
    BL18 tonifies LR Yin, also subdues LR Yang.
    SP6, KI3; BL17, 20, 23 tonify Blood.

Liver Yin/Heart Yin deficiency—absence seizures

GV14, 16, GB20 to subdue internal Wind.
ST40 to dispel Phlegm.
P6 to resolve Phlegm from the Heart, clear orifices.
KI6 to tonify Kidney Yin, the basis of all Yin.
HT7 to tonify Heart Yin, calm the Mind.
BL44, Shentang, to calm Shen.
LR3 to tonify Liver Yin, subdue Liver Yang.
BL47, Hunman, to settle the Ethereal Soul.
SP6 to tonify Yin, dispel Phlegm.
Avoid excess sour and bitter foods, including bitter medications and herbs.

Spleen Yang deficiency. Spleen deficiency can be responsible for both generalized convulsions and absence seizures. Generalized tonic-clonic seizures with gurgling noises or foaming at the mouth during acute attacks are pathognomonic of this type of seizure with the presence of Phlegm.

Treatment is directed toward tonifying Spleen, resolving Phlegm, and opening orifices:
Acute tonic-clonic seizures can be treated with GV26 and KI1.
Prophylactic treatment:
    Decrease Phlegm-producing, sweet, and greasy foods.
    Vigorously tonify Spleen using the Five-Element, Four-Point protocol:
        Tonify SP2, HT8; sedate SP1, LR1.
    ST40, SP6 resolve Phlegm.
    P5 resolves Phlegm from the Heart.
    P6, HT9 clears Heart, opens orifices.
    ST25 is an important point for Phlegm misting the Mind: it regulates the Stomach, opens the Mind's orifices.
    BL15, BL44 tonifies Heart, tonifies Shen.
    GV20 clears the Mind.
    LI4, LU7 regulate ascending of Clear Qi, descending of turbid Qi in the head, thus clearing the Mind.
    GV16, GB20 subdues Wind.
    Modify lifestyle to decrease excess mental activities, achieve a balance between rest and study, and minimize stressful situations that cause worry and anxiety.

Partial/focal seizures

Focal seizures are most often caused by head trauma causing localized Blood stasis.

Treatment

Emergent treatment with GV26, KI1.

SP6, BL17 to move Blood.

P6 moves Blood, calms the Mind.

HT7 calms the Mind.

LR14, BL18 Liver Mu-Shu points to move LR Blood.

Aromatherapy

The effect of essential oils for treatment of epilepsy has not been well studied; however, essential oils have been recommended to aid in relaxation and stress reduction as a method to reduce the frequency of seizures.[1] In this author's experience, essential oils can be a useful adjunct as part of a stress management program for children in which seizure activity increases with stress. Essential oils generally used for calming and relaxation, such as lavender *(Lavandula angustifolia)*, sweet orange *(Citrus sinensis)*, and bergamot *(Citrus bergamia)*, given by inhalation or with massage, are beneficial.

A nonsystematic and nonrandomized pilot study of 100 volunteer subjects was conducted during a 10-year period. Subjects all had epilepsy; the majority had complex partial seizures with secondary generalized tonic-clonic attacks. The ages of subjects were not stipulated. Subjects self-selected into three groups: aromatherapy massage only, hypnosis only, and aromatherapy massage with hypnosis. Whole-body massage was provided. Essential oils chosen by subjects were jasmine *(Jasminum grandiflorum)*, ylang-ylang *(Cananga odorata)*, lavender *(L. angustifolia)*, chamomile (type not noted), bergamot *(C. bergamia)*, and marjoram *(Origanum majorana)*. There was no control group. The goal of the study was to determine whether subjects could pair the smell of the essential oil with becoming relaxed and thereby prevent seizure onset. One third of subjects who had either aromatherapy massage or aromatherapy massage and hypnosis were seizure free at 1 year. At the 2-year period, some subjects relapsed (number not specified). There was little standardization in the number of treatments subjects received and in the personnel providing the intervention. The author of the study notes that this was a difficult intervention to provide because it was time consuming and labor intensive.[2]

Magnet Therapy

For health maintenance treatment in children with petite mal–type seizures, apply a 9000-G Accuband REC magnet with the designated bionorth side (the side with the indentation) facing the skin to acupuncture point KD6 and another 9000-G Accuband REC magnet with the opposite side facing the skin on KD27.[1] Leave the magnets in place for 15 minutes at a time and treat once per week. This type of magnet is available from OMS (800-323-1839) or AHSM (800-635-7070).

Osteopathy

The osteopathic literature is littered with reports concerning the efficacy of osteopathic manipulation in the treatment of seizures. In his earliest writings, A.T. Still, the founder of osteopathy, described the successful treatment of patients with grand mal–type seizures.[1,2] William Sutherland, who pioneered cranial osteopathy, described a technique applied to the temporal bones and cranial base that could be used to abort a seizure.[3] H.H. Fryette and P.T. Wilson each published a study in the mid 1900s; however, neither study was randomized or controlled. Wilson's study followed 92 children with cerebral palsy, 20 of whom had seizure disorder. All of the children with seizure disorder showed some improvement after 6 to 12 months of osteopathic treatment.[4] Fryette described four patients with seizure activity following trauma, three of whom were children. All four patients had resolution of seizure activity with osteopathic treatment.[5] Lippincott, Tessien, Capobianco, and Frymann have each reported cases or studies demonstrating improvement or alleviation of seizure activity with osteopathic treatment.[6-9] None of these were randomized or controlled. However, Frymann's study, which also used a reported improvement in developmental parameters, attempted a crossover by making one group wait 8 weeks for onset of treatment; unfortunately, there was not a true control group in the study.

Osteopathic manipulative treatment of children with seizure disorder has two goals. The first involves treating compensatory dysfunction resulting from the seizures. In a child with intractable seizures, secondary muscle hypertonicity, joint contractures, fascial strain, and other types of somatic dysfunction increase the child's level of discomfort, interfere with normal function, and may even exacerbate or lower the child's tolerance to the seizure activity. Techniques aimed at correcting or improving these compensatory strains will help the child's overall functional capacity.

The second aspect involves the principles of osteopathy in the cranial field, whereby balance of the cranial mechanism and its related tissues is thought to optimize normal activity in the brain. In some of the literature, the seizure foci has been described as a functional scar[10] around which the cranial mechanism must function. Alterations in tissue or fluid mechanics, which interfere with the brain's ability to adapt to this new fulcrum, may exacerbate the seizure activity. Cranial techniques that address the fluid and potency characteristics of the cranial mechanism are most commonly used in these children. Although adverse effects have been rarely reported, they do exist.[11,12] Consequently, it is recommended that this approach be done only by a trained physician who can deal with any untoward outcomes.

Osteopathic manipulative treatment of children with seizure disorder must always be done with judicious consideration of the child's current pharmacotherapeutic regimen and complementary course of therapy. The body's response to osteopathic treatment may alter the child's response and tolerance to medication, homeopathic remedies, and herbal compounds. Consequently, good communication between all practitioners is paramount. The osteopathic physician may manage the child's pharmacotherapeutic agents and administer osteopathic manipulative treatment concurrently, or the osteopath may work in a complementary role, consulting with the managing physician. Whatever the arrangement, any change in the child's therapeutic regimen should be made slowly, with caution and vigilance to the child's response.

References

Pediatric Diagnosis and Treatment

1. Shinnar S, Pellock JM: Update on the epidemiology and prognosis of pediatric epilepsy, *J Child Neurol* 17(Suppl 1):S4-S17, 2002.

2. Behrman RE, Kliegman RM, Jenson HB, editors: *Nelson's textbook of pediatrics*, ed 17, Philadelphia, 2004, Saunders.

3. Morton LD, Pellock JM: Overview of childhood epilepsy and epileptic syndromes and advances in therapy, *Curr Pharm Des* 6: 879-900, 2000.

4. Managing childhood epilepsy, *Drug Ther Bull* 39:11-16, 2001.

5. Jensen FE: Acute and chronic effects of seizures in the developing brain: experimental models, *Epilepsia* 40(Suppl 1):S51-S58, 1999; discussion S64-S66.

6. Thiele EA, Gonzalez-Heydrich J, Riviello JJ Jr: Epilepsy in children and adolescents, *Child Adolesc Psychiatric Clin North Am* 8: 671-694, 1999.

7. Arnold ST, Dodson WE: Epilepsy in children, *Baillieres Clin Neurol* 5:783-802, 1996.

8. Swaiman K: *Pediatric neurology, principles and practice*, St Louis, 1989, Mosby.

9. Barron T: The child with spells, *Pediatr Clin North Am* 38: 711-724, 1991.

10. Engelborghs S, D'Hooge R, De Deyn PP: Pathophysiology of epilepsy, *Acta Neurol Belg* 100:201-213, 2000.

11. Appleton RE: Treatment of childhood epilepsy, *Pharm Ther* 67:419-431, 1995.

12. Baumann RJ, Duffner PK: Treatment of children with simple febrile seizures: the AAP practice parameter. American Academy of Pediatrics, *Pediatr Neurol* 23:11-17, 2000.

13. Rajadhyaksha S, Shah KN: Controversies in febrile seizures, *Indian J Pediatr* 67(1 Suppl):S71-S79, 2000.

14. Baumann RJ: Prevention and management of febrile seizures, *Paediatr Drugs* 3:585-592, 2001.

15. Knudsen FU: Febrile convulsions, treatment and prognosis [in Danish], *Ugeskr Laeger* 163:1098-1102, 2001 (abstract).

16. Bettis DB, Ater SB: Febrile seizures: emergency department diagnosis and treatment, *J Emerg Med* 2:341-348, 1985.

17. Korinthenberg R: Grand mal epilepsy in childhood [in German], *Monatsschr Kinderheilkd* 140:614-618, 1992 (abstract).

18. Hirtz D, Ashwal S, Berg A: Practice parameter: evaluating a first nonfebrile seizure in children, *Neurology* 55:615-623, 2000.

19. Dam M: Children with epilepsy: the effect of seizures, syndromes, and etiological factors on cognitive functioning, *Epilepsia* 31 (Suppl 4):S26-S29, 1990.

20. Cavazzuti GB: Discontinuing of antiepileptic therapy [in Italian], *Pediatr Med Chir* 20:317-322, 1998 (abstract).

21. Nordli DR Jr, Kelley KR: Selection and evaluation of children for epilepsy surgery, *Pediatr Neurosurg* 34:1-12, 2001.

22. Olson DM: Evaluation of children for epilepsy surgery, *Pediatr Neurosurg* 34:159-165, 2001.

23. Dulac O: Benign epilepsies of childhood—distinct syndromes and overlap, *Epileptic Disord* 2(Suppl 1):S41-S43, 2000.

24. Mirsky AF, Duncan CC, Myslobodsky MS: Petit mal epilepsy: a review and integration of recent information, *J Clin Neurophysiol* 3:179-208, 1986.

25. Duncan JS: Idiopathic generalized epilepsies with typical absences, *J Neurol* 244:403-411, 1997.

26. Porter RJ: The absence epilepsies, *Epilepsia* 34(Suppl 3):S42-S48, 1993.

27. Robinson R, Taske N, Sander T et al: Linkage analysis between childhood absence epilepsy and genes encoding GABAA and GABAB receptors, voltage-dependent calcium channels, and the ECA1 region on chromosome 8q, *Epilepsy Res* 48:169-179, 2000.

28. Costeff H, Groswasser Z, Goldstein R: Long-term follow-up review of 31 children with severe closed head trauma, *J Neurosurg* 73:684-687, 1990.

29. Sullivan MG: Parents may seek alternative epilepsy medicines, *Pediatr News* 39:32, 2005.

Acupuncture

1. Lai CW, Lai YH: History of epilepsy in Chinese traditional medicine, *Epilepsia* 32:299-302, 1991.

2. Chen KY, Chen GP, Feng X: Observation of immediate effect of acupuncture on electroencephalograms in epileptic patients, *J Tradit Chinese Med* 3:121-124, 1983.

3. Liu A: Clinical application of moxibustion over point dazhui, *J Tradit Chinese Med* 19:283-286, 1999.

4. Yang J: Treatment of status epilepticus with acupuncture, *J Tradit Chinese Med* 10:101-102, 1990.

5. Shi ZY, Gong BT, Jia YW et al: The efficacy of electro-acupuncture on 98 cases of epilepsy, *J Tradit Chinese Med* 7:21-22, 1987.

6. Gross-Tsur V, Lahad A, Shalev RS: Use of complementary medicine in children with attention deficit hyperactivity disorder and epilepsy, *Pediatr Neurol* 29:53-55, 2003.

7. Xiang L, Wang H, Li Z: TCD observation on cerebral blood flow dynamics inference of cerebral palsy with scalp therapy [in Chinese], *Zhen Ci Yan Jiu* 21:7-9, 1996 (abstract).

8. Wu Y, Shen Q, Zhang Q: The effect of acupuncture on high oxygen pressure-induced convulsion and its relationship to the brain GABA concentration in mice [in Chinese], *Zhen Ci Yan Jiu* 17:104-109, 1992 (abstract).

9. Zhao P, Huang ZN, Chen G et al: Electro-acupuncture attenuates nitric oxide release from rat striatum after transient middle cerebral artery occlusion, *Acupunct Electrother Res* 25:101-107, 2000.

10. Yang R, Huang ZN, Cheng JS: Anticonvulsion effect of acupuncture might be related to the decrease of neuronal and inducible nitric oxide synthases, *Acupunct Electrother Res* 25: 137-143, 2000.

11. Shu J, Liu RY, Huang XF: The effects of ear-point stimulation on the contents of somatostatin and amino acid neurotransmitters in brain of rat with experimental seizure, *Acupunct Electrother Res* 29:43-51, 2004.

12. Loo M: *Pediatric acupuncture*, London, 2002, Elsevier.

Aromatherapy

1. Betts T: The fragrant breeze: the role of aromatherapy in treating epilepsy, *Aromatherapy Q* 51:25-27, 1996.

2. Betts T: Use of aromatherapy (with or without hypnosis) in the treatment of intractable epilepsy—two-year follow-up study, *Seizure* 12:534-538, 2003.

Magnet Therapy

1. Loo M: *Pediatric acupuncture*, London, 2002, Elsevier.

Osteopathy

1. Still AT: *Philosophy of osteopathy*, Kirksville, Mo, 1899, AT Still.

2. Still AT: *Principles and practice of osteopathy*, ed 2, Kirksville, Mo, 1905, AT Still.

3. Sutherland WG: *The cranial bowl*, ed 2, 1939, Sutherland.

4. Wilson P: Cerebral palsy: a study of 92 cases, *Osteopath Prof* 21: 11-15, 1954.

5. Fryette HH: Epilepsy: correction of second dorsal believed effective in treatment of epilepsy, *Osteopath Prof* 16:20-47, 1949.

6. Lippincott H: Case of birth injury or cranial trauma, *AAO J* 3:15, 1993.

7. Tessien RM: OMT: a standby in children's seizures, *J Am Osteopath Assoc* 75:264, 1975.

8. Capobianco A: The cranial base under strain: causes and consequences: the first of two parts, *Cranial Letter* 56:10-16, 2003.

9. Frymann VM, Carney RE, Springall P: Effect of osteopathic medical management on neurological development in children, *J Am Osteopathic Assoc* 92:729-744, 1992.

10. Wales AL: *Osteopathic treatment of children with epilepsy*. Personal communication, 1991.

11. Greenman PE, McPartland JM: Cranial findings and iatrogenesis from craniosacral manipulation in patients with traumatic brain syndrome, *J Am Osteopathic Assoc* 95:182-191, 1995.

12. Sutherland WG: *Teachings in the science of osteopathy*, Portland Ore, 1990, Rudra Press.

Epistaxis

Acupuncture | May Loo

Homeopathy | Janet L. Levatin

Magnet Therapy | Agatha P. Colbert, Deborah Risotti

✳ PEDIATRIC DIAGNOSIS AND TREATMENT

Epistaxes, or nosebleeds, are rare in infancy and common in childhood.[1,2] Their incidence decreases after puberty.[2] Epistaxis often causes great anxiety in patients, parents, and clinicians.[3]

The most common site of bleeding is the Kiesselbach plexus, an area in the anterior septum with rich vasculature and thin mucosa.[2,4]

Epistaxis results from the interaction of multiple factors that damage the nasal mucosal lining, affect the vessel walls, or alter the coagulability of the blood. The causes may be categorized as environmental (e.g., digital or other nasal trauma, foreign bodies, dry air); local (e.g., nasal polyps or other intranasal growths such as hemangiomas or tumors); systemic (e.g., upper respiratory infection, allergies, coagulopathies, vascular anomalies); or pharmacological (e.g., chronic use of nasal steroid sprays, aspirin ingestion related).[2,3,5-7] In many children a family history of childhood epistaxis is common.[2,7] Recurrent idiopathic epistaxis in children is repeated nasal bleeding in patients < age 16 years for which no specific cause has been identified.[1]

Fortunately, most nosebleeds are self-limiting or respond to simple measures, such as manual compression with the child's head tilted forward to avoid blood trickling back into the throat; packing with a piece of cotton; or cold compresses applied to the nose.[1,2,4] If these measures do not stop the bleeding, local application with various agents, such as a solution of oxymetazoline (Afrin), Neo-Synephrine (0.25% to 1%), petroleum jelly, or an antiseptic cream, or electrical cauterization of the nasal septum may be necessary.[2,4,8,9] During the winter or in a dry environment, a room humidifier, saline drops, and petrolatum cream can be used to prevent nosebleeds. In severe or repeated epistaxis, otolaryngological and hematological evaluation may be necessary for making a definitive diagnosis, and hospitalization or surgical intervention may also be indicated.[2]

✳ CAM THERAPY RECOMMENDATIONS

Acupuncture

Epistaxis or nosebleeds can be stopped by using a combination of local and distal points. The most common local points are:
GV23[1]
LI20[1]

Bailao (MHN14) at the highest point of the nasolabial groove[2]
Yintang (MHN3) at the midpoint between the medial extremities of the eyebrows[2]
A powerful distal point is: SP1.[2]
For severe nosebleed that does not stop, BL54 can be added.[1]

Homeopathy

Before using this section, please see Appendix A, Homeopathy, for definitions of practitioner expertise categories and general information on prescribing homeopathic medicines.

Clinical Expertise Category 1

Category 1 includes uncomplicated epistaxis.

There are no controlled clinical trials of homeopathic treatment for epistaxis, although the homeopathic literature contains evidence for its use in the form of accumulated clinical experience.[1] Uncomplicated epistaxis can often be treated effectively with homeopathy. It is safe to use homeopathic treatment for epistaxis, either alone or in combination with other therapies and measures to stop the bleeding. In any case in which bleeding is heavy or cannot be stopped, emergency care should be sought without delay.

The goal in treating epistaxis homeopathically is to determine the single homeopathic medicine whose description in the materia medica most closely matches the symptom picture of the patient. Sometimes mental and emotional states, in addition to physical symptoms, are considered. Once the medicine has been selected, it can be given orally or sublingually in the 30C potency every 10 to 15 minutes. In more serious situations, higher potencies such as 200C may be required. If the medicine has not helped within four to five doses, then another homeopathic medicine should be tried or some other form of therapy should be instituted as needed. Once symptoms have begun to resolve, the medicine can be given less frequently or stopped. It can be repeated again for a relapse of symptoms.

The following is a list of homeopathic medicines commonly used to treat patients with epistaxis. It must be emphasized that this list is partial and represents some of the probable choices from the homeopathic materia medica. If the symptoms of a given patient are not represented here, a search of the homeopathic literature would be needed to find the simillimum.

Arnica montana

Arnica montana is the medicine to consider when the nosebleed occurs after a trauma. If indicated, treatment at an emergency care facility should be sought.

Belladonna

Belladonna is used to treat the sudden onset of epistaxis with a profuse discharge of hot, bright red blood. The patient may be feverish or have a red face. If indicated, treatment at an emergency care facility should be sought.

Drosera rotundifolia

The use of *Drosera rotundifolia* should be considered when the nosebleed occurs in a patient with a severe cough. If indicated, treatment at an emergency care facility should be sought.

Phosphorus

Children who need *Phosphorus* have a tendency to have nosebleeds producing bright-red blood that does not clot easily, leading to a prolonged episode of bleeding. The nosebleed may occur after blowing the nose. The child is fearful and desires consolation. If indicated, treatment at an emergency care facility should be sought.

Magnet Therapy

First, massage SP1 on the same side as the bleeding nostril for 1 minute.[1] If the bleeding persists, place a 9000-G Accuband REC magnet with the designated bionorth (the side with indentation) on SP1. If bleeding still continues, add another 9000-G Accuband REC magnet, with the side opposite the side with the indentation (biosouth side) facing the skin to the ipsilateral LR1.[1] Leave the magnet in place for 5 minutes. This type of magnet is available from OMS (800-323-1839) or AHSM (800-635-7070).

References

Pediatric Diagnosis and Treatment

1. Burton MJ, Doree CJ: Interventions for recurrent idiopathic epistaxis (nosebleeds) in children, *Cochrane Database Syst Rev* (1): CD004461, 2004.
2. Behrman RE, Kliegman RM, Jenson HB, editors: *Nelson's textbook of pediatrics,* ed 17, Philadelphia, 2004, Saunders, pp 1387-1388.
3. Middleton PM: Epistaxis, *Emerg Med Australas* 16:428-440, 2004.
4. Francois M: Epistaxis in children [in French], *Arch Pediatr* 3: 806-813, 1996.
5. Giridharan W, Belloso A, Pau H et al: Epistaxis in children with vascular malformations—commentary of two cases and literature review, *Int J Pediatr Otorhinolaryngol* 65:137-141, 2002.
6. Brown NJ, Berkowitz RG: Epistaxis in healthy children requiring hospital admission, *Int J Pediatr Otorhinolaryngol* 68:1181-1184, 2004.
7. Sandoval C, Dong S, Visintainer P et al: Clinical and laboratory features of 178 children with recurrent epistaxis, *J Pediatr Hematol Oncol* 24:47-49, 2002.
8. Loughran S, Spinou E, Clement WA et al: A prospective, single-blind, randomized controlled trial of petroleum jelly/Vaseline for recurrent paediatric epistaxis, *Clin Otolaryngol* 29:266-269, 2004.
9. Kubba H, MacAndie C, Botma M et al: A prospective, single-blind, randomized controlled trial of antiseptic cream for recurrent epistaxis in childhood, *Clin Otolaryngol* 26:465-468, 2001.

Acupuncture

1. O'Connor J, Bensky D, editors: *Acupuncture, a comprehensive text,* Seattle, 1981, Eastland Press.
2. Deadman P, Al-Khafaji M: *A manual of acupuncture,* East Sussex, United Kingdom, 1998, Journal of Chinese Medicine Publications.

Homeopathy

1. *ReferenceWorks Pro 4.2,* San Rafael, Calif, 2008, Kent Homeopathic Associates.

Magnet Therapy

1. Loo M: *Pediatric acupuncture,* London, 2002, Elsevier.

Fever

Acupuncture | May Loo

Chiropractic | Anne Spicer

Herbs—Chinese | Catherine Ulbricht, Jennifer Woods, Mark Wright

Herbs—Western | Alan D. Woolf, Paula M. Gardiner, Lana Dvorkin-Camiel, Jack Maypole

Homeopathy | Janet L. Levatin

Naturopathy | Matthew I. Baral

✳ PEDIATRIC DIAGNOSIS AND TREATMENT

Human beings are homeothermic, which means that body temperature is normally maintained within a relatively narrow range despite wide variations in energy intake and expenditure and environmental temperature.[1] The thermoregulatory center, located in the anterior hypothalamus,[2] responds to changes in blood temperature and to cold and warm receptors in the skin. Thermosensitive responses include redirecting blood to or from cutaneus vascular beds, increased or decreased sweating, extracellular fluid volume regulation, and behavioral responses.[3]

Fever is typically defined as rectal temperature greater than 38° C (100.4° F), tympanic temperature greater than 38° C (100.4° F), oral temperature greater than 37.8° C (100° F), and axillary temperature greater than 37.2° C (99° F).[4] Diurnal variation indicates lower body temperatures in the early morning and as much as 1° C (1.8° F) higher in the late afternoon or early evening.[3,4]

Fever remains one of the most common reasons parents seek medical attention for their child. It is the primary complaint of 30% of patients seen by pediatricians in practice and the cause of as many as 50% of after-hour calls.[4] Parents seek advice from a myriad of resources in addition to their pediatricians, as evidenced recently by almost 600,000 citations on www.google.com for the entry "fever and children."

The physiology of the fever response is mediated endogenously and exogenously. Endogenous pyrogen, produced by immunological cells such as polymorphonuclear leukocytes and phagocytic cells, include the cytokines interleukin (IL)-α and IL-6, tumor necrosis factor-α (TNF-α), and interferon (IFN). Stimulated leukocytes and other cells produce lipids that also serve as endogenous pyrogens. The best-studied lipid mediator is prostaglandin E2 (PGE2).[3-5] Exogenous pyrogen such as microbes, bacterial endotoxin, or other products of microbes and drugs produce fever by stimulating macrophages and circulating leukocytes and other cells to produce endogenous pyrogens. Endotoxin is one of the few substances that can directly affect thermoregulation in the hypothalamus as well as stimulate endogenous pyrogen agents.[1,3,4] In children, infection is the most common cause of acute febrile episode, and inflammatory diseases account for recurrent and persistent temperature elevation.[6]

A rise in the hypothalamic set-point triggers the cold response—characterized by shivering, vasoconstriction, and decreased peripheral perfusion—which is a mechanism to maintain the body in homeostasis. The cold response decreases heat loss from the body, allowing temperature to rise to the new set-point, resulting in fever.[4]

Fever can be managed with conservative measures such as extra fluids and cooling measures such as tepid sponge bathing in warm water (not alcohol). To date, the risks and benefits of antipyretic therapy remain controversial. Parents and caregivers often manifest "fever phobia"[7]—believing that fever can cause brain damage and other serious consequences, such that they are quick to administer antipyretics at the first sign of a fever.[4]

Arguments against giving antipyretics include the protective effect of fever, the intrinsic homestatic control, and the side effects of antipyretics. Fever is an adaptive, protective mechanism that generates acute phase reactants; accelerates a variety of immunological responses such as phagocytosis, leukocyte migration, and lymphocyte transformation; and increases inflammatory response, resulting in decreased microbial reproduction.[1,4] Some studies have demonstrated that antipyretic therapy may actually prolong influenza A infection.[8]

Fever engenders certain physiological changes. Each centigrade of fever increases the basal metabolic rate by 10% to 12% and increases basal cellular oxygen consumption by about 13%, with a proportionate increase in carbon dioxide production and requirements for fluid and calories.[1] Very high fever can impair the immunological response. Interestingly, however, in the absence of hyperthermic insults (e.g., dehydration, being in a closed, hot automobile) and in neurologically normal children, the body does not allow fever to rise to a potentially lethal level by producing cryogens that act as natural antipyretic substances to keep temperature in a homeostatic balance. Without a hyperthermic insult, a child's temperature very rarely exceeds 41.1° C (106° F),[4] so it is questionable whether the core temperatures during the febrile state ever reach intrinsically noxious level that merit antipyretic intervention or when, if ever, fever's adaptive metabolic changes are more physiologically detrimental than beneficial.[9,10]

Acetaminophen and ibuprofen, two of the most common antipyretics given to children,[9-12] are used to control fever and for symptomatic relief, such as of myalgia and headache. Both drugs are inhibitors of hypothalamic cyclooxygenase, thus inhibiting PGE2 synthesis. Prolonged use of acetaminophen may produce renal injury, and massive overdose may produce hepatic failure. Ibuprofen may cause dyspepsia, gastrointestinal bleeding, reduced renal blood flow, and rarely, aseptic meningitis, hepatic toxicity, or aplastic anemia. Serious injury from ibuprofen overdose is unusual. The decline of body temperature after antipyretic therapy does not distinguish serious bacterial from less serious viral diseases. There is no evidence that alternating acetaminophen and ibuprofen can achieve faster antipyresis; however, it may lead to dosing errors.[4]

Aspirin should never be given to children and teenagers because of the risk of Reye syndrome.

The other nonsteroidal antiinflammatory drugs have a limited role in pediatrics.[13] Dosage of medication should be carefully calculated according to both the age and weight of the child. However, children are frequently given improper doses, resulting in toxicity or inadequate symptomatic improvement.[12]

Fever can precipitate febrile seizures in the susceptible child between 6 months and 5 or 6 years of age.[14] However, there is no evidence that antipyretics can prevent febrile seizures even in children with a history of febrile convulsions. When febrile convulsion occurs, pediatricians in general reassure parents that they are benign and self-limiting and that long-term prognosis in the vast majority of cases is good.[15]

Treatment of fever is indicated (1) in children with cardiovascular or pulmonary diseases, because febrile illnesses increase oxygen consumption and these children may already have an increase in carbon dioxide production; (2) in a seriously ill child with diminished oral intake, such that the marked increase in insensible water loss and increase in cellular energy expenditure predisposes the patient to dehydration and utilization of substrates contained within body tissues[1]; (3) in immunocompromised children in whom fever may indicate more serious illness; and (4) in children younger than 3 months. Hyperpyrexia (>41° C) indicates greater risk of severe infection, hypothalamic disorders, or central nervous system (CNS) hemorrhage and should always be treated with antipyretics.[3]

Specific treatment should be directed toward the disorder that caused the fever, such as antibiotics for an ear infection or an antiinflammatory drug for chronic inflammatory bowel disease (IBD).

At this time, there are no conventional modalities to increase the child's natural immunity to prevent further susceptibility to febrile illness. Various complementary and alternative medicine (CAM) modalities can increase immunity and manage fever with minimal adverse effects.

✳ CAM THERAPY RECOMMENDATIONS

Acupuncture

Traditional Chinese medicine (TCM) defines fever as Heat accumulation caused by external pathogenic invasion or internal organ imbalances. Historical evidence indicates that acupuncture was used in the plague epidemic in Guangzhou (Canton) in 1894.[1] Current data are generally positive for the antipyretic effect of acupuncture. Recent animal studies have elucidated the possible biochemical mechanisms of acupuncture on fever. An early study from China using acupuncture on points corresponding to human GV14 and LI11 revealed no change on Wind-Heat fever in rabbits induced with bacterial endotoxins.[2] However, subsequent animal studies have shown more favorable results.

An animal study from Russia showed that the opioid antagonist naloxone administered intravenously reduced the intensity and duration of the antipyretic action of acupuncture, thus suggesting that the antipyretic mechanism of acupuncture involves the same endogenous opioid system as in pain relief.[3] In an animal study from Japan, fever was induced in rats by injecting either lipopolysaccharide (LPS), IL-1β, or PGE2. Electroacupuncture (EA) stimulation applied for 30 minutes at the site equivalent to Quchi (LI11) acupoint suppressed fever and reduced the concentrations of both brain and serum levels of PGE2, which suggests that EA stimulation produces an antipyretic effect through the inhibition of the action of PGE2.[4] An animal study from Korea injected LPS into rats and stimulated acupoints Shaofu (HT8), Zutonggu (BL66), or Xingjian (LR2). The results showed that each acupoint significantly reduced fever induced by LPS injection. LPS increased hypothalamic messenger ribonucleic acid (mRNA) levels of IL-6 and IL-1β, which were reduced to normal levels by acupuncture stimulation on BL66. These results suggest that acupuncture stimulation may be effective for reducing elevated body temperature induced by bacterial inflammation, and part of its action may be mediated through the suppression of hypothalamic production of proinflammatory cytokines.[5] An animal study from Russia indicates that when an antipyretic medication is used in combination with acupuncture, its effect is potentiated and lasts longer.[6]

A clinical review from Russia indicates that acupuncture exerts antipyretic effects by triggering adaptive mechanisms that are directed toward correction of disturbances in the homeostatic systems of the body.[7] A clinical study from China suggests that acupuncture stimulation of LI11 and LI4 lowered body temperature through decreasing metabolic heat production and cutaneous vasodilatation.[8] Other major antifebrile points studied clinically include GV14 and ST36.[9] One study in China reports that when fever due to Wind-Cold invasion was treated with acupuncture on Dazhui (GV14), Fengchi (GB13), and Quchi (LI11), in addition to significant drop in axillary temperature of sometimes more than 1° C, respiratory rate, pulse, and blood pressure also decreased; symptoms were reduced; and the percentage of T lymphocytes increased.[10] A clinical observation in China of pasting herbs on acupuncture points in 72 ill infants revealed that an increase in humoral immune substances such as IgA, IgM, IgG; this treatment was better as a preventive measure and prophylaxis for fever.[11] Acupressure can be considered a potential modality for fever management at home.

TCM posits that Heat accumulation in fever is due to either excess Heat or excess Yang with Yin deficiency. Children are constitutionally Yin deficient and have relative abundance of Yang. They are also vulnerable to frequent febrile illnesses, which further deplete Yin. The acute fevers are due to external pathogens. Wind-Cold invasion—viral infection—begins to manifest fever in the Shao Yang stage, whereas Wind-Heat invasion—bacterial infection—can manifest fever from the very beginning during the Wei Qi level. Heat due to hot weather is also considered an external pathogen because it can deplete Yin. Chronic Heat can be due to any disorder that causes Yin deficiency, to continuous consumption of Hot energy foods, or to excess emotions that causes Qi stagnation and may also be due to familial or constitutional predisposition to chronic conditions with underlying Heat disturbance, such as chronic inflammatory diseases.

Treatment Recommendations

Chinese fever treatment[12] focuses on expelling pathogen, symptomatic lowering of fever, and tonify Yin and the immune system.

Symptomatic treatment

Lowering of fever due to any cause: GV14, LI11.

ST36 can be used to lower fever and increase immunity.

Conventional cooling measures such as tepid baths (children should take baths with lukewarm and not cold water, as the sudden chill would cause the child to shiver, which causes compensatory increases in metabolism and further elevation of temperature).

Eliminate Hot energy foods; increase fluid intake.

Expel pathogen according to stage or level of invasion.

Five-Element, Four-Point Heat treatment if specific organ is identified, such as Lung Heat for respiratory illness, Large Intestine Heat for bacterial diarrhea or IBD.

Tonify Yin.

Tonify immune system.

Chiropractic

Fever is a symptom and not a disease. To date there is no chiropractic literature citing outcomes of chiropractic management of the febrile child. There is, however, ample evidence that the chiropractic adjustment positively affects the immune system.[1]

The chiropractic adjustment influences natural killer cell production and autonomic balance,[2] B-cell lymphocyte count,[3] polymorphonuclear neutrophils and monoctyes,[4] and even CD4 counts.[5]

Fever is recognized by the chiropractor as an elevation in body temperature in response to CNS feedback. Fever is commonly a normal and beneficial immune response to disease, interfering with proliferation of bacteria and killing existing bacteria.[6] In fact, lack of fever may be seen as a sign of poor prognosis.[7,8]

Chiropractic management of the child with fever is oriented toward determining the source of the fever, which will facilitate a decision as to whether conservative management is both safe and indicated and whether the body requires aid from external sources. In the traditional medical fashion, the chiropractor would endeavor to rule out life-threatening illness from various body systems and dehydration. The McCarthy Scale of Illness Severity is simple and serves as a useful adjunct to the chiropractor (Table 36-1). When determined to be safe, the chiropractic approach would be to assess the nervous system at the spinal level to eliminate any obstruction to vital body function. The chiropractic adjustment that eliminates subluxation will restore internal feedback mechanisms and enhance immune function.[6]

This author has found that the most useful adjustment for stabilization of body temperature is the Logan Basic technique. This adjustment is gentle, safe, and comfortable. It is performed on the side of the anteriorly displaced sacrum by making a contact with a gloved thumb on the sacrotuberous ligament, midway between its attachments at the sacral apex and the ischial tuberosity. Lifting the ligament in a 45-degree posterior and 45-degree lateral direction will allow the sacrum to shift back to a neutral position. The free hand very lightly massages the sacroiliac joints and paraspinals where tension is found. The contact is maintained until such time as complete relaxation occurs at the sacrotuberous ligament and the sacrum has reestablished its normal functional position.

Adjusting the upper cervical spine is also advantageous.

TABLE 36-1

McCarthy Scale of Illness Severity

ITEM	NORMAL = 1	MODERATE IMPAIRMENT = 3	SEVERE IMPAIRMENT = 5
Quality of cry	Strong cry with normal tone or is content/not crying	Whimpering or sobbing	Weak or moaning or high-pitched cry
Reaction to parental stimulation	Cries briefly, then stops or is content/not crying	Cries on and off	Continual cry or hardly responsive
State variation	Stays awake or, if asleep, wakes easily when stimulated	Eyes close briefly/awake or if asleep; wakes with prolonged stimulation	Falls asleep or, if asleep, will not wake
Color	Pink	Pale extremities or acrocyanosis	Pale, cyanotic, or ashen
Hydration	Skin and eyes normal, mucous membranes moist	Skin and eyes normal, mouth slightly dry	Skin doughy or tented, mucous membranes dry, sunken eyes
Response to social overtures	Smiles or alerts	Brief smile or alerts briefly	No smile, face anxious, dull, expressionless, or no alerting

From McCarthy PL, Sharpe MR, Spiesel SZ et al: Observation scales for febrile children, *Pediatrics* 70:802-809, 1982.

Although the chiropractic adjustment is not applied as an antipyretic but instead as a balancing influence to the autonomic nervous system, it is not unusual for the fever to drop several degrees within 20 minutes of the chiropractic adjustment.

The following minimal emergency referral criteria for the chiropractor are suggested:

- McCarthy score > 10
- Acute weight loss > 7.5% of body weight
- Persistent bile-stained vomiting
- Convulsion
- Apnea
- Respiratory grunting or central cyanosis
- Petechial rash
- Bloody stool
- Fever lasting 3+ days while taking antibiotics[9]

Referral for medical care does not preclude the continuation of chiropractic management, provided that it remains safe.

Parents are advised to monitor the child's temperature every 2 hours to capture any rapid change in status that requires reassessment.

Adequate hydration is essential.

Consumption of garlic has a mild germicidal effect.

Omega-3 fatty acids (eicosapentaenoic acid [EPA]/docosohexonic acid [DHA]) have an antiinflammatory effect.[10]

Vitamin C may also be a useful support measure in managing inflammatory processes.

Echinacea and goldenseal have immune-boosting effects on the body.

Peppermint tea or oil may assist in fever reduction.

Herbs—Chinese

The Chinese herb Qing Hao (above and below-ground parts of *Artemisia annua* L. and *Artemisia apiacea* Hance) is used to help reduce fever and treat symptoms of malaria.[1] The decoction Sho-saiko-to (its Kampo name), or Xiao Chai Hu Tang (its Chinese name), is also used to treat fever/malaria. Sho-saiko-to comprises root of *Bupleurum chinense* DC. (Chai Hu), root of *Scutellaria baicalensis* Georgi (Huang Qin), tuber of *Pinellia ternata* (Thunb.) Breitenb. (Ban Xia), root of *Panax ginseng* C.A. Mey. (Ren Shen), fresh rhizome of *Zingiber officinale* (Willd.), Roscoe (Sheng Jiang), fruit of *Ziziphus jujuba* Mill. var. *inermis* (Bunge) Rehder (Da Zao), and root of Fisch (Gan Cao).[2] Well-designed clinical trials are needed before a recommendation can be made.

The Chinese and Thai herbal medicine systems have also incorporated *Andrographis,* renowned in these traditions mostly for its "bitter" properties as a treatment for digestive problems and as a treatment for a variety of febrile illnesses.[3]

Herbs—Western

Fever bark *(Alstonia constricta)* belongs to the Apocynaceae family. Historically, fever bark has been used for the treatment of fever, but there is no sufficient reliable scientific information to support the use of this plant for fever. The toxic effects of the plant attributed to reserpine and yohimbine constituents far outweigh the benefits of using it. (See Chapter 39, Headache, discussion of the use of willowbark.)

Homeopathy

Before using this section, please see Appendix A, Homeopathy, for definitions of practitioner expertise categories and general information on prescribing homeopathic medicines.

Practitioner Expertise Category 1

Category 1 includes fever associated with self-limited viral illnesses.

Practitioner Expertise Categories 2 or 3

Categories 2 and 3 includes fever associated with serious viral illnesses, bacterial illnesses, malignancies, or chronic conditions.

There are no controlled clinical trials of classical homeopathic treatment for fever, although the homeopathic literature contains much evidence to support its use in the form of accumulated clinical experience.[1] Acute fevers usually occur as the body's response to an infection, either viral or bacterial. Sometimes a fever is the only sign of a viral illness, especially at the onset of the illness, and sometimes fever is one sign among several. It is not necessary to treat a relatively well-appearing child with a fever that is low or mid-range and is not producing significant discomfort, unless the child is subject to febrile seizures or is 2 months of age or younger. If treatment for a mild febrile illness is needed, it is safe to use a homeopathic medicine either alone or in conjunction with conventional antipyretics or other alternative measures such as herbs or hydrotherapy. Any child with a fever must be observed closely over time and, when clinically indicated, conventional medical evaluation and treatment should be sought.

The goal in treating fever homeopathically is to determine the single homeopathic medicine whose description in the materia medica most closely matches the symptom picture of the patient. It may be necessary to study several sections of a homeopathic repertory, such as the cough, throat inflammation, inner ear inflammation, stomach (vomiting), and rectum (diarrhea) sections, in addition to the section on fever. Often mental and emotional states in addition to physical symptoms are considered in the homeopathic analysis of fever. Once the medicine has been selected, it can be given orally or sublingually in the 30C potency three to four times daily. In more acute situations a higher potency, such as 200C or 1M (1000C), given two to three times daily, might be needed to effectively treat the patient. If the medicine has not helped after six doses, then another homeopathic medicine should be tried and/or another form of therapy should be instituted. Once symptoms have begun to resolve, the medicine can be given less frequently or stopped. It can be repeated again for a relapse of symptoms. For any of the medicines listed here, the patients described might also require additional care such as a medical evaluation or antibiotic therapy.

The following list contains some of the many homeopathic medicines used to treat patients with fever. It must be emphasized that this list is partial and represents some of the probable choices from the homeopathic materia medica. If the symptoms of a given patient are not represented here, further research in the homeopathic literature would be needed to find the simillimum.

Aconitum napellus

Aconitum napellus (aconite) is needed when a fever develops suddenly, especially if it occurs after the patient has been exposed to cold weather, especially a cold dry wind. *Aconitum napellus* is also indicated when a fever develops after a frightening or shocking experience. The fever is worst in the evening and at night. It may be preceded by a chill. The patient is usually restless, anxious, and fearful but can be sad and tearful. He is overly sensitive to pain. The face is red and congested, and the patient may perspire. There is a marked thirst. If given at the beginning of an illness, *Aconitum napellus* can often stop an illness from progressing. This medicine be used to treat the initial stages of croup, urinary tract infection, scarlatiniform viral exanthems, otitis media, and influenza, among other conditions. Other treatment, such as an antibiotic, might also be indicated.

Belladonna

Belladonna is given at the onset of a febrile illness, before any suppuration has occurred. The patient is usually dry, but he or she may also perspire. The eyes appear bright, and the pupils are dilated. The face is very hot, whereas the hands and feet are cold. Any pains, such as headache, feel throbbing or bursting. The fever is worst at 3 PM and at night. The patient is excitable and may even become delirious or violent. *Belladonna* can be used to treat scarlatiniform exanthems, otitis media (without suppuration), early pneumonia, and tonsillitis, among other conditions. Other treatment, such as an antibiotic, might also be indicated.

Chamomilla vulgaris

The use of *Chamomilla vulgaris* should be considered when a fever occurs during teething. The child is hot and red (often just on one cheek) and often perspires. The fever is worst at 9 AM or 9 PM. The child is very irritable and possibly inconsolable. Being carried around may soothe the child temporarily.

Arsenicum album

The fever that is responsive to *Arsenicum album* (arsenic) has a marked chill phase, which is especially noted any time from midnight to 3 AM. The patient is very chilly and feels better in a warm room and after warm drinks. He or she is anxious, restless, and fearful and may alternately appear weak and collapsed. He or she is thirsty for small sips of water. *Arsenicum album* can be used to treat influenza, pneumonia, and diarrheal illnesses, among other conditions.

Bryonia alba

The patient requiring *Bryonia alba* has a fever that has a gradual onset and increases in severity over time. He or she has heat alternating with chills. The fever is worse at 9 PM. Any pains is exacerbated by motion, even very slight motion. He or she does not perspire and is very thirsty for large amounts of liquid. He or she is irritable and wishes to be left alone. *Bryonia alba* can be used to treat influenza, pneumonia, pleurisy, and bronchitis, among other conditions.

Ferrum phosphoricum

Ferrum phosphoricum can be used at the beginning of many viral illnesses when there are few signs and symptoms of a specific illness. The face is flushed, although the fever is usually not too high. There is usually not a marked chill phase.

Naturopathy

In the field of naturopathy, the normal development of fever is thought to serve many beneficial functions. Unfortunately, the general trend has been toward suppressing this very helpful but often uncomfortable symptom. The urgency surrounding fever reduction seems unnecessary in most cases as long as the temperature remains below 106° F (41° C) and the child is well hydrated. Fevers have effects on the body that impede microbial growth and stimulate the immune system, such as increasing white blood cell count and activity, stimulating IFN production,[1,2] and enhancing the action of cytokines.[3,4] Its effect seems so helpful that reputable facilities such as the Duke University Medical Center use hyperthermia treatment as a complementary treatment for cancer, supported by the National Cancer Institute. Other uses that have been explored in research is the use of hyperthermia treatment in patients with human immunodeficiency virus or acquired immune deficiency syndrome (HIV/AIDS), which can decrease levels of HIV RNA.[5] It may be postulated that this antiviral effect may extend to more common viral infections found in the pediatric population. Other studies show that antipyretics may suppress the production of antibodies, further prolonging infection.[6]

Treatments

Physical medicine

Hydrotherapy is a safe and effective treatment for fever and is less suppressive than antipyretic therapy. Examples include tepid sponge baths, wet socks, and wet sheet wrap.

Tepid sponge bath: The child may be gently bathed with a washcloth dipped in room-temperature water, not cold water. Evaporation will allow gradual cooling without a chilling effect.

Wet socks: This treatment is not limited to fevers but can be used for head colds and other infections that have congestion as a main component. A pair of cotton socks dipped in ice-cold water is wrung out and put on the feet, covered by a pair of thick, dry wool socks. An unexplained effect occurs, decreasing congestion in the head as well as lowering fevers.

Wet sheet wrap: A cotton sheet dipped in room-temperature water and wrung out may be wrapped around the child. This may be used for higher fevers that need to be brought down quickly.

Botanical medicine

Several botanicals are useful in treating fevers. Administering these either orally as a tea or as an enema can have beneficial effects. The enema will have a quicker cooling effect than oral preparations and also serves as a rehydration therapy, especially if the child is averse to consuming the tea orally or is too listless to drink. A combination tea of elderberry (*Sambucus nigra),* yarrow *(Achillea millefolium),* and peppermint *(Mentha piperita)* in equal parts is a popular combination. If using the tinctures, the combination may be used in the same ratio, and ½ droppersful per hour is suggested. *S. nigra* can cause urticaria in some patients, so a testing dose such as ⅛ teaspoon orally with the tincture for tolerability is suggested.

Warming botanical combination is used with a lower-grade or prolonged fever that never reaches 101° F. The intent is to produce a therapeutic fever to break a chronic cycle. Combine equal parts ginger root *(Zingiber officinale),* cayenne *(Capsicum frutescens),* cinnamon *(Cinnamomum),* angelica *(Angelica archangelica),* or prickly ash *(Xanthoxylum americanum)* for a total of 2 to 5 mL in a 30-mL bottle of either juice or tea and sip slowly.

Fasting

The natural tendency of animals and humans is to decrease food consumption when they are ill. One might deduce that this inborn preference gives the body a chance to focus on fighting infection rather than expending energy on digestion. Interestingly, fasting has been shown to improve the bactericidal activity of neutrophils[7] and increase monocyte bactericidal activity and natural killer cell cytolytic activity.[8] Furthermore, fasting deprives the body of iron, upon which bacteria and viruses thrive. The inclination of humans to reject food high in iron such as meat when they are sick reinforces this concept.

References

Pediatric Diagnosis and Treatment

1. Feigin RD, Cherry JD: *Textbook of pediatric infectious diseases,* ed 3, Philadelphia, 1992, Saunders.
2. Cranston WI: Central mechanisms of fever, *Fed Proceed* 38: 49-51, 1979. In Feigin RD, Cherry JD: *Textbook of pediatric infectious diseases,* ed 3, Philadelphia, 1992, Saunders.
3. Behrman RE, Kliegman RM, Jenson HB, editors: *Nelson textbook of pediatrics,* ed 17, Philadelphia, 2004, Saunders.
4. Crocetti MT, Serwint JR: Fever, separating fact from fiction, *Contemp Pediatr* 22:34-42, 2005.
5. Mackowiak PA: Physiological rationale for suppression of fever, *Clin Infect Dis* 31(Suppl 5):S185-S189, 2000.
6. Bourrillon A: Management of prolonged fever in infants [in French], *Arch Pediatr* 6:330-335, 1999 (abstract).
7. Crocetti M, Moghbeli N, Serwint J: Fever phobia revisited: have parental misconceptions about fever changed in 20 years? *Pediatrics* 107:1241-1246, 2001.
8. Plaisance KI, Kudaravalli S, Wasserman SS et al: Effect of antipyretic therapy on the duration of illness in experimental influenza A, *Shigella sonnei,* and *Rickettsia rickettsii* infections, *Pharmacotherapy* 20:1417-1422, 2000.
9. Mackowiak PA, Plaisance KI: Benefits and risks of antipyretic therapy, *Ann N Y Acad Sci* 856:214-223, 1998.
10. Greisman LA, Mackowiak PA: Fever: beneficial and detrimental effects of antipyretics, *Curr Opin Infect Dis* 15:241-245, 2002.
11. McErlean MA, Bartfield JM, Kennedy DA et al: Home antipyretic use in children brought to the emergency department, *Pediatr Emerg Care* 17:249-251, 2001.
12. Li SF, Lacher B, Crain EF: Acetaminophen and ibuprofen dosing by parents, *Pediatr Emerg Care* 16:394-397, 2000.
13. Stamm D: Paracetamol and other antipyretic analgesics: optimal doses in pediatrics [in French], *Arch Pediatr* 1:193-201, 1994 (abstract).

14. Rajadhyaksha S, Shah KN: Controversies in febrile seizures, *Indian J Pediatr* 67(1 Suppl):S71-S79, 2000.
15. Knudsen FU: Febrile convulsions, treatment and prognosis [in Danish], *Ugeskr Laeger* 163:1098-1102, 2001 (abstract).

Acupuncture

1. Lai W, Li Y: Research on the plague epidemic in Guangzhou (Canton) in 1894 [in Chinese], *Zhonghua Yi Shi Za Zhi* 29: 207-210, 1999 (abstract).
2. Kuang X, Liang C, Liang Z et al: The effect of acupuncture on rabbits with fever caused by endotoxin [in Chinese], *Ci Yan Jiu* 17:212-216, 1992 (abstract).
3. Nezhentsev M, Aleksandrov S: Effect of naloxone on the antipyretic action of acupuncture [in Russian], *Pharmacology* 46: 289-293, 1993 (abstract).
4. Fang JQ, Guo SY, Asano K et al: Antipyretic action of peripheral stimulation with electroacupuncture in rats, *In Vivo* 12:503-510, 1998.
5. Son YS, Park HJ, Kwon OB et al: Antipyretic effects of acupuncture on the lipopolysaccharide-induced fever and expression of interleukin-6 and interleukin-1 beta mRNAs in the hypothalamus of rats, *Neurosci Lett* 319:45-48, 2002.
6. Nezhentsev MV, Aleksandrov SI: Evaluation of the antipyretic action of psychotropic drugs and their effect on the antipyretic effect of acupuncture therapy [in Russian], *Biull Eksp Biol Med* 115:262-264, 1993 (abstract).
7. Nezhentsev MV, Aleksandrov SI: The current concepts of the humoral mechanisms of the analgetic and antipyretic actions of acupuncture (a review of the literature) [in Russian], *Sprava* Mar-Apr:39-42, 1994 (abstract).
8. Lin MT, Chandra A, Chen-Yen SM et al: Stimulation of acupuncture loci Chu-Chih (LI-11) and Ho-Ku (LI-4) hypothermia effects and analgesia in normal adults, *J Tradit Chin Med* 9:74-83, 1981.
9. Rogers PA, Schoen AM, Limehouse J: Acupuncture for immune-mediated disorders. Literature review and clinical applications, *Probl Vet Med* 4:162-193, 1992.
10. Tan D: Treatment of fever due to exopathic wind-cold by rapid acupuncture, *J Tradit Chin Med* 12:267-271, 1992.
11. Yu P, Hao X, Zhao R et al: Pasting acupoints with Chinese herbs applying in infant acute bronchitis and effect on humoral immune substances [in Chinese], *Zhen Ci Yan Jiu* 17:110-112, 1992 (abstract).
12. Loo M: *Pediatric acupuncture,* London, 2002, Elsevier.

Chiropractic

1. Allen JM: The effects of chiropractic on the immune system: a review of the literature, *Chiropractic J Austr* 23:132-135, 1993.
2. Leach RA, Burgess SC: Neuroimmune hypothesis. In Leach RA, editor: *The chiropractic theories,* Baltimore, 2004, Lippincott, Williams and Wilkins.
3. Brennan PC, Kokjohn K, Triano JJ et al: Immunologic correlates of reduced spinal mobility: preliminary observations in a dog model. In Wold S, editor: *Proceedings of the 1991 International Conference on Spinal Manipulation,* Arlington, Va, 1991, Foundation for Chiropractic Education and Research.
4. Brennan PC, Kokjohn K, Kaltinger CL et al: Enhanced phagocytic cell respiratory burst induced by spinal manipulation: potential role of substance P, *J Manipulative Physiol Ther* 12:289, 1989.
5. Selano JL, Hightower BC, Pfleger B et al: The effects of specific upper cervical adjustments on the CD4 counts of HIV positive patients, *Chiro Res J* 3:32-39, 1994.

6. Fallon JM: The role of subluxation in fever and febrile seizures, *Today Chiropractic* Mar/Apr:64-66, 1996.

7. Grossman M: Fever, In Rudolph AM, Hoffman JE, Rudolph DC, editors: *Rudolph's pediatrics,* ed 20, Stanford, Conn, 1996, Appleton and Lange.

8. Soliman SE, Plaugher G, Alcantara J: The febrile child. In Anrig C, Plaugher G, editors: *Pediatric chiropractic,* Baltimore, 1998, Williams and Wilkins.

9. Davies N: *Chiropractic pediatrics,* London, 2000, Churchill Livingstone.

10. Hall BS: Allergy, endocrine and metabolic diseases in childhood. In Davies NJ, editor: *Chiropractic pediatrics,* London, 2000, Churchill Livingstone.

Herbs—Chinese

1. Trevett A, Lalloo D: A new look at an old drug: artemesinin and qinghaosu, *P N G Med J* 35:264-269, 1992.

2. *Xiao-chai-hu-tang.* Available at http://tcm.health-info.org/formulas/singles/Xiao-chai-hu-tang.htm. Accessed August 2005.

3. Natural Standard Research Collaboration. Available at www.naturalstandard.com. Accessed 2005.

Homeopathy

1. *ReferenceWorks Pro 4.2,* San Rafael, Calif, 2008, Kent Homeopathic Associates.

Naturopathy

1. Downing JF, Martinez-Valdez H, Elizondo RS et al: Hyperthermia in humans enhances interferon-gamma synthesis and alters the peripheral lymphocyte population, *J Interferon Res* 8:143-150, 1988.

2. Downing JF, Taylor MW, Wei KM et al: In vivo hyperthermia enhances plasma antiviral activity and stimulates peripheral lymphocytes for increased synthesis of interferon-gamma, *Interferon Res* 7:185-193, 1987.

3. Leroux E, Auzenne E, Weidner D et al: Febrile and acute hyperthermia enhance TNF-induced necrosis of murine L929 fibrosarcoma cells via caspase-regulated production of reactive oxygen intermediates, *J Cell Physiol* 187:256-263, 2001.

4. Pritchard MT, Wolf SF, Kraybill WF et al: The anti-tumor effect of interleukin-12 is enhanced by mild (fever-range) thermal therapy, *Immunol Invest* 34:361-380, 2005.

5. Steinhart CR, Ash SR, Gingrich C et al: Effect of whole-body hyperthermia on AIDS patients with Kaposi's sarcoma: a pilot study, *J Acquir Immune Defic Syndr Hum Retrovirol* 11:271-281, 1996.

6. White L, Mavor S: *Kids, herbs, and health,* Loveland, Colo 1998, Interweave Press.

7. Uden AM, Trang L, Venizelos N et al: Neutrophil functions and clinical performance after total fasting in patients with rheumatoid arthritis, *Ann Rheum Dis* 42:45-51, 1983.

8. Wing EJ, Stanko RT, Winkelstein A et al: Fasting-enhanced immune effector mechanisms in obese subjects, *Am J Med* 75:91-96, 1983.

Fifth Disease

Chiropractic | Anne Spicer

✳ PEDIATRIC DIAGNOSIS AND TREATMENT

Erythema infectiosum, also known as *fifth disease* or *slapped cheek disease,* is a benign, common childhood exanthema.[1] It was the fifth in a classification scheme of childhood exanthems, after measles, scarlet fever, rubella and Filatov-Dukes disease (an atypical scarlet fever).[2] It is caused by parvovirus B$_{19}$, a small deoxyribonucleic acid (DNA) virus. It is most prevalent in primary school–aged children[3] and can occur in epidemics, with seasonal peaks in late winter and spring; sporadic infections occur throughout the year.

Transmission is primarily by the respiratory route, presumably via large droplets spread from nasopharyngeal viral shedding. The incubation period ranges from 4 to 28 days (average 16 to 17 days). The prodromal phase is mild and consists of low-grade fever, headache, and symptoms of mild upper respiratory tract infection. The hallmark is the characteristic rash, often described as having a "slapped cheek" appearance.[3,4] Arthritis and arthralgia may occur in older adolescents.[2]

Diagnosis is made primarily by history and clinical examination. In high-risk children, such as those who are immunocompromised, serological diagnosis can be done with the demonstration of viral DNA using the polymerase chain reaction test in various body fluids or tissue biopsy.[4]

Erythema infectiosum is usually a mild, self-limiting illness in children that does not require specific treatment. Parents often give antipyretics for fever. Children are not routinely excluded from school or childcare.[1]

✳ CAM THERAPY RECOMMENDATIONS

Chiropractic

Although there is an absence of literature related to chiropractic management of fifth disease specifically, this disease would be addressed similar to any other infectious disease. The approach would be to remove any interference to normal immune function and support any additional burden placed on the system by the active disease.

Evidence exists that the chiropractic adjustment has influence over natural killer cell production and autonomic balance,[1] B-cell lymphocyte count,[2] polymorphonuclear neutrophils and monoctyes,[3] and even CD4 counts.[4] Therefore the chiropractic adjustment of a subluxation complex would be a priority.

Supplementation with immune-enhancing nutrients may provide the body with necessary resources to manage an acute infection. Commonly recommended nutrients include zinc and vitamin A[5]; zinc is available in liquid formulations and is vital to normal immune function. Vitamin C may be given to the young infant in the form of rose hip syrup and should be dosed within gut tolerance.[6,7] An initial dose of 250 mg is a good starting place. Gut microflora will support the immune function, as will omega-3 fatty acid (eicosapentaenoic acid [EPA]/docosahexaenoic acid [DHA]), which also has antiinflammatory actions.[8] Vitamin E has antioxidant as well as antiinflammatory properties.[9]

Echinacea purpurea is recommended to stimulate the immune system.[6] Use is recommended for a period not to exceed 2 consecutive weeks, as the body may develop a tolerance level with prolonged use. Although echinacea is safe, allergic reactions have been reported in children with a history of allergies, particularly to plants in the daisy family.

Adequate rest and hydration will contribute to recovery.

Exacerbations of the condition subsequent to the initial disease are managed similarly with chiropractic, supplementation, and lifestyle changes.

References

Pediatric Diagnosis and Treatment

1. Frydenberg A, Starr M: Slapped cheek disease. How it affects children and pregnant women, *Austr Fam Physician* 32:589-592, 2003.
2. Balkhy HH, Sabella C, Goldfarb J: Parvovirus: a review, *Bull Rheum Dis* 47:4-9, 1998.
3. Behrman RE, Kliegman RM, Jenson HB, editors: *Nelson textbook of pediatrics,* ed 17, Philadelphia, 2004, Saunders.
4. Broliden K, Tolfvenstam T, Papadogiannakis N et al: Parvovirus B19 infection—an incidious chameleon [in Swedish], *Tidsskr Nor Laegeforen* 120:455-458, 2004 (abstract).

Chiropractic

1. Leach RA, Burgess SC: Neuroimmune hypothesis. In Leach RA, editor: *The chiropractic theories,* Baltimore, 2004, Lippincott Williams and Wilkins.
2. Brennan PC, Kokjohn K, Triano JJ et al: Immunologic correlates of reduced spinal mobility: preliminary observations in a dog model. In Wold S, editor: *Proceedings of the 1991 International Conference on Spinal Manipulation,* Arlington, Va, 1991, Foundation for Chiropractic Education and Research.
3. Brennan PC, Kokjohn K, Kaltinger CL, et al: Enhanced phagocytic cell respiratory burst induced by spinal manipulation: potential role of substance P, *J Manipulative Physiol Ther* 14:399-408, 1989.

4. Selano JL, Hightower BC, Pfleger B et al: The effects of specific upper cervical adjustments on the CD4 counts of HIV positive patients, *Chiro Res J* 3:32-39, 1994.

5. Ghandari N et al: Effect or routine zinc supplementation on pneumonia in children aged 6 months to 3 years: randomized controlled trial in an urban slum, *Br Med J* 324:1358-1361, 2002.

6. Davies N: *Chiropractic pediatrics,* London, 2000, Churchill Livingstone.

7. Forastiere F, Pistelli R, Sestini P et al: Consumption of fresh fruit rich in vitamin C and wheezing symptoms in children, *Thorax* 55: 283-288, 2000.

8. Stevens LJ, Zentall SS, Abate ML et al: Omega-3 fatty acids in boys with behavior, learning and health problems, *Physiol Behav* 59:915-920, 1996.

9. Heffner JE, Repine JE: Pulmonary strategies of antioxidant defense, *Am Rev Resp Dis* 140:531-554, 1989.

CHAPTER 38

Gastroesophageal Reflux

Acupuncture | May Loo

Chiropractic | Anne Spicer

Herbs—Western | Alan D. Woolf, Paula M. Gardiner, Lana Dvorkin-Camiel, Jack Maypole

Magnet Therapy | Agatha P. Colbert, Deborah Risotti

Osteopathy | Jane Carreiro

✳ PEDIATRIC DIAGNOSIS AND TREATMENT

Gastroesophageal reflux disease (GERD), the retrograde movement of gastric contents across the lower esophageal sphincter (LES) into the esophagus, is the most common esophageal disorder in children of all ages[1] but occurs mostly in infants because of immaturity of the esophagus and stomach and higher liquid intake.[2]

The symptoms of infantile GERD usually consist of regurgitation (especially postprandially), signs of esophagitis (irritability, arching, choking, gagging, feeding aversion), and resulting failure to thrive.[1] The respiratory (extraesophageal) presentations in infants may manifest as obstructive apnea, stridor, or as lower airway disease in which reflux complicates primary airway disease such as laryngomalacia or bronchopulmonary dysplasia.[1] Older children, in contrast, may have regurgitation during the preschool years; complaints of heartburn supervene during later childhood and adolescence; and extraesophageal, airway manifestations as asthma or as otolaryngological disease such as laryngitis or sinusitis.[1,3]

In some children, ear-nose-throat or respiratory symptoms may be the only manifestion of GERD.[3] A French study of 72 children revealed that GERD is an important etiology in pediatric otolaryngological diseases.[4] A prospective, double-blind study of 595 children in Italy with difficult-to-treat respiratory symptoms revealed 47% presented with asthma as the main symptom of GERD.[5]

Although the majority of infantile GERD peaks at about 4 months and resolves spontaneously by 12 months of age, as the lower esophageal sphincter mechanism matures,[1,6] symptoms in older children tend to be chronic, waxing and waning, and completely resolving in no more than half. A genetic predisposition as an autosomal dominant form is located on chromosome 13q14 and chromosome 9.[1,2]

The initial diagnosis consists of a thorough history, which may include standardized questionnaires (e.g., the Infant Gastroesophageal Reflux Questionnaire [I-GERQ]), and physical examination.[1] To date, no single tool alone has proved to be diagnostic in these patients.[5] Laboratory evaluation includes contrast studies of the esophagus and upper gastrointestinal (GI) tract, esophageal pH monitoring, intraesophageal impedance and Bravo wireless pH monitoring, endoscopy, radionucleotide scintigraphy, esophageal manometry, and laryngotracheobronchoscopy.[1,3,6] Early detection and treatment of gastroesophageal reflux (GER) in children may result in a better long-term outcome, improved quality of life, and a reduction in overall healthcare burden.[7]

Infantile GERD can be managed conservatively with positioning, thickening of formula, varied feeding volumes, and hypoallergenic diet.[1,2] The American Academy of Pediatrics and the North American Society of Pediatric Gastroenterology and Nutrition recommend non-prone positioning during sleep. During awake periods when the infant is observed, prone position and upright carried position may be used to minimize reflux.[1]

Conservative therapy and lifestyle modification form the foundation of GERD therapy for older children. They are counseled to avoid acidic foods (e.g., tomatoes, chocolate, mint) and beverages (e.g., juices, carbonated and caffeinated drinks). However, when symptoms persist, acid suppression is the mainstay of management.[7]

There is increasing evidence that older children with GERD need higher dosages of acid suppressive therapy to achieve clinical response.[3] Chronic antacid therapy is not recommended.[2] Other medical management consists of histamine-2-receptor antagonists (H2Ras), proton pump inhibitors (PPIs), and prokinetic agents.[1,6]

The PPIs are well tolerated by infants and children,[2] but their efficacy and safety need to be evaluated.[8,9]

Surgery, usually fundoplication, is indicated for intractable GERD in children, particularly those with refractory esophagitis or strictures, and those with supraesophageal symptoms who are at risk for significant morbidity from chronic pulmonary disease.[1,5] Fundoplication should be avoided before 2 to 3 years of age if possible,[2] but is indicated in the infant who has apneic episodes secondary to documented GER.[6] Long-term clinical follow-up of children with GERD is necessary because of persistence of symptoms and the risk of complications.[10]

✳ CAM THERAPY RECOMMENDATIONS

Acupuncture

There are no studies on acupuncture treatment of GER. From the Chinese medicine standpoint, the pathophysiology of GER is similar to vomiting: reversal of the flow of stomach Qi.

The same treatments for vomiting can be applied here, using acupressure or magnets to treat infants:

P6

ST36

ST44—also chosen for its harmonizing, cooling, and calming effect[1]

Chiropractic

Chiropractic research in the area of GERD is lacking at present. However, the chiropractic approach to the management of GERD is to restore optimum function to the body. Particular attention is paid to the spinal nerves that affect the upper GI system. Chiropractors may look to C4-C5, the origin of the phrenic nerve, as facilitation may cause abnormal tone at the diaphragm,[1] which may in turn increase the occurrence of reflux. Attention would also be paid to T3-T7 for the neurological influence at the esophagus and upper portions of the stomach.[2,3] The vagus nerve, which rests adjacent to and is affected by the cervical spine alignment and musculature, also has influence at the LES.[4] Abnormal tone at the LES may also increase the occurrence of reflux. Reduction of the subluxation complex (SC) at these corresponding spinal segments enhances autonomic balance, allowing the tissues to maintain a more normal tone, position, and responsiveness during the developmental extension of the esophagus caudally into the abdomen in the first 18 months of life.

Because of the influence of normal developmental predispositions in the infant (e.g., short esophagus, incomplete myelination of GI-related nerves, incomplete digestive capacity, prone posture and high fluid intake), this author finds that a high frequency of care is sometimes required to manage the recurrent viscerosomatic SC resultant of persistent reflux.

A hiatal herniation of the stomach through the diaphragm is a fundamental or contributory factor in many cases. When this hiatal herniation is present, manual reduction is effective in reducing or eliminating reflux.

Omega-3 fatty acids are useful in providing the raw material for maturation of healthy nerves and therefore may hasten the progress of the vagal, phrenic, and spinal nerve myelination.

Supplementation with vitamins A, E and B complex, probiotics, and lecithin may also prove useful.[5] Aloe vera taken orally may help heal the mucosal lining of the gut while supplementation with pancreatic digestive enzymes aids in digestion.[6] A chewable (pulverized if necessary) calcium/magnesium/vitamin D supplement may help buffer acid, but should be taken in small amounts to avoid rebound hyperacidity.

Deep focal massage may reflexively reduce gastric acidity when applied at the left fifth intercostal space adjacent to the sternum and at the fifth thoracic intertransverse space on the left side.[7]

Food intolerances may cause symptoms that mimic GERD; therefore an evaluation of food allergies/sensitivities may prove useful.[8] Persistence of symptoms after a trial of chiropractic management suggests an increased likelihood of food sensitivity, and a 6-week trial of complete dairy elimination may be beneficial.[9] The older child and the mother of a breastfeeding infant with GERD should avoid citrus, tomatoes, spearmint or peppermint oils, garlic, onion, whole milk, high-fat foods, coffee (caffeine), carbonated beverages, and chocolate.[10,11] Other common foods that may be contributing factors include soy and wheat. Patients should be sure to consume enough protein and carbohydrate. Caution should be taken not to overfeed.

Although cereal-thickened formulas are often recommended, some digestive enzymes do not become prominent until the eruption of primary teeth around 6 months of age, making digestion of grains more difficult for the infant. This may be evidenced by increased diarrhea in those infants fed thickened formulas.[12] When formulas are thickened with indigestible carbohydrates, bioavailability of iron, zinc, and calcium is reduced.[13]

An infant who lies flat on the back or in a side-lying posture is more likely to have reflux episodes, although a supine inclined position may reduce irritation. Prolonged use of infant car seats or "bouncy" seats may actually make the reflux worse.[14] The older child may find comfort in a left side–lying position with the head of the bed elevated. The prone position results in the lowest production of reflux episodes in infancy. Infants may find comfort when held prone over a caregiver's forearm. Prone sleep posture is not recommended because of increased risk of sudden infant death syndrome; however, this risk may be reduced by using a new firm mattress with thin, flat bedding.

Care must be taken by the chiropractor to monitor for signs of gastroesophageal erosion and development of anemia, slowed growth, and apnea as well as respiratory aspiration conditions. Any indication of these conditions would warrant a prompt referral to a gastroenterologist.

Herbs—Western

Herbs used to treat GERD are similar to those used to treat abdominal pain, dyspepsia, and nausea, such as ginger, licorice *(Glycyrrhiza)*, and mucilaginous herbs such as slippery elm *(Ulmus)* and marshmallow. There are no herbal clinical studies on the treatment of GERD for children. Patients with GERD should avoid peppermint, as it may decrease the tone in the esophageal sphincter, making their symptoms worse.[1]

Magnet Therapy

Gently massage acupuncture point Yintang. Then use two ¾-inch Neodymium nylon-coated magnets on two other acupuncture points, CV15 and CV16.[1] The two magnets will have opposite sides facing the skin at these two points. Place the side designated north on CV15 and a similar magnet with the opposite side facing the skin on CV16. Leave magnets in place for 1 hour. Neodymium nylon-coated Spot magnets (1-inch, ¾-inch, and ½-inch sizes) may be obtained from Painfree Lifestyles (800-480-8601).

Osteopathy

GER is a condition in which acidic secretions and gastric contents flow backward from the stomach into the esophagus. Although some amount of reflux occurs in almost everyone, it is usually asymptomatic, sporadic, and clinically irrelevant. Reflux is particularly prevalent in infants and young children owing in part to conditions of immaturity in the GI tract.[1] In the mature gut, three mechanisms inhibit or control reflux.

First, an area of increased pressure at the gastroesophageal junction, known as the HPZ (high-pressure zone), prevents reflux of gastric contents into the esophageal lumen. Second, esophageal peristalsis clears the esophagus by moving the refluxed secretions back into the stomach. Third, increased production of saliva, in response to lowered esophageal pH, acts as a buffer, neutralizing the acidity of gastric secretions. Although no conclusive studies have evaluated the efficacy of osteopathic manipulation in the treatment of GERD, much has been written about it.

The HPZ of the lower esophagus is probably the most potent antireflux mechanism present. In the adult the HPZ is 3 to 4 cm long. In the newborn it is considerably smaller. In the premature and term newborn, pressures at the HPZ are lower than in adults, with the lowest pressures in the most premature patients. As might be expected, pressures in the HPZ increase as the infant matures.[2] The lower esophageal HPZ is created through the concerted efforts of the LES, the crura of the diaphragm, and the phrenoesophageal ligament. Oscillations in pressure at the HPZ correlate with respiratory cycles.[3,4] From an osteopathic perspective, patients with reflux typically present with altered mechanics in the muscles of respiration and the thoracic cage. Tissue strains that alter the relationships between the structures creating the HPZ may also impede its function. Most osteopathic texts discuss normalizing the structural relationships of the thoracic cage using rib raising, myofascial, and balancing techniques to address these areas.[5] Many children with reflux have areas of obvious tenderness that may respond to counterstrain or myofascial approaches.

From an osteopathic perspective, GER in children is often associated with one or more of the following: diaphragmatic restrictions, strains at the thoracolumbar junction, altered respiratory mechanics in the thorax, strains at the craniocervical junction, and cranial findings suggestive of vagal irritation. Concurrent with these findings are the presence of viscerosomatic reflexes. Although the primary area of tissue dysfunction in children with reflux is the thoracic cage and lumbar areas, findings of somatic dysfunction that may also contribute to the child's symptoms are found at the cranial base, cervical spine, and pelvis. Osteopaths have reported a strong association between cranial base dysfunction and GERD in children.[6-8] Interestingly, vagal stimulation seems to be involved in both inhibition and excitation of smooth muscle activity of the LES. Muscular, fascial, and articular strains in the cervical area—specifically C3, C4, and C5—are also commonly found.[1,7] The increase in spinal cord activity and/or altered sensory input at those levels may affect phrenic nerve function, altering diaphragmatic mechanics. Restricted diaphragm motion, regardless of its etiology, will affect the relationship of the phrenoesophageal ligament to the esophagus and possibly the acuity of the angle of His. This may compromise the ability of both to contribute to the HPZ. Furthermore, if diaphragmatic mechanics are altered, functional isolation of the crura from costal portions, an important component in HPZ control, may be undermined. Altered respiratory mechanics may be a result of biomechanical strain in any part of the thoracic cage, the diaphragm, or the crura. Each of these may affect competency of the HPZ.

Infants with reflux often have viscerosomatic reflexes on osteopathic structural examination. These areas of somatic dysfunction are found in the paraspinal muscles between the fifth and seventh thoracic vertebrae. They may arise secondary to the esophageal irritation, but they may also contribute to it via nociceptive input into the spinal cord.[9,10] Some children may also have Chapman's reflexes, which are areas of tissue changes that represent neurolymphatic reflexes. These findings may be associated with imbalances between parasympathetic and sympathetic input. Normally, increases in intraabdominal pressure trigger a vagally mediated contraction of the smooth muscle at the LES proportional to the increase in gastric pressure. This reflex is immature in the infant. Consequently, the prolonged transit times of the infant stomach cause gastric distention, which increases the incidence of transient relaxation of the sphincter. This is thought to contribute to the reflux.[11,12] In general, the intensity and duration of reflux is inversely correlated with the transit time through the stomach. Viscerosomatic reflexes can be treated with gentle inhibition techniques; rib raising, balancing, and other indirect techniques may be used to address tissue strains at the costovertebral junction.

Because reflux may be exacerbated by immune sensitivity, osteopathic physicians will often recommend dietary changes. If the baby is breastfeeding, the mother may need to try an elimination diet to deduce which substances may be aggravating the clinical picture. Antigens from cow's milk, peanut mold, and other foods cross into breastmilk. If the baby is bottle-fed, other less antigenic formulas should be tried.

References

Pediatric Diagnosis and Treatment

1. Behrman RE, Kliegman RM, Jenson HB, editors: *Nelson textbook of pediatrics*, ed 17, Philadelphia, 2004, Saunders.

2. Cezard JP: Managing gastro-oesophageal reflux disease in children, *Digestion* 69(Suppl 1):3-8, 2004.

3. Strople J, Kaul A: Pediatric gastroesophageal reflux disease—current perspectives, *Curr Opin Otolaryngol Head Neck Surg* 11:447-451, 2003.

4. van den Abbeele T, Couloigner V, Faure C et al: The role of 24 h pH-recording in pediatric otolaryngologic gastro-esophageal reflux disease, *Int J Pediatr Otorhinolaryngol* 67(Suppl 1):S95-S100, 2003.

5. Mattioli G, Sacco O, Repetto P et al: Necessity for surgery in children with gastrooesophageal reflux and supraoesophageal symptoms, *Eur J Pediatr Surg* 14:7-13, 2004.

6. Spitz L, McLeod E: Gastroesophageal reflux, *Semin Pediatr Surg* 12:237-240, 2003.

7. Gold BD: Review article: epidemiology and management of gastro-oesophageal reflux in children, *Aliment Pharmacol Ther* 19(Suppl 1):22-27, 2004.

8. Rudolph CD: Are proton pump inhibitors indicated for the treatment of gastroesophageal reflux in infants and children? *J Pediatr Gastroenterol Nutr* 37(Suppl 1):S60-S64, 2003.

9. Colletti RB, Di Lorenzo C: Overview of pediatric gastroesophageal reflux disease and proton pump inhibitor therapy, *J Pediatr Gastroenterol Nutr* 37(Suppl 1):S7-S11, 2003.

10. Semeniuk J, Kaczmarski M, Sidor K et al: Long-term clinical observation of infants with gastroesophageal reflux [in Polish], *Pol Merkuriusz Lek* 16:208-212, 2004.

Acupuncture

1. Eyssalet J: Personal communication, 2005.

Chiropractic

1. Stoner F: *The eclectic approach to chiropractic,* ed 2, Las Vegas, 1976, FHS.
2. Netter F: *Upper digestive tract,* Summit, NJ, 1978, Ciba.
3. DeBoer KF, Schultz M, McKnight ME: Acute effects of spinal manipulation on gastrointestinal myoelectric activity in conscious rabbits, *Manual Med* 3:85-94, 1988.
4. Moore KL: *Clinically oriented anatomy,* ed 5, Baltimore, 2006, Lippincott Williams and Wilkins.
5. Anderson FM: *The physician's practical guide to nutritional therapy,* Atlanta, 1979, Symmes Systems.
6. Thomas RJ: Gastrointestinal disorders. In Lawrence D, editor: *Fundamentals of chiropractic diagnosis and management,* Baltimore, 1991, Williams and Wilkins.
7. Chaitow L: *Palpation skills: assessment and diagnosis through touch,* New York, 1977, Churchill Livingstone.
8. Castell DO: Diet and the lower esophageal sphincter, *Am J Clin Nutr* 28:1296-1298, 1975.
9. Beattie RM: Managing gastro-oesophageal reflux in infants and children, *J Fam Health Care* 13:98-101, 2003.
10. Jackson SB: Gastroesophageal reflux disease, *Top Clin Chiropractic* 2:24-29, 1995.
11. Babka JC, Castell DO: On the genesis of heartburn, *Am J Dig Dis* 18:391, 1973.
12. Iacono G, Vetrano S, Cataldo F et al: Clinical trial with thickened feeding for treatment of regurgitation in infants, *Digest Liver Dis* 34:532-534, 2002.
13. Bosscher D, Van Caillie-Bertrand M, Van Dyck K et al: Thickening infant formula with digestible and indigestible carbohydrate: availability of calcium, iron and zinc in vitro, *J Pediatr Gastroenterol Nutr* 30:373-378, 2000.
14. Orenstein SR, Whittington PF, Orenstein DM: The infant seat as treatment for gastroesophageal reflux, *N Engl J Med* 309:760-763, 1983.

Herbs—Western

1. Mills S, Bone K, editors: *The essential guide to herbal safety,* St Louis, 2005, Elsevier.

Magnet Therapy

1. Loo M: *Pediatric acupuncture,* London, 2002, Elsevier.

Osteopathy

1. Carreiro JE: *An osteopathic approach to children,* London, 2003, Churchill Livingstone.
2. Milla PJ: The ontogeny of intestinal motor acti. In Walker WA, Durie PR, Hamilton JR et al, editors: *Pediatric gastrointestinal disease,* St Louis, 1996, Mosby.
3. Mittal RK, Fisher MJ: Electrical and mechanical inhibition of the crural diaphragm during transient relaxation of the lower esophageal sphincter, *Gastroenterology* 99:1265-1268, 1990.
4. Welch RW, Gray JE: Influence of respiration on recordings of lower esophageal sphincter pressure in humans, *Gastroenterology* 83:590-594, 1982.
5. Ward RC, Hruby RJ, Jerome JA et al: *Foundations for osteopathic medicine,* Philadelphia, 2003, Lippincott Williams and Wilkins.
6. Magoun HIS: *Osteopathy in the cranial field,* ed 3, Kirksville, Mo, 1976, The Journal Printing Company.
7. Kuchera ML, Kuchera WA: *Osteopathic considerations in systemic disease,* Columbus, OH, 1994, Greydon Press.
8. Frymann VM: Relation of disturbances of craniosacral mechanism to symptomatology of the newborn, *J Am Osteopathic Assoc* 65:1059-1075, 1966.
9. Salmenpera L, Perheentupa J, Pakarinen P et al: Zinc supplementation of infant formula, *Am J Clin Nutr* 59:985-989, 1994.
10. Aihara Y, Nakamura H, Sato A et al: Neural control of gastric motility with special reference to cutaneo-gastric reflexes. In Brooks C, editor: *Integrative functions of the autonomic nervous system,* New York, 1979, Elsevier.
11. Gupta M, Brans YW: Gastric retention in neonates, *Pediatrics* 62:26-29, 1978.
12. Holloway RH, Hongo M, Berger K et al: Gastric distention: a mechanism for postprandial gastroesophageal reflux, *Gastroenterology* 89:779-784, 1985.

CHAPTER 39

Headache

Acupuncture | May Loo

Aromatherapy | Maura A. Fitzgerald

Chiropractic | Anne Spicer

Herbs—Western | Alan D. Woolf, Paula M. Gardiner, Lana Dvorkin-Camiel, Jack Maypole

Massage Therapy | Mary C. McLellan

Mind/Body | Timothy Cuthbert, Lynda Richtsmeier Cyr

Nutrition | Joy A. Weydert

Osteopathy | Jane Carreiro

Psychology | Anna Tobia

✳ PEDIATRIC DIAGNOSIS AND TREATMENT

Headaches occur in about 40% of preschool children and as many as 70% of school-aged children.[1,2] The criteria provided in the 55-page International Headache Society (IHS) handbook are widely used in classifying headaches in childhood and adolescence. However, there is growing concern that the criteria need to be modified to increase sensitivity for pediatric headaches.[3-8] Childhood headaches can be broadly classified as acute or chronic. Acute headaches in children are mostly due to viral illnesses, sinusitis,[9] mild head trauma,[10] caffeine-induced from consumption of large amount of caffeinated drinks,[11] and a small percentage due to bacterial sepsis and meningitis, central nervous system (CNS) abnormalities such as brain tumor, and serious head trauma.[1,12]

The majority of chronic headaches in school-aged children are idiopathic, which means that no specific etiology exists, and the pain is the main symptom and the primary disease entity itself. A small percentage of chronic headaches are secondary to a definite medical condition such as hypoglycemia.[2] Idiopathic headaches in childhood fall into the migraine, migrainous disorder, and tension-type categories.[4,13-15] Stress was the most frequently cited precipitating factor in all types of idiopathic headaches, whereas weather, environmental factors, and some foods also play a role.[16]

Migraine is considered the most common headache in childhood,[4,13-15] affecting as many as 5% to 10% of all children,[17] and may represent up to 54% of pediatric headaches.[18] The acute episodes can be triggered by numerous factors: emotional upset; stress such as school pressure or lack of sleep; sensory stimulation such as loud noise or bright light; and sympathetic stimulation such as sports or physical exercise.[19] Headache is sometimes preceded by a visual or sensory aura. The characteristic attack consists of severe, throbbing, or pulsating pain—usually unilateral but often bilateral in children—frequently accompanied by digestive symptoms (e.g., nausea, vomiting, abdominal pain) and sometimes hypersensitivity to light and sound.[19] The duration is 4 to 72 hours in adults and 2 to 48 hours in children younger than 15 years.[3]

Various hypotheses have been proposed for pathophysiology of migraine, but the precise mechanism is still poorly understood. The headache appears to involve both central and peripheral structures. There is vasodilatation and vasoconstriction of the neurovascular system,[3] possibly due to inflammation of cerebral arteries.[20,21] There may be altered neuronal excitability in the CNS.[22] Recent evidence suggests involvement of catecholamines,[23,24] serotonin,[25] and some neuropeptides.[26,27] There is increasing focus on the role of dopamine, both in the prodromal symptoms (e.g., nausea, vomiting, drowsiness) and in the headache phase with pain perception and cerebral blood flow.[28,29] Migraine in children is often associated with abdominal pain[30] and cyclical vomiting.[31,32] Strong family history is supported by the finding of a dopamine receptor gene locus in migrainous patients with aura.[20,28]

Separation of migraine without aura from episodic tension-type headache may be difficult. The most important differential characteristics of migraine are the intensity of pain, association with emotions, aggravation by physical activity, and presence of nausea and vomiting.[13] Adolescents usually have migraine with aura and tension headaches, whereas younger children tend to present with migrainelike headaches aggravated by physical activity and sometimes accompanied by photophobia.[5]

Much has been written about the "migraine personality," the emotional makeup of the headache sufferers. These patients have a high prevalence of various neurotic and even psychotic symptoms[33]: excessive striving for tidiness and for perfection in performance,[34] and exaggerated tendency in pain perception, self-criticism,[35] and symbiotic attachment to their own families.[34] They are at increased risk for comorbid affective and anxiety disorder: generalized anxiety disorder, panic disorder, obsessive-compulsive disorder, phobic disorder,[36] and depression.[34,36] Pediatric and adolescent patients have been found to be emotionally rigid with a tendency to repress anger and aggression.[37]

Migraine in children and adolescents is extremely disabling, causing loss of school days and extracurricular activities.[17,38] Rest and often sleep bring relief. Western treatment is mainly with medication, ranging from over-the-counter (OTC) analgesics to specific oral and intramuscular injection of antimigraine medications for acute attacks and daily prophylactic pharmacotherapy. No panacea is available.

In November 2004 the American Academy of Pediatrics endorsed the practice parameter of pharmacological treatment of migraine headache in children and adolescents, put forth by the American Academy of Neurology Quality Standards Subcommittee and the Practice Committee of the Child Neurology Society. After reviewing 166 studies, the committees concluded that for treatment of acute migraine, ibuprofen and probably acetaminophen are effective for children older than 6 years, and sumatriptan (a specific and selective 5-hydroxytryptamine receptor agonist nasal spray) can be considered for adolescents older than 12 years.[39] The side effects include hot flushes, nausea, vomiting, fatigue, and drowsiness but are usually minor and transient.[12] For preventive therapy, flunarizine is probably effective but is not available in the United States. The committees further indicate that data are conflicting or insufficient to make any other recommendations and that the lack of evidence is disappointing.[40] Migraine headaches increase in frequency with age through adolescence.[41] The youngest child reported to have developed migraine was 1 year old,[12] and the incidence in children 3 to 7 years of age is 3%, which increases to 4% to 11% (age 7 to 11 years) and 8% to 23% (age 11 to 15+ years), with the mean age at onset being 7.2 years for boys and 10.9 years for girls.[30,42] Safe and effective treatment for both acute episodes and for prevention are therefore urgently needed.

Diagnosis and differentiation of headaches can be difficult, especially in the very young.[43] Conventional medicine recommends systematic evaluations with careful history taking and neurological examination to identify the primary etiology[4,44,45] and diagnostic testing based on individual findings and indications.[46] Although very few studies have evaluated therapy of headache in young patients,[46] medical practitioners generally agree that medications are first-line treatment for acute symptoms.[18,19] Appropriate medications are more limited in young children, with older children and adolescents having more options.[47] Emphasis on nonpharmacological modalities is growing.[46,47] Partially because of concern of the undesirable side effects of drugs and the possibility of development of chemical dependency, many centers are turning to complementary and alternative medicine (CAM) therapies such as relaxation,[48] acupuncture,[49] biofeedback, and hypnosis.[12]

Because the etiology of headache can range from a benign, transient condition associated with a viral infection to serious, life-threatening brain tumor, it would be advisable to have an integrative approach in children. A proper neurological evaluation can be helpful for ruling out significant pathology. In non–life-threatening headaches, CAM diagnoses and treatment can be used either as a primary modality or as an adjunctive therapy to medication or can be incorporated in multidisciplinary approaches that may include relaxation training, change in lifestyle, and diet. CAM would be especially helpful in the management of "idiopathic" headaches that do not have explanation in western medicine but can be described as energetic disturbances from either internal or external causes. For those headaches that do have clear conventional diagnoses, CAM can offer a complementary energetic perspective that can add another dimension to diagnosis and treatment.

✳ CAM THERAPY RECOMMENDATIONS

Acupuncture

After a proper neurological evaluation has ruled out significant pathology, Traditional Chinese Medicine (TCM) diagnoses and acupuncture treatment can be used as a primary modality, as an adjunctive therapy, or as part of a multidisciplinary approach for non–life-threatening headaches.

Although recent reviews and meta-analyses of adult data support acupuncture for the treatment of headaches, the majority of the studies are considered to be substandard or scientifically flawed.[1] There is a paucity of information on children.

Reports of clinical improvement with acupuncture range from 20%[2] to approximately 67%[3] to as high as 95.6%.[4] Case reports from China indicate that SI17 is effective for vascular headaches,[5] and the extra point Sishencong[6] and Dazhui[7] also have analgesic effects for headaches. A randomized controlled trial (RCT) of acupuncture for chronic daily headache in 74 adults indicated that when medical management is supplemented with acupuncture, health-related quality of life improved and patients perceived that they suffered less from headaches.[8]

This author proposes a classification that incorporates information from classical references, adult acupuncture books, and the author's own experience in integrating conventional and TCM pediatrics. This integrated approach broadly categorizes pediatric headaches as Acute Causes due to External pathogens and Chronic, Recurrent Causes due to Internal imbalances.

Acupuncture assessment and treatment recommendations for headache are discussed in the following sections.[9]

Acute/External Causes of Headaches

The acute headaches are due to external pathogenic invasions and to acute head trauma.

Wind Cold—viral syndrome
Wind Heat—bacterial infection
Wind Damp—associated with dampness
Blood stasis—head trauma

Chronic/Internal Causes of Headaches

The chronic headaches are associated with internal organ imbalance due to various causes: stress, emotional excesses, lifestyle aberrations, dietary imbalance, or constitutional vulnerability. They are best classified according to location of headaches in relation to distribution of meridians.

Taiyang—occipital headache
Shaoyang—lateral side of head and neck; migraines
Yangming—forehead
Shaoyin—inside the brain
Taiyin—heavy and tight sensation as though head is tightly wrapped with a band

Jueyin—vertex
Variable location with history of head trauma

Acute Headaches

Wind-Cold invasion

Because Wind tends to affect the top of the body, headache is a frequent manifestation of both Wind-Cold (viral) and Wind-Heat (bacterial) conditions. Wind-Heat Headache can be sharp and generalized.

Wind Damp

Wind-Damp headache is characterized by a sensation of heaviness, often associated with exposure to dampness or rainy weather.

Blood stasis—head trauma

A blow to the head causes Blood stasis in the area of the trauma. Acute head trauma is best evaluated with the help of Western evaluation and technology. Head injury with abnormal neurological examination and positive laboratory substantiation, such as findings on skull radiographs, computed tomography scans, or magnetic resonance imaging scans of the head, usually indicates serious trauma and the child often needs to be hospitalized for close observation and further interventions.

Chronic, Recurrent Headaches Caused by Internal Imbalances

Chronic, recurrent headaches are due to impairment of Qi and Blood flow to the internal organ. The various causes include stress, emotional excesses, lifestyle aberrations, dietary imbalance, or constitutional vulnerability. Headache manifests along the path of the meridians to the head, such that the location of the headache would indicate pathogenic imbalance.

History is important to elicit six specific categories of information for assessing chronic headaches, as follows:

1. Location
2. Characteristics: for example, sharp, throbbing, presence of aura, relief with rest, aggravated by activity (Yang type); dull, achy, relief with activity (Yin type)
3. Relationship to food: types of food, manner of eating
4. Association with emotions that correspond to specific organs
5. Initial episode that precipitated the headache, such as exposure to viral infection or trauma
6. Evolution of headache: It is important to map the relationship between the initial episode and the current complaint.

The acupuncture treatment needs to address the *root* or the initiating factor as well as correct the current imbalances.

Chronic Headaches Classified According to Location

Taiyang

Taiyang headache occurs along the BL Taiyang channel, often at the back of the neck, that correlate to the Western diagnosis of tension headaches, which occur in as many as one third of childhood headaches,[10] and may present as sharp attacks that are sometimes difficult to distinguish from migraine without aura. Taiyang headaches are usually less intense, do not have emotional components, and usually do not have

gastrointestinal (GI) symptoms such as nausea, vomiting, or abdominal pain.

Shaoyang headache/migraine

Shaoyang type are the typical migranous throbbing headache along the lateral side of head and neck. Reports on acupuncture treatment are usually favorable for adult migraines. The few studies that include children also appear to show promise of acupuncture as a pediatric treatment modality. Several studies propose the possible biochemical effects of acupuncture on migraine as normalizing levels of serotonin[11] and affecting the serum catecholamine levels.[4,11] Needling LR3 alone has been demonstrated to affect breakdown of catecholamine.[12] Increased activity of the opioid system has also been demonstrated.[13] An animal study posits that efficacy of SI17 lies in its antiinflammatory effects on blood vessels of dura mater; it brings about inhabitation of the neurongenic inflammation on the affected side.[14] Acupuncture has been shown to be effective for both acute migraine attacks[15,16] and prophylaxis.[16-19] When TCM principles are used to differentiate headaches, acupuncture can significantly improve symptoms and even cure migraines.[20] The long-term effect of reduction in frequency, duration, and intensity after treatment can persist for months and even many years,[21,22] or with up to 50% decrease in drug intake.[19] The effect of acupuncture is comparable to some of the potent antimigraine medications but does not cause any negative side effects.[18] In a well-controlled randomized study of childhood migraine, acupuncture treatment significantly reduced both migraine frequency and intensity.[13] A multidisciplinary approach that included acupuncture, dietary changes, medication, physical therapy, and lifestyle adaptations was effective in treating the majority of patients with various types of migraine-related dizziness and vertigo.[23] Age, sex, social status, and expectations of benefit did not show any relation to treatment efficacy, but those with fewer emotional issues reported a better response.[24]

Acupuncture has been demonstrated to be efficacious even for "German migraine." Germany is a unique country in which 12% to 25% of the population is reported to be afflicted with migraine.[25] The symptoms tend to be severe: sudden onset of usually unbearable headache that can last as long as 72 hours, be accompanied by vegetative symptoms,[26] and occur frequently. Patients often take numerous analgesics for symptomatic relief but suffer various side effects. Acupuncture has been successful both for amelioration of acute symptoms and for prophylactic treatment.[25,26]

A German RCT of 302 adults with migraines revealed that both real and sham acupuncture were more effective than no treatment in reducing headaches.[27]

A U.S. RCT evaluated the effect of 12 acupuncture treatments on 401 adults with chronic headache disorder, predominantly migraine, in a primary care setting. The study suggests that acupuncture was beneficial and cost-effective.[28] A German RCT of 91 patients with migraine, episodic, or chronic tension-type headache, who were treated for 4 weeks in the hospital with TCM, revealed lasting improvement in the majority of patients. The most frequently used points were GB20, GB14, ExHN5, LI4, LI20, CV20, and LR3.[29]

Yangming headache—frontal headache

According to Western medicine, frontal headache is usually associated with sinusitis[30] and occurs in older children after the frontal sinuses are formed. In TCM, headache located on the forehead generally indicates Yangming Stomach imbalance, usually caused by dietary indiscretions such as eating too much red meat, eating spicy and fried foods, overeating, or eating too quickly or eating while studying.

Migraine in children is frequently characteristically Yangming: frontal location accompanied by abdominal pain.[31] In recent years, Yangming headache has been diagnosed with increasing frequency in children who spend long hours in front of a computer monitor. The eyestrain and continuous electromagnetic stimulation to Yintang point can lead to frontal headaches. Dull, achy frontal headache is caused by a deficiency of ST Yin, which occurs when children eat irregularly or eat very late at night.

Taiyin headache

Taiyin headache is characterized by a heavy and tight sensation, as though the head were wrapped with a band. The pain is usually dull and achy and can be generalized or localized to the forehead. Western medicine reports that when patients regularly take analgesics, this type of headache occurs with drug withdrawal.[32] TCM attributes the cause of Taiyin headache to SP deficiency with accumulation of Dampness in the head. Other Spleen deficiency signs may be present, such as poor muscle tone, fatigue, and digestive problems. Predisposing factors include a strong, positive family history; dampness either from living in a Damp environment or from eating excess Phlegm-producing foods (e.g., milk products; greasy, fried foods; peanuts; sweets; white sugar); and engaging in excess mental activities.

Shaoyin—headache "inside" the brain

Children frequently describe the headache as just "pain inside the whole head." Western medicine does not have a diagnosis for this nonspecific type of pain, but TCM considers these as Shaoyin headaches due to Kidney and Heart deficiency.

Jueyin

The typical Jueyin headache occurs at the vertex, the top of the head. This is most often due to metabolic imbalances, such as hypoglycemia, or when children adhere to a strict diet or are anorexic.

Variable locations with history of head trauma

Chronic headaches can be due to severe accidents and falls that cause Blood stasis in a particular area of the head.

Treatment

The treatment for headache can be general or specific.

General treatment for all types of headaches

GB20, Fengchi, is the most important point for headaches and can be chosen as the first point for headaches of any type.[33]
GV16 is indicated for "hundred diseases of the head."

LU7 is a special point for any type of headache.[34]
LI4 is a very strong dispersing point for headache and should be used with care in children who are deficient.
Local tender points on the head are important in treating headaches.[33]
A combination of local and distal points are very effective in the treatment of headaches.[33,35]
Needle treatment:
   Simple needling: Reducing method on the local points for sedation; tonification method for distal points.
   Ion pumping cords: Connect the black clamp to the local point and the red clamp to the distal point.
Magnet treatment:
   Place the bionorth (−) pole facing down on the local point and the biosouth (+) pole facing down on the distal point. Place the black clamp on the local point, and connect it with the red clamp on the distal point.
Specific treatment recommendations are outlined next. These are very brief recommendations; for detailed protocols, see Acupuncture reference 9.

Acute/External pathogens

Keep the child's occiput and back of the neck warm with a scarf or a hooded coat during cold and rainy weather.
Three major Wind acupoints to expel Wind in the head: GV16, GB20, BL12.
Use the Five-Element protocol to dispel Cold from the Taiyang Bladder channel:
   Tonify BL60, SI5; sedate BL66.
Or Heat from the Taiyang Bladder channel:
   Tonify BL66; sedate BL60, SI5.
GV14, LI11 to dispel Heat.
Wind-Damp:
ST8 combined with SP3 or SP6.
Dispel Wind-Damp acupoints: SP9, ST40.
Use the Five-Element, Four-Point protocol to tonify the Spleen (see Appendix B).
Yintang as local point if forehead headache is also present.
Blood stasis:
Acupuncture treatment should be instituted for head trauma headaches only if neurological examination and laboratory evaluations are negative for skull fracture or CNS bleed. These headaches can occur anywhere, depending on the site of trauma. Treatment can begin with any tender points as local points, followed by a distal point along the channel that connects to the local point.
BL17, SP10: general treatment for Blood stasis.
Taiyang for headache in the temple region.
TB18 for occipital headache.

Chronic recurrent headaches

Taiyang headache treatment
Use the Five-Element protocol to dispel Cold from the Taiyang Bladder channel:
   Tonify BL60, SI5; sedate BL66.
Modify lifestyle to reduce stress.
Use local points: BL10, GV16, GB20 combined with BL60 as a distal point.

Shaoyang migraine headache treatment

Use the Five-Element, Four-Point protocol to dispel Liver Heat:
Tonify LR2, KI10; sedate LR8, HT8.

GB 20.

GB41 combined with TB5.

LR3.[36]

Taiyang is a local, temporal point; it also helps to subdue liver Yang.

LR2 controls Liver Fire.

SP6.

LU7.

BL18.

SI17 on the affected side of migraine.[14]

Decrease sour and greasy foods in the diet.

Modify lifestyle to diminish stress.

Teach the child calming Qigong exercises.

Yangming/frontal headache

Use the Five-Element, Four-Point protocol to dispel Stomach Heat:
Tonify ST44, BL66; sedate ST41, SI5.

Local points: Yingtang, BL2, ST8, GV23 combined with distal points along ST and BL meridian:
ST34, ST40, ST44, BL60.

CV12.[37]

Decrease energetically Hot foods, greasy/fried foods in the diet.

Taiyin headache

Use the Five-Element, Four-Point protocol to tonify Spleen:
Tonify SP2, HT8; sedate SP1, LR1.

ST40, ST44, SP6, CV12.

Modify the child's lifestyle, especially if there are excess mental activities and insufficient rest.

Decrease Phlegm-producing and artificially sweetened foods in the diet.

Shaoyin headache

Kidney deficiency

GV20 and especially Sishencong are very beneficial for KI deficiency headaches.[6]

Super Mingmen treatment: GV4, BL23, BL52.

KI3, CV4, SP6, GB19.

Use the Five-Element, Four-Point protocol to tonify both Kidney Yin and Kidney Yang:
Tonify KI7, LU8; sedate KI3, SP3.

Decrease excess salt in diet.

Heart deficiency Shaoyin headache

HT7, KI3.

P6.

Decrease bitter foods and medications.

BL15 back shu point for Heart.

Jueyin:

Metabolic disorders should be properly diagnosed and treated by Western evaluation with acupuncture instituted for pain relief.

GV20 as a local point combined with KI1, BL67, or LR3 as distal points.

Blood stasis:

Acupuncture treatment for chronic, localized headache with history of head trauma should be instituted only when neurological examination and laboratory evaluation results are negative for the presence of CNS hematoma or abnormalities. The treatment can be the same as those for acute Blood stasis headache: combining local tender points with distal points along the same channel, and Blood moving and invigorating points: BL17, SP10.

Local points such as:
Taiyang for Blood stasis in the temple region.
GV20 or Sishencong for Blood stasis in the vertex.[9]

Aromatherapy

Essential oils are often suggested for the treatment of headache. The mechanism of analgesia is uncertain but may be related to modulation of pain perception by inhibiting nociceptive impulses or by activating the endogenous opioid system, which suppresses the pain impulses.[1] Secondarily the essential oils may affect a mental state of increased relaxation, thereby decreasing the effects of anxiety on the pain-anxiety cycle.[2]

A series of experiments were conducted on 32 healthy adult male subjects that mimicked the possible mechanisms of headache and then tested the effect of peppermint and eucalyptus essential oils. The situations were: (1) increasing pressure applied to the scalp and the middle finger of the right hand, (2) thermal pain induced by an electrical voltage, and (3) ischemic pain produced by applying a collar around the head and inflating it while the subject rhythmically bit on an object. Four different preparations were applied with a sponge to the large areas of the subjects' forehead and temples. Preparations were applied for a period of 3 minutes. Preparations tested were 10 g peppermint *(Mentha piperita)* with 5 g eucalyptus *(Eucalyptus* sp.) in 90% ethanol, 10 g peppermint with trace eucalyptus in ethanol, 5 g eucalyptus with trace peppermint in ethanol, and a placebo of traces of peppermint and eucalyptus in ethanol. Measurements included electromyographic (EMG) activity of the temporal muscle, electroencephalography (ECG), self-report of pain on a 0-50 scale, and current mood state. Peppermint and the combination of peppermint and eucalyptus showed significance in a number of areas. Peppermint and eucalyptus oil had a stronger impact on muscle relaxation and pain and on performance-related activity and concentration. Sensitivity to pressure was not reduced by any preparation, but peppermint was the strongest in reducing ischemic pain. Eucalyptus alone and the ethanol placebo resulted in no significant reductions.[1]

Essential oils of angelica *(Angelica archangelica),* bergamot *(Citrus bergamia),* sandalwood *(Santalum album),* sweet marjoram *(Origanum marjorana),* lavender *(Lavandula angustifolia),* peppermint, and eucalyptus by topical application are all described as useful for headache reduction in case reports.[3,4] Additionally, rosemary *(Rosmarinus officinalis)* and Roman chamomile *(Chamaemelum nobile)* are often cited as useful for headache pain.[5] The essential oils are applied topically, and the site of application depends on the type of headache. For stress or tension headaches, application to the back of the neck and shoulders helps relieve muscle tension leading to headache pain. In the author's experience, essential oils that are rubefacients or have a "feel" of warmth when applied, such as rosemary or sweet marjoram, are most beneficial for tension headaches. For headaches that are experienced in the forehead and facial areas, such as sinus headaches or migraines, application of essential oil to the temples is useful; lavender or peppermint are often used in this way. The essential oil is applied at the start of the headache and can be used periodically throughout its duration. Peppermint is recommended for migraine patients who also experience nausea, as it is useful for both pain and nausea.

Chiropractic

The chiropractic approach to the child with headaches is to evaluate the body for evidence of interference to normal neuromuscular function. There are several quality studies regarding headaches in adults; however, few case studies are reported involving children with headaches. Given the similarities in headache patterns (as well as case reports on chiropractic) in adults and children, adult studies can likely be extrapolated to children.

It is understood that headaches have multiple causes. A range of precipitating or aggravating factors may produce varied headache types in the same individual.[1-3] Tension-type, cervicogenic, and migraine headaches are the most common headache forms in children and are all managed similarly by the chiropractor with the adjustment of the subluxation complex (SC) at the center of any treatment protocol.

Anatomical associations may help to explain the effect of chiropractic on headaches. The trigeminocervical nucleus mediates noxious stimulation from the trigeminal nerve and afferents from the first three vertebral segments of the upper neck, the head, many intracranial blood vessels, and the throat.[4] Efferents from the first three vertebrae in the neck also innervate the dura, parts of the scalp, and the suboccipital musculature.[5] Therefore cervical spine joint and tissue abnormalities are associated with headache.[6] In support of this, surgical release of the C2 nerve root has been associated with a reduction in headache, nausea, vomiting, photophobia, and phonophobia.[7] Chronic irritation of the cervical sympathetic chain ganglion or of the sympathetic fibers to the vertebrals and carotids may lead not only to headache, but also to diverse autonomically based regional symptoms. It has been suggested that cervicogenic, tension-type, and migraine headache all have some degree of cervical spine involvement.[8,9]

An RCT compared amitriptyline with chiropractic adjustments in the management of muscle tension headaches. Both the chiropractic group and the pharmaceutical group showed similar improvement in headache symptoms during the 6-week trial. However, at a 4-week followup, only the chiropractic group maintained improvement in headaches.[10]

An RCT demonstrated a 69% reduction in headaches in those receiving chiropractic adjustments as compared with a 37% reduction in those receiving soft tissue massage and low-level laser therapy. Headache intensity decreased 36% in the chiropractic group and 17% in the soft tissue group. Only the chiropractic group had a reduction in the use of OTC analgesics.[11]

A case series analysis was completed that involved 11 adult males with chronic tension headaches. The participants were prohibited from utilizing headache-related pharmaceuticals or other intervention during the 10-week study. The chiropractic management included spinal adjustments (primarily to the cervical spine) as well as moist hot packs and trigger point therapy to the cervical and thoracic spine. The average pretreatment headache frequency was 6.4 episodes per 2 weeks, and the average post-treatment frequency was 3.1 episodes in the same period.[12]

An RCT of 127 people, each with an average of 18 years of chronic migraine, was conducted in New South Wales, Australia. Two months of data collection occurred both before and after a 2-month treatment interval, which included a maximum of 16 chiropractic adjustments. Results demonstrated a statistically significant reduction in migraine frequency and associated disability. In fact, a significant number of the experimental group were able to eliminate use of pharmaceuticals by the end of the study.[13]

The same author who evaluated satisfaction of adult headache patients undergoing chiropractic care completed both a retrospective and a prospective headache study. In the retrospective study involving 15 adults, the satisfaction rating was nearly 90% after an average of 12 visits. In the prospective study, the post-treatment satisfaction of 18 subjects was 90% after 9 visits.[14] In the majority of subjects, satisfaction was derived from reduction of headache symptoms.

A study of 22 adult headache sufferers found reduced headache symptoms after cervical manipulation and soft tissue massage, but no change in EMG or skin temperature of the dominant hand. The authors suggest a cortical response resulting in an autonomic shift as being responsible for the decrease in headache pain.[15]

Ninety-three percent of 332 headache study participants found favorable results after an average of 8.6 cervical adjustments.[16]

In a 2-year follow-up study of migraine patients, 87 migraine sufferers were provided spinal adjustments until spinal function was normalized. This took between 1 and 74 adjustments at an average of weekly intervals. At the 2-year follow-up, one third of subjects reported no further headache symptoms, slightly more than 41% reported marked improvement in migraine symptoms, 20% reported no change, and 4.6% reported worsening of the migraines.[17] Permanent recovery from migrainous-type headaches is not typically expected, and intermittent evaluation for the SC is advised along with indicated dietary and lifestyle changes.

A reported case study involved a 6-year-old girl with headaches and neck pain during the past 2 months along with bruxism of a daily frequency during the previous 2 years. After two adjustments to the first cervical vertebrae, all symptoms resolved and had not returned by the 4-month follow-up.[18]

A compilation of five pediatric headache cases was recorded by a single author in the chiropractic literature.[19] A 7-year-old with near daily headaches during the previous 2 years became pain free after 6 weeks of chiropractic management. The second case was an 8-year-old whose migraine headaches were eliminated after 6 weeks of chiropractic management. The third case was an 8-year-old with frontal headaches that woke her from sleep. She experienced only two headaches within a 4-month period after her initial chiropractic adjustment. In the fourth case, a 14-year-old with a 5-year history of migraine headaches had relief within the first 2 weeks of care. The final case involved a 15-year-old with a 10-month history of generalized headaches. After 2 weeks of care, the medication that had been required several times per week for pain control was no longer utilized. Within 3 months of care, the headaches were rare and mild. In two of these cases, headaches returned after physical trauma and again responded to the chiropractic management.

A 13-year-old girl presented with a 1-year history of headaches and neck pain. After 2 weeks of chiropractic care, she no longer had headaches or neck pain.[20]

A 10-year-old male with a 3-year history of migraine headaches received chiropractic adjustments to the neck and upper back. Within the first month of care, no migraine headaches occurred, although he did experience two prodromal episodes.[21]

An interesting report was made of a 14-year-old with headaches who was also noted to have a limited field of vision. She received chiropractic adjustments to the cervical and thoracic spine seven times. Her headaches resolved, and her visual acuity and field of vision returned to normal.[22]

Thirty-one headache subjects underwent cervical evaluation. It was found that 100% had abnormal fixation of motion at the C0-C1 unit, 75% at the C7-T1, and 25% at C1-C3.[23] In this same study, 84% of headache subjects had abnormal motion at two or more upper cervical segments. This appears consistent with other studies reported here. Evaluation of non-headache subjects reveals a substantially lower incidence of cervical fixation, with only 5% having fixation at C0-C1.[24] Other areas associated with headaches in children are the temporomandibular joint and the lumbosacral junction.

According to the author of *Chiropractic Pediatrics*:
- Pain in the frontal region is often associated with C0-C1 or C2-C3.
- Pain in the retroorbital region is often associated with C2-C3.
- Pain in the temporosphenoidal or occipital region is often associated with C1-C2.
- Pain in the suboccipital region or into the neck is often associated with lower cervical spine, the thoracolumbar junction, or the lumbosacral junction.[25]
- Postural retraining may be a necessary component in thoroughly addressing headaches in children. Adult headache subjects are more likely to show an abnormally reduced cervical lordosis and more rounded shoulders than their non-headache counterparts.[26] These distortions may be associated with muscle hypertonicity and tenderness, commonly found in headache sufferers at the occipital groups, cervical paraspinals, trapezius, and levators.[27]
- Cranial adjustments may provide headache relief where spinal adjustments alone cannot.[28]
- Pinching-type pressure at the deep web of the thumb may reduce headache pain.
- Biofeedback has been found to be an effective tool in reducing headache symptoms.[29,30] Simple relaxation techniques are useful for various stress-related symptoms in children. Directly addressing (or avoiding if possible) stressful situations with the child may eliminate stress-related headaches.
- Rubbing lavender oil into the temples during a tension-type headache may bring about relief. Taking feverfew orally has been shown to reduce frequency of migraine headaches over time.
- Constipation has been known to be a factor in some headaches and may relate to hydration. Careful attention to adequate hydration and GI function is always a prudent measure when addressing vital body health.
- Headaches that are related to toxicity/allergy would be addressed with dietary or lifestyle changes. An elimination trial of caffeine, chocolate, MSG, and artificial sweeteners may prove a fruitful place to start.
- A wholesome diet plentiful in fresh fruits and vegetables and free of trans fats or simple sugars may also reduce headaches related to poor diet. Maintaining adequate hydration may minimize or eliminate headaches.
- Headaches related to sinus congestion must be managed as an infective or allergic process.
- Headaches as a result of intracranial bleed, brain tumor, or intracranial inflammation established in the thorough history and examination are referred for urgent medical attention.

Herbs—Western

Headaches are a common phenomenon of childhood and become even more widespread during adolescence. Evaluation and management of headaches in children requires careful history taking combined with physical and neurological assessment. Consideration of acuity, past medical history, patterns of discomfort, and potential triggers may have an impact on recommended therapies. In terms of herbs and dietary supplements, it is particularly important to consider potential interactions and side effects of therapies used in children and adolescents.

Treatment

Traditionally, willowbark has been considered a safe and effective treatment for headaches in adults and children. However, a number of reasons suggest otherwise: willowbark contains salicin and is not recommended for oral intake due to the large amount (liters) needed for effectiveness. Moreover, its use is contraindicated for use in children with viral infection due to potential concern of Reye syndrome.[1] Peppermint oil may be an effective treatment for headache in children 8 years or older when applied topically or orally. In particular, combination products containing peppermint oil and menthol may aid in muscle relaxation for tension headache. However, oral or topical application of peppermint oil is considered unsafe for infants and small children because of its association with bronchospasm and respiratory arrest.[2,3] Furthermore, many topically-applied products that contain peppermint oil also contain menthol, which may also contribute to respiratory or CNS toxicity, including respiratory arrest and seizures.[3]

Prevention

The leaf of the feverfew plant *(Tanacetum parthenium)*, when applied orally, may be effective herbal therapy for migraine headache prevention in adults. However, available evidence suggests that it is ineffective for children. Limited data are available for effects and risks associated with long-term use (> 4 months). Most studies have used feverfew products standardized to contain 0.2% to 0.35% of the parthenolide constituent, the putative pharmacoactive ingredient. However, research suggests that standardized doses do not appear to be linked to its effectiveness.[4-6] Furthermore, caution is advised because of feverfew's association with inhibition of platelet function.

While investigating the treatment of migraines in adolescents, the use of olive oil containing oleic acid as a placebo was found to be a possibly effective treatment. This regimen investigated taking olive oil containing oleic acid, 1382 mg daily, over a 2-month period to reduce the frequency, duration, and severity of migraine headaches. (Olive oil is classified partially per its acid content, which is measured as free oleic acid. Extra-virgin olive oil contains a maximum of 1% free oleic acid, virgin olive oil contains 2%, and ordinary olive oil contains 3.3%. Unrefined olive oils with more than 3.3% free oleic acid are considered "unfit for human consumption.")[4,7,8] Other herbal therapies used include garlic, ginger, gingko, lemon balm, milk thistle, and turmeric. However, there is not enough evidence to recommend using these therapies to treat or prevent headaches in adults or children.[4]

Massage Therapy

Myofascial trigger point pain is a common cause of regional, cervicogenic headaches,[1] tension headaches, tinnitus, and temporomandibular joint pain.[2] Myofascial trigger points are discrete, focal, hyperirritable spots located in taut bands of skeletal muscle that may have developed from trauma or repetitive use.[2] The taut bands may be related to excessive release of acetylcholine in abnormal motor endplates and the associated response to sensitized nerve fibers.[3]

Specific trigger points that can cause regional ocular pain may be located in the sternoclaviculomastoid, masseter, orbicularis oculi, and zygomaticum major muscles; occipital pain from the occipitalis, suboccipitalis, and sternocleidomastoid muscles; frontal pain from the frontalis muscle; and jaw pain from the temporalis and masseter muscles.[4] Pressure may be applied to myofascial trigger points to help decrease pain and sensitivity related to the specific trigger point. Once a trigger point is identified, it is relatively easy to teach a patient to perform self-trigger point application for pain prevention and reduction. Myofascial trigger points may feel like unexplainable denser tissue upon palpation—almost the difference between cold versus room-temperature butter. When a trigger point has been palpated, gentle to moderate pressure can be applied to confirm the point in which the patient may feel anywhere from a tender sensation such as pushing upon a bruise to a completely reproducible referral pain. It is best to apply gradual pressure during the process so that patients may have better control over their pain experience. Often when a trigger point is successfully palpated, the patient will respond, "Yes, that is my headache," but as soon as pressure has been removed from the site, the pain will stop. Trigger point "maps" are readily available to indicate where the common trigger points are located and to where they refer pain, which may be incredibly useful to a practitioner wishing to gain experience in palpating and treating trigger points.

A study on the home effectiveness of self-application of trigger point pressure followed by stretching over a 5-day period was more effective than active range of motion in decreasing pain intensity and trigger point sensitivity.[5] Use of massage therapy with exercise was found to be more effective than ultrasound treatment for the management of trigger point pain and in reducing the number and intensity of points.[6]

Other massage modalities may be utilized to help reduce headache pain. A pilot study of adults with chronic headaches who received Trager treatments over a 6-week period had a 44% reduction in analgesic use, decreased frequency of headaches, and improvement in quality of life indicators compared with controls using only medication for headache management.[7] The Trager method is a structural integration technique that balances the body within gravity through techniques involving manual soft tissue manipulation, joint mobilization, stretching, and exercises. Another RCT reported adult patients with chronic headache or migraine who received massage had decreased pain intensity, fewer somatic symptoms, lower anxiety and headache scores, increased number of hours slept, greater percentage of headache-free days, and fewer days with mild headache pain when compared with the controls.[8] An uncontrolled study of adult patients with chronic tension headache had decreased headache frequency and duration when compared with their premassage baseline.[9]

Other studies have concluded that massage is an effective therapy for the management of chronic and acute pain. Research has shown elevated plasma β-endorphin levels after massage therapy,[10] which may explain some of its pain-reducing properties. Theorists have postulated that massage therapy may decrease substance P levels during massage treatment, but controlled studies have yet to be done. A systematic review of 22 articles on the effects of massage therapy on relaxation and comfort indicated that 8 of 10 significantly decreased anxiety or perception of tension; 7 of 10 produced physiological relaxation; and 3 studies demonstrated it was effective at reducing pain.[11] Another systematic review of 23 articles suggested there is evidence that massage therapy is a useful approach to pain relief in numerous chronic, nonmalignant pain conditions, specifically musculoskeletal complaints.[12] The efficacy of massage therapy to decrease pain scores in acute postoperative pain management has also been demonstrated.[13-17]

Massage therapy may be an effective adjunct in the management of headache pain. Teaching patients the location of their trigger points and effective self-treatment may be a cost-effective method to help patients manage their headache symptoms.

Mind/Body

Mind/body techniques have a well-established track record in the treatment of headaches (tension type and migraine) and arguably represent first-line treatments of choice for many children and adolescents.[1-3]

The biofeedback literature has been very clear that both in short- and long-term follow-up, thermal biofeedback and bifrontal surface EMG biofeedback are both quite effective in reducing the frequency and severity of pediatric headaches.[4]

Meta-analysis[5] has indicated medium to large effect sizes for thermal biofeedback compared with pharmacological treatments for childhood migraine. Biofeedback appears to be both time- and cost-efficient. A pilot study indicated good success with an abbreviated protocol that involved a single "live" biofeedback session followed by home practice and telephone follow-up.[5] However, more intensive therapeutic intervention is often needed for significant improvements in functioning. Neurofeedback (measuring and feeding back information about electrical brain activity in real time) is being developed as a treatment option for adults with migraine, as is hemo-encephalographic biofeedback (measuring and feeding back information about local cerebral blood flow activity).[6]

Relaxation, stress management, and cognitive-behavioral interventions are also quite effective in all types of pediatric headache and should be an important foundation of most headache treatment plans.[7] A Cochrane database systematic review from 2003 concluded that relaxation and cognitive-behavioral techniques are effective in the management of chronic/recurrent pediatric headache pain.[8]

In one study in Hungary,[9] women with tension-type and mixed headaches who were taught a specific relaxation technique called "autogenics" (which involves repetitive self-suggestions about muscle relaxation, such as "My right arm is warm and heavy") were able to significantly reduce analgesic use. The authors' clinical experience suggests this to be a useful technique for children and adolescents as well.

Although the authors could find no RCTs specific to pediatric headache, other mind/body techniques such as yoga and meditation may have a place in the treatment of children with muscle tension or migraine headache. Certainly clinical experiences and case studies from the adult literature are suggestive of a potential benefit from practice of these techniques, which would be reasonable to extrapolate to children and adolescents.[10]

In the authors' experience, mind/body techniques can be blended with massage, bodywork, and acupuncture in a multimodality approach; however, in general, some from of self-regulation/relaxation skill training is viewed as a relative treatment priority.

Hypnosis also has a strong track record in the treatment of childhood headache. In a prospective randomized controlled study, 30 children with frequent migraine episodes were randomized to propranolol, placebo, or training in self-hypnosis. The frequency of migraine episodes in the propranolol or placebo group did not change. Children who learned and practiced self-hypnosis had a reduction of 60% in frequency of migraine episodes over the first 3 months and more than 90% as they continued practice for 1 year of follow-up.[11]

Olness led another study designed to assess a possible mechanism of self-hypnosis efficacy in the prevention of juvenile migraine. Mast cells are increased in adults, and this study hypothesized that children with recurrent migraines who learn and practice self-hypnosis will have evidence of decreased mast cell activation when compared with juvenile migraineurs who have not learned and practiced self-hypnosis. Thirty children between ages 6 and 12 years provided 24-hour urine collections for assessment of mast cell products (tryptase and histamine). Children were randomized to training in self-hypnosis or to a waiting control group. Children in the self-hypnosis group were also provided biofeedback via temperature and galvanic skin resistance. Children in the self-hypnosis group had

a reduction of 60% in frequency of migraine episodes during the initial 12 weeks of follow-up and continued with further reductions through a total of 24 weeks of follow-up. There was an association between the reduction of migraine episodes and reduction in urine tryptase levels, which suggests that regular practice of self-hypnosis suppressed mast cell activation.[12]

Nutrition

Discussion

Therapies used to treat headaches often attempt to target the underlying process—vasodilatation, vasoconstriction, inflammatory response, or muscle tension, to name a few. Many of these processes may also be addressed and attenuated with nutrition or nutritional supplements.

Dehydration is a common but often unrecognized culprit of headache pain. The brain is more than 75% water, and when it detects a shortage of available fluids, it implements a water rationing process by producing histamines, thus directing certain subordinate water regulators to redistribute the amount of water in circulation. This system helps move water to areas where it is needed for basic metabolic activity and survival. When histamine and its subordinate regulators come across pain-sensing nerves in the body, they cause strong and continual pain.

Food allergies or triggers may precipitate headache pain for some people. Caffeine, wine, aged cheeses, processed meats, chocolate, aspartame, and MSG are just a few of the foods or food additives that may be problematic. These contain amines/histamines, nitrates, or substrates that stimulate blood vessel reactivity or activate pain nerve fibers. Recognizing and eliminating hidden sources of these foods or additives in the diet may help reduce the incidence of headache.

Magnesium is vital for proper muscle contraction and nerve conduction. Low magnesium levels have been implicated in the cause of both migraine and tension-type headaches. Many studies have shown the effectiveness of supplemental magnesium for preventing and treating migraine and tension-type headaches.[1,2] Magnesium appears to affect the *N*-methyl-D-aspartate (NMDA) receptors that play a crucial role in pain perception. In deficient states, NMDA receptors develop a hypersensitivity to pain. Magnesium acts as an NMDA receptor antagonist, much in the same way that ketamine does, to reduce pain.

A deficit of mitochondrial energy metabolism is thought to play a role in headache pathogenesis. The B vitamins are essential in certain metabolic reactions, particularly the conversion of carbohydrates into sugar, which is "burned" to produce energy, and in the breakdown of fats and protein; to maintain muscle tone; and to promote the health of the nervous system. Riboflavin (vitamin B$_2$) is the precursor of flavin mononucleotide and flavin adenine dinucleotide, which are required for the electron transport chain activity that produces energy. Clinical studies have shown the effectiveness of high-dose riboflavin as an option for migraine prophylaxis.[3]

Supplementation with omega-3 fatty acids was found to be effective in the management of recurrent migraines in adolescents.[4] Use of the supplements reduced the frequency, severity, and duration of headache experience by both male and female adolescents. Omega-3 fatty acids are naturally occurring anti-inflammatory agents used to reduce inflammation that may be causing vascular constriction.

Fasting may contribute to headache, as this may be a stressor to already hyperactive brain cells. One observational study noted an increased incidence of headache in subjects during Ramadan, a time of fasting and prayer in the Muslim faith.[5] This relative state of hypoglycemia would essentially provide less glucose to the brain for energy.

Treatment

Nutritional management of headaches might include the following recommendations:

- Assure proper hydration with water.
- Eliminate foods known to trigger headaches. Look for hidden sources of caffeine, MSG, or asparatame as food additives.
- Prevent hypoglycemia by encouraging a low glycemic load diet, avoiding processed carbohydrates and refined sugar, and eating small, frequent meals balanced in the sources of carbohydrates, fats, and protein.
- Supplement with magnesium in the form of glycinate, gluconate, aspartate, or oxide in a dose of 500 mg twice per day. Dietary sources of magnesium include avocado, pork, milk, clams, mushrooms, spinach, barley, quinoa, and sunflower and pumpkin seeds.
- Supplement with riboflavin (vitamin B_2) 400 mg per day. Dietary sources for vitamin B_2 include brewer's yeast, almonds, organ meats, whole grains, wheat germ, mushrooms, wild rice, broccoli, spinach, and milk.
- Provide daily sources of omega-3 fatty acids, either through supplementation with fish oil, flax seed oil, or hemp oil at 1000 mg per day, or with dietary sources including salmon, mackerel, herring, flax seeds, hemp seeds, or walnuts. Omega-3 fatty acids have natural antiinflammatory qualities to help reduce pain. Make sure the fish sources are free of heavy metal (mercury) and pesticide contamination.
- Drink chamomile tea, which has natural calming effects on the nervous system and relaxes smooth muscles.

Osteopathy

Headaches may have many etiologies, but the most common appears to be tension-type or cervicogenic headaches. These headaches usually begin as a vague ache in the occipital area, base of the head, or top of the neck. Within hours it may progress to involve the entire head. The child may complain of pain behind the eyes or show signs of photosensitivity. The headaches usually worsen as the day goes on and improve with sleep. When severe, they may trigger migraine-type symptoms of nausea, photophobia, and even vomiting. These signs of vagal irritation can be present in any severely painful headaches and are not limited to migraine.

The patient with cervicogenic cephalgia often complains of chronic low-grade headache, pressure or ache, and stiffness at the base of the head or upper neck, which then exacerbates into the severe headache. Children may have several episodes per week that require them to see the school nurse or miss class.

Frequently there is no predisposing history or precipitating event. This headache pattern may be exacerbated by stress, desk or computer work for a prolonged period of time, or activities that require prolonged extension and shortening of the craniocervical tissues. Studies have shown that cervicogenic cephalgia can be generated by irritation of musculoskeletal components of the cervical spine and craniocervical area,[1] hence the name. The pathophysiology of cervicogenic cephalgia involves spinal facilitation of dorsal horn cells at the level of the midbrain, where trigeminal input summates on cells that also receive input from the anterolateral system of the upper cervical spine.[1-3]

Cervicogenic cephalgia is generated by irritation to structures in the upper cervical or craniocervical areas. On physical examination there is usually extension of the occiput on the atlas and significant restriction of mechanics at the craniocervical junction, involving the suboccipital tissues. Trigger points in the extensor muscles of the head and neck may or may not be present[4]; however, tender points are commonly found. There is marked compression and restriction of normal mechanics in the cranial base with apparent secondary restriction in the vault.[3] In some children, tender points over the lambdoidal and occipitomastoid sutures will reproduce the pain pattern and a feeling of light-headedness. SBS compression is frequently palpated in these patients[5] and may be primary or secondary to the strain. Fascial restriction throughout the cervical and upper thoracic area is also present. In those patients in whom the headache has a tendency to evolve into a migraine, there is often paraspinal muscle spasm between T1 and T4, the area of origin of the sympathetic innervation of the intracranial vasculature.[6] Similar findings in the head and upper neck may be present in children with headaches arising from mechanical strain at the occipitoatlantal junction. Strains in this area may produce tissue tensions in the rectus capitis posterior minor muscle. This small muscle attaches to the intracranial dura mater[7] and is a potential pain generator.

Osteopaths will use a variety of techniques to treat the aforementioned findings. An emphasis would be placed on techniques appropriate to the cranium and neck. Sutherland techniques, indirect techniques, and muscle energy are commonly employed. An older child may be taught to abort an evolving headache using self-employed myofascial, counterstrain, or muscle energy techniques.

Osteopathic physicians consider the role of vision in maintaining postural strains. Most children with headaches that do not resolve with osteopathic treatment may benefit from evaluation by a functional optometrist. Likewise, nutritional aspects need to be considered. Food sensitivities manifest as headaches in some children. Osteopathic treatment may help reduce muscle spasm in those children whose headache presentation includes clenching or grinding of their teeth. In some such cases, a consultation with a dentist who understands the relationship of the bite to head and neck biomechanics will often facilitate osteopathic treatment.

Psychology

Most psychological interventions for headaches focus on teaching relaxation techniques and developing self-monitoring skills so that children will be more aware of a problem before it escalates and be able to alter their physiology to minimize the impact of a headache. Biofeedback has demonstrated effectiveness for both migraine and tension headaches in children. There are no risk or safety issues for children with headaches who use this procedure. For children with migraines without aura, 10 sessions of biofeedback resulted in decreased number of days with migraines per month and lessened migraine duration.[1] Another study focused on thermal biofeedback (teaching hand warming) combined with stress management and deep breathing techniques for children with migraines.[2] With four 1-hour sessions, headache intensity and number of days with headaches significantly decreased. Evaluation at the 6-month follow-up revealed that 100% of the treated children demonstrated clinical improvement.

A literature review on pediatric migraine and biofeedback concluded that thermal biofeedback is highly successful in alleviating headaches and that more than two thirds of children in most studies could be classified as treatment successes using a criterion of 50% symptom reduction.[3] The authors noted a difference between biofeedback that used a few therapist-guided sessions with the remainder of treatment in a home-based self-administered format compared with entirely therapist-guided, in-clinic treatment. Home-based biofeedback yielded less improvement (e.g., 69% improved) compared with clinic-based biofeedback (e.g., most studies 100% improved). Finally, combining parent training in behavior management strategies with biofeedback is also beneficial.[4] Children whose parents received training had significantly greater reductions in headache frequency, were more likely to experience clinically significant improvements, were more likely to be headache free, and had better adaptive functioning both during treatment and at 3-month follow-up compared with children who received biofeedback alone.

Tension headaches are also successfully treated using biofeedback; however, there are fewer studies evaluating its effectiveness.[3] Six sessions of thermal biofeedback were found to be effective in treating tension headaches, and at the 6-month follow-up, four of the five participants were headache free.[5] EMG biofeedback yields success rates of about 80% to 90% for tension headaches and is currently the most promising treatment approach.[3]

Relaxation skills are an important component to reducing and managing headaches. One element common to relaxation programs is the tensing and relaxing of muscle groups. This allows the patient to be more aware of the tension being held in different muscles and teaches the skills to relax the tightness and tension. By practicing these relaxation exercises several times per week, when no headache is present, the child will be more adept at shifting his or her physiology from tensed to relaxed. Then, at the beginning stages of a headache, the child can reduce the muscle tightness that contributes to maintaining the headache and pain.[6]

A sample relaxation script is as follows:

Today we are going to practice some special exercises that will help you learn to relax and will even help you control your pain. These are called Relaxation Exercises, and you can do them anytime to make yourself feel better. In order for you to feel your best from these exercises there are three rules to follow. First, you must do what I say, even if it sounds silly. Second, try hard to pay attention to how you muscles feel when they are tense and tight and then when they are loose and relaxed. Third, you must practice this at home with mom or dad so you can learn to do it whenever you want.

Let's shake all the wiggles out first. Now, get as comfortable as you can in the chair and let your arms and legs be loose and relaxed. Close your eyes. Follow what I say carefully and pay close attention to your body and what you feel.

Breathe in and out slowly. Imagine your lungs are two red balloons that you have to fill up with air as slowly as possible. Picture them slowly pumping up. Now when they are full, let the air slowly go out of the balloons. It's time to fill up the balloons again. They are filling up nice and slow, almost full, now nice and full. And let the air out slowly. The balloon is deflating, letting all its air out.

Now try to squeeze your eyes closed as tight as you can to keep all the light out. Make it as dark as you can. Feel how tight your eyes are, and scrunch up your nose to make your eyes even tighter. And now relax your eyes and nose. Feel how heavy and relaxed your face feels. Now make it as dark as you can. Squeeze your eyes shut and scrunch up your nose. Hold it tight. A little bit tighter. Now let your face relax. Notice how good it feels to relax. Your face is smooth and relaxed.

You have a giant jawbreaker bubble gun in your mouth in your favorite flavor. It's very hard to chew, but you want the sweet flavor. Bite down on it. Use your lips and neck muscles. Make your whole mouth tight as you chew it. Now relax. Let your jaw hang lose and your mouth be a little bit open with your tongue nice and relaxed inside. Now you want the yummy taste again, so you chew it up. Work as hard as you can. Squeeze your mouth to get all the taste. Good. Now relax your mouth and your whole face and neck. You've beaten the bubble gum. Make yourself as loose as you can.

Now pretend you are a turtle sitting in a field of green grass. It is so nice to be relaxing in the warm sun. Feel how relaxed you feel with the warm sun on your face and the soft grass underneath you. Uh oh, you sense danger. Pull yourself inside the shell. Pull your shoulders up to your ears and your head down into your shoulders. Hold it tight. Make your arms tense and hold them close to your sides. Hold it tight—as long as you can. And the danger is gone and you can relax. Come back out of your home and into the warm sun. Notice how warm your body feels laying there in the soft grass. It is so peaceful. Your arms and legs feel heavy and relaxed. Watch out now. Danger is back. Get back in your shell quickly—close in, making everything tight. Hold your arms tight and your shoulders up. Pull your head down and feel the tension making your muscles tight. Now you are safe and you can come out. The danger is all gone. You can relax in the sun with nothing to be afraid of. Feel how warm and relaxed your body feels. You are heavy and relaxed. Notice how good you feel laying in the soft grass with the warm sun in your face.

Stay as relaxed as you can. Let your whole body go limp and all of your muscles completely relax. Notice how heavy your body feels in the chair. It might be hard to tell where the chair ends and your body begins. You can have this relaxed and warm feeling whenever you want. Just practice like we did today, making yourself tight and then relaxing, and you will feel more and more relaxed. I will count backward from five to one, and when I get to one you can open your eyes but you will keep the relaxed, warm, feeling with you. Five, four, you mind becoming more awake, three, noticing the sounds around you, two, your body waking up but still peaceful and relaxed, and one, you can open your eyes when you are ready.

References

Pediatric Diagnosis and Treatment

1. Swaiman KF: *Pediatric neurology, principles and practice*, St Louis, 1989, Mosby.
2. Szczepanik E: Idiopathic headache in children [in Polish], *Med Wieku Rozwoj* 4:185-195, 2000 (abstract).
3. Cano A, Palomeras E, Alfonso S et al: Migraine without aura and migrainous disorder in children; International Headache Society (HIS) and revised HIS criteria, *Cephalalgia* 20:617-620, 2000.
4. Winner P, Martinez W, Mate L et al: Classification of pediatric migraine: proposed revision to the HIS criteria, *Headache* 35:407-410, 1995.
5. Wober-Bingol C, Wober C, Wagner-Ennsgraber C et al: IHS criteria for migraine and tension-type headache in children and adolescents, *Headache* 36:231-238, 1996.
6. Metsahonkala L, Sillanpaa M: Migraine in children—an evaluation of the HIS criteria, *Cephalalgia* 14:285-290, 1994.
7. Seshia SS, Wolstein JR, Adams C et al: International headache society criteria and childhood headache, *Develop Med Child Neurol* 36:419-428, 1994.
8. Sanin LC, Mathew NT, Bellmeyer LR et al: The International Headache Society (IHS) headache classification as applied to a headache clinic population, *Cephalalgia* 14:443-446, 1994.
9. Burton LJ, Quinn B, Pratt-Cheney JL et al: Headache etiology in a pediatric emergency department, *Pediatr Emerg Care* 13:1-4, 1997.
10. Kan L, Nagelberg J, Maytal J: Headaches in a pediatric emergency department: etiology, imaging, and treatment, *Headache* 40:25-29, 2000.
11. Hering-Hanit GN: Caffeine-induced headaches in children and adolescents, *Cephalagia* 23:332-335, 2003.
12. Behrman RE, Kliegman RM, Jenson HB, editors: *Nelson textbook of pediatrics*, ed 17, Philadelphia, 2004, Saunders.
13. Wober-Bingol C, Wober C, Karwautz A et al: Diagnosis of headache in childhood and adolescence: a study in 437 patients, *Cephalalgia* 15:13-21, 1995.
14. Abbas A: Headache, *Practitioner* 233:1081-1082, 1084, 1989.
15. Zebenholzer K, Wober C, Kienbacher C et al: Migrainous disorder and headache of the tension-type not fulfilling the criteria: a follow-up study in children and adolescents, *Cephalalgia* 20:611-616, 2000.
16. Niczyporuk-Turek A: Factors contributing to so-called idiopathic headaches [in Polish], *Neurol Neurochir Pol* 31:895-904, 1997 (abstract).
17. Annequin D, Dumas C, Tourniaire B et al: Migraine and chronic headache in children [in French]], *Rev Neurol (Paris)* 156:4S68-4S74, 2000 (abstract).
18. Gallai V, Sarchielli P, Carboni F et al: Applicability of the 1988 IHS criteria to headache patients under the age of 18 years attending 21 Italian headache clinics. Juvenile Headache Collaborative Study Group, *Headache* 35:146-153, 1995.
19. Annequin D, Tourniaire B, Dumas C: Migraine, misunderstood pathology in children [in French], *Arch Pediatr* 7:985-990, 2000 (abstract).
20. Peroutka SJ: Dopamine and migraine, *Neurology* 49:650-656, 1997.
21. Spierings EL: Mechanism of migraine and action of antimigraine medications, *Med Clin North Am* 85:943-958, vi-vii, 2001.
22. Del Zompo M: Dopaminergic hypersensitivity in migraine: clinical and genetic evidence, *Function Neurol* 15(Suppl 3):163-170, 2000.
23. Di Piero V, Bruti G, Venturi P et al: Aminergic tone correlates of migraine and tension-type headache: a study using the tridimensional personality questionnaire, *Headache* 41:63-71, 2001.
24. Markelova VF, Tauleuv AM, Belitskaia RA et al: Effect of reflexotherapy on catecholamine excretion in migraine [in Russian], *Sov Med* (2):59-63, 1982 (abstract).
25. Markelova VF, Vesnina VA, Malygina SI et al: Changes in blood serotonin levels in patients with migraine headaches before and after a course of reflexotherapy [in Russian], *Zh Nevropatol Psikhiatr Im S S Korsakova* 84:1313-1316, 1984 (abstract).
26. Peroutka SJ: Beyond monotherapy: rational polytherapy in migraine, *Headache* 38:18-22, 1998.
27. Ferrari MD: Biochemistry of migraine, *Pathol Biol (Paris)* 40:287-292, 1992.
28. Mascia A, Afra J, Schoenen J: Dopamine and migraine: a review of pharmacological, biochemical, neurophysiological, and therapeutic data, *Cephalalgia* 18:174-182, 1998.
29. Fanciullacci M, Alessandri M, Del Rosso A: Dopamine involvement in the migraine attack, *Function Neurol* 15(Suppl 3):171-181, 2000.
30. Stewart WF, Linet MS, Celentano DD et al: Age and sex-specific incidence rates of migraine with and without visual aura, *Am J Epidemiol* 34:1111-1120, 1991.
31. Barth N, Riegels M, Hebebrand J et al: "Cyclic vomiting" in childhood and adolescence [in German], *Z Kinder Jugendpsychiatr Psychother* 28:109-117, 2000 (abstract).
32. Rashed H, Abell TL, Familoni BO et al: Autonomic function in cyclic vomiting syndrome and classic migraine, *Dig Dis Sci* 44(8 Suppl):74S-78S, 1999.
33. Guitera V, Gutierrez E, Munoz P et al: Personality changes in chronic daily headache: a study in the general population [in Spanish], *Neurologia* 16:11-16, 2001 (abstract).
34. Schafer ML, Lautenbacher S, Postberg-Flesch C: New investigations on the melancholic type personality structure in migraine patients [in German], *Nervenarzt* 71:573-579, 2000 (abstract).
35. Hassinger HJ, Semenchuk EM, O'Brien WH: Appraisal and coping responses to pain and stress in migraine headache sufferers, *J Behav Med* 22:327-340, 1999.
36. Guillem E, Pelissolo A, Lepine JP: Mental disorders and migraine: epidemiologic studies [in French], *Encephale* 25:436-442, 1999 (abstract).
37. Lanzi G, Zambrino CA, Ferrari-Ginevra O et al: Personality traits in childhood and adolescent headache, *Cephalalgia* 21:53-60, 2001.
38. Linder SL, Winner P: Pediatric headache, *Med Clin North Am* 85:1037-1053, 2001.
39. American Academy of Pediatrics Statement of Endorsement: pharmacological treatment of migraine headache in children and adolescents, *Pediatrics* 115:1107, 2005.
40. Lewis D, Ashwal S, Hershey A et al: American Academy of Neurology Quality Standards Subcommittee; Practice Committee of the Child Neurology Society: Practice parameter: pharmacological treatment of migraine headache in children and adolescents: report of the American Academy of Neurology Quality Standards Subcommittee and the Practice Committee of the Child Neurology Society, *Neurology* 63:2215-2224, 2004.
41. Lipton RB, Silberstein SD, Stewart WF: An update on the epidemiology of migraine, *Headache* 34:319-328, 1994.
42. Sewart WF, Lipton RB, Celentano DD et al: Prevalence of migraine headaches in the United States, *J Am Med Assoc* 267:64-69, 1992.
43. Gervil M: Headache in children [in Danish], *Ugeskr Laeger* 159:2680-2685, 1997.
44. Silberstein SD: Twenty questions about headaches in children and adolescents, *Headache* 30:716-724, 1990.

45. Lipton RB, Goadsby P, Silberstein SD: Classification and epidemiology of headache, *Clin Cornerstone* 1:1-10, 1999.

46. Wober C, Wober-Bingol C: Clinical management of young patients presenting with headache, *Functional Neurol* 15(Suppl 3): 89-105, 2000.

47. Winner PK: Headaches in children. When is a complete diagnostic workup indicated? *Postgrad Med* 101: 81-85, 89-90, 1997.

48. Fichtel A, Larsson B: Does relaxation treatment have differential effects on migraine and tension-type headache in adolescents? *Headache* 41:290-296, 2001.

49. Bischko JJ: Acupuncture in headache, *Res Clin Studies Headache* 5:72-85, 1978.

Acupuncture

1. Melchart D, Linde K, Fischer P, et al: Acupuncture for idiopathic headache (Cochrane Review), Cochrane Database 1:CD001218, 2001.

2. Dowson DI, Lewith GT, Machin D: The effects of acupuncture versus placebo in the treatment of headache, *Pain* 21:35-42, 1985.

3. Loh L, Nathan PW, Schott GD et al: Acupuncture versus medical treatment for migraine and muscle tension headaches, *J Neurol Neurosurg Psychiatry* 47:333-337, 1984.

4. Vesnina VA: Current methods of migraine reflexotherapy [in Russian], *Zh Nevropatol Psikhiatr Im S Korsakova* 80:703-709, 1980.

5. Zhang X, Li Y, Ren S et al: Efficacy and effect of SI17 therapy on pancreatic polypeptide in vascular and tension-type headache, *J Tradit Chin Med* 20:206-209, 2000.

6. Liu H: Illustrative cases treated by the application of the extra point sishencong, *J Tradit Chin Med* 18:111-114, 1998.

7. Wu JS: Observation on analgesic effect of acupuncturing the dazhui point, *J Tradit Chin Med* 9:240-242, 1989.

8. Coeytaux RR, Kaufman JS, Kaptchuk TJ et al: A randomized, controlled trial of acupuncture for chronic daily headache, *Headache* 45:1113-1123, 2005.

9. Loo M: *Pediatric acupuncture*, London, 2002, Elsevier.

10. Gallai V, Sarchielli P, Carboni F et al: Applicability of the 1988 IHS criteria to headache patients under the age of 18 years attending 21 Italian headache clinics. Juvenile Headache Collaborative Study Group, *Headache* 35:146-153, 1995.

11. Markelova VF, Vesnina VA, Malygina SI et al: Changes in blood serotonin levels in patients with migraine headaches before and after a course of reflexotherapy [in Russian], *Zh Nevropatol Psikhiatr Im S S Korsakova* 84:1313-1316, 1984 (abstract).

12. Riederer P, Tenk H, Werner H et al: Manipulation of neurotransmitters by acupuncture (A preliminary communication), *J Neural Transm* 37:81-94, 1975.

13. Pintov S, Lahat E, Alstein M et al: Acupuncture and the opioid system: implications in management of migraine, *Pediatr Neurol* 17:129-133, 1997.

14. Yu S, Kuang P, Zhang F et al: Anti-inflammatory effects of tianrong acupoint on blood vessels of dura mater, *J Tradit Chin Med* 15:209-213, 1995.

15. Duo X: 100 cases of intractable migraine treated by acupuncture and cupping, *J Tradit Chin Med* 19:205-206, 1999.

16. Reilly R: Acute and prophylactic treatment of migraine, *Nurs Times* 90:35-36, 1994.

17. Massiou H: Prophylactic treatments of migraine, *Rev Neurol (Paris)* 156(Suppl 4):4S79-4S86, 2000.

18. Hesse J, Mogelvang B, Simonsen H: Acupuncture versus metoprolol in migraine prophylaxis: a randomized trial of trigger point inactivation, *J Intern Med* 235:451-456, 1994.

19. Baischer W: Acupuncture in migraine: long-term outcome and predicting factors, *Headache* 35:472-474, 1995.

20. Gao S, Zhao D, Xie Y: A comparative study on the treatment of migraine headache with combined distant and local acupuncture points versus conventional drug therapy, *Am J Acupunct* 27:27-30, 1999.

21. Vincent CA: A controlled trial of the treatment of migraine acupuncture, *Clin J Pain* 5:305, 1989.

22. Liguori A, Petti F, Bangrazi A et al: Comparison of pharmacological treatment versus acupuncture treatment for migraine without aura—analysis of socio-medical parameters, *J Tradit Chin Med* 20:231-240, 2000.

23. Johnson GD: Medical management of migraine-related dizziness and vertigo, *Laryngoscope* 108:1-28, 1998.

24. Baischer W: Psychological aspects as predicting factors for the indication of acupuncture in migraine patients [in German], *Wien Klin Wochenschr* 105:200-203, 1993 (abstract).

25. Chrubasik S, Kress W: Value of acupuncture in treatment of migraine [in German], *Anaesthesiol Reanim* 20:150-152, 1995 (abstract).

26. Hu J: Acupuncture treatment of migraine in Germany, *J Tradit Chin Med* 18:99-101, 1998.

27. Linde K, Streng A, Jurgens S et al: Acupuncture for patients with migraine: a randomized controlled trial, *J Am Med Assoc* 293: 2118-2125, 2005.

28. Vickers AJ, Rees RW, Zollman CE et al: Acupuncture of chronic headache disorders in primary care: randomised controlled trial and economic analysis, *Health Technol Assess* 8:iii, 1-35, 2004.

29. Melchart D, Hager S, Hager U et al: Treatment of patients with chronic headaches in a hospital for traditional Chinese medicine in Germany. A randomised, waiting list controlled trial, *Complement Ther Med* 12:71-78, 2004.

30. Seiden AM, Martin VT: Headache and the frontal sinus, *Otolaryngol Clin North Am* 34:227-241, 2001.

31. Annequin D, Tourniaire B, Dumas C: Migraine, misunderstood pathology in children [in French], *Arch Pediatr* 7:985-990, 2000 (abstract).

32. Diener HC, Dichgans J, Scholz E et al: Analgesic-induced chronic headache: long-term results of withdrawal therapy, *J Neurol* 236: 9-14, 1989 (abstract).

33. Hu J: Headache, *J Tradit Chin Med* 14:237-240, 1994.

34. Maciocia G: *The foundations of Chinese medicine, a comprehensive text for acupuncturists and herbalists*, London, 1989, Churchill Livingstone.

35. Zhu Z, Wang X: Clinical observation on the therapeutic effects of wrist-ankle acupuncture in treatment of pain of various origins, *J Tradit Chin Med* 18:192-194, 1998.

36. Rao X: Clinical application of taichong acupoint, *J Tradit Chin Med* 20:38-39, 2000.

37. Lin B: Treatment of frontal headache with acupuncture on zhongwan—a report of 110 cases, *J Tradit Chin Med* 11:7-8, 1991.

Aromatherapy

1. Gobel H, Schmidt G, Soyka D: Effect of peppermint and eucalyptus oil preparations on neurophysiological and experimental algesimetric headache parameters, *Cephalalgia* 14:228-234, 1994.

2. Ching M: Contempory therapy: aromatherapy in the management of acute pain? *Contemp Nurse* 8:146-151, 1999.

3. Germaine M: Aromatherapy for migraines, *Aromatherapy Summer*:2-3, 1999.

4. Mauskop A: The role of alternative therapies in headache, *NHF Headlines* Nov/Dec:1-3, 5, 2002.

5. Battaglia S: *The complete guide to aromatherapy*, Virginia, Queensland, Australia, 1995, The Perfect Potion.

Chiropractic

1. Tuchin PJ, Bonello R: Classic migraine or not classic migraine, that is the question, *Austr J Chiropractic Osteopath* 5:66-74, 1996.
2. Kidd R, Nelson C: Musculoskeletal dysfunction of the neck in migraine and tension headache, *Headache* 33:566-569, 1993.
3. Marcus DA: Migraine and tension type headaches: the questionable validity of current classification systems, *Pain* 8:28-36, 1992.
4. Bogduk N: The anatomical basis for cervicogenic headache, *J Manipulative Physiol Ther* 15:67-70, 1992.
5. Tuchin PJ: The efficacy of chiropractic spinal manipulative therapy (SMT) in the treatment of migraine—a pilot study, *Austr Chiropractic Osteopath* 6:41-47, 1997.
6. Curl DD: Chiropractic aspects of headache as a somatovisceral problem. In Masarsky CS, Todres-Masarsky M, editors: *The somatovisceral aspects of chiropractic*, Philadelphia, 2001, Churchill Livingstone.
7. Pikus HJ, Phillips JM: Outcome of surgical decompression of the second cervical root for cervicogenic headache, *Neurosurg* 39:63-71, 1996.
8. Balduc H: Neurological system. In Lawrence DJ, editor: *Fundamentals of chiropractic diagnosis and management*, Baltimore, 1991, Williams and Wilkins.
9. Nelson CF: The tension headache, migraine headache continuum: a hypothesis, *J Manipulative Physiol Ther* 17:156-167, 1994.
10. Boline PD, Kassak K, Bronfort G et al: Spinal manipulation vs. amitriptyline for the treatment of chronic tension-type headaches: a randomized clinical trial, *J Manipulative Physiol Ther* 18:148-154, 1995.
11. Nillson N, Christensen HW, Hartvigsen J: The effect of spinal manipulation in the treatment of cervicogenic headache, *J Manipulative Physiol Ther* 20:326-330, 1997.
12. Mootz RD, Dhami MSI, Hess JA et al: Chiropractic treatment of chronic episodic tension type headache in male subjects: a case series analysis, *J Can Chiropractic Assoc* 38:152-159, 1994.
13. Tuchin PJ, Pollard H, Bonello R: A randomized controlled trial of chiropractic spinal manipulative therapy for migraine, *J Manipulative Physiol Ther* 23:91-95, 2000.
14. Vernon H: Chiropractic manipulative therapy in the treatment of headaches: a retrospective and prospective study, *J Manipulative Physiol Ther* 5:109-112, 1982.
15. Hoyt WH, Shaffer F, Bard DA et al: Osteopathic manipulation in the treatment of muscle-contraction headache, *J Am Osteopath Assoc* 78:49-52, 1979.
16. Droz JM, Crot F: Occipital headaches, *Ann Swiss Chiropractic Assoc* 8:127-135, 1986.
17. Wright JS: Migraine: a statistical analysis of chiropractic treatment, *J Chiropractic* 12:63-67, 1978.
18. Knutson GA: Vectored upper cervical manipulation or chronic sleep bruxism, headache, and cervical spine pain in a child, *J Manipulative Physiol Ther* 26:1-3, 2003.
19. Anderson-Peacock ES: Chiropractic care of children with headaches: five case reports, *J Clin Chiropractic Pediatr* 1:18-26, 1996.
20. Hewitt EG: Chiropractic care of a 13-year old with headache and neck pain: a case report, *J Can Chiropractic Assoc* 38:160-162, 1994.
21. Cochran JA: Chiropractic treatment of childhood migraine headache: a case study, *Proceed Natl Conf Chiropractic Pediatr* 85-90, 1994.
22. Stephns D, Gorman F: The prospective treatment of visual perception deficit by chiropractic spinal manipulation: a report on two juvenile patients, *Chiropractic J Austr* 26:82-86, 1996.
23. Vernon HT: Spinal manipulation and headaches of cervical origin: a review of literature and presentation of cases, *Manual Med* 6:73-79, 1991.
24. Dwyer A, Aprill C, Bogduk N: Cervical zygopophyseal joint pain patterns: a study in normal volunteers, *Spine* 15:453-457, 1990.
25. Davies N: *Chiropractic pediatrics*, London, 2000, Churchill Livingstone.
26. Nagasawa A, Sakakibara T, Takahashi A: Roentgenographic findings of the cervical spine in tension-type headache, *Headache* 33:90-95, 1993.
27. Hagino CC, Steiman I, Vernon HT: Cervicogenic dysfunction in muscle contraction headache and migraine, *J Manipulative Physiol Ther* 15:418-429, 1992.
28. Magoun HI: Trauma: a neglected cause of cephalgia, *J Am Osteopath Assoc* 74:400-410, 1975.
29. Chapman SL: A review and clinical perspective on the use of EMG and thermal biofeedback for chronic headaches, *Pain* 27:1-43, 1986.
30. Collett L, Cottraux J, Juenet C: GSR feedback and Shultz relaxation in tension headaches: a comparative study, *Pain* 25:205-213, 1986.

Herbs—Western

1. McKevoy GK, editor: *AHFS drug information*, Bethesda, Md, 1998, American Society of Health-System Pharmacists.
2. Peppermint. Available at www.naturaldatabase.com. Accessed Jan 18, 2005.
3. Blumenthal M, Goldberg A, Brinckmann J, editors: *Herbal Medicine Expanded Commission E Monographs*, Newton, Mass, 2000, Integrative Medicine Communications.
4. Headaches. Available at www.naturaldatabase.com. Accessed Jan 18, 2005.
5. Awang DVC: Prescribing therapeutic feverfew (*Tanacetum parthenium* (L.) Schultz Bip., syn. *Chrysanthemumparthenium* (L.) Bernh), *Int Med* 1:11-13, 1998.
6. de Weerdt GJ, Bootsman HPR, Hendriks H: Herbal medicines in migraine prevention. Randomized double-blind, placebo-controlled, crossover trial of a feverfew preparation, *Phytomedicine* 3:225-230, 1996.
7. Harel Z, Gascon G, Riggs S et al: Supplementation with omega-3 polyunsaturated fatty acids in the management of recurrent migraines in adolescents, *J Adolesc Health* 31:154-161, 2002.
8. *Olive oil*. Available at www.naturaldatabase.com. Accessed Mar 25, 2005.

Massage Therapy

1. Borg-Stein J: Cervical myofascial pain and headaches, *Curr Pain Headache Rep* 6:324-330, 2002.
2. Alvarez DJ, Rockwell PG: Trigger points: diagnosis and management, *Am Fam Physician* 68:653-660, 2002.
3. Hong CZ, Simons DG: Pathophysiologic and electrophysiologic mechanisms of myofascial trigger points, *Arch Phys Med Rehabil* 79:863-872, 1998.
4. Simons DG, Travel JG, Simons LS et al: *Travell & Simons' myofascial pain and dysfunction: the trigger point manual*, ed 2, vols 1 and 2, Baltimore, 1998, Lippincott, Williams and Wilkins.
5. Hanten WP, Olson SL, Butts NL et al: Effectiveness of a home program of ischemic pressure followed by sustained stretch for treatment of myofascial trigger points, *Phys Ther* 81:1059-1060, 2001.
6. Gam AN, Warming S, Larsen LH et al: Treatment of myofascial trigger-points with ultrasound combined with massage and exercise—a randomized controlled trial, *Pain* 77:73-79, 1998.
7. Foster KA, Liskin J, Cen S et al: The Trager approach in the treatment of chronic headache: a pilot study, *Altern Ther Health Med* 10:40-46, 2004.

8. Hernandez-Reif M, Dieter J, Field T et al: Migraine headaches are reduced by massage therapy, *Int J Neurosci* 96:1-11, 1998.

9. Quinn C, Chandler C, Moraska A: Massage therapy and frequency of chronic tension headaches, *Am J Pub Health* 92:1657-1661, 2002.

10. Kaada B, Torsteinbo O: Increase of plasma endorphins in connective tissue massage, *Gen Pharmacol* 20:487-489, 1989.

11. Richards KC, Gibson R, Overton-McCoy AL: Effect of massage in acute and critical care: *AACN Clin Issues* 11:77-96, 2000.

12. Tsao JC: Effectiveness of massage therapy for chronic, non-malignant pain: a review, *Evid Based Complement Alternat Med* 4:165-179, 2007.

13. LeBlanc-Louvry I, Costaglioli B, Boulon C et al: Does mechanical massage of the abdominal wall after colectomy reduce postoperative pain and shorten the duration of ileus? Results of a randomized study, *J Gastrointest Surg* 6:43-49, 2002.

14. Piotrowski MM, Paterson C, Mitchinson A et al: Massage as adjunctive therapy in the management of acute postoperative pain: a preliminary study in men, *J Am Coll Surg* 197:1037-1046, 2003.

15. Taylor AG, Galpner DI, Taylor P et al: Effects of adjunctive Swedish massage and vibration therapy on short-term postoperative outcomes: a randomized, controlled trial, *J Altern Complement Med* 9:77-89, 2003.

16. van der Dolder PA, Roberts DL: A trial into the effectiveness of soft tissue massage in the treatment of shoulder pain, *Austr J Physiother* 49:183-188, 2003.

17. Mitchinson AR, Kim HM, Rosenberg JM et al: Acute postoperative pain management using massage as an adjuvant therapy: a randomized trial, *Arch Surg* 142:1158-1167, 2007.

Mind/Body

1. Hermann C, Kim M, Blanchard E: Behavioral and prophylactic pharmacological intervention studies of pediatric migraine: an exploratory meta-analysis, *Pain* 20:239-256, 1995.

2. Holden E, Deichmann M, Levy J: Empirically supported treatments in pediatric psychology: recurrent pediatric headache, *J Pediatr Psychol* 24:91-109, 1999.

3. Hermann C, Blanchard E: Biofeedback in the treatment of headache and other childhood pain, *Appl Psychophysiol Biofeedback* 27:143-162, 2002.

4. Andrasik F, Schwartz M: Pediatric headache, In Schwartz M, Andrasik F, editors: *Biofeedback: a practitioner's guide*, New York, 2003, Guilford Press.

5. Powers W, Mitchell M, Byars K et al: A pilot study of one-session biofeedback training in pediatric headache, *Neurology* 56:133, 2001.

6. Culbert T, Banez G. Pediatric applications other than headache. In Schwartz M, Andrasik F: *Biofeedback: a practitioner's guide*, ed 3, New York, 2003, Guilford Press.

7. McGrath P, Hillier L: Recurrent headache: triggers, causes, and contributing factors. In McGrath P, Hillier L, editors: *The child with headache: diagnosis and treatment*, Seattle, 2003, IASP Press.

8. Eccleston C, Yorke L, Morley S, et al: Psychological therapies for the management of chronic and recurrent pain in children and adolescents, *Cochrane Data System Rev* 1:CD003968, 2003.

9. Zsombok T, Juhasz G, Budavari A et al: Effect of autogenic training on drug consumption in patients with primary headache: an 8-month follow-up study, *Headache* 43:251-257, 2003.

10. Astin J, Beckner M, Soeken K et al: Psychological interventions in rheumatoid arthritis: a meta-analysis of randomized controlled trials, *Arthritis Rheum* 47:291-302, 2002.

11. Olness K, MacDonald J, Uden D: A prospective study comparing self hypnosis, propranolol and placebo in management of juvenile migraine, *Pediatrics* 79:593-597, 1987.

12. Olness K, Theoharides T, Hall H et al: Mast cell activation in child migraine patients before and after training in self regulation, *Headache* 41:130-138, 1999.

Nutrition

1. Wang F, Van Den Eeden SK, Acherson LM et al: Oral magnesium oxide prophylaxis of frequent migrainous headache in children: a randomized, double-blind, placebo-contolled trial, *Headache* 32:601-610, 2003.

2. Altura BM, Altura BT: Tension headaches and muscle tension: is there a role for magnesium? *Med Hypothesis* 57:705-713, 2001.

3. Schoenen J, Jacquy J, Lenaerts M: Effectiveness of high-dose riboflavin in migraine prophylaxis. A randomized controlled trial, *Neurology* 50:466-469, 1998.

4. Harel Z, Gason G, Riggs S et al: Supplementation with omega-3 polyunsaturated fatty acids in the management of recurrent migraines in adolescents, *J Adolesc Health* 31:154-161, 2002.

5. Karaagaoglu N, Yucecan S: Some behavioural changes observed among fasting subjects, their nutritional habits, and energy expenditure in Ramadan, *Int J Food Sci Nutr* 51:125-134, 2000.

Osteopathy

1. Bogduk N: The anatomical basis for cervicogenic headache, *J Manipulative Physiol Ther* 15:67-70, 1992.

2. Bogduk N: The clinical anatomy of the cervical dorsal rami, *Spine* 7:319-330, 1982.

3. Carreiro JE: Neurology. In Carreiro JE: *An osteopathic approach to children*, London, 2003, Churchill Livingstone.

4. Fitzgerald RTD: Observations on trigger points, fibromyalgia, recurrent headache and cervical syndrome, *J Man Med* 6:124-129, 1991.

5. Magoun HIS: *Osteopathy in the cranial field*, ed 3, Kirksville, Mo, 1976, The Journal Printing Company.

6. Willard FH: Autonomic nervous system. In Ward R, editor: *Foundations for osteopathic medicine*, ed 2, Philadelphia, 2003, Lippincott Williams and Wilkins.

7. Hack GD, Kortizer RT, Robinson WL et al: Anatomic relation between the rectus capitus posterior minor muscle and the dura mater, *Spine* 20:2484-2486, 1995.

Psychology

1. Siniatchkin M, Hierundar A, Kropp P et al: Self-regulation of slow cortical potentials in children with migraine: an exploratory study, *Appl Psychophysiol Biofeedback* 25:13-32, 2000.

2. Scharff L, Marcus DA, Masek BJ: A controlled study of minimal-contact thermal biofeedback treatment in children with migraine, *J Pediatr Psychol* 27:109-119, 2002.

3. Hermann C, Blanchard E: Biofeedback in the treatment of headache and other childhood pain, *Appl Psychophysiol Biofeedback* 27:143-162, 2002.

4. Allen K, Shriver M: Role of parent-mediated pain behavior management strategies in biofeedback treatment of childhood migraines, *Behav Ther* 29:477-490, 1998.

5. Andorfer R, Allen K: Extending the efficacy of a thermal biofeedback treatment package to the management of tension-type headaches in children, *Headache* 41:183-192, 2001.

6. Severson H, Eisenberg R: *Relaxation and self-esteem tape for children. An audiocassette tape for children aged 5-10*, Eugene, Ore, 1989, Rainbow Production.

CHAPTER 40

Heat Rash

Acupuncture | May Loo

Herbs—Western | Alan D. Woolf, Paula M. Gardiner,
Lana Dvorkin-Camiel, Jack Maypole

✳ PEDIATRIC DIAGNOSIS AND TREATMENT

Heat rash, or miliaria rubra, is a disorder of the eccrine glands. Sweat glands are found over nearly the entire skin surface and provide the primary means, through evaporation of the water in sweat, for cooling the body. These glands can become occluded by keratinous plugs in the sweat duct and become unable to clear sweat during hot and humid weather. The retained sweat manifests as miliaria rubra—erythematous, minute papulovesicles that may impart a prickling sensation.

The lesions are most commonly localized to sites of occlusion or flexural areas, such as the neck, groin, and axillae, where friction may contribute to their pathogenesis. Involved skin may become macerated and eroded. Severe, extensive miliaria rubra may result in disturbance of heat regulation. Lesions of miliaria rubra may become infected, particularly in malnourished or debilitated infants.

Miliaria rubra is generally reversible, responding dramatically to cooling measures such as air conditioning, gentle breeze from a fan, or removal of excessive clothing. Lightweight, soft cotton clothing is advisable for summer wear, as cotton is very absorbent and keeps moisture away from the skin. Topical agents such as powders, creams, and ointments are usually ineffective and may exacerbate the eruption by keeping the skin warm and further occluding the pores. Supplemental vitamin C may help restore normal sweating in refractory cases.[1-4]

✳ CAM THERAPY RECOMMENDATIONS

Acupuncture

In Chinese medicine the skin and sweat glands are functionally part of the Lung. Heat rash is therefore a manifestation of Lung Heat. The easiest treatment is dispersing Lung Heat:
Two-Point protocol: Tonify LU5; sedate LU10.
Four-Point protocol: Tonify LU5; sedate LU10; tonify KI10; sedate HT8.

Needling tonification/sedation of a point can be carried out by turning the needle clockwise (with the child as the clock) for tonification and counterclockwise for sedation.

Acumassage tonification/sedation of a point can be carried out by massaging the point clockwise (with the child as the clock) for tonification and counterclockwise for sedation.

Magnets can be easily applied to children of all ages:
South pole down on points for tonification: on LU5, KI10.
North pole down for sedation: on LU10, HT8.

General points for Heat dispersion can also be incorporated:
GV14 (Dazhui), LI11 (Quchi)

The child should drink extra fluids and avoid thermodynamically hot foods.

Herbs—Western

Heat rash is a skin irritation marked by redness, small raised bumps, chafing, and a burning or itching sensation. It is self-limited and responds to exposure of the affected skin to cooler, dry air temperature.

References

Pediatric Diagnosis and Treatment

1. In Behrman RE, Kliegman RM, Jenson HB, editors: *Nelson textbook of pediatrics*, ed 17, Philadelphia, 2004, Saunders.
2. Sato K, Kang WH, Saga K et al: Biology of sweat glands and their disorders. II. Disorders of sweat gland function, *J Am Acad Dermatol* 20:713-726, 1989.
3. Sato K, Kang WH, Saga K et al: Biology of sweat glands and their disorders, *J Am Acad Dermatol* 20:537-563, 1989.
4. Hart JA: Babies and heat rashes; rash—child under 2 years. In *MedlinePlus Medical Encyclopedia*, National Institutes of Health, Department of Health & Human Services. Available at www.nlm.nih.gov/medlineplus. Accessed July 2, 2005.

CHAPTER 41

Hiccups

Acupuncture | May Loo
Chiropractic | Anne Spicer

Magnet Therapy | Agatha P. Colbert, Deborah Risotti
Osteopathy | Jane Carreiro

✳ PEDIATRIC DIAGNOSIS AND TREATMENT

Hiccups are due to brief, powerful involuntary spasm and contraction of the diaphragm and the auxiliary respiratory muscles during inspiration, followed by glottic closure. The movement of inspiratory air is rushed, producing a typical "hiccupping" sound.[1,2] *Chronic hiccup* is defined as recurrent episodes of hiccups or a duration exceeding 48 hours.[2] Hiccups is a physiological gastrointestinal (GI) reflex that already exists in utero[2] and appears to still occur frequently in young infants.[1] Possible etiology includes gastroesophageal reflux[2] or is secondary to feeding gastrostomy,[3] tracheostomy,[2] intubation,[1] and as side effects to medications, such as diazepam, a medication for treating seizures.[3] Although the physiological effect from hiccups is generally considered negligible,[2] upper airway obstruction has been found in unintubated, young infants[1] and respiratory alkalosis in tracheostomy[2] and gastrostomy[4] patients.

The majority of acute episodes of hiccups are self-limiting. Numerous remedies have been reported over the centuries, but no single "cure" stands out as being the most effective.[5] Various home remedies include telling the child to hold his or her breath for as long as possible or breathing in and out of a paper bag (a confined space)—both of which induce elevated levels of pCO_2 to stimulate respiration. Chronic and recurrent hiccups may be treated with medication, the most common being Baclofen.[2,4] More aggressive treatments in adults, such as calcium channel blocker Nifedipine[6] crushing of the phrenic nerve or microvascular decompression of the vagus nerve,[7] are not indicated in children.

✳ CAM THERAPY RECOMMENDATIONS

Acupuncture

In Chinese medicine,[1] hiccups are due to rebellious Stomach Qi that disrupts the downward movement of Lung Qi during inspiration. Various causes that are applicable in children include improper eating and diet, such as eating too fast[2] or eating excessive Cold and raw foods[2,3]; Liver Qi stagnation, such as from emotional disturbances; and prolonged illnesses that result in insufficient Qi in the digestive system.[3] Body points[2-5] auriculopoints,[6-8] and other microsystem points[9,10] have all been used for treatment of hiccups.

Treatment

Because children are not usually seen for acute episode of hiccups, acupressure of body points can be taught to the parents to administer during an attack. If the child is seen for recurrent or chronic hiccups, south pole tonification magnets can be applied to the body points, and pellets can be applied to microsystem ear points.

Main points: P6, CV17, ST36[3,4]

"Hiccup relieving point" is located at the middle of the posterior border of the sternocleidomastoid muscle, at the anatomical point where the phrenic nerve crosses the anterior scalenus muscle.[2]

Auxiliary points include: CV14, LI4,[3] ST25,[10] Middle Sifeng (extra point 29)[11] of the middle finger.

Auricular points: Shenmen, Point Zero, ST, Hiccups point.[6-8]

In the rare, severe cases, needling of LI18 (Futu) as a Yangming point[12] or electroacupuncture stimulation of the "hiccup relieving point" may be tried in children.[2]

Chiropractic

The chiropractic approach to management of hiccups would be to identify and correct any interference to normal neurological function by correction of the subluxation complex (SC). Because of the relatively long length of the phrenic nerve and immature myelination status, hiccups occur frequently in utero as well as in the first few months of life. The medulla oblongata controls respiration and passes into the area of the cervical cord at C1. If an SC is present in the area of C1 or C3-C5, there could be irritation to the respiratory control centers or the phrenic nerve resulting in abnormal frequency or protracted hiccups.

A single case report of an adult involving chiropractic management of intractable hiccups may be extrapolated to pediatric patients. A 58-year-old female had a 10-day history of hiccups precipitated by a case of pneumonia.[1] She experienced 15-minute hiccup paroxysms every 30 minutes. She had chiropractic adjustments to the cervical and thoracic spine along with soft tissue mobilization in the neck two times on the first day and subsequently reported 45-minute intervals without a single hiccup. She was able to sleep that night after only intermittent sleep in the past 2 weeks, and she awoke without hiccups. She was adjusted four more times in the next 2 weeks and never had a return of her hiccup symptoms.

Direct stimulation of the phrenic nerve may be useful.[2,3] This may be performed manually by applying compressive pressure to the phrenic nerve as it courses along the posterior aspect of the SCM muscle at the level of the cricoid cartilage. This should be performed bilaterally with sustained pressure for approximately 15 seconds and repeated as necessary.

A trigger point technique involves lifting the uvula. This is done with an instrument or manually with equal benefit.[4] In some cases, massaging the base of the uvula may provide more lasting effects.[5]

Similar to this technique is the use of a cotton-tipped swab to stimulate the palate.[6] In this procedure, the point of stimulation is on the midline, just posterior to the junction of the hard and soft palates, and the recommended duration of stimulation is 1 minute.

Another technique, as outlined by Travell, is to apply manual sustained protraction on the tongue of the patient with hiccups.[7]

An unresolved case of hiccups and chronic recurrent SC may indicate a viscerosomatic reflex from an underlying organic disease process and should be investigated or referred as such.

Magnet Therapy

Gently massage the area on the child's mid back between BL17 and BL22.[1] If this seems to be helping, place Neodymium nylon-coated Spot magnets of suitable size for the child (1-inch, ¾-inch, or ½-inch size), on the most significant point(s) between BL17 and BL22. These magnets may be obtained from Painfree Lifestyles (800-480-8601). If the hiccups persist and the child is younger than 2 years, add 800-G Accuband magnet with the designated bionorth side (the side with a tiny protrusion) to acupuncture points ST36 and ST41[1] on one side. If the child is older than 2 years and hiccups persist, add two 9000-G Accuband REC magnets. The designated north pole of this magnet (side with the indentation) should be placed on ST36 and the designated south pole (opposite side of the magnet) on ST41. The 9000-G Accuband REC magnets may be obtained from OMS (800-323-1839) or AHSM (800-635-7070).

Osteopathy

Persistent hiccups can be irritating to both infant and parent. From a traditional osteopathic perspective, the recurrence of persistent hiccups may be due to irritation to the diaphragm or phrenic nerve.[1,2] Irritation to the phrenic nerve may occur either as the nerve passes through the deep tissues of the anterior neck or through irritation to the cervical roots at the level of the third, fourth, or fifth cervical vertebrae. Diaphragmatic irritation may also be responsible for persistent hiccups. Diaphragmatic irritation may be caused by alterations in the biomechanical relationship of the crura and dome of the diaphragm. This may be associated with a slight increase in respiratory rate and decreased diaphragm excursion. Indirect and functional osteopathic techniques used to address somatic dysfunction in the cervical spine, anterior neck, and/or lower thoracic area have been described as being effective in halting the hiccups in adults.[1-3] However, there are no controlled studies evaluating the efficacy of osteopathic manipulation in the management of hiccups in children.

References

Pediatric Diagnosis and Treatment

1. Brouillette RT, Thach BT, Abu-Osba YK et al: Hiccups in infants: characteristics and effects on ventilation, *J Pediatr* 96:219-225, 1980.
2. Federspil PA, Zenk J: Hiccup [in German], *HNO* 47:867-875, 1999.
3. Behrman RE, Kliegman RM, Jenson HB, editors: *Nelson textbook of pediatrics*, ed 17, Philadelphia, 2004, Saunders.
4. Johnson BR, Kriel RL: Baclofen for chronic hiccups, *Pediatr Neurol* 15:66-67, 1996.
5. Lewis JH: Hiccups: causes and cures, *J Clin Gastroenterol* 7:539-592, 1985.
6. Lipps DC, Jabbari B, Mitchell MH et al: Nifedipine for intractable hiccups, *Neurology* 40:531-532, 1990.
7. Johnson DL: Intractable hiccups: treatment by microvascular decompression of the vagus nerve. Case report, *J Neurosurg* 78:813-816, 1993.

Acupuncture

1. Loo M: *Pediatric acupuncture*, London, 2002, Elsevier.
2. Yan LS: Treatment of persistent hiccupping with electroacupuncture at "hiccup-relieving" point, *J Tradit Chin Med* 8:29-30, 1988.
3. Zhao CX: Acupuncture and moxibustion treatment of hiccup, *J Tradit Chin Med* 9:182-183, 1989.
4. Deadman P, Al-Khafaji M: *A manual of acupuncture*, East Sussex, United Kingdom, 1998, Journal of Chinese Medicine Publications.
5. Cui S: Clinical application of acupoint tianshu, *J Tradit Chin Med* 12:52-54, 1992.
6. Oleson TD: *Auriculotherapy manual, Chinese and Western systems of ear acupuncture*, Los Angeles, 1992, Health Care Alternatives.
7. Li X, Yi J, Qi B: Treatment of hiccough with auriculo-acupuncture and auriculo-pressure—a report of 85 cases, *J Tradit Chin Med* 10:257-259, 1990.
8. Li F, Wang D, Ma X: Treatment of hiccoughs with auriculoacupuncture, *J Tradit Chin Med* 11:14-16, 1991.
9. Yoo TW: *Koryo hand acupuncture*, vol 1, Seoul, 1977, Korea, Eum Yang Mek Jin.
10. Schlager A: Korean hand acupuncture in the treatment of chronic hiccups, *Am J Gastroenterol* 93:2312-2313, 1998.
11. Qi Y: Treatment of hiccough with acupuncture on middle sifeng, *J Tradit Chin Med* 13:202, 1993.
12. Jiang YG: Clinical applications of point futu, *J Tradit Chin Med* 6:6-8, 1986.

Chiropractic

1. Diamond MF, Ouzounian PM: Chiropractic hiccup resolution: a case report, *J Am Chiro Assoc* May:46-50, 2001.
2. Aravot DJ, Wright G, Rees A et al: Non-invasive phrenic nerve stimulation for intractable hiccups, *Lancet* 2:1047, 1989.
3. Bhargava RP, Datta S, Badgaiya R: A simple technique to stop hiccups, *Ind J Physiol Pharmacol* Jan-Mar:58, 1985.
4. Travell J: A trigger point for hiccup, *J Am Osteop Assoc* 77:308-312, 1977.
5. Smolders J: Trigger points: myofacial treatment for persistent hiccups: a case report, *Dynamic Chiropractic* 5:3, 1987.
6. Goldsmith S: A treatment for hiccups, *J Am Med Assoc* 249:1566, 1983.
7. Adams M: Ambulance rider, *Woman's J* Jan 28, 1927.

Magnet Therapy

1. Loo M: *Pediatric acupuncture*, London, 2002, Elsevier.

Osteopathy

1. Armstrong WC: *Technique for hiccoughs*, 1941.

2. Sutherland WG: *Teachings in the science of osteopathy*, Portland, Ore, 1990, Rudra Press.
3. LePere JH: Halting hiccups with phrenic nerve pressure, *J Am Osteopath Assoc* 77:741, 1978.

CHAPTER 42

Hives

Acupuncture | May Loo

Herbs—Western | Alan D. Woolf, Paula M. Gardiner, Lana Dvorkin-Camiel, Jack Maypole

✳ PEDIATRIC DIAGNOSIS AND TREATMENT

Acute urticaria are hives with less than 6 weeks' duration,[1] and they occur frequently in children,[2-4] especially in infants and young children.[5] The most common causes are foods and drugs, inhaled and contact allergens, and infections.[1] Pathophysiological reaction can be either immunoglobulin (Ig)-E mediated or non–IgE mediated. IgE-mediated acute urticaria can be due to systemically absorbed allergens such as foods, drugs (particularly antibiotics), and stinging insect venoms, as well as contact urticaria such as from latex gloves. Non–IgE-mediated acute urticaria includes allergic reaction to radiocontrast agents, viruses such as hepatitis B and Epstein-Barr virus, opiates, and nonsteroidal antiinflammatory agents.[1,3,6,7]

Diagnosis begins with a careful history, especially searching for the association of onset of urticaria with any offending agent.[6] Confirmation can be made by elimination of specific foods and drugs, provocative skin tests, and challenge with suspected foods.[1,7,8] Acute urticaria is a frequent manifestation of food allergy,[8-10] with the most common foods being milk, egg, peanuts, soy, wheat, tree nuts, fish, and shellfish.[7,11] Inhaled allergens can be evaluated with tests for IgE (i.e., prick skin tests, radioallergosorbent tests).[1,3,11] Allergy to multiple foods and chronic allergic diseases, such as asthma or atopic dermatitis, would complicate the evaluation. In non–IgE-mediated hives, such as gastrointestinal (GI) food allergies, testing is not helpful. Well-devised elimination diets followed by physician-supervised oral food challenges are critical in proper identification.[11] Evaluation for infectious etiology should include appropriate cultures or serology.[1]

In addition to elimination of allergenic foods, oral food challenges should be an integral part of the long-term pediatric management, as children often outgrow food allergies.[11] Nonsedative antihistamines are the drugs of choice and generally provide substantial symptom relief until spontaneous remission occurs.[3] Newer antihistamines have better efficacy and are better tolerated by children.[5] Epinephrine is administered in the event of a serious reaction.[7] Twenty percent to 30% of acute urticaria cases will become chronic or recurrent.[12]

✳ CAM THERAPY RECOMMENDATIONS

Acupuncture

Acupuncture has been used worldwide to treat acute and chronic urticaria, but its usage is more prevalent in the Asian countries. The acute condition is considered to be Wind types that come and go quickly. Wind-Heat urticaria tends to be red, sometimes feels warm to the touch, and can be intensely pruritic. The child may have other Heat symptoms such as red cheeks and restlessness. Wind-Cold urticaria is lighter red or even white and the skin feels cold. The lesions improve with warm weather. Rashes associated with GI symptoms such as nausea, vomiting, or loose stools have Heat in the intestinal tract and may recur or become chronic. When light-colored urticaria occurs in a weak and pale child, the rash is due to deficiency of Blood, Qi, or both. This may occur especially after a child has had an illness and often recurs or becomes chronic, especially each time the child is ill or weak.[1-4]

Evidence-Based Information

There are no data on acupuncture treatment of hives in children. Clinical research has demonstrated that acupuncture decreases blood eosinophil and serum IgE in allergic conditions.[5]

Clinical observations from Taiwan indicate that acute urticaria is often easily and effectively treated with four acupoints: LI11 (Quchi), SP10 (Xuehai), SP6 (Sanyinjiao), and ST36 (Zusanli). A clinical study from China indicates that acupuncture can be effective against urticaria.[7]

Treatment Recommendations:

Treatment recommendations include the following[1-3,4,8]:
General treatment for itching: ST15, GB31.[1]
General treatment without pattern differentiation: LI11, SP10, SP6, ST36.[6]
Treatment according to pattern differentiation:
   Wind-Heat: GB20 to eliminate Wind.
   LI11 to expel Heat.
   Disperse Heat from the Lung meridian (Lung is associated with the skin):
      Tonify LU5; sedate LU10.
   Wind-Cold: GB20 to eliminate Wind.
   Expel Cold from the Lung meridian: Sedate LU5; tonify LU10.

Urticaria with GI symptoms:

SP6, ST36 to tonify SP, harmonize Stomach.

Disperse ST heat: Tonify ST44; sedate ST41.

Urticaria in a weak and deficient child:

SP10 to tonify Blood.

KI3, SP6 to tonify KI, SP.

ST36 to increase immunity.

This child should be monitored closely and be treated regularly to boost immunity and strengthen the overall system.

Herbs—Western

Itching associated with hives is best managed with oral diphenhydramine. Triggering of hives is best prevented by the avoidance of the offending irritant or allergen. The application of aloe vera gel may be helpful for reducing inflammation, but there are no studies to support its effectiveness for hives.

References

Pediatric Diagnosis and Treatment

1. Behrman RE, Kliegman RM, Jenson HB, editors: *Nelson textbook of pediatrics*, ed 17, Philadelphia, 2004, Saunders.
2. Baxi S, Dinakar C: Urticaria and angioedema, *Immunol Allergy Clin North Am* 25:353-367, 2005.
3. Hestholm F, Morken T, Skadberg BT et al: Urticaria and angioedema in children [in Norwegian], *Tidsskr Nor Laegeforen* 122:610-614, 2002 (abstract).
4. Greaves M: Management of urticaria, *Hosp Med* 61:463-469, 2000.
5. Richard MA, Grob JJ: Urticaria in the child [in French], *Arch Pediatr* 8:1383-1391, 2001 (abstract).
6. Greaves MW, Hussein SH: Drug-induced urticaria and angioedema: pathomechanisms and frequencies in a developing country and in developed countries, *Int Arch Allergy Immunol* 128:1-7, 2002.
7. Sicherer SH: Manifestations of food allergy: evaluation and management, *Am Fam Physician* 59:415-424, 429-430, 1999.
8. Burks W: Skin manifestations of food allergy, *Pediatrics* 111: 1617-1624, 2003.
9. Drouet M: Acute or chronic food allergy: adapted therapeutic and diagnostic procedure [in French], *Allerg Immunol (Paris)* 29: 15-20, 1997 (abstract).
10. Le Sellin J: Clinical signs of food allergy [in French], *Allerg Immunol (Paris)* 29:11-14, 1997 (abstract).
11. Sicherer SH: Food allergy: when and how to perform oral food challenges, *Pediatr Allergy Immunol* 10:226-234, 1999.
12. Mortureux P, Leaute-Labreze C, Legrain-Lifermann V et al: Acute urticaria in infancy and early childhood: a prospective study, *Arch Dermatol* 134:319-323, 1998.

Acupuncture

1. Deadman P, Al-Khafaji M: *A manual of acupuncture*, Ann Arbor, Mich, 1998, Journal of Chinese Medicine Publications.
2. Maciocia G: *The foundations of Chinese medicine, a comprehensive text for acupuncturists and herbalists*, London, 1989, Churchill Livingstone.
3. O'Connor J, Bensky D, editors: *Acupuncture, a comprehensive text*, Seattle, 1981, Eastland Press.
4. Diagnosis and treatment of gynecology and pediatrics. In *Chinese Zhenjiuology, a series of teaching videotapes*, Beijing, 1990, coproduced by Chinese Medical Audio-Video Organization and Meditalent Enterprises.
5. Lau BH, Wong DS, Slater JM: Effect of acupuncture on allergic rhinitis: clinical and laboratory evaluations, *Am J Chin Med (Gard City N Y)* 3:263-270, 1975.
6. Chen CJ, Yu HS: Acupuncture treatment of urticaria, *Arch Dermatol* 134:1397-1399, 1998.
7. Lai X: Observation on the curative effect of acupuncture on type I allergic diseases, *J Tradit Chin Med* 13:243-248, 1993.
8. Loo M: *Pediatric acupuncture*, London, 2002, Elsevier.

Immune System

Acupuncture | May Loo

Aromatherapy | Maura A. Fitzgerald

Chiropractic | Anne Spicer

Herbs—Chinese | Catherine Ulbricht, Jennifer Woods, Mark Wright

Herbs—Western | Alan D. Woolf, Paula M. Gardiner, Lana Dvorkin-Camiel, Jack Maypole

Magnet Therapy | Agatha P. Colbert, Deborah Risotti

Massage Therapy | Mary C. McLellan

Nutrition | Joy A. Weydert

Osteopathy | Jane Carreiro

✳ PEDIATRIC DIAGNOSIS AND TREATMENT

The human immune response is an extremely complex cascade of events that involves numerous different types of immune factors and biochemical mediators. The immune system can be broadly divided into humoral and cellular compartments. The *humoral response* refers to complement and immunoglobulin (Ig) antibody-mediated B-cell system. The *cellular response* refers to delayed hypersensitivity mediated via T cells, which consist of a wide variety of cells that include leukocytes, polymorphonuclear neutrophils (PMNs), eosinophils, mast cells, macrophages, and natural killer (NK) cells. This classification is not precise, as there is a great deal of interaction and crossover of functions. Recent studies have focused in depth on the proinflammatory mediators, such as cytokines and leukotrienes. These mediators are a heterogeneous group of biochemical compounds produced by a gamut of cells that includes epithelial cells, fibroblasts, PMNs, and macrophages. They trigger or orchestrate an immune response by acting as signals between cells of the immune system, leading to inflammatory responses against pathogens. Neurotransmitters in the central nervous system and nutrition also actively participate in the immune response. Although immune reactions can be protective to the host, a hyperimmune response can be destructive by damaging normal structures such that the regulatory process is necessary to prevent "immunological runaway."[1]

Immune deficiency is associated with recurrent infections, malnutrition, trauma, and immaturity of the immune system. Children with recurrent infections often manifest immune insufficiency.[2,3] Abnormalities of the local defense mechanisms of the upper airways are very common.[4] Poor nutrition, especially diet low in protein, can cause both humoral and cellular deficiencies. Iron, trace minerals, and vitamin deficiencies can all affect the child's immune system.[5-11] Trauma can induce a potent inflammatory response.[12,13] Even hemorrhage alone may be a sufficient stimulus to activate the immune system.[14] Infants and young children have immature immune systems and are at greater risk for infections.[6,15] The neonates especially have very inadequate immune systems such that they are vulnerable to infections and often respond poorly to vaccines.[16-20]

Although inadequate immune response predisposes children to illnesses and infections, current data also suggest that hyperactive immune or inflammatory response possibly due to poor regulatory control results in destruction of normal tissues. Asthma, inflammatory bowel disease (IBD), juvenile rheumatoid arthritis (JRA), cardiovascular disease, diabetes, and cancer are some of the chronic disorders attributed to uncontrolled hyperimmune response to an initial stimulus. Evidence suggests that JRA is caused by T cell infiltration of the synovial membrane.[21,22] Cardiovascular diseases in children, such as rheumatic heart disease, are secondary immune response to infections.[23] The presence of proinflammatory mediators in diabetes suggests that hyperinflammatory response to an infection causes pancreatic β-cell destruction.[24,25] Increased levels of mediators have also been found in cancer.[26] Recognition of the significance of proinflammatory mediators has generated fervent development of immune modulatory treatments. These treatments are costly, and only a few are approved for usage in children. There is no medication that induces natural immune defense or regulation.

Western medicine also considers skin, lungs, and liver as immune organs. The skin is a protective organ. The lungs have important B-cell secretion of antibodies and T cell–mediated immune responses to foreign antigens.[27] The liver hepatocytes produce acute phase proteins and complement in bacterial infections. Many cells participate in T-cell immune response against bacterial infections and hematogenous tumor metastases.[28]

✳ CAM THERAPY RECOMMENDATIONS

Acupuncture

Traditional Chinese medicine (TCM) traditionally incorporates strengthening of the immune system as part of the treatment of children. In TCM, Wei Qi is the Defensive Qi that circulates outside the channels and in the skin and connective tissues, controls the opening and closing of the pores, and acts like a "shield" to protect the body against external pathogens.

Acupuncture stimulates both humoral and cellular immune response as a protective mechanism and also exerts regulatory effect on hyperinflammation by modulating the synthesis and release of proinflammatory mediators. Current hypotheses suggest that a common pathway connects opioids and the immune system. The immune function is discussed in detail in Chapter 6 in the section on acupuncture.

A simple immune tonification or strengthening protocol is suggested here for general health maintenance: stimulating these points regularly with needles or noninvasive acupuncture or acupressure to prevent illnesses. During an acute illness, it is important not to use this protocol while the child is still ill, or still has the "bug," so the priority would be to expel the pathogen and then tonify the child. Otherwise, strengthening the ill child would also strengthen and "trap" the pathogens inside.[1] In chronic illnesses such as IBD, the priority of treatment is to first balance the internal organs and add immune tonification points as adjunctive therapy.

Simple, General Immune Tonification Protocol for Children

ST36

LI4 if used together with ST36

Shu points associated with Wei Qi production and movement:

BL13: Lung Shu

BL18: Liver Shu

BL20: Spleen Shu

BL21: Stomach Shu

BL23: Kidney Shu[1]

Other immunostimulant points include LI11, SP6, GV14, BL11, and CV12.

Reactive Back Shu and Front MU points are useful in organic diseases.[2]

Aromatherapy

Aromatherapy is thought to improve or support immune function by a direct effect on the immune system; its effect on mood, fatigue, and sleep; improvement in pain management; and its antiseptic properties.[1,2] A direct effect on the immune system by an essential oil is postulated but unproved. Aromatherapy researchers and authors have proposed that particular oils, including clove (*Syzygium aromaticum*), lemon verbena (*Lippis citriodora*), thyme (*Thymus vulgaris*), lavender (*Lavandula angustifolia*), and lemon (*Citrus limon*), affect immune functions such as production of white blood cells or immunogloblins.[2] However, research in this area is in early stages and often on animal models.

Alexander postulates that it may be possible to condition a positive immune response by successive exposures to an essential oil.[3] For example, if an essential oil is used in the successful treatment of a chronically recurring infection, such as herpes, the next time it is used the condition may respond quicker because the aroma triggers an immune response based on memory. The mild effect of the essential oil is enhanced through successive exposures that trigger an increasingly stronger physiological effect. Conditioning occurs because the essential oil has a perceptible odor (and taste), making it easy to recognize and associate. This principle was also the basis of a study on aromatherapy and epilepsy (see Chapter 34, Epilepsy) and could be applied to other situations in which a physiological response is desired, such as initiating the relaxation response or inducing sleep.[3]

Because of the complex relationship among immune function, chronic illness, and fatigue or rest, the most valuable role for aromatherapy in immune functioning may be in providing supportive treatment for symptoms and side effects. For example, aromatherapy that relieves anxiety or pain and enhances sleep improves the child's physical condition and his or her ability to withstand infection. Additionally, because most essential oils have antiseptic properties, diffusion in the area in which the child is spending time may reduce the number of airborne pathogens. A popular way to achieve this is to mix essential oils in a spray bottle and spray periodically in a room. Many essential oils have antibacterial or antiviral properties, including lemon (*C. limon*), lemon balm (*Melissa officinalis*), spike lavender (*Lavandula spica*), ravensara (*Ravensara aromatica*), rosemary (*Rosmarinus officinalis*), eucalyptus (*Eucalyptus* sp.), sandalwood (*Santalum album*), and peppermint (*Mentha piperita*).[2]

In a randomized controlled trial on alopecia areata, a condition often caused by autoimmune reaction, 86 adults were randomly assigned to two groups: scalp massage only or scalp massage with addition of essential oils. The essential oils were combined as thyme (*T. vulgaris*), 2 drops; lavender (*L. angustifolia*), 3 drops; rosemary (*R. officinalis*), 3 drops; and cedar (*Cedrus atlantica*), 2 drops, in a carrier oil composed of 3 mL jojoba and 20 mL grapeseed oils. The massage-only group used the carrier oil combination without the essential oils. Subjects were instructed to perform scalp massage nightly for a minimum of 2 minutes and to wrap a warm towel around the head after the massage. Subjects were not blinded to smell. Assessment of change in hair coverage was made by objective measures and the review of pre- and post-photographs by dermatologists who were blinded to the intervention groups. The aromatherapy massage group improved to a greater degree than the massage-alone group.[5]

Chiropractic

The effect of the chiropractic adjustment was posed by the founder to be a reduction in the tension on the nerves, thereby allowing normal transmission of nerve energy.[1] Although this has not been disproved, other physiological effects that take place following an adjustment may more closely answer the question of immune impact by chiropractic. It is well understood that increased stress reactions play a suppressive role in immune function and participate in disease processes.[2] Studies demonstrate that the chiropractic adjustment is followed by decreased stress reaction as seen in decreased cortisol levels[3] and increased endorphin levels.[4,5] Inflammatory cytokines also decrease after chiropractic adjustments.[6] Adjustments to the spine also augment IgA, IgG, and IgM[7], whereas fixations at the spinal joints induce immunosuppression.[8] A study that involved twice-weekly adjustments of radiographically established subluxation complex found a substantial increase in B-lymphocytes by the end of the 1-month trial.[9] In a randomized controlled trial (RCT), subjects receiving chiropractic adjustments to the thoracic spine had significant increases in both PMNs and monocytes as compared with pretreatment status and with control groups.[10] A study involving patients with active acquired immune deficiency syndrome (AIDS) resulted in a remarkable 48% increase in CD4 counts after chiropractic adjustments to the upper cervical spine, compared with a decrease of 7.96% in the control group.[11] More frequently, researchers are identifying a significant, if not primary, role of the nervous system in moderating immune function[12-16] Normalizing nerve function at the spinal level is the major goal of the chiropractic spinal adjustment.

Diet also plays an extremely important role in body physiology.[17,18] Wherever possible, the chiropractor recommends organic foods that minimize the toxic load on the body from substances such as pesticides, herbicides, and chemical ripening agents. Any foods that enhance antiinflammatory function should be added to or increased in the daily diet, particularly fresh fruits and vegetables. Proinflammatory foods, such as those with sugars, processed grains, and trans fats, should be avoided.

Eicosapentaenoic acid (EPA)/docosahexaenoic acid (DHA) supplementation has been shown to enhance immune activity in the body.[19]

Zinc is vital for normal immune function.

Vitamin A is particularly useful in minimizing the manifestations of infectious disease.

Herbs—Chinese

The root and rhizome of *Ligusticum sinense* Oliv. (Gao Ben), root of *Panax ginseng* C.A. Mey. (Ren Shen), fruit of *Schisandra chinensis* (Turcz.) Baill. (Wu Wei Zi), and root of *Astragalus membranaceus* (Fisch.) Bunge (Huang Qi), four commonly used Chinese herbs, may boost the human immune system based on the results of several animal and human studies.[1,2]

Huang Qi is often used in the treatment of numerous ailments, including heart, liver, and kidney diseases, as well as cancer, viral infections, and immune system disorders.[2] Also, paeonol, believed to be the active ingredient in rootbark of *Paeonia suffruticosa* Andrews (Mu Dan Pi), has been shown to have some therapeutic effects in resisting many species of fungi and bacteria. However, the mechanism of such effects remains unclear, and more research is needed.[3,2]

From the TCM perspective, the Spleen most closely correlates with the Western concept of the immune system. In other words, patients presenting with weak immune response are generally considered to be Spleen Qi deficient in TCM. In practice, patients who repeatedly catch colds are often treated either with Yu Ping Feng San or Bu Zhong Yi Qi Tang (see Chapter 10, Allergies). Both these formulations contain a combination of herbs that are regarded as able to fend off or actively treat colds (e.g., root of *Saposhnikovia divaricata* [Turcz.] Schischk. and fresh rhizome of *Zingiber officinale* [Willd.] Roscoe) on the one hand, and on the other hand as supplementing the Spleen Qi (i.e., boosting the immune system) (e.g., root of *A. membranaceus* [Fisch.] Bunge, rhizome of *Atractylodes macrocephala* [Koidz.]).

Work suggests that root of *A. membranaceus* promotes lymphocyte transformation, induces interferon (IFN) production, and promotes Ig production. Although rhizome of *A. macrocephala* enhances phagocytosis of neutrophils, roots of *P. ginseng* C.A. Mey. (RenShen) and *Codonopsis pilosula* (Franch.) Nannf. are reported to increase the number of leukocytes.[4]

Herbs—Western

The foundation of a healthy immune system in children involves healthy nutrition and lifestyle. In Western and Chinese herbal healing traditions, some herbs are used as a "tonic," with the goal of boosting immunity. Astragalus is also known as *A. membranaceus,* synonym *Phaca membranacea, Astragalus mongholicus,* and is classified as Fabaceae/Leguminosae or of the Papilionaceae family.

Some evidence exists that astragalus may stimulate and improve immune system function in conditions such as the common cold, blood disorders, cancer, and human immunodeficiency virus (HIV)/AIDS. Further research is necessary in this area. Even though there are no reported toxicities, immunosuppression can occur with doses larger than 28 grams.[1]

Echinacea (see also Chapter 15, Bronchiolitis) has been studied intravenously alone and in combination preparations for immune system stimulation (including in patients with leukopenia receiving cancer chemotherapy). It remains unclear whether clinically significant benefits exist. More evidence is needed to rate echinacea for these uses.[2]

Goldenseal (*Hydrastis canadensis,* Ranunculaceae family) is sometimes suggested to be an immune system stimulant, and it has been used historically for the treatment of common cold and other upper respiratory tract infections, nasal congestion, allergic rhinitis, fever, pneumonia, whooping cough, earache, conjunctivitis, and many other disorders. Goldenseal is an endangered plant today. Unfortunately, the evidence in this area is insufficient, so in order to make a conclusion for its therapeutic use, additional research is needed. Long-term use of the plant can cause digestive disorders, constipation, excitatory states, hallucinations, and occasionally delirium. In addition, overdoses can induce cardiac abnormalities, seizure, paralysis, and even death.[3]

Maitake mushroom (*Grifola frondosa,* Polyporaceae family) has been consumed as food in Asia for thousands of years. This mushroom has been used for numerous conditions such as cancer, HIV/AIDS, chronic fatigue syndrome (CFS), hepatitis, and chemotherapy support. Animal and laboratory studies suggest that β-glucan extracts from maitake may alter the immune system. However, no reliable studies in humans are available. Thus far, no adverse reactions have been associated with the use of the mushroom.[4]

Bromelain, or the common pineapple, is also known as *Ananas comosus* (and synonyms *Ananas ananas, Ananas duckei, Ananas sativus, Bromelia ananas, Bromelia comosa,* of the *Bromeliaceae* family). Some historical indications of bromelain include allergic rhinitis, enhanced antibiotic absorption, and cancer prevention. There is not enough information to recommend for or against the use of bromelain in urinary tract infections. Bromelain may cause gastrointestinal (GI) disturbances and IgE-mediated allergic reactions. Cross-allergenicity may also occur with members of the Asteraceae/Compositae plant family.[5]

Magnet Therapy

Depending on the age of the child, use either an 800-G Accuband magnet or a 9000-G Accuband REC magnet. For children younger than 2 years, tape the designated biosouth side (smooth side) of the 800-Gauss Accuband magnet facing the skin on the "Immune Point." The Immune Point is located while the child is lying supine with arms placed along the side of the body, dorsal side up and slightly bent at the elbow. Palpate for a tender point around LI11 and TH10.[1] This point will be very sensitive to palpation. Children older than 2 years should have the biosouth side (side with no indentation) of a 9000-G Accuband REC magnet taped on the Immune Point. These magnets may be left in place for 1 hour per day, and treatments may be done daily for 2-4 weeks. The magnets may be obtained from OMS (800-323-1839) or AHSM (800-635-7070).

Massage Therapy

Recent RCTs report that massage therapy may improve immune system health. Two different RCTs of HIV-positive children reported that patients who received massage were less stressed and had enhanced immune function including increased NK cell number as well as increased or stable CD4 compared with the control group, prior baseline levels, and patients who received progressive muscle relaxation.[1,2] In addition, one of the studies reported a significant increase in the number of activation markers (CD4CD25[+] cells)[2] and the other study showed increased CD4/CD8 ratio and CD4 ratios.[1]

A study of adult men receiving daily massages for 1 month showed significantly increased NK cell number and cytotoxicity, soluble CD8, and the cytotoxic subset of CD8 cells compared with their baseline. Two thirds of the subjects were HIV positive and experienced no changes in their HIV disease progression markers.[3] To compare the effect of relaxation modalities on immune function in HIV-positive adults, another study compared the effects of massage therapy, massage plus exercise, and massage plus biofeedback versus a control group. There was no statistically significant difference in CD4[+] or CD8 leukocytes among the groups, but the massage and massage plus biofeedback groups reported improved quality of life indicators.[4] A pilot and subsequent RCT of women with breast cancer demonstrated a statistically significant increase in NK cells and lymphocytes in the massage group compared with the control group.[5,6]

A pilot study of healthy volunteers reported increased salivary IgA levels following massage treatment.[7]

In addition to promoting opportunities for relaxation, receiving massage therapy on a regular basis decreases anxiety.[3,5,6,8-24] Decreasing stress and anxiety can benefit overall immune health through decreased cortisol levels. Massage therapy studies report decreased blood and salivary cortisol levels following massage treatments.[3,10-14,25-27]

Massage treatments for immunocompromised children can be tailored based on the need of the child. If musculoskeletal complaints exist, a massage modality may be chosen to treat that specific complaint. If there are no specific complaints, a massage modality to induce relaxation, such as Swedish massage or any of the energetic therapies, could be beneficial. The massage practitioner should assess the child for presence of contraindications that may be common for children being treated for an impaired immune system. For example, if any permanent vascular access devices exist for infusion therapies, those indwelling lines should be avoided. If patients are receiving medication that may put them at risk for thrombocytopenia, a light-touch massage modality should be utilized (i.e., Swedish massage, energy modalities).

A recent study reported increased bacterial counts present on massage therapists' palms following a massage session, even after hand washing, while simultaneously bacterial counts were decreased on the clients' skin.[28] If a massage provider is treating other clients as well as an immune-suppressed patient, extra care must be taken to thoroughly wash the hands prior to treating the immune-suppressed patient in order to protect that patient from pathogens. Ideally, treating these patients prior to other clients may help decrease their exposure to pathogens. Many massage providers can utilize well-fitting, disposable, nonlatex gloves in conjunction with vegetable-based massage oils to provide massage to this patient population while further protecting the patient from disease. If a massage provider (i.e., parent) wears artificial nails, the use of gloves should be strongly considered, as artificial nails may have high bacteria counts present. Removing all jewelry prior to treatment is also recommended, as bacteria may be present beneath rings and stones.

Nutrition

Discussion

Nutrition is vitally important in developing the body's resistance to infection. In the absence of good quality foods with all their essential nutrients, the body is impaired owing to the lack of these nutrients that nourish cells and drive the biochemical reactions. Many of the modern-day illnesses, such as asthma, eczema, chronic viral illnesses, and autoimmune diseases, are a result of a dysregulated immune system. More frequently, research is pointing to dietary deficiencies as a cause of this dysregulation—specifically the shift to Th2 dominance—which promotes the production of IgE and self-antibodies and stimulates mast cells and eosinophils. Anything that shifts the Th1/Th2 ratio to a Th2 predominance increases the incidence of viral illness and chronic disease. Factors that induce Th2 cytokines and suppress cell-mediated immunity (Th1) include processed vegetable oils with trans fatty acids, refined sugar, alcohol (all products of the typical Western diet), chronic antibiotic use, environmental pollutants, tobacco, prednisone, stress (increased cortisol production), heavy metals, circulating immune complexes, and pathogens.

Zinc deficiency causes an imbalance between Th1 and Th2 responses. In experimental human models, interleukin-2 (Il-2) and IFN-γ, both products of Th1, were decreased in zinc-deficient states.[1] NK cell activity and thymulin, a thymus-specific hormone, were also decreased. Once zinc was supplemented, these functions returned to normal, which indicates that zinc has specific effects on T-cell proliferation and function. In another study, vitamins C, E, and B$_6$ all were found to enhance Th1 function. Folate deficiency was found to impair Th1 function.[2] Vitamin E increased cell-mediated immunity in elderly subjects, thus reducing the risk of acquiring upper respiratory illnesses.[3] Vitamin E's mechanism of action was to increase gene expression of Il-2 (Th1) and decrease the expression of Il-4 (Th2). Similar findings were seen with supplementations of selenium, glutathione, probiotics, and β-1,3-D-glucan derived from the medicinal mushroom *Lentinus edodes*.[4] Mixed results were seen in studies using omega-3 fatty acids, with no specific effect on either Th1 or Th2 responses. Decreased Th1 and Th2-like responses were observed, which resulted in a balance with overall antiinflammatory effects.[5]

Treatment

Nutritional recommendations to support the immune system might include the following:

- Encourage a healthy diet of whole grains, fresh fruits, and vegetables to provide important sources of vitamins, minerals, and phytochemicals. Food sources for specific nutrients include:
  - Zinc—oysters, herring, legumes, wheat bran
  - Selenium—nuts, seafood, animal protein
  - Vitamin E—wheat germ, sunflower seeds, green leafy vegetables, avocado
  - Vitamin C—fruits, melons, strawberries, tomatoes, peppers
  - Glutathione—asparagus, broccoli, avocado, spinach, garlic, fresh meats
  - Folate—leafy vegetables, beets, wheat, dry beans
  - β-1,3-D-glucan—Reishi and shiitake mushrooms, bakers yeast, barley, oats
- Reduce intake of processed and refined foods that contain sugar, partially hydrogenated vegetable oils, and trans fats. Sugar impairs white blood cell function and depletes zinc from the body.
- Use probiotics that will give 1 to 10 billion viable bacteria per day, implementing a variety of strains of beneficial bacteria. Foods that contain live cultures of these beneficial bacteria often do not have enough in a typical serving to reach the recommended dose.
- Increase intake of omega-3 fatty acids either through dietary sources including salmon, mackerel, herring, flax seeds, hemp seeds, or walnuts or through supplementation with fish oil, flax seed oil, or hemp oil at 1000 mg per day. Make sure the fish sources are free of heavy metal (mercury) and pesticide contamination.

Osteopathy

Two osteopathic perspectives should be considered when treating children with immune system dysfunction. The first concerns facilitating lymphatic function through various lymphatic techniques. Although no such techniques have been tested on children, studies of adults have shown improvements in a variety of immune components.[1-6] The second consideration has to do with the influence of the musculoskeletal system on the hormonal and neurological factors that affect immune function. Immune system components such as IL, NK cells, IFN, and tumor necrosis factor, as well as the cells of the immune system, are part of a neuroendocrine immune network that responds to neural, hormonal, and immune influences. The hypothalamus-pituitary-adrenal (HPA) axis provides a strong measure of control on the neuroendocrine-immune network. Cortisol is one of the most potent inhibitors of interleukins and T-cell function. Increased sympathetic tone elevates levels of norepinephrine in the lymph nodes, which alters the production rate of β-cells. Both cortisol and norepinephrine levels rise in response to increased hypothalamic activity. The allostatic load described by McEwen[7-11] is a measurement of chronic adaptive changes in this axis. Nociception is one of the prime escalators of HPA activity.[12-15] Depending upon the patient, nociception may be a conscious phenomenon, pain, or an unconscious phenomenon. Nociception may also result in spinal facilitation and increased activity in the interneuronal pool. Clinically this presents as changes in visceral function, somatic muscle tone, vasomotor tone, and fluid balance. Signs or symptoms of hyperalgesia and inflammation usually accompany these changes. Early osteopaths described the osteopathic lesion as an area of tissue texture changes, asymmetry, restricted range of motion, and tenderness. These are all signs of spinal facilitation. From an osteopathic perspective, areas of somatic dysfunction are potential generators of nociceptive drive to the HPA axis. No single finding is more or less likely to escalate hypothalamic tone. Rather, it is the "somatic load," the overall level of somatic dysfunction that will summate, increasing hypothalamic activity and potentially contributing to altered immune system function in the child.[16] This perspective is well suited to the philosophy of osteopathy, which views osteopathic manipulation as a tool used to facilitate health in the child.

References

Pediatric Diagnosis and Treatment

1. Feigin RD, Cherry JD: *Textbook of pediatric infectious diseases*, ed 3, Philadelphia, 1992, Saunders.
2. Herrod HG: Follow-up of pediatric patients with recurrent infection and mild serologic immune abnormalities, *Ann Allergy Asthma Immunol* 79:460-464, 1997.
3. Gross TG, Steinbuch M, DeFor T et al: B cell lymphoproliferative disorders following hematopoietic stem cell transplantation: risk factors, treatment and outcome, *Bone Marrow Transplant* 23:251-258, 1999.
4. Jorissen M: Differential diagnosis of local defense mechanism diseases in ENT, *Acta Otorhinolaryngol Belg* 54:413-415, 2000.
5. Chandra RK: Nutrition and immunology: from the clinic to cellular biology and back again, *Proceed Nutr Soc* 58:681-683, 1999.
6. Beisel WR: Nutrition in pediatric HIV infection: setting the research agenda. Nutrition and immune function: overview, *J Nutr* 126(10 Suppl):2611S-2615S, 1996.
7. Bhaskaram P: Nutritional modulation of immunity to infection, *Indian J Pathol Microbiol* 35:392-400, 1992.
8. Martin TR: The relationship between malnutrition and lung infections, *Clin Chest Med* 8:359-372, 1987.
9. Keusch GT: Nutritional effects on response of children in developing countries to respiratory tract pathogens: implications for vaccine development, *Infect Dis* 13(Suppl 6):S486-S491, 1991.
10. Dhur A, Galan P, Hercberg S: Iron status, immune capacity and resistance to infections, *Comp Biochem Physiol A* 94:11-19, 1989.

11. Oppenheimer SJ: Iron and its relation to immunity and infectious disease, *J Nutr* 131(2S-2):616S-633S, 2001; discussion 633S-635S.

12. Harris BH, Gelfand JA: The immune response to trauma, *Semin Pediatr Surg* 4:77-82, 1995.

13. Koller M, Wick M, Muhr G: Decreased leukotriene release from neutrophils after severe trauma: role of immature cells, *Inflammation* 25:53-59, 2001.

14. Harris BH, Gelfand JA: The immune response to trauma, *Semin Pediatr Surg* 4:77-82, 1995.

15. Crowe JE Jr: Immune responses of infants to infection with respiratory viruses and live attenuated respiratory virus candidate vaccines, *Vaccine* 16:1423-1432, 1998.

16. Bot A: DNA vaccination and the immune responsiveness of neonates, *Int Rev Immunol* 19:221-245, 2000.

17. Dekaris D: Characteristics of immunoreactivity in neonates and young children. Review of the literature [in Romanian], *Lijec Vjesn* 120:65-72, 1998 (abstract).

18. Wolach B: Neonatal sepsis: pathogenesis and supportive therapy, *Semin Perinatol* 21:28-38, 1997.

19. Haeney M: Infection determinants at extremes of age, *J Antimicrob Chemother* 34(Suppl A):1-9, 1994.

20. Fleer A, Gerards LJ, Verhoef J: Host defence to bacterial infection in the neonate, *J Hosp Infect* 11(Suppl A):320-327, 1988.

21. Sakkas LI, Platsoucas CD: Immunopathogenesis of juvenile rheumatoid arthritis: role of T cells and MHC, *Immunol Res* 14:218-236, 1995.

22. Tucker LB: Juvenile rheumatoid arthritis, *Curr Opin Rheumatol* 5:619-628, 1993.

23. Kolbas V: Immunology of cardiovascular diseases in children [in Serbo-Croatian], *Lijec Vjesn* 112:404-407, 1990 (abstract).

24. Fohlman J, Friman G: Is juvenile diabetes a viral disease? *Ann Med* 25:569-574, 1993.

25. Rogers PA, Schoen AM, Limehouse J: Acupuncture for immune-mediated disorders. Literature review and clinical applications, *Probl Vet Med* 4:162-193, 1992.

26. Pahwa S, Morales M: Interleukin-2 therapy in HIV infection, *AIDS Patient Care STDS* 12:187-197, 1998.

27. Bellanti JA: Recurrent respiratory tract infections in paediatric patients, *Drugs* 54(Suppl 1):1-4, 1997.

28. Seki S, Habu Y, Kawamura T et al: The liver as a crucial organ in the first line of host defense: the roles of Kupffer cells, natural killer (NK) cells and NK1.1 Ag+ T cells in T helper 1 immune responses, *Immunol Rev* 174:35-46, 2000.

Acupuncture

1. Loo M: *Pediatric acupuncture*, London, 2002, Elsevier.

2. Rogers PA, Schoen AM, Limehouse J: Acupuncture for immune-mediated disorders. Literature review and clinical applications, *Probl Vet Med* 4:162-193, 1992.

Aromatherapy

1. Battaglia S: *The complete guide to aromatherapy*, Virginia, Queensland, Australia, 1995, Perfect Potion.

2. Buckle J: *Clinical aromatherapy: essential oils in practice*, ed 2, Edinburgh, 2003, Churchill Livingstone.

3. Alexander M: Part IV modulating immunity with aromatherapy: conditioning, suppression and stimulation of the immune system, *Int J Aromatherapy* 12:49-56, 2002.

4. Betts T: Use of aromatherapy (with or without hypnosis) in the treatment of intractable epilepsy—two-year follow-up study, *Seizure* 12:534-538, 2003.

5. Hay IC, Jamieson M, Ormerod AD: Randomized trial of aromatherapy: successful treatment for alopecia areata, *Arch Dermatol* 134:1349-1352, 1998.

Chiropractic

1. Palmer DD: *The science, art and philosophy of chiropractic*, Portland, Ore, 1910, Portland Printing House.

2. Leach RA, Burgess SC: Neuroimmune hypothesis. In Leach RA, editor: *The chiropractic theories: a textbook of scientific research*, Baltimore, 2004, Lippincott Williams and Wilkins.

3. Rosner A: Endocrine disorders. In Masarsky CS, Todres-Masarsky M, editors: *The somatovisceral aspects of chiropractic*, Philadelphia, 2001, Churchill Livingstone.

4. Vernon HT, Dhami MS, Howley TP, et al: Spinal manipulation and beta-endorphin: a controlled study of the effect of a spinal manipulation on plasma beta-endorphin levels in normal males, *J Manipulative Physiol Ther* 9:115-123, 1986.

5. Christian GF, Stanton GJ, Sissons D et al: Immunoreactive ACTH, beta-endorphin, and cortisol levels in plasma following spinal manipulative therapy, *Spine* 13:1411-1417, 1988.

6. Teodorczyk Injeyan JA, Injeyan S, Ruegg R: Spinal manipulative therapy reduces inflammatory cytokines but not substance P production in normal subjects, *J Manipulative Physiol Ther* 29:14-21, 2006.

7. Alcorn SM: Antibodies and antigens—their definition, source and relevant function, *J Aust Chiropractic Assoc* 11:18-37, 1978.

8. Brennan PC, Kokjohn K, Triano JJ, et al: Immunologic correlates of reduced spinal mobility: preliminary observations in a dog model. In Wold S, editor: *Proceedings of the 1991 International Conference on Spinal Manipulation*, Arlington Va, 1991, Foundation for Chiropractic Education and Research.

9. Vora GS, Bates HA: The effects of spinal manipulation on the immune system (a preliminary report), *ACA J Chiropractic* 14:S103-S105, 1980.

10. Brennan PC, Kokjohn K, Kaltinger CJ et al: Enhanced phagocytic cell respiratory burst induced by spinal manipulation: potential role of substance P, *J Manipulative Physiol Ther* 14:399-408, 1991.

11. Selano JL, Hightower BC, Pfleger B, et al: The effects of specific upper cervical adjustments on the CD4 counts of HIV positive patients, *Chiropractic Res J* 3:32-39, 1994.

12. Budgell BS: Reflex effects of subluxation: the autonomic nervous system, *J Manipulative Physiol Ther* 23:104-106, 2000.

13. Brooks WH, Cross RJ, Roszman TL et al: Neuroimmunomodulation: neural anatomical basis for impairment and facilitation, *Ann Neurol* 12:56-61, 1982.

14. Solomon GF, Amkraut AA: Psychoneuroendocrinological effects on the immune response, *Annu Rev Micorbiol* 35:155-184, 1981.

15. Bulloch K, Moore RY: Innervation of the thymus gland by brain stem and spinal cord in mouse and rat, *Am J Anat* 162:157-166, 1981.

16. Leach RA, Burgess SC: Neuroimmune hypothesis. In Leach RA, editor: *The chiropractic theories: a textbook of scientific research*, Baltimore, 2004, Lippincott, Williams and Wilkins.

17. Isolaure E, Slaminen S, Sandholm-Mattila T: New functional foods in the treatment of food allergy, *Ann Med* 31:299-302, 1999.

18. Isolauri E, Rebeiro H, Gibson G et al: Functional foods and probiotics: Working Group Report of the First World Congress of Pediatric Gastroenterology, Hepatology and Nutrition, *J Pediatr Gastroenterol Nutr* 35:S106-S109, 2002.

19. Hall BS: Allergy, endocrine and metabolic diseases in childhood. In Davies NJ, editor: *Chiropractic pediatrics*, London, 2000, Churchill Livingstone.

Herbs—Chinese

1. Sinclair S: Chinese herbs: a clinical review of Astragalus, Ligusticum, and Schisandra, *Altern Med Rev* 3:338-344, 1998.
2. Natural Standard Research Collaboration. Available at www.naturalstandard.com. Accessed 2005.
3. Li FC, Zhou XL, Mao HL: A study of paeonol injection on immune functions in rats, *Zhongguo Zhong Xi Yi Jie He Za Zhi* 14:37-38, 1994.
4. Weibo L: Treatment of AIDS by traditional Chinese medicine and materia medica, *J Tradit Chin Med* 11:249-252, 1991.

Herbs—Western

1. Upton R, editor: *Astragalus root: analytical, quality control, and therapeutic monograph*, Santa Cruz, Calif, 1999, American Herbal Pharmacopoeia, pp 1-25.
2. Melchart D, Clemm C, Weber B et al: Polysaccharides isolated from *Echinacea purpurea herba* cell cultures to counteract undesired effects of chemotherapy—a pilot study, *Phytother Res* 16:138-142, 2002.
3. Gruenwald J, Brendler T, Jaenicke C: PDR for herbal medicines, ed 1, Montvale, NJ, 1998, Medical Economics.
4. McGuffin M, Hobbs C, Upton R, et al, editors: *American Herbal Products Association's botanical safety handbook*, Boca Raton, Fla, 1997, CRC Press.
5. Nettis E, Napoli G, Ferrannini A et al: IgE-mediated allergy to bromelain, *Allergy* 56:257-258, 2001.

Magnet Therapy

1. Loo M: *Pediatric acupuncture*, London, 2002, Elsevier.

Massage Therapy

1. Diego MA, Field T, Hernandez-Reif M et al: HIV adolescents show improved immune function following massage therpy, *Int J Neurosci* 106:35-45, 2001.
2. Shor-Posner G, Hernandez-Reif M, Miguez MJ et al: Impact of a massage therapy clinical trial on immune status in young Dominican children infected with HIV-1, *J Altern Complement Med* 12:511-516, 2006.
3. Ironson G, Field T, Scafidi F et al: Massage therapy is associated with enhancement of the immune system's cytotoxic capacity, *Int J Neurosci* 84:205-217, 1996.
4. Birk TJ, McGrady A, MacArthur RD et al: The effects of massage therapy alone and in combination with other complementary therapies on immune system measures and quality of life in human immunodeficiency virus. *J Alern Complement Med* 6:405-414, 2000.
5. Hernandez-Reif M, Ironson G, Field T et al: Breast cancer patients have improved immune and neuroendocrine functions following massage therapy, *J Psychosom Res* 57:45-52, 2004.
6. Hernandez-Reif M, Field T, Ironson G et al: Natural killer cells and lymphocytes increase in women with breast cancer following massage therapy, *Intern J Neuroscience*, 115:495-510, 2005.
7. Groër M, Mozingo J, Droppleman P et al: Measures of salivary secretory immunoglobulin A and state anxiety after a nursing back rub, *J Adv Nurs* 7:2-6, 1994.
8. Hernandez-Reif M, Field T, Krasnegor J et al: Lower back pain is reduced and range of motion increased after massage therapy, *Int J Neurosci* 106:131-145, 2001.
9. Fraser J, Kerr JR: Psychophysiological effects of back massage on elderly institutionalized patients, *J Adv Nurs* 18:238-245, 1993.
10. Field T, Ironson G, Scafidi F et al: Massage therapy reduces anxiety and enhances EEG patterns of alertness and math computations, *Int J Neurosci* Sep:197-205, 1996.
11. Field T, Peck M, Krugman S et al: Burn injuries benefit from massage therapy, *J Burn Care Rehabil* 19:241-244, 1998.
12. Moyer CA, Rounds J, Hannum JW: A meta-analysis of massage therapy research, *Psychol Bull* 130:3-18, 2004.
13. Field T, Morrno C, Valdeon C et al: Massage reduces anxiety in child and adolescent psychiatric patients, *J Am Acad Adolesc Psychiatry* 31:125-131, 1992.
14. Field T, Sunshine W, Hernandez-Reif M et al: Chronic fatigue syndrome: massage therapy effects of depression and somatic symptoms in chronic fatigue, *J Chronic Fatigue Syndrome* 3:43-51, 1997.
15. Post-White J, Kinney ME, Savik K et al: Therapeutic massage and healing touch improve symptoms in cancer, *Integr Caner Ther* 2:332-344, 2003.
16. Schachner L, Field T, Hernandez-Reif M et al: Atopic dermatitis decreased in children following massage therapy, *Pediatr Dermatol* 15:390-395, 1998.
17. Field T, Peck M, Sed et al: Post-burn itching, pain, and psychological symptoms are reduced with massage therapy, *J Burn Care Rehabil* 21:189-193, 2000.
18. Rexilius SJ, Mundt C, Erikson Megel M et al: Therapeutic effects of massage therapy and handling touch on caregivers of patients undergoing autologous hematopoietic stem cells, *Oncol Nurs Forum* 29:E35-E44, 2002.
19. Ferrell-Tory AT, Glick OJ: The use of therapeutic massage as a nursing intervention to modify anxiety and the perception of cancer pain, *Cancer Nurs* 16:93-101, 1993.
20. Cassileth BR, Vickers AJ: Massage therapy for symptom control: outcome study at a major cancer center, *J Pain Symptom Manage* 28:3, 2004.
21. Mehling WE, Jacobs B, Acree M et al: Symptom management with massage and acupuncture in postoperative cancer patients: a randomized controlled trial, *J Pain Symptom Manage* 33:258-266, 2007.
22. Wilkinson SM, Love SB, Westcombe AM et al: Effectiveness of aromatherapy massage in the management of anxiety and depression in patients with cancer: a multi-center randomized controlled trial, *J Clin Oncol* 25:532-538, 2007.
23. Phipps S: Reduction of distress associated with pediatric bone marrow transplant: complementary health promotion interventions, *Pediatr Rehabil* 5:223-234, 2003.
24. Diego MA, Field T, Hernandez-Reif M: Vagal activity, gastric motility, and weight gain in massaged preterm neonates, *J Pediatr* 147:50-55, 2005.
25. Field T, Henteleff T, Hernandez-Reif M et al: Children with asthma have improved pulmonary functions after massage therapy, *J Pediatr* 132:854-858, 1998.
26. Field T, Hernandez-Reif M, Seligman S et al: Juvenile rheumatoid arthritis benefits from massage therapy, *J Pediatr Psychol* 22:607-617, 1997.
27. Ironson G, Field T, Scafidi F et al: Massage therapy is associated with enhancement of the immune system's cytotoxic capacity, *Int J Neurosci* 84:205-217, 1996.
28. Donoyama N, Wakuda T, Tanitsu T et al: Washing hands before and after performing massages? Changes in bacterial survival count on skin of a massage therapist and a client during massage therapy, *J Altern Complement Med* 10:684-686, 2004.

Nutrition

1. Prasad AS: Effects of zinc deficiency on Th1 and Th2 cytokine shifts, *J Infect Dis* 182(Suppl 1):S62-S68, 2000.
2. Long KZ, Santos JI: Vitamins and the regulation of the immune response, *Pediatr Infect Dis J* 18:283-290, 1999.
3. Meydani SN, Barklund MP, Liu S et al: Vitamin E supplementation enhances cell-mediated immunity in healthy elderly subjects, *Am J Clin Nutr* 52:557-563, 1990.
4. Kidd P: Th1/Th2 balance: the hypotheses, its limitations, and implications for health and disease, *Altern Med Rev* 8:223-246, 2003.
5. Kankaanpaa P, Sutas Y, Salminen S et al: Dietary fatty acids and allergy, *Ann Med* 31:282-287, 1999.

Osteopathy

1. Steele TF: Utilization of osteopathic lymphatic pump in the office and home for treatment of viral illnesses and after vaccine immunizations, *Fam Physician* 2:8-11, 1998.
2. Mesina J, Hampton D, Evans R et al: Transient basophilia following the application of lymphatic pump techniques: a pilot study [see comments], *J Am Osteopath Assoc* 98:91-94, 1998.
3. Paul RT, Stomel RJ, Broniak FF et al: Interferon levels in human subjects throughout a 24-hour period following thoracic lymphatic pump manipulation, *J Am Osteopath Assoc* 86:92-95, 1986.
4. Measel JW: The effect of the lymphatic pump on the immune response: I. Preliminary studies on the antibody response to pneumococcal polysaccharide assayed by bacterial agglutination and passive hemagglutination, *J Am Osteopath Assoc* 82:28-31, 1982.
5. Dugan EP, Lemley WW, Roberts CA et al: Effect of lymphatic pump techniques on the immune response to influenza vaccine, *J Am Osteopath Assoc* 101:472, 2001.
6. Jackson KM, Steele TF, Dugan EP et al: Effect of lymphatic and splenic pump techniques on the antibody response to hepatitis B vaccine: a pilot study, *J Am Osteopath Assoc* 98:155-160, 1998.
7. McEwen BS, Stellar E: Stress and the individual: mechanisms leading to disease, *Arch Intern Med* 153:2093-2101, 1993.
8. McEwen BS: Stress, adaptation, and disease: allostasis and allostatic load, *Ann N Y Acad Sci* 840:33-44, 1998.
9. McEwen BS, Seeman T: Protective and damaging effects of mediators of stress. Elaborating and testing the concepts of allostasis and allostatic load, *Ann N Y Acad Sci* 896:30-47, 1999.
10. Seeman TE, Singer BH, Rowe JW et al: Price of adaptation—allostatic load and its health consequences. MacArthur studies of successful aging, *Arch Intern Med* 157:2259-2268, 1997.
11. McEwen BS: The neurobiology of stress: from serendipity to clinical relevance, *Brain Res* 886:172-189, 2000.
12. Esterling B: Stress-associated modulation of cellular immunity. In Willard FH, Patterson M, editors: *Nociception and the neuroendocrine-immune connection*, Indianapolis, 1992, American Academy of Osteopathy, pp 275-294.
13. Donnerer J: Nociception and the neuroendocrine-immune system. In Willard FH, Patterson M, editors: *Nociception and the neuroendocrine-immune connection*, Indianapolis, 1992, American Academy of Osteopathy, pp 260-273.
14. Willard FH, Mokler DJ, Morgane PJ: Neuroendocrine-immune system and homeostasis. In Ward RC, editor: *Foundations for osteopathic medicine*, Baltimore, 1997, Williams and Wilkins.
15. Van Buskirk RL: Nociceptive reflexes and the somatic dysfunction: a model, *J Am Osteopath Assoc* 90:792-809, 1990.
16. Carreiro JE: *An osteopathic approach to children*, London, 2003, Churchill Livingstone.

Impetigo

Chiropractic | Anne Spicer

Herbs—Chinese | Catherine Ulbricht, Jennifer Woods, Mark Wright

✳ PEDIATRIC DIAGNOSIS AND TREATMENT

Impetigo is the most common bacterial skin infection of children.[1-3] It represents approximately 10% of all pediatric skin problems[4] and has an increased incidence in the homeless[5] and in refugee and immigrant children.[6] It is more common during the summer.[1-3]

Impetigo is a superficial bacterial infection of the epidermis.[8] There are two classic forms: nonbullous and bullous. The nonbullous variety accounts for more than 70% of cases[4] and is caused predominantly by *Staphylococcus aureus* and group A β-hemolytic streptococci (GABHS).[9-11] Bullous impetigo is mainly an infection of infants and young children and is always caused by coagulase-positive *S. aureus*.[4,7,12]

Lesions frequently occur on the face, especially around the nose, because nasal bacteria spread onto the skin when the child has an upper respiratory tract infection or a break in the skin.[1-3] The infection can spread by the fingers, clothing, and towels.

Lesions that occur in other areas of the body may be preceded by insect bites, abrasions, lacerations, chickenpox, scabies, pediculosis, or burns. Regional adenopathy is found in up to 90% of cases, and leukocytosis is present in approximately 50% of patients.[4]

Impetigo is typically diagnosed by clinical presentation.[8] The most effective treatment, or indeed the question of whether treatment is necessary, is uncertain.[2,13] Most cases seem to resolve spontaneously within approximately 2 weeks even without treatment.[4] A Cochrane Systematic review and meta-analysis demonstrated that although topical antibiotics are more effective than placebo, evidence is weak for the superiority of topical antibiotics over some oral antibiotics such as erythromycin or penicillin.[2,13] Most clinicians manage mild or moderately severe impetigo with débridement and a topical agent that is usually an antibiotic ointment.[3,4,9,12] The decision to treat systemically with a β-lactamase–resistant oral antibiotic should weigh the risk of medication side effects and the possibility for emergence of resistant organisms versus the potential of development of serious complications such as osteomyelitis, septic arthritis, pneumonia, septicemia, nephritis, and carditis.[3,4]

✳ CAM THERAPY RECOMMENDATIONS

Chiropractic

Although chiropractic management of impetigo has not been reported in the literature, the chiropractor would manage the child with this condition by removing interference to normal body function. There is evidence that the chiropractic adjustment has influence over natural killer cell production and autonomic balance,[1] immunoglobulin (IgA, IgG, and IgM) levels and B-cell lymphocyte count,[2] polymorphonuclear neutrophils and monoctyes,[3] and even CD4 counts.[4] Therefore the chiropractic adjustment of a subluxation complex would be a priority.

Supplementation with immune-enhancing nutrients may provide the body with necessary resources to manage an acute infection. Commonly recommended nutrients include zinc and vitamin A[5]; zinc is available in liquid formulations and is vital to normal immune function. Vitamin C may be given to the young infant in the form of rose hip syrup and should be dosed within gut tolerance.[6,7] An initial dose of 250 mg is a good starting place. Gut microflora will support the immune function, as will omega-3 fatty acids (eicosapentaenoic acid [EPA]/docosahexaenoic acid [DHA]), which also have antiinflammatory actions.[8] Vitamin E has antioxidant as well as antiinflammatory properties.[9]

Echinacea purpurea is recommended as a stimulant to the immune system.[6] Use is recommended for a period not to exceed 2 consecutive weeks, as the body may develop a tolerance level with prolonged use. Although echinacea is quite safe, allergic reactions have been recorded in children with a history of allergies, particularly to plants in the daisy family.

Topical application of colloidal silver or tea tree oil may have antibacterial effects. Topical application of a goldenseal powder may also be useful, although a reputable product must be used to avoid exposure to contaminants that may interfere with complete healing.

Careful hygiene is essential to minimize spread of the infection.

Referral is recommended in the presence of accompanying fever or sore throat.

Herbs—Chinese

Western medicine understands impetigo as being caused by *Streptococcus* spp. or *Staphylococcus* spp. infection. Traditional Chinese medicine (TCM) names it variously "pustular nest cutaneous lesion" and "yellow water cutaneous lesion." It is considered to be due to an attack of "toxic Heat." In cases of restricted spread, TCM treatment can be topical with herbs such as rhizome of *Coptis chinensis* Franch. (Huang Lian), bark of *Phellodendron amurense* Rupr. (Huang Bai), or flowers of *Chrysanthemum morifolium* Ramat. (Ju Hua) and of *Lonicera japonica* Thunb. (Jin Yin Hua). Huang Lian and Huang Bai both contain the alkaloid berberine, which has been shown to be bacteriostatic with *Streptococcus hemolyticus* and *S. aureus*.[1] Similarly, in vitro, aqueous extract of Jin Yin Hua and Ju Hua dramatically inhibits *S. aureus* and *S. hemolyticus*.[1,2]

Any of these four herbs can be prepared as a decoction for application locally by swabbing lesions. Some texts recommend grinding Huang Lian and Huang Bai with sesame oil or petroleum jelly (Vaseline) for local application as an ointment. The idea behind this is that the herbs are actually held in place on the lesions, which does not occur when aqueous swabbing is used. Patients should be warned that preparations containing berberine are intensely yellow staining.

In the event of widespread lesions and systematic signs such as enlarged lymph nodes and fever, oral dosing of decoctions using these herbs, as well as others, are preferred. When the condition has substantially abated in severity and extent of spread, topical applications can again be used.

No scientific data of in vivo outcomes for patients have been found, but the in vitro observations of the effects of these herbs on the causative organisms supports the traditional claim of perhaps being effective.

References

Pediatric Diagnosis and Treatment

1. Wenk C, Itin PH: Epidemiology of pediatric dermatology and allergology in region of Aargau, Switzerland, *Pediatr Dermatol* 20:482-487, 2003.
2. Koning S, Verhagen AP, van Suijlekom-Smit LW et al: Interventions for impetigo, *Cochrane Database Syst Rev* (2):CD003261, 2004.
3. Hedrick J: Acute bacterial skin infections in pediatric medicine: current issues in presentation and treatment, *Paediatr Drugs* 5(Suppl 1):35-46, 2003.
4. Behrman RE, Kliegman RM, Jenson HB, editors: *Nelson textbook of pediatrics*, ed 17, Philadelphia, 2004, Saunders.
5. Raoult D, Foucault C, Brouqui P: Infections in the homeless, *Lancet Infect Dis* 1:77-84, 2001.
6. Pedersen FK, Moller NE: Diseases among refugee and immigrant children [in Danish], *Ugeskr Laeger* 162:6207-6209, 2000 (abstract).
7. Johnston GA: Treatment of bullous impetigo and the staphylococcal scalded skin syndrome in infants, *Expert Rev Anti Infect Ther* 2:439-446, 2004.
8. Stulberg DL, Penrod MA, Blatny RA: Common bacterial skin infections, *Am Fam Physician* 66:119-124, 2002.
9. Sharma S, Verma KK: Skin and soft tissue infection, *Indian J Pediatr* 68(Suppl 3):S46-S50, 2001.
10. Brook I, Frazier EH, Yeager JK: Microbiology of nonbullous impetigo, *Pediatr Dermatol* 14:192-195, 1997.
11. Darmstadt GL, Lane AT: Impetigo: an overview, *Pediatr Dermatol* 11:293-303, 1994.
12. Sanfilippo AM, Barrio V, Kulp-Shorten C et al: Common pediatric and adolescent skin conditions, *J Pediatr Adolesc Gynecol* 16:269-283, 2003.
13. George A, Rubin G: A systematic review and meta-analysis of treatments for impetigo, *Br J Gen Pract* 53:480-487, 2003.

Chiropractic

1. Leach RA, Burgess SC: Neuroimmune hypothesis. In Leach RA, editor: *The chiropractic theories*, Baltimore, 2004, Lippincott Williams and Wilkins.
2. Brennan PC, Kokjohn K, Triano JJ et al: Immunologic correlates of reduced spinal mobility: preliminary observations in a dog model. In Wold S, editor: *Proceedings of the 1991 International Conference on Spinal Manipulation*, Arlington, Va, 1991, Foundation for Chiropractic Education and Research.
3. Brennan PC, Kokjohn K, Kaltinger CL et al: Enhanced phagocytic cell respiratory burst induced by spinal manipulation: potential role of substance P, *J Manipulative Physiol Ther* 12:289-XXX, 1989.
4. Selano JL, Hightower BC, Pfleger B et al: The effects of specific upper cervical adjustments on the CD4 counts of HIV positive patients, *Chiropractic Res J* 3:32-XX, 1994.
5. Bhandari N, Bahr R, Taneja S et al: Effect or routine zinc supplementation on pneumonia in children aged 6 months to 3 years: randomized controlled trial in an urban slum, *Br Med J* 324: 1358-1361, 2002.
6. Davies N: *Chiropractic pediatrics*, London, 2000, Churchill Livingstone.
7. Forastiere R, Pistelli P, Sestini C et al: Consumption of fresh fruit rich in vitamin C and wheezing symptoms in children, *Thorax* 55:283-288, 2000.
8. Stevens LJ, Zentall SS, Abate ML et al: Omega-3 fatty acids in boys with behavior, learning and health problems, *Physiol Behav* 59:915-920, 1996.
9. Heffner JE, Repine JE: Pulmonary strategies of antioxidant defense, *Am Rev Resp Dis* 140:531-554, 1989.

Herbs—Chinese

1. *Xin Bian Zhong Yao Da Ci Dian [Newly compiled Chinese official dictionary]*, Taipei, 1984, Xin Wen Feng Chu Ban Gong Si.
2. Natural Standard Research Collaboration. Available at www.naturalstandard.com. Accessed Month, 2005.

Inflammatory Bowel Disease

Acupuncture | May Loo

Aromatherapy | Maura A. Fitzgerald

Chiropractic | Anne Spicer

Homeopathy | Janet L. Levatin

Massage Therapy | Mary C. McLellan

Mind/Body | Timothy Culbert, Lynda Richtsmeier Cyr

Naturopathy | Matthew I. Baral

Nutrition | Joy A. Weydert

Probiotics | Russell H. Greenfield

✳ PEDIATRIC DIAGNOSIS AND TREATMENT

Chronic inflammatory bowel disease (IBD), which comprises ulcerative colitis (UC) and Crohn's disease (CD), is now being recognized with increasing frequency in children of all ages[1] and has become one of the most significant chronic diseases affecting children and adolescents.[2] IBD presents unique challenges for diagnosis and management because physically and psychosocially developing children often do not present with the classic symptoms.[3] The most common time of onset of IBD is during adolescence and young adulthood, between 15 and 25 years of age. Twenty-five percent to 30% of all patients with CD and 20% of those with UC present before age 20.[4] In North America, the incidence for 10 to 19 year olds is approximately 2:100,000 for UC and 3.5:100,000 for CD,[5] but the condition may begin as early as the first year of life.[6] Four percent of pediatric IBD occurs before the age of 5 years, with a peak age of onset in the late adolescent years.[3] The incidence of IBD is worldwide,[7] primarily occurring in industrialized countries with well-nourished populations.[8]

UC and CD are syndromes rather than single entities,[9] because they share many similarities in epidemiological, immunological, clinical, and therapeutic characteristics.[8] The Rome Diagnostic Criteria, previously known as the "Manning criteria," is a standardized guideline to differentiate irritable bowel syndrome (IBS) from organic intestinal disease. The criteria consist of the following:

At least 3 months of continuous or recurrent symptoms of:
Abdominal pain or discomfort that is:
  a. Relieved with defecation; and/or
  b. Associated with a change in frequency of stool; and/or
  c. Associated with a change in consistency of stool; and
Two or more of the following, at least on one fourth of occasions or days:
  a. Altered stool frequency (more than three bowel movements each day or fewer than three bowel movements each week);
  b. Altered stool form (lumpy/hard or loose/watery stool);
  c. Altered stool passage (straining, urgency, or feeling of incomplete evacuation);
  d. Passage of mucus; and/or
  e. Bloating or feeling of abdominal distention.[10,11]

Both genetic and environmental influences are involved in the pathogenesis of IBD.[6] There is strong evidence for genetic influence, and specific loci on chromosomes have been identified, especially for CD.[12,13] The risk of IBD in family members of an affected individual has been reported to be in the range of 7% to 22%; a child whose parents both have IBD has a greater than 35% chance of acquiring the disorder.[6]

The possible environmental risks include lack of breastfeeding or early weaning, perinatal infections, and "Western diet" with high fatty acid (FA) intake.[8] Infectious gastroenteritis may be a triggering event,[3] but no specific infectious agent has been reproducibly associated with IBD.[6] Currently, the dominant view of IBD pathophysiology is hyperactive immune response of the gastrointestinal (GI) mucosa to triggering factors present in the gut lumen, resulting in chronic inflammation and ensuing tissue injury.[8]

Colonic malignancy is a major complication of both UC and CD patients with pancolitis beginning in childhood.[14] The chronic, lifelong disease process also leads to significant psychosocial impact on the child and adolescent.[15]

Crohn's Disease

CD has an equal incidence in boys and girls.[5] Thirty percent of children have a positive family history.[5] In the last 15 years, huge advances have been made in the understanding of immunopathogenesis of CD. Patients with CD frequently have a mutation of the NOD2/CARD15 gene, which normally is associated with the innate recognition of microbial products and the provision of epithelial barrier function. Dysregulated interactions between the innate immune system and enteric bacteria can therefore lead to chronic intestinal inflammation in CD.[16-23]

In addition to the environmental triggers for IBD, tobacco smoking increases the risk for CD.[24] The enteric pathology in CD is transmural inflammation, which is characteristically asymmetrical and segmental with skip areas. Granulomas are pathognomonic for the disorder. Any segment of the bowel may be involved: aphthous ulcerations can occur in the mouth, esophagus, stomach, or duodenum,[8] and perianal lesions including skin tags, fissures, fistulas, and abscesses[1] can occur in 15% of pediatric patients with CD.[25] The majority of children (50% to 70%) with CD have involvement in the terminal ileum, and more than half of these patients also have inflammation in variable segments of the colon, usually the ascending colon.[8,26] Ten percent to 20% of children have isolated colonic disease, and 10% to 15% have diffuse small bowel disease involving the more proximal ileum or jejunum.[1]

The clinical presentation of CD depends on the part of the GI tract involved. Usually the child presents with small intestine symptoms consisting of recurrent, poorly localized abdominal pain; chronic diarrhea; lassitude; low-grade fever in the late afternoon and evening; anorexia; and weight loss of several months' duration.[1,8] CD involving the colon may be clinically indistinguishable from UC, with symptoms of bloody mucopurulent diarrhea, crampy abdominal pain, and urgency to defecate.[8]

Growth failure, seen in 30% of pediatric CD,[3] is a disconcerting problem in young children,[27,28] especially in those children afflicted with CD before age 5, who usually have both weight and linear growth failure at the time of presentation.[29] In older children, growth deceleration is usually insidious and may precede the onset of intestinal symptoms by years,[29] thereby delaying diagnosis.[30] Inadequate nutrient intake, anorexia, malabsorption, increased losses, and increased metabolic demands all contribute to poor growth.[1] In the adolescent, sexual development may be delayed.[3]

The transmural inflammation leads to bacterial overgrowth and the formation of fistulas and strictures that can cause obstruction. The risk of adenocarcinoma of the colon for Crohn's colitis is 4 to 20 times that of the general population.[1] Perianal disease may precede the appearance of the intestinal manifestations of CD by years and is seen most commonly in patients with colitis. When perianal disease does not respond to medical therapy, surgical management is necessary.

Ulcerative Colitis

UC is a diffuse, chronic inflammation restricted to the mucosal lining of the rectum and large intestine and extends proximally in a symmetrical, uninterrupted pattern to involve parts or all of the large intestine.[31] The rectum is involved in more than 95% of cases.[8] In addition to the environmental triggers for IBD, UC patients report a higher incidence of cow's milk allergy.[5] Unlike CD, smoking has a protective effect for UC.[32,33]

The most common presenting symptoms are rectal bleeding, diarrhea, and abdominal pain. Children usually have more extensive disease at the time of diagnosis than adults.[31] Mild disease is seen in 50% to 60% of UC and is characterized by increased mucosal blood flow with erythema and mucosal edema, which can lead to granularity and friability, resulting in spontaneous bleeding. The disease is usually confined to the distal colon, and the child does not have any systemic signs and symptoms.

Thirty percent of pediatric patients present with moderate disease characterized by bloody diarrhea, cramps, urgency to defecate, and abdominal tenderness. Systemic signs such as anorexia, low-grade fever, and mild anemia may be present. Fifteen percent of pediatric UC patients have growth failure.

Severe colitis occurs in approximately 10% of patients, presenting with more than six bloody stools per day, abdominal tenderness, fever, anemia, leukocytosis, and hypoalbuminemia. In less than 5% of pediatric patients, UC may appear with extraintestinal manifestations such as arthropathy, skin manifestations, or liver disease.[8,34]

The major GI complications of UC are massive bleeding, toxic megacolon, and carcinoma. Toxic megacolon is rare in young patients but is a medical and surgical emergency because of the high risk for colonic perforation, gram-negative sepsis, and massive hemorrhage.[37] Children who develop UC before 14 years of age have a cumulative colorectal cancer incidence rate of 5% at 20 years and 40% at 35 years.[38] Children who develop the disease between 15 and 39 years of age have a cumulative incidence rate of 5% at 20 years and 30% at 35 years. Therefore it is estimated that there is an 8% risk of dying from colon cancer 10 to 25 years after diagnosis of colitis if the disease symptoms are not controlled.[37]

Extraintestinal Manifestations

Twenty-five percent to 35% of patients with CD or UC have at least one extraintestinal manifestation, which may be diagnosed before, concurrently with, or after the diagnosis of IBD is made.[38] Skin manifestations, aphthous ulcers in the mouth; ocular findings such as uveitis, arthritis (occurring in 7% to 25% of pediatric patients), hepatobiliary disease, urological complications including renal stones (which occur in approximately 5% of children with IBD), and hydronephrosis have been reported.[1] Rarely, arthritis can be the first and sometimes only initial symptom for months to years in children with IBD.[3] CD also have characteristic erythema nodosum—raised, red, tender nodules that appear primarily on the anterior surfaces of the leg and affect 3% of children.[39] It is estimated that 75% of patients with erythema nodosum ultimately develop arthritis.[40]

Diagnostic Evaluation

Physical examination and initial laboratory evaluations can all be nonspecific. Once infectious causes have been ruled out, it is best to refer the child to a pediatric gastroenterologist for further diagnostic evaluation, which would include flexible colonoscopy with colonic and terminal ileal biopsy specimens. The flexible, small-caliber endoscopes allow colonoscopic evaluation of pediatric patients of all ages, including infants,[41] by direct visualization and biopsy of the colon and terminal ileum. An upper GI with small bowel follow-through x-ray contrast study is performed on younger children, whereas double-contrast radiography (enteroclysis) is the state-of-the-art technique for examining fine mucosal details to detect early ulceration in the small bowel in older children. When abscesses and fistulas in CD are suspected, computed tomography and ultrasonography are useful additional studies.[1] The pediatric CD activity index, which includes growth parameters, was developed in 1990 and validated at 12 pediatric GI centers as a scoring system for diagnosing CD. At this time, a disease activity index is being developed for pediatric UC.[42]

Management

The general goals of treatment for children with IBD are to achieve control of the inflammatory process, to promote growth through adequate nutrition, and to permit the child to function as normally as possible, such as attending school or participating in sports.[1] Nutrition is a very important part of management, because growth failure is a major concern.[3] Recommendations for nutritional therapy include an increase in energy and protein intake to 150% of recommended daily allowances for height and age. Some studies recommend nocturnal nasogastric infusion as supplements of daily intake. Nutritional support has been shown to be as effective as steroids in achieving remission of disease in children.[3,28,43]

The genetically impaired mucosal antibacterial activity is consistent with the benefit from antibiotic or probiotic treatment in CD.[22]

Omega-3 FAs have been shown to reduce relapse rates.[44] Various pharmacological agents are being used in IBD. Recently, immunosuppressive therapies are increasingly preferred[8,45-47] for controlling the hyperactive mucosal immune system. Steroids are used in acute flare-ups but are usually not beneficial in maintaining long-term remission in CD.[48,49] Growth retardation can occur in children even with small doses of steroids and is not overcome by administration of growth hormone.[49] Other immunosuppressive drugs also have significant toxicities that include potential risks of infection and malignancy such that they should not be used indiscriminately,[50] especially in children.

Refractory IBD can be treated by surgery.[47] Various surgical endorectal pull-through procedures have been used to treat UC. CD is often more difficult to manage because surgery does not cure the disease. It is considered only for uncontrollable bleeding, stenotic bowel, or fistulas unresponsive to medical therapy.[1,48]

✳ CAM THERAPY RECOMMENDATIONS

Acupuncture

Acupuncture has been used for various GI conditions[1] and has traditionally been used in the treatment of IBD in China.[2] Although there is a tremendous amount of information regarding the physiological effects of acupuncture on pain and on the digestive system, well-designed, prospective, randomized controlled clinical trials are still lacking. Clinically, complementary and alternative medicine (CAM) has been increasingly used by patients with IBD.[3] An international survey of North American and European patients revealed 51% of 289 IBD patients used some form of alternative medicine, including acupuncture.[4] Fear of side effects of conventional therapy and the perceived safety of CAM are two of the most common reasons cited for the use of CAM.[3,5] Some also turn to CAM as a complement to conventional medicine.[6]

Clinical studies and reports have demonstrated some general response for acupuncture treatment in IBD. A randomized controlled trial (RCT) in China of 62 patients with chronic colitis comparing acupuncture and moxibustion at acupoints such as Tianshu (ST25) and Guanyuan (CV4) with Western drugs showed that acupuncture and moxibustion had a marked curative effective with few side effects.[7]

The mechanism of acupuncture efficacy in IBD can be summarized as exerting effects on GI physiology and immunology, improving blood circulation, and controlling pain. Extensive research in animal models and human subjects indicate that acupoint stimulation leads to changes in gastric acid secretion,

GI motility, neurohormonal changes, and changes in sensory thresholds,[1,8] possibly mediated through opioid and other neural pathways.[9]

The pathogenesis of IBD may involve both local and systemic immunological abnormalities. There is convincing evidence of acupuncture's amelioration of the hyperimmune response in IBD. A prospective, randomized, single-blind clinical trial from Germany demonstrated that acupuncture treatment resulted in improvements in well-being and quality of life and decrease in α-(1)-acid glycoprotein, a serum marker of inflammation, in active CD.[2] Cytokines, especially interleukin (IL)-1β and IL-6 messenger ribonucleic acid (mRNA), are important inflammatory factors and immune regulators in the pathogenesis of UC. Many studies showed increased IL-1β and IL-6 mRNA levels in the colonic mucosa and peripheral blood of patients with UC. An animal study from China demonstrated that acupuncture and moxibustion greatly inhibited the expression of IL-1β and IL-6 mRNA cytokines in the experimental UC rats, thus reducing immunocyte response to inflammation, which led to diminished inflammation with reparation of tissue.[8] One researcher proposed that a possible immunosuppressive action of acupuncture is in controlling the release of neuropeptides from nerve endings and subsequent vasodilative and antiinflammatory effects through calcitonin gene-related peptide.[6]

An animal study from the Netherlands demonstrated that artificially induced colitis in mice is associated with microcirculatory disturbances in the colon.[10] Acupuncture is well known for increasing blood flow[11] and especially in improving microcirculation.[12-14]

One clinical report from China suggests that strong moxibustion at ST25, CV4, BL23 can theoretically improve microcirculation of the intestinal mucosa.[15] Finally, acupuncture can be implemented in IBD for its well-known chronic pain control effect mediated through neuropeptides such as endorphins.[16-26]

TCM Differentiation and Treatment Suggestions

Several possible traditional TCM differentiations[27] correlate with Western diagnosis of IBD, as follows:

Spleen deficiency: This is usually associated with other signs of Spleen deficiency, such as fatigue, pallor, or abdominal distention.

Damp Heat in the Intestines: CD correlates to Damp-Heat in the Small Intestines, and UC correlates to Damp-Heat and Blood stasis in the Large Intestines, manifesting as bloody diarrhea and severe abdominal pain.

Liver Qi stagnation: Emotional disturbances such as anger and frustration are often present.

Kidney deficiency: This correlates to the strong genetic predisposition in IBD. It is often associated with watery stools or diarrhea at dawn and is more serious and therefore more difficult to treat.

Treatment suggestions

Spleen deficiency
ST40 to expel Damp.

SP3, SP6, BL20 to tonify the Spleen.

Vigorous tonification of the Spleen with the Five-Element, Four-Point protocol(see Appendix B):

Tonify SP2, HT8; sedate SP1, LR1.

CV12 tonifies the Middle Energizer.

Decrease intake of sweets, greasy/fried foods, and Phlegm-producing foods.

Damp-Heat in the Intestines

Eliminate or decrease energetically Hot foods, greasy/fried foods, excessive sweets, and Phlegm-producing foods.

LI11 to clear overall Heat.

TB6 to clear Heat from the Intestines and promote bowel movements.

CV10 to resolve Dampness and stimulate descending of Qi in the intestines.

Resolve Dampness:

    ST44 to resolve Dampness.

    SP9 to resolve Damp-Heat.

ST25 to stop diarrhea.

CV6 to tonify the Lower Burner.

Tonify the Spleen:

    Strong moxibustion on ST25, CV4, BL23.[15]

    Moxa on ST25 and CV4.[7]

Additional treatment for CD

Use the Five-Element, Four-Point protocol for clearing Heat from the Small Intestine(see Appendix B):

    Tonify SI2, BL66; sedate ST5, TB6.

Additional treatment for UC

ST25, BL25, the Large Intestine Mu-Shu points, stimulate LI Qi and alleviate diarrhea and pain.

ST37, Lower Sea point for the Large Intestine, to stop diarrhea.

Also treat Blood stasis and bleeding:

    SP1 to stop acute bleeding.

    SP10, BL17 to remove Blood stasis.

Use the Five-Element, Four-Point protocol for clearing Heat from the Large Intestine:

    Tonify LI2, BL66; sedate LI5, SI5.

Liver Qi stagnation

CV12, P6 for feeling of stuffiness in the epigastrium.[28]

Explore issues that caused emotional disturbance. Teach the child calming exercises.

Massage Yintang for calming effect.

Avoid excess sour foods and medications.

Resolve Liver Qi stagnation.

LR14 promotes smooth flow of Liver Qi.

LR13 harmonizes LR and SP.

LR3 to tonify LR Yin, move Liver Qi.

CV6, GB34 together to move Qi in the abdomen and diminish abdominal pain.

Tonify the Spleen:

    CV12, ST36, BL20 to tonify the Spleen.

    Use the Four-Point protocol: Tonify SP2, HT8; sedate SP1, LR1.

Clear Heat from the Small Intestine or Large Intestine, depending on symptoms.

Kidney deficiency

GV4, BL23 to warm the fire of Mingmen and invigorate Kidney Yang.

CV6 to warm lower Burner to stop diarrhea.

KI6, SP6 to tonify KI Yin.

Strong moxibustion at ST25, CV4, BL23.

Aromatherapy

Pittler and Ernst did a review and meta-analysis of studies of oral essential oil of peppermint *(Mentha piperita)* for the treatment of IBS. They reviewed 8 RCTs. Three trials demonstrated a significant difference in favor of the peppermint essential oil intervention, two trials did not, and three trials were not included because of missing information about methodology. The source of peppermint essential oil was Colpermin or Elanco LOK caps; the dosage was 0.2 to 0.4 mL administered three times per day. The reviewers found a number of problems with study design in this series, including the lack of use of common diagnostic criteria (Manning Criteria) for identification of subjects with IBS, the short time period used for evaluation, and the lack of a wash-out period between the crossover. The authors of the review concluded that the role of peppermint was not well established and more research was needed.[1]

More recently a randomized, double-blind, control trial was done with 42 children. Subjects were 8 years or older, and all met the Manning or Rome criteria for IBS. Subjects received either peppermint oil in an enteric capsule (Colpermin, which contains 187 mg of peppermint oil/capsule) or a placebo for a period of 2 weeks. Subjects weighing more than 45 kg received 2 capsules three times per day, and those weighing between 30 and 45 kg received 1 capsule three times per day. The children receiving the peppermint showed significant improvement in severity of pain and no significant difference in other GI symptoms such as abdominal rumbling, distention, belching, or gas. No adverse drug reactions were reported. The investigators concluded that peppermint oil is useful for the treatment of pain related to IBS in children.[2] Essential oil of peppermint is sold over the counter, usually in enteric-coated capsules of 0.2 mL.

Chiropractic

In addressing the child with IBD, the chiropractic management approach will likely be similar whether there is a diagnosis of UC or CD. The goal of management is to improve the hormonal and autonomic balance through improving neurological function at the spinal level. Chiropractors pay particular attention to the L1 and L2 spinal segments, as adjustments have been reported to benefit those with IBS, perhaps via the inferior mesenteric ganglion.[1]

In a study of 17 patients with Crohn's disease, a common area of chiropractic subluxation complex was noted at the low thoracic spine.[2] In this study, all 17 individuals receiving chiropractic care experienced a reduction in gastrointestinal symptoms with 12 showing long-term, stable remissions. The authors postulate that the displacement of the vertebrae causes a narrowing of the intervertebral foramen that disrupts the reciprocal innervation between the brain and the viscera. A case study of a 25-year-old woman with a 5-year history of IBS was reported to have symptomatic resolution after her first visit for chiropractic adjustments. She remained symptom-free through 2 years of follow-up.[3]

In a study population of 11 men with uncomplicated ulcerous disease, pain relief was established after chiropractic adjustments an average of 10 days earlier than with traditional pharmaceutical therapy.[4] Improvement in gastric symptoms with the chiropractic adjustment may be more notable when there is a concomitant presence of mid back pain.[5]

Multiple case studies related to pelvic pain and organic dysfunction (PPOD) have shown benefit in women with pelvic pain and bowel disturbances among their most prominent symptoms.[6-10] Although these cases may not be classical IBS, the somatovisceral mechanism behind the functional improvement would likely carry over.

The chiropractor would supplement the necessary spinal adjustment with related dietary alterations, such as increasing protein and fluids while decreasing sugars, trans fats, and allergenic suspects. Supplementation with vitamin A, B complex, probiotics, and lecithin may also prove useful.[1]

Peppermint oil (in capsule form) taken after meals may inhibit smooth muscle contraction and slow diarrhea.[11]

Herbs—Western

IBS is a complicated condition to treat, as there are various symptoms from abdominal pain, diarrhea, and constipation. Chamomile *(Matricaria chamomilla)* is a commonly recommended herb in IBS owing to its carminative, antiinflammatory, antispasmodic, and nervine properties.[1,2] No clinical trials have addressed chamomile as a single agent in IBS in adults and children. However, Iberogast is a combination of fresh plant extract of *Iberis amara* and extracts of eight other dried herbal drugs *(Chelidonii herba, Cardui mariae fructus, Melissae folium, Carvi fructus, Liquiritiae radix, Angelicae radix, Matricariae flos,* and *Menthae piperitae folium).*[3] Experimental and clinical studies indicated that the extracts of the dried herbal drugs have mainly spasmolytic properties; the fresh plant extract of *I. amara* has a tonic effect on the GI tract.[4] Clinical trials in adults have demonstrated a positive effect for its treatment of dyspepsia and IBS in adults.[4-7] There are no trials of Iberogast for children with IBS. Iberogast was found to be toxicologically safe in therapeutically effective doses, and adverse events are rare.[3,4]

Peppermint *(M. piperita)* is used to treat a variety of digestive complaints such as colic in infants, flatulence, diarrhea, indigestion, nausea and vomiting, morning sickness, and IBS.[1,2,8] Several studies have demonstrated the variable efficacy of peppermint oil in adults with IBS,[9,10] yet a meta-analysis concluded that the "role of peppermint oil in IBS has not been established beyond a reasonable doubt."[11] A multicenter, double-blind RCT that investigated the efficacy and clinical usefulness of peppermint oil capsules (Colpermin) in the treatment of IBS symptoms in children found a statistically significant difference compared with placebo. No side effects were reported.[12] Adverse reactions to enteric-coated peppermint oil capsule are rare but can include hypersensitivity reaction, contact dermatitis, abdominal pain, heartburn, perianal burning, bradycardia, and muscle tremor.[8,13]

Homeopathy

Before using this section, please see Appendix A, Homeopathy, for definitions of practitioner expertise categories and general information on prescribing homeopathic medicines.

Practitioner Expertise Category 3

There are no controlled clinical trials of homeopathic treatment for IBD, although the homeopathic literature contains evidence for its use in the form of accumulated clinical experience.[1] Homeopathic treatment can be used safely for IBD, either alone or in combination with other treatment modalities, both alternative and conventional. Because IBD is a complex medical problem with a high likelihood of attendant morbidity, successful homeopathic treatment usually requires extensive training in the art and science of homeopathy. Any one of many homeopathic medicines may be used to treat IBD, depending on the characteristics of the patient being treated; sophisticated homeopathic analysis and long-term follow-up are required. For these reasons, specific medicines for treating IBD will not be presented here. Interested readers are referred to the homeopathic literature for further study.[1]

Massage Therapy

Adult patients have reported use of massage therapy to help with symptom management for IBD[1,2] despite the lack of any evidence to the efficacy of this modality for this disease progress. One study investigated specifically the use of reflexology (a massage modality where pressure is applied to reflex areas on the feet, hands, and ears that correspond to other body parts and organs[3]) for the symptom management of IBS. This single-blind trial of adult IBS patients who received either reflexology foot massage or non-reflexology massage had no change in their abdominal pain, bowel pattern, or abdominal distention.[4]

Stimulation of the parasympathetic nervous system increases stomach gastrin levels, intestinal peristalsis, and circulation to the GI tract.[5] Direct application of massage to the abdomen assists with the mechanical action of peristalsis. Perhaps during acute episodes of IBD, massage therapy treatments could be suspended to prevent increased motility during sessions.

Massage could be beneficial to some of the psychological implications of chronic disease, as receiving massage therapy on a regular basis decreased anxiety[6-17] and depression scores in a large number of RCTs.[8,11,12,15,17-22] Massage therapy studies report decreased blood and salivary cortisol levels following massage treatments* which suggests physical evidence of reduced stress levels within the body. Decreasing overall stress levels, anxiety, and depression may be helpful for patients suffering from IBD, as patients may report increased acute episodes during times of stress. Massage therapy has been shown to be an effective adjunctive therapy for pain management (see Chapter 21) in patients with acute and chronic pain.

Mind/Body

Stress may be a significant mediating factor in exacerbating or inhibiting recovery from IBD, and therefore mind/body therapies can play an important adjunctive role in treatments plans for individuals with CD or UC.[1] Thermal biofeedback training as a component of a behavioral intervention package has been described as being beneficial in adults with IBD. The authors'

---

*References 8,9,11,12,19,23-26.

clinical experience suggests that various forms of biofeedback, diaphragmatic breathing, meditation, and other relaxation approaches are useful adjuncts for children with IBD, particularly as an "emotional regulation" and stress management tool. Mind/body skills training and support groups for teens with IBD have also been helpful in our clinical experience. There is some support for this approach in adult IBD patients.[2] However, to date there is no published literature in pediatrics on this topic.

IBS is sometimes classified in this category as well. IBS is likely strongly, if not primarily, a psychophysiological disorder, and so mind/body therapies play a frontline role in restoring and maintaining optimal states of autonomic nervous system balance.

Motion Sickness (Nausea and Vomiting)

Motion sickness is characterized by symptoms of nausea and vomiting and underlying autonomic nervous system arousal. Most studies on mind/body approaches for motion sickness have been done in adults, the majority of the subjects being Air Force pilots. Experience suggests that these same approaches may be adaptable to pediatric clients. Nausea associated with motion sickness seems to respond well to controlled breathing techniques.[3] Adding music to the breath control training may be additionally beneficial.[4] Although the overall effectiveness of controlled breathing and music intervention are not as effective as pharmacological interventions, they do offer an alternative treatment that is free of adverse side effects. Biofeedback training as a way to maintain a more controlled, optimum state of autonomic nervous balance can be helpful in reducing nausea associated with motion sickness. Adult studies suggest that autogenics training[5] and a combination of biofeedback and cognitive-behavioral interventions are also useful for motion sickness control.[6,7]

The authors teach a version of this by having the child or adolescent breathe in through the nose to the count of 3 seconds and then exhale through the mouth to the count of 6 seconds, keeping the shoulders relaxed and the belly soft. Nausea and vomiting of other etiologies (chemotherapy associated, postoperative) may also respond to similar mind/body approaches. Mind/body techniques can be combined with accupoint stimulation (P6) and clinical aromatherapy (essential oil of peppermint, spearmint, ginger, or fennel) for excellent nausea control.

Naturopathy

Diet

It seems common sense to seriously consider diet when discussing diseases of the GI tract. The symptoms of CD may be alleviated, if not eliminated, using natural treatments and diet changes. Ideally, a patient with CD should avoid all allergens, especially those that are most commonly implicated in IBD: wheat, chocolate, dairy, corn, artificial sweeteners, eggs, and yeast.[1,2] In fact, antibodies to yeast have been found in patients with CD, whereas none were found in healthy subjects.[3,4] Patients with CD also have higher blood levels of IgE antibodies,[5] which are involved in allergic reactions, and may represent an overall hyperreactive immune system. It should also be noted that patients with CD seem to have a higher prevalence of lactose sensitivity.[6] Carrageenan is another food additive that should be eliminated, as it can induce colonic ulcerations in animal models.[7,8]

An elimination diet may be considered as part of treatment, as it has successfully kept patients in remission for up to 51 months, with only a 10% relapse rate,[9] and has proven to be more effective in terms of remission rates when compared with corticosteroid treatment.[10]

However, the elimination diet is not practical for a child living in the everyday world of social events and school. Removing the top offenders may be the best approach. Patients with CD were found to consume more refined carbohydrates and sugars than their healthy counterparts.[11,12] Therefore patients with CD should adopt a diet high in complex carbohydrates and fiber and low in sugar and refined carbohydrates, as this has been found in the literature to be the least aggravating.[13,14] The use of a high-fiber diet resulted in significantly fewer hospital visits.[15] The Gotschall diet, otherwise known as the Specific Carbohydrate Diet, may be useful in treatment of IBD. It eliminates the use of specific disaccharides such as all grain products, yams, parsnips, bean sprouts, chickpeas, potatoes, soy, dairy and lactose, and sugar with the exception of honey.

Gut Colonization

Reseeding of the gut with beneficial bacteria such as *Lactobacillus acidophilus* and *Saccharomyces boulardii* may benefit patients, because the bacterial environment may be abnormal in those with CD.[16,17] Healthy gut flora can also inhibit overgrowth of certain organisms such as *Candida albicans*. Neutrophils in patients with CD seem to have an impaired ability to fight against *C. albicans*.[18,19] That patients may be sensitized to probiotic organisms if given during acute flare-ups is of theoretical concern.

Lifestyle and Healthy Habits

Patients who may be at risk for tobacco use should be screened, because it is associated with CD.[20-22] Smoking also increases the rate of recurrence of the disease, even after surgery.[23] Patients with CD may be susceptible to bone demineralization due to calcium and vitamin D malabsorption. In addition, corticosteroid treatment has a negative effect on bone mineralization.[24] Weight-bearing exercise will have a beneficial effect on bone strength, and low-impact exercise programs increase bone mineral density in these patients.[25]

Nutritional Supplements

Many nutrients seem to be deficient in patients with CD. This may be a result of malabsorption or an increased requirement for antioxidant nutrients due to their increased oxidative stress.[26] Antioxidants in general (β-carotene, vitamin C, vitamin E, selenium, zinc, magnesium, and vitamin D) were found to be deficient in patients with CD.[27]

Vitamin C

Levels of vitamin C in patients with CD were found to be lower than those in healthy patients.[28-30] Patients were also found to have fewer antioxidant defenses in their intestines, making them more susceptible to oxidative damage. This further supports the use of antioxidants such as vitamin C.[31]

Zinc

Zinc is often deficient in CD and is of particular concern because it can lead to dermatological problems as well as visual complications, which both can be successfully treated with zinc supplementation.[32-35] In addition, growth problems in patients with CD have been linked to low zinc levels.[36] Severity of sequellae may be related to zinc levels, as CD patients with fistula formation were found to have lower levels of zinc than CD patients without this complication.[37] Patients may be given 15 to 30 mg twice daily, which should always be balanced with 2 to 4 mg of copper per day.

Selenium

Selenium levels have been shown to be low, so supplementation may have a protective effect from oxidative damage.[38,39] In particular, patients who have undergone small bowel resection are particularly susceptible to selenium deficiency.[40]

Vitamin A

Patients with CD were found to have low levels of vitamin A and carotenoids.[41,42] There was a significant correlation between low vitamin A and zinc status and activity of disease in patients with CD.[43] A dose of 10,000 to 25,000 IU per day is safe.

Vitamin E

Vitamin E should be considered for its antioxidative properties. An appropriate dose is 400 to 800 IU per day.

Folate and other B vitamins

Folate, along with vitamin B_1, B_2, and B_6, were all found to be depleted in patients with CD.[44,45] Those patients who are on total parenteral nutrition should definitely consider folate supplementation, as parenteral nutrition can result in very low folate status.[46] An appropriate dose is 400 to 800 μg folate per day and 1000-μg intramuscular vitamin B_{12} per week.

Essential FAs

Patients with IBD may have decreased levels of essential FAs,[47] and fish oils rich in omega-3 FAs can help maintain remission in CD.[48-50]

Magnesium

An increased intake of magnesium was correlated to a reduced risk for the development of IBD.[51] Patients with IBD often show decreased magnesium status, which can lead to additional complications such as cramps, bone pain, delirium, acute crises of tetany, fatigue, depression, cardiac abnormalities, urolithiasis, impaired healing, and colonic motility disorders.[52,23] Those patients who have undergone resection of the small bowel are particularly susceptible to magnesium deficiency, which can present clinically as muscle fatigue.[54] At least 200 mg per day of magnesium citrate, orotate, aspartate, or a combination of the three is recommended.

L-Glutamine

The amino acid glutamine is the preferred fuel for GI epithelial cells and supplementation may be helpful. A typical dose is 1 to 3 g/day.

Botanical Medicine

Quercetin is a bioflavonoid derived from onions and used for its mast cell–stabilizing abilities as well as antioxidant properties. A typical dose is ¼ teaspoon taken 20 minutes before meals.

Robert's formula is a herbal combination traditionally used by naturopathic physicians for IBD. Goldenseal (*Hydrastis canadensis*) and wild indigo (*Baptisia tinctoria*) are used for their antimicrobial properties, *Echinacea angustfolia* for its immune-stimulating effects, and slippery elm (*Ulmus fulva*) and marshmallow (*Althea officinalis*) are used for their mucilage content and can help soothe the intestinal lining. Poke root (*Phytolacca americana*) and cabbage powder (*Brassica oleracea*) are included for their abilities to heal ulcers. Cranesbill root (*Geranium maculatum*) has styptic properties that can decrease intestinal bleeding. During acute aggravations, 4 to 6 capsules taken three times per day may be used, and a maintenance dose of 2 capsules three times per day is recommended.[55]

Stress Management

Stress management can decrease symptomology in patients with CD.[56]

Other Therapies

Dehydroepiandrosterone (DHEA) levels should be measured in CD patients. DHEA levels were found to be low in patients with IBD.[57] A typical dose is 20 to 30 mg per day.

Butyrate enema may be of benefit because it decreases inflammatory reactions that occur in the bowels of patients with CD.[58]

Nutrition

Discussion

Nutritional interventions in IBD are very important, as these patients commonly manifest malnutrition and deficiencies of the essential vitamins, minerals, and FAs. As a result of the intestinal inflammation, absorption of these nutrients and actual loss through exudative processes are problems. Nutritional therapy can target the deficiencies due to these losses and additionally can help heal the inflamed mucous membranes, thus lessening the disease process.

It is increasingly evident that the Western diet, which is high in saturated fats and refined carbohydrates and low in fiber, may contribute to the incidence of IBD by increasing inflammation. There is also growing concern that certain foods may act as antigens, therefore aggravating and promoting the inflammatory process.[1] Identifying these potential allergens through IgG- and IgE-specific food sensitivity panels may help to determine which foods to eliminate. It has been hypothesized that the advent of refrigeration may have increased the incidence of CD in modern times. Certain bacteria, such as *Yersinia* and *Listeria* species, continue to grow at low levels despite refrigeration. Biopsies of patients with CD found traces of these bacteria in the lesions, which suggests that refrigeration of these contaminated foods allows consumers to be exposed to these bacteria chronically, therefore contributing to ongoing inflammation.[2] Eating a diet that is rich in whole foods and consists of fresh fruits and vegetables and protein derived from fish and plant sources would provide all the essential nutrients and fiber and be less inflammatory overall. It is also important to avoid all foods containing carrageenan, a food additive used to stabilize milk proteins in processed foods. This additive is used by researchers experimentally to induce UC in animals.[3]

Probiotics have multiple beneficial effects on the intestinal mucosa and often compete with the less beneficial bacteria that adhere to and promote destruction of the cellular mucosa. In one study, a probiotic mixture helped induce remission in patients with active UC.[4] Another study in children with CD showed decrease in disease activity and in steroid use with *Lactobacillus* GG.[5] Probiotics, in the form of germinated barley foodstuff (GBF) that provided the short-chain FA butyrate, were used in a multicenter open trial in patients with UC. Disease activity decreased significantly in those who received GBF compared with those who did not. Both groups remained on baseline treatments of 5-aminosalicylic acid (5-ASA) or steroids.[6]

Supplementation with fish oil in adults with UC resulted in a reduction of clinical symptoms and disease activity on sigmoidoscopy exam in two double-blind, placebo-controlled studies.[7,8] Supplementation with fish oil or flax seed oil provides the essential omega-3 FAs α-linolenic acid (ALA) and EPA, which are natural antiinflammatory agents.

Supplementation with multiple vitamins and essential minerals is important to replace those lost from inflammation and malabsorption. Patients with IBD have been found to have elevated homocysteine levels and low 5-methyl-tetrahydrofolate levels, indicating poor folate status. These patients typically are also deficient in calcium, vitamin D, vitamin B$_{12}$, zinc, iron, and magnesium, leading to other clinical symptoms of osteopenia, growth delay, and skin disorders.

Treatment

Nutritional management of IBD might include the following recommendations:

- A diet of fresh, whole foods high in fruits and vegetables to provide adequate complex carbohydrates and fiber. Vegetables that are steamed rather than raw will have less roughage and be easier to digest. Encourage vegetable protein and fish and decrease intake of animal proteins that are high in saturated fats.
- Eliminate food allergens identified by IgG- and IgE-specific food sensitivity panels.
- Use probiotics that will give 1 billion to 10 billion viable bacteria per day, implementing a number of strains of beneficial bacteria. Foods that contain live cultures of these beneficial bacteria often do not have enough in a typical serving to reach the recommended dose.
- Increase intake of omega-3 FAs, either through dietary sources including salmon, mackerel, herring, flax seeds, hemp seeds, or walnuts or through supplementation with fish oil, flax seed oil, or hemp oil at 1000 mg per day. Make sure the fish sources are free of heavy metal (mercury) and pesticide contamination.
- In addition to healthy eating habits, supplement the diet with these nutrients:
  Folic acid: 1 mg per day
  Calcium: 1000 to 1500 mg per day
  Vitamin D: 2000 IU per day

Vitamin B$_{12}$: 400 µg per day
Zinc: 15 to 20 mg per day
Iron: 30 mg per day (Absorption is improved when taken with a source of Vitamin C.)
Magnesium: 500 to 1000 mg per day (in the form of gluconate, glycinate, or aspartate for better absorption)

Probiotics

CD and UC are inflammatory disorders of the GI tract in which pathophysiology appears tightly associated with the resident intestinal microbiota, perhaps even an abnormal immune response to that flora.[1] This idea is partly supported by the fact that CD occurs in sites with the highest concentration of luminal bacteria[2] and that antibiotic therapy is often effective in the treatment of CD. It is known that people with UC have lower intestinal mucosal counts of lactobacilli in inflamed tissue on biopsy[3] and people with CD have reduced fecal levels of bifidobacteria as compared with those with normal GI tracts.[4,5]

Data supporting the use of probiotic therapy for people with IBD are compelling, specifically as relate to its use as an adjunct to conventional medical care for maintaining remission in IBD and pouchitis,[6] but are not conclusive. Fourteen children with CD developed a higher number of IgA-secreting cells, as well as upregulation of IL-10 (an antiinflammatory cytokine), after 10 days of oral therapy with 10 billion colony-forming units (CFU) of *Lactobacillus* GG.[7] Using a nonpathogenic strain of *Escherichia coli*, researchers have shown therapeutic benefits essentially equivalent to use of 500 mg mesalazine with respect to induction and maintenance of remission of UC.[8,9] A study using *S. boulardii* with mesalazine, or mesalazine alone, for people with CD showed significantly decreased relapse rates in the supplemented group.[10] A preparation of eight different microbes, VSL#3, that contained 900 billion organisms (including *Bifidobacterium longum*, *Bifidobacterium infantis*, *Bifidobacterium breve*, *Lactobacillus acidophilus*, *Lactobacillus casei*, *Lactobacillus bulgaricus*, *Lactobacillus plantarum*, and *Streptococcus thermophilus*) was shown to enhance maintenance of remission of pouchitis[11-12] and UC.[13] Yet not all studies have been positive: One study that evaluated the use of *Lactobacillus* GG after curative resection for CD reported no impact on recurrence,[14] and another that used *Lactobacillus* GG showed no effect as primary therapy for pouchitis.[15]

This author has witnessed positive results using microbes such as *Lactobacillus* GG, *Lactobacillus reuteri*, and bifidobacteria. A 2- to 3-month trial of therapy that employs well-studied organisms shown to be safe and potentially effective should be offered to children with persistent IBD symptoms. Dosing guidelines to consider are 10 billion CFU for children < 12 kg and 20 billion CFU for children > 12 kg. To date this author has no experience using the VSL#3 product, but existing data strongly suggest the potential for benefit.

Treatment with probiotics is extremely well tolerated, and palatability is an infrequent issue because the capsules can be opened and mixed into drinks or soft foods. Sometimes the agents are available as a powder as well. If effective, treatment can continue indefinitely. Use with extreme caution, if at all, for those children at risk for infectious complications (immunosuppression or use of immunosuppressive agents, presence of central venous catheter, prematurity).

References

Pediatric Diagnosis and Treatment

1. Baldassano RN, Piccoli DA: Inflammatory bowel disease in pediatric and adolescent patients, *Gastroenterol Clin North Am* 28: 445-458, 1999.

2. Farmer RG, Michener WM: Prognosis of Crohn's disease with onset in childhood or adolescence, *Dig Dis Sc* 24:752, 1979.

3. Buller HA: Problems in diagnosis of IBD in children [in Dutch], *Neth J Med* 50:S8-S11, 1997 (abstract).

4. Mendeloff AI, Calkins BM: The epidemiology of idiopathic inflammatory bowel disease. In Kirsner JB, Shorter RG, editors: *Inflammatory bowel disease*, Philadelphia, 1988, Lea and Febiger.

5. Calkins BM, Lilienfield AM, Garland CG et al: Tends in incidence rates of ulcerative colitis and Crohn's disease, *Dig Dis Sci* 29:913, 1984 (abstract).

6. Behrman RE, Kliegman RM, Jenson HB, editors: *Nelson textbook of pediatrics*, ed 17, Philadelphia, 2004, Saunders.

7. Andres PG, Friedman LS: Epidemiology and the natural course of inflammatory bowel disease, *Gastroenterol Clin North Am* 28: 255-281, vii, 1999.

8. Roy CC, Silverman A, Alagille D: *Pediatric clinical gastroenterology*, ed 4, New York, 1995, Mosby.

9. Scholmerich J: Future developments in diagnosis and treatment of inflammatory bowel disease, *Hepatogastroenterology* 47:101-114, (abstract) 2000.

10. Tibble JA, Sigthorsson G, Foster R et al: Use of surrogate markers of inflammation and Rome criteria to distinguish organic from nonorganic intestinal disease, *Gastroenterology* 123:450-460, 2002.

11. Schuster MM: Defining and diagnosing irritable bowel syndrome, *Am J Manag Care* 7(8 Suppl):S246-S251, 2001.

12. Duerr RH, Barmada MM, Zhang L et al: Linkage and association between inflammatory bowel disease and a locus on chromosome 12, *Am J Hum Genet* 63:95-100, 1998.

13. Duerr RH, Barmada MM, Zhang L et al: High-density genome scan in Crohn disease shows confirmed linkage to chromosome 14q11-12, *Am J Hum Genet* 66:1857-1862, 2000.

14. Devroede GJ, Taylor WF, Sauer J et al: Cancer risk and life expectancy of children with ulcerative colitis, *New Engl J Med* 289:491, 1973.

15. Casati J, Toner BB: Psychosocial aspects of inflammatory bowel disease, *Biomed Pharmacother* 54:388-393, 2000.

16. Macdonald TT, Disabatino A, Gordon JN: Immunopathogenesis of Crohn's disease, *JPEN J Parenter Enteral Nutr* 29(4 Suppl): S118-S125, 2005.

17. Griffiths AM: Enteral nutrition in the management of Crohn's disease, *JPEN J Parenter Enteral Nutr* 29(4 Suppl):S108-S117, 2005.

18. Ferreira AC, Almeida S, Tavares M et al: NOD2/CARD15 and TNFA, but not IL1B and IL1RN, are associated with Crohn's disease, *Inflamm Bowel Dis* 11:331-339, 2005.

19. Wehkamp J, Schmid M, Fellermann K et al: Defensin deficiency, intestinal microbes, and the clinical phenotypes of Crohn's disease, *J Leukoc Biol* 77:460-465, 2005.

20. Kobayashi KS, Chamaillard M, Ogura Y et al: Nod2-dependent regulation of innate and adaptive immunity in the intestinal tract, *Science* 307:731-734, 2005.

21. Mascheretti S, Schreiber S: Genetic testing in Crohn disease: utility in individualizing patient management, *Am J Pharmacogenomics* 5:213-222, 2005.

22. Wehkamp J, Fellermann K, Stange EF: Human defensins in Crohn's disease, *Chem Immunol Allergy* 86:42-54, 2005.

23. Pierik M, Yang H, Barmada MM et al; IBD International Genetics Consortium: The IBD International Genetics Consortium provides further evidence for linkage to IBD4 and shows gene-environment interaction, *Inflamm Bowel Dis* 11:1-7, 2005.

24. Lindberg E, Tysk C, Andersson K et al: Smoking and inflammatory bowel disease. A case control study, *Gut* 29:352-357, 1988.

25. Markowitz J, Daum F, Algar M, et al: Perianal disease in children and adolescents with Crohn's disease, *Gastroenterology* 86:829, 1984 (abstract).

26. Griffiths AM: Crohn's disease, *Rec Adv Pediatr* 10:145ff, 1992.

27. Goulet O: Inflammatory bowel disease in children [in French], *Rev Prat* 48:403-409, 1998, (abstract).

28. Booth IW: The nutritional consequences of gastrointestinal disease in adolescence, *Acta Pediatr Scand* 373(Suppl):91-102, 1991.

29. Mamula P, Telega GW, Markowitz JE et al: Inflammatory bowel disease in children 5 years of age and younger, *Am J Gastroenterol* 97:2005-2010, 2002.

30. Hildebrand H, Karlberg J, Kristiansson B: Longitudinal growth in children and adolescents with inflammatory bowel disease, *J Pediatr Gastroenterol Nutr* 18:165-173, 1994 (abstract).

31. Langholz E, Munkholm P, Krasilnikoff PA: Inflammatory bowel disease with onset in childhood [in Swedish], *Scand J Gastroenterol* 32:139-147, 1997 (abstract).

32. Tysk C, Jarnerot G. Has smoking changed the epidemiology of ulcerative colitis? *Scand J Gastroenterol* 27:508-512, 1992.

33. Lindberg E, Tysk C, Andersson K et al: Smoking and inflammatory bowel disease. A case control study, *Gut* 29:352-357, 1998.

34. Grand RJ, Homer DR: Inflammatory bowel disease in childhood and adolescence, *Pediatr Clin North Am* 22:835, 1975 (citation).

35. Binder SC, Patterson JF, Glotzer DJ: Toxic megacolon in ulcerative colitis, *Gastroenterology* 66:1088, 1974 (citation).

36. Ekbom A, Helmick C, Zack M et al: Ulcerative colitis and colorectal cancer: a population-based study, *N Engl J Med* 323:1228-1233, 1990 (abstract).

37. Griffiths AM, Sherman PM: Colonoscopic surveillance for cancer in ulcerative colitis: a critical review, J Pediatr Gastroenterol Nutr 24:202-210, 1997 (citation).

38. Danzi JT: Extraintestinal manifestations of idiopathic inflammatory bowel disease, *Arch Intern Med* 148:297, 1988 (abstract).

39. Gryboski JD, Spiro HM: Prognosis in children with Crohn's disease, *Gastroenterology* 74:807, 1978 (abstract).

40. Winesett M: Inflammatory bowel disease in children and adolescents, *Pediatr Ann* 26:227-234, 1997.

41. Hassall E, Barclay GN, Ament ME: Colonoscopy in childhood, *Pediatrics* 73:594, 1984 (abstract).

42. Hyams JS, Ferry GD, Mandel FS et al: Development and validation of a pediatric Crohn's Disease Activity Index, *J Pediatr Gastroenterol Nutr* 12:439, 1991 (abstract).

43. Oliva MM, Lake AM: Nutritional considerations and management of the child with inflammatory bowel disease, *Nutrition* 12:151-158, 1996.

44. Belluzzi A, Brignola C, Campieri M et al: Effect of enteric-coated fish oil preparation on relapses in Crohn's disease, *N Engl J Med* 334:1557-1560, 1996 (abstract).

45. Aranda R, Horgan K: Immunosuppressive drugs in the treatment of inflammatory bowel disease, *Semin Gastrointest Dis* 9:2-9, 1998.

46. Haller C, Markowitz J: A perspective on inflammatory bowel disease in the child and adolescent at the turn of the millennium, *Curr Gastroenterol Rep* 3:263-271, 2001.

47. Kozarek RA: Review article: immunosuppressive therapy for inflammatory bowel disease, *Aliment Pharmacol Ther* 7:117-123, 1993.

48. Lofberg R, Rutgeerts P, Malchow H et al: Budesonide prolongs time to relapse in ileal ileocecal Crohn's disease: a placebo controlled one year study, *Gut* 39:82-86, 1996 (abstract).
49. Stotland BR, Lichtenstein GR: Newer treatments for inflammatory bowel disease, *Primary Care* 23:577-608, 1996.
50. Choi PM, Targan SR: Immunomodulator therapy in inflammatory bowel disease, *Dig Dis Sci* 39:1885-1892, 1994.

Acupuncture

1. Diehl DL: Acupuncture for gastrointestinal and hepatobiliary disorders, *J Altern Complement Med* 5:27-45, 1999.
2. Joos S, Brinkhaus B, Maluche C et al: Acupuncture and moxibustion in the treatment of active Crohn's disease: a randomized controlled study, *Digestion* 69:131-139, 2004.
3. Quattropani C, Ausfeld B, Straumann A et al: Complementary alternative medicine in patients with inflammatory bowel disease: use and attitudes, *Scand J Gastroenterol* 38:277-282, 2003.
4. Rawsthorne P, Shanahan F, Cronin NC et al: An international survey of the use and attitudes regarding alternative medicine by patients with inflammatory bowel disease, *Am J Gastroenterol* 94:1298-1303, 1999.
5. Moum B: Medical treatment: does it influence the natural course of inflammatory bowel disease? *Eur J Intern Med* 11:197-203, 2000.
6. Zijlstra FJ, van den Berg-de Lange I, Huygen FJ et al: Anti-inflammatory actions of acupuncture, *Mediators Inflamm* 12:59-69, 2003.
7. Yang C, Yan H: Observation of the efficacy of acupuncture and moxibustion in 62 cases of chronic colitis, *J Tradit Chin Med* 19:111-114, 1999.
8. Wu HG, Zhou LB, Pan YY et al: Study of the mechanisms of acupuncture and moxibustion treatment for ulcerative colitis rats in view of the gene expression of cytokines, *World J Gastroenterol* 5:515-517, 1999.
9. Li Y, Tougas G, Chiverton SG et al: The effect of acupuncture on gastrointestinal function and disorders, *Am J Gastroenterol* 87:1372-1381, 1992.
10. Garrelds IM, Heiligers JP, Van Meeteren ME et al: Intestinal blood flow in murine colitis induced with dextran sulfate sodium, *Dig Dis Sci* 47:2231-2236, 2002.
11. Kuo TC, Lin CW, Ho FM: The soreness and numbness effect of acupuncture on skin blood flow, *Am J Chin Med* 32:117-129, 2004.
12. Liu Q: Effects of acupuncture on hemorheology, blood lipid content and nail fold microcirculation in multiple infarct dementia patients, *J Tradit Chin Med* 24:219-223, 2004.
13. Litscher G: Cerebral and peripheral effects of laser needle-stimulation, *Neurol Res* 25:722-728, 2003.
14. Litscher G, Wang L, Huber E et al: Changed skin blood perfusion in the fingertip following acupuncture needle introduction as evaluated by laser Doppler perfusion imaging, *Lasers Med Sci* 17:19-25, 2002.
15. Zhang X: 23 cases of chronic nonspecific ulcerative colitis treated by acupuncture and moxibustion, *J Tradit Chin Med* 18:188-191, 1998.
16. Kaptchuk TJ: Acupuncture: theory, efficacy, and practice, *Ann Intern Med* 136:374-383, 2002.
17. Han JS: Acupuncture and endorphins, *Neurosci Lett* 361:258-261, 2004.
18. Carlsson C: Acupuncture mechanisms for clinically relevant long-term effects—reconsideration and a hypothesis, *Acupunct Med* 20:82-99, 2002.
19. Cao X: Scientific bases of acupuncture analgesia, *Acupunct Electrother Res* 27:1-14, 2002.

20. Shen J: Research on the neurophysiological mechanisms of acupuncture: review of selected studies and methodological issues, *J Altern Complement Med* 7(Suppl 1):S121-S127, 2001.
21. Gollub RL, Hui KK, Stefano GB: Acupuncture: pain management coupled to immune stimulation, *Zhongguo Yao Li Xue Bao* 20:769-777, 1999.
22. Ulett GA, Han J, Han S: Traditional and evidence-based acupuncture: history, mechanisms, and present status, *South Med J* 91:1115-1120, 1998.
23. Ulett GA, Han S, Han JS: Electroacupuncture: mechanisms and clinical application, *Biol Psychiatry* 44:129-138, 1998.
24. Sher L: The role of the endogenous opioid system in the effects of acupuncture on mood, behavior, learning, and memory, *Med Hypotheses* 50:475-478, 1998.
25. Andersson S, Lundeberg T: Acupuncture—from empiricism to science: functional background to acupuncture effects in pain and disease, *Med Hypotheses* 45:271-281, 1995.
26. Smith FW Jr: Neurophysiologic basis of acupuncture, *Probl Vet Med* 4:34-52, 1992.
27. Loo M: *Pediatric acupuncture*, London, 2002, Elsevier.
28. Chen Z: Treatment of ulcerative colitis with acupuncture, *J Tradit Chin Med* 15:231-233, 1995.

Aromatherapy

1. Pittler MH, Ernst E: Peppermint oil for irritable bowel syndrome: a critical review and meta-analysis, *Am J Gastroenterol* 93:1131-1135, 1998.
2. Kline RM, Kline JJ, Di Palma J et al: Enteric-coated, pH-dependent peppermint oil capsules for the treatment of irritable bowel syndrome in children, *J Pediatr* 138:125-128, 2001.

Chiropractic

1. Thomas RJ: Gastrointestinal disorders. In Lawrence D, editor: *Chiropractic diagnosis and management*, Baltimore, 1991, Williams and Wilkins.
2. Takeda Y, Arai S, Touichi H: Long term remission and alleviation of symptoms in allergy and crohn's disease patients following spinal adjustment for reduction of vertebral subluxations, *J Vertebral Sublux Res* 4:129-141, 2002.
3. Wagner T: Irritable bowel syndrome and spinal manipulation: a case report, *Chiropractic Technique* 7:139-140, 1995.
4. Pikalov AA, Kharin VV: The use of spinal manipulative therapy in the treatment of duodenal ulcer: a pilot study, *J Manipulative Physiol Ther* 17:310-313, 1994.
5. Bryner P, Staerker PG: Indigestion and heartburn: a descriptive study of prevalence in persons seeking care from chiropractors, *J Manipulative Physiol Ther* 19:317-323, 1996.
6. Browning JE: Pelvic pain and organic dysfunction is a patient with low back pain, response to distractive manipulation: a case presentation, *J Manipulative Physiol Ther* 10:116-121, 1987.
7. Browning JE: Chiropractic distractive decompression in treating pelvic pain and multiple system pelvic organic dysfunction, *J Manipulative Physiol Ther* 12:265-274, 1989.
8. Browning JE: Mechanically induced pelvic pain and organic dysfunction in a patient without low back pain, *J Manipulative Physiol Ther* 13:406-411, 1990.
9. Browning JE: Uncomplicated mechanically induced pelvic pain and organic dysfunction in low back pain patients, *J Can Chiropractic Assoc* 35:149-155, 1991.
10. Polk JR: A new approach to pelvic pain management, *Today's Chiropractic* 20:42-46, 1991.
11. Anderson FM: *The physician's practical guide to nutritional therapy*, Atlanta, 1979, Symmes Systems.

Herbs—Western

1. Blumenthal M: *The complete German Commission E monographs: therapeutic guide to herbal medicines*, 1998.
2. Mills S, Bone K: *Principles and practice of phytotherapy, modern herbal medicine*, New York, 2000, Churchill Livingstone.
3. Barret M: *The handbook of clinically tested herbal remedies*, New York, 2004, Haworth Press.
4. Saller R, Pfister-Hotz G, Iten F et al: Iberogast: a modern phytotherapeutic combined herbal drug for the treatment of functional disorders of the gastrointestinal tract (dyspepsia, irritable bowel syndrome)—from phytomedicine to "evidence based phytotherapy." A systematic review [in German], *Forschende Komplementarmedizin und Klassische Naturheilkunde* 9(Suppl 1):1-20, 2002.
5. Madisch A, Holtmann G, Plein K et al: Treatment of irritable bowel syndrome with herbal preparations: results of a double-blind, randomized, placebo-controlled, multi-centre trial, *Aliment Pharmacol Ther* 19:271-279, 2004.
6. Reichling J, Saller R: *Iberis amara* L. (bitter candytuft)—profile of a medicinal plant [in German], *Forschende Komplementarmedizin und Klassische Naturheilkunde* 9(Suppl 1):21-33, 2002.
7. Madisch A, Melderis H, Mayr G et al: Commercially available herbal preparation and its modified dispense in patients with functional dyspepsia. Results of a double-blind, placebo-controlled, randomized multicenter trial [in German], *Zeitschrift fur Gastroenterologie* 7:511-517, 2001.
8. Mills S, Bone K, editors: *The essential guide to herbal safety*, St Louis, 2005, Elsevier.
9. Madisch A, Heydenreich CJ, Wieland V et al: Treatment of functional dyspepsia with a fixed peppermint oil and caraway oil combination preparation as compared to cisapride. A multicenter, reference-controlled double-blind equivalence study, *Arzneimittelforschung* 49:925-932, 1999.
10. Liu JH, Chen GH, Yeh HZ et al: Enteric-coated peppermint-oil capsules in the treatment of irritable bowel syndrome: a prospective, randomized trial, *J Gastroenterol* 32:765-768, 1997.
11. Pittler MH, Ernst E: Peppermint oil for irritable bowel syndrome: a critical review and metaanalysis, *Am J Gastroenterol* 93:1131-1135, 1998.
12. Kline RM, Kline JJ, Di Palma J et al: Enteric-coated, pH-dependent peppermint oil capsules for the treatment of irritable bowel syndrome in children, *J Pediatr* 138:125-128, 2001.
13. Blumenthal M: *The ABC clinical guide to herbs*, Austin, 2003, The American Botanical Council.

Homeopathy

1. *ReferenceWorks Pro 4.2* San Rafael, Calif, 2008, Kent Homeopathic Associates.

Massage Therapy

1. Burgmann T, Rawsthorne P, Bernstein CN: Predictors of alternative and complementary medicine use in inflammatory bowel disease: do measures of conventional health care utilization relate to use? *Am J Gastroenterol* 99:889-893, 2004.
2. Rawsthorne P, Shanahan F, Cronin NC et al: An international survey of the use and attitudes regarding alternative medicine by patients with inflammatory bowel disease, *Am J Gastroenterol* 94:1298-1303, 1999.
3. Association of Reflexologists. Available at www.reflexology.org/index.html. Accessed April 30, 2008.
4. Tovey P: A single-blind trial of reflexology for irritable bowel syndrome, *Br J Gen Pract* 52:19-23, 2002.
5. Diego MA, Field T, Hernandez-Reif M: Vagal activity, gastric motility, and weight gain in massaged preterm neonates, *J Pediatr* 147:50-55, 2005.
6. Hernandez-Reif M, Field T, Krasnegor J et al: Lower back pain is reduced and range of motion increased after massage therapy, *Int J Neurosc* 106:131-145, 2001.
7. Fraser J, Kerr JR: Psycho-physiological effects of back massage on elderly institutionalized patients, *J Adv Nurs* 18:238-245, 1993.
8. Field T, Ironson G, Scafidi F et al: Massage therapy reduces anxiety and enhances EEG patterns of alertness and math computations, *Int J Neurosci* 3:197-205, 1996.
9. Field T, Peck M, Krugman S et al: Burn injuries benefit from massage therapy. *J Burn Care Rehabil* 19:241-244, 1998.
10. Moyer CA, Rounds J, Hannum JW: A meta-analysis of massage therapy research, *Psychol Bull* 130:3-18, 2004.
11. Field T, Morrno C, Valdeon et al: Massage reduces anxiety in child and adolescent psychiatric patients, *J Am Acad Adolesc Psychiatry* 31:125-131, 1992.
12. Field T, Sunshine W, Hernandez-Reif M et al: Chronic fatigue syndrome: massage therapy effects of depression and somatic symptoms in chronic fatigue, *J Chronic Fatigue Syndrome* 3:43-51, 1997.
13. Post-White J, Kinney ME, Savik K et al: Therapeutic massage and healing touch improve symptoms in cancer, *Integr Cancer Ther* 2:332-344, 2003.
14. Ferrell-Tory AT, Glick OJ: The use of therapeutic massage as a nursing intervention to modify anxiety and the perception of cancer pain, *Cancer Nurs* 16:93-101, 1993.
15. Cassileth BR, Vickers AJ: Massage therapy for symptom control: outcome study at a major cancer center, *J Pain Symptom Manage* 28:3, 2004.
16. Mehling WE, Jacobs B, Acree M et al: Symptom management with massage and acupuncture in postoperative cancer patients: a randomized controlled trial, *J Pain Symptom Manage* 33:258-266, 2007.
17. Hernandez-Reif M, Field T, Ironson G et al: Natural killer cells and lymphocytes increase in women with breast cancer following massage therapy, *Intern J Neuroscience,* 115:495-510, 2005.
18. Schachner L, Field T, Hernandez-Reif M et al: Atopic dermatitis decreased in children following massage therapy, *Pediatr Dermatol* 15:390-395, 1998.
19. Field T, Peck M, Sed et al: Post-burn itching, pain, and psychological symptoms are reduced with massage therapy, *J Burn Care Rehabil* 21:189-193, 2000.
20. Rexilius SJ, Mundt C, Erikson Megel M et al: Therapeutic effects of massage therapy and handling touch on caregivers of patients undergoing autologous hematopoietic stem cells, *Oncol Nurs Forum* 29:E35-E44, 2002.
21. Wilkinson SM, Love SB, Westcombe AM et al: Effectiveness of aromatherapy massage in the management of anxiety and depression in patients with cancer: a multi-center randomized controlled trial, *J Clin Oncol* 25:532-538, 2007.
22. Hernandez-Reif M, Ironson G, Field T et al: Breast cancer patients have improved immune and neuroendocrine functions following massage therapy, *J Psychosom Res* 57:45-52, 2004.
23. Field T, Henteleff T, Hernandez-Reif M et al: Children with asthma have improved pulmonary functions after massage therapy, *J Pediatr* 132:854-858, 1998.
24. Field T, Hernandez-Reif M, Seligman S et al: Juvenile rheumatoid arthritis benefits from massage therapy, *J Pediatr Psychol* 22:607-617, 1997.
25. Ironson G, Field T, Scafidi F et al: Massage therapy is associated with enhancement of the immune system's cytotoxic capacity, *Int J Neurosci* 84:205-217, 1996.

26. Sunshine W, Field T, Quintino O et al: Fibromyalgia benefits from massage therapy and transcutaneous electrical stimulation, *J Clin Rheumatol* 2:18-22, 1996.

Mind/Body

1. Anton P: Stress and mind-body impact on the course of inflammatory bowel diseases, *Semin Gastrointest Dis* 10:14-19, 1999.
2. Maunder R, Esplen J: Supportive-expressive group psychotherapy for persons with inflammatory bowel disease, *Can J Psychiatry* 46:622-626, 2001.
3. Yen Pik Sang FD, Golding JF, Gresty MA: Suppression of sickness by controlled breathing during madly nauseogenic motion, *Aviat Space Environ Med* 74:998-1002, 2003.
4. Yen Pik Sang FD, Billar JP, Golding JF et al: Behavioral methods of alleviating motion sickness: Effectiveness of controlled breathing and a music audiotape, *J Travel Med* 10:108-111, 2003.
5. Cowings PS, Toscano WB, Cowings PS: Autogenic-feedback training exercise is superior to promethazine for control of motion sickness symptoms, *J Clin Pharmacol* 40:1154-1165, 2000.
6. Jones DR, Levy RA, Gardner L et al: Self-control of psychophysiologic response to motion stress: using biofeedback to treat airsickness, *Aviat Space Environ Med* 56:1152-1157, 1985.
7. Giles DA, Lochridge GK: Behavioral airsickness management program for student pilots, *Aviat Space Environ Medicine* 56:991-994, 1985.

Naturopathy

1. Workman EM, Alun Jones V, Wilson AJ et al: Diet in the management of Crohn's disease, *Hum Nutr Appl Nutr* 38:469-473, 1984.
2. Joachim G: The relationship between habits of food consumption and reported reactions to food in people with inflammatory bowel disease—testing the limits, *Nutr Health* 13:69-83, 1999.
3. Barclay GR, McKenzie H, Pennington J et al: The effect of dietary yeast on the activity of stable chronic Crohn's disease, *Scand J Gastroenterol* 27:196-200, 1992.
4. McKenzie H, Main J, Pennington CR et al: Antibody to selected strains of *Saccharomyces cerevisiae* (baker's and brewer's yeast) and *Candida albicans* in Crohn's disease, *Gut* 31:536-538, 1990.
5. Levo Y, Shalit M, Wollner S et al: Serum IgE levels in patients with inflammatory bowel disease, *Ann Allergy* 56:85-87, 1986.
6. Meryn S: Role of nutrition in acute and long-term therapy of chronic inflammatory bowel diseases, *Wien Klin Wochenschr* 98:774-779, 1986.
7. Kitsukawa Y, Saito H, Suzuki Y et al: Effect of ingestion of eicosapentaenoic acid ethyl ester on carrageenan-induced colitis in guinea pigs, *Gastroenterology* 102:1859-1866, 1992.
8. Marcus AJ, Marcus SN, Marcus R et al: Rapid production of ulcerative disease of the colon in newly-weaned guinea-pigs by degraded carrageenan, *J Pharm Pharmacol* 41:423-426, 1989.
9. Jones VA, Dickinson RJ, Workman E et al: Crohn's disease: maintenance of remission by diet, *Lancet* 2:177-180, 1985.
10. Riordan AM, Hunter JO, Cowan RE et al: Treatment of active Crohn's disease by exclusion diet: East Anglian multicentre controlled trial, *Lancet* 342:1131-1134, 1993.
11. Martini GA, Brandes JW: Increased consumption of refined carbohydrates in patients with Crohn's disease, *Klin Wochenschr* 54:367-371, 1976.
12. Thornton JR, Emmett PM, Heaton KW: Diet and Crohn's disease: characteristics of the pre-illness diet, *Br Med J* 2:762-764, 1979.
13. Riemann JF, Kolb S: Low-sugar and fiber-rich diet in Crohn disease, *Fortschr Med* 102:67-70, 1984.

14. Brandes JW, Lorenz-Meyer H: Sugar free diet: a new perspective in the treatment of Crohn disease? Randomized, control study, *Z Gastroenterol* 19:1-12, 1981.
15. Heaton KW, Thornton JR, Emmett PM: Treatment of Crohn's disease with an unrefined-carbohydrate, fibre-rich diet, *Br Med J* 2:764-766, 1979.
16. Neut C, Colombel JF, Guillemot F et al: Impaired bacterial flora in human excluded colon, *Gut* 30:1094-1098, 1989.
17. Keighley MR, Arabi Y, Dimock F et al: Influence of inflammatory bowel disease on intestinal microflora, *Gut* 19:1099-1104, 1978.
18. Curran FT, Youngs DJ, Allan RN et al: Candidacidal activity of Crohn's disease neutrophils, *Gut* 32:55-60, 1991.
19. Tonnesmann E, Burkle PA, Schafer B et al: The immune competence of patients with Crohn's disease, *Klin Wochenschr* 57: 1097-1107, 1979.
20. Rubin DT, Hanauer SB: Smoking and inflammatory bowel disease, *Eur J Gastroenterol Hepatol* 12:855-862, 2002.
21. Thomas GA, Rhodes J, Green JT et al: Role of smoking in inflammatory bowel disease: implications for therapy, *Postgrad Med J* 76:273-279, 2000.
22. Cosnes J, Carbonnel F, Carrat F et al: Effects of current and former cigarette smoking on the clinical course of Crohn's disease, *Aliment Pharmacol Ther* 13:1403-1411, 1999.
23. Yamamoto T, Keighley MR: Smoking and disease recurrence after operation for Crohn's disease, *Br J Surg* 87:398-404, 2000.
24. Kocian J, Kocianova J: Disorders of bone mineralization and their treatment in Crohn's disease, *Vnitr Lek* 44:162-165, 1998.
25. Robinson RJ, Krzywicki T, Almond L et al: Effect of a low-impact exercise program on bone mineral density in Crohn's disease: a randomized controlled trial, *Gastroenterology* 115:36-41, 1998.
26. Kruidenier L, Kuiper I, Lamers CB et al: Intestinal oxidative damage in inflammatory bowel disease: semi-quantification, localization, and association with mucosal antioxidants, *Pathol* 201:28-36, 2003.
27. Geerling BJ, Badart-Smook A, Stockbrugger RW et al: Comprehensive nutritional status in patients with long-standing Crohn disease currently in remission, *Am J Clin Nutr* 67:919-926, 1998.
28. Hoffenberg EJ, Deutsch J, Smith S et al: Circulating antioxidant concentrations in children with inflammatory bowel disease, *Am J Clin Nutr* 65:1482-1488, 1997.
29. Buffinton GD, Doe WF: Altered ascorbic acid status in the mucosa from inflammatory bowel disease patients, *Free Radic Res* 22: 131-143, 1995.
30. Hughes RG, Williams N: Leucocyte ascorbic acid in Crohn's disease, *Digestion* 17:272-274, 1978.
31. Buffinton GD, Doe WF: Depleted mucosal antioxidant defenses in inflammatory bowel disease, *Free Radic Biol Med* 19:911-918, 1995.
32. Myung SJ, Yang SK, Jung HY et al: Zinc deficiency manifested by dermatitis and visual dysfunction in a patient with Crohn's disease, *J Gastroenterol* 33:876-879, 1998.
33. Krasovec M, Frenk E: Acrodermatitis enteropathica secondary to Crohn's disease, *Dermatology* 193:361-363, 1996.
34. Rath HC, Caesar I, Roth M et al: Nutritional deficiencies and complications in chronic inflammatory bowel diseases, *Med Klin* 93:6-10, 1998.
35. Penny WJ, Mayberry JF, Aggett PJ et al: Relationship between trace elements, sugar consumption, and taste in Crohn's disease, *Gut* 24:288-292, 1983.
36. Nishi Y, Lifshitz F, Bayne MA et al: Zinc status and its relation to growth retardation in children with chronic inflammatory bowel disease, *Am J Clin Nutr* 33:2613-2621, 1980.

37. Kruis W, Rindfleisch GE, Weinzierl M: Zinc deficiency as a problem in patients with Crohn's disease and fistula formation, *Hepatogastroenterology* 32:133-134, 1985.

38. Reimund JM, Hirth C, Koehl C et al: Antioxidant and immune status in active Crohn's disease. A possible relationship, *Clin Nutr* 19:43-48, 2000.

39. Rannem T, Ladefoged K, Hylander E et al: Selenium depletion in patients with gastrointestinal diseases: are there any predictive factors? *Scand J Gastroenterol* 33:1057-1061, 1998.

40. Rannem T, Ladefoged K, Hylander E et al: Selenium status in patients with Crohn's disease, *Am J Clin Nutr* 56:933-937, 1992.

41. Rumi G Jr, Szabo I, Vincze A et al: Decrease of serum carotenoids in Crohn's disease, *J Physiol Paris* 94:159-161, 2000.

42. Bousvaros A, Zurakowski D, Duggan C et al: Vitamins A and E serum levels in children and young adults with inflammatory bowel disease: effect of disease activity, *J Pediatr Gastroenterol Nutr* 26:129-135, 1998.

43. Schoelmerich J, Becher MS, Hoppe-Seyler P et al: Zinc and vitamin A deficiency in patients with Crohn's disease is correlated with activity but not with localization or extent of the disease, *Hepatogastroenterology* 32:34-38, 1985.

44. Kuroki F, Iida M, Tominaga M et al: Multiple vitamin status in Crohn's disease. Correlation with disease activity, *Dig Dis Sci* 38:1614-1618, 1993.

45. Elsborg L, Larsen L: Folate deficiency in chronic inflammatory bowel diseases, *Scand J Gastroenterol* 14:1019-1024, 1979.

46. Tominaga M, Iida M, Aoyagi K et al: Red cell folate concentrations in patients with Crohn's disease on parenteral nutrition, *Postgrad Med J* 65:818-820, 1989.

47. Siguel EN, Lerman RH: Prevalence of essential fatty acid deficiency in patients with chronic gastrointestinal disorders, *Metabolism* 45:12-23, 1996.

48. Tsujikawa T, Satoh J, Uda K et al: Clinical importance of n-3 fatty acid-rich diet and nutritional education for the maintenance of remission in Crohn's disease, *J Gastroenterol* 35:99-104, 2000.

49. Miura S, Tsuzuki Y, Hokari R et al: Modulation of intestinal immune system by dietary fat intake: relevance to Crohn's disease, *J Gastroenterol Hepatol* 13:1183-1190, 1998.

50. Belluzzi A, Brignola C, Campieri M et al: Effect of an enteric-coated fish-oil preparation on relapses in Crohn's disease, *N Engl J Med* 334:1557-1560, 1996.

51. Reif S, Klein I, Lubin F et al: Pre-illness dietary factors in inflammatory bowel disease, *Gut* 40:754-760, 1997.

52. Galland L: Magnesium and inflammatory bowel disease, *Magnesium* 7:78-83, 1988.

53. Main AN, Morgan RJ, Russell RI et al: Mg deficiency in chronic inflammatory bowel disease and requirements during intravenous nutrition, *J Parenter Enteral Nutr* 5:15-19, 1981.

54. Hessov I, Hasselblad C, Fasth S et al; Magnesium deficiency after ileal resections for Crohn's disease, *Scand J Gastroenterol* 18:643-649, 1983.

55. Alshuler L: *Gastroenterology,* Seattle, 1999, Bastyr University.

56. Milne B, Joachim G, Niedhardt J: A stress management programme for inflammatory bowel disease patients, *J Adv Nurs* 11:561-567, 1986.

57. de la Torre B, Hedman M, Befrits R: Blood and tissue dehydroepiandrosterone sulphate levels and their relationship to chronic inflammatory bowel disease, *Clin Exp Rheumatol* 16:579-582, 1998.

58. Segain JP, de la Bletiere DR, Bourreille A et al: Butyrate inhibits inflammatory responses through NFκB inhibition: implications for Crohn's disease, *Gut* 47:397-403, 2000.

Nutrition

1. Lutz RB: Inflammatory bowel disease. In Rakel D, editor: *Integrative medicine*, Philadelphia, 2003, Saunders.

2. Hugot JP, Alberti C, Berrebi D et al: Crohn's disease: the cold chain hypothesis, *Lancet* 362:2012-2015, 2003.

3. Pizzorno LU, Pizzorno JE, Murray MT: *Natural medicine: instructions for patients*, London, 2002, Churchill Livingstone/Elsevier.

4. Bibiloni R, Fedorak RN, Tannock GW et al: VSL#3 probiotic-mixture induced remission in patients with active ulcerative colitis, *Am J Gastroenterol* 100:1539-1546, 2005.

5. Gupta P, Andrew H, Kirschner BS et al: Is *Lactobacillus* GG helpful in children with Crohn's disease? Results of a preliminary, open-label study, *J Pediatr Gastroent Nutr* 31:453-457, 2000.

6. Kanauchi O, Mitsuyama K, Homma T, et al: Treatment of ulcerative colitis patients by long-term administration of germinated barley foodstuff: multi-center open trial, *Int J Mol Med* 12:701-704, 2003.

7. Aslan A, Triadafilopoulos G: Fish oil fatty acid supplementation in active ulcerative colitis: a double-blind, placebo-controlled, crossover study, *Am J Gastroenterol* 87:432-437, 1992.

8. Stenson WF, Cort D, Rodgers J et al: Dietary supplementation with fish oil in ulcerative colitis, *Ann Intern Med* 116:609-614, 1992.

Probiotics

1. Schultz M, Sartor RB: Probiotics and inflammatory bowel diseases, *Am J Gastroenterol* 95(Suppl):S19, 2000.

2. Giaffer MH, Holdsworth CD, Duerden BI: The assessment of facial flora in patients with inflammatory bowel disease by a simplified bacteriological technique, *J Med Microbiol* 35:238, 1991.

3. Pathmakanthan S, Thornley JP, Hawkey CJ: Mucosally associated bacterial flora of the human colon: Quantitative and species specific differences between normal and inflamed colonic biopsies, *Microbial Ecol Health Dis* 11:169, 1999.

4. van de Merwe JP, Schroder AM, Wensinck F et al: The obligate anaerobic fecal flora of patients with Crohn's disease and their first-degree relatives, *Scand J Gastroenterol* 23:1125, 1988.

5. Favier C, Neut C, Mizon C et al: Fecal β-d-galactosidase production and bifidobacteria are decreased in Crohn's disease, *Dig Dis Sci* 42:817, 1997.

6. Markowitz JE, Bengmark S: Probiotocs in health and disease in the pediatric patient, *Pediatr Clin North Am* 49;127, 2002.

7. Malin M, Suomalainen H, Saxelin M et al: Promotion of IgA immune response in patients with Crohn's disease by oral bacteriotherapy with *Lactobacillus* GG, *Ann Nutr Metab* 40:137, 1996.

8. Kruis W, Schutz E, Fric P et al: Double-blind comparison of an oral *Escherichia coli* preparation and mesalazine in maintaining remission of ulcerative colitis, *Aliment Pharmacol Ther* 11:853, 1997.

9. Rembacken BJ, Snelling AM, Hawkey PM et al: Non-pathogenic *Escherichia coli* versus mesalazine for the treatment of ulcerative colitis: a randomized trial, *Lancet* 354:635, 1999.

10. Guslandi M, Mezzi G, Sorghi M et al: *Saccharomyces boulardii* in maintenance treatment of Crohn's disease, *Dig Dis Sci* 45:1462, 2000.

11. Gionchetti P, Rizzello F, Venturi A et al: Maintenance therapy of chronic pouchitis: a randomized, placebo-controlled, double blind trial with a new probiotic preparation, *Gastroenterology* 114:A4037, 1998.

12. Gionchetti P, Rizzello F, Helwig U et al: Prophylaxis of pouchitis with probiotic therapy: a double-blind, placebo-controlled trial, *Gastroenterology* 124:1202, 2003.

13. Gionchetti P, Rizzello F, Matteuzzi D et al: Microflora in the IBD pathogenesis. Possible therapeutic use of probiotics, *Gastroenterol Int* 11:108, 1998.

14. Pranatera C, Scribano ML, Falasco G et al: Ineffectiveness of probiotics in preventing recurrence after curative resection for Crohn's disease: a randomized controlled trial with *Lactobacillus* GG, *Gut* 51:405, 2002.

15. Kuisma J, Mentula S, Jarvinen H et al: Effect of *Lactobacillus rhamnosus* GG on ileal pouch inflammation and microbial flora, *Aliment Pharmacol Ther* 17:509, 2003.

CHAPTER 46

Motion Sickness

Acupuncture | May Loo

Aromatherapy | Maura A. Fitzgerald

Chiropractic | Anne Spicer

Herbs—Chinese | Catherine Ulbricht, Jennifer Woods, Mark Wright

Herbs—Western | Alan D. Woolf, Paula M. Gardiner, Lana Dvorkin-Camiel, Jack Maypole

Homeopathy | Janet L. Levatin

Mind/Body | Timothy Culbert, Lynda Richtsmeier Cyr

Osteopathy | Jane Carreiro

✳ PEDIATRIC DIAGNOSIS AND TREATMENT

Motion sickness is defined as the discomfort experienced when perceived motion disturbs the organs of balance. Symptoms may include nausea, vomiting, pallor, cold sweats, hypersalivation, hyperventilation, and headaches.[1] Surveys conducted on school-aged children (9 to 18 years old) revealed significantly greater motion sickness for female as compared with male subjects, and there was little relation between an individual's level of physical activity and susceptibility to motion sickness.[2]

The control and prevention of motion sickness symptoms have included pharmacological, behavioral, and complementary therapies. Sometimes a simple intervention, such as seating the child with forward external vision, can significantly reduce symptoms.[3] Pharmaceutical management includes antihistamines, calcium channel antagonists, and scopolamine. A Cochrane Database Systematic Review of scopolamine for preventing motion sickness in 901 subjects revealed scopolamine as more effective than placebo, superior to methscopolamine, and equivalent to antihistamines as a preventive agent.[1] All medications can cause side effects such as drowsiness, blurring of vision or dizziness, or dry mouth and can usually function only as preventive agents, not as treatment for established symptoms of motion sickness.

✳ CAM THERAPY RECOMMENDATIONS

Acupuncture

The major acupuncture point for controlling nausea and vomiting from motion sickness is P6,[1,2] which is easily accessible on the arm for massage while the child is in the car or on the airplane.

ST36 can also be used together with P6 for a powerful combination of points.[2]

Aromatherapy

Aromatherapy is often recommended for nausea of any type, including motion sickness and postoperative or chemotherapy-related nausea. Research has focused on postoperative nausea.

In a randomized, placebo controlled trial of 33 adult postoperative ambulatory surgery patients, subjects were exposed to 2 × 2 gauze pads prepared with 2 mL peppermint essential oil *(Mentha piperita)*, 1 mL isopropyl alcohol 70%, or 2 mL isotonic saline. The researchers found that nausea scores were reduced in all three groups. There was no significant difference among groups.[1] Alternatively, in a smaller randomized, placebo controlled study of 18 women postoperative for gynecological surgery, a statistically significant reduction in nausea was observed in the group receiving peppermint essential oil as compared with the control (no treatment) and placebo (peppermint essence) groups. Subjects were given a bottle of 5 mL peppermint essential oil or essence. Most subjects inhaled directly from the bottle.[2]

It is the author's experience that essential oils of peppermint, spearmint *(Mentha spicata)*, ginger *(Zingiber officinalis)*, and lemon *(Citrus limon)* can be helpful to children experiencing nausea. The choice of the oil should be left to the child, as a scent that is unpleasant to the child is not likely to be tolerated. The essential oils are administered by applying 1 to 2 drops to a tissue or cotton ball and having the child inhale. The cotton ball can be placed in a plastic sandwich bag to contain the scent. Older children or adolescents may choose to inhale directly from the bottle; however, this is usually too strong for younger children.

Chiropractic

There are no case studies or clinical trials on chiropractic as it pertains to the management of motion sickness. However, the chiropractic approach to the person with motion sickness is to remove the subluxation complex (SC) impediment to normal postural function. Cervical intersegmental joints affect perception of spatial orientation and posture through abundant afferent input to the higher centers.[1,2] An SC in the cervical region may mimic prolonged postural instability and produce symptoms of dizziness, vertigo, and nausea.[3] It is now understood that weakened postural stability is a precursor to motion sickness symptoms, not just a product of such a phenomenon.[4,5] Cervical adjustments have been demonstrated to restore postural stability.[6] Because postural deficiencies also result in pathological changes in the spinal segments, discs, ligaments, and myofascial supports of the spine, it is recommended by this author that any child with symptoms of motion sickness be evaluated by a chiropractor. The goal of the chiropractic management is to restore proper spatial orientation and posture to prevent degenerative consequences, although reduction of motion sickness can certainly be a treatment effect as well.

It has also been found that vestibular neurons course through the brainstem[7,8] and have projections that converge with the dorsal motor nucleus of the vagus.[9,10] Vestibular function is also intimately tied to the sympathetic and parasympathetic systems.[11,12] These findings suggest a more systemic effect of the postural deficiencies secondary to the SC.

This author has found that C0-C1 is the most commonly affected area in people with motion sickness or nausea and dizziness.

Chiropractors may also stimulate the acupressure point on the anterior wrist, located two finger widths superior to the palmar margin between the palmaris longus and flexor carpi radialis tendons.

Eating ginger has been known to decrease the sensation of nausea and may decrease the intensity of the symptoms during travel.[13,14]

Herbs—Chinese

Ginger rhizome of *Z. officinalis* (Willd.) Roscoe has long been used to prevent motion sickness. The herb is commonly used in Chinese herbal medicine. Mostly it is used orally in decoctions, but it can also be taken as crystallized ginger or as candy. It is sometimes used in massage as a rubefacient. For antinausea applications, it would be taken orally. Studies show that ginger significantly reduces nausea associated with motion sickness by preventing the development of gastric dysrhythmias and the elevation of plasma vasopressin.[3-7]

One randomized controlled clinical trial studied the effects of ginger in the treatment of motion sickness. The study included 13 volunteers who had motion sickness. The volunteers were given a dose of ginger (1 or 2 g), and motion sickness was induced. The study found that pretreatment with ginger reduced the nausea, increased the time before the onset of nausea, and shortened the recovery time after nausea induction caused by circular movement. Ginger had no effect on nausea induced by injecting vasopressin. The results of this research are not clear, and further study is needed before conclusions can be drawn.[7]

Acupressure at Nei Guan (P6) is generally regarded as helpful for motion sickness (adults and children alike).

Herbs—Western

The most common and long-used herbs used for the treatment of motion sickness, nausea, and vomiting include ginger root, peppermint, chamomile, fennel, and other carmative herbs. Ginger *(Z. officinale)* has been used as a remedy for dyspepsia and nausea for centuries. The authoritative German Commission E Monograph approves the use of ginger root as a treatment for dyspepsia and prophylactic against motion sickness.[1] Several randomized controlled trials and meta analyses show mixed support for ginger's use as an antiemetic for nausea secondary to several conditions: morning sickness,

chemotherapy-associated nausea, postoperative nausea, and motion sickness.[2-7] In one clinic trial on motion sickness, 28 children aged 4 to 8 years received standardized preparation of ginger root (Zintona capsules) 30 minutes before the start of the 2-day trip and every 4 hours thereafter as necessary or 12.5 to 25 mg dimenhydrate 30 minutes before the start of the 2-day trip and every 4 hours thereafter as necessary. The physician rated the ginger as having good effectiveness in 100% of the children and rated dimenhydrate as having good effectiveness in 30.8% of the children. The dimenhydrate group reported more side effects (vertigo, increased salivation, stomach ache, nausea, dry mouth, pallor, and cold sweats), whereas the ginger root group reported none.[6] Ginger is well tolerated but in large doses may cause abdominal discomfort, heartburn, or diarrhea.

Homeopathy

Before using this section, please see Appendix A, Homeopathy, for definitions of practitioner expertise categories and general information on prescribing homeopathic medicines.

Practitioner Expertise Category 1

There are no controlled clinical trials of classical homeopathy for treatment of motion sickness, although the homeopathic literature contains evidence for its use in the form of accumulated clinical experience.[1] Motion sickness can often be treated effectively with homeopathy. For uncomplicated motion sickness, it is safe to try homeopathic treatment alone or in combination with other therapies, either conventional (e.g., antiemetics) or alternative (e.g., herbs, acupressure).

The goal in treating motion sickness homeopathically is to determine the single homeopathic medicine whose description in the materia medica most closely matches the symptom picture of the patient. Often mental and emotional states, in addition to physical symptoms, are considered. Once the medicine has been selected, it can be given orally or sublingually, in the 30C potency, 30 to 60 minutes prior to any activity that might induce motion sickness. It can then be repeated every 15 to 30 minutes as needed. If the medicine does not help on one occasion, then another homeopathic medicine should be tried the next time the patient engages in an activity that is known to cause motion sickness.

The following is a list of homeopathic medicines commonly used to treat patients with motion sickness. It must be emphasized that this list is partial and represents only some of the probable choices from the homeopathic materia medica. If the symptoms of a given patient are not represented here, a search of the homeopathic literature would be needed to find the simillimum.

Cocculus indicus

Cocculus indicus is one of the most commonly used medicines for motion sickness, including carsickness and seasickness. Patients are dizzy and have a headache. They may vomit or experience diarrhea. They will feel weak, tremulous, empty, or hollow. The thought or smell of food exacerbates the condition. The sitting position and exposure to fresh air tend to aggravate the condition, whereas lying down provides relief.

Tabacum

Tabacum should be considered for the patient with seasickness or carsickness when the nausea is constant and very severe or incapacitating. The patient is cold, sweaty, and pale.

Petroleum

Petroleum is a medicine to think of for air, car, or seasickness that is ameliorated by eating. *Petroleum* is used to treat patients with eczema who suffer from motion sickness.

Borax veneta (Sodium borate)

Borax veneta is a medicine for airsickness (and other forms of motion sickness) when the patient becomes ill during the descent.

Mind/Body

Motion sickness is characterized by symptoms of nausea and vomiting and underlying autonomic nervous system arousal. Most of the studies on mind/body approaches for motion sickness have been done in adults, the majority of the subjects being U.S. Air Force pilots. Experience suggests that these same approaches may be adaptable to pediatric clients. Nausea associated with motion sickness seems to respond well to controlled breathing techniques.[1] Adding music to the breath control training may be additionally beneficial.[2] Although the overall effectiveness of controlled breathing and music intervention are not as effective as pharmacological interventions, they do offer an alternative treatment that is free of adverse side effects. Biofeedback training as a way to maintain a more controlled, optimum state of autonomic nervous balance can be helpful in reducing nausea associated with motion sickness. Adult studies suggest that autogenics training[3] and a combination of biofeedback and cognitive-behavioral interventions are also useful for motion sickness control.[4,5]

The authors teach a version of this by having the child or adolescent breathe in through the nose to the count of 3 seconds and then exhale through the mouth to the count of 6 seconds, keeping the shoulders relaxed and the belly soft. Nausea and vomiting of other etiologies (chemotherapy associated, postoperative) may also respond to similar mind/body approaches. Mind/body techniques can be combined with acupoint stimulation (P6) and clinical aromatherapy (essential oil of peppermint, spearmint, ginger, or fennel) for excellent nausea control.

Osteopathy

From an osteopathic perspective, motion sickness may be related to problems in one of three areas: the vestibular system, the proprioceptive system, or the extraocular muscles. An individual's sense of balance and stability arise through an orchestrated interaction involving input from these three sensory systems and complex cerebral processing. This mechanism is capable of detecting the constantly changing external environment and adjusting the musculoskeletal system to meet its demands. Motion sickness or vertigo arises when there is a discrepancy among the inputs from these three systems. With a mild discrepancy, the child might feel lightheaded and unsteady; when the discrepancy reaches a sufficient threshold, the chemotactic trigger zone is activated and the child feels nauseous and may even vomit. Within the osteopathic concept of structure and function, motion sickness may result from mechanical dysfunction affecting one or more of the sensory inputs into this system.

On a simplified level, one component of balance involves a comparison of information sent from the labyrinth systems located in the petrous portion of each temporal bone. Tissue strains and imbalances in the cranial base, the cranial cervical junction or its stabilizing muscles has the potential to affect the relative positions of the temporal bones[1] and thus the semicircular canals contained within them.[2-4] This would alter the information being sent to the cortex, potentially creating a "contradiction" between the two systems. Dural strains may influence temporal bone mechanics and/or produce venous congestion in the vascular plexus traveling with the eighth cranial nerve as it traverses the facial canal.[3,5] Within the osteopathic concept, either of these could result in alterations in the function of the vestibular nerve.[4] Although there are no efficacy studies in children, cranial techniques have been reported to be beneficial in treating vertiginous symptoms in adults.[6,7]

Biomechanical strains in the cervical area may predispose the child to motion sickness by altering proprioceptive input from that area.[8,9] Trigger points in the sternocleidomastoid muscle have been reported to be associated with motion sickness.[4,10] Osteopathic approaches such as balanced membranous tension, functional, and myofascial techniques are usually used to treat these findings in younger children. Muscle energy techniques may be added in older children who can cooperate with instructions.

Visual inputs must also be considered in children with motion sickness. This may present as frank strabismus or as a more functional problem that affects head and neck posturing. The principles of osteopathy in the cranial field can be used to diagnose altered postural mechanics in the head and neck that arise from visual imbalances. The myopia of young children can be overcorrected with lenses that are too strong. This results in strain in the extraocular muscles and intraocular tissues as well as alterations in head and neck posturing as the child tries to bring the target into focus.[11,12] The chronic stress on the cervical tissues alters biomechanical relations and resting tissue tone. This is turn may present as symptoms of lightheadedness, nausea, and aversion to rapid visual processing. As the symptoms worsen or are prolonged, these children will often develop headache. The symptoms are exacerbated when the child is trying to visually focus. In these cases osteopathic physicians will work in conjunction with functional optometrists to find the corrective lenses best suited to the child's needs by evaluating postural accommodation and muscle tone changes associated with different lens prescriptions. Children wearing prism lenses may also be more susceptible to motion sickness.

References

Pediatric Diagnosis and Treatment

1. Spinks AB, Wasiak J, Villanueva EV, et al: Scopolamine for preventing and treating motion sickness, *Cochrane Database Syst Rev* (3):CD002851, 2004.
2. Dobie T, McBride D, Dobie T Jr. et al: The effects of age and sex on susceptibility to motion sickness, *Aviat Space Environ Med* 72:13-20, 2001.

3. Turner M, Griffin MJ: Motion sickness in public road transport: the relative importance of motion, vision and individual differences, *Br J Psychol* 90:519-530, 1999.

Acupuncture

1. Deadman P, Al-Khafaji M: *A manual of acupuncture*, Ann Arbor, Mich, 1998, Journal of Chinese Medicine Publications.
2. O'Connor J, Bensky D, editors: *Acupuncture, a comprehensive text*, Seattle, 1981, Eastland Press.

Aromatherapy

1. Anderson LA, Gross JG: Aromatherapy with peppermint, isopropyl alcohol or placebo is equally effective in relieving postoperative nausea, *J PeriAnesth Nurs* 19:29-35, 2004.
2. Tate S: Peppermint oil: a treatment for postoperative nausea, *J Adv Nurs* 26:543-549, 1997.

Chiropractic

1. Bovim G, Schrader H, Sand T: Neck pain in the general population, *Spine* 19:1307-1309, 1994.
2. Dwyer A, Aprill C, Bogduk N: Cervical zygapophyseal joint pain patterns I: a study in normal volunteers, *Spine* 15:453-457, 1986.
3. Smart LJ, Smith DL: Postural dynamics: clinical and empirical implications, *J Manipulative Physiol Ther* 24:340-349, 2001.
4. Ricco GE, Stofregen TA: An ecological theory of motion sickness and postural instability, *Ecological Psychol* 3:195-240, 1991.
5. Stoffregen TA, Smart LJ: Postural instability precedes motion sickness, *Brain Res Bull* 47:437-438, 1998.
6. Hospers LA: EEG and CEEG studies before and after upper cervical of SOT category II adjustment in children after head trauma, in epilepsy and in "hyperactivity," *Proc Natl Conf Chiropractic* Nov:84-139, 1992.
7. Yates BJ, Yagamat Y: Convergence of cardiovascular and vestibular input on neurons in the medullary paramedian reticular formation, *Brain Res* 513:166-170, 1990.
8. Yates BJ: Vestibular influences on the sympathetic nervous system, *Brain Res Rev* 17:51-59, 1992.
9. Balaban CD, Beryozkin G: Vestibular nucleus projection to nucleus tractus soltarius and the dorsal motor nucleus of the vagus nerve: potential substrates for vestibulo-autonomic interactions, *Exp Brain Res* 98:200-212, 1994.
10. Yates BJ, Grélot L, Kerman IA et al: The organization of vestibular inputs to nucleus tractus solitarius (NTS) and adjacent structures in the cat brainstem, *Am J Physiol* 267:974-983, 1994.
11. Porter JD, Balaban CD: Connections between medial and spinal vestibular nuclei with brain stem regions that mediate autonomic function in the rat, *Abstr 18 Midwinter Res Meet Assoc Res Otolaryngol* p 401, 1995.
12. Yates BJ, Balaban CD, Miller AD et al: Vestibular inputs to the lateral tegmental field of the cat: potential role in autonomic control, *Brain Res* 689:197-206, 1995.
13. Grant KL, Lutz RB: Alternative therapies: ginger, *Am J Health-Syst Pharm* 57:945-947, 2000.
14. Grøntved A, Brask T, Kambskard J et al: Ginger root against seasickness: a controlled trial on the open sea, *Acta Otolaryngol* 105:45-49, 1982.

Herbs—Chinese

1. Pei JS, Tong BL, Chen KJ et al: Experimental research on antimotion sickness effects of Chinese medicine "pingandan" pills in cats, *Chin Med J (Engl)* 195:322-327, 1992.

2. Chen KJ, Li CS, Zhang GX: Clinical and experimental studies of royal made ping an dan on treatment of motion sickness, *Zhongguo Zhong Xi Yi Jie He Za Zhi* 12:469-472, 1992.
3. Lien HC, Sun WM, Chen YH et al: Effects of ginger on motion sickness and gastric slow-wave dysrhythmias induced by circular vection, *Am J Physiol Gastrointest Liver Physiol* 284:G481-G489, 2003.
4. Wood CD, Manno JE, Wood MJ et al: Comparison of efficacy of ginger with various antimotion sickness drugs, *Clin Res Pr Drug Regul Aff* 6:129-136, 1988.
5. Stewart JJ, Wood MJ, Wood CD et al: Effects of ginger on motion sickness susceptibility and gastric function, *Pharmacology* 42: 111-120, 1991.
6. Holtmann S, Clarke AH, Scherer H et al: The anti-motion sickness mechanism of ginger. A comparative study with placebo and dimenhydrinate, *Acta Otolaryngol* 108:168-174, 1989.
7. Natural Standard Research Collaboration. Available www.naturalstandard.com. Accessed 2005.

Herbs—Western

1. Blumenthal M, editor: *The complete German Commission E monographs: therapeutic guide to herbal medicines*, Austin, 1998, American Botanical Council.
2. Arfeen Z, Owen H, Plummer JL et al: A double-blind randomized controlled trial of ginger for the prevention of postoperative nausea and vomiting, *Anaesth Intensive Care* 23:449-452, 1995.
3. Visalyaputra S, Petchpaisit N, Somcharoen K et al: The efficacy of ginger root in the prevention of postoperative nausea and vomiting after outpatient gynaecological laparoscopy, *Anaesthesia* 53: 506-510, 1998.
4. Aikins Murphy P: Alternative therapies for nausea and vomiting of pregnancy, *Obstet Gynecol* 91:149-155, 1998 (review, with 36 references).
5. Ernst E, Pittler MH: Efficacy of ginger for nausea and vomiting: a systematic review of randomized clinical trials, *Br J Anaesth* 84:367-371, 2000 (review, with 36 references).
6. Careddu P: Motion sickness in children: results of a double-blind study with ginger (Zintona) and dimenhydrinate, *Eur Phytother* 6:102-107, 1999.
7. Jewell D, Young G: Interventions for nausea and vomiting in early pregnancy [see comment] [update in Cochrane Database Syst Rev (4):CD000145, 2003; PMID: 14583914] [update of Cochrane Database Syst Rev (2):CD000145, 2000; PMID: 10796155], Cochrane Database System Rev (1):CD000145, 2002. [Review, with 59 references.]

Homeopathy

1. *ReferenceWorks Pro 4.2*, San Rafael, Calif, 2008. Kent Homeopathic Associates.

Mind/Body

1. Yen Pik Sang FD, Golding JF, Gresty MA: Suppression of sickness by controlled breathing during madly nauseogenic motion, *Aviat Space Environ Med* 74:998-1002, 2003.
2. Yen Pik Sang FD, Billar JP, Golding JF et al: Behavioral methods of alleviating motion sickness: effectiveness of controlled breathing and a music audiotape, *Jf Travel Med* 10:108-111, 2003.
3. Cowings PS, Toscano WB, Cowings PS: Autogenic-feedback training exercise is superior to promethazine for control of motion sickness symptoms, *J Clin Pharmacol* 40:1154-1165, 2000.
4. Jones DR, Levy RA, Gardner L et al: Self-control of psychophysiologic response to motion stress: using biofeedback to treat airsickness, *Aviat Space Environ Med* 56:1152-1157, 1985.

5. Giles DA, Lochridge GK: Behavioral airsickness management program for student pilots, *Aviat Space Environ Med* 56:991-994, 1985.

Osteopathy

1. Hruby RJ: The total body approach to the osteopathic management of temporomandibular joint dysfunction, *J Am Osteopath Assoc* 85:502-510, 1985.
2. Sutherland WG: *Teachings in the science of osteopathy*, Portland, Ore, 1990, Rudra Press.
3. Magoun HIS: *Osteopathy in the cranial field*, ed 3, Kirksville, MO, 1976, The Journal Printing Company.
4. Kuchera ML, Kuchera WA: *Osteopathic considerations in systemic disease*, Columbus, Ohio, 1994, Greydon Press.
5. Carreiro JE: Neurology. In *An osteopathic approach to children*, London, 2003, Churchill Livingstone.

6. Korr IM: *The neurobiological mechanisms in manipulative therapy*, New York, 1977, Plenium Press.
7. Cole W: Disorders of the nervous system, In Hoag JM, editor: *Osteopathic medicine*, New York, 1969, McGraw-Hill.
8. Norre ME: Head extension effect in static posturography, *Ann Otol Rhinol Laryngol* 104:570-573, 1995.
9. Ghez C: The control of movement, In Kandel ER, Schwartz JH, Jessell TM, editors: *Principles of neural science*, New York, 1991, Elsevier.
10. Travell JG, Simons DG: *Myofascial pain and dysfunction; the trigger point manual*, Baltimore, 1983, Williams and Wilkins.
11. Carreiro JE: *Ophthalmology: an osteopathic approach to children*, London, 2003, Churchill Livingstone.
12. Treganza A, Frymann VM: Explorations into posture and body mechanics, *Acad Ther* 8:339-344, 1973.

Night Terror

Acupuncture | May Loo

Homeopathy | Janet L. Levatin

Mind/Body | Timothy Culbert, Lynda Richtsmeier Cyr

✳ PEDIATRIC DIAGNOSIS AND TREATMENT

Night terrors (pavor nocturnus) are common in children.[1,2] They occur in 1% to 3% of children, particularly in boys between 5 and 7 years of age.[1]

Typically, night terror occurs suddenly early in the sleep period,[3] during stage 3 or 4 of slow-wave stage.[1,2] The child sits up, screams, appears frightened with dilated pupils, hyperventilates, and may thrash violently but cannot be consoled and is unaware of parents or surroundings. Night terror usually lasts 10 to 15 minutes, and the child falls asleep calmly. The next morning the child has total amnesia, which is a diagnostic feature of night terror. Approximately one third of children with night terrors experience somnambulism.[1,2]

Both constitutional and neurophysiological factors appear to play a role in night terror. At a cross-sectional examination of 20 children with pavor nocturnus, 14 exhibited sharp waves and one slow wave. The electroencephalographic (EEG) findings indicate that this condition is not related to epilepsy but hint at constitutional delay of cerebral maturation, and therefore the child outgrows night terrors with age.[4,5] It has also been hypothesized that night terror disorder and panic disorder involve a similar constitutional vulnerability to dysregulation of brainstem-altering systems.[6] Studies of twin cohorts and families with sleep terror suggest genetic involvement of parasomnias.[7]

Treatment is generally with reassurance to the parents. An underlying emotional disorder should be explored in children with persistent and prolonged night terrors. Evaluation of family dynamics and a short course of diazepam or imipramine may be considered for treatment of protracted cases.[1]

✳ CAM THERAPY RECOMMENDATIONS

Acupuncture

There are no data on acupuncture treatment of night terror. Chinese medicine interprets sleep as a time when the Eternal Soul, the Hun, leaves the physical body to visit the Eternal Soul world. Dreams are images brought back from the Soul world.[1-3]

KI6 is a point discussed in Chinese classics as having a calming effect on the "spirits" and can be used to treat sleep disorders and nightmares.

SP6 also calms the spirit and can be used to treat "sudden fright disorder" in children.[4]

Homeopathy

Before using this section, please see Appendix A, Homeopathy, for definitions of practitioner expertise categories and general information on prescribing homeopathic medicines.

Practitioner Expertise Category 1 or 2

There are no controlled clinical trials of homeopathy for treatment of night terrors, although the homeopathic literature contains evidence for its use in the form of accumulated clinical experience.[1] Night terrors can often be treated quickly and effectively with homeopathy. Homeopathy is especially effective when used in combination with measures such as stress reduction, normalization of bedtime and sleep routines, and counseling, either family or individual, when it is appropriate for the case.

The goal in treating night terrors homeopathically is to determine the single homeopathic medicine whose description in the materia medica most closely matches the symptom picture of the patient. It is important to understand the patient's mental and emotional state and sleep habits; additionally, any physical symptoms or pathology should be considered. Once the medicine has been selected, it can be given orally, sublingually in the 30C potency once or twice daily for 4 or 5 days. In some cases, a higher potency, such as 200C of 1M (1000C), may be necessary for successful treatment. If the medicine has not helped in 2 to 3 weeks (after being given for 4 to 5 days and then waiting and observing for 1 or 2 weeks), then another homeopathic medicine should be tried or some other form of therapy should be instituted as needed. Once symptoms have begun to resolve, the medicine can be given less frequently or stopped. It can be repeated again for a relapse of symptoms.

The following is a list of homeopathic medicines commonly used to treat patients with night terrors. It must be emphasized that this list is partial and represents some of the probable choices from the homeopathic materia medica. If the symptoms of a given patient are not represented here, a search of the homeopathic literature would be needed to find the simillimum.

Calcarea carbonica

The child needing *Calcarea carbonica* may have lots of anxieties and fears, including anxiety about his health and fear of dogs, darkness, and storms. He or she is adversely affected by hearing bad news. This child is a hard worker with a strong sense of responsibility for his or her age. The anxieties, fears, and overly responsible nature can carry over into his sleep and cause nightmares or night terrors. This child may complain of seeing frightening faces or having disagreeable thoughts when trying to go to sleep.

Cina maritima

The child needing *Cina maritima* has a variety of sleep disturbances including talking, screaming, or crying out during sleep; grinding the teeth; and night terrors. The child may be seen on her hands and knees while asleep. In general, children needing cina maritima are very irritable. They are subject to gastrointestinal difficulties, including worm infestations. Night terrors may be worse until the worms are diagnosed and treated (in addition to giving the patient cina maritima, conventional antihelminthic treatment should be prescribed).

Kali bromatum

The child needing *Kali bromatum* is fearful at night and suffers from insomnia, especially when left alone. There may be sleepwalking and tooth grinding in addition to night terrors. He or she can suffer from attacks of rage and manic behavior. This is also a medicine for some autistic or mentally retarded children.

Stramonium

Stramonium is an important medicine for night terrors. The child needing stramonium experiences a combination of fears and violent behavior (the violence is usually a later development). Oftentimes the night terrors start after a frightening experience, such as a dog bite or a car accident, or a neurological illness such as meningitis or encephalitis. The child has many fears, including fear of animals in general, dogs, water, mirrors, diseases, and ghosts. Nightmares and night terrors develop. Rages and violent behavior may later occur. The patient may have tics, chorea, stuttering, or frank convulsions (the patient with convulsions will need conventional care in addition to homeopathic treatment). During the night terror the child shrieks, has dilated pupils, and looks terror stricken. In the office the child may not exhibit troublesome behaviors. Early treatment with stramonium can help prevent this child's condition from becoming chronic.

Mind/Body

Stress, anxiety, and excess autonomic arousal can all interfere with normal sleep patterns for children and adolescents. As a subset of sleep disorders, night terrors are common, and evidence supports a psychophysiological dimension. Cognitive-behavioral strategies may be helpful as an overall approach in counseling families about nighttime fears in general, as these are often very frightening events for parents.[1] Biofeedback approaches have also been reported as successful in lowering autonomic nervous system arousal and improving sleep in children with a variety of sleep issues.[2] Kohen et al.[3] described four children, ages 8 to 12 years, with severe night terrors who responded well to a combined treatment approach utilizing imipramine (20 to 60 mg at bedtime, which was later discontinued during the study) together with training in relaxation and mental imagery (self-hypnosis). Again, although strong evidence-based information is lacking, meditation, hypnosis, and yoga would seem to afford potentially similar benefits and could be considered as reasonable options as well as part of a comprehensive integrative approach.

The authors find that mental imagery (favorite place or safe place), autogenics training (a form of relaxation involving repetitive self-suggestions about warm and relaxed muscles), music/nature sounds, clinical aromatherapy, and good, consistent nighttime sleep routines can all be quite helpful in initiating and maintaining sleep. Children are encouraged to use these techniques to assist them in falling asleep in a positive emotional "frame," reduce nighttime fears, and settle the body, all of which can facilitate faster, better sleep.

References

Pediatric Diagnosis and Treatment

1. Behrman RE, Kliegman RM, Jenson HB, editors: *Nelson textbook of pediatrics*, ed 17, Philadelphia, 2004, Saunders.
2. Smeyatsky N, Baldwin D, Botros W et al: The treatment of sleep disorders, *S Afr Med J* May(Suppl):1-8, 1992.
3. Pagel JF: Nightmares and disorders of dreaming, *Am Fam Physician* 61:2037-2042, 2044, 2000.
4. Fehlow P: Significance of EEG findings in pavor nocturnus [in German], *Kinderarztl Prax* 58:561-565, 1990.
5. Thiedke CC: Sleep disorders and sleep problems in childhood, *Am Fam Physician* 63:277-284, 2001.
6. Garland EJ, Smith DH: Simultaneous prepubertal onset of panic disorder, night terrors, and somnambulism, *J Am Acad Child Adolesc Psychiatry* 30:553-555, 1991.
7. Guilleminault C, Palombini L, Pelayo R et al: Sleepwalking and sleep terrors in prepubertal children: what triggers them? *Pediatrics* 111:e17-e25, 2003.

Acupuncture

1. Loo M: *Pediatric acupuncture*, London, 2002, Elsevier.
2. Maciocia G: *The foundations of Chinese medicine, a comprehensive text for acupuncturists and herbalists*, London, 1989, Churchill Livingstone.
3. Maciocia G: *The practice of Chinese medicine, the treatment of diseases with acupuncture and Chinese herbs*, London, 1994, Churchill Livingstone.
4. Deadman P, Al-Khafaji M: *A manual of acupuncture*, Ann Arbor, Mich, 1998, Journal of Chinese Medicine Publications.

Homeopathy

1. *ReferenceWorks Pro 4.2*, San Rafael, Calif, 2008, Kent Homeopathic Associates.

Mind/Body

1. Barowsky E, Moskowitz J, Zweig J: Biofeedback for disorders of initiating and maintaining sleep, *Ann N Y Acad Sci* 602:97-103, 1990.
2. Gordon J, King, N: Children's night-time fears: an overview, *Counsel Psychol Quart* 15:121-132, 2002.
3. Kohen D, Mahowald M, Rosen G: Sleep-terror disorder in children: the role of self-hypnosis in management, *Am J Clin Hypnosis* 34:233-244, 1992.

Obesity

Acupuncture | May Loo

Chiropractic | Anne Spicer

Herbs—Chinese | Catherine Ulbricht, Jennifer Woods, Mark Wright

Herbs—Western | Alan D. Woolf, Paula M. Gardiner, Lana Dvorkin-Cameil, Jack Maypole

Homeopathy | Janet L. Levatin

Naturopathy | Matthew I. Baral

✳ PEDIATRIC DIAGNOSIS AND TREATMENT

Obesity in childhood and adolescence is increasing in the United States and worldwide[1-3] in epidemic proportions,[4,5] with an upward trend of 0.2 kg increase in body weight/year at any given age.[6] It has become a major pediatric health issue.[7] The National Center for Health Statistics (NCHS) at the Centers for Disease Control and Prevention (CDC) reports an alarming trend of overweight in children. From 1963-1970 to 1999-2002, the prevalence of overweight among children aged 6 to 11 years quadrupled, from approximately 4% to 16%. During the same time period, the prevalence among adolescents aged 12 to 19 years increased more than threefold from approximately 5% to 16%. Among 6- to 19-year-old boys, the prevalence continues to show disparities among racial/ethnic groups, with significantly higher overweight among Mexican Americans (25.5%) versus non-Hispanic blacks (17.9%) versus non-Hispanic whites (14.3%). Among Mexican-American, non-Hispanc black, and non-Hispanic white girls, the prevalence was 18.5%, 23.2%, and 12.9%, respectively.[8] Obesity is usually evident by age 5 to 6 years.[9]

Obesity in children is difficult to define, as it is influenced by age, developmental stage, physical fitness, and individual variations in caloric needs. The CDC defines *overweight* as increased body weight in relation to height when compared with an acceptable weight standard[10] and is related to health risks and problems in children and adolescents. Skinfold thickness is difficult to apply to children.[11] In general, a body mass index (BMI; in kg/m^2) between the 85th and 95th percentiles indicates a risk of being overweight; a BMI greater than the 95th percentile indicates being overweight[4]; and children whose weight exceeds 120% of that expected for their height are considered overweight. Because obese children are at increased risk of becoming obese adults and developing obesity-related complications later in life, early identification and treatment is of utmost importance.[2,4,5,12] The potential for persistence of obesity into adulthood increases with obesity at an early age or in adolescence, with severity, and with parental obesity.[13] The risk of adult obesity is greater if at least one parent is obese and especially when the child is obese before 10 years of age.[14]

Etiology

Endogenous obesity such as metabolic or hormonal disorders, or syndromes such as Prader-Willi, are uncommon in children.[9,15] A comprehensive history and examination can usually elicit any medical causes of obesity.[1] The majority of obesity cases in children are exogenous because of a disproportionate intake of calories to expenditure.[9] Genetic factors influence the inheritance of obese phenotype, the major affectors of body fat content, energy intake and expenditure, and responsiveness to dietary intervention.[5,11] Obesity is most likely a complex polygenic trait.[16]

The most important issue in exogenous obesity is the balance of energy intake with energy expenditure. The major determinants of energy expenditure are basal metabolism, the metabolic response to food, physical activity, and growth. These are age related in children.[9] The traditional view that obesity occurs when intake exceeds expenditure or in individuals with lower metabolic rate is now controversial, especially with respect to the pediatric population. Studies have demonstrated that obese individuals can have metabolism comparable to non-obese individuals[17] and that some obese people in fact can have higher metabolic rates.[16] Obese and non-obese individuals often have similar energy intakes and expenditures.[4,11] This implies that the difference between obesity and non-obesity can result from very small imbalances of energy intake and expenditure,[4,11] possibly due to very small differences in basal metabolic rate or the thermic effects of food.[11] In addition, children go through distinct developmental periods with different energy needs, such as early infancy and adolescence. Because of the inherent individual requirement for energy[9] and susceptibility to the balance in energy[4] and because changes in intake or expenditure in children may occur concomitantly with physiological changes, such as hormonal levels in adolescence, weight gain especially during critical developmental periods is not always directly related to energy expenditure.[4]

The hypothalamus is the center for regulation of energy balance. It integrates neural, hormonal, and nutrient messages from the gut and circulation and sends signals to higher centers, leading to feelings of hunger or satiety. The hypothalamus also controls energy expenditure via the autonomic nervous system (ANS) and pituitary hormones. The hypothalamus nuclei contain more than 40 neurotransmitters that affect food intake and thermogenesis. Those that stimulate appetite, such as opioids and neuropeptide Y, suppress sympathetic nervous system activity and thus reduce energy expenditure, whereas the neurotransmitters that inhibit food intake, such as serotonin, dopamine, and choelcystokinin, have the reverse effect of decreasing appetite and stimulating energy expenditure. There is evidence that hormones such as insulin and the concentrations of nutrients such as glucose and amino acids all play a role. Leptin is a recently discovered hormone that is synthesized in fat and acts on the hypothalamus to suppress food intake and increase energy expenditure. Its concentration is high in nearly all obese people, and it falls with weight loss, which possibly suggests some resistance to the central effects of leptin in obesity.[4]

Obesity in children is often associated with high intake of sweets and fattening foods, which is often underreported by children.[17] This, coupled with an increasing sedentary lifestyle in children,[11] increase in television viewing,[17] and decrease in regular physical activity,[17] especially in prepubertal girls,[4] result in development of obesity in the pediatric population.

Complications

Obese children are predisposed to developing physical and psychoemotional complications. The physical complications include hypertension,[19,20] cardiovascular disease[15,21] (autopsy findings reveal progression of atherosclerotic plaques can begin in the very young[4]), and fatty liver, which can occur without correlation to severity of obesity.[9] One of the most dramatic and disturbing findings in the past decade is the tremendous increase in the incidence of type II diabetes in children and adolescents with obesity.[4,22,23] Other physical complications include orthopedic problems due to increased weight on the hips and knees[15] and obstructive sleep apnea with symptoms of snoring and difficult breathing during sleep.[24] Psychologically, the obese child carries emotional burdens[25] such as low self-esteem, resulting in less social interaction with peers and less participation in team sports.[9] The negative psychosocial effect can be long term, as women who were overweight adolescents are less likely to marry, have lower-paying jobs, and complete fewer years of school. Overweight men are also less likely to marry.[4] Currently, approximately 15% of children and adolescents aged 6 to 19 years are at risk for developing these complications.[26]

Treatment

The best treatment of obesity is prevention. The American Academy of Pediatrics (AAP) issued a policy statement in 2003 with the following recommendations: Identify and track patients at risk by virtue of family history, birth weight, or socioeconomic, ethnic, cultural, or environmental factors; calculate and plot BMI once a year in all children and adolescents; use change in BMI to identify rate of excessive weight gain relative to linear growth; encourage, support, and protect breastfeeding; and encourage parents and caregivers to promote healthy eating patterns by offering nutritious snacks such as vegetables and fruits, low-fat dairy foods, and whole grains; encouraging children's autonomy in self-regulation of food intake and setting appropriate limits on choices; and modeling healthy food choices. Routinely promote physical activity, including unstructured play at home, in school, in childcare settings, and throughout the community. Recommend limitation of television and video time to a maximum of 2 hours per day; and recognize and monitor changes in obesity-associated risk factors for adult chronic disease, such as hypertension, dyslipidemia, hyperinsulinemia, impaired glucose tolerance, and symptoms of obstructive sleep apnea syndrome.[27]

Although the AAP policy recommendations are stated clearly, their clinical implementation is difficult for the primary care pediatrician, who is still in the uncomfortable position of needing to do something for the overweight child and is at the same time uncertain about the nature of the disease and has no cure.[28] Although BMI is the best clinically available measure of overweight, its application to individual patients is uncertain because of limited knowledge of the current and future health effect of BMI and the possible limits in the applicability of current BMI cutoff points, particularly for minority race/ethnicity.[26] The U.S. Preventive Services Task Force (USPSTF) found insufficient evidence for the effectiveness of behavioral counseling or other preventive intervention with overweight children and adolescents that can be conducted in the primary care setting.[26]

When available, overweight children are referred to weight-loss centers, where a multidisciplinary team consisting of a pediatrician, a nutritionist, a psychotherapist, and other ancillary personnel—the number increases with the level of academic involvement of the clinic—devise an appropriate treatment regimen. Diet and exercise remain the cornerstones in Western management of obesity.[16] Weight management usually involves trying to set reasonable weight-loss goals[13,15] consisting of a combination of healthy diet and physical activities to change the sedentary lifestyle.[1,15] The theory is that a reduction of 500 kcal/day would result in the loss of 1 lb of fat per week.[9]

The specialists recognize that family involvement is crucial in management of childhood obesity.* Children's food preferences and physical activity (or inactivity) are often influenced by parents.[17] Family readiness to change would also influence therapy.[13] Long-term success requires parental support to motivate the child in continuing the healthier lifestyle and eating habits.[17] Anorexic medications have significant side effects such as heart disease and pulmonary hypertension and are not approved by the U.S. Food and Drug Administration for use in pediatric populations. Gastric bypass surgery for premorbid obese adults should at best be considered as experimental in children and adolescents.[13]

❉ CAM THERAPY RECOMMENDATIONS

Acupuncture

Although data are abundant regarding the efficacy of acupuncture in treatment of obesity, most studies are of poor quality and are rejected by the medical community. A U.K. systematic

*References 1, 7, 13, 15, 17, 29.

review of randomized controlled trials (RCTs) up to January 2004 of complementary therapies that included acupuncture concluded that evidence for complementary and alternative medicine (CAM) in obesity is not convincing.[1] A review of seven RCTs conducted in China concluded that the methodology quality of the studies of acupuncture for obesity was too poor to provide strong evidence for clinical practice.[2]

Although numerous clinical reports of acupuncture treatment of obesity in adults are available, only a few are on children. A clinical trial from China treated 101 children with simple obesity using a photo-acupuncture apparatus and found that the obesity indexes lowered significantly and levels of blood lipids, glucose, cortisol, and triiodothyronine all improved markedly.[3] A clinical report from Russia indicated electroacupuncture of 62 children reduced body mass, decreased fatty tissue content, increased performance of cardiovascular function, and normalized blood serum lipids.[4] A clinical study from China of 16 adults with primary obesity treated with transcutaneous electrical stimulation on acupoints revealed a moderate but significant weight reduction.[5] A clinical study from Poland of 69 obese perimenopausal and postmenopausal women found that when acupuncture treatment was added to a low-calorie diet, more lowering of BMI and body weight was observed. The acupoints used were GV20 (Baihui), CV12 (Zhongwan), ST36 (Zusanli), ST21 (Liangmen), ST25 (Tianshu), LIV3 (Taichong), LIV13 (Zhangen), P6 (Neiguan), H7 (Shenmen), and ear points Shenmen and Stomach.[6] The same group used laser acupuncture combined with low-calorie diet to treat postmenopausal obesity and found that the combination was more effective in lowering body weight, BMI, and waist:hip ratio.[7]

Several possible mechanisms have been proposed in both human and animal studies of the effect of acupuncture in obesity. Existing data indicate that acupuncture affects lipid and carbohydrate metabolism and regulates salt, fluids, and endocrine functions. Acupuncture has been shown to regulate hyperlipidemia,[8] cholesterol, and high-density lipoprotein metabolism[9] and increases cyclical adenosine monophosphate (cAMP), which can activate lipase and promote decomposition of lipid.[10] The previously mentioned Russian study on 62 children showed decreasing fatty tissue content and normalization of serum lipids with acupuncture.[4] Acupuncture treatment can also have a positive effect on carbohydrate metabolism, with a decrease in serum glucose and an increase in lactic dehydrogenase (LDH).[11] Acupuncture has been shown to decrease edema in obesity by regulating water and salt metabolism through lowering serum sodium and aldosterone levels.[12]

Acupuncture has been shown to exert impressive effects on the hypothalamus and ANS in weight control. A clinical study of 19 year olds that measured fasting blood glucose, noradrenaline, dopamine, adrenalin, and cortisol levels indicated that patients with simple obesity had hypofunctioning of the sympathetic-adrenal system and the hypothalamus-pituitary-adrenal system. Acupuncture treatment enhanced the functions of both the sympathetic-adrenal system and the hypothalamus-pituitary-adrenal systems to bring about weight loss.[13] Recent animal studies from China have attempted to elucidate the biochemical effects of acupuncture in the hypothalamus.

One study using electroacupuncture stimulation at ST36 and ST44 evaluated electrical activity in the ventromedial nucleus of hypothalamus (VMH) in rats and showed that acupuncture can produce weight reduction by increasing excitability of the satiety center.[14]

One study reported in 2000 indicated that the levels of noradrenaline (NA) in the lateral hypothalamic area (LHA) of obese rats were higher than those in the normal, non-obese rats, but that the level of serotonin (5-HT) and the activity of adenosine triphosphatase (ATPase) in LHA of obese rats were lower than those of the normal rats. After acupuncture treatment, weight reduction occurred, accompanied by a reduction in the level of NA in LHA and an increase in the 5-HT and activity of ATPase, leading the researchers to conclude that antiobesity mechanism of acupuncture may lie in effective regulation of LHA.[15] The same group of researchers reported 1 year later that the levels of tyrosine (Tyr) and dopamine (DA) were lower, the 5-hydroxytryptamine (5-HT) and 5-hydroxyindole acetic acid (5-HIAA) were higher, and the frequency of the spontaneous discharge of nerve cells in the VMH was lower in obese rats as compared with normal, non-obese rats. After acupuncture treatment, weight reduction occurred; the frequency of spontaneous discharges of nerve cells in the VMH were markedly increased; the levels of Tyr, DA, and tryptamine (Typ) and 5-HT:5-HIAA ratio were elevated; and the 5-HT level decreased. The researchers suggested that acupuncture exerted a regulatory effect on the VMH for weight reduction.[16] A more recent animal study from China found that the levels of tryptophan (Trp) and 5-HIAA were increased, whereas the 5-HT level and 5-HT:5-HIAA ratio were decreased in the raphe nuclei of obese rats compared with non-obese rats. Acupuncture treatment produced weight reduction, increased the 5-HT level and 5-HT:5-HIAA ratio, and decreased the contents of Trp and 5-HIAA, which suggests that acupuncture regulates the monoamine neurotransmitters in the raphe nuclei in weight control.[17]

Acupuncture was also effective in preventing complications of obesity by reducing the arteriosclerotic index, the indicator for development of cardiovascular disease,[18] and by lowering blood pressure.[10] Even when acupuncture fails to reduce weight, it can improve the psychological outlook of the obese patient.[19]

Auricular or ear acupuncture has been found to be effective in obesity either used alone or in conjunction with other approaches. One clinical report indicates pressure on auricular points was effective for weight reduction.[20] A Japanese single-blind sham treatment using bilateral auricular acupuncture stimulation reduced body weight even in non-obese subjects.[21] The mechanism of auriculoacupuncture in obesity may be suppression of appetite. One theory posits that this is mediated through stimulation of the auricular branch of the vagal nerve and elevation of serotonin levels, both of which have been shown to increase tone in the smooth muscle of the stomach, thus suppressing appetite.[22] A Japanese animal study indicates that auriculoacupuncture modulates feeding-related hypothalamic neuronal activity and most likely influences satiation.[23] Auricular and body points seem to work synergistically to reduce cholesterol and triglycerides with resultant weight loss.[24] A clinical report from China indicated that body acupuncture plus ear acupuncture was effective in the treatment of simple obesity in 195 adults.[25] An integrated approach with auricular acupuncture, diet control, and aerobic exercise resulted in 86.7% success in weight reduction.[26]

Chinese Medicine Differentiation and Treatment of Obesity

Traditional Chinese medicine (TCM)[27] considers a variety of Qi imbalances as the cause of obesity, each requiring a specific treatment regimen. Through energetic balance of the internal viscera, acupuncture treatment has been successful in reducing weight, often with long-lasting effects. The primary organs of dysfunction in obesity are the Stomach, Spleen, Liver, and Kidney. Current acupuncture thinking posits three major obesity syndromes that are applicable in children:

Spleen and Stomach Qi deficiency/Stomach excess Heat
Liver Yang excess/Liver Qi stagnation
Kidney Qi or Yin deficiency

Spleen and Stomach Qi deficiency/Stomach excess Heat

Spleen and Stomach Qi deficiency/Stomach excess Heat is the most common TCM syndrome for obesity in pediatrics. Stomach Heat children have increased appetite and gain weight easily, with a tendency to "stuff their faces" under stress. Spleen Qi deficiency results in poor appetite. In both cases, the children would not respond to a Western dietary regimen.

These children tend to be sedentary owing to weight and to muscle weakness with Spleen deficiency and Dampness; are easily fatigued; and tend to worry, which can lead to obsession, especially about their weight. Successful treatments are directed toward dispersing Heat, resolving Dampness, and harmonizing the Middle Energizer. Acupuncture treatments of the Spleen and Stomach have been shown to decrease weight by having a positive effect on carbohydrate metabolism, with a decrease in serum glucose and an increase in lactic dehydrogenase LDH,[11] and by reducing cholesterol and triglyceride levels.[28]

Evaluation. History and physical examination would reveal signs of Spleen Qi deficiency in the presence of Heat and Dampness.

Treatment
To disperse Heat:
Eliminate Hot spices and foods from the diet; decrease Warm foods; increase Cooling foods.
Use the Five-Element, Four-Point system to disperse Heat from the Stomach (see Appendix B):
Tonify ST44, BL66; sedate ST41, SI5.
LI11 to disperse Heat overall.
To resolve Dampness:
Eliminate or decrease artificially sweetened foods, specifically candies, cookies, and cakes.
ST40 to resolve Damp.
To tonify the Spleen and Stomach and harmonize the Middle Energizer:
Tonify the Spleen with the Four-Point protocol: tonify SP2, HT8; sedate SP1, LR1 (see Appendix B).
Tonify the Middle Energizer: CV12.
Tonify the Stomach: tonify ST41, SI5; sedate ST43, GB41.
Specific "big points": ST25, ST36, ST37, ST40, ST44, SP6, SP9.

Treat auriculopoints:
Shenmen, Point Zero, Hunger, Mouth, Esophagus, Stomach, Spleen, Sanjiao, Endocrine.
Exercise:
No increased physical activities should be done at the beginning of treatment, as the child would become discouraged with his or her inability to perform. Exercise or increased physical activities can be added to the treatment regimen once the child has shown some response to the treatment, such as fewer Heat and Dampness signs, less Spleen Qi deficiency, or some weight loss. The activities need to be increased slowly as tolerated.

Liver Yang excess/Liver Qi stagnation

These children may respond to lower-calorie diets, as greasy and fattening foods are injurious to the Liver. Excess medications may also cause Liver imbalance. These children are sedentary, easily fatigued and frustrated, irritable, can have smoldering anger, and sometimes withdraw or appear depressed yet are resistant to psychiatric intervention.

Successful managements in the studies have involved moving Qi, subduing Liver Yang, and tonifying Liver Yin.

Treatment
Diet:
Eliminate greasy and fattening foods; diminish sour foods. Decrease intake of medications, especially over-the-counter drugs, which tend to be taken indiscriminately.
Treat Liver Yang excess:
LR3, LR13 to move Liver Qi.
Yintang for overall calming effect.
Diminish stress that precipitates frustration and anger.
Tonify Liver Yin:
LR3, LR8 to tonify LR Yin.
BL47, Hunmen, Gate of Ethereal Soul, to settle the Ethereal Soul.
HT7 to tonify Heart Yin, calm the Mind.
BL44, Shentang, Hall of the Shen, to settle the Shen.
KI6 to nourish Kidney Yin.
Auriculopoints:
Shenmen, Point Zero, Liver, Heart, Spleen, Kidney.
Exercise:
Same principle as SP Qi deficiency: gradual increase of physical activities as tolerated.

Kidney Qi or Yin deficiency

Kidney Qi or Yin deficiency obesity usually has onset in infancy or early childhood before 6 years of age and has a strong family history of obesity with one or both parents being overweight. The child tends to continue to have the baby physique: short and chubby with puffy face, hands, and feet.

The Kidney in TCM correlates to both the kidney and adrenals, as well as the hypothalamus and ANS.

These obese children can be sad, fearful, or angry; have difficulty with concentration; and lack will power or motivation to "stick to a diet." They easily become short of breath and start coughing when they do anything physically strenuous. Hypertension and cardiovascular complications would be the most common in this group. These obese children are the most difficult to manage.

Evaluation. The early onset of obesity and positive family history would point toward Kidney deficiency.

Treatment

Diet—for the whole family:

Eliminate any excess salt in foods: no extra added salt; no salty foods such as pretzels or chips.

Presence of Liver Yin symptoms: eliminate or decrease sour foods; decrease medications.

For Heart Fire symptoms: eliminate bitter foods in the diet; also be careful in taking medications, which are usually bitter.

For Spleen deficiency: eliminate artificially sweetened foods; some medications for children also contain artificial sweeteners.

For Lung deficiency: eliminate spicy foods.

Tonify Kidney Yin and Kidney Qi:

If there is no Liver Yang excess, the Kidney can be tonified overall with the Four-Point protocol:

Tonify KI7, LU8; sedate KI3, SP3.

BL52 to increase Will power; diminish Fear.

In treating any secondary organ dysfunction, always include some Kidney points:

KI3 to tonify both Kidney Yin and Yang, *or*

KI6 to tonify Kidney Yin; KI7 to tonify KI Yang.

Treat the specific secondary organs:

Tonify the Spleen with the Four-Point protocol.

Add ST40 to disperse Damp.

Tonify the Lung with the Four-Point protocol:

Tonify LU9, SP3; sedate LU10, HT8.

Tonify the Heart with the Four-Point protocol:

Tonify HT9, LR1; sedate HT3, KI10.

BL44 to settle Shen.

Treat emotional problems with the respective "Soul" points.

Modify lifestyle to minimize situations that precipitate frustration and anger; or fear; or sadness. Acupuncture treatment can be provided concomitantly with individual or family therapy.

Auricular points:

Shenmen, Point Zero, Kidney, Adrenals, Sanjiao, hypothalamus, and pituitary.

Add specific organ points in the ear accordingly: SP, LR, LU, HT.

Chiropractic

The chiropractic approach to obesity is simply to address the basics of diet and exercise. Certainly prevention is preferable. When healthy eating habits are established in early childhood, the dividends are paid in a lifetime of greater health. Obesity is often a family issue, even if it affects only a single member. Approaching management from a family perspective is more likely to succeed and is consistent with the holistic natural approach that is a mainstay in chiropractic.

Good family eating habits are preferably started prior to conception, but certainly as early as infancy. Parental administration of eating is more controlled in a bottle-fed baby, as the parents are able to precisely measure the child's intake.

This may cause parents to restrict or force food intake based on some arbitrary measure. (Overfeeding is the more common circumstance.) The infant may then distrust internal signals of hunger or satiety. The recommendation with bottle feeding is to pay careful attention to the infant's feeding behaviors so as to feed only when hungry and to withdraw food when the infant is satisfied. Breastfeeding is thus recommended as a preferable means of feeding an infant and serves to lower the risk of obesity.[1,2]

As toddlers, children begin to decide more strongly which foods they prefer and which they dislike. This is perhaps the most difficult time for the parent. Children often train their parents to feed them only their favorite foods through tantrums, fasting, and behavioral reinforcements. Parents are instructed to offer only excellent-quality foods (e.g., fresh vegetables, fruits, lean meats/legumes, whole grain products) and allow the child to eat as much or as little as the child sees fit. No child will intentionally starve. He or she may choose not to eat that meal in an effort to persuade the parent to offer lesser quality foods, which, if offered, will invite the child to reject future offerings of superior foods. It is helpful for the parents to know that it may take 10 or more episodes of exposure to a new food before the child will accept it. If the child rejects peas one day, they should be tried again in a few weeks.

Infancy is also the most common time that parents begin to use food as reward and punishment. This habit may be well intentioned but certainly sends the wrong message about healthy consumption of food.[3]

The necessity and benefit of establishing healthy diet and exercise habits early in life was exposed in a recent comprehensive qualitative study.[4] It was observed that by the time children are 8 years old, they may have developed a negative attitude about health if they see it as prohibiting them from eating favorite foods or forcing them to eat fruits and vegetables. Also, those who are not athletically adept tend to avoid exercise to escape the risk of peer harassment. Children in this study expressed a need for help in making changes in eating and activity levels, whereas parents found it difficult to take on the "battle" of making those changes in children who were trying to exert their own independence from their parent. The parents often just hoped that the children would outgrow the overweight. It is also noted that in some cases, the parents did not recognize the presence of the overweight.[3]

By the time of adolescence, children assert much greater control over their own consumption habits. Skipping breakfast is a common bad habit that may contribute to obesity at this age.[5] Intake of fast foods and empty-calorie foods is highest at this age. Adolescents are aware of the hazards of poor nutrition but may not be able to discern which foods qualify as poor-quality foods.[6]

The family is encouraged to go grocery shopping together. Each member of the family gets a turn to choose any fruit or vegetable that the entire family has to taste-test. Families are invited to try new recipes. Where possible, planting a vegetable or two in a garden or deck planter can be a healthy family activity. These ideas stimulate a curiosity about foods and create a festive attitude about family dining.

Parents must be advised to rid the home of unhealthy foods. These are primarily simple carbohydrates, processed and fried foods, and those foods with saturated or hydrogenated/trans fats. Soft drinks and fruit juices should also be avoided. If these foods remain available, the child *will* consume them. The older the child, the more likely they are to find a hidden stash of wayward foods.

School lunch programs that have decreased the sodium and fat composition have been found to be at least as palatable as their less healthy counterparts.[7] Social pressure by families and physicians can instigate a change in school lunch programs.

Parental role modeling is critical, both for eating and for exercise behaviors. Behaviors that include the parents or the entire family are more likely to succeed. Family meals together with the television turned off provide a healthier setting for appropriate intake and family bonding. A variety of foods should be encouraged in meal preparation. Meals made from scratch are generally more likely to be healthy. A pilot study introducing a diet of low-glycemic-index foods suggests its usefulness in children with obesity.[8]

Parents are more likely to identify diet as a contributor to their child's obesity than lack of exercise. The chiropractor must be able to educate the family on the need for a balance between diet and physical activity to improve health and weight status.

Television, computer, and video game usage should be decreased to no more than 2 hours per day. This alone may decrease obesity substantially.[9] Requiring the child to spend at least an equal amount of time in a physical activity as they do in a "screen" activity (television screen, computer screen, video screen) may provide a motivation to be active. A television in a child's bedroom is a risk factor for obesity.

The family should be encouraged to take a walk or bike ride after dinner, though less strenuous activities may be a more acceptable way to start. A game of horseshoes or croquet in the yard is a casual alternative to television. Setting goals that are incremental and attainable are most likely to succeed. Small successes provide the reinforcement needed to continue the diet and lifestyle changes. Fun and variety are key to ongoing participation by the child.

Families are encouraged to keep individual diaries of food intake and physical activity. The obese child should be weighed in the chiropractic office approximately one time per month. Support groups with other families may provide added enthusiasm and assistance.

Adequate hydration aids digestion and may improve energy levels.

Omega-3 fatty acid supplementation can counteract some of the negative impact of trans-fat consumption.

Choline, inositol, and methionine may be used in combination for adolescent or teen obesity to moderate blood sugar and enhance carbohydrate metabolism.

Licorice root helps to reduce sugar cravings and has a sweet taste itself. It can be taken in tea, tincture, or chewable form.

Daily doses of niacin may be helpful in reducing hyperlipidemia.

The chiropractor must be prepared to evaluate the obese adolescent for type II diabetes mellitus.

Because chiropractic has its own unit within the American Public Health Association, chiropractors are encouraged by some to participate in efforts to shape policy regarding issues such as childhood obesity,[10] especially as they may relate to school lunch programs.

Herbs—Chinese

Obesity, which is one of the leading causes of metabolic syndrome, may be treated by inhibiting fatty acid synthase (FAS). One study found that the Chinese herbs root of *Polygonum multiflorum* Thunb. (He Shou Wu), stem and branch of *Loranthus parasiticus* (L.) Merr. (Sang Ji Sheng), and green tea leaf significantly reduced the body weight of rats by inhibiting FAS. Although more studies are needed, the researchers concluded that their results are promising for the development of future nontoxic and low-cost weight-reducing substances from these herbs.[1]

Strong evidence suggests that the Chinese herb Ma Huang (stem of *Ephedra sinica* Stapf), also known as *ephedra*, may also promote weight loss, although traditionally it has not been used for such an application. Although the herb is proven to be effective in treating obesity when used with caffeine, research indicates that it also has severe adverse effects and may even lead to death in users. It has therefore been banned in the United States.[2] Traditionally, Ma Huang was used almost exclusively as a diaphoretic. In use, it was decocted separately from other herbs, with the froth being removed from the surface 10 or so times, before finally adding it to the rest of the separately decocting herbs compose the whole prescription. This recommendation dates from a text written in 500 CE, which states that the herb should be prepared this way, as the froth provokes restless agitation in people. In addition to this need for special preparation, tight constraints to use of the herb have been recorded. For example, the *Lei Gong Pao Zhi Yao Xing Fu* (*Lei Gong's Nature of Prepared Officinals in Verse*) (Anon., *ca.* fourteenth century) states:

> It should not be used lightly (i.e. flippantly) in summer and autumn. It can be used only for true-cold (i.e. externally contracted cold) pernicious factors at the surface [of the body]. If there is no cold pernicious factor, or the cold factor is inside [the body], or the patient has an internal deficiency syndrome, or fever [arising from] deficient Yin and fear of cold, yet there is an absence of headache, body aches and tension and the six pulses are not floating and tense, then it cannot be used. Further, even when there is a syndrome suited to diaphoresis, it should not be taken very much. Sweat is the Heart's fluid. If there is a syndrome in which diaphoresis should not be used, yet it is nevertheless used, or a syndrome which can be sweated, but which is sweated excessively, then the Heart Blood will become agitated. This may lead to desertion of Yang, or unceasing nosebleed. Further doses still may result in a serious illness.

Classical recommendations on constraints to use should be kept in mind when judging herb-induced problems reported in current times.

Herbs—Western

In the treatment of pediatric obesity, it is clear that diet and exercise are the most safe and clinically studied interventions. Several large-scale systematic reviews of the use of herbal products in the treatment of adult obesity caution the use of herbal products in the treatment of obesity due to a lack of evidence or safety concerns.[1-3] Herbs found in weight-loss products include herbal stimulants such as green tea, guarana (high in caffeine), and bitter orange, which contains synephrine and octopamine and acts similar to epinephrine and norepinephrine. Another stimulant, Ma Huang *(E. sinica)* is currently banned in weight-loss products in the United States. Ephedrine, the primary constituent of ephedra, has shown some efficacy in clinical trial for adult weight loss but the concern of side effects such as high blood pressure, tachycardia, and irritability make ephedra contraindicated as a weight-loss product for children. Other herbal products may include herbal diuretics such as dandelion root or an herbal laxative such as senna or cascara sagrada.

Homeopathy

Before using this section, please see Appendix A, Homeopathy, for definitions of practitioner expertise categories and general information on prescribing homeopathic medicines.

Practitioner Expertise Category 3

There are no controlled clinical trials of homeopathic treatment for obesity, although the homeopathic literature contains evidence for its use in the form of accumulated clinical experience.[1] Most patients with obesity need a comprehensive treatment plan including a variety of treatment modalities. Homeopathy can be used effectively and safely in combination with other treatment modalities, both alternative and conventional. Because obesity is a complex and multifaceted problem, successful homeopathic treatment usually requires extensive training in the art and science of homeopathy. Any one of many homeopathic medicines may be used to treat obesity, depending on the characteristics of the patient being treated; sophisticated homeopathic analysis and long-term follow-up are required. For these reasons, specific medicines for treating obesity will not be presented here. Interested readers are referred to the homeopathic literature for further study.[1]

Naturopathy

Unfortunately, the obesity epidemic has now spilled over into the pediatric population. It is estimated that more than 1 in 5 children are overweight or obese.[1]

Consideration of family history when assessing these patients is crucial, as obese children younger than 3 years old have less chance of becoming obese as adults if their parents are not obese. However, in older children with obesity, the risk for becoming an obese adult increases regardless of the parents' statures. Children with obese parents have an obesity development risk twice as high as those without obese parents.[2]

Recently a study of 344 children and adolescents showed that children who have more body fat have bones that are less dense.[3] This is of particular concern because teens gain 50% of their skeletal mass during puberty,[4] so obesity can therefore have a direct effect on the development of osteoporosis later in life. The list of concomitant conditions found in obese children includes orthopedic problems, polycystic ovaries, menstrual irregularities, gallstones, asthma, and sleep apnea. High blood pressure is present in 20% to 30% of overweight children 5 to 11 years old,[5] and they are more likely to have

hypertension as adults.[6,7] Long-term studies reveal that children who are overweight are twice as likely to develop heart disease and hypertension and three times as likely to develop diabetes.[8]

Etiologies
Sedentary lifestyle

Because this dilemma has many long-term effects on society as a whole, researchers and medical professionals have desperately tried to find the reasoning behind childhood obesity. One hypothesis is that the amount of television viewing among children today is higher than ever. Ten years ago, studies showed that 67% of children watched more than 2 hours of television per day.[9] This figure has no doubt grown exponentially in the past decade with the addition of video games. The amount of sedentary time spent in front of the television is concerning because of its direct relationship to weight problems in young people.[10] Only 2% of pediatricians frequently recommended television reduction.[11] However, it may serve as a useful component to the treatment of childhood obesity.[12]

Food quality

An additional factor involved with the relationship between obesity and television is snacking on high-sugar foods during viewing. The effects of product advertising during children's programs no doubt contributes to this issue, as more than 90% of foods advertised on television are high in fat, sugar, or salt.[13] Another contributing factor is the standard American diet. The fast food industry has directed much of its efforts toward marketing its products to children. With the growing prevalence of double-income homes, families are finding less time to prepare home-cooked meals, and fast food is often the answer. The high-fat, high-sodium, and high-sugar foods purchased at the drive-through have little nutritional value or fiber and directly contribute to the growing number of overweight children.

When a meal of high sugar or high carbohydrate is consumed, insulin levels rise sharply, contributing to fat storage. Adding several other components to meals, such as fat, fiber, and protein, can help blunt the insulin response. Decreasing serum levels of insulin may have a compounding impact on satiety and weight loss, as insulin is an appetite stimulant. Consuming more than the average three meals per day in smaller quantities can also have a beneficial effect on insulin levels. Decreased levels are related to increased feeding frequency.[14]

Metabolism

It has been postulated that lower metabolic rate causes obesity. Although this may be true to a small extent, research demonstrates that obese and nonobese adolescents gain weight at the same rate when overfed.[15] The issue may lie more in the abnormal regulation of appetite, which can result in the development of obesity over a longer period of time.

Treatment

- Decreased television viewing can help prevent childhood obesity.[12]
- Consume small, frequent meals throughout the day.
- Consume meals that contain fat, fiber, and protein.

Fiber has a reduced caloric density but increases satiety, and foods rich in soluble fiber modulate insulin response to the ingested carbohydrate, resulting in a flattening of postprandial glucose and insulin responses. Decreasing serum levels of insulin may have an additional impact on satiety, as insulin is an appetite stimulant.[16]

Medium-chain triglycerides

Medium chain triglycerides (MCTs) seem to increase diet-induced thermogenesis when added to the diet[17,18] and more quickly induce satiety.[19] MCTs are derived from coconut oil and can be safely added into the diet. Pizzorno et al.[20] suggests 1 to 2 tbsp per day.

Chromium

Chromium has been used successfully for aiding weight loss because it seems to help increase the sensitivity of cells to insulin,[21] lowering serum glucose levels[22] and lowering the response of insulin to an oral glucose load.[23] A sedentary lifestyle, refined carbohydrates, and a diet high in sugar can all reduce an individual's levels of chromium. Chromium has also been shown to increase the levels of lean muscle mass in individuals who are physically active. This may have an additive effect on weight loss, as muscle tissue requires more calories to function and grow, and adipose cells can supply that energy. An added benefit of chromium is that it may decrease blood lipid and cholesterol levels,[24] further decreasing the not-uncommon risk of hyperlipidemia in obese children. Supplementation with chromium has virtually no side effects and may be used in a multifaceted weight-loss program. A typical adult dose is 200 to 400 µg/day.

Vitamin C

A double-blind, placebo-controlled study of obese adults showed that supplementation of 3 g vitamin C per day resulted in increased weight loss compared with the control group. The belief is that vitamin C may increase cellular energy consumption by increasing sodium pump activity.[25,26]

5-Hydroxytryptophan/vitamin B₆

Serotonin has direct effects on food consumption. Eating a high-carbohydrate meal makes tryptophan available to the brain to serve as a crucial ingredient for the manufacture of serotonin, and serotonin levels in the blood and brain drop dramatically during dieting.[27,28] It is possible that binge carbohydrate consumption comes from low levels of serotonin in the brain. This can cause strong cravings, which may explain why most diets are not successful. 5-hydroxytryptophan (5-HTP) is converted to serotonin, and vitamin B₆ is essential for this conversion to occur. There is some evidence that supplementation of 5-HTP may prove a powerful treatment tool in childhood obesity.[29,30] Side effects reported include nausea and, in isolated cases, eosinophilia-myalgia syndrome from very high doses (1400 mg/day) and a confirmed contaminated batch.[31,32] A reasonable dose is 50 mg three times per day to start in children 6 years and older. The adult dose is typically 300 to 900 mg/day. 5-HTP should not be combined with monoamine oxidase inhibitors or selective serotonin reuptake inhibitors because of the risk of serotonin syndrome. A safe upper limit adult dose of pyridoxine is 250 mg/day.

References

Pediatric Diagnosis and Treatment

1. Proimos J, Sawyer S: Obesity in childhood and adolescence, *Austr Fam Physician* 29:321-327, 2000.
2. Stettler N: Obesity in children and adolescents [in German], *Ther Umsch* 57:532-536, 2000 (abstract).
3. Troiano RP, Flegal KM, Kuczmarski RJ: Overweight prevalence and trends for children and adolescents, *Arch Pediatr Adolesc Med* 149:1085-1091, 1995.
4. Goran MI: Metabolic precursors and effects of obesity in children: a decade of progress, 1990-1999, *Am J Clin Nutr* 73:158-171, 2001.
5. Perusse L, Bouchard C: Role of genetic factors in childhood obesity and in susceptibility to dietary variations, *Ann Med* 31(Suppl 1):19-25, 1999.
6. Freedman DS, Srinivasan SR, Valdez RA et al: Secular increases in relative weight and adiposity among children over two decades: the Bogalusa Heart Study, *Pediatrics* 99:420-426, 1997 (abstract).
7. Rudloff LM, Feldmann E: Childhood obesity: addressing the issue, *J Am Osteopath Assoc* 99(4 Suppl):S1-S6, 1999.
8. Centers for Disease Control and Prevention: *Prevalence of overweight and obesity among children and adolescents: United States, 1999-2002.* Available at www.cdc.gov/nchs/pressroom/04facts/obesity.htm. Accessed August 30, 2005.
9. Roy CC, Silverman A, Alagille D: *Pediatric clinical gastroenterology*, ed 4, St Louis, 1995, Mosby.
10. Centers for Disease Control and Prevention: *Defining overweight and obesity*, Atlanta, 2004, Centers for Disease Control and Prevention. Available at: www.cdc.gov/nccdphp/dnpa/obesity/defining.htm. Accessed: August 30, 2005.
11. Klish WJ: Childhood obesity: pathophysiology and treatment, *Acta Paediatr Japan* 37:1-6, 1995.
12. Berenson GS, Wattigney WA, Tracy RE et al: Atherosclerosis of the aorta and coronary-arteries and cardiovascular risk-factors in persons aged 6 to 30 years and studied at necropsy (The Bogalusa Heart Study), *Am J Cardiol* 70:851-858, 1992.
13. Dietz W: How to tackle the problem early? The role of education in the prevention of obesity, *Int J Obes Relat Metab Disord* 23(Suppl 4):S7-S9, 1999.
14. Whitaker RC, Wright JA, Pepe MS et al: Predicting obesity in young adulthood from childhood and parental obesity, *N Engl J Med* 337:869-873, 1997.
15. Moran R: Evaluation and treatment of childhood obesity, *Am Fam Physician* 59:861-873, 1999.
16. Wilding J: Science, medicine, and the future: obesity treatment, *Br Med J* 315:997-1000, 1997.
17. Strauss R: Childhood obesity, *Curr Probl Pediatr* 29:1-29, 1999.
18. Andersen RE, Crespo CJ, Bartlett SJ et al: Relationship of physical activity and television watching with body weight and level of fatness in children, *J Am Med Assoc* 279:938-942, 1998.
19. Feld LG, Springate JE, Waz WR: Special topics in pediatrics: hypertension, *Semin Nephrol* 18:295-303, 1998.
20. Bartosh SM, Aronson AJ: Childhood hypertension. An update on etiology, diagnosis, and treatment, *Pediatr Clin North Am* 46:235-252, 1999.
21. Bronfin DR, Urbina EM: The role of the pediatrician in the promotion of cardiovascular health, *Am J Med Sci* 310(Suppl 1):S42-S47, 1995.
22. Pinhas-Hamiel O, Dolan LM, Daniels SR et al: Increased incidence of non-insulin-dependent diabetes mellitus among adolescents, *J Pediatr* 128:608-615, 1996.

23. Libman I, Arslanian SA: Type II diabetes mellitus: no longer just adults, *Pediatr Ann* 28:589-593, 1999.

24. Marcus CL, Loughlin GM: Obstructive sleep apnea in children, *Semin Pediatr Neurol* 3:23-28, 1996.

25. Holtz C, Smith TM, Winters FD: Childhood obesity, *J Am Osteopath Assoc* 99:366-371, 1999.

26. Whitlock EP, Williams SB, Gold R et al: Screening and interventions for childhood overweight: a summary of evidence for the US Preventive Services Task Force, *Pediatrics* 116:125-144, 2005.

27. American Academy of Pediatrics, Committee on Nutrition: Prevention of pediatric overweight and obesity, *Pediatrics* 112: 424-430, 2003.

28. Charney E: Childhood obesity: the measurable and the meaningful, *J Pediatr* 132:193-195, 1998.

29. Keller C, Stevens KR: Assessment, etiology, and intervention in obesity in children, *Nurse Pract* 21:31-42, 1996.

Acupuncture

1. Pittler MH, Ernst E: Complementary therapies for reducing body weight: a systematic review, *Int J Obes Relat Metab Disord* 29: 1030-1038, 2005.

2. Liu XM, Zhang MM, Du L: Quality of methodology and reporting of randomized controlled trials of acupuncture for obesity [in Chinese], *Zhongguo Yi Xue Ke Xue Yuan Xue Bao* 26:192-194, 2004 (abstract).

3. Yu C, Zhao S, Zhao X: Treatment of simple obesity in children with photo-acupuncture [in Chinese], *Zhongguo Zhong Xi Yi Jie He Za Zhi* 18:348-350, 1998 (abstract).

4. Gadzhiev AA, Mugarab-Samedicinei VV, Isaev II et al: Acupuncture therapy of constitution-exogenous obesity in children [in Russian], *Probl Endokrinol (Mosk)* 39:21-24, 1993 (abstract).

5. Tian D, Li X, Shi Y, Liu Y et al: Study on the effect of transcutaneous electric nerve stimulation on obesity [in Chinese], *Beijing Da Xue Xue Bao* 35:277-279, 2003 (abstract).

6. Wozniak P, Oszukowski P, Stachowiak G et al: The effectiveness of low-calorie diet or diet with acupuncture treatment in obese peri- and postmenopausal women [in Polish], *Ginekol Pol* 74: 102-107, 2003 (abstract).

7. Wozniak P, Stachowiak G, Pieta-Dolinska A et al: Laser acupuncture and low-calorie diet during visceral obesity therapy after menopause, *Acta Obstet Gynecol Scand* 82:69-73, 2003.

8. Liu Z: Effects of acupuncture on lipid, TXB2, 6-keto-PGF, alpha in simple obese patients complicated with hyperlipidemia [in Chinese], *Zhen Ci Yan Jiu* 21:17-21, 1996 (abstract).

9. Liu Z: Effect of acupuncture and moxibustion on the high density lipoprotein cholesterol in simple obesity [in Chinese], *Zhen Ci Yan Jiu* 15:227-231, 1990 (abstract).

10. Liu ZC, Sun FM, Shen DZ: Effect of acupuncture and moxibustion on antiobesity in the variation of plasma cyclic nucleotide and the function of vegetative nervous system [in Chinese], *Zhong Xi Yi Jie He Za Zhi* 11:67-68. 83-86, 1991 (abstract).

11. Zhao Y: Effect of acupuncture on carbohydrate metabolism in patients with simple obesity, *J Tradit Chin Med* 12:129-132, 1992.

12. Sun F: The antiobesity effect of acupuncture and its influence on water and salt metabolism [in Chinese], *Zhen Ci Yan Jiu* 21:19-24, 1996 (abstract).

13. Liu Z, Sun F, Li J et al: Effect of acupuncture on weight loss evaluated by adrenal function, *J Tradit Chin Med* 13:169-173, 1993.

14. Zhao M, Liu Z, Su J: The time-effect relationship of central action in acupuncture treatment for weight reduction, *J Tradit Chin Med* 20:26-29, 2000.

15. Liu Z, Sun F, Han Y: Effect of acupuncture on level of monoamines and activity of adenosine triphosphatase in lateral hypothalamic area of obese rats [in Chinese], *Zhongguo Zhong Xi Yi Jie He Za Zhi* 20:521-523, 2000 (abstract).

16. Liu Z, Sun F, Su J et al: Study on action of acupuncture on ventromedial nucleus of hypothalamus in obese rats, *J Tradit Chin Med* 21:220-224, 2001.

17. Wei Q, Liu Z: Effects of acupuncture on monoamine neurotransmitters in raphe nuclei in obese rats, *J Tradit Chin Med* 23: 147-150, 2003.

18. Liu Z, Sun F, Li J et al: Prophylactic and therapeutic effects of acupuncture on simple obesity complicated by cardiovascular diseases, *J Tradit Chin Med* 12:21-29, 1992.

19. Mazzoni R, Mannucci E, Rizzello SM et al: Failure of acupuncture in the treatment of obesity: a pilot study, *Eat Weight Disord* 4: 198-202, 1999.

20. Zhan J: Observations on the treatment of 393 cases of obesity by semen pressure on auricular points, *J Tradit Chin Med* 13:27-30, 1993.

21. Shiraishi T, Onoe M, Kojima TA et al: Effects of bilateral auricular acupuncture stimulation on body weight in healthy volunteers and mildly obese patients, *Exp Biol Med (Maywood)* 228: 1201-1207, 2003.

22. Richards D, Marley J: Stimulation of auricular acupuncture points in weight loss, *Austr Fam Physician*(Suppl 2):S73-S77, 1998.

23. Asamoto S, Takeshige C: Activation of the satiety center by auricular acupuncture point stimulation, *Brain Res Bull* 29:157-164, 1992.

24. Sun Q, Xu Y: Simple obesity and obesity hyperlipemia treated with otoacupoint pressure and body acupuncture, *J Tradit Chin Med* 13:22-26, 1993.

25. Qunli W, Zhicheng L: Acupuncture treatment of simple obesity, *J Tradit Chin Med* 25:90-94, 2005.

26. Huang MH, Yang RC, Hu SH: Preliminary results of triple therapy for obesity, *Int J Obesity Related Metabol* 20:830-836, 1996.

27. Loo M: *Pediatric acupuncture*, London, 2002, Elsevier.

Chiropractic

1. Von Kries, Koletzko B, Sauerwald T et al: Breast-feeding and obesity: cross sectional study, *Br Med J* 319:147-150, 1999.

2. Gilman MW, Rifas-Shiman SL, Camargo CA Jr et al: Risk of overweight among adolescents who were breastfed as infants, *J Am Med Assoc* 285:2461-2467, 2001.

3. Sherry B, Birch LL, Cook FH et al: Attitudes, practices and concerns about child feeding and child weight status among socioeconomically diverse white, Hispanic and African-American mothers, *J Am Dietetic Assoc* 104:215-221, 2004.

4. Borra ST, Kelly L, Shirreffs MB et al: Developing health messages: qualitative studies with children, parents, and teachers help identify communications opportunities for healthful lifestyles and the prevention of obesity, *J Am Dietetic Assoc* 103:721-728, 2003.

5. Siega-Riz A, Popkin B, Carson T: Trends in breakfast consumption for children in the United States from 1965-1991, *Am J Clin Nutr* 67:748-756, 1998.

6. Glanz K: Nutrition education for risk-factor reduction and patient education: a review, *Prev Med* 14:721-752, 1985.

7. Whittaker RC, Wright JA, Finch AJ et al: An environmental intervention to reduce dietary fat in school lunches, *Pediatrics* 91: 1107-1111, 1993.

8. Young P, West K, Oriz J et al: A pilot study to determine the feasibility of the low glycemic index diet as a treatment for overweight children in primary care practice, *Ambul Pediatr* 4: 28-33, 2004.

9. Anderson RE, Crespo CJ, Bartlett SJ et al: Relationship of physical activity and television watching with body weight and level of fatness among children: results from the Third National Health and Nutrition Examination Survey, *J Am Med Assoc* 279:938-942, 1998.

10. Baird R: Public health and chiropractic: meeting somewhere in the middle, *J Am Chiropractic Assoc* Jun:9-14, 2002.

Herbs—Chinese

1. Tian WX, Li LC, Wu XD et al: Weight reduction by Chinese medicinal herbs may be related to inhibition of fatty acid synthase, *Life Sci* 74:2389-2399, 2004.

2. Natural Standard Research Collaboration. Available at www.naturalstandard.com. Accessed 2005.

Herbs—Western

1. Saper RB, Eisenberg DM, Phillips RS: Common dietary supplements for weight loss, *Am Fam Physician* 70:1731-1738, 2004.

2. Lenz TL, Hamilton WR: Supplemental products used for weight loss, *J Am Pharm Assoc (Wash DC)* 44:59-67, 2004.

3. Hahn A, Strohle A, Wolters M: [Dietary supplements and functional food for weight reduction—expectations and reality], *MMW Fortschr Med* 145:40-45, 2003.

Homeopathy

1. *ReferenceWorks Pro 4.2*, San Rafael, Calif, 2008, Kent Homeopathic Associates.

Naturopathy

1. Troiano RP, Flegal KM, Kuczmarski RJ et al: Overweight prevalence and trends for children and adolescents: the National Health and Nutrition Examination Surveys, 1963 to 1991, *Arch Pediatr Adolesc Med* 149:1085-1091, 1995.

2. Whitaker RC, Wright JA, Pepe MS et al: Predicting obesity in young adulthood from childhood and parental obesity, *N Engl J Med* 337:869-873, 1997.

3. Horlick M: St. Luke's Hospital, N.Y., *USA Today* December 10, 2002.

4. Venkateswaran R: Nutrition for youth, *Clin Fam Pract* 2:791-822, 2000.

5. Figueroa-Colon R, Franklin FA, Lee JY et al: Prevalence of obesity with increased blood pressure in elementary school-age children, *South Med J* 90:806-813, 1997.

6. Lauer RM, Clarke WR: Childhood risk factors for high adult blood pressure: the Muscatine Study, *Pediatrics* 84:633-641, 1984.

7. Srinvasan SR, Bao W, Wattigney WA et al: Adolescent overweight is associated with adult overweight and related multiple cardiovascular risk factors: the Bogalusa Heart Study, *Metabolism* 45:235-240, 1996.

8. Mossberg H: 40-year follow-up of overweight children, *Lancet* 2:491-493, 1989.

9. Goran MI, Gower BA, Nagy TR et al: Developmental changes in energy expenditure and physical activity in children: evidence for a decline in physical activity in girls prior to puberty, *Pediatrics* 101:887-891, 1998.

10. Andersen RE, Crespo CJ, Bartlett SJ et al: Relationship of physical activity and television watching with body weight and level of fatness among children, *J Am Med Assoc* 279:938-942, 1998.

11. Price JH, Desmond SM, Ruppert ES et al: Pediatricians' perceptions and practices regarding childhood obesity, *Am J Prev Med* 5:95-103, 1989.

12. Robinson TN: Reducing children's television viewing to prevent obesity: a randomized controlled trial, *J Am Med Assoc* 282:1561-1567, 1999.

13. Taras HL, Gage M: Advertised foods on children's television, *Arch Pediatr Adolesc Med* 149:649-652, 1995.

14. Louis-Sylvestre J, Lluch A, Neant F et al: Highlighting the positive impact of increasing feeding frequency on metabolism and weight management, *Forum Nutr* 56:126-128, 2003.

15. Bandini LG, Schoeller DA, Edwards I et al: Energy expenditure during carbohydrate overfeeding in obese and nonobese adolescents, *Am J Physiol* 256:E357-E367, 1989.

16. Kimm SY: The role of dietary fiber in the development and treatment of childhood obesity, *Pediatrics* 96:1010-1014, 1995.

17. Hill JO, Peters JC, Yang D et al: Thermogenesis in humans during overfeeding with medium-chain triglycerides, *Metabolism* 38:641-648, 1989.

18. St-Onge MP, Ross R, Parsons WD et al: Medium-chain triglycerides increase energy expenditure and decrease adiposity in overweight men, *Obes Res* 11:395-402, 2003.

19. St-Onge MP, Jones PJ: Physiological effects of medium-chain triglycerides: potential agents in the prevention of obesity, *J Nutr* 132:329-332, 2002.

20. Pizzorno J, Murray M: *Textbook of natural medicine*, ed 2, Edinburgh, 1999, Churchill Livingstone.

21. Mertz W: Chromium in human nutrition: a review, *J Nutr* 123:626-633, 1993.

22. Anderson RA, Polansky MM, Bryden NA et al: Chromium supplementation of human subjects: effects on glucose, insulin, and lipid variables, *Metabolism* 32:894-899, 1983.

23. Grant KE, Chandler RM, Castle AL et al: Chromium and exercise training: effect on obese women, *Med Sci Sports Exerc* 29:992-998, 1997.

24. Press RI, Geller J, Evans GW: The effect of chromium picolinate on serum cholesterol and apolipoprotein fractions in human subjects, *West J Med* 152:41-45, 1990.

25. Werbach M: *Nutritional influences on illness*, ed 2, Tarzana, Calif, 1996, Third Line Press.

26. Naylor GJ, Grant L, Smith C: A double blind placebo controlled trial of ascorbic acid in obesity, *Nutr Health* 4:25-28, 1985.

27. Goodwin GM, Cowen PJ, Fairburn CG et al: Plasma concentrations of tryptophan and dieting, *Br Med J* 300:1499-1500, 1990.

28. Anderson IM, Parry-Billings M, Newsholme EA et al: Dieting reduces plasma tryptophan and alters brain 5-HT function in women, *Psychol Med* 20:785-791, 1990.

29. Cangiano C, Ceci F, Cascino A et al: Eating behavior and adherence to dietary prescriptions in obese adult subjects treated with 5-hydroxytryptophan, *J Clin Nutr* 56:863-867, 1992.

30. Ceci F, Cangiano C, Cairella M et al: The effects of oral 5-hydroxytryptophan administration on feeding behavior in obese adult female subjects, *J Neural Transm* 76:109-117, 1989.

31. Sternberg EM, Van Woert MH, Young SN et al: Development of a scleroderma-like illness during therapy with L-5-hydroxytryptophan and carbidopa, *N Engl J Med* 303:782-787, 1980.

32. Michelson D, Page SW, Casey R et al: An eosinophilia-myalgia syndrome related disorder associated with exposure to L-5-hydroxytryptophan, *J Rheumatol* 21:2261-2265, 1994.

Otitis Externa and Otitis Media

Acupuncture | May Loo
Chiropractic | Anne Spicer
Herbs—Chinese | May Loo

Homeopathy | Janet L. Levatin
Magnet Therapy | Agatha P. Colbert, Deborah Risotti
Naturopathy | Matthew I. Baral

✳ OTITIS EXTERNA: PEDIATRIC DIAGNOSIS AND MANAGEMENT

Otitis externa (OE) is a common occurrence in the pediatric age group.[1,2] The predominant symptom of acute OE is ear pain, often severe, and sometimes accompanied by clumpy otorrhea. Chronic OE may result in conductive hearing loss and often presents symptomatically with itching as a precursor of pain.[1-3]

Evaluation consists of a thorough history, adequate débridement, and a careful otological examination.[1,2,4] Edema of the ear canal, erythema, and thick otorrhea are prominent physical signs of the acute disease. Other physical findings may include palpable and tender lymph nodes in the periauricular region and erythema and swelling of the pinna and periauricular skin.[3] Predisposing risk factors to the development of OE include external trauma, maceration of the skin from water or humidity, excessive dryness (dry canal skin and lack of cerumen), presence of skin pathology (e.g., eczema), and glandular obstruction.[3,5,6] A recent study (1999 to 2001) of 87 children (ages 3.5 to 12 years) diagnosed with OE in Israel revealed that cleaning the ears with a cotton-tipped applicator was a leading cause of OE.[6] Children with tympanostomy tubes are especially at high risk for suppurative complications.[2]

The most common organisms are *Pseudomonas aeruginosa* and *Staphylococcus aureus*; less common are *Enterobacter aerogenes, Proteus mirabilis, Klebsiella pneumoniae,* streptococci, coagulase-negative staphylococci, and diphtheroids; and fungi such as *Candida* spp. and *Aspergillus* spp. may also be isolated.[3,5] Management of patients with acute OE includes débridement, topical therapy with acidifying and antimicrobial agents, and systemic antimicrobial therapy is sometimes indicated.[5] Topical otic preparations that contain neomycin (active against gram-positive organisms and some gram-negative organisms, notably *Proteus* species) with either colistin or polymyxin (active against gram-negative bacilli, notably *Pseudomonas* species) and corticosteroids are effective in treating most forms of acute external otitis.[3] Ofloxacin otic preparation combines polymyxin/neomycin with hydrocortisone and has been advocated as being effective for acute OE and safe for children because of its lack of ototoxicity.[7] However, an increase in incidence of fungal infections of the ear was found after widespread use of ofloxacin began.[8] The management of patients with chronic OE includes cleansing and débridement accompanied by topical acidifying and drying agents. Occasionally, surgery is necessary to allow cleansing, aeration, and/or removal of scarred tissue in chronic OE.[5]

Prevention of OE is necessary in children susceptible to recurrences, such as swimmers. The most effective prophylaxis is instillation of dilute 70% alcohol or acetic acid (2%) immediately after swimming or bathing. Trauma to the ear should be minimized, such as decreasing cleansing with cotton-tipped applicators. During an acute episode of OE, patients should not swim and the ears should be protected from water during bathing.[2,3,5]

✳ OTITIS EXTERNA: CAM RECOMMENDATIONS

Acupuncture

Currently there are no data on acupuncture treatment of OE.

A commonly used protocol is treatment of the local ear points: GB2, SI19, TB21. Parents can be taught to massage these points.

Magnet treatment can be applied by "pulling down" the inflammation by using an ion pumping cord connecting local and distal points: place the bionorth (–) downward on GB2 and biosouth (+) downward on BL60, and connect with a black clamp on the GB2 magnet and a red clamp on BL60.

Chiropractic

Although OE case studies or clinical trials are absent in the chiropractic literature, the chiropractic management would be directed at removing interference to normal body function. Evidence exists that the chiropractic adjustment has influence over natural killer cell production and autonomic balance,[1] immunoglobulin (IgA, G, and M) levels and B-cell lymphocyte count,[2] polymorphonuclear neutrophils and monoctyes,[3] and even CD4 counts.[4]

Supplementation with immune-enhancing nutrients may provide the body with necessary resources to manage an acute infection. Commonly recommended nutrients include zinc and vitamin A,[5] vitamin C,[6] and omega-3 fatty acids (eicosapentaenoic acid [EPA]/docosahexaenoic acid [DHA]).[7]

Echinacea purpurea is recommended as a stimulant to the immune system.[8] Use is recommended for a period not to exceed 2 consecutive weeks, as the body may develop a tolerance level with prolonged use. Although echinacea is quite safe, allergic reactions in children with a history of allergies, particularly to plants in the daisy family, have been recorded.

Topical application of colloidal silver is effective at reducing surface bacterial proliferation. Mullein/garlic oil can be administered into the ear canal to reduce bacterial growth and provide mild anesthetic relief.

Herbs—Chinese

Several Chinese medicine pediatric formulas have been designed to treat ear infections.

The most specific of these is the Children's Ear Formula (Golden Flower Herbs). This formula of 13 herbs is designed to clear Heat, resolve toxins, dispel Dampness, and relieve pain. Of the formula, herbs used to transform Phlegm and drain Dampness account for 49%; Wind-clearing herbs account for 21%; and antimicrobial herbs account for 16%.

The Children's Ear Formula comes in a powdered form, which is reconstituted with hot water when the formula is needed. The formula can be used for infants or children up to 6 years old. Give 1 mL (cc) of herb plus 1 mL for each year of the child's age. An infant would receive 1 mL; a 1 year old would receive 2 mL, and so on, up to 5 or 6 mL as a maximum dose. One eyedropper squeeze (about half the dropper) equals 1 mL. Give a dose every 2 hours until pain is relieved. It will also reduce accompanying fever. Usually, the child will need one to three doses to control the event. In some cases, the pain may last several days, in which case one dose is given every 3 or 4 hours.

The second specific formula created at the Shengzhou Chinese Medical Hospital is the Bupleurum and Angelica Formula (Blue Poppy Herbs). This combination of 13 herbs is designed to clear heat and transform Phlegm, disperse stagnation, quiet the Spirit, and relieve pain. It is a modified version of the classical formula Xiao Chai Hu Tang. The herbs are prepared in a 12:1 extract in a glycerin tincture. Dosage for babies is 1 to 2 droppersful every 2 hours until pain is relieved, then less frequent dosing; for 2 to 4 year olds, the dosage is 2 to 3 droppersful in the same regimen.

The third pediatric formula, less specific, but generally useful for ear infections and other upper respiratory illnesses in children is the Windbreaker, a formula of 21 herbs (Chinese Modular Solutions). This formula clears Wind, Heat, and Phlegm, treating the acute inflammatory stage of ear infections as well as any lingering congestion and middle ear effusion. The formula comes as a liquid alcohol extract. The alcohol can be removed by placing the drops in a small amount of hot water and allowing them to cool before administration. Dosage is 1 dropperful every 3 hours in babies and 2 to 3 droppersful for children 2 years and older.

Xiao Chai Hu Tang (Minor Bupleurum) is another formula frequently used for ear infections, especially when the ear infections become recurrent. This formula cools Liver Heat, transforms Phlegm, and tonifies Spleen Qi. Strengthening the Spleen and eliminating Dampness will support the intestines and digestive function, which have often been damaged by previous antibiotics.[1]

Homeopathy

Practitioner Expertise Category 1

Category 1 includes simple, acute OE.

Practitioner Expertise Category 2

Category 2 includes chronic or recalcitrant OE.

There are no controlled clinical trials of homeopathic treatment for treatment of OE, although the homeopathic literature contains evidence for its use in the form of accumulated clinical experience.[1] OE can often be treated effectively with homeopathy. It is safe to use homeopathic treatment for OE, either alone or in combination with other therapies, both alternative and conventional. Homeopathy may be of particular benefit in cases of recurrent OE or cases that are recalcitrant to other forms of treatment, as simple acute cases are usually easily treated with local measures.

The goal in treating OE homeopathically is to determine the single homeopathic medicine whose description in the materia medica most closely matches the symptom picture of the patient. Sometimes mental and emotional states, in addition to physical symptoms, are considered. Once the medicine has been selected, it can be given orally or sublingually in the 30C potency two to three times daily. If the medicine has not helped in four to five doses in acute cases, or in 3 to 4 days in more chronic cases, then another homeopathic medicine should be tried or some other form of therapy should be instituted as needed. Once symptoms have begun to resolve, the medicine can be given less frequently or stopped. It can be repeated again for a relapse of symptoms.

Topical homeopathic treatment can also be tried for OE, either alone or as an adjunct to systemic homeopathic treatment. One brand of ear drops that is available over the counter is Similasan. Similasan "Ear Wax Relief" contains Causticum 12X, Graphites 15X, and Lachesis 12X and can be instilled in the ear(s) if impacted wax has caused the ear canal to become irritated. Similasan "Earache Relief" contains *Chamomilla* 10X, Mercurius solubilis 15X, and sulphur 12X and can be instilled in the ear(s) for typical symptoms of OE.

The following is a list of homeopathic medicines commonly used to treat patients with OE. It must be emphasized that this list is partial and represents some of the probable choices from the homeopathic materia medica. If the symptoms of a given patient are not represented here, a search of the homeopathic literature would be needed to find the simillimum.

Fluoricum acidum

Fluoricum acidum is a remedy for OE with copious discharge. The ear is itchy and, when scratched, has a burning sensation. There may be ringing in the ears and a feeling of numbness in the bones around the ears. The patient is warm blooded.

Graphites

The child needing *Graphites* has a chronic tendency for thick ear discharges. The left ear is more likely to be affected. The skin behind the ears has a tendency to crack or have rashes. There may be associated otitis media and/or tinnitus. The condition may become worse if the discharge is suppressed with conventional medicines.

Picricum Acidum

Picric acidum is for OE cases in which a furuncle or boil has formed in the ear canal. There is a burning sensation in the ear and pain behind the right ear that radiates down the lateral neck. The patient may be worse from exertion, either physical or mental. If clinically indicated, the patient may also need to seek conventional treatment to have the boil removed.

Pulsatilla Nigricans

OE with severe pain and swelling of the canal calls for pulsatilla. There is a purulent discharge, and the patient may report a sensation of something crawling out of the ear. The ear lobe may be bright red and swollen, and other tissues around the ear may also be swollen. The pains are worse at night. The condition may develop after a viral syndrome, and associated otitis media may be present. If clinically indicated, the patient may need to seek conventional treatment.

Magnet Therapy

Palpate three separate acupuncture points just in front of the ear (TH21, SI19, GB2) for tenderness (see Appendix B). For children younger than 2 years, tape an 800-G Accuband magnet with the designated bionorth side (side with tiny protrusion) facing the skin on the identified tender point. For children older than 2 years, tape a 9000-G Accuband REC magnet on the most tender point. Leave the 9000-G magnet in place for 10 to 15 minutes. The 800-G magnet can be left in place for several hours.

✳ OTITIS MEDIA: PEDIATRIC DIAGNOSIS AND MANAGEMENT

Otitis media, infection of the middle ear, can occur in children as acute otitis media (AOM) and as two types of chronic otitis: chronic suppurative otitis media and chronic serous otitis media (CSOM). Next to the common cold, AOM is the most commonly diagnosed illness of children in the United States. It is most prevalent in young children 6 to 18 months of age, and 86% of children will experience at least one episode of AOM by age 1 year.[1] AOM decreases with age, occurring infrequently in adolescents.[2]

The majority of ear infections are caused by upper respiratory tract viruses and bacteria. The most common viral culprits are respiratory syncytial virus (RSV),[3] rhinovirus,[4] and influenza virus.[5] Viruses cause ear infection by directly invading the middle ear and disrupting eustachian tube function[6] or by inducing inflammatory injury that facilitates attachment of bacteria to respiratory epithelial cells.[7,8]

Approximately 65% to 75% of middle ear infections are due to bacteria.[4] The predominant organisms are pneumococcus, *Haemophilus influenzae, Moraxella catarrhalis,*[9-12] and group B *Streptococcus.*[13] Bacterial pathogens adhere to mucous membranes, and colonization ensues. The severity of infection or response to the invading bacteria depends on the health of the child's immune system.[11] The humoral system is especially significant in protecting the middle ear cavity from disease, and the nasopharyngeal lymphoid tissues are the first line of defense against bacterial colonization.[14] The sterility of the eustachian tube and tympanic cavity depends on the mucociliary system and secretion of antimicrobial molecules, such as lysozyme, lactoferrin, and β-defensins.[15] Evidence exists that many children with recurrent episodes of AOM have minor immunological defects.[14] Pneumococci are by far the most virulent of AOM bacteria. Prior to the advent of the vaccine, it caused approximately 6 million cases of otitis media annually in the United States.[16] Uncontrolled pneumococcal otitis can lead to meningitis.[17] Pneumolysin, the pneumococcal toxin, is especially injurious to the cell wall and can induce severe tissue injury.[17] The 7-valent pneumococcal conjugate vaccine, approved in 2000 for use in the United States, covers the seven serotypes that account for about 80% of invasive infections in children younger than 6 years.[18] The goal of using pneumococcal vaccine is to prevent symptomatic infections in the middle ear and prevent colonization of pneumococci that can cause subsequent middle ear infection.[19]

The vaccine was demonstrated to have more than 90% efficacy[16,20] and has resulted in a modest reduction of total episodes of AOM.[21] A Finnish study of 1662 infants revealed a decrease of more than 50% of infection by the vaccine cross-reactive serotypes but an increase of 33% of infection by other pneumococcal serotypes and an increase of 11% in infection by *H. influenzae.*[22] Other etiological agents include *Mycoplasma* spp., *Chlamydia* spp.,[23] and allergens.[4] Incidence of AOM is higher in winter and early spring.

The pathogenesis of otitis media is mediated primarily through eustachian tube dysfunction. The eustachian tube protects the middle ear from nasopharyngeal secretions, provides drainage into the nasopharynx of secretions produced within the middle ear, and permits equilibration of air pressure with atmospheric pressure in the middle ear. Infants and children are vulnerable to developing middle ear infection for several reasons. First, their eustachian tubes are shorter and more horizontal such that drainage of the middle ear is impaired. Second, children are prone to developing congestion from acute upper respiratory tract infection (URI), cigarette smoke, or environmental allergens and pollutants.[11,24,25] The congestion generates a negative middle ear pressure, resulting in intermittent obstruction of the eustachian tube[25] that can lead to bacterial colonization.[23] Third, children have inadequate mucociliary function necessary for maintaining eustachian tube sterility.[26]

The diagnosis of AOM, particularly in infants and young children, is often made with a degree of uncertainty. The clinical history of fever, otalgia (or pulling of the ear in an infant), and irritability or excessive crying in an infant or toddler are nonspecific and frequently overlap those of an uncomplicated viral upper respiratory infection.[5,6,27,28] The American Academy of Pediatrics (AAP) policy statement indicates that to diagnose AOM accurately, the clinician should confirm a history of acute onset, identify signs of middle ear effusion (MEE) and evaluate for the presence of signs and symptoms of middle ear inflammation.[29] MEE is more common than AOM. It is often difficult for the pediatrician to discriminate between MEE and AOM.[17,18,30,31] MEE may accompany viral upper respiratory infections, be a prelude to AOM, or be a sequela of AOM.[25] The tympanic membrane of AOM on otoscopic examination varies from hyperemia with preservation of landmarks to a bright-red, tense, bulging, distorted appearance. In advanced stage of suppuration, the tympanic membrane ruptures with a gush of purulent or blood-tinged fluid from the ear.[23]

Traditionally AOM is treated with antibiotics. A clinical trial of 223 children with AOM, ranging in age from 6 months to 12 years, who were randomized to antibiotic treatment (ABX) and watchful waiting (WW) revealed 66% of subjects in the WW group completed study without antibiotic treatment. Compared with WW, ABX treatment was associated with decreased numbers of treatment failures and improved symptom control but increased ABX-related adverse events and a higher percent carriage of multidrug-resistant *S. pneumoniae* strains in the nasopharynx.[32] Although few community pediatricians practice initial observation without antibiotics, this modality is increasingly accepted by educated parents who feel included in medical decisions.[33]

More important, the new AAP clinical practice guideline for AOM gives the option of allowing selected children to fight an ear infection on their own before initiating antibiotic treatment. These children would initially receive analgesics (because most episodes of AOM are associated with pain, assessment and reduction of pain must be an integral part of AOM management), whereas antibiotics are reserved for those whose conditions worsen or fail to improve within 48 to 72 hours.[29] Although new to many U.S. physicians, the observation option for AOM is an official policy in the Netherlands, Sweden, and now New York State.[34] By offering the observation option, the new guideline changes the central AOM management decision from the question of which antibiotic should be given[35] to whether an antibiotic should be given at all.[36]

The paradigm shift is imperative because 5.2 million AOM episodes are diagnosed each year[37]; in 2000 there were 16 million office visits for otitis media, with 802 antibacterial prescriptions per 1000 visits given for a total of more than 13 million prescriptions[38] or 60% of all antibiotics written for children.[39-41] In 1995 the estimated direct cost and indirect cost of AOM were $1.96 billion and $1.02 billion, respectively.[37]

The widespread use of antibiotics has resulted in worldwide increase in the number of multidrug-resistant bacterial pathogens,[9,11,42] including the dramatic increase in resistance of pneumococcus to penicillin.[43-48] Up to 10% of pediatric AOM cases are recalcitrant to antibiotic therapy.[49] The prevalence of resistant organisms tends to increase in the winter months.[50] In addition, antimicrobials suppress normal flora, which is beneficial to the host because it is able to interfere with and therefore prevent pathogenic infections and may enhance recovery from URI.[50] On the other hand, since the advent of antibiotics, complications such as mastoiditis and intracranial infections have significantly decreased.[23]

If a decision is made to treat with an antibacterial agent, both the Centers for Disease Control Prevention (CDC) and the AAP recommend high-dose amoxicillin (80 to 90 mg/kg/day) to treat uncomplicated AOM in children at high risk for infection with unsusceptible penumococcus.[18,29] A double-blind

study from Costa Rica revealed single-dose azithromycin (Zithromax) to be more effective and have better patient compliance and fewer adverse effects.[51]

The best treatment for AOM would be prevention. In addition to pneumococcal vaccine, another preventive measure is breastfeeding, which confers lifelong protection against infectious illness, including otitis.[52,53] An effective RSV vaccine for the infant and young child could markedly decrease otitis media disease.[3] Intranasal spray of attenuated viruses is currently under investigation in the hope that early antiviral therapy would reduce the risk of otitis media following respiratory tract infections.[5,8]

Chronic Otitis Media

Chronic otitis media is divided into two categories: chronic suppurative otitis media and chronic otitis media with effusion (OME). Chronic suppurative otitis media is not temporally related to acute otitis, as the pathological changes in the middle ear are different. The classic symptoms of established chronic suppurative otitis are otorrhea and deafness or some form of hearing loss.[23] Chronic suppurative otitis media can lead to the formation of cholesteatoma, a cyst that contains desquamated epithelial cells, which can cause local bone erosion and lead to retention of infected material.[23]

OME is one of the most common diseases in childhood.[24] It is related to infection, eustachian tube obstruction, allergic or immunological disorders, and enlarged adenoids.[23] The serous fluid in CSOM contains bacteria such as *H. influenzae* and pneumococcus and is therefore predisposed to the development of OME.[54] OME has been implicated to be an immune-mediated disease,[18] as immune complexes have been demonstrated in MEE[55,56] and highly organized lymphatic tissue has been found in the middle ear mucosa.[57]

The rationale for treating OME is prevention of recurrence of AOM. Currently, once-daily antibiotic regimen is the recommended prophylaxis. The benefit is also weighed against the increasing risk of emergence of resistant bacteria.[53] When antibiotics fail to control recurrent otitis, a short trial of prednisone is sometimes prescribed.[49] Surgery is recommended when medical treatment fails,[49] especially when the child has hearing loss.[10] Tympanostomy tubes appear to be beneficial in OME but are of less value in chronic suppurative otitis.[53] Increase in hearing loss has been reported with insertion of ventilation tubes.[58] Adenoidectomy is sometimes recommended,[7] especially after tympanostomy tube failure,[53] although a recent randomized trial from the Netherlands of 217 children aged 12 to 48 months found that adenoidectomy does not significantly reduce the incidence of otitis media in conjunction with the insertion of tympanostomy tubes in children younger than 4 years.[59]

Although recognizing that increasing numbers of parents and caregivers use various forms of complementary and alternative medicine (CAM) for their children, the AAP makes no recommendations for CAM treatment of AOM, stating that data are currently limited and controversial. The AAP does recommend, however, that clinicians become more informed about CAM, ask whether CAM treatments are being used, and be ready to discuss potential benefits or risks.[29]

✳ OTITIS MEDIA: CAM THERAPY RECOMMENDATIONS

Acupuncture

Recent acupuncture data on treatment of otitis media in children are completely lacking. Only one clinical trial was reported in 1985.[2] Traditional Chinese medicine (TCM) diagnoses correlate well with Western categorizations of acute and chronic otitis media.

Acute Otitis Media: Wind-Cold and Wind-Heat Invasion, Dampness

AOM correlates to the Shao Yang stage of Wind-Cold invasion and to the Wei Qi level of Wind-Heat invasion. Dampness—the Western medicine congestion and fluid accumulation in the eustachian tube—predisposes the child to external invasions, and suppuration correlates to TCM diagnosis of Damp-Heat. An integrative approach would be beneficial, both with diagnosis using otoscopic examination and with follow-up audiologic evaluations such as tympanograms and other hearing tests. Acupuncture treatment can be given concomitantly with antibiotics, as TCM's goal in expelling the pathogens and tonifying the immune system complements the Western regimen.

Treatment

Treat the local ear points: GB2, SI19, TB21.

Parents can be taught to massage these points.

Can "pull down" the inflammation by using an ion pumping cord to connect local and distal points: Connect the black clamp to GB2 local point and the red clamp to BL60. If using magnets, place the bionorth (−) side downward on GB2 and the biosouth (+) side downward on BL60, and connect with the black clamp on the GB2 magnet and the red clamp on BL60.

Use Shaoyang protocol:

GB16, GB20 to dispel Wind.

LI4 + KI7 to cause sweating.

GV14 if fever is present.

Prophylactically tonify the Stomach and LI to prevent further progression into the Yangming stage (mastoiditis).

If Cold is present, use the Four-Point protocol to dispel Cold from the GB channel (see Appendix B):

Tonify GB38, SI5; sedate GB43, BL66.

In infants and young children, use two points: Tonify GB38; sedate GB43.

If Heat is present, use the Four-Point protocol to disperse Heat from the GB channel:

Tonify GB43, BL66; sedate GB38, SI5.

In infants and young children, use two points: Tonify GB43, sedate GB38.

If Damp is present, resolve Damp:

GB34 transforms Shaoyang Damp.

SP9 clears Damp Heat.

ST40 resolves Damp.

Tonify the Spleen: SP3, SP6; or use the Four-Point protocol.

After the ear infection has resolved, tonify the immune system.

Prophylactic treatment

Because AOM is prevalent during winter and early spring, the TCM principle of "winter disease, summer cure" would be prophylactically tonifying Wei Qi or the immune system, treating the local ear points, or tonifying the Shaoyang Gallbladder channel during the summer months.

Tonify Gallbladder: Tonify GB43, BL66; sedate GB44, LI1.

Tonify Kidney Yin:

Because the ears are the external orifice for Kidney, tonification of Kidney Yin during an acute invasion is comparable to prevention of suppurative complications.

KI 6 tonifies KI Yin.

Chronic Otitis Media with Effusion

Spleen Qi deficiency

The lingering effusion is indicative of Dampness due to Spleen deficiency. Children are constitutionally Spleen Qi deficient. They may become more Spleen deficient owing to inheritance of weak pre-Heaven Spleen Qi, such as a strong family of Spleen Qi deficiency, Spleen deficiency in both parents during conception, or in the mother during pregnancy; a diet with excessive sweets, dairy, and greasy foods; chronic illnesses; or living in a Damp environment. Spleen Qi deficiency results in Dampness accumulation. Chronic Dampness would in turn further injure the Spleen. Spleen corresponds with the emotions of worry and obsession and with excess mental activities. A careful history would uncover any situations that would predispose to worry, such as academic overload or lack of rest due to school or extracurricular activities.

Treatment

Treat the local ear points: GB2, SI19, TB21.

Treat local-distal points as indicated in acute treatment.

Avoid artificially sweetened foods.

Vigorously tonify the Spleen with the Four-Point protocol.

Modify lifestyle to allow the child to feel less pressure from school work and other activities and to minimize worry.

Shaoyang Heat

Shaoyang Heat tends to affect children in the Wood phase of development when the Gallbladder is vulnerable. Heat in the Gallbladder channel may be due to lingering pathogenic Heat from previous illnesses that were not completely expelled or consumption of excess greasy foods or medications that injure the Wood element. Although the Liver is the "general" that directs Qi, the Gallbladder has the important function of carrying out the decisions. This child then would have chronic otitis with other Heat symptoms and indecisiveness.

Treatment

Treat local and distal points.

Avoid greasy or sour foods. Minimize medications.

Gallbladder Heat: Tonify GB43, BL66; sedate GB38, SI5.

Two points: Tonify GB43; sedate GB38.

Chronic suppurative otitis media: Kidney Yin deficiency/Spleen Damp

The hearing loss associated with chronic suppurative otitis media is indicative of injury to the Kidney Yin, Kidney Essence, with persistence of Spleen Damp.

Treatment
Treat local and distal points.
Avoid excess salty foods.
KI 6 tonifies Kidney Yin.
Tonify the Spleen with the Four-Point protocol.
Transform Damp.

Prophylactic treatment
During periods of remission, tonify the immune system.

Chiropractic

Chiropractic management of the child with otitis media is to restore normal neurological function through elimination of the subluxation complex (SC) and correct any chemical or lifestyle influences. There is evidence that the chiropractic adjustment has influence over natural killer cell production,[1] immunoglobulin (IgA, IgG, and IgM) levels and β-cell lymphocyte count,[2] polymorphonuclear neutrophils and monocytes,[3] and even CD4 counts,[4] thus allowing improved ability of the immune system to resolve infective processes.

In addition, highly viscous or profuse fluid accumulation in the middle ear may occur in response to a chemical sensitization. Middle ear congestion due to lack of adequate patency of the eustachian tube may occur from muscular imbalance. Lack of adequate lymph drainage may occur from cervical muscular compression on the lymph due to hypertonicity. This hypertonicity may be secondary to the SC.

In an unscientific survey of children raised under a chiropractic model of care versus a medical model of care, 80% of the medically raised children had at least one episode of otitis media, compared with only 31% of the chiropractically raised children.[5]

A retrospective study of 46 children who presented to a chiropractic office with complaints of ear symptoms was conducted. The 46 children had a total of 95 episodes of ear symptoms. Based on parental report and observation by the chiropractor, 93% of children were reported as improved.[6]

A case series of five children with otitis media who presented for chiropractic care was conducted. All patients had lasting resolution of symptoms with no residual morbidity or other complications.[7]

A prospective study involving 332 children with otitis media was performed by a New York chiropractor. Tympanometric evaluations were performed on these children in addition to the customary chiropractic examination and otoscopy. The average number of chiropractic adjustments provided was 4.09. Otoscopic examination returned to normal by an average of 7.65 days, and tympanometric examination returned to normal by an average of 9.26 days. The overall rate of recurrence within 6 months was 15.56%.[8]

Multiple case studies also support the benefits of the chiropractic adjustment in the wellness of the child with otitis media.[9-12]

The most common spinal regions to be adjusted include the C0-C4 and C215 vertebral segments.

The chiropractor would utilize cranial adjusting as indicated, especially including a temporal rocking technique, to ease the middle ear congestion.[14,15]

An auricular adjustment may be used. This involves grasping the ear with the thumb and index finger and applying traction in all directions. An optional method is to grasp the ear and rapidly tug the ear away from the head and anteriorly.[16] The latter is sometimes painful and not tolerated well by younger children.

Temporomandibular dysfunction may also be a part of the development of the condition.[15,17]

Because the eustachian tube is partially controlled via muscular attachments, the tensor veli palatini (TVP) muscle may be the subject of some attention by the chiropractor. The easily accessible origin of the TVP is at the posterior lateral margin of the hard palate. The chiropractor will gently digitally manipulate this muscle in an effort to exercise a stretch on the TVP. The goal of this oral sweep maneuver is to cause a slight pumping action on the eustachian tube in an effort to enhance drainage from the middle ear.[18]

Alternatively, endonasal massage of the deep lateral pharyngeal wall at the outlet of the eustachian tube may also enhance drainage of the middle ear.[19,20]

Older children may find some relief with chewing gum, as the same nerve that activates the TVP innervates the muscles of mastication.

Lymphatic stimulation is also commonly used by the chiropractor because of the possibility of lymphatic congestion secondary to muscular imbalance and SC.[13] This can be accomplished by gently stroking along the anterior and posterior margins of the sternocleidomastoid from superior to inferior.

Tapping on the mid-sternum may increase thymus activity to help fight infection.[14]

Mullein and garlic eardrops can be applied topically to the middle ear for anesthesia and bacterial suppression.

Application of a heat pack over the affected ear may provide additional pain relief.[21]

As with any infective process, avoiding empty calories or proinflammatory foods is advisable. The chiropractor is concerned with ensuring a diet rich in fresh fruits and vegetables, whole grains, lean meats, and fish.

Supplementation with immune-enhancing nutrients may provide the body with necessary resources to manage an acute infection. Commonly recommended nutrients include zinc, vitamins A and C, and omega-3 fatty acids (eicosapentaenoic acid [EPA]/docosahexaenoic acid [DHA]).

Echinacea purpurea is recommended as a stimulant to the immune system.[15] Use is recommended for a period not to exceed 2 consecutive weeks, as the body may develop a tolerance level with prolonged use. Although echinacea is quite safe, allergic reactions in children with a history of allergies, particularly to plants in the daisy family, have been recorded.

As many as 80% of children with ear infections have food sensitivities, especially to dairy and wheat. In a 1-month trial of elimination of the offending food, improvement in otitis media was demonstrated.[22,23] Reintroduction of the offending food should be accompanied by monitoring of the middle ear for reemergence of fluid. Because dairy has a tendency to cause mucous production even in the absence of allergy, it is recommended that all dairy products be excluded from the diet until the episode of otitis media is resolved.

Steam inhalation may be useful, particularly if essential oils such as pine menthol and camphor are added to the water. This technique may be utilized in school-aged children.[15]
Avoid second-hand smoke exposure.
Avoid use of pacifiers.
Children may find some pressure release from inflating balloons.[16]

Homeopathy

Before using this section, see Appendix A, Homeopathy, for definitions of practitioner expertise categories and for general information on prescribing homeopathic medicines.

Practitioner Expertise Categories 1 and 2

• AOM in patients 6 months of age or older

Practitioner Expertise Categories 2 and 3

• AOM in patients under 6 months of age, and chronic or recurrent otitis media

Otitis media is one of the conditions most frequently treated by homeopathic practitioners. In a 1992 survey of medical doctors using homeopathy in their practices, otitis media was reported as the illness treated third most frequently.[1] There is a small body of research evidence to support the use of homeopathic medicine for AOM.[2-5] Although the studies do not provide definitive evidence because of methodological concerns, including small sample size,[2,4] lack of blinding,[2,3] and lack of rigorous diagnostic criteria,[4] positive effects were seen in the treatment groups. The most consistent findings in these studies were a reduction in the duration of pain by at least one day in the treatment groups[2,4,5] and fewer recurrences of otitis media in the treatment groups for at least one year after completion of the studies.[2,3] These findings suggest that homeopathy can be a useful form of therapy for otitis media. Larger, more rigorous trials are needed to confirm this hypothesis. In addition to the aforementioned research evidence, the homeopathic literature contains much evidence in the form of accumulated clinical experience to support the use of homeopathic treatment for otitis media.[6]

Because of concerns about the overuse of antibiotics and the emergence of resistant microorganisms, and because research data indicate that many children recover from AOM without treatment, it has been suggested that patients with AOM who meet certain criteria be observed and be given symptomatic treatment for up to 72 hours before being given antimicrobial therapy. Inclusion and exclusion criteria for this "observation option" are summarized in Box 49-1. These recommendations are summarized by Rosenfeld.[7]

Because it is accepted practice to wait before treating many cases of otitis media with antimicrobial therapy, and because there is some evidence that homeopathy helps with the acute symptoms of AOM, children who fall within the guidelines for the observation option are ideal candidates for homeopathic treatment. During the waiting period homeopathic treatment

Box 49-1

Inclusion and Exclusion Criteria for Observing Patients before Beginning Antimicrobial Therapy for AOM

Inclusion criteria

• 6 months of age or older
• No prior AOM treatment failures
• No AOM diagnosis in the previous month

Exclusion criteria

• Younger than 6 months of age
• Severe episode of otitis media
• Coexisting bacterial sinusitis or streptococcal pharyngitis
• History of immune deficiency disease
• Craniofacial anomalies, such as cleft palate

AOM, Acute otitis media.

can provide more relief of symptoms than can be provided with conventional analgesics and decongestants alone. Homeopathic treatment may be curative and preventive in some cases. Homeopathy is safe to use in infants and children of all ages for treatment of otitis media and can be used in conjunction with other treatment modalities—conventional and alternative.

The goal of treating otitis media homeopathically is to determine the single homeopathic medicine whose description in the materia medica most closely matches the symptom picture of the patient. Often mental and emotional states, in addition to physical symptoms, are considered. Once the medicine has been selected, it can be given orally or sublingually in the 30C potency every 2 to 3 hours, or two to three times daily, depending on the severity of the symptoms. For more severe symptoms, a 200C potency can be given two to three times daily. If the medicine has not helped in five to six doses, then another homeopathic medicine should be tried or some other form of therapy should be instituted, as needed. Once symptoms have begun to resolve, the medicine can be given less frequently or stopped. It can be repeated again for a relapse of symptoms.

The following is a list of homeopathic medicines commonly used to treat patients with AOM. It must be emphasized that this list is partial and represents some of the probable choices from the homeopathic materia medica. If the symptoms of a given patient are not represented here, further research in the homeopathic literature would be needed to find the simillimum.

Pulsatilla nigricans

Pulsatilla nigricans is the most frequently indicated homeopathic medicine for acute and chronic ear infections. Usually the infection is preceded by an upper respiratory tract infection with discharge of thick yellow or green nasal mucus. A child who is old enough to describe the symptoms will complain of full or bursting feelings in the ear, and may also describe a pulsing or throbbing sensation. The symptoms are worse in the evening and when the child is overheated; they are better with gentle motion (such as being carried around) and in cool or open air. The child is warm and flushed. He or she is weepy and needs a lot of attention.

Belladonna

Belladonna is used early in the course of AOM when the child experiences the sudden onset of intense, throbbing ear pain, especially on the right side. The infection is accompanied by a high fever with redness of the face and tympanic membranes, dilated pupils, and possibly signs of delirium (see Chapter 36, Fever). The symptoms are worse at 3 PM and after midnight. The child feels worse lying down, on exposure to noise or drafts, and if his or her body is jarred.

Chamomilla vulgaris

Chamomilla vulgaris is an excellent medicine for acute and chronic otitis media. Consider *Chamomilla vulgaris* in cases in which OM occurs with teething. Diarrhea with green stools may accompany the infection. The child is sensitive to the pain of the infection, is extremely irritable and irascible, and has an aversion to being examined or watched. Carrying the child around or going for a ride may be the only way to pacify him or her. The typical patient needing *Chamomilla vulgaris* is hot, red, and thirsty. Often one cheek is hot and red, while the other is pale and cool. Symptoms are worst from 9 to 10 AM and 9 to 10 PM.

Hepar sulphuris calcareum

The child needing *Hepar sulphuris calcareum* is chilled and wants to be covered, especially over the ears. The ear pain is described as "sticking" or "splinterlike." Often there is an accompanying sore throat. Symptoms are worse late at night and are exacerbated by exposure to cold. The child is sensitive to pain and may shriek with the pain. The child hates to be touched or examined.

Mercurius solubilis hahnemanni

The child needing *Mercurius solubilis hahnemanni* alternates between fever with sweating and chills. The ear infection may be accompanied by sore throat, sinusitis, or bronchitis. Thick nasal discharge, a coated tongue, and foul-smelling breath may be noted. The patient is worse at night and from becoming overheated and feels better from the application of cold compresses.

Naturopathy

Ear infections are one of the most common reasons for pediatric visits to a naturopathic physician. It is also the most common condition that is treated with antibiotics in the United States.[1] In the Netherlands, antimicrobial therapy is not the first line treatment for otitis media, and this has resulted in lower rates of bacterial resistance.[2,3] Parents are becoming increasingly wary of the use of antibiotics as they are concerned with antibiotic resistance, antibiotic-induced diarrhea, and in some cases the addition of yet another medication to their child's regimen. The naturopathic approach examines why the child is getting frequent infections and aims to support their inherent healthy nature, not to wait until they develop a problem and then address the bacterial cause. The vulnerability to infection may be a result of several factors that can have profound effects on the immune system. Suboptimal levels of vitamins or minerals,

emotional stressors, diet, lifestyle, and the microbial milleu of the patient must all be considered. Otitis media is a condition that may be treated successfully with natural means without putting the child at significant risk for sequelae or from side effects of the alternative treatments.

Systemic Treatments

Food intolerance/allergy

It is difficult to debate the role that allergies play in the development of otitis media. There is ample research on the connection between the generally atopic child and the frequency of otitis media. In particular, it is the allergic component to otitis media with effusion[4,5] that predisposes one to acute suppurative otitis. In this author's experience, avoidance of one or several of the foods found to be most allergenic, such as wheat, dairy, eggs, soy, peanuts, fish, corn, tomatoes, and citrus, has produced significant reductions in frequency of otitis and upper respiratory infections. The most common scenario is a pertinent history of symptoms arising once a child was provided either milk or milk-based formula. Increased infections, diarrhea or constipation, chronic rhinitis, colic, wheezing, and rash have all been associated with food intolerance, and diary products seem to be the most frequently offending food for the large majority of these patients. Testing by a specialty lab that measures IgG in addition to IgE can help to identify an offending food. Elimination of that food for at least 1 month will provide the best results. If improvements are seen with the elimination, it is suggested to either remove that food from the diet or rotate consumption to every several days.

Probiotics

The flora of the upper respiratory and alimentary tracts has specific immune enhancing effects as well as local antiinfectious qualities. In particular, alpha-hemolytic streptococcus, a common inhabitant of the upper respiratory tract found in healthy patients, has been shown to prevent recurrences of otitis media because of its abilities to inhibit infections caused by common respiratory pathogens such as *Haemophilus* spp. and *Streptococcus pneumoniae*.[6,7,8]

Interestingly, patients with recurrent otitis media have fewer of the protective alpha-hemolytic streptococci and more of *Haemophilus* spp. and *S. pneumoniae* inhabiting their mucosa than controls, which may be caused by antibiotic use.[9,10] The development of other conditions that can lead to or complicate otitis media, such as recurrent adenotonsillitis and obstructive adenoid hypertrophy, may also affect or be affected by the microbiology of the upper respiratory tract.[11] These facts emphasize the concern of antibiotic overuse compounded by neglecting to replace important protective flora. In this author's experience, patients who have been treated with antibiotics for frequent bouts of otitis media also have a strong history of recurrent sinusitis, tonsillitis, and upper respiratory tract infections. It is possible that by repeatedly treating these conditions with antibiotics and not replacing the indigenous flora, a cycle of infection susceptibility is being encouraged. Unfortunately, the potential promise of replacing alpha-hemolytic streptococcus has yet to prove itself, as it was not found to decrease occurrences of acute otitis media when applied as a nasal spray.[12] However, oral administration of a probiotic supplement containing *Lactobacillus GG*, *Streptococcus thermophilus*, *Lactobacillus acidophilus*, and *Bifidobacterium* spp. resulted in decreased levels in the upper respiratory tract of bacteria that are known causes of otitis media. As a result, this treatment may serve as a very effective method of prevention.[13]

Lactobacillus GG in particular was shown to protect against sinusitis, bronchitis, and otitis media.[14] The majority of bacteria in the gut of a breast-fed infant are bidfidobacteria. Formula-fed infants have considerably lower levels of this crucial microbe, which may explain higher rates of atopy in children consuming primarily formula. It is essential that these children are provided a probiotic supplement that contains bifidobacteria. The levels of bifidobacteria in breast-fed children are also known to decrease once solid foods or cow's milk are introduced into the diet, so it should be part of any combination supplement given to a patient regardless of their main source of food. Dosage can vary, and most quality supplements have at least 2 billion CFUs per serving. Serving sizes are typically 1 capsule or ¼ to ½ teaspoon. Capsules may be opened and put in food or drink or put directly into the mouth of the infant, applied with a wet finger. The dose is one serving per day, and the only adverse effects that have been noted are mild gas and bloating that discontinues when dosing is reduced.

Breastfeeding

Breastfeeding provides strong protection against otitis media.[15] Infants may have up to two times the increased risk of both acute otitis media and otitis media with effusion if they are exclusively fed formula.[16] The optimal duration for breastfeeding has not been elucidated, but there is evidence to show that breastfeeding for at least 4 to 6 months can defend against frequent bouts of otitis.[17,18,19] The protection seems to be so effective that this inhibition can last up to four months after discontinuing breastfeeding. Once children have been weaned off breast milk for 12 months, the susceptibility to developing otitis rises to the same levels as those who were never breast fed.[20] This finding may indicate that attempting to breast feed children as long as possible is the most prudent choice.

Without question, the diet of the breastfeeding mother needs to be considered when looking at otitis frequency in the pediatric patient. Even when a child is exclusively breast fed, they may still produce antibodies to cow's milk,[21] presumably owing to exposure to antigens in breast milk. Therefore it is important to examine the mother's diet to screen for potentially allergenic foods, and a rotation diet or total elimination of the offending food should be adopted and followed with close observation of symptoms.

Vitamin/Mineral status and supplementation

It is well documented in the literature that vitamin and mineral status can affect the immune status of children. Those in particular that have antioxidant properties should be considered,[22] as increased free radical production has been noted in the middle ears of human patients and animal models that have otitis media with effusion.[23,24] Vitamin A deficiency can result in a reduction in mucus-secreting cells and a replacement of columnar epithelial cells by thick layers of stratified epithelium known as *keratinization*. Protection from infections is decreased with keratinization, so vitamin A supplementation could potentially increase infection resistance at the mucosal level. However, one study found that low serum vitamin A levels and those of other carotenoids did not correlate with otitis susceptibility,[25] whereas another study reported fewer otitis occurrences in patients with measles who received supplemental vitamin A.[26]

Antioxidants are directly involved in the antimicrobial processes of the immune system, and children with acute infections such as otitis media and tonsillitis have a higher level of oxidative stress.[27] As a result, these patients also have lower serum levels of vitamins A, C, and E, and beta-carotene.[28] Supplementation may benefit these patients. In addition, multivitamin administration has been shown to decrease rates of otitis in children.[29] There is also intriguing evidence of the protective potential for antioxidants in the pregnant mother's diet, because children of mothers who consume a diet high in vitamin C have a decreased otitis risk. Vitamin C supplementation, however, does not affect this risk.[30]

Selenium is a potent antioxidant mineral that seems to have significant immunostimulatory effects[31-34] and should be considered as a supplemental agent when treating children with chronic upper respiratory tract infections, including otitis. A reasonable dosage for selenium in infants and children is difficult to assess. Adult recommended daily allowances (RDAs) for selenium are 55 µg/day for men and women. A tolerable upper threshold for intake has been established at 400 µg/day by the Food and Nutrition Board.[35]

Naturopathic physicians often use several treatments for disease to maximize effectiveness. It is worth noting that successful treatments for other upper respiratory tract diseases should be considered when searching for effective otitis management. Sinusitis, which is often found as a concomitant condition with otitis, may be treated with multivitamin and mineral supplementation along with essential fatty acids such as cod liver oil.[36] Essential fatty acids can have favorable effects on inflammatory processes, which are increased in patients with otitis. This same treatment combination has shown favorable results in the prevention of otitis media,[37] but larger studies are necessary. Multivitamin and mineral supplements should contain a broad base of antioxidant nutrients such as selenium, vitamins A, C, and E, and zinc. Essential fatty acid supplements (EFAs) should contain approximately equal amounts of eicosapentaenoic acid (EPA) and docosahexaenoic acid (DHA). High-quality companies have stringent processes for purifying the oils, to remove contaminants such as polychlorinated biphenyls or heavy metals. EFA products should also contain vitamin E, as it prevents oxidation and rancidity. Before considering a fatty acid, its purification standards should be researched. The dose may be approximately 1 to 2 g total EPA/DHA combination. Most companies provide this amount in 1 to 2 teaspoons. Side effects may include loose stools that will resolve once the dose is decreased.

Local treatments
Ear drops

Probably the most common naturopathic topical treatment for otitis media are herbal ear drops, which often contain a combination of St. John's Wort *(Hypericum perforatum)*, garlic

(Allium sativum), mullein *(Verbascum thapsus),* and marigold *(Calendula officinalis).* The use of these drops has demonstrated promising results. When compared with anesthetic ear drops, naturopathic ear drops were found to be equally effective.[38] Another study demonstrated that patients treated only with the herbal drops improved in the shortest time when compared to those treated with anesthetic ear drops or antibiotics.[39] In fact, those patients treated only with antibiotics experienced the longest recovery period. Theories used to explain why antibiotics may be counter-productive include encouraging the growth of resistant organisms and inhibition of the local immune system, particularly bactericidal-permeability increasing protein, which is known to be inhibited in otitis.[40]

It is possible that the effectiveness of these ear drops are due to several factors. *H. perforatum* has purported antiviral effects,[41] mainly against human immunodeficiency and hepatitis C viruses.[42] *H. perforatum* may have other general antiviral effects that would be useful in otitis treatment. The antimicrobial effects of garlic are also well documented,[43] which adds to the therapeutic benefits of these combinations. The antiedematous and wound-healing effects of *C. officinalis* may explain the success of this therapy.[44,45] It is thought that these botanical medicines are well absorbed and have local immunostimulatory abilities. The ratio of herbs in most ear drops is approximately equal among the ingredients. Dosage is 3 to 5 drops in the affected ear 2 to 3 times per day.

For severe pain, anecdotal evidence exists for the use of two other specific botanicals that may be added to the formulation mentioned above: 1 to 5 drops of the tinctures of *Aconite napellus* or *Gelsemium sempervirens* may be added to 1 ounce of the ear drops. Dosing for this formulation may be the same as the herbal ear drops mentioned previously. Apply several times a day, 3 to 5 drops each time.

Contraindications to the use of any herbal ear drops include a perforated tympanic membrane.

Physical Medicine

Local therapies may also consist of treatments that include delivery of massage, heat, cold, and moisture. There is a limited amount of research on these methods, but the anecdotal evidence is convincing. Applying a hot compress to the affected ear has been effective in treating pain for otitis. An old folk remedy called the *onion poultice* has been helpful in this author's practice. An onion is cut in half and placed in a microwave oven for 20 to 40 seconds or a conventional oven for several minutes until warm to the touch (testing on the inside of the parent's wrist is a good assessment). The child lies down with the affected ear up and the onion is then placed on the ear and covered with towels to contain the heat. Once the onion cools, it may be reheated and used again several times in that treatment period. Another technique called *contrast hydrotherapy* involves applying a cycle of hot and cold compresses to the ear, which alleviates pain and helps cycle new and old blood to and from the site, including necessary immune cells. The hot compress may either be a hot water bottle or washcloth soaked in hot water and wrung out. The cold compress may be ice wrapped in a moist towel or a towel dipped in ice cold water. A general rule of 2 minutes hot and 30 seconds cold can be used, ending on the cold portion of the therapy. At least three cycles are recommended per treatment, several times a day.

References

Otitis Externa

Pediatric Diagnosis and Management

1. Leung AK, Fong JH, Leong AG: Otalgia in children, *J Natl Med Assoc* 92:254-260, 2000.
2. Ramsey AM: Diagnosis and treatment of the child with a draining ear, *J Pediatr Health Care* 16:161-169, 2002.
3. Behrman RE, Kliegman RM, Jenson HB, editors: *Nelson textbook of pediatrics,* ed 17, Philadelphia, 2004, Saunders.
4. Schroeder A, Darrow DH: Management of the draining ear in children, *Pediatr Ann* 33:843-853, 2004.
5. Brook I: Treatment of otitis externa in children, *Paediatr Drugs* 1:283-289, 1999.
6. Nussinovitch M, Rimon A, Volovitz B et al: Cotton-tip applicators as a leading cause of otitis externa, *Int J Pediatr Otorhinolaryngol* 68:433-435, 2004.
7. Ruben RJ: Efficacy of ofloxacin and other otic preparations for otitis externa, *Pediatr Infect Dis J* 20:108-110, 2001; discussion 120-122.
8. Martin TJ, Kerschner JE, Flanary VA: Fungal causes of otitis externa and tympanostomy tube otorrhea, *Int J Pediatr Otorhinolaryngol* 69:1503-1508, 2005.

Chiropractic

1. Leach RA, Burgess SC: Neuroimmune hypothesis, In Leach RA, editor: *The chiropractic theories,* Baltimore, 2004, Lippincott Williams and Wilkins.
2. Brennan PC, Kokjohn K, Triano JJ et al: Immunologic correlates of reduced spinal mobility: preliminary observations in a dog model, In Wold S, editor: *Proceedings of the 1991 International Conference on Spinal Manipulation,* Arlington, Va, 1991, Foundation for Chiropractic Education and Research.
3. Brennan PC, Kokjohn K, Kaltinger CJ et al: Enhanced phagocytic cell respiratory burst induced by spinal manipulation: potential role of substance P, *J Manipulative Physiol Ther* 14:399-408, 1991.
4. Selano JL, Hightower BC, Pfleger B et al: The effects of specific upper cervical adjustments on the CD4 counts of HIV positive patients, *Chiropractic Res J* 3:32-39, 1994.
5. Bhandari N, Bahl R, Taneja S et al: Effect or routine zinc supplementation on pneumonia in children aged 6 months to 3 years: randomized controlled trial in an urban slum, *Br Med J* 324:1358-1361, 2002.
6. Forastiere R, Pistelli R, Sestini P et al: Consumption of fresh fruit rich in vitamin C and wheezing symptoms in children, *Thorax* 55:283-288, 2000.
7. Stevens LJ, Zentall SS, Abate ML et al: Omega-3 fatty acids in boys with behavior, learning and health problems, *Physiol Behav* 59:915-920, 1996.
8. Davies N: *Chiropractic pediatrics,* London, 2000, Churchill Livingstone.

Herbs—Chinese

1. Neustaedter R: Personal communication, August 2005.

Homeopathy

1. *ReferenceWorks Pro 4.2,* San Rafael, Calif, 2008, Kent Homeopathic Associates.

Otitis Media

Pediatric Diagnosis and Management

1. Block SL, Harrison CH, Hedrick J et al: Restricted use of antibiotic prophylaxis for recurrent acute otitis media in the era of penicillin non-susceptible *Streptococcus pneumoniae, Int J Pediatr Otorhinolaryngol* 61:47-60, 2001.
2. White CB, Foshee WS: Upper respiratory tract infections in adolescents, *Adolesc Med* 11:225-249, 2000.
3. Anderson LJ: Respiratory syncytial virus vaccines for otitis media, *Vaccine* 19(Suppl 1):S59-S65, 2000.
4. Behrman RE, Kliegman RM, Jenson HB, editors: *Nelson textbook of pediatrics*, ed 17, Philadelphia, 2004, Saunders.
5. Hayden FG: Influenza virus and rhinovirus-related otitis media: potential for antiviral intervention, *Vaccine* 19(Suppl 1):S66-S70, 2000.
6. Heikkinen T: The role of respiratory viruses in otitis media, *Vaccine* 19(Suppl 1):S51-S55, 2000.
7. Jund R, Grevers G: Rhinitis, sore throat and otalgia... benign common cold or dangerous infection? [in German], *MMW Fortschr Med* 142:32-36, 2000 (abstract).
8. Glezen WP: Prevention of acute otitis media by prophylaxis and treatment of influenza virus infections, *Vaccine* 19(Suppl 1): S56-S58, 2000.
9. Ruoff G: Upper respiratory tract infections in family practice, *Pediatr Infect Dis J* 17(8 Suppl):S73-S78, 1998.
10. Oh HM: Upper respiratory tract infections—otitis media, sinusitis and pharyngitis, *Singapore Med J* 36:428-431, 1995.
11. Cappelletty D: Microbiology of bacterial respiratory infections, *Pediatr Infect Dis J* 17(8 Suppl):S55-S61, 1998.
12. St Geme JW 3rd: The pathogenesis of nontypable *Haemophilus influenzae* otitis media, *Vaccine* 19(Suppl 1):S41-S50, 2000.
13. Pichichero ME: Group A beta-hemolytic streptococcal infections, *Pediatr Rev* 19:291-302, 1998.
14. Rynnel-Dagoo B, Agren K: The nasopharynx and the middle ear. Inflammatory reactions in middle ear disease, *Vaccine* 19(Suppl 1): S26-S31, 2000.
15. Park K, Lim DJ: Development of secretory elements in murine tubotympanum: lysozyme and lactoferrin immunohistochemistry, *Ann Otol Rhinol Laryngo* 102:385-395, 1993.
16. Zimmerman RK: Pneumococcal conjugate vaccine for young children, *Am Fam Physician* 63:1991-1998, 2001.
17. Tuomanen EI: Pathogenesis of pneumococcal inflammation: otitis media, *Vaccine* 19(Suppl 1):S38-S40, 2000.
18. Centers for Disease Control and Prevention: *Vaccine information*. Available at www.cdc.gov/vaccines/vpd-vac/pneumo/default.htm. Accessed August 15, 2005.
19. Briles DE, Hollingshead SK, Nabors GS et al: The potential for using protein vaccines to protect against otitis media caused by *Streptococcus pneumoniae, Vaccine* 19(Suppl 1):S87-S95, 2000.
20. Overturf GD: The American Academy of Pediatrics Committee on Infectious Diseases. Technical report: prevention of pneumococcal infections, including the use of pneumococcal conjugate vaccine in children, *Pediatrics* 106:367-376, 2000.
21. Pelton SI: Acute otitis media in the era of effective pneumococcal conjugate vaccine: will new pathogens emerge? *Vaccine* 19(Suppl 1): S96-S99, 2000.
22. Eskola J, Kilpi T, Palmu A et al: Finnish Otitis Media Study Group: efficacy of a penumococcal conjugate vaccine against acute otitis media, *N Engl J Med* 344:403-409, 2001.
23. Feigin R, Cherry JD: *Textbook of pediatric infectious diseases*, ed 3, Philadelphia, 1992, Saunders.
24. Dunne AA, Werner JA: Status of the controversial discussion of the pathogenesis and treatment of chronic otitis media with effusion in childhood [in German], *Laryngorhinootologie* 80:1-10, 2001.
25. Knight LC, Eccles R: The relationship between nasal airway resistance and middle ear pressure in subjects with acute upper respiratory tract infection, *Otolaryngology* 113:196-200, 1993.
26. Lim DJ, Chun YM, Lee HY et al: Cell biology of tubotympanum in relation to pathogenesis of otitis media—a review, *Vaccine* 19(Suppl 1):S17-S25, 2000.
27. Niemela M, Uhari M, Jounio-Ervasti K et al: Lack of specific symptomatology in children with acute otitis media, *Pediatr Infect Dis J* 13:765-768, 1994.
28. Kontiokari T, Koivunen P, Niemela M et al: Symptoms of acute otitis media, *Pediatr Infect Dis J* 17:676-679, 1998.
29. Diagnosis and management of acute otitis media—Subcommittee on Management of Acute Otitis Media—AAP Policy, *Pediatrics* 113:1451-1465, 2004.
30. Pichichero ME, Poole MD: Assessing diagnostic accuracy and tympanocentesis skills in the management of otitis media, *Arch Pediatr Adolesc Med* 155:1137-1142, 2001.
31. Pichichero ME: Diagnostic accuracy, tympanocentesis training performance, and antibiotic selection by pediatric residents in management of otitis media, *Pediatrics* 110:1064-1070, 2002.
32. McCormick DP, Chonmaitree T, Pittman C et al: Nonsevere acute otitis media: a clinical trial comparing outcomes of watchful waiting versus immediate antibiotic treatment, *Pediatrics* 115: 1455-1465, 2005.
33. Finkelstein JA, Stille CJ, Rifas-Shiman SL et al: Watchful waiting for acute otitis media: are parents and physicians ready? *Pediatrics* 115:1466-1473, 2005.
34. New York Regional Otitis Project: *Observation option toolkit for acute otitis media*, Albany, NY, 2002, New York Department of Health, Publication 4894.
35. Dowell SF, Butler JC, Giebink GS et al: Acute otitis media management and surveillance in an era of pneumococcal resistance: a report from the Drug-Resistant *Streptococcus pneumoniae* Therapeutic Working Group, *Pediatr Infect Dis* 18:1-9, 1999.
36. Rosenfeld RM: Observation option toolkit for acute otitis media, *Int J Pediatr Otorhinolaryngol* 58:1-8, 2001.
37. Marcy M, Takata G, Shekelle P et al: *Management of acute otitis media: evidence report/technology assessment 15*, Rockville, Md, 2001, Agency for Healthcare Research and Quality, Agency for Healthcare Research and Quality Publication 01-#010.
38. Schappert SM: Office visits for otitis media: United States, 1975–90, *Adv Data* 214:1-18, 1992.
39. Finkelstein JA, Davis RL, Dowell SF et al: Reducing antibiotic use in children: a randomized trial in 12 practices, *Pediatrics* 108:1-7, 2001.
40. Cherry DK, Woodwell DA: National ambulatory medical care survey: 2000 summary, *Adv Data* 328:1-32, 2002.
41. McCaig LF, Besser RE, Hughes JM: Trends in antimicrobial prescribing rates for children and adolescents, *J Am Med Assoc* 287:3096-3102, 2002.
42. Dagan R, Leibovitz E, Greenberg D et al: Dynamics of pneumococcal nasopharyngeal colonization during the first days of antibiotic treatment in pediatric patients, *Pediatr Infect Dis J* 17:880-885, 1998.
43. Dowell SF, Marcy SM, Phillips WR et al: Principles of judicious use of antibacterial agents for pediatric upper respiratory tract infections, *Pediatrics* 101:163-165, 1998.
44. Georgraphic variations in penicillin resistance in *Streptococcus pneumoniae*—selected sites, United States, 1997, *MMWR Morb Mortal Wkly Rep* 48:656-661, 1999.

45. Jacobs MR: Increasing antibiotics resistance among otitis media pathogens and their susceptibility to oral agents based on pharmacodynamic parameters, *Pediatr Infect Dis J* 19:S47-S56, 2000.

46. Porat N, Arguedas A, Spratt BG et al: Emergence of penicillin-nonsusceptible *Streptococcus pneumoniae* clones expressing serotypes not present in the antipneumococcal conjugate vaccine, *J Infect Dis* 190:2154-2161, 2004.

47. Lieberman JM: Appropriate antibiotic use and why it is important: the challenges of bacterial resistance, *Pediatr Infect Dis J* 22:1143-1151, 2003.

48. Jacobs MR: Worldwide trends in antimicrobial resistance among common respiratory pathogens in children, *Pediatr Infect Dis J* 22(Suppl):S109-S119, 2003.

49. Middleton DB: Pharyngitis, *Primary Care* 23:719-739, 1996.

50. Brook I: Microbial factors leading to recurrent upper respiratory tract infections, *Pediatr Infect Dis J* 17(8 Suppl):S62-S67, 1998.

51. Arguedas A, Emparanza P, Schwartz RH et al: A randomized, multicenter, double blind, double dummy trial of single dose azithromycin versus high dose amoxicillin for treatment of uncomplicated acute otitis media, *Pediatr Infect Dis J* 24:153-161, 2005.

52. Heinig MJ: Host defense benefits of breastfeeding for the infant. Effect of breastfeeding duration and exclusivity, *Pediatr Clin North Am* 48:105-123, 2001.

53. Giebink GS: Otitis media prevention: non-vaccine prophylaxis, *Vaccine* 19(Suppl 1):S129-S133, 2000.

54. Cabenda SI, Peerbooms PG, van Asselt GJ et al: Serous otitis media (S.O.M.). A bacteriological study of the ear canal and the middle ear, *Int J Pediatr Otolaryngol* 16:119-124, 1998.

55. Maxim PE, Veltri RW, Sprinkle PM et al: Chronic serous otitis media: an immune complex disease, *Trans Am Acad Ophthalmol Otolaryngol* 84:234-238, 1977.

56. Prellner K, Nilsson NI, Johnson U et al: Complement and C1q binding substances in otitis media, *Ann Otol Rhinol Laryngol Suppl* 89:129-132, 1980.

57. Van der Baan S, Seldenrijk CA, Henzen-Logmans SC et al: Serous otitis media and immunological reactions in the middle ear mucosa, *Acta Otolaryngol* 106:428-434, 1988.

58. Gundersen T, Tonning FM, Kveberg KH: Ventilating tubes in the middle ear. Long-term observations, *Arch Otolaryngol* 110:783-784, 1984.

59. Hammaren-Malmi S, Saxen H, Tarkkahen J et al: Adenoidectomy does not significantly reduce the incidence of otitis media in conjunction with the insertion of tympanostomy tubes in children who are younger than 4 years: a randomized trial, *Pediatrics* 116:185-189, 2005.

Acupuncture

1. Loo M: *Pediatric acupuncture*, London, 2002, Elsevier.
2. Tian ZM: Acupuncture treatment for aerotitis media, *J Tradit Chin Med* 5:259-260, 1985.

Chiropractic

1. Leach RA, Burgess SC: Neuroimmune hypothesis, In Leach RA, editor: *The chiropractic theories*, Baltimore, 2004, Lippincott Williams and Wilkins.

2. Brennan PC, Kokjohn K, Triano JJ et al: Immunologic correlates of reduced spinal mobility: preliminary observations in a dog model, In Wold S, editor: *Proceedings of the 1991 International Conference on Spinal Manipulation*, Arlington, Va, 1991, Foundation for Chiropractic Education and Research.

3. Brennan PC, Kokjohn K, Kaltinger CJ et al: Enhanced phagocytic cell respiratory burst induced by spinal manipulation: potential role of substance P, *J Manipulative Physiol Ther* 14:399-408, 1991.

4. Selano JL, Hightower BC, Pfleger B et al: The effects of specific upper cervical adjustments on the CD4 counts of HIV positive patients, *Chiropractic Res J* 3:32-39, 1994.

5. van Breda WM, van Breda JM: A comparative study of the health status of children raised under the health care models of chiropractic and allopathic medicine, *J Chiropractic Res* 5:101-103, 1989.

6. Froehle RM: Ear infection: a retrospective study examining improvement from chiropractic care and analyzing for influencing factors, *J Manipulative Physiol Ther* 19:169-177, 1996.

7. Fysh PN: Chronic recurrent otitis media: case series of five patients with recommendations for case management, *J Clin Chiropractic Pediatr* 1:66-78, 1996.

8. Fallon J: The role of the chiropractic adjustment in the care of 332 children with otitis media, *J Clin Chiropractic Pediatr* 2:167-183, 1997.

9. Fallon J: Acute otitis media in a 3-year-old: a case report, *Chiropractic Pediatr* 2:1-3, 1994.

10. Burnier A: The side effects of the chiropractic adjustment, *Chiropractic Pediatr* 1:22-24, 1995.

11. Peet JB: Case study: chiropractic results with a child with recurring otitis media accompanied by effusion, *Chiropractic Pediatr* 2:8-12, 1996.

12. Hough DW: Chiropractic care for otitis media patients, *Today Chiropractic* Nov-Dec:54-57, 1999.

13. Fysh PN: *Chiropractic care for the pediatric patient*, Arlington, Va, 2002, International Chiropractors Association Council on Chiropractic Pediatrics.

14. Bilgrai Cohen K: Clinical management of infants and children, Santa Cruz, Calif, 1988 Extension Press.

15. Davies N: *Chiropractic pediatrics*, London, 2000, Churchill Livingstone.

16. Lamm L, Ginter L: Otitis media: a conservative chiropractic management protocol, *Topic Clin Chiropractic* 5:18-28, 1998.

17. Tanaka ST, Martin CJ, Thibodeau P: Clinical neurology, In Anrig C, Plaugher G, editors: *Pediatric chiropractic*, Baltimore, 1998, Williams and Wilkins.

18. Hendricks CL, Larkin-Their SM: Otitis media in young children, *J Chiropractic Res Study Clin Investigation* 2:9-13, 1989.

19. Swenson R: Pediatric disorders, In Lawrence DJ, editor: *Fundamentals of chiropractic diagnosis and management*, Baltimore, 1991, Williams and Wilkins.

20. Todd NW, Feldman CM: Allergic airway disease and otitis media in children, *Int J Pediatr Otorhinolaryngol* 10:27-35, 1985.

21. Mendelsohn R: *How to raise a healthy child in spite of your doctor*, Chicago, 1990, Balantine Books.

22. Nisouli TM, Nsouli SM, Linde RE et al: Role of food allergy in serous otitis media, *Ann Allergy* 73:215-219, 1994.

23. Kohl M: Otitis media: treating an effect when you do not know the cause, *Altern Complement Ther* 2:68-70, 1996.

Homeopathy

1. Jacobs J, Chapman EH, Crothers D: Patient characteristics and practice patterns of physician using homeopathy, *Arch Fam Med* 7:537-540, 1998.

2. Friese KH, Druse S, Moeller H: Acute otitis media in children: a comparison between conventional and homeopathic therapy, *H N O* 44:462-466, 1996.

3. Harrison H, Fixsen A, Vickers A: A randomized comparison of homoeopathic and standard care for the treatment of glue ear in children, *Comp Ther Med* 7:132-135, 1999.

4. Jacobs J, Springer DA, Crothers D: Homeopathic treatment of acute otitis media in children: a preliminary randomized placebo-controlled trial, *Pediatr Inf Dis J* 20:177-183, 2001.

5. Frei H, Thurnesen A: Homeopathy in acute otitis media in children: treatment effect or spontaneous resolution? *Brit Hom J* 90:180-182, 2001.

6. *ReferenceWorks Pro 4.2*, San Rafael, Calif, 2008, Kent Homeopathic Associates.

7. Rosenfeld RM: Clinical pathway for acute otitis media, In Rosenfeld RM, Bluestone CD, editors: *Evidence-based otitis media*, ed 2, Hamilton, Ont, 2003, BC Decker.

Naturopathy

1. Froom J, Culpepper L, Jacobs M et al: Antimicrobials for acute otitis media? A review from the International Primary Care Network, *Br Med J* 315:98-102, 1997.

2. Machka K, Braveny I, Dabernat H et al: Distribution and resistance patterns of *Haemophilus influenzae*: a European cooperative study, *Eur J Clin Microbiol Infect Dis* 7:14-24, 1988.

3. Goettsch WG, Goossens H, de Neeling AJ et al: Infections and bacterial resistance in the community, *Ned Tijdschr Geneeskd* 143:1296-1299, 1999.

4. Bernstein JM, Lee J, Conboy K et al: Further observations on the role of IgE-mediated hypersensitivity in recurrent otitis media with effusion, *Otolaryngol Head Neck Surg* 93:611-615, 1985.

5. Bernstein JM, Doyle WJ: Role of IgE-mediated hypersensitivity in otitis media with effusion: pathophysiologic considerations, *Ann Otol Rhinol Laryngol Suppl* 163:15-19, 1994.

6. Roos K, Holm S: The use of probiotics in head and neck infections, *Curr Infect Dis Rep* 4:211-216, 2002.

7. Tagg JR, Dierksen KP: Bacterial replacement therapy: adapting "germ warfare" to infection prevention, *Trends Biotechnol* 21:217-223, 2003.

8. Tano K, Grahn-Hakansson E, Holm SE et al: Inhibition of OM pathogens by alpha-hemolytic streptococci from healthy children, children with SOM and children with rAOM, *Int J Pediatr Otorhinolaryngol* 56:185-190, 2000.

9. Bernstein JM, Sagahtaheri-Altaie S, Dryja DM et al: Bacterial interference in nasopharyngeal bacterial flora of otitis-prone and non-otitis-prone children, *Acta Otorhinolaryngol Belg* 48:1-9, 1994.

10. Bernstein JM, Faden HF, Dryja DM et al: Micro-ecology of the nasopharyngeal bacterial flora in otitis-prone and non-otitis-prone children, *Acta Otolaryngol* 113:88-92, 1993.

11. Brook I, Shah K, Jackson W: Microbiology of healthy and diseased adenoids, *Laryngoscope* 110:994-999, 2000.

12. Tano K, Grahn Hakansson E, Holm SE et al: A nasal spray with alpha-haemolytic streptococci as long term prophylaxis against recurrent otitis media, *Int J Pediatr Otorhinolaryngol* 62:17-23, 2002.

13. Gluck U, Gebbers JO: Ingested probiotics reduce nasal colonization with pathogenic bacteria (*Staphylococcus aureus, Streptococcus pneumoniae*, and beta-hemolytic streptococci), *Am J Clin Nutr* 77:517-520, 2003.

14. Hatakka K, Savilahti E, Ponka A et al: Effect of long term consumption of probiotic milk on infections in children attending day care centres: double blind, randomised trial, *Br Med J* 322:1327, 2001.

15. Sheard NF: Breast-feeding protects against otitis media, *Nutr Rev* 51:275-277, 1993.

16. Duffy LC, Faden H, Wasielewski R et al: Exclusive breastfeeding protects against bacterial colonization and day care exposure to otitis media, *Pediatrics* 100:E7, 1997.

17. Duncan B, Ey J, Holberg CJ et al: Exclusive breast-feeding for at least 4 months protects against otitis media, *Pediatrics* 91:867-872, 1993.

18. Shaaban KM, Hamadnalla I: The effect of duration of breast feeding on the occurrence of acute otitis media in children under three years, *East Afr Med J* 70:632-634, 1993.

19. Aniansson G, Alm B, Andersson B et al: A prospective cohort study on breast-feeding and otitis media in Swedish infants, *Pediatr Infect Dis J* 13:183-188, 1994.

20. Sassen ML, Brand R, Grote JJ: Breast-feeding and acute otitis media, *Am J Otolaryngol* 15:351-357, 1994.

21. Tainio VM, Savilahti E, Arjomaa P et al: Plasma antibodies to cow's milk are increased by early weaning and consumption of unmodified milk, but production of plasma IgA and IgM cow's milk antibodies is stimulated even during exclusive breast-feeding, *Acta Paediatr Scand* 77:807-811, 1988.

22. Karabaev KE, Antoniv VF, Bekmuradov RU: Pathogenetic validation of optimal antioxidant therapy in suppurative inflammatory otic diseases in children [in Russian] *Vestn Otorinolaringol* (1): 5-7, 1997.

23. Doner F, Delibas N, Dogru H et al: The role of free oxygen radicals in experimental otitis media, *J Basic Clin Physiol Pharmacol* 13: 33-40, 2002.

24. Yariktas M, Doner F, Dogru H et al: The role of free oxygen radicals on the development of otitis media with effusion, *Int J Pediatr Otorhinolaryngol* 68:889-894, 2004.

25. Durand AM, Sabino H Jr., Masga R et al: Childhood vitamin A status and the risk of otitis media, *Pediatr Infect Dis J* 16:952-954, 1997.

26. Ogaro FO, Orinda VA, Onyango FE et al: Effect of vitamin A on diarrhea and respiratory complications of measles, *Trop Geogr Med* 45:283-286, 1993.

27. Cemek M, Caksen H, Cemek F et al: Investigation of antioxidant status in children with acute otitis media and tonsillitis, *Int J Pediatr Otorhinolaryngol* 68:1381-1385, 2004.

28. Cemek M, Dede S, Bayiroglu F et al: Oxidant and antioxidant levels in children with acute otitis media and tonsillitis: a comparative study, *Int J Pediatr Otorhinolaryngol* 69:823-827, 2005.

29. Dobo M, Czeizel AE: Long-term somatic and mental development of children after periconceptional multivitamin supplementation, *Eur J Pediatr* 157:719-723, 1998.

30. Daly KA, Brown JE, Lindgren BR et al: Epidemiology of otitis media onset by six months of age, *Pediatrics* 103:1158-1166, 1999.

31. Kiremidjian-Schumacher L, Roy M, Wishe HI et al: Regulation of cellular immune responses by selenium, *Biol Trace Elem Res* 33:23-35, 1992.

32. Kiremidjian-Schumacher L, Roy M, Wishe HI et al: Supplementation with selenium augments the functions of natural killer and lymphokine-activated killer cells, *Biol Trace Elem Res* 52:227-239, 1996.

33. Kiremidjian-Schumacher L, Roy M: Selenium and immune function, *Z Ernahrungswiss* 37(Suppl 1):50-56, 1998.

34. Kiremidjian-Schumacher L, Roy M: Effect of selenium on the immunocompetence of patients with head and neck cancer and on adoptive immunotherapy of early and established lesions, *Biofactors* 14:161-168, 2001.

35. Food and Nutrition Board, Institute of Medicine: *Dietary reference intakes*, Washington, DC, 2000, National Academy Press.

36. Linday LA, Dolitsky JN, Shindledecker RD: Nutritional supplements as adjunctive therapy for children with chronic/recurrent sinusitis: pilot research, *Int J Pediatr Otorhinolaryngol* 68:785-793, 2004.

37. Linday LA, Dolitsky JN, Shindledecker RD et al: Lemon-flavored cod liver oil and a multivitamin-mineral supplement for the secondary prevention of otitis media in young children: pilot research, *Ann Otol Rhinol Laryngol* 111:642-652, 2002.

38. Sarrell EM, Mandelberg A, Cohen HA: Efficacy of naturopathic extracts in the management of ear pain associated with acute otitis media, *Arch Pediatr Adolesc Med* 155:796-799, 2001.

39. Sarrell EM, Cohen HA, Kahan E: Naturopathic treatment for ear pain in children, *Pediatrics* 111:e574-579, 2003.

40. Nell MJ, Koerten HK, Grote JJ: Bactericidal/permeability-increasing protein prevents mucosal damage in an experimental rat model of chronic otitis media with effusion, *Infect Immun* 68:2992-2994, 2000.

41. Barnes J, Anderson LA, Phillipson JD: St. John's wort (*Hypericum perforatum* L.): a review of its chemistry, pharmacology and clinical properties, *J Pharm Pharmacol* 53:583-600, 2001.

42. Kubin A, Wierrani F, Burner U et al: Hypericin: the facts about a controversial agent, *Curr Pharm Des* 11:233-253, 2005.

43. Yoshida H, Katsuzaki H, Ohta R et al: An organosulfur compound isolated from oil-macerated garlic extract, and its antimicrobial effect, *Biosci Biotechnol Biochem* 63:588-590, 1999.

44. Zitterl-Eglseer K, Sosa S, Jurenitsch J et al: Anti-oedematous activities of the main triterpendiol esters of marigold (*Calendula officinalis* L.), *J Ethnopharmacol* 57:139-144, 1997.

45. Lavagna SM, Secci D, Chimenti P et al: Efficacy of *Hypericum* and *Calendula* oils in the epithelial reconstruction of surgical wounds in childbirth with caesarean section, *Farmaco* 56: 451-453, 2001.

CHAPTER 50

Pharyngitis

Acupuncture | May Loo
Aromatherapy | Maura A. Fitzgerald
Herbs—Chinese | May Loo
Homeopathy | Janet L. Levatin

Magnet Therapy | Agatha P. Colbert, Deborah Risotti
Osteopathy | Jane Carreiro
Probiotics | Russell H. Greenfield

✳ PEDIATRIC DIAGNOSIS AND TREATMENT

Acute pharyngitis and tonsillitis are common in healthy children and adolescents. The tonsils and adenoids, located at the portal of entry of many airborne and alimentary antigens, prevent bacterial colonization and form antibodies. They influence both local and systemic immunity and are often considered the first line of defense against respiratory infections.[1,2]

The majority of pharyngitis cases have viral etiology such as rhinovirus, adenovirus, Epstein-Barr virus (mononucleosis), and influenza A and B.[3,4] Younger children have frequent episodes, whereas adolescents experience an average of two to four nasopharyngeal infections annually.[5] Bacterial pharyngitis occurs when the pathogens adhere to and colonize in the mucous membranes. The extent of pathogenic injury varies according to the host's immune system. In a healthy individual, only mild edema and swelling may occur.[6] The most important bacterial agent is group A β-hemolytic streptococcus (GABHS).[7] The incidence of GABHS in children ranges from 5%[8] to 20%[9-12] to 35%.[12-15] Even during the peak streptococcal infection seasons of winter and early spring,[3] GABHS occurs in less than 40% of pharyngitis cases.[16] GABHS is primarily a disorder of children between 5 and 15 years of age.[3] The clinical presentation of GABHS consists of sudden onset of sore throat, fever, and pain on swallowing.[3,17] Headache, nausea, vomiting, and abdominal pain may also be present in children.[3,18] Physical examination reveals tonsillopharyngeal erythema with or without exudates and tender anterior cervical adenoapthy.[3,17] However, only about 15% to 30% of children present with classic clinical signs,[17,18] such that clinically viral pharyngitis and GABHS are often indistinguishable,[3] making it difficult for even experienced physicians to reliably diagnose GABHS pharyngitis solely on the basis of clinical presentation.[7,19]

Infrequently other infectious agents produce sore throat, including non–group A *Streptococcus* spp., *Arcanobacterium haemolyticum*, *Haemophilus influenzae*, *Mycoplasma* spp., *Chlamydia* spp., *Neisseria* spp., *Moraxella catarrhalis*, and *Corynebacterium diphtheriae*. They can be distinguished from GABHS because they are usually accompanied by other concomitant clinical illness.[14,15,20,21] Because of the prevalence of viral pharyngitis and unreliable clinical findings, the Infectious Diseases Society of America[3] and the American Academy of Pediatrics (AAP) Principles on Management of Common Office Infections[22] recommend throat culture and/or rapid

group A strep antigen detection test (RADT) to precisely diagnose GABHS.[7,8,12-14,17] Generally, throat cultures are less expensive but considered as an effective diagnostic tool[11,12]; the more expensive RADTs are preferred by some clinicians because they provide results faster, have a high specificity (95% or greater), and have greater sensitivity such that they are attributed to reduce the risk of spread of GABHS, to allow patients to return to school or work sooner, and may reduce the acute morbidity of this illness.[19] Newer immunoassays and nucleic acid techniques being developed will be more sensitive and specific.[23]

Viral pharyngitis is benign and self-limiting, needing only symptomatic care without antibiotics.[3,24,25] The 1995 statement by the AAP; the Committee on Rheumatic Fever, Endocarditis, and Kawasaki Disease of the Council on Cardiovascular Disease in the Young; and the American Heart Association recommends the proper identification and adequate antibiotic treatment of GABHS tonsillopharyngitis as the primary prevention of acute rheumatic fever. Penicillin remains the treatment of choice because of its cost effectiveness, its narrow spectrum of activity, and its long-standing proven efficacy.[26] Remarkably, GABHS have never developed resistance to any of the penicillins.[27] Alternative therapy (e.g., with cephalosporin or erythromycin) is given for penicillin allergy, noncompliance, and treatment failure.[3,7,14,17,25]

A 10-day course of oral penicillin or an intramuscular injection of penicillin G benzathine is considered equivalent treatment. Early antibiotic therapy is reported to reduce the duration of pharyngitis and minimize formation of peritonsillar retropharyngeal and parapharyngeal abscesses.[5,17,28] The primary objective for antibiotic therapy of GABHS infection, however, is the prevention of rheumatic fever.[18] The incidence of rheumatic fever has declined in industrialized countries since the 1950s and now has an annual incidence of around 0.5 cases per 100,000 school-aged children. In developing countries it remains an endemic disease, with annual incidences ranging from 100 to 200 per 100,000 school-aged children, and is a major cause of cardiovascular mortality. The risk of developing rheumatic fever following untreated tonsillopharyngitis is 1%.[9,10] The current understanding is that a genetically determined predisposition[29] results in the host's autoimmune response to GABHS.[9,10] In France and most of Europe, it is tacitly agreed that all cases of pharyngitis and tonsillitis should be treated with antibiotics without identification of the causal agent.[9,10]

As many as 35% of children may experience recurrence,[6,13,18,23] with increased prevalence in children younger than 8 years.[15] Explanations for recurrence include poor compliance with taking medication due to frequent dosing for 10 days and/or poor palatability of the liquid formulation,[30,31] co-colonization by other organisms, and reacquisition from a family member or peer.[14,18] Compliance can be improved with a more convenient twice-daily dosing (b.i.d.), which has been found to be as efficacious as a more frequent regimen,[32] and by using shorter-course non-penicillin antibiotics, which tend to be broader spectrum and are often more expensive,[33] although they may have fewer gastrointestinal (GI) side effects.[34] Currently, routine laboratory evaluation or treatment of close household contacts is not recommended.[3]

Although literature in support of antibiotic treatment abounds, it remains controversial. Four Cochrane reviews indicate that antibiotic use seems to be discretionary rather than mandatory for pharyngitis, as symptomatic relief is only about 16 hours faster compared with placebo, and that serious complications such as rheumatic fever and glomerulonephritis are now rare in developed countries.[35] There is also concern that antibiotics can suppress natural immune response via eradication of normal pharyngeal flora that act as natural host defenses[14] by interfering with pathogenic activities and preventing infection.[25] Evidence is mounting that antibiotics may have little impact on the duration of sore throat symptoms, regardless of etiology. Complications of sore throat are now so rare that an adverse drug reaction from antibiotic therapy is more likely.[36] Tonsillectomy and adenoidectomy for recurrent pharyngitis remains controversial.[1,37] There is no good evidence of long-term benefit from surgical interventions.[38]

✳ CAM THERAPY RECOMMENDATIONS

Acupuncture

At this time, there are very few data on acupuncture[1] treatment of pharyngitis.

In a randomized, double-blind, sham-controlled study in Korea of 150 adult patients scheduled to undergo abdominal hysterectomy, the use of capsicum plaster on the Korean hand acupuncture point KA20 significantly reduced postoperative sore throat.[2]

Traditional Chinese medicine (TCM) diagnoses can correlate to Western categories of acute and recurrent pharyngitis. The best approach would be to integrate Western diagnosis and treatment with TCM: examining the throat and palpating for cervical adenopathy is much easier than Chinese pulse taking and tongue diagnosis in children. Laboratory confirmation of GABHS is important.

Acute Pharyngitis
Wind-Cold invasion

Wild-Cold invasion correlates to viral pharyngitis with negative laboratory findings for GABHS. The mild sore throat indicates that the invasion is beginning to enter the Yangming stage involving the Stomach organ and meridian.

Treatment
Extra fluids to prevent dehydration.
GV16, GB20 to expel Wind.
LU7, LI4, BL12 to expel Cold.
Add CV22, KI27 as specific points for throat treatment.
Dazhui point, GV14, can be used to treat pain[3] or for any fever.
Tonify the immune system after infection has resolved.

Wind-Heat invasion

Wild-Heat invasion correlates to bacterial pharyngitis, including GABHS.

The Wind-Heat invasion or bacterial infection is much more virulent than the Wind-Cold invasion and enters quickly into the Qi level, which in this case correlates to deep penetrating of the Yangming organs and meridians. Acupuncture treatment can be given concomitantly with antibiotics.

Treatment
Extra fluids to prevent dehydration.
GV16, GB20 to expel Wind.
Add CV22, KI27 as specific points for throat treatment.
Dazhui point, GV 4, can be used to treat pain[3] and for fever.
Use either the Two-Point or Four-Point protocol to disperse Yangming Stomach Heat:
Tonify ST44; sedate ST 41.
Tonify ST44, BL66; sedate ST41, SI5.
GI side effects of antibiotics can be minimized with tonification of SP.

Stomach Heat

In addition to Wind invasions that cause Yangming Heat, TCM also posits that the sensation of soreness in the throat can be due to Stomach Heat derived from excess consumption of energetically Hot foods, sweet foods, or greasy and fried foods. Because Western medicine does not recognize the relationship between sore throat and foods, the negative culture in this case would be diagnosed as viral pharyngitis. One distinguishing feature is that these children often complain of abdominal pain that may be temporally related to eating.

Treatment
Eliminate excess Heat foods, sweets, and greasy and fried foods.
Clear Stomach Heat with the Five-Element, Four-Point protocol:
Tonify ST44, BL66; sedate ST41, SI5.
SP6, CV12 to tonify Stomach Yin.

Chronic, Recurrent Pharyngitis
Yin deficiency

Two conditions can predispose to chronic pharyngitis with Yin deficiency: pathogenic Heat that lingers and accumulates when Heat is not adequately expelled in acute invasions, and continual consumption of excess Heat foods. Both of these can cause a chronic state of Heat that exhausts Yin. Because Kidney Yin is the foundation of all Yin, tonification of KI6 has been found to be important for treating recurrent sore throat.[4]

Treatment
Eliminate excess Heat foods, sweets, and greasy and fried foods.
Use the Four-Point protocol to clear Stomach Heat.
KI6 to tonify KI Yin.

SP6, CV12 to tonify Stomach Yin.

Immune protocol to increase immunity.

Parents can be taught to do acupressure on CV22, KI27 for acute symptoms and SP6, KI6 for tonification of SP and KI Yin in chronic, recurrent pharyngitis. Although the current Western approach is to not treat close family contacts with medication, acupressure can be used as a preventive measure because it does not encompass antibiotic concerns of potential side effects and overuse.

Aromatherapy

Generally essential oils that have analgesic and/or antiseptic properties are recommended for pharyngitis.[1,2] Among these oils are frankincense *(Boswellia carteri)*, lavender *(Lavandula angustifolia)*, lemon *(Citrus limon)*, tea tree *(Melaleuca alternifolia)*, and eucalyptus *(Eucalyptus* sp.). Essential oils for pharyngitis are administered by steaming or inhalation. In an observational study of 39 children (ages 9 to 15 years) with chronic pharyngitis, subjects received a treatment that combined ultrasound inhalations with essential oils (unfortunately the essential oils used were not specified in the English language abstract of this Russian study). Inhalations were done for 5 to 10 minutes daily for 10 days. Subjects reported improvement after 8 to 10 procedures.[3]

Herbs—Chinese

Windbreaker is a nonspecific formula for upper respiratory infection, including sore throat. It is a formula of 21 herbs (Chinese Modular Solutions) designed to clear Wind, Heat, and Phlegm, treating the acute inflammatory stage of colds as well as lingering congestion. The formula comes as a liquid alcohol extract. The alcohol can be removed by placing the drops in a small amount of hot water and allowing it to cool before administration. Dosage is 1 dropperful every 3 hours in babies and 2 to 3 dropperful for children 2 years and older (See Appendix C).

CQ Jr. (Blue Poppy Herbs) is a formula of 16 herbs that combine the two classical formulas, Xiao Chai Hu Tang and Si Wu Tang. It is designed to dispel Wind, clear Heat, resolve toxins, and harmonize the Liver-Spleen, eliminating Dampness. The herbs are prepared in a 10:1 extract in a glycerin tincture. The dosage for babies is 1 to 2 dropperful every 2 hours until pain is relieved, and then less frequent dosing. For 2 to 4 year olds, the dosage is 2 to 3 dropperful in the same regimen.[1]

Homeopathy

Before using this section, please see Appendix A, Homeopathy, for definitions of practitioner expertise categories and general information on prescribing homeopathic medicines.

Practitioner Expertise Category 1 or 2

Category 1 or 2 includes acute, uncomplicated pharyngitis or tonsillitis.

Practitioner Expertise Category 3

Category 3 includes chronic or recurrent pharyngitis or tonsillitis.

To date there has been one study comparing homeopathic treatment and antibiotic treatment for acute rhinopharyngitis in children.[1] Two groups of French children (499 total), aged 18 months to 4 years, who had at least five bouts of acute rhinopharyngitis in 1999 were compared in 2000 in a post hoc analysis on the following measures: medical effectiveness of the treatment (homeopathic or antimicrobial), episodes of complications after treatment, a quality of life scale, and direct and indirect medical costs. The results are summarized in Table 50-1.

The homeopathic group performed significantly better on all measures. Limitations of this study include lack of control of the use of other medications, such as decongestants and antipyretics, given during the study period; possible bias in the two groups (including differences in passive smoke exposure and attendance at daycare); and lack of blinding. Additionally, the medicines prescribed were not mentioned, nor were throat cultures performed on the children. Further research is indicated to investigate the potential of homeopathy for treating sore throats. In addition to the aforementioned preliminary research results, the homeopathic literature contains much

---

⁕ **TABLE 50-1**

Outcomes in Children after Homeopathic and Antimicrobial Therapy for Rhinopharyngitis

	HOMEOPATHIC GROUP	ANTIBIOTIC GROUP	P VALUE
Medical effectiveness (number of illness episodes after treatment)	2.71	3.97	<0.001
Number of complications (complications not specified)	1.25	1.95	<0.001
Quality of life score	21.38	30.43	<0.001
Direct medical costs	88 (euros)	99 (euros)	<0.05
Indirect medical costs (percentage of parents needing sick leave to care for a sick child after entry into study)	9.5%	31.6%	<0.001

From Trichard M, Chaufferin G, Nicoloyannis N: Pharmacoeconomic comparison between homeopathic and antibiotic treatment strategies in recurrent acute rhinopharyngitis in children, *Homeopathy* 94:3-9, 2005.

evidence in the form of accumulated clinical experience to support the use of homeopathic treatment for sore throats.[2]

Sore throat (pharyngitis and/or tonsillitis) is a common complaint in the pediatric population. Most sore throats are caused by viral or nonharmful bacterial pathogens, and no specific conventional treatment is needed. In such cases, homeopathic treatment can be used to provide symptom relief and may play a role in preventing recurrences. When a sore throat is caused by GABHS, antimicrobial therapy is indicated, as infection with this bacterium is highly contagious and can have negative sequelae including glomerulonephritis and complications of rheumatic fever. In case of GABHS throat infections, homeopathic treatment can be used in conjunction with an antibiotic for symptom relief. Homeopathy also can be used in cases of recurrent GABHS infection, between infections, with the goal of preventing recurrences by altering the child's susceptibility. In this section, treatment of acute sore throats will be discussed. With more experience and training, interested clinicians can begin treating chronic and recurrent sore throats.

The goal in treating sore throats homeopathically is to determine the single homeopathic medicine whose description in the materia medica most closely matches the symptom picture of the patient. Often mental and emotional states, in addition to physical symptoms, are considered. Once the medicine has been selected, it can be given orally or sublingually in the 30C potency every 2 to 3 hours, or two to three times daily, depending on the severity of the symptoms. For more severe symptoms, a 200C potency can be given two to three times daily. If the medicine has not helped in five to six doses, then another homeopathic medicine should be tried or some other form of therapy should be instituted as needed. Once symptoms have begun to resolve, the medicine can be given less frequently or stopped. It can be repeated again for a relapse of symptoms.

The following is a list of homeopathic medicines commonly used to treat patients with sore throats. It must be emphasized that this list is partial and represents some of the probable choices from the homeopathic materia medica. If the symptoms of a given patient are not represented here, further research in the homeopathic literature would be needed to find the simillimum.

Belladonna

Belladonna is needed when the sore throat is of sudden onset. The throat is red and swollen and feels hot. Often the inflammation is on the right side. The patient feels worse with motion, such as turning the head, and when swallowing liquids. A "strawberry" tongue may be present, especially in cases of scarlet fever. The patient has a high fever with a flushed face and dilated pupils and may be delirious.

Hepar sulphuris calcareum

The sore throat pain responsive to *Hepar sulphuris calcareum* is sticking in quality. Exudate may be present on the tonsils. The patient is quite chilly and feels worse from exposure to cold air or drinking cold liquids and better from keeping warm and drinking warm drinks. The pain is referred to the ear on swallowing. The patient is quite irritable.

Lachesis muta

The patient who needs *Lachesis muta* usually has a left-sided sore throat or a sore throat that begins on the left side and moves to the right. The tonsils are swollen and may appear very dark. The patient may feel as though a lump is in the throat. They do not tolerate tight collars or having their neck touched. The throat feels worse from drinking warm liquids and better from drinking cold liquids. The pain is worse at night or on waking in the morning.

Mercurius solubilis hahnemanni

Patients who need *Mercurius solubilis hahnemanni* often have sore throats with exudates on the tonsils and/or a swollen, coated tongue. The patient has increased salivation and often has foul-smelling breath and a metallic taste in the mouth. The anterior cervical glands are swollen and painful. The patient alternates between feeling too hot and too cold. He may be sweaty, especially at night.

Gelsemium sempervirens

The patient needing *Gelsemium sempervirens* has a slowly developing symptom picture. Often the sore throat is part of an influenza-like illness with myalgias, chills, a dull headache, and generalized weakness. The throat pain extends to the ear when the patient swallows.

Phytolacca decandra

The patient needing *Phytolacca decandra* has a throat that feels hot and sore, especially in the area of the tonsils or the root of the tongue. The tonsils appear dark. There is a sensation of narrowing in the throat. The anterior cervical glands are hard and painful. The patient feels worse from drinking warm liquids and better from drinking cold liquids.

Magnet Therapy

Ask the child to point to the area on the neck where he or she feels the throat pain, and apply a ¾-inch Neodymium nylon-coated 3950-G magnet with the designated north side facing the skin. Leave the magnet in place for 1 to 2 hours. Magnets may be obtained from Painfree Lifestyles (800-480-8601).

Osteopathy

The goal of osteopathic manipulation in the treatment of the child with acute uncomplicated pharyngitis is to improve lymphatic and venous drainage of cellular waste products from the area; facilitate arterial delivery of oxygen, nutrients, and therapeutic agents; and decrease pain and discomfort. Vascular and lymphatic flow occurs via the vessels in the posterior pharyngeal wall, which pass through the prevertebral fascias and into the thorax. Hemodynamics can be improved by addressing respiratory mechanics in the thorax, altered function in the cranial mechanism, and tissue strains in the fascias of the deep neck and mediastinum, specifically those that support the hyoid bone. Thickened pharyngeal secretions and vasoconstriction are thought to result from increased sympathetic input. Rib raising techniques and techniques to influence the cervical ganglion are thought to decrease sympathetic tone.[1] Pain and discomfort may be relieved by treating the corresponding Chapman's reflexes[2,3] found in the neck.

Chronic pharyngitis may be a symptom of allergy, sinus infection, gastroesophageal reflux, or mouth breathing. Each of these conditions would be approached differently. The osteopathic findings differ for each condition, and in some cases osteopathic examination may be used to help establish the correct diagnosis. Allergies and gastroesophageal reflux are discussed in Chapters 10 and 38, respectively. Sinus infection and mouth breathing will be discussed here.

In recurrent or chronic sinusitis the child's inability to respond to antibiotics and other therapies may be due to multiple factors. Within the osteopathic concept these factors include impaired function of cranial and facial mechanics.[4-6] According to Sutherland's model, under normal conditions a gentle pumping motion in the tissues of the face, head, and neck influences drainage of the sinuses.[7,8] Recurrent or chronic infections may occur when the sinus is unable to drain properly and cilia and cellular function are thus impaired. Altered biomechanical function in the tissues of the face and pharynx may also impede lymphatic drainage through the pharyngeal lymph nodes, further compounding the problem. Osteopathic manipulation would be directed at improving sinus drainage, decreasing inflammation, and facilitating lymphatic function.

Some children with chronic pharyngitis may be obligate mouth breathers. Mouth breathing dries the pharyngeal mucous membrane. In response, the secretory cells become active but the viscosity of the secretions changes, producing a thicker mucus. The factors associated with obligate mouth breathing are numerous. Several examples that would potentially respond to osteopathic treatment include altered or asymmetrical jaw occlusion, a high arched palate, deviated nasal septum, and strains in the neck that produce hyperextension of the head.

Chronic, Recurrent Pharyngitis

In children with chronic, recurrent, or unexplained sore throat, there is often somatic dysfunction involving the anterior cervical tissues or facial mechanics. An older child may be able to localize the discomfort to the front of the throat and describe the symptoms as worse with swallowing and as a "pressure-like" sensation or "tightness" as opposed to a scratchy feeling. The child may also describe a feeling of something "caught" in the throat. In these cases there may be dysfunction in the mechanics of the hyoid bone, mandible, tongue, and supporting tissues.[9,10] A history of shoulder, arm, or neck trauma may or may not be present. Balancing techniques can be applied to the hyoid, anterocervical, and intraoral tissues to provide relief to the child.[11] Cranial techniques are used to address the cranial base and facial components.

Sore throat may result from tissue congestion in the posterior pharynx. Venous and lymphatic drainage from this area occurs via the posterior pharyngeal tissues into the prevertebral area and the thorax. Tissue strains that affect the functional mechanics of the cranium, prevertebral tissues, thorax, or mediastinum may impede proper drainage from the posterior pharynx, resulting in posterior lymphoid hyperplasia, pharyngeal irritation, and inflammation. On physical exam the posterior pharynx has a cobbled appearance without evidence of postnasal drainage. Osteopathic evaluation often reveals somatic dysfunction involving the cranial base, specifically the sphenobasilar area, with fascial strains extending into the deep neck and upper thorax. Myofascial, cranial, and balancing techniques can be used to address these findings.

Postnasal drainage from the sinuses may also play a role in symptoms of sore throat. Within the context of the principles of osteopathy in the cranial field, proper drainage from the paranasal sinuses is dependent upon normal facial mechanics and balance in the autonomic control of the secretory glands.[1] Somatic dysfunction in the face, head, or neck may interfere with this mechanism. The area of the sphenopalatine fossa has also been described as being important in maintaining autonomic nervous system balance[8,12] in the sinuses and upper respiratory tissues. Many connective tissues of the pharynx have their attachments near the sphenopalatine fossa. Strains in these tissues may interfere with the venous and arterial structures supplying the area.

Probiotics

The primary use of probiotics for children with pharyngitis is to lessen side effects associated with antibiotic use, most notably antibiotic-associated diarrhea. Antibiotic therapy destroys bacteria nonselectively and thus has a considerable effect on equilibrium of the intestinal flora. Repeated antibiotic treatments can significantly impair homeostasis, leading to immune system imbalances and the emergence of infectious, inflammatory, or allergic disorders.[1]

From the perspective of prevention, data suggest that interfering bacteria, such as α-streptococci, can hinder growth of pathogenic organisms and subsequent development of infection in the head and neck region.[2]

One study evaluated children aged 1 to 6 years with acute bacterial infections who received antibiotics.[3] Subjects were randomized to receive a fruit-flavored drink, a nutritional supplement, or a nutritional supplement plus a symbiotic (combination of prebiotic and probiotic). Those children who received the synbiotic experienced greater weight gain and a trend toward improved response to antibiotic therapy.

Guidance with respect to choice of specific organisms and duration of therapy is sorely lacking. To further complicate matters, there seems little rationale behind the variety of dosages or combination of microbes employed in published studies. Oftentimes similar dosages have been utilized for distinct microbes, whereas widely disparate dosages have been employed by researchers studying the same probiotic. At this time, dosage recommendations are far from set in stone.

This author recommends using probiotic therapy during the course of antibiotic administration and for 1 to 2 weeks thereafter. Well-studied organisms shown to be safe, such as *Lactobacillus* GG, *Lactobacillus reuteri*, or *Lactobacillus acidophilus* should be employed. Dosing guidelines to consider are 10 billion colony-forming units (CFU) for children weighing less than 12 kg and 20 billion CFU for children weighing more than 12 kg. Treatment is extremely well tolerated, and palatability is an infrequent issue, as the capsules can be opened and mixed into drinks or soft foods. Sometimes the agents are available as a powder as well. If effective, treatment can continue indefinitely. Use with extreme caution, if at all, for those children at risk for infectious complications (e.g., immunosuppression or use of immunosuppressive agents, presence of central venous catheter, prematurity).

References

Pediatric Diagnosis and Treatment

1. Paulussen C, Claes J, Claes G et al: Adenoids and tonsils, indications for surgery and immunological consequences of surgery, *Acta Otorhinolaryngol Belg* 54:403-408, 2000.
2. Rynnel-Dagoo B, Agren K: The nasopharynx and the middle ear. Inflammatory reactions in middle ear disease, *Vaccine* 19(Suppl 1):S26-S31, 2000.
3. Bisno AL, Gerber MA, Gwaltney JM Jr. et al: Diagnosis and management of group A streptococcal pharyngitis: a practice guideline. Infectious Diseases Society of America, *Clin Infect Dis* 25:574-583, 1997.
4. Peter J, Ray CG: Infectious mononucleosis, *Pediatr Rev* 19:276-279, 1998.
5. White CB, Foshee WS: Respiratory tract infections in adolescents, *Adolesc Med* 11:225-249, 2000.
6. Cappelletty D: Microbiology of bacterial respiratory infections, *Pediatr Infect Dis J* 17(8 Suppl):S55-S61, 1998.
7. Leung AK, Kellner JD: Group A beta-hemolytic streptococcal pharyngitis in children, *Adv Ther* 21:277-287, 2004.
8. Hayes CS, Williamson H Jr: Management of group A beta-hemolytic streptococcal pharyngitis, *Fam Physician* 63:1557-1564, 2001.
9. Olivier C: Rheumatic fever—is it still a problem? *J Antimicrob Chemother* 45(Suppl):13-21, 2000.
10. Olivier C: Acute articular rheumatism in the child in 1997 [in French], *Pathol Biol (Paris)* 46:802-812, 1998 (abstract).
11. Pichichero M: Cost-effective management of sore throat: it depends on the perspective, *Arch Pediatr Adolesc Med* 153:672-674, 1999.
12. Tsevat J, Kotagal UR: Management of sore throats in children: a cost-effectiveness analysis, *Arch Pediatr Adolesc Med* 153:681-688, 1999.
13. Guggenbichler JP: Cefetamet pivoxil in the treatment of pharyngitis/tonsillitis in children and adults, *Drugs* 47(Suppl 3):27-33, 1994; discussion 34.
14. Pichichero ME: Group A streptococcal tonsillopharyngitis: cost-effective diagnosis and treatment, *Emerg Med* 25:390-403, 1995.
15. Pichichero ME, Green JL, Francis AB et al: Recurrent group A streptococcal tonsillopharyngitis, *Pediatr Infect Dis J* 17:809-815, 1998.
16. Pichichero ME: Sore throat after sore throat after sore throat. Are you asking the critical questions? *Postgrad Med* 101:205-206, 209-212, 215–218, 1997.
17. Kiselica D: Group A beta-hemolytic streptococcal pharyngitis: current clinical concepts, *Am Fam Physician* 49:1147-1154, 1994.
18. Pichichero ME: Group A beta-hemolytic streptococcal infections, *Pediatr Rev* 19:291-302, 1998.
19. Shulman ST, Gerber MA: Rapid diagnosis of pharyngitis caused by group A streptococci, *Clin Microbiol Rev* 17:571-580, 2004.
20. Ruoff G: Upper respiratory tract infections in family practice, *Pediatr Infect Dis J* 17(8 Suppl):S73-S78, 1998.
21. Behrman RE, Kliegman RM, Jenson HB, editors: *Nelson textbook of pediatrics*, ed 17, Philadelphia, 2004, Saunders.
22. Hover AR, Cornwell V, Stevenson S et al: Evaluation of the American Academy of Pediatrics Principles on Management of Common Office Infections in a managed care setting, *Medicine* 97:541-544, 2000.
23. Garcia-de-Lomas J, Navarro D: New directions in diagnostics, *Pediatr Infect Dis J* 16(3 Suppl):S43-S48, 1997.
24. Middleton DB: Pharyngitis, *Primary Care* 23:719-739, 1996.
25. Oh HM: Upper respiratory tract infections—otitis media, sinusitis and pharyngitis, *Singapore Med J* 36:428-431, 1995.
26. Dajani A, Taubert K, Ferrieri P et al: Treatment of acute streptococcal pharyngitis and prevention of rheumatic fever: a statement for health professionals. Committee on Rheumatic Fever, Endocarditis, and Kawasaki Disease of the Council on Cardiovascular Disease in the Young, the American Heart Association, *Pediatrics* 96:758-764, 1995.
27. Shulman ST, Gerber MA: So what's wrong with penicillin for strep throat? *Pediatrics* 113:1816-1819, 2004.
28. Jund R, Grevers G: Rhinitis, sore throate and otalgia… benign common cold or dangerous infection? *Fortschr Med* 142:32-36, 2000. [Abstract. Article in German.]
29. Bezold LI, Bricker JT: Acquired heart disease in children, *Curr Opin Cardiol* 9:121-129, 1994.
30. Dajani AS: Adherence to physicians' instructions as a factor in managing streptococcal pharyngitis, *Pediatrics* 97:976-980, 1996.
31. Block SL: Short-course antimicrobial therapy of streptococcal pharyngitis, *Clin Pediatr (Phila)* 42:663-671, 2003.
32. Bass JW, Person DA, Chan DS: Twice-daily oral penicillin for treatment of streptococcal pharyngitis: less is best, *Pediatrics* 105:422-423, 2000.
33. Gerber MA, Tanz RR: Approaches to the treatment of group A streptococcal pharyngitis, *Opin Pediatr* 13:51-55, 2001.
34. Adam D: Short-course antibiotic therapy for infections with a single causative pathogen, *Intern Med Res* 28(Suppl 1):13A-24A, 2000.
35. Arroll B: Antibiotics for upper respiratory tract infections: an overview of Cochrane reviews, *Respir Med* 99:255-261, 2005.
36. Wolter JM: Management of a sore throat. Antibiotics are no longer appropriate, *Austr Fam Physician* 27:279-281, 1998.
37. Bicknell PG: Role of adenotonsillectomy in the management of pediatric ear, nose and throat infections, *Pediatr Infect Dis J* 13(Suppl 1):S75-S78, 1994; discussion S78-S79.
38. Harris C: Childhood ENT disorders. When to refer to specialists, *Austr Fam Physician* 31:701-704, 716, 2002.

Acupuncture

1. Loo M: *Pediatric acupuncture*, London, 2002, Elsevier.
2. Park HS, Kim KS, Min HK et al: Prevention of postoperative sore throat using capsicum plaster applied at the Korean hand acupuncture point, *Anaesthesia* 59:647-651, 2004.
3. Wu JS: Observation on analgesic effect of acupuncturing the dazhui point, *J Tradit Chin Med* 9:240-242, 1989.
4. Lu F: Experience in the clinical application of acupoint zhaohai (K 6), *J Tradit Chin Med* 15:118-121, 1995.
5. Deadman P, Al-Khafaji M: *A manual of acupuncture*, Ann Arbor, Mich, 1998, Journal of Chinese Medicine Publications.
6. Maciocia G: *The foundations of Chinese medicine, a comprehensive text for acupuncturists and herbalists*, London, 1989, Churchill Livingstone.
7. Maciocia G: *The practice of Chinese medicine, the treatment of diseases with acupuncture and Chinese herbs*, London, 1994, Churchill Livingstone.

Aromatherapy

1. Battaglia S: The complete guide to aromatherapy, Virginia, Queensland, Australia, 1995, The Perfect Potion.
2. Price S, Parr PP: *Aromatherapy for babies and children*, San Francisco, 1996, Thorsons.
3. Shevrygin BV, Fedorova TV, Pekli FF: Natural ether oils in the treatment of chronic pharyngitis in children in pediatric practice [in Russian], *Vestn Otorinolaringol* 2:52-53, 1999.

Herbs—Chinese

1. Neustaedter R: Personal communication, August 2005.

Homeopathy

1. Trichard M, Chaufferin G, Nicoloyannis N: Pharmacoeconomic comparison between homeopathic and antibiotic treatment strategies in recurrent acute rhinopharyngitis in children, *Homeopathy* 94:3-9, 2005.
2. *ReferenceWorks Pro 4.2*, San Rafael, Calif, 2008, Kent Homeopathic Associates.

Osteopathy

1. Hoyt W: Current concepts in the management of sinus disease, *J Am Osteopath Assoc* 90:913-919, 1990.
2. Owen C: *An endocrine interpretation of Chapman's reflexes*, ed 2, Boulder, Colo, 1963, American Academy of Osteopathy.
3. Ward RC, Hruby RJ, Jerome JA et al: *Foundations for osteopathic medicine*, Philadelphia, 2003, Lippincott.
4. Frymann VM: Manipulative treatment of sinus infection. In *The collected papers of Viola Frymann*, Indianapolis, 1998, American Academy of Osteopathy.
5. Sept KE: AAO case study—"sinusitis", *AOAJ* 4:20-21, 1994.
6. Hoyt W: Current concepts in the management of sinus disease, *J Am Osteopath Assoc* 90:913-919, 1990.
7. Sutherland WG: *Teachings in the science of osteopathy*, Portland, Ore, 1990, Rudra Press.
8. Magoun HIS: *Osteopathy in the cranial field,* ed 3, Kirksville, Mo, 1976, The Journal Printing Company.
9. Carreiro JE: *An osteopathic approach to children*, London, 2003, Churchill Livingstone.
10. Magoun HIS: *Osteopathy in the cranial field,* Kirksville, MO, 1951, The Journal Printing Company.
11. Kuchera ML, Kuchera WA: *Osteopathic considerations in systemic disease*, Columbus, Ohio, 1994, Greydon Press.
12. Sutherland WG: *The cranial bowl,* ed 2, 1939, Sutherland.

Probiotics

1. Isolauri E, Sutas Y, Kankaanpaa P et al: Probiotics: effects on immunity, *Am J Clin Nutr* 73(Suppl):S444, 2001.
2. Roos K, Holm S: The use of probiotics in head and neck infections, *Curr Infect Dis Rep* 4:211-216, 2002.
3. Schrezenmeir J, Heller K, McCue M et al: Benefits of oral supplementation with and without synbiotics in young children with acute bacterial infections, *Clin Pediatr* 43:239, 2004.

CHAPTER 51

Pinworms

Homeopathy | Janet L. Levatin
Magnet Therapy | Agatha P. Colbert, Deborah Risotti

✳ PEDIATRIC DIAGNOSIS AND MANAGEMENT

Pinworm infection, or enterobiasis, is caused by *Enterobius vermicularis*, a small (1 cm in length), white, threadlike round-worm that typically inhabits the cecum, adjacent areas of the ileum, ascending colon, and appendix. It is the most common helminth infection in the United States[1] and is also prevalent throughout the world.[2-5] Infection occurs by ingestion of embryonated eggs that are carried on fingernails, clothing, bedding, or house dust.[1]

Pinworm infection is prevalent in temperate climates, occurs in individuals of all ages (especially in children), and in all socioeconomic levels. The highest incidence is in younger children from preschool to first grade,[3,4] an age group of children who still suck their fingers.[6] Transmission increases in school,[7] in large families,[8] in poorer communities with overcrowding, in areas where scarcity of water results in inadequate personal and community hygiene,[2,9] and in institutional residences.[1]

Gravid females migrate at night to the perianal and peri-neal regions where they deposit eggs.[1] *Enterobius* spp. infection causes symptoms by mechanical stimulation and irritation, allergic reactions, and migration of the worms to anatomical sites where they become pathogenic.[1] The most common complaints include itching and restless sleep secondary to nocturnal peri-anal or perineal pruritus.[10] Scratching may cause skin irritation and, in more serious cases, eczematous dermatitis, hemorrhage, or secondary bacterial infections.[9] Complicated perianal lesions are unusual.[11] Aberrant migration to ectopic sites occasionally may lead to appendicitis,[12-14] chronic salpingitis, peritonitis, hepatitis, and ulcerative lesions in the large or small bowel.[1,9]

Clinical diagnosis can be easily made by a history of nocturnal perianal pruritus in children. Definitive diagnosis can be established by using the "cellophane tape test": pressing the tape against the perianal region to see the worms or eggs.[10] The starting point for treatment is good hygiene by instructing the children to wash hands at home and in school.[8,15] Anthel-mintic drugs include mebendazole, albendazole, and pyrantel pamoate, which should be administered to infected individuals and all family members. A single oral dose of mebendazole (100 mg by mouth for all ages), repeated in 2 weeks, results in cure rates of 90% to 100%.[1]

✳ CAM THERAPY RECOMMENDATIONS

Homeopathy

Before using this section, please see Appendix A, Homeopathy, for definitions of practitioner expertise categories and general information on prescribing homeopathic medicines.

Clinician Expertise Category 1

There are no controlled clinical trials of homeopathic treatment for pinworms, although the homeopathic literature contains evidence for its use in the form of accumulated clinical experience.[1] Although it is safe to use homeopathic treatment for pinworms, either alone or in combination with other therapies (conventional or alternative), because pinworms tend to spread among children fairly easily, it is advisable to use some other form of treatment in addition to homeopathy to assure that the worms are eradicated. Homeopathy may be of most use in cases of recurrent pinworms, where it may alter the patient's susceptibility and increase resistance to recurrent infections.

The goal in treating pinworms homeopathically is to determine the single homeopathic medicine whose description in the materia medica most closely matches the symptom picture of the patient. Sometimes mental and emotional states, in addition to physical symptoms, are considered. Once the medicine has been selected, it can be given orally or sublingually in the 30C potency two times daily for 3 to 5 days. If the medicine has not helped after several days, then another homeopathic medicine should be tried or some other form of therapy should be instituted as needed. As mentioned previously, it is advisable to combine homeopathy with some other form of treatment known to be efficacious in eradicating pinworms. Once symptoms have begun to resolve, the homeopathic medicine can be given less frequently or stopped. It can be repeated again for a relapse of symptoms.

The following is a list of homeopathic medicines commonly used to treat patients with pinworms. It must be emphasized that this list is partial and represents some of the probable choices from the homeopathic materia medica. If the symptoms of a given patient are not represented here, a search of the homeopathic literature would be needed to find the simillimum.

Cina maritima

Cina maritima is the main homeopathic medicine for pinworms. The child with pinworms who needs cina maritima is restless, irritable, and angry and has an extremely itchy anus. There may be tantrums and shrieking and a tendency for convulsions.

Spigelia anthelmia

Consider using *Spigelia anthelmia* for pinworms and other types of worms when the symptoms include itching, tickling, and a sensation of crawling in the rectum. There may be stools consisting of only mucus. *Spigelia anthelmia* is also known as a medicine for nerve pain with severe sharp pains in the affected area.

Teucrium marum verum

The child with pinworms who needs *Teucrium marum varum* will have the most anal itching after passing stools. *Teucrium marum varum* is also known as a medicine for nasal polyps.

Magnet Therapy

Tape four ¾-inch Neodymium nylon-coated magnets around the anus, during the hours of sleep, in a pattern of alternating bionorth/biosouth polarity. Magnets may be obtained from Painfree Lifestyles (800-480-8601).

References

Pediatric Diagnosis and Management

1. Behrman RE, Kliegman RM, Jenson HB, editors: *Nelson textbook of pediatrics,* ed 17, Philadelphia, 2004, Saunders.
2. Acosta M, Cazorla D, Garvett M: Enterobiasis among schoolchildren in a rural population from Estado Falcon, Venezuela, and its relation with socioeconomic level [in Spanish], *Invest Clin* 43:173-181, 2002.
3. Lee KJ, Ahn YK, Ryang YS: *Enterobius vermicularis* egg positive rates in primary school children in Gangwon-do (province), Korea, *Korean J Parasitol* 39:327-328, 2001.
4. Fan PC: Review of enterobiasis in Taiwan and offshore islands, *J Microbiol Immunol Infect* 31:203-210, 1998.
5. Gan Y, Wu Q, Ou F et al: Studies on the efficacy of albendazole candy for treatment of intestinal nematode infections [in Chinese], *Zhongguo Ji Sheng Chong Xue Yu Ji Sheng Chong Bing Za Zhi* 12:147-149, 1994 (abstract).
6. Herrstrom P, Fristrom A, Karlsson A et al: *Enterobius vermicularis* and finger sucking in young Swedish children, *Scand J Prim Health Care* 15:146-148, 1997.
7. Yang YS, Kim SW, Jung SH et al: Chemotherapeutic trial to control enterobiasis in schoolchildren, *Korean J Parasitol* 35:265-269, 1997.
8. Blake J: An action plan to prevent and combat threadworm infection, *Nurs Times* 99:18-19, 2003.
9. St Georgiev V: Chemotherapy of enterobiasis (oxyuriasis), *Expert Opin Pharmacother* 2:267-275, 2001.
10. Kucik CJ, Martin GL, Sortor BV: Common intestinal parasites, *Am Fam Physician* 69:1161-1168, 2004.
11. Mattia AR: Perianal mass and recurrent cellulitis due to *Enterobius vermicularis*, *Am J Trop Med Hyg* 47:811-815, 1992.
12. Saxena AK, Springer A, Tsokas J et al: Laparoscopic appendectomy in children with *Enterobius vermicularis*, *Surg Laparosc Endosc Percutan Tech* 11:284-286, 2001.
13. Chernysheva ES, Ermakova GV, Berezina EI: The role of helminthiasis in the etiology of acute appendicitis [in Russian], *Khirurgiia (Mosk)* 10:30-32, 2001.
14. Dahlstrom JE, Macarthur EB: *Enterobius vermicularis*: a possible cause of symptoms resembling appendicitis, *Austr N Z J Surg* 64:692-694, 1994.
15. Ibarra J: Threadworms: a starting point for family hygiene, *Br J Community Nurs* 6:414-420.

Homeopathy

1. *ReferenceWorks Pro 4.2,* San Rafael, Calif, 2008, Kent Homeopathic Associates.

Primary Teeth Eruption

Homeopathy | Janet L. Levatin

Magnet Therapy | Agatha P. Colbert, Deborah Risotti

✳ PEDIATRIC DIAGNOSIS AND MANAGEMENT

Teething is the normal process of eruption of teeth through the gums.[1,2] Primary (baby) teeth are formed during pregnancy.[1] Timing of eruption of teeth depends on heredity,[1] but in general the first tooth appears between 5 and 7 months of age, and all the primary teeth usually appear by age 3 years.[1,2] The first permanent molars usually erupt at about age 6 years.[3]

Teething can lead to intermittent localized discomfort in the area of eruption. Although some children have no apparent difficulties,[3] many infants manifest a variety of nonspecific symptoms, such as crying, restlessness, feeding or sleeping difficulties, drooling, irritability, and low-grade fever.[1-3] Parents can become quite anxious when confronted with a distressed baby and worry whether the symptoms signify more serious conditions. A simple rubbing of the gum can reveal whether a tooth is close to erupting.[1] Severe systemic symptoms such as diarrhea, fever, rashes, or seizures usually do not occur with teething.[4,5] Occasionally, an eruption cyst can occur within the mucosa overlying an erupting tooth. This should be referred to a dentist to distinguish it from a dentigerous cyst.[6]

Treatment modalities for teething have been diverse throughout the ages, frequently depending on the tenets of the medical profession and lay people, but usually are directed toward symptomatic pain relief.[4] Current conventional treatment includes home remedies such as chewing on ice rings and over-the-counter medications such as oral analgesic and anesthetic gels that can be applied directly to the gums to relieve pain and inflammation.[2,3]

✳ CAM THERAPY RECOMMENDATIONS

Homeopathy

Before using this section, please see Appendix A, Homeopathy, for definitions of practitioner expertise categories and general information on prescribing homeopathic medicines.

Practitioner Expertise Category 1

There are no controlled clinical trials of homeopathy for treatment of problematic primary teeth eruption (referred to in homeopathic materia medica books as "slow dentition" and "difficult dentition"), although the homeopathic literature contains evidence for its use in the form of accumulated clinical experience.[1] Teething problems can often be treated effectively with homeopathy. It is safe to use homeopathic treatment for teething problems, either alone or in conjunctions with other treatment modalities such as conventional analgesics or herbs.

The goal in treating teething problems homeopathically is to determine the single homeopathic medicine whose description in the materia medica most closely matches the symptom picture of the patient. Sometimes mental and emotional states and developmental markers, in addition to physical symptoms, are considered. Once the medicine has been selected, it can be given orally, sublingually, or in dilute liquid form in the 30C potency once every 30 to 60 minutes for acute pain or two to four times daily for less acute pain. If the medicine has not helped in five to six doses, then another homeopathic medicine should be tried or some other form of therapy should be instituted as needed. Once symptoms have begun to resolve, the medicine can be given less frequently or stopped. It can be repeated again for a relapse of symptoms.

The following is a list of homeopathic medicines commonly used to treat patients with teething problems. It must be emphasized that this list is partial and represents some of the probable choices from the homeopathic materia medica. If the symptoms of a given patient are not represented here, a search of the homeopathic literature would be needed to find the simillimum.

Chamomilla vulgaris

Chamomilla vulgaris is the most commonly indicated homeopathic medicine for painful teething. The infant is extremely irritable and fussy. The gums are swollen and red, and the infant is generally hot and thirsty. One cheek is hot and red; the other is pale and cool. The child seems to want many things but rejects them when they are offered. Being carried about is the only way to calm the child. The teething problems may accompany an ear infection or diarrhea with green stools.

Calcarea carbonica

Calcarea carbonica is a medicine to consider for slow, difficult teething. The child also may be slow in other areas of development, such as learning to walk or talk. He or she is a plump child with a large head and abdomen. Children needing *Calcarea carbonica* are often sweaty, and the sweat may smell sour. The child may also be constipated and have a weak resistance to infections such as viral illnesses.

Calcarea phosphorica

The infant needing *Calcarea phosphorica* also has slow, difficult teething. The child is irritable and whiny and demanding of attention, but much less so than the child needing *Chamomilla vulgaris*. This child may be pale and thin.

Silica terra

Children needing *Silica terra* can have slow and difficult teething. Consider this medicine for children with decay or breakage of a primary tooth or an infection or abscess of the gum around a primary tooth. The infant may be thin and delicate and have a weak immune system. In addition to problems with teeth and teething, there also may be difficulties with the skin or nails.

MagnetTherapy

Gently rub a domino-sized 3950-G ceramic magnet in a counterclockwise manner on the skin over the site of the erupting tooth for 2 to 3 minutes. Repeat three to four times per day. Magnets may be obtained from Painfree Lifestyles (800-480-8601) or AHSM (800-635-7070).

References

Pediatric Diagnosis and Management

1. Beard LM: Teething/toothache, *Pediatr News* Jan:32-33, 2005.
2. Jones M: Teething in children and the alleviation of symptoms, *J Fam Health Care* 12:12-13, 2002.
3. Behrman RE, Kliegman RM, Jenson HB, editors: *Nelson textbook of pediatrics,* ed 17, Philadelphia, 2004, Saunders.
4. McIntyre GT, McIntyre GM: Teething troubles? *Br Dent J* 192:251-255, 2002.
5. Leung AK: Teething, *Am Fam Physician* 39:131-134, 1989.
6. Bodner L, Goldstein J, Sarnat H: Eruption cysts: a clinical report of 24 new cases, *J Clin Pediatr Dent* 28:183-186, 2004.

Homeopathy

1. ReferenceWorks Pro 4.2, San Rafael, Calif, 2008, Kent Homeopathic Associates.

CHAPTER 53

Ringworm

Aromatherapy | Maura A. Fitzgerald

Herbs—Western | Alan D. Woolf, Paula M. Gardiner, Lana Dvorkin-Camiel, Jack Maypole

Magnet Therapy | Agatha P. Colbert, Deborah Risotti

Massage Therapy | Mary C. McLellan

✳ PEDIATRIC DIAGNOSIS AND MANAGEMENT

Dermatophytoses, commonly known as ringworm or tinea, represent superficial fungal infections of the glabrous skin[1] caused by dermatophytes.[2] Tinea corporis is very common in childhood.[3] The sex distribution is about equal in preadolescents, but males predominate among adolescents.[4] The infection can be acquired by direct contact with infected children or by contact with infected scales or hairs. A single dermatophyte lesion can cause vast dissemination.[5]

The typical clinical lesion begins as a dry, mildly erythematous, elevated, scaly papule or plaque that spreads centrifugally as it clears centrally to form the characteristic annular lesion, the "ringworm" appearance. However, central clearing does not always occur,[5] which sometimes complicates clinical diagnosis of the lesion. Diagnosis should always be confirmed with microscopic examination of potassium hydroxide (KOH) wet-mount preparations and fungal cultures.[3,5] Tinea corporis usually does not fluoresce with a Wood lamp.[5]

Most lesions clear spontaneously within several months, but some may become chronic.[5] Tinea corporis usually responds to treatment with a topical antifungal agent.[1,5] Combination antifungal/corticosteroid preparations, such as clotrimazole 1%/betamethasone diproprionate 0.05% cream (Lotrisone, Schering, Kenilworth, N.J.) are widely used by nondermatologists in the treatment of superficial fungal infections in patients of all ages, often for children younger than 4 years of age.[6] However, Lotrisone is approved by the U.S. Food and Drug Administration (FDA) for the treatment of tinea only in adults and children older than 12 years and for a maximum of 4 weeks.[7] Treatment failure[6] and steroid-related side effects such as striae distensae, hirsutism, and growth retardation have been associated with Lotrisone, making it contraindicated in young children and in immunosuppressed patients.[2,7] Oral griseofulvin is the current systemic drug of choice for immunosuppressed children.[3,8] Local and environmental measures to prevent transmission must accompany pharmaceutical treatment for successful eradication of the infection.[3]

✳ CAM THERAPY RECOMMENDATIONS

Aromatherapy

In vitro and in vivo studies have been conducted to establish the antifungal properties of a number of essential oils. The mechanisms of action include disruption of cell membrane, inhibition of growth, and inhibition of cellular respiration.[1] Laboratory and animal testing of the essential oils of cinnamon bark (*Cinnamomum zeylanicum*), lemongrass (*Cymbopogon citratus*), thyme (*Thymus vulgaris*), perilla (*Perilla frutescens*), lavender (*Lavandula angustifolia*), tea tree (*Melaleuca alternifolia*), and wormseed (*Chenopodium ambrosioides* [Note: This essential oil is listed as dangerous in many texts and is not recommended for use with children.]) showed anti-*Trichophyton* activity to varying degrees.[2,3] Price and Parr recommend a topical application of 4 drops tea tree, 2 drops geranium (*Pelargonium graveolens*), and 2 drops sweet thyme mixed in 50 mL of lotion.[4]

Herbs—Western

Tinea capitis, or ringworm, is caused by a superficial infection by a fungus, and it is often treated by the use of an antifungal shampoo. Avoidance of the sharing of hats, combs, and hairbrushes is also recommended. In vitro studies of tea tree oil have demonstrated its effectiveness as an antifungal agent; however, there are few studies of its topical use for the relief of tinea in children.

Magnet Therapy

Apply the designated north pole of a ¾-inch Neodymium nylon-coated magnet directly over the skin and leave it in place for 12 hours. Repeat daily. Magnets may be obtained from Painfree Lifestyles (800-480-8601).

Massage Therapy

Massage should be avoided over skin conditions considered contagious thorough contact to avoid further spread of the disease to the child or the massage practitioner.[1-3] A recent study demonstrated increased bacterial counts on massage therapists' hands during and after massage treatments, although counts were lower on the clients' skin.[4]

R

References

Pediatric Diagnosis and Management

1. Gupta AK, Cooper EA, Ryder JE et al: Optimal management of fungal infections of the skin, hair, and nails, *Am J Clin Dermatol* 5:225-237, 2004.
2. Erbagci Z: Topical therapy for dermatophytoses: should corticosteroids be included? *Am J Clin Dermatol* 5:375-384, 2004.
3. Rudy SJ: Superficial fungal infections in children and adolescents, *Nurse Pract Forum* 10:56-66, 1999.
4. Zienicke HC, Korting HC, Lukacs A et al: Dermatophytosis in children and adolescents: epidemiological, clinical, and microbiological aspects changing with age, *J Dermatol* 18:438-446, 1991.
5. Behrman RE, Kliegman RM, Jenson HB, editors: *Nelson textbook of pediatrics*, ed 17, Philadelphia, 2004, Saunders.
6. Alston SJ, Cohen BA, Braun M: Persistent and recurrent tinea corporis in children treated with combination antifungal/corticosteroid agents, *Pediatrics* 111:201-203, 2003.
7. Greenberg HL, Shwayder TA, Bieszk N et al: Clotrimazole/betamethasone/diproprionate: a review of costs and complications in the treatment of common cutaneous fungal infections, *Pediatr Dermatol* 19:78-81, 2002.
8. Elewski BE: Cutaneous mycoses in children, *Br J Dermatol* 134(Suppl 46):7-11, 1996; discussion 37-38.

Aromatherapy

1. Harris R: Progress with superficial mycoses using essential oils, *Int J Aromather* 12:83-91, 2002.
2. Inouye S, Uchida K, Yamaguchi H: In-vitro and in-vivo anti-*Trichophyton* activity of essential oils by vapour contact, *Mycoses* 44:99-107, 2001.
3. Kishore N, Chansouria JP, Dubey NK: Antidermatophytic action of the essential oil of *Chenopodium ambrosioides* and an ointment prepared from it, *Phytother Res* 10:453-455, 1996.
4. Price S, Parr PP: *Aromatherapy for babies and cildren,* San Francisco, 1996, Thorsons.

Massage Therapy

1. Tappan F: *Healing massage techniques: holistic, classic, and emerging methods,* Norwalk, Conn, 1988, Appleton & Lange.
2. Fritz S: *Mosby's fundamentals of therapeutic massage,* ed 3, St Louis, 2005, Mosby.
3. American Massage Therapy Association: *Massage therapy facts for physicians,* Evanston, Ill, 2005, AMTA. Available at www.amtamassage.org/pdf/FactsForPhysicians.pdf. Accessed April 30, 2008.
4. Donoyama N, Wakuda T, Tanitsu T et al: Washing hands before and after performing massages? Changes in bacterial survival count on skin of a massage therapist and client during massage therapy, *J Altern Complement Med* 10:684-686, 2004.

CHAPTER 54

Roseola

Chiropractic | Anne Spicer

✳ PEDIATRIC DIAGNOSIS AND MANAGEMENT

Roseola infantum is also known as *exanthema subitum* or *sixth disease* according to the childhood exanthem classification after measles, scarlet fever, rubella, Filatov-Dukes disease (an atypical scarlet fever), and erythema infectiosum (fifth disease). The cause is usually human herpesvirus (HHV)-6 and, less frequently, HHV-7 β-herpesviruses. These large, double-stranded deoxyribonucleic acid (DNA) lymphotropic viruses are ubiquitous,[1] tend to infect infants during the first year of life, and usually cause lifelong latency.[2,3]

Clinically the infection may be silent or may manifest as roseola,[4] a mild febrile, exanthematous illness with upper respiratory prodromal symptoms followed by 3 to 5 days of high temperature, usually ranging from 37.9° to 40° C (101° to 106° F), with an average of 39° C (103° F) although the child usually appears well. Fever then abruptly resolves, followed by a rash within 12 to 24 hours of fever resolution. The classic rash of roseola is rose colored, as the name implies, and is fairly distinctive, beginning as discrete, small (2 to 5 mm), slightly raised pink lesions on the trunk and usually spreading to the neck, face, and proximal extremities. The rash is not usually pruritic, and no vesicles or pustules develop. Febrile convulsions may occur in 5% to 10% of children during the high fever period.[1,5,6,7] Of the two distinct variants of HHV-6, type B causes more than 99% of HHV-6–associated roseola cases.[8] More than 90% of children are seropositive by age 3 years.[6]

Diagnosis is usually clinical, based on history and examination. Laboratory tests for diagnosing active HHV-6 and HHV-7 infections (if needed, as in immunocompromised children) include serological evaluation, virus culture, and polymerase chain reaction of cell-free biological fluid.[4,6] These viruses have been associated with substantial morbidity among infants and children, such as convulsions and encephalitis,[8,9] and with hepatitis, pneumonitis, and hemophagocytosis syndrome[7]; may play a role in the etiology of Hodgkin disease and other malignancies[8]; and may accelerate the progression of human immunodeficiency virus infection.[3]

Treatment is usually symptomatic and supportive in the prodromal phase and with antipyretics and fluids in the febrile phase. Most children have excellent prognoses without significant sequelae. Children with complications such as encephalitis and pneumonitis and immunocompromised children should be referred for specialist management and treatment.[4] HHV-6 is inhibited by several antiviral drugs but not acyclovir. Treatment trials so far have been inconclusive for antiviral management.[6,7]

✳ CAM THERAPY RECOMMENDATIONS

Chiropractic

Although literature specifically related to chiropractic management of roseola is lacking, this disease would be addressed like any other infectious disease. The approach would be to remove any interference to normal immune function and support any additional burden placed on the system by the active disease.

There is evidence that the chiropractic adjustment has influence over natural killer cell production and autonomic balance,[1] immunoglobulin (IgA, G, and M) levels and β-cell lymphocyte count,[2] polymorphonuclear neutrophils and monoctyes,[3] and even CD4 counts.[4] Therefore the chiropractic adjustment of a subluxation complex would be a priority.

The chiropractic adjustment that eliminates subluxation will restore internal feedback mechanisms and enhance immune function.[5] The adjustment may stimulate internal regulation of fever, serving as a useful comfort and healing measure in the early febrile stage of roseola. Fever is recognized by the chiropractor as an elevation in body temperature in response to feedback from the central nervous system. Fever is commonly a normal and beneficial immune response to disease, interfering with proliferation of antigens and killing off existing infection.[5] In fact, lack of fever may be seen as a sign of poor prognosis.[6,7]

Supplementation with immune-enhancing nutrients may provide the body with necessary resources to manage an acute infection. Commonly recommended nutrients include zinc and vitamin A[8]; zinc is available in liquid formulations and is vital to normal immune function. A calcium supplement may also prove useful in cases of roseola.[9] Vitamin C may be given to the young infant in the form of rose hip syrup and should be dosed within gut tolerance.[9,10] An initial dose of 250 mg is a good starting place. Gut microflora will support the immune function, as will omega-3 fatty acids (eicosapentaenoic acid [EPA]/docosahexaenoic acid [DHA]), which also have antiinflammatory actions.[11] Vitamin E has antioxidant as well as antiinflammatory properties.[12]

Echinacea purpurea is recommended as a stimulant to the immune system.[9] Use is recommended for a period not to exceed 2 consecutive weeks, as the body may develop a tolerance level with prolonged use. Although echinacea is safe, allergic reactions in children with a history of allergies, particularly to plants in the daisy family, have been recorded.

Adequate rest and hydration will contribute to recovery.

References

Pediatric Diagnosis and Management

1. Caserta MT, Hall CB: A practitioner's guide to human herpesvirus-6 (HHV-6) and human herpesvirus-7 (HHV-7), *AIDS Patient Care STDS* 12:833-842, 1998.
2. Krueger GR, Klueppelberg U, Hoffmann A et al: Clinical correlates of infection with human herpesvirus-6, *In Vivo* 8:457-485, 1994.
3. Lusso P, Gallo RC: Human herpesvirus 6, *Baillieres Clin Haematol* 8:201-223, 1995.
4. Leach CT: Human herpesvirus-6 and -7 infections in children: agents of roseola and other syndromes, *Curr Opin Pediatr* 12: 269-274, 2000.
5. Kleinschmidt-DeMasters BK, Gilden DH: The expanding spectrum of herpesvirus infections of the nervous system, *Brain Pathol* 11:440-451, 2001.
6. Galama JM: Human herpes viruses type 6 and 7; causative agents of, among others, exanthema subitum [in Dutch], *Ned Tijdschr Geneeskd* 140:124-128, 1996 (abstract).
7. Behrman RE, Kliegman RM, Jenson HB, editors: *Nelson's textbook of pediatrics*, Philadelphia, 2004, Saunders.
8. Braun DK, Dominguez G, Pellett PE: Human herpesvirus 6, *Clin Microbiol Rev* 10:521-567, 1997.
9. Bale JF Jr: Human herpesviruses and neurological disorders of childhood, *Semin Pediatr Neurol* 6:278-287, 1999.

Chiropractic

1. Leach RA, Burgess SC: Neuroimmune hypothesis. In Leach RA, editor: *The chiropractic theories*, Baltimore, 2004, Lippincott Williams and Wilkins.
2. Brennan PC, Kokjohn K, Triano JJ et al: Immunologic correlates of reduced spinal mobility: preliminary observations in a dog model. In Wold S, editor: *Proceedings of the 1991 International Conference on Spinal Manipulation*, Arlington, Va, 1991, Foundation for Chiropractic Education and Research.
3. Brennan PC, Kokjohn K, Kaltinger CJ et al: Enhanced phagocytic cell respiratory burst induced by spinal manipulation: potential role of substance P, *J Manipulative Physiol Ther* 14:399-408, 1991.
4. Selano JL, Hightower BC, Pfleger B et al: The effects of specific upper cervical adjustments on the CD4 counts of HIV positive patients, *Chiropractic Res J* 3:32-39, 1994.
5. Fallon JM: The role of subluxation in fever and febrile seizures, *Today's Chiropractic* Mar/Apr:64-66, 1996.
6. Grossman M: Fever. In Rudolph AM, Hoffman JE, Rudolph DC, editors: *Rudolph's pediatrics*, ed 20, Stanford, Conn, 1996, Appleton & Lange.
7. Soliman SE, Plaugher G, Alcantara J: The febrile child. In Anrig C, Plaugher G, editors: *Pediatric chiropractic*, Baltimore, 1998, Williams and Wilkins.
8. Bhandari N, Bahl R, Taneja S et al: Effect or routine zinc supplementation on pneumonia in children aged 6 months to 3 years: randomized controlled trial in an urban slum, *Br Med J* 324: 1358-1361, 2002.
9. Davies N: *Chiropractic pediatrics*, London, 2000, Churchill Livingstone.
10. Forastiere R, Pistelli R, Sestini P et al: Consumption of fresh fruit rich in vitamin C and wheezing symptoms in children, *Thorax* 55:283-288, 2000.
11. Stevens LJ, Zentall SS, Abate ML et al: Omega-3 fatty acids in boys with behavior, learning and health problems, *Physiol Behav* 59:915-920, 1996.
12. Heffner JE, Repine JE: Pulmonary strategies of antioxidant defense, *Am Rev Resp Dis* 140:531-554, 1989.

Rubella

Chiropractic | Anne Spicer

✳ PEDIATRIC DIAGNOSIS AND MANAGEMENT

Rubella, also known as *German measles,* is an acute viral illness characterized by mild constitutional symptoms, a rash similar to that of mild rubeola or scarlet fever, and enlargement and tenderness of the postoccipital, retroauricular, and posterior cervical lymph nodes.[1,2] Rubella in early pregnancy can cause congenital rubella syndrome (CRS), a devastating disease that affects multiple systems in the fetus, resulting in microcephaly, deafness, mental retardation, and heart, liver, and spleen damage.[1-3] Autism has also been associated with in utero exposure to rubella.[4] Infants with CRS can shed large quantities of virus from body secretions for as long as 1 year and can therefore transmit the disease to anyone caring for them who are susceptible, especially a pregnant woman.[3]

Before the advent of rubella vaccines, rubella epidemics occurred every 6 to 9 years. During the 1962 to 1965 worldwide rubella epidemic, an estimated 12.5 million cases of rubella occurred in the United States, resulting in 2000 cases of encephalitis, 11,250 fetal deaths, 2100 neonatal deaths, and 20,000 infants born with CRS.[1,3] The economic impact of this epidemic in the United States was estimated at $1.5 billion.[5]

In 1969, live, attenuated, noncommunicable rubella vaccines were first licensed in the United States,[6] and a vaccination program was established with the goal of preventing congenital infections, including CRS. By 1979, rubella vaccination had eliminated the characteristic 6- to 9-year epidemic cycle of rubella in the United States.[7] Substantial declines in rubella and CRS continued to take place during the following 2 decades. Since 2001, fewer than 25 rubella cases have been reported each year; vaccination coverage among school-aged children is at least 95% and population immunity is estimated at 91%. In October 2004, the Centers for Disease Control and Prevention (CDC) concluded that rubella is no longer endemic in the United States. As of 2004, a total of 43 of 44 countries and territories in the Western hemisphere have included rubella vaccine in their routine immunization programs.[1]

✳ CAM THERAPY RECOMMENDATIONS

Chiropractic

Although literature specifically related to chiropractic management of rubella is lacking, this disease would be addressed like any other infectious disease. The approach would be to remove any interference to normal immune function and support any additional burden placed on the system by the active disease.

There is evidence that the chiropractic adjustment has influence over natural killer cell production and autonomic balance,[1] immunoglobulin (IgA, G, and M) levels and β-cell lymphocyte count,[2] polymorphonuclear neutrophils and monoctyes,[3] and even CD4 counts.[4] Therefore the chiropractic adjustment of a subluxation complex would be a priority. Neil Davies, author of the text *Chiropractic Pediatrics,* states that it may be necessary to assess and adjust the child as often as three times per day during the height of the acute febrile stage.[5]

Supplementation with immune-enhancing nutrients may provide the body with necessary resources to manage an acute infection. Commonly recommended nutrients include zinc and vitamin A[6]. Zinc is available in liquid formulations and is vital to normal immune function. A calcium supplement may also prove useful in cases of rubella.[5] Vitamin C may be given to the young infant in the form of rose hip syrup and should be dosed within gut tolerance.[5,7] An initial dose of 250 mg is a good starting place. Gut microflora will support the immune function, as will omega-3 fatty acids (eicosapentaenoic acid [EPA]/docosahexaenoic acid [DHA]), which also have antiinflammatory actions.[8] Vitamin E has antioxidant as well as antiinflammatory properties.[9]

Echinacea purpurea is recommended as a stimulant to the immune system.[5] Use is recommended for a period not to exceed 2 consecutive weeks, as the body may develop a tolerance level with prolonged use. Although echinacea is quite safe, allergic reactions in children with a history of allergies, particularly to plants in the daisy family, have been recorded.

References

Pediatric Diagnosis and Management

1. Achievements in public health: elimination of rubella and congenital rubella syndrome—United States, 1969-2004, *MMWR Morbid Mortal Wkly Rep* Mar 21:1-4, 2005.
2. Behrman RE, Kliegman RM, Jenson HB, editors: *Nelson textbook of pediatrics,* ed 17, Philadelphia, 2004, Saunders.
3. Epidemiology and prevention of vaccine-preventable diseases. In: *The pink book,* ed 6, Waldorf, Md, 2001, Public Health Foundation.
4. Measles-mumps-rubella vaccine and autistic spectrum disorder: report from the New Challenges in Childhood Immunizations Conference, Oak Brook, Ill, 2000, *Pediatrics* 207:E84, 2001.
5. Centers for Disease Control and Prevention: *Rubella surveillance report 1,* Atlanta, 1969, CDC.

6. Preblud SR, Serdula MK, Frank JA Jr et al: From the Center for Disease Control: current status of rubella in the United States, 1969-1979, *J Infect Dis* 142:776-779, 1980.

7. Williams NM, Preblud SR: Current epidemiology of rubella in the United States, *Proc 19th Natl Immun Conf* 11-17, 1984.

Chiropractic

1. Leach RA, Burgess SC: Neuroimmune hypothesis, In Leach RA, editor: *The chiropractic theories,* Baltimore, 2004, Lippincott, Williams and Wilkins.

2. Brennan PC, Kokjohn K, Triano JJ et al: Immunologic correlates of reduced spinal mobility: preliminary observations in a dog model. In Wold S, editor: *Proceedings of the 1991 International Conference on Spinal Manipulation,* Arlington, Va, 1991, Foundation for Chiropractic Education and Research.

3. Brennan PC, Kokjohn K, Kaltinger CJ et al: Enhanced phagocytic cell respiratory burst induced by spinal manipulation: potential role of substance P, *J Manipulative Physiol Ther* 14:399-408, 1991.

4. Selano JL, Hightower BC, Pfleger B et al: The effects of specific upper cervical adjustments on the CD4 counts of HIV positive patients, *Chiropractic Res J* 3:32, 1994.

5. Davies N: *Chiropractic pediatrics,* London, 2000, Churchill Livingstone.

6. Bhandari N, Bahl R, Taneja S et al: Effect or routine zinc supplementation on pneumonia in children aged 6 months to 3 years: randomized controlled trial in an urban slum, *Br Med J* 324: 1358-1361, 2002.

7. Forastiere R, Pistelli R, Sestini P et al: Consumption of fresh fruit rich in vitamin C and wheezing symptoms in children, *Thorax* 55:283-288, 2000.

8. Stevens LJ, Zentall SS, Abate ML et al: Omega-3 fatty acids in boys with behavior, learning and health problems, *Physiol Behav* 59:915-920, 1996.

9. Heffner JE, Repine JE: Pulmonary strategies of antioxidant defense, *Am Rev Resp Dis* 140:531-554, 1989.

CHAPTER 56

Scabies

Herbs—Western | Alan D. Woolf, Paula M. Gardiner, Lana Dvorkin-Camiel, Jack Maypole

Massage Therapy | Mary C. McLellan

✳ PEDIATRIC DIAGNOSIS AND MANAGEMENT

Scabies is a skin disorder caused by a parasite, *Sarcoptes scabiei* var. *hominis,* which colonizes the human epidermis. It is a highly contagious condition found in children throughout the world and occurs more frequently in lower socioeconomic populations,[1-3] in homeless children,[4] and in institutions such as orphanages.[5]

Clinically, children can present with extensive pruritus and characteristic skin lesions.[6,7] Erythematous papules with burrowing is pathognomonic for scabies. These lesions are often excoriated.[8] In the immunocompromised child, the rash may include vesicles, pustules, or nodules.[9] The diagnosis of common scabies is generally based on clinical findings. Atypical forms can be diagnosed by microscopic examination of skin scrapings for parasites.[6,10]

Treatment of scabies in infants and children is the subject of worldwide concern because of the risks and benefits of the variety of scabicides.[1] Topical treatments are usually advocated.[9,11]

Standard therapy is the application of permethrin 5% cream (Elimite) or 1% lindane cream or lotion to the entire body from the neck down, with particular attention to intensely involved areas. The medication is left on the skin for 8 to 12 hours; if necessary, it may be reapplied in 1 week for another 8- to 12-hour period. Lindane 1% cream is less expensive than permethrin, but extreme caution must be exercised in prescribing it for infants because percutaneous absorption may result in toxic side effects that consist of nausea, vomiting, weakness, tremors, irritability, disorientation, seizures, and even respiratory compromise. The entire family should be treated, as should caretakers of the infested child. Clothing, bed linens, and towels should be thoroughly laundered.[10]

Although numerous countries have used oral ivermectin for both adults and children,[6,9,12-16] the U.S. Food and Drug Administration has not yet approved oral ivermectin for the treatment of scabies infection. The safety of oral ivermectin in young children has yet to be established.[17]

Prevention of recurrence is also an integral part of treatment. Aggressive health educational programs, community motivation, and improvement of the hygiene and socioeconomic status of at-risk populations are all important in reducing the incidence of scabies.[2,3,9]

✳ CAM THERAPY RECOMMENDATIONS

Herbs—Western

Permethrin-containing creams are the scabicide often used first for the treatment of scabies. Although tea tree oil has also been used as a pesticide,[1] its efficacy for the relief of scabies in children has not been proven.

Massage Therapy

Massage therapy is contraindicated in the setting of scabies, as it may help transmit the parasites elsewhere on the body or to the therapist.

References

Pediatric Diagnosis and Management

1. Singalavanija S, Limpongsanurak W, Soponsakunkul S: A comparative study between 10 per cent sulfur ointment and 0.3 per cent gamma benzene hexachloride gel in the treatment of scabies in children, *J Med Assoc Thai* 86(Suppl 3):S531-S536, 2003.
2. Wong LC, Amega B, Connors C et al: Outcome of an interventional program for scabies in an indigenous community, *Med J Austr* 175:367-370, 2001.
3. Inanir I, Sahin MT, Gunduz K et al: Prevalence of skin conditions in primary school children in Turkey: differences based on socioeconomic factors, *Pediatr Dermatol* 19:307-311, 2002.
4. Estrada B: Ectoparasitic infestations in homeless children, *Semin Pediatr Infect Dis* 14:20-24, 2003.
5. Pruksachatkunakorn C, Damrongsak M, Sinthupuan S: Sulfur for scabies outbreaks in orphanages, *Pediatr Dermatol* 19:448-453, 2002.
6. Diagnosis and treatment of scabies in 2002: rapid diagnosis and proper management limit the risk of spread, *Prescrire Int* 11:152-155, 2002.
7. Pfutzner W: Infectious skin diseases in childhood. 1: Bacteria and fungi [in German], *MMW Fortschr Med* 144:24-28, 30, 2002 (abstract).
8. Arya V, Molinaro MJ, Majewski SS et al: Pediatric scabies, *Cutis* 71:193-196, 2003.
9. Flinders DC, De Schweinitz P: Pediculosis and scabies, *Am Fam Physician* 69:341-348, 2004.
10. Behrman RE, Kliegman RM, Jenson HB, editors: *Nelson's textbook of pediatrics,* Philadelphia, 2004, Saunders.
11. Sanfilippo AM, Barrio V, Kulp-Shorten C et al: Common pediatric and adolescent skin conditions, *J Pediatr Adolesc Gynecol* 16:269-283, 2003.

12. Micali G, Lacarrubba F, Tedeschi A: Videodermatoscopy enhances the ability to monitor efficacy of scabies treatment and allows optimal timing of drug application, *J Eur Acad Dermatol Venereol* 18:153-154, 2004.

13. del Mar Saez-De-Ocariz M, McKinster CD, Orozco-Covarrubias L et al: Treatment of 18 children with scabies or cutaneous larva migrans using ivermectin, *Clin Exp Dermatol* 27:264-267, 2002.

14. Victoria J, Trujillo R: Topical ivermectin: a new successful treatment for scabies, *Pediatr Dermatol* 18:63-65, 2001.

15. Usha V, Gopalakrishnan Nair TV: A comparative study of oral ivermectin and topical permethrin cream in the treatment of scabies, *J Am Acad Dermatol* 42:236-240, 2000.

16. Marliere V, Roul S, Labreze C et al: Crusted (Norwegian) scabies induced by use of topical corticosteroids and treated successfully with ivermectin, *J Pediatr* 135:122-124, 1999.

17. Santoro AF, Rezac MA, Lee JB: Current trend in ivermectin usage for scabies, *J Drugs Dermatol* 2:397-401, 2003.

Herbs—Western

1. Walton SF, McKinnon M, Pizzutto S et al: Acaricidal activity of *Melaleuca alternifolia* (tea tree) oil: in vitro sensitivity of *Sarcoptes scabiei* var *hominis* to terpinen-4-ol, *Arch Dermatol* 140:563-566, 2004.

CHAPTER 57

Stuttering

Acupuncture | May Loo
Homeopathy | Janet L. Levatin

Mind/Body | Timothy Culbert, Lynda Richtsmeier Cyr
Osteopathy | Jane Carreiro

✳ PEDIATRIC DIAGNOSIS AND MANAGEMENT

Language development occurs most rapidly between 2 and 5 years of age. Vocabulary increases from 50 to 100 words to more than 2000. Sentence structure advances from telegraphic phrases ("Baby cry") to sentences that incorporate all the major grammatical components.[1]

About 5 percent of children develop dysfluency and stuttering during the period of rapid language acquisition. Stuttering is involuntary, with up to 80% natural, spontaneous recovery,[2] often within 6 months.[3]

The precise etiology is unknown and may be multifactorial; inappropriate reactions by parents, caretakers, or unqualified physicians and psychosocial problems in the child's surroundings may consolidate the disorder.[3]

Treatment involves guidance to parents to reduce pressures associated with speaking. Early identification of stuttering is advisable because this disorder may progress to lifelong communicative impairments that can have both social and occupational impact.[3,4] The Individuals with Disabilities Education Act (IDEA) of 1997 is the federal mandate that provides speech-language pathologists with specific guidelines for evaluating stuttering in children and in determining eligibility for speech-language services in schools.[5,6]

However, a recent review indicates that speech therapy has never "cured" stuttering. The best interventions appear to be directed toward "efficient" and "effective" symptom reduction.[2]

The Lidcombe Program has been found to be an effective and safe treatment method for early intervention in preschool children,[7] but therapists must weight the natural course of children outgrowing the stuttering versus the benefit of early intervention.[8] A U.S. study evaluated self-contained ear-level devices delivering altered auditory feedback (AAF) in adolescents who stutter and found that stuttering was reduced and the speech produced was more natural when the device was used compared with when it was not used.[9] A German clinical trial that involved children from ages 9 to 19 in a stuttering therapy summer camp for children and adolescents, where participants learned a more open handling of their stuttering and acquired basics for a fluent speech, resulted in an average reduction of stuttering frequency from 22.2% to 9.5%.[10] Children with other disorders, such as attention-deficit hyperactivity disorder, present special challenges for evaluation and treatment.[11,12]

✳ CAM THERAPY RECOMMENDATIONS

Acupuncture

There are no data on acupuncture treatment of stuttering in children. A single case report from Australia of two adults treated with acupuncture showed no change in the stuttering frequency or the speech rate. However, the low subject numbers involved suggest caution in concluding that acupuncture is not a successful intervention for stuttering.[1] Future research is needed on this topic.

Classical acupuncture has utilized the point HT5 for treatment of stuttering. The tongue is the sensory organ of the heart. HT5 has major functions for stuttering: it exerts a calming effect, is the Luo-connecting point of the Heart channel, has a direct connection to the root of the tongue, and therefore has been indicated for treatment of various speech difficulties, including stuttering.[2]

Homeopathy

Before using this section, please see Appendix A, Homeopathy, for definitions of practitioner expertise categories and general information on prescribing homeopathic medicines.

Practitioner Expertise Category 2

Category 2 includes simple stuttering.

Practitioner Expertise Category 3

Category 3 includes stuttering as part of a symptom complex or syndrome.

There are no controlled clinical trials of homeopathic treatment of stuttering, although the homeopathic literature contains evidence for its use in the form of accumulated clinical experience.[1] Stuttering that is time limited is a frequent occurrence in children at certain stages in the development of their speech and language skills. This type of stuttering usually resolves spontaneously and requires no treatment. Persistent stuttering that is pathological can sometimes be treated effectively with homeopathy. It is safe to try homeopathic treatment for persistent stuttering, either alone or in combination with other therapies. Because stuttering is a neurological problem, it may occur as part of a larger symptom complex or syndrome. To increase the likelihood of successful homeopathic treatment, the entire case, not just the stuttering, should be considered and researched in the homeopathic literature.

The goal in treating stuttering homeopathically is to determine the single homeopathic medicine whose description in the materia medica most closely matches the symptom picture of the patient. Often mental and emotional states, in addition to physical symptoms, are considered. Once the medicine has been selected, it can be given orally or sublingually in the 200C potency once weekly for 1 or 2 months. The patient should be observed for a few weeks or months to determine whether any improvement has occurred. If the stuttering has not improved, then another homeopathic medicine can be tried or some other form of treatment can be instituted as needed. Once symptoms have begun to resolve, the medicine can be given less frequently or stopped. It can be repeated again for a relapse of symptoms.

The following is a list of homeopathic medicines commonly used to treat patients with stuttering. It must be emphasized that this list is partial and represents only some of the probable choices from the homeopathic materia medica. If the symptoms of a given patient are not represented here, a search of the homeopathic literature would be needed to find the simillimum.

Bovista lycoperdon

Bovista lycoperdon can be used when stuttering occurs in a patient who is awkward in general and tends to drop things. Stammering and mistakes in speech are present. The patient may have changeable moods.

Causticum hahnemanni

Causticum hahnemanni can be tried for patients who are most likely to stutter when they are excited. Tics, tremors, twitches, or even seizures may occur. Children needing causticum are very sensitive and emotional. They may also be quite fearful, particularly of animals, darkness, and/or ghosts.

Mercurius solubilis hahnemanni

Mercurius solubilis hahnemanni is a remedy for stuttering when the patient is very slow to respond in conversation. The child may have a sensitive nature with strong emotions or may seem shy and withdrawn. Typically the child also suffers from recurrent infections, such as otitis media, throat, or intraoral infections.

Stramonium

In addition to stuttering, children needing *Stramonium* may suffer from tics, chorea, seizures, and other neurological problems. There will usually be some history of nightmares or night terrors, strong fears, and/or violent behavior. Often the onset of the problems follows a frightening traumatic event or a severe illness, such as meningitis, that has affected the nervous system.

Mind/Body

The research on mind/body therapies for stuttering in pediatric populations is limited. Relaxation and breath work training have been utilized within a broader cognitive-behavioral treatment approach.[1,2] Waterloo and Gotestam[3] conducted a randomized controlled trial to assess the efficacy of the regulated-breathing method for stuttering. This method includes training in diaphragmatic breathing, general relaxation, and behavioral habit reversal approaches. Thirty-two subjects were randomly assigned to treatment and wait-list control groups. Breath work training occurred during a 2- to 3-hour treatment session. At 8-month follow-up, stuttering in the treatment group was significantly less compared with both pretreatment and the control group.

Electromyographic (EMG) biofeedback has been used to reduce speech muscle tension in pediatric patients. Craig and Cleary[4] used a single-subject design method that measured baseline stuttering, treatment of EMG biofeedback, withdrawal of treatment, and then reintroduction of treatment. Results from this study suggest that EMG biofeedback may be effective in reducing stuttering.

Osteopathy

From an osteopathic perspective, stuttering and other impediments of speech may result from mechanical strains in the face, cranium, neck, and jaw. The mandible is in two parts at birth and fuses at mental sometime around age 6 years. Stress and dysfunctions in the cranial base and temporal bones of submandibular tissues may create strains and torsions at the site of ossification. This may influence the position of the tongue and its ability to articulate with the teeth appropriately during speech. The tongue is stabilized below by the hyoid bone, which is suspended from the digastric, stylohyoid, omohyoid, thyrohyoid, and sternohyoid muscles. Mechanical strains that affect the position of the hyoid will alter the position of the tongue. Fascial and muscular strains in the genioglossus, hyloglossus, and geniohyoid will also interfere with tongue mechanics,[1,2] potentially affecting speech.

A. A. Tomatis, a French otolaryngologist, described stuttering as a problem with dominance of the external auditory system.[3] Tomatis explained that alterations in the timing of the passage of sound waves through the external auditory canal or the delivery of auditory signals from the cochlea will influence how the individual interprets the timing of syllables. Within the osteopathic concept of structure and function, the shape of the external auditory canal and middle ear may play a role in how sound and auditory signals are transmitted. The temporal bone is in three parts at birth. Ossification of the cartilaginous areas among the three parts is not complete until age 7 or 8 years.[4] Various authors have described the presence of intraosseous strains in the temporal bone that affect the function of the middle ear and auditory canal in children.[5-7] Cranial techniques may be employed to address these strains and improve temporal bone and oropharyngeal function. Although no controlled studies exist, osteopathic evaluation should be considered in children with a history of stuttering following head, neck, or face trauma.

References

Pediatric Diagnosis and Management

1. Behrman RE, Kliegman RM, Jenson HB, editors: *Nelson textbook of pediatrics*, ed 17, Philadelphia, 2004, Saunders.
2. Kalinowski J, Saltuklaroglu T: The road to efficient and effective stuttering management: information for physicians, *Curr Med Res Opin* 20:509-515, 2004.

3. Koester M, Nekham-Heis D, Matthaus J: My child stutters! Which speech disorders are to be treated by a specialist? [in German], *MMW Fortschr Med* 144:46-48, 2002.
4. Baker BM, Blackwell PB: Identification and remediation of pediatric fluency and voice disorders, *J Pediatr Health Care* 18:87-94, 2004.
5. Olson ED, Bohlman P: IDEA '97 and children who stutter: evaluation and intervention that lead to successful, productive lives, *Semin Speech Lang* 23:159-164, 2002.
6. Whitmire K, Dublinske S: Provision of speech-language services in the schools: working with the law, *Semin Speech Lang* 24:147-153, 2003.
7. Jones M, Onslow M, Harrison E, Packman A: Treating stuttering in young children: predicting treatment time in the Lidcombe Program, *J Speech Lang Hear Res* 43:1440-1450, 2000.
8. Kingston M, Huber A, Onslow M et al: Predicting treatment time with the Lidcombe Program: replication and meta-analysis, *Int J Lang Commun Disord* 38:165-177, 2003.
9. Stuart A, Kalinowski J, Rastatter M et al: Investigations of the impact of altered auditory feedback in-the-ear devices on the speech of people who stutter: initial fitting and 4-month follow-up, *Int J Lang Commun Disord* 39:93-113, 2004.
10. Baumeister H, Caspar F, Herziger F: Treatment outcome study of the stuttering therapy summer camp 2000 for children and adolescents [in German], *Psychother Psychosom Med Psychol* 53:455-463, 2003.
11. Healey EC, Reid R: ADHD and stuttering: a tutorial, *J Fluency Disord* 28:79-92, 2003; quiz 93.
12. Monfrais-Pfauwadel MC, Lacombe I: Attention deficits in the school aged stuttering child: constituent trait or comorbidity [in French], *Rev Laryngol Otol Rhinol (Bord)* 123:291-295, 2002.

Acupuncture

1. Craig AR, Kearns M: Results of a traditional acupuncture intervention for stuttering, *J Speech Hear Res* 38:572-578, 1995.
2. Deadman P, Al-Khafaji M: *A manual of acupuncture*, East Sussex, United Kingdom, 1998, Journal of Chinese Medicine Publications.

Homeopathy

1. *ReferenceWorks Pro 4.2*, San Rafael, Calif, 2008, Kent Homeopathic Associates.

Mind/Body

1. Elliott A, Miltenberger R, Rapp J et al: Brief application of simplified habit reversal to treat stuttering in children, *J Behav Ther Exp Psychiatry* 29:289-302, 1998.
2. Wagaman J, Miltenberger R, Arndorfer R: Analysis of a simplified treatment for stuttering in children, *J Appl Behav Anal* 26:53-61, 1993.
3. Waterloo K, Gotestam K: The regulated-breathing method for stuttering: an experimental evaluation, *J Behav Ther Exp Psychiatry* 19:11-19, 1988.
4. Craig A, Cleary P: Reduction of stuttering by young male stutterers using EMG feedback, *Biofeed Self Reg* 7:241-255, 1982.

Osteopathy

1. Carreiro JE: *An osteopathic approach to children,* London, 2003, Churchill Livingstone.
2. Miller E: Treating the tongue, 2002 [unpublished work].
3. Tomatis AA: *The conscious ear*, Barrytown, NY, 1991, Station Hill Press.
4. Bosma JF: *Anatomy of the infant head,* Baltimore, 1986, Johns Hopkins University Press.
5. Infants and children. In Magoun HIS, editor: *Osteopathy in the cranial field*, Kirksville, Mo, 1951, CJ Krehbiel.
6. Sutherland WG: *Teachings in the science of osteopathy,* Portland, Ore, 1990, Rudra Press.
7. Sutherland WG: *The cranial bowl,* ed 2, 1939, Sutherland.

Thrush

Aromatherapy | Maura A. Fitzgerald
Homeopathy | Janet L. Levatin

✳ PEDIATRIC DIAGNOSIS AND MANAGEMENT

Oral candidiasis, commonly known as *oral thrush*, is a superficial mucous membrane infection usually caused by the yeast *Candida albicans*.[1] It is the most common oral fungal infection. Approximately 2% to 5% of normal newborns acquire *Candida* spp. from their mothers at delivery and remain colonized. Thrush may develop as early as 7 to 10 days of age and appears often within the first year of life from antibiotic treatment[2] or from pacifier use, which can contribute to the colonization and proliferation of yeast in the oral cavity.[3] Oral thrush appears infrequently in older children as an adverse effect of antibiotics or inhaled or topically applied corticosteroids.[4] Incidence of oral candidiasis in hospitals is increasing, with hundreds more strains identified in the neonatal intensive care unit and newborn nursery.[5]

Persistent or recurrent thrush with no obvious predisposing reason, such as recent antibiotic treatment, warrants investigation of an underlying condition such as diabetes mellitus or immunodeficiency, especially vertically transmitted human immunodeficiency virus (HIV) infection. Worldwide reports indicate that oropharyngeal candidiasis is the most common and frequently one of the first signs of HIV infection in children and can be used as a marker for disease progression or for response to treatment.[6-13]

The lesions are usually found as plaques on the surface of the tongue, buccal mucosa, palate, cheeks, and lips.[14] Diagnosis is by clinical presentation. Confirmation of diagnosis can be made by gently removing or scraping the plaques, which causes mild punctate areas of bleeding from the *Candida* spp. lesions.[2]

Thrush may be mild and asymptomatic, requiring no treatment. The baby may be fussy or may decrease intake of nutrients because of pain and discomfort from infection.

The most commonly prescribed antifungal agent is nystatin. Therapeutic agents found to be effective include (in decreasing order of efficacy) miconazole gel, amphotericin B suspension, gentian violet, and nystatin suspension.[2] Resistant strains of *Candida* spp. are emerging in HIV-positive children, making treatment difficult.[15]

✳ CAM THERAPY RECOMMENDATIONS

Aromatherapy

A 2% solution of tea tree oil (*Melaleuca alternifolia*) as a mouthwash has been shown to be effective in older children for oral thrush secondary to immunosuppression.[1]

The solution should be swished around the mouth and then spit out. Although the mouthwash cannot be used in infants, Price and Parr recommend a sterilization solution of 4 drops of tea tree oil in 480 mL (1 pint) of boiled water.[2] Pacifiers and feeding equipment should be soaked for 30 minutes and rinsed well before use.

Homeopathy

Before using this section, please see Appendix A, Homeopathy, for definitions of practitioner expertise categories and general information on prescribing homeopathic medicines.

Practitioner Expertise Category 1

Category 1 includes uncomplicated thrush.

There are no controlled clinical trials of homeopathic treatment for thrush, although the homeopathic literature contains evidence to support its use in the form of accumulated clinical experience.[1] It is safe to use homeopathic treatment for thrush, either alone or in combination with other therapies. Yeast infections may require a combination of systemic and local treatment (herbal, conventional, and/or nutritional).

The goal in treating thrush homeopathically is to determine the single homeopathic medicine whose description in the materia medica most closely matches the symptom picture of the patient. Sometimes mental and emotional states, in addition to physical symptoms, are considered. Once the medicine has been selected, it can be given orally or sublingually in the 30C potency two to three times daily for 3 to 5 days. If the medicine has not helped after several days, then another homeopathic medicine should be tried or some other form of therapy should be instituted as needed. Once symptoms have begun to resolve, the medicine can be given less frequently or stopped. It can be repeated again for a relapse of symptoms.

The following is a list of homeopathic medicines commonly used to treat patients with thrush. It must be emphasized that this list is partial and represents some of the probable choices from the homeopathic materia medica. If the symptoms of a given patient are not represented here, a search of the homeopathic literature would be needed to find the simillimum.

Borax veneta

Borax veneta is the most commonly used homeopathic medicine for thrush. The typical white patches of thrush will be seen inside the mouth. The gums are inflamed and may bleed easily. They child may exhibit fear of downward motion, such as being lowered into a crib.

Mercurius solubilis hahnemanni

Thrush that requires *Mercurius solubilis hahnemanni* will be accompanied by drooling and a bad odor emanating from the mouth. The gums may bleed easily, and the tongue is thickly coated. The child alternates between feeling chilly and feeling hot and may be very sweaty. There may be an increased thirst for cold drinks.

Sulphur

The patient needing sulphur has lips and gums that are red and swollen. The tongue is white in the center and red on the sides and tip. The child is warm and has an increased thirst. Symptoms may be worse at 5 AM.

References

Pediatric Diagnosis and Management

1. Vazquez JA, Sobel JD: Mucosal candidiasis, *Infect Dis Clin North Am* 16:793-820, 2002.
2. Behrman RE, Kliegman RM, Jenson HB, editors: *Nelson textbook of pediatrics,* ed 17, Philadelphia, 2004, Saunders.
3. Mattos-Graner RO, de Moraes AB, Rontani RM et al: Relation of oral yeast infection in Brazilian infants and use of a pacifier, *ASDC J Dent Child* 68:10, 33-36, 2001.
4. Ellepola AN, Samaranayake LP: Inhalational and topical steroids, and oral candidosis: a mini review, *Oral Dis* 7:211-216, 2001.
5. Muriel MA, Vizcaino MJ, Bilbao R et al: Identification of yeast and sensitivity in vitro against different antifungal agents [in Spanish], *Enferm Infecc Microbiol Clin* 18:120-124, 2000 (abstract).
6. Ramos-Gomez F: Dental considerations for the paediatric AIDS/HIV patient, *Oral Dis* 8(Suppl 2):49-54, 2002.
7. Birnbaum W, Hodgson TA, Reichart PA et al: Prognostic significance of HIV-associated oral lesions and their relation to therapy, *Oral Dis* 8(Suppl 2):110-114, 2002.
8. Karande S, Bhalke S, Kelkar A et al: Utility of clinically-directed selective screening to diagnose HIV infection in hospitalized children in Bombay, India, *J Trop Pediatr* 48:149-155, 2002.
9. Gaitan-Cepeda L, Cashat-Cruz M, Morales-Aguirre JJ et al: Prevalence of oral lesions in Mexican children with perinatally acquired HIV: association with immunologic status, viral load, and gender, *AIDS Patient Care STDS* 16:151-156, 2002.
10. Vazquez JA: Therapeutic options for the management of oropharyngeal and esophageal candidiasis in HIV/AIDS patients, *HIV Clin Trials* 1:47-59, 2000.
11. Flaitz CM, Baker KA: Treatment approaches to common symptomatic oral lesions in children, *Dent Clin North Am* 44:671-696, 2000.
12. Korting HC, Schaller M: New developments in medical mycology [in German], *Hautarzt* 52:91-97, 2001.
13. Nicolatou O, Theodoridou M, Mostrou G et al: Oral lesions in children with perinatally acquired human immunodeficiency virus infection, *J Oral Pathol Med* 28:49-53, 1999.
14. Arkell S, Shinnick A: Update on oral candidosis, *Nurs Times* 99:52-53, 2003.
15. Pelletier R, Peter J, Antin C et al: Emergence of resistance of *Candida albicans* to clotrimazole in human immunodeficiency virus-infected children: in vitro and clinical correlations, *J Clin Microbiol* 38:1563-1568, 2000.

Aromatherapy

1. Buckle J: *Clinical aromatherapy: essential oils in practice,* ed 2, Edinburgh, 2003, Churchill Livingstone.
2. Price S, Parr PP: *Aromatherapy for babies and children,* San Francisco, 1996, Thorsons.

Homeopathy

1. *ReferenceWorks Pro 4.2,* San Rafael, Calif, 2008, Kent Homeopathic Associates.

CHAPTER 59

Umbilical Hernia

Homeopathy | Janet L. Levatin

✳ PEDIATRIC DIAGNOSIS AND MANAGEMENT

Umbilical hernias are extremely common in infancy and childhood.[1-3] The hernia is caused by imperfect closure or weakness of the umbilical ring, where protrusion of intraabdominal contents may occur during crying, coughing, or straining and can be reduced easily through the fibrous ring at the umbilicus.[1] Predisposing factors include black race and low birthweight.[4] The incidence is 1.9% to 18.5% in white (Caucasian) children.[1] The occurrence of an umbilical hernia during infancy is congenital. The diagnosis is easily made by physical examination.[2,5]

The size of the defect varies from less than 1 cm in diameter to as much as 5 cm, but large hernias are rare. The great majority of pediatric umbilical hernias are asymptomatic, although they may occasionally cause intermittent umbilical or abdominal pain.[1] Most congenital hernias disappear spontaneously by 1 year of age.[2] Incarceration and strangulation are uncommon. Rupture of umbilical hernia with resultant evisceration is extremely rare. Strapping neither improves nor accelerates closure.[1]

Surgery is not advised unless the hernia persists to age 4 or 5 years, enlarges, causes symptoms, or becomes strangulated or unless the fascial defect becomes progressively larger after the age of 1 to 2 years. Defects exceeding 2 cm are less likely to close spontaneously.[1,4]

✳ CAM THERAPY RECOMMENDATIONS

Homeopathy

Before using this section, please see Appendix A, Homeopathy, for definitions of practitioner expertise categories and general information on prescribing homeopathic medicines.

Clinician Expertise Category 1

Category 1 includes simple umbilical hernia that is not strangulated and is unassociated with other anatomical defects.

There are no controlled clinical trials of homeopathy for treatment of umbilical hernia, although the homeopathic literature contains evidence for its use in the form of accumulated clinical experience.[1] It is safe to try homeopathic treatment for umbilical hernia unassociated with other anatomical defects and unaccompanied with strangulation, prior to beginning conventional therapy (surgery); however, homeopathy is less likely to be effective for an anatomical problem such as umbilical hernia than it is for a functional or energetic problem.

The goal in treating umbilical hernia homeopathically is to determine the single homeopathic medicine whose description in the materia medica most closely matches the symptom picture of the patient. Often mental and emotional states, in addition to physical symptoms, are considered. Once the medicine has been selected, it can be given orally or sublingually in the 30C or 200C potency once daily for 3 days. This regimen could be repeated once every 3 to 4 weeks until some other course of treatment is chosen, if needed. Once the hernia has begun to resolve, the medicine can be given less frequently or stopped.

The following is a list of homeopathic medicines referenced in the homeopathic literature as medicines for patients with umbilical hernia.[1] It must be emphasized that this list is partial and represents some of the probable choices from the homeopathic materia medica. If the symptoms of a given patient are not represented here, a search of the homeopathic literature would be needed to find the simillimum.[1]

Aurum metallicum

The child with an umbilical hernia who needs *Aurum metallicum* is usually observed to be a serious, introverted, responsible child. Crampy abdominal pains may be associated with the hernia. Aurum metallicum may also be tried for inguinal hernias when they occur in a child similar in nature to the one described here.

Calcarea carbonica

Calcarea carbonica is a medicine to consider when the inguinal hernia is present in a child whose abdominal wall muscles seem thin and weak. The child may have low muscle tone in general.

Nux vomica

Nux vomica should be considered when the umbilical hernia occurs in a child or infant with constipation and straining at stool. The patient is colicky and has an irritable, oversensitive nature.

Sulphur

The child with an umbilical hernia who needs *Sulphur* is usually a robust, warm-blooded child.

Veratrum album

The child with an umbilical hernia who needs *Veratrum album* will usually be precocious, restless, and overstimulated. He or she may be prove to bouts of gastroenteritis.

References

Pediatric Diagnosis and Management

1. Marinkovic S, Bukarica S: Umbilical hernia in children [in Serbian], *Med Pregl* 56:291-294, 2003.
2. Graf JL, Caty MG, Martin DJ et al: Pediatric hernias, *Semin Ultrasound CT MR* 23:197-200, 2002.
3. Scherer LR 3rd, Grosfeld JL: Inguinal hernia and umbilical anomalies, *Pediatr Clin North Am* 40:1121-1131, 1993.
4. Behrman RE, Kliegman RM, Jenson HB, editors: *Nelson textbook of pediatrics,* ed 17, Philadelphia, 2004, Saunders.
5. Armstrong O: Umbilical hernia [in French], *Rev Prat* 53:1671-1676, 2003.

Homeopathy

1. *ReferenceWorks Pro 4.2,* San Rafael, Calif, 2008, Kent Homeopathic Associates.

CHAPTER 60

Upper Respiratory Tract Infection

Acupuncture | May Loo
Aromatherapy | Maura A. Fitzgerald
Herbs—Chinese | May Loo

Herbs—Western | Alan D. Woolf, Paula M. Gardiner,
Lana Dvorkin-Camiel, Jack Maypole
Massage Therapy | Mary C. McLellan

PEDIATRIC DIAGNOSIS AND MANAGEMENT

Upper respiratory tract infection (URI), or the common cold, is the most frequent infection in children in the United States and throughout the industrialized world. It is the major cause for visits to pediatrician.[1] A preschool-aged child has an average of 6 to 10 colds per year, and 10% to 15% of school-aged children have at least 12 infections per year. The greatest incidence is from early fall until the late spring,[2] resulting in frequent absences from school.

The clinical symptoms vary greatly without any correlation with specific viruses.[3] The majority of the symptoms are mild, consisting of rhinorrhea, sneezing, nasal congestion and obstruction, postnasal drip, and cough. Additional symptoms of low-grade fever, sore throat, clear eye discharge, digestive discomfort, and general malaise may also be present.[4,5] Some common viruses that cause URI include rhinovirus, coronavirus, adenovirus, respiratory syncytial virus (RSV), influenza, and parainfluenza virus.[3,6,7] Transmission varies with different viruses. RSV spreads primarily through contact with symptomatic children and contaminated objects; influenza spreads mainly via airborne droplets. The precise route of transmission for rhinovirus remains controversial.[6]

The viruses gain entry into host cells through specific viral surface proteins, which cause tissue injury and result in clinical disease.[8] For example, parainfluenza viruses bind to cell surface receptors and then fuse directly with the cell membrane to release the viral replication machinery into the host cell's cytoplasm.[9] Recent studies suggest that it is the host's response to the virus, not the virus itself, that determines the pathogenesis and severity of common cold. Proinflammatory mediators, especially the cytokines, appear to be the central component of the response by infected cells.[10-12]

The virulence of rhinovirus is strongest in infants younger than 1 year (median age 6.5 months)[13] and in immunocompromised children.[14] Wheezing is associated with RSV in children younger than 2 years and with rhinovirus in those older than 2 years.[15] Influenza has an annual attack rate between 15% and 42% in preschool- and school-aged children.[16,17]

Simultaneous infection by more than one virus, such as RSV and adenovirus together, can also occur frequently in the pediatric population.[13] Many children can also have associated bacterial infection, such as *Haemophilus influenzae* conjunctivitis.[13]

Specific viral diagnosis is not necessary, both because of the benign, self-limiting nature of the disease[18] and also because the prevalence of different viruses overlaps from fall to spring, such that it is very difficult to determine precisely which virus or viruses are causing the symptoms.[3] Current medical management of URI remains symptomatic, controversial, and in most cases ineffective. Fluid, rest, humidifier, and saline nose drops constitute the mainstay of nonpharmacological treatment. The role of vitamin C both in prevention and in treatment of the common cold remains controversial.[19,20] Topical adrenergic agents do not have systemic side effects, but overuse can result in rebound congestion.[21]

Systemic medications are primarily used for symptomatic relief of congestion and cough, and most have limited efficacy.[11] Antihistamine and combinations of antihistamine with decongestants are the ingredients in at least 800 over-the-counter (OTC) cold remedies. The majority of studies in the past decade,[5,21-23] as well as recent meta-analyses, continue to conclude that antihistamines and OTC medicines are of marginal or no benefit in treating cold symptoms.[24-26] First-generation antihistamines can cause untoward side effects such as sedation in children.[26] Dextromethorphan is an antitussive that is abundant in OTC formulations. Although this medication is reportedly safe when taken in the recommended dosages, cases of recreational use by teenagers and deaths by overdose have been reported.[27] A 2007 study, which was based on a report by the Centers for Disease Control and Prevention (CDC), reported that three infants died from the toxic effects of cough and cold medicines in 2005, and more than 1500 children younger than 2 years were treated in emergency departments for adverse events related to cough and cold medicines in 2004 and 2005.[27a] As a result, the U.S. Food and Drug Administration issued a statement recommending cough and cold products not be given to children younger than 2 years unless directed by a healthcare provider.

Codeine is ineffective in controlling URI cough.[28] Antibiotics are never indicated for the common cold[5,29,30] but continue to be injudiciously overprescribed, leading to the emergence of more resistant strains of bacteria, higher healthcare costs, and increased risk of side effects.[31-37] During the influenza season, the number of antimicrobial courses prescribed to children increases by 10% to 30%.[17]

Research for new medical therapies for the common cold is directed toward increasing resistance to or immunity against the viruses. Interferons are proteins that can induce a nonspecific resistance to viral infection. However, the usual route of administration is by intramuscular injection, usually given on a daily basis because its blood concentration decreases sharply within 24 hours. In view of the self-limiting nature of URI and the trauma of daily injections, it is unlikely that interferon would be used to treat URI in children.[38] Histamine antagonists are not indicated in the common cold.[39] Antiinflammatory mediators[11] and specific antiviral agents[40] may be promising. Although viral URI is a benign illness of short duration, it can lead to bacterial complications—otitis media, sinusitis and lower respiratory tract infections, or even mastoiditis and meningitis—that have much more significant consequences in children.[41,42] Younger infants are especially susceptible to development of more serious bacterial infections.

The best treatment is prevention. Parents and family members should be educated about washing hands, cleaning environmental surfaces, isolating infants and children with infection, and avoiding crowded places such as busy daycare centers.[22] The American Academy of Pediatrics (AAP) recommends that RSV intravenous immune globulin (RSV-IGIV) and palivizumab, a humanized murine monoclonal antibody, be administered as prophylaxis for prevention of RSV URI, which can lead to severe lower respiratory tract infections in high-risk infants, children younger than 24 months with chronic lung disease, certain preterm infants, and children with congenital heart disease.[43] The CDC has marked vaccine development for RSV "a high priority."[44] The AAP also recommends annual influenza immunization for all children with high-risk conditions who are 6 months of age and older, healthy children 6 through 24 months of age, household contacts and out-of-home caregivers of children younger than 24 months of age, and healthcare professionals.[45] The World Health Organization is attempting to develop and distribute effective vaccines to prevent and/or reduce key viral respiratory diseases.[46]

Development of one single vaccine effective against the common cold is unlikely because of the large number of viral serotypes.[4] Rhinovirus, for example, has at least 100 different immunotypes.[12] The goals of a vaccination program for viral URI are the prevention of lower respiratory tract infections and the prevention of infection-associated morbidities, hospitalization, and mortality.

✳ CAM THERAPY RECOMMENDATIONS

Acupuncture

Traditional Chinese medicine (TCM) defines URI as Wind-Cold, which is similar to but a different description of the Western concept of virus infection as the external cold pathogen transmitted via wind or airborne droplets. Along with symptomatic treatment and home management, TCM also focuses simultaneously on "eliminating the pathogenic factors by supporting the healthy energy,"[1] which translates in biochemical terms as improving the immunity and general health of the child. This is especially important in URI because the host response is of primary importance in pathogenesis of URI and because recurrent URIs are more likely to lead to complications. Because URI,

like asthma, is seasonal, TCM often adopts the tenet of "winter disease, summer cure," advocating the stimulation of pertinent acupoints, such as Wind points, during the summer to prevent URI occurrence during cold weather.[2]

Current reports support efficacy of acupuncture for treating the common cold.[3-6] URI occurs at the most superficial stage of Wind-Cold invasion. Treatment of BL points can be beneficial even in infants.[7] Symptomatic improvement can be substantiated by positive physiological changes. Acupuncture stimulation of LI20 and LI4 has been shown to increase the velocity of the nasal mucociliary transport in chronic rhinitis patients[4]; a pilot study showed change in nasal airway resistance, although the results were not statistically significant.[8]

Although there is a paucity of studies on acupuncture treatment of URI in children, as these children are usually kept at home for observation, results from studies of lower respiratory tract infection, allergic rhinitis, and adult studies can be extrapolated for URI in improvement of immune function and alleviation of symptoms. A clinical report using herbal paste to stimulate acupuncture points in 72 infants with acute bronchitis demonstrated high clinical cure and improvement rate, while laboratory findings revealed an increase in humoral immune substances such as immunoglobulin (Ig)-M, IgG, complement C3, and especially IgA.[9] A double-blind, randomized, placebo-controlled trial from Hong Kong of 85 children treated for persistent allergic rhinitis demonstrated acupuncture as being effective in decreasing acute symptoms and increasing the symptom-free days with no serious adverse effects.[10] Needling general Wind-Cold points in adults—Dazhui (GV14), Fengchi (GB20), and Quchi (LI11)—resulted in decrease in temperature, respiratory rate, pulse, and blood pressure with a simultaneous increase in the percentage of T-lymphocytes.[11] Even massaging local acupoints was effective in relieving symptoms and enhancing immune functions, with increases in immune indices that persisted for at least 6 months.[1] One report of acumassage of Yingxiang LI20 for only 30 seconds resulted in clinical relief from nasal congestion, even though no change in nasal airway resistance or airflow occurred.[12] These reports are encouraging for parents, as acupressure can be easily learned by nonprofessionals; is well tolerated by children of all ages, including infants; has no side effects; and costs nothing.

Acupuncture can be used to treat URI complications such as otitis media or sinusitis. In a clinical study of chronic maxillary sinusitis that included children as young as 3 years, acupuncture treatment resulted in significant improvement of symptoms. However, because of the danger of rapid progression to more serious sequelae, the author recommends that antibiotics still be considered for acute sinusitis.[13]

Treatment

Acupuncture treatment protocol for URI is as follows[14]:
Increase fluid intake.
Decrease Cold energy foods.
General treatment to Dispel Wind—major points BL12, GB20.
Local points for rhinitis: LI20, Yintang, ST2:
    Connect with ion pumping cord: black on LI20 or ST2; red on distal point BL60.

If using magnets, place bionorth (–) pole facing down on LI20 or ST2 and biosouth (+) pole facing down on BL60, and connect with ion pumping cord as previously described.

Use the Five-Element, Four-Point Cold treatment to eliminate Cold from the Bladder channel:

Tonify BL60, SI5; sedate BL66.

ST40 to transform Phlegm.

GV14, LI11 to clear Heat if fever is present.

Tonify immune system.

Home massage program:

Teach parents to massage LI20 for symptomatic relief.

Massage BL meridian for general tonification and improvement of immunity.

Aromatherapy

URI occurs commonly in children. The aromatherapy approach is twofold, using essential oils as preventatives and as treatment for an existing condition. To prevent URI, antiseptic essentials oils can be diffused into common spaces or bedrooms to decrease airborne microorganisms. An effective way to do this is to make a disinfectant room spray. Kelville and Green recommend this mixture: 3 drops eucalyptus (*Eucalyptus* sp.), 1 drop peppermint (*Mentha piperita*), 2 drops pine (*Pinus sylvestris*), 1 drop tea tree (*Melaleuca alternifolia*), and 2 drops bergamot (*Citrus bergamia*) in 1 ounce of water.[1] This should be shaken just before spraying, as the essential oils tend to separate from the water.

Once a child has an URI, essential oils can play a role in reducing symptoms and shortening the course of the illness. Essential oils can continue to be defused in the room, administered by steam inhalation or applied as a chest rub in which case the essentials oils will be both absorbed and inhaled. Essential oils that are antiviral include thyme (*Thymus vulgaris*), rosemary (*Rosmarinus officinalis*), peppermint (*M. piperita*), ravensare (*Ravensara aromatica*), tea tree (*M. alternifolia*), eucalyptus (*Eucalyptus* sp.), and bergamot (*C. bergamia*).[1-3] Price and Parr suggest a mixture of 4 drops tea tree, 2 drops lemon (*Citrus limon*), and 2 drops rose otto (*Rosa damascena*) in 50 mL carrier oil for a cold.[4] They also suggest a mixture of 3 drops sandalwood (*Santalum album*), 2 drops sweet marjoram (*Origanum majorana*), and 2 drops sweet thyme in 50 mL carrier oil if the child has a cough.[4]

A mixture of aromatic oils, camphor, menthol, and eucalyptus in a petroleum base, (Vick's VapoRub, Proctor & Gamble, Cincinnati, Ohio) was studied in a randomized, single-blind, placebo-controlled, crossover design study of 12 adult subjects with chronic bronchitis. In this study, 7.5 grams of the product were inuncted or rubbed on the chest and then covered with a cloth, and the control was the petroleum ointment without aromatic oils. Subjects were randomly assigned to groups and crossed over to the other treatment at a subsequent appointment. There was a significantly enhanced clearance of mucus at 30 minutes and 60 minutes in subjects exposed to the active substance, with no difference during the subsequent 5 hours.[5]

Herbs—Chinese

Windbreaker is a formula of 21 herbs (Chinese Modular Solutions) designed to clear Wind, Heat, and Phlegm, treating the acute inflammatory stage of colds as well as lingering congestion. The formula is available as a liquid alcohol extract. The alcohol can be removed by placing the drops in a small amount of hot water and allowing it to cool before administration. The dose is 1 dropperful every 3 hours in babies and 2 to 3 droppersful for children 2 years and older (see Appendix C).[1]

Herbs—Western

Echinacea, a member of the Asteraceae/Compositae family, may be found or used in a variety of species, including *Echinacea angustifolia*, *Echinacea purpurea*, and *Echinacea pallida*.

Taking echinacea orally might help reduce severity of symptoms and duration of the common cold in adults by about 10% to 30%[1-9] or may show no benefit, according to results of other trials.[10-12] Research conducted with *E. purpurea* juice extract in children aged 2 to 11 years suggested lack of effectiveness for the treatment of cold symptoms.[13] In this study, *E. purpurea* 3.75 mL or 5 mL was taken twice daily based on age. Children in the treatment group were more likely to develop a rash than children taking placebo.[13] The best time to take echinacea is not prophylactically, but rather at the initial stages of symptoms, continuing the therapy for 7 to 10 days. Some common side effects reported with the use of echinacea include allergic reactions and gastrointestinal symptoms.

A combination of echinacea, propolis, and vitamin C—an herbal preparation (Chizukit) containing 50 mg/mL echinacea, 50 mg/mL propolis, and 10 mg/mL vitamin C—has been reported to reduce the number and duration of cold episodes in children.[14] Unfortunately, overall prevention research has not been well designed; therefore additional research must be conducted before making conclusions and clear recommendations.

Massage Therapy

In 1998, Children's Hospital Boston established the Center for Holistic Pediatric Education and Research (CHPER) to provide complementary and alternative medicine (CAM) consultations and education to inpatients at this hospital. Between 1999 and 2004, 762 consults were provided to patients on the Pulmonary Service; the chief complaints initiating the consultation were pain in the back, upper body, chest, and neck as well as anxiety. During acute or chronic respiratory infections, chest, shoulder, neck, and back discomfort may develop from persistent cough.[1-3] This pain or discomfort could lead to ineffective cough and deep breathing as a result of splinting.[1-3] To help decrease the musculoskeletal pain associated with coughing, children experiencing respiratory infections could benefit from back, shoulder, and anterior chest wall massage therapy with particular attention to the intercostals, scalenes, serratus, pectorals, and trapezius. Should cough-related pain or discomfort extend to the abdomen, massage to the intercostals and external obliques may also be helpful. If children are splinting with cough or laughter or indicating it hurts too much to laugh, this would be a good indication to try some massage to improve their comfort level. Children experiencing respiratory illness may feel more comfortable in an upright position during treatment rather than lying down. To treat the child in an upright position, he or she can be positioned in a chair with the head supported by a table-top pillow or seated upright in the parent's lap with the head resting on the parent's chest or shoulder. Infants and young children can readily be treated while cradled on their parent's shoulder or chest.

In addition to massage being helpful for cough-related pain, massage can also help relax or calm the child or infant who may be experiencing increased work of breathing or intermittent bronchospasms due to illness. Controlled studies have demonstrated decreased anxiety levels in children with asthma or cystic fibrosis who receive parental Swedish massage.[4,5] These studies have also demonstrated increased peak flow readings and improved pulmonary function tests in the massage-treated children compared with controls. Small studies in adult populations with pulmonary disease have also demonstrated improved peak flows[6,7] as well as decreased respiratory rate and increased chest wall expansion.[7]

Chest physiotherapy (CPT), which incorporates percussion and vibration, originated from use of massage in postoperative patients in the seventeenth century.[8] CPT has become a standard of care in hospital settings to prevent and treat atelectasis, ineffective cough, and respiratory secretion management.

References

Pediatric Diagnosis and Management

1. Pitrez PM, Pitrez JL: Acute upper respiratory tract infections: outpatient diagnosis and treatment [in Portuguese], *J Pediatr (Rio J)* 79(Suppl 1):S77-S86, 2003.
2. Behrman RE, Kliegman RM, Jenson HB, editors: *Nelson textbook of pediatrics*, ed 17, Philadelphia, 2004, Saunders.
3. Freymuth F, Vabret A, Gouarin S et al: Epidemiology of respiratory virus infections [in French], *Allergy Immunol (Paris)* 33:66-69, 2001 (abstract).
4. Kirkpatrick GL: The common cold, *Primary Care* 23:657-675, 1996.
5. Middleton DB: An approach to pediatric upper respiratory infections, *Am Fam Physician* 44(5 Suppl):33S-40S, 46S-47S, 1991.
6. Goldmann DA: Transmission of viral respiratory infections in the home, *Pediatr Infect Dis J* 19(10 Suppl):S97-S102, 2000.
7. El-Sahly HM, Atmar RL, Glezen WP et al: Spectrum of clinical illness in hospitalized patients with "common cold" virus infections, *Clin Infect Dis* 31:96-100, 2000.
8. Walker TA, Khurana S, Tilden SJ: Viral respiratory infections, *Pediatr Clin North Am* 41:1365-1381, 1994.
9. Moscona A: Entry of parainfluenza virus into cells as a target for interrupting childhood respiratory disease, *J Clin Invest* 115:1688-1698, 2005.
10. Stickler GB, Smith TF, Broughton DD: The common cold, *Eur J Pediatr* 144:4-8, 1985.
11. Turner RB: Epidemiology, pathogenesis, and treatment of the common cold, *Ann Allergy Asthma Immunol* 78:531-539, 1997.
12. Hendley JO: Clinical virology of rhinoviruses, *Adv Virus Res* 54:453-466, 1999.
13. Pierres-Surer N, Beby-Defaux A, Bourgoin A et al: Rhinovirus infections in hospitalized children: a 3-year study [in French], *Arch Pediatr* 5:9-14, 1998 (abstract).
14. Pitkaranta A, Hayden FG: Rhinoviruses: important respiratory pathogens, *Ann Med* 30:529-537, 1998.
15. Rakes GP, Arruda E, Ingram JM et al: Rhinovirus and respiratory syncytial virus in wheezing children requiring emergency care: IgE and eosinophil analyses, *Am J Resp Crit Care Med* 159:785-790, 1999.
16. Glezen WP, Couch RB: Interpandemic influenza in the Houston area, 1974–76, *N Engl J Med* 298:587-592, 1978.
17. Neuzil KM, Zhu Y, Griffin MR et al: Burden of interpandemic influenza in children younger than 5 years: a 25-year prospective study, *J Infect Dis* 185:147-152, 2002.
18. Nahmias A, Yolken R, Keyserling H: Rapid diagnosis of viral infections: a new challenge for the pediatrician, *Adv Pediatr* 32:507-525, 1984.
19. Kasa RM: Vitamin C: from scurvy to the common cold, *Am J Med Tech* 49:23-26, 1983.
20. Hemila H: Vitamin C supplementation and common cold symptoms: problems with inaccurate reviews, *Nutrition* 12:804-809, 1996.
21. Fireman P: Pathophysiology and pharmacotherapy of common upper respiratory diseases, *Pharmacotherapy* 13:101S, 143S, 1993.
22. Luks D, Anderson MR: Antihistamines and the common cold: a review and critique of the literature, *J Gen Intern Med* 11:240-244, 1996.
23. Smith MB, Feldman W: Over the counter cold medications: a critical review of clinical trials between 1950 and 1991, *J Am Med Assoc* 269:2258, 1993.
24. Schroeder K, Fahey T: Over-the-counter medications for acute cough in children and adults in ambulatory settings, *Cochrane Database Syst Rev* (4):CD001831, 2004.
25. Schroeder K, Fahey T: Should we advise parents to administer over the counter cough medicines for acute cough? Systematic review of randomised controlled trials, *Arch Dis Child* 86:170-175, 2002.
26. Sutter AI, Lemiengre M, Campbell H et al: Antihistamines for the common cold, *Cochrane Database Syst Rev* (3):CD001267, 2003.
27. Murray S, Brewerton T: Abuse of over-the-counter dextromethorphan by teenagers, *South Med J* 86:1151-1153, 1993.
27a. Traynor K: Nonprescription cold remedies unsafe for children, FDA advisers say, *Am J Health Syst Pharm* 64:2408-2410, 2007.
28. Eccles R. Codeine, cough and upper respiratory infection, *Pulmon Pharmacol* 9:293-297, 1996.
29. Dowell SF, Schwartz B, Phillips WR: Appropriate use of antibiotics for URIs in children: part I. Otitis media and acute sinusitis. The Pediatric URI Consensus Team, *Am Fam Physician* 58:1113-1118, 1123, 1998.
30. Dowell SF, Schwartz B, Phillips WR: Appropriate use of antibiotics for URIs in children: part II. Cough, pharyngitis and the common cold. The Pediatric URI Consensus Team, *Am Fam Physician* 58:1335-1342, 1345, 1998.
31. Mainous AG III, Hueston WJ, Clark JR: Antibiotics and upper respiratory infection: do some folks think there is a cure for the common cold? *J Fam Practice* 42:357, 1996.
32. English JA, Bauman KA: Evidence-based management of upper respiratory infection in a family practice teaching clinic, *Fam Med* 29:38, 1997.
33. Nambiar S, Schwartz RH, Sheridan MJ: Are pediatricians adhering to principles of judicious antibiotic use for upper respiratory tract infections? *South Med J* 95:1163-1167, 2002.
34. Gonzales R, Malone DC, Maselli JH et al: Excessive antibiotic use for acute respiratory infections in the United States, *Clin Infect Dis* 33:757-762, 2001.
35. Gaur AH, Hare ME, Shorr RI: Provider and practice characteristics associated with antibiotic use in children with presumed viral respiratory tract infection, *Pediatrics* 115:635-642, 2005.
36 Jelinski S, Parfrey P, Hutchinson J: Antibiotic utilisation in community practices: guideline concurrence and prescription necessity, *Pharmacoepidemiol Drug Saf* 14:319-326, 2005.
37. Fakih MG, Hilu RC, Savoy-Moore RT et al: Do resident physicians use antibiotics appropriately in treating upper respiratory infections? A survey of 11 programs, *Clin Infect Dis* 37:853-856, 2003. Epub 2003 Aug 27.

38. Houglum JE: Interferon: mechanisms of action and clinical value, *Clin Pharmacol* 2:20-28, 1983.

39. Seidenberg J: Antihistamines in pediatrics [in German], *Monatsschr Kinderheilkd* 137:54-56, 1989 (abstract).

40. Saroea HG: Common colds. Causes, potential cures, and treatment, *Can Fam Physician* 39:2215-2216; 2219–2220, 1993.

41. Pitkaranta A, Hayden FG. Rhinoviruses: important respiratory pathogens, *Ann Med* 30:529-537, 1998.

42. Isaacson G: Sinusitis in childhood, *Pediatr Clin North Am* 436:1297, 1996.

43. AAP Policy Statement: revised indications for the use of palivizumab and respiratory syncytial virus immune globulin intravenous for the prevention of respiratory syncytial virus infections—Committee on Infectious Diseases and Committee on Fetus and Newborn, *Pediatrics* 112:1442-1446, 2003.

44. Centers for Disease Control and Prevention: *The Advisory Committee on Immunization Practices national immunization program, 2004.* Available at www.cdc.gov/vaccines/recs/acip/downloads/min-archive/min-june04.rtf. Accessed August 15, 2005.

45. AAP Policy Statement: Recommendations for influenza immunization of children—Committee on Infectious Diseases, *Pediatrics* 113:1441-1447, 2004.

46. World Health Organization: *Communicable diseases.* Available at www.searo.who.int/ LinkFiles/ RC_54_WorkofWHO. pdf. Accessed August 15, 2005.

Acupuncture

1. Zhu S, Wang N, Wang D et al: A clinical investigation on massage for prevention and treatment of recurrent respiratory tract infection in children, *J Tradit Chin Med* 18:285-291, 1998.

2. Chen K, Li S, Shi Z et al: Two hundred and seventeen cases of winter diseases treated with acupoint stimulation in summer, *J Tradit Chin Med* 20:198-201, 2000.

3. Hu J: Acupuncture treatment of common cold, *J Tradit Chin Med* 20:227-230, 2000.

4. Xu J: Influence of acupuncture on human nasal mucociliary transport [in Chinese], *Zhonghua Er Bi Yan Hou Ke Za Zhi* 24:90-91, 127, 1989.

5. Yu S, Cao J, Yu Z: Acupuncture treatment of chronic rhinitis in 75 cases, *J Tradit Chin Med* 13:103-105, 1993.

6. Oskolkova MK, Podgalo DA, Briazgunov IP et al: Acupuncture and electropuncture in the overall therapy of diseases in children [in Russian], *Pediatriia* Mar:53-56, 1980 (abstract).

7. Long X, Chang Q, Shou Q: Clinical observation on 46 cases of infantile repeated respiratory tract infection treated by mild-moxibustion over acupoints on back, *J Tradit Chin Med* 21:23-26, 2001.

8. Davies A, Lewith G, Goddard J et al: The effect of acupuncture on nonallergic rhinitis: a controlled pilot study, *Altern Ther Health Med* 4:70-74, 1998.

9. Yu P, Hao X, Zhao R et al: Pasting acupoints with Chinese herbs applying in infant acute bronchitis and effect on humoral immune substances [in Chinese], *Zhen Ci Yan Jiu* 17:110-112, 1992 (abstract).

10. Ng DK, Chow PY, Ming SP et al: A double-blind, randomized, placebo-controlled trial of acupuncture for the treatment of childhood persistent allergic rhinitis, *Pediatrics* 114:1242-1247, 2004.

11. Tan D: Treatment of fever due to exopathic wind-cold by rapid acupuncture, *J Tradit Chin Med* 12:267-271, 1992.

12. Takeuchi H, Jawad MS, Eccles R: The effects of nasal massage of the "yingxiang" acupuncture point on nasal airway resistance and sensation of nasal airflow in patients with nasal congestion associated with acute upper respiratory tract infection, *Am J Rhinol* 13:77-79, 1999.

13. Pothman R, Yeh HL: The effects of treatment with antibiotics, laser and acupuncture upon chronic maxillary sinusitis in children, *Am J Chin Med* 10:55-58, 1982.

14. Loo M: *Pediatric acupuncture*, London, 2002, Elsevier.

Aromatherapy

1. Keville K, Green M: *Aromatherapy: a complete guide to the healing art*, Berkeley, Calif, 1995, The Crossing Press.

2. Buckle J: *Clinical aromatherapy: essential oils in practice*, ed 2, Edinburgh, 2003, Churchill Livingstone.

3. Price S, Price L: *Aromatherapy for health professionals*, Edinburgh, 1995, Churchill Livingstone.

4. Price S, Parr PP: *Aromatherapy for babies and children*, San Francisco, 1996, Thorsons.

5. Hasani A, Pavia D, Toms N et al: Effect of aromatics on lung mucociliary clearance in patients with chronic airways obstruction, *J Altern Complement Med* 9:243-249, 2003.

Herbs—Chinese

1. Neustaedter R: Personal communication, August 2005.

Herbs—Western

1. Brinkeborn RM, Shah DV, Degenring FH: Echinaforce and other Echinacea fresh plant preparations in the treatment of the common cold. A randomized, placebo controlled, double-blind clinical trial, *Phytomedicine* 6:1-6, 1999.

2. Barrett B, Vohmann M, Calabrese C: Echinacea for upper respiratory infection, *J Fam Pract* 48:628-635, 1999.

3. Lindenmuth GF, Lindenmuth EB: The efficacy of echinacea compound herbal tea preparation on the severity and duration of upper respiratory and flu symptoms: a randomized, double-blind, placebo-controlled study, *J Altern Complement Med* 6:327-334, 2000.

4. Dorn M, Knick E, Lewith G: Placebo-controlled, double-blind study of *Echinacea pallida* radix in upper respiratory tract infections, *Complement Ther Med* 5:40-42, 1997.

5. Henneicke-von Zepelin H, Hentschel C, Schnitker J et al: Efficacy and safety of a fixed combination phytomedicine in the treatment of the common cold (acute viral respiratory tract infection): results of a randomised, double blind, placebo-controlled, multicentre study, *Curr Med Res Opin* 15:214-227, 1999.

6. Giles JT, Palat CT III, Chien SH et al: Evaluation of echinacea for treatment of the common cold, *Pharmacother* 20:690-697, 2000.

7. Melchart D, Linde K, Fischer P, et al: Echinacea for preventing and treating the common cold, *Cochrane Database Syst Rev* 2: CD000530, 2000.

8. Schulten B, Bulitta M, Ballering-Bruhl B et al: Efficacy of *Echinacea purpurea* in patients with a common cold. A placebo-controlled, randomised, double-blind clinical trial, *Arzneimittelforschung* 51:563-568, 2001.

9. Goel V, Lovlin R, Barton R et al: Efficacy of a standardized echinacea preparation (Echinilin) for the treatment of the common cold: a randomized, double-blind, placebo-controlled trial, *J Clin Pharm Ther* 29:75-83, 2004.

10. Grimm W, Muller HH: A randomized controlled trial of the effect of fluid extract of *Echinacea purpurea* on the incidence and severity of colds and respiratory infections, *Am J Med* 106:138-143, 1999.

11. Barrett BP, Brown RL, Locken K et al: Treatment of the common cold with unrefined echinacea. A randomized, double-blind, placebo-controlled trial, *Ann Intern Med* 137:939-946, 2002.

12. Yale SH, Liu K: *Echinacea purpurea* therapy for the treatment of the common cold: a randomized, double-blind, placebo-controlled clinical trial, *Arch Intern Med* 164:1237-1241, 2004.

13. Taylor JA, Weber W, Standish L et al: Efficacy and safety of echinacea in treating upper respiratory tract infections in children: a randomized controlled trial, *J Am Med Assoc* 290:2824-2830, 2003.

14. Cohen HA, Varsano I, Kahan E et al: Effectiveness of an herbal preparation containing echinacea, propolis, and vitamin C in preventing respiratory tract infections in children: a randomized, double-blind, placebo-controlled, multicenter study, *Arch Pediatr Adolesc Med* 158:217-221, 2004.

Massage Therapy

1. Boat TF: Cystic fibrosis. In Behrman RE, Kliegman R, Jenson HB, editors: *Nelson textbook of pediatrics,* ed 17, Philadelphia, 2004, Saunders.

2. Shafer TH, Wolfson MR, Bhutani VK: Respiratory muscle function, assessment and training, *Phys Ther* 61:1711-1723, 1983.

3. Warren A: Mobilization of the chest wall, *Phys Ther* 48:582-585, 1968.

4. Field T, Henteleff T, Hernandez-Reif M et al: Children with asthma have improved pulmonary functions after massage therapy, *J Pediatr* 132:854-858, 1998.

5. Hernandez-Reif M, Field T, Krasnegor J et al: Children with cystic fibrosis benefit from massage therapy, *J Pediatr Psychol* 24: 175-181, 1999.

6. Beeken JE, Parks D, Cory J et al: The effectiveness of neuromuscular release massage therapy in five individuals with chronic obstructive lung disease, *Clin Nurs Res* 7:309-325, 1998.

7. Witt P, MacKinnon J: Psychological integration: a method to improve chest mobility of patients with chronic lung disease, *Phys Ther* 66:214-217, 1986.

8. Fritz S: *Mosby's fundamentals of therapeutic massage,* ed 3, St Louis, 2005, Mosby.

Urinary Tract Infection

Acupuncture | May Loo

Chiropractic | Anne Spicer

Herbs—Western | Alan D. Woolf, Paula M. Gardiner,
Lana Dvorkin-Camiel, Jack Maypole

Homeopathy | Janet L. Levatin

Osteopathy | Jane Carreiro

Probiotics | Russell H. Greenfield

✳ PEDIATRIC DIAGNOSIS AND MANAGEMENT

Urinary tract infection (UTI)* occurs frequently in the pediatric population,[1-3] affecting an estimated 6.5% of girls and 3.3% of boys in their first year of life.[3] Approximately 3% to 5% of all girls and 1.0% of all boys have at least one UTI between infancy and late teenage years.[4] There is a striking female preponderance after 1 to 2 years of age, with a 10:1 female-to-male ratio.[2,4] UTI in children is often underdiagnosed. Both diagnosis and treatment, especially in infants and young children, are challenging to the general pediatrician.

The risk factors for developing UTI vary according to the age of the child. Congenital anomalies that cause obstruction and reflux are the major factors predisposing infants and young children to UTI. School-aged children often hold back urine and delay urination for an extended period of time, especially when they are on the playground. Sexual activity is often associated with UTI in the adolescent.[6] Local immunological impairment of the urinary tract (e.g., presence of P1 blood group antigen, increased urothelial colonization) also contribute to development of UTI.[2] The overall health and immune status of the child is also important in determining severity of infection.[7] The highest incidence for first-time UTI is found in infants younger than 1 year.[8] UTI in infants and young children less than 2 years old is a special challenge for several reasons: (1) the manifestations of UTI in this age group tend to be nonspecific and often manifest as unexplained high fever,[8] such that the diagnosis can be easily missed and prevalence underestimated[7]; (2) it is difficult to obtain a clean, midstream urine in the diapered population; and (3) the young kidney is most vulnerable to infection,[9] such that the early infections often rapidly progress to pyelonephritis.[8] Circumscision[9,10] and breastfeeding[9] seem to offer some protection against UTI in babies.

In 1999, the Urinary Tract Subcommittee of the American Academy of Pediatrics (AAP) Committee on Quality Improvement developed an evidence-based practice parameter on the diagnosis, treatment, and evaluation of an initial UTI in febrile infants and young children between the ages of 2 months and 2 years. The recommendations included emphasis of the need

for culturing appropriately collected specimens: transurethral catheterization or suprapubic bladder tap are needed to obtain an uncontaminated urine specimen in this age group.[3,11]

The classic signs and symptoms of urinary cystitis in older children include dysuria (burning sensation or pain with urination), increased frequency, nocturnal enuresis, abdominal and suprapubic pain, urgency, and cloudy (pyuria) or bloody urine (hematuria).[12]

Diagnosis is based on a properly collected urine culture with more than 100,000 colonies of a single pathogen. The most common organism in children is *Escherichia coli*,[4] which accounts for 90% of first episodes of acute cystitis in children and 75% of recurrent infections.[11] The pathogenic virulence of *E. coli* in UTI is in its ability to adhere to uroepithelial cells and red blood cells.[11] *Klebsiella* spp. and *Proteus* spp. are more preponderant in girls, whereas gram-positive organisms occur more frequently in boys. *Staphylococcus saprophyticus* occurs in both sexes. Viral infections, especially adenovirus,[4] fungal, and parasitical infections, may also cause UTI.[13]

The AAP recommends that all infants with documented UTI undergo complete imaging studies to include ultrasonography and either voiding cystourethrogram (VCUG) or radionuclide cystourethrography in order to assess the abnormalities that predispose children to reflux and pyelonephritis and to assess the extent of renal involvement during infection.[3,14] Although many clinicians still advocate ultrasound as the imaging modality of choice,[15] some clinicians recently consider sonography to be of little value and the utility of VCUG, especially in children older than 1 year, to require review.[16] There is no agreement on the most appropriate combination of studies in older children, because subjecting the child to an invasive procedure is weighed against the low possibility of finding a congenital anomaly.[14]

Prompt diagnosis and treatment are important to prevent pyelonephritic scarring, especially in the first year of life. Renal scarring is associated with development of hypertension in about 10% of children and accounts for approximately 20% of children with end-stage renal disease who require dialysis or even renal transplant.[17] The severity of renal scarring is directly related to delay in diagnosis.[18] The treatment is with antibiotics, both for its bactericidal effect and also (probably) for reducing adhesion capability of bacteria to the urothelium.[4,19] The AAP has recommended treatment for 7 to 14 days if an appropriate clinical response is observed,[3] although many clinicians currently

---

*In this discussion, *urinary tract infection* refers only to urinary cystitis, or bladder infection.

consider a shorter course of 2 to 4 days as sufficient for uncomplicated infection.[16] A repeat microbiological examination 48 to 72 hours after institution of treatment and a follow-up culture within 1 week after cessation of therapy are recommended.[4]

Prophylaxis has been considered important in pediatric UTI; children who are found to have vesicoureteric reflux are often managed with a single daily dose of antibiotics for 3 to 6 months to prevent recurrence.[12,17] However, whether such treatment is advantageous in these children is questionable. Although prophylaxis does prevent recurrence, there is no evidence that it improves long-term outcome.[16] Children with underlying genitourinary abnormalities such as congenital anomalies or obstructive uropathy need to be treated for at least 1 year.[12] High-risk children, such as siblings, should be investigated for reflux.[18] Adolescents should be counseled about the relationship between sexual activities and the development of UTI.[6]

Asymptomatic bacteriuria has been a topic of concern for pediatricians. At this time, screening for bacteriuria in healthy infants and children does not appear necessary. Although bacteriuria may be found in 1% to 2% of the pediatric population, asymptomatic children have a very high rate of spontaneous clearing of the bacteriuria, which in itself does not destroy the renal parenchyma.[4,20]

✳ CAM THERAPY RECOMMENDATIONS

Acupuncture

There are no data at this time on acupuncture treatment[1] of UTI in children. In a three-arm randomized controlled trial of 67 adult Scandinavians that compared real acupuncture, sham acupuncture, and an untreated control group, acupuncture was found to significantly prevent recurrent lower UTI at 6-month follow-up: 85% of the acupuncture group had zero recurrence of cystitis compared with 58% in the sham group and 36% in the control group.[2]

Because of scarring and renal complications, an integrative approach to urinary cystitis would be important, especially in infants and young children. Western laboratory confirmation should be used both to make a definitive diagnosis and for follow-up evaluation. Acupuncture can be an adjunctive therapy with antibiotics for acute episodes and as prophylaxis to prevent recurrences.

Traditional Chinese medicine defines urinary cystitis primarily as Damp-Heat in the Bladder. This can occur as an acute Damp-Heat invasion or as a chronic, recurrent condition due to Spleen deficiency, Liver and Gallbladder Heat, or Kidney Yin deficiency.

Acute infections are due to invasion of Heat combined with Dampness in the Bladder. Spleen deficiency predisposes the child to chronic, recurrent infections.

Acute urinary cystitis—Damp-Heat invasion

Treatment recommendations. The Damp-Heat in the urinary system obstructs the water passages, so the treatment for all bladder infections needs to expel Heat and dispel Dampness from the Bladder and open water passages.

Increase fluid intake, and encourage the child to empty the bladder whenever it feels full.

Decrease energetically Hot foods and Phlegm-producing foods.

ST40 to disperse Dampness.

Expel Heat from Bladder using the Five-Element, Four-Point protocol:
    Tonify BL66; sedate BL60, SI5.

Treat CV3, BL28, the Mu and Shu points of Bladder, to clear Heat and drain Dampness.

BL22, Back Shu of Triple Heater, promotes the transformation of fluids and the separation of clear from turbid in the Lower Burner; drains Dampness from the Lower Burner.

SP9 drains Damp-Heat from the Lower Burner.

BL63 stops pain in the BL channel.

LU7 is the confluent point of the Conception vessel and regulates Water passages, especially in descending fluids to the Bladder.

Tonify Spleen with either SP3, meridian tonification, or Five-Element, Four-Point protocol:
    Tonify SP2, HT8; sedate SP1, LR1.

After the acute infection clears, strengthen the child with the immune protocol.

Chronic, recurrent cystitis

Spleen Qi deficiency

Because both acute and chronic cases of urinary cystitis have Damp-Heat in the Bladder, the acute treatments are also applicable for chronic cystitis.

Avoid artificially sweetened foods.

Vigorously tonify the Spleen with the Four-Point protocol.

Modify lifestyle to allow the child to feel less pressure from schoolwork and other activities and to minimize worry.

Liver and Gallbladder Heat. Liver and Gallbladder Heat is rarely seen in babies and very young children, and it tends to affect children in the Wood phase of development when the Liver and Gallbladder are vulnerable.

Treatment as listed for acute UTI.

Avoid greasy or sour foods.

LR3 and LR13 to move Liver Qi.

Disperse Heat in the Liver and Gallbladder channels with Four-Point protocol:
    Liver Heat: Tonify LR2, KI10; sedate LR8, HT8.
        Two points: Tonify LR2; sedate LR8.
    Gallbladder Heat: Tonify GB43, BL66; sedate GB38, SI5.
        Two points: Tonify GB43; sedate GB38.

Modify lifestyle to diminish stress that causes frustration and irritability.

Decrease medications, especially excessive over-the-counter medications.

Tonify Spleen.

Kidney deficiency. *Kidney deficiency* can refer to UTI during infancy or in children with congenital renal anomalies.

Treatment as listed for acute UTI.

Avoid salty foods.

Tonify Kidney Yin and Kidney Yang:
    KI3 tonifies KI Yin, Essence, and KI Yang.

Overall Kidney tonification with Four-Point protocol:
Tonify KI7, LU8; sedate KI3, SP3.

Modify lifestyle to minimize fearful situations. Family or individual therapy may be needed if a great deal of family dysfunction or other factors that precipitate Fear in the child are present.

Chiropractic

The chiropractic approach to the child with UTI would be to remove any interference to normal neurological and physiological function. Particular attention would be addressed to the T9-L2 spinal segments.[1]

Sharon Vallone, DC, reports a case of a 7-year-old girl who sustained an injury to the lumbosacral junction (without lasting pain) and shortly thereafter developed UTIs. Twenty-one infections occurred during the next 24 months. Treatments included antibiotics, homeopathy, and hygiene alterations without resolution. Chiropractic adjustments were given two times per week for 3 weeks with complete resolution of symptoms and infection. There was no recurrence of the infection at a 9-week follow-up.[2]

Focal, deep tissue massage at the superior ramus of the pubis at the midline and at the upper edges of the bilateral transverse processes of L2 may reflexively reduce bladder pain.[3]

Unsweetened cranberry juice may create an increased resistance to bacteria within the lining of the bladder.[1]

Consumption of garlic, either fresh in foods or in capsule form, has a mild bacteriocidal effect.

Increase fluid intake.

Avoid caffeine and sugar.

Teas made of couchgrass and/or cornsilk are soothing diuretics.[4] Bearberry has astringent and antiseptic qualities but must be used with caution because prolonged use irritates the urinary tract.[5] A 3-day course should be sufficient to control the infection.

Soaking in a hot tub may relieve some of the pain intensity and relax agitated muscle.

Allergy must be ruled out, as persistence or recurrence of UTIs may be associated with detrusor spasm secondary to allergy.[6]

Referral to a licensed acupuncturist may relieve symptoms.

Medical referral for antibiotic therapy must be considered if symptomatic improvement is not noted after a brief trial of conservative care.

Supplementation with probiotics to restore normal flora is a necessary course of management after any course of antibiotic therapy.

Herbs—Western

Cranberry, or *Vaccinium macrocarpon*, has multiple synonyms, including *Oxycoccus macrocarpos*, *Vaccinium oxycoccos*, *Oxycoccus hagerupii*, *Oxycoccus microcarpus*, *Oxycoccus palustris*, *Oxycoccus quadripetalus*, *Vaccinium hagerupii*, *Vaccinium microcarpum*, and *Vaccinium palustre*. It belongs to the Ericaceae family. Cranberry juice consumed on a daily basis (300 mL) appears to prevent UTIs in young and elderly women. The studies have been primarily sponsored by Ocean Spray, a juice manufacturer.[1-3]

Unfortunately, cranberry juice or extract does not seem to prevent UTIs associated with neurogenic bladder in adults and children.[4-6]

It appears that cranberry may be helpful for the treatment of UTIs only when it is used as an adjunct therapy to treatments such as antibiotics. There are no well-designed trials supporting the use of cranberries alone for UTIs, and in vitro research does not prove cranberry's effectiveness when used alone.

This plant is generally well tolerated, but in large doses (>3 to 4 L/day) it can cause gastrointestinal upset and diarrhea. Use of doses >1 L per day on a long-term basis might increase risk of uric acid kidney stone formation.[7]

Peppermint may be found as *Mentha piperita* or *Mentha lavanduliodora* and is of the Lamiaceae/Labiatae family. Currently peppermint tea is not recommended alone for the treatment of UTI, as there is no clear evidence supporting its effectiveness for the treatment of this condition because of limited study of peppermint tea and other therapies.

Homeopathy

Before using this section, please see Appendix A, Homeopathy, for definitions of practitioner expertise categories and general information on prescribing homeopathic medicines.

Practitioner Expertise Category 1

Category 1 includes bladder infections/urinary cystitis unassociated with urosepsis or pyelonephritis.

Practitioner Expertise Category 3

Category 3 includes recurrent, chronic, or complex bladder infections/urinary cystitis.

There are no controlled clinical trials of homeopathic treatment of bladder infections, although the homeopathic literature contains much evidence for its use in the form of accumulated clinical experience.[1] Acute bladder infections unassociated with urosepsis, pyelonephritis, or other complications can often be treated effectively with homeopathy in children old enough to report their symptoms (approximately 4 years of age or older). If a bacterial infection is suspected, a urinalysis and urine culture should be obtained. While culture results are pending, it is safe to try homeopathic treatment in a clinically stable patient for 1 or 2 days prior to beginning antibiotic therapy. Homeopathy could also be used in conjunction with antibiotic therapy if the urinalysis is suggestive of a bacterial infection for which antibiotic treatment would be helpful or if the patient's clinical condition warrants antibiotic treatment. If antibiotic treatment is used, concurrent use of probiotics may help offset any disruption of the normal intestinal flora.

The goal in treating cystitis homeopathically is to determine the single homeopathic medicine whose description in the materia medica most closely matches the symptom picture of the patient. Often mental and emotional states, in addition to physical symptoms, are considered. Once the medicine has been selected, it can be given orally or sublingually in the 30C potency every 2 to 3 hours. If it has not helped in four to five doses, then another homeopathic medicine should be tried or some other form of therapy should be instituted as needed. Once symptoms have begun to resolve, the medicine can be given less frequently or stopped. It can be repeated again for a relapse of symptoms.

The following is a list of homeopathic medicines commonly used to treat patients with bladder infections. It must be emphasized that this list is partial and represents some of the probable choices from the homeopathic materia medica. If the symptoms of a given patient are not represented here, a search of the homeopathic literature would be needed to find the simillimum.

Cantharis vesicatoria

Cantharis vesicatoria is one of the main homeopathic medicines for bladder infections or urethritis. The infection may be mild or more severe, including hemorrhagic cystitis. There is frequent urgency to urinate, although often the output is scanty. Intense burning pain occurs with urination before, during, and after the urine is voided. Urination may be so painful that it causes the patient to shriek. The child may grab or rub at the genital area because of the pain.

Sarsaparilla officinalis

Sarsaparilla officinalis is another commonly used homeopathic medicine for bladder infections. Urination is more copious than it is in Cantharis patients, and the pain occurs at the end of urination, often with the last few drops. The urine may contain a reddish sediment.

Pulsatilla nigricans

A patient who needs *Pulsatilla nigricans* will often have changeable symptoms. The urge to urinate is strong and sudden, even when there is little urine in the bladder. Pain increases the longer the urine is withheld, and there may be involuntary loss of urine. Sharp pains occur after urination.

Nux vomica

The main symptom of the patient who needs *Nux vomica* is frequent urgency to urinate, although only small amounts of urine are passed. There may be painful retention of urine and spasms of the urethral sphincter. The patient is aggravated by being cold and is often irritable.

Osteopathy

The goals of osteopathic treatment of children with UTI include decreasing discomfort and urinary frequency and addressing factors that may delay bladder emptying, exacerbate vesicular reflux, or alter urethral peristalsis. Dysfunction or strains of the tissues in the pelvic floor, especially the pubic symphysis, may cause urethral irritation, leading to symptoms of dysuria and frequency.[1] The urethra runs beneath the pubic symphysis, suspended in a fascial hammock. The pubic symphysis is cartilaginous and capable of small movements throughout most of life. Slight alterations in the relation between the two pubic rami creates tension and strain in the fascial hammock, potentially irritating the urethra. This may be the etiology of dysuria in cases of aseptic cystitis. Young women using diaphragm contraception may also experience cystitis due to either the irritating force of the diaphragm or mechanical dysfunction at the pubic symphysis. Gymnasts and equestrians may experience similar symptoms due to biomechanical dysfunction at the pubic symphysis.

From an osteopathic perspective, the cramping pain sometimes associated with UTI can be aggravated by congestion in the pelvic tissues. Somatic dysfunction of the lumbosacral and sacroiliac areas may exacerbate the child's discomfort. This dysfunction may occur secondary to the infection as part of a somatic response to pain. Conversely, in children with recurrent cystitis, the somatic findings may predispose them to ongoing problems by adversely affecting lymphatic and venous drainage from the pelvic area.

Musculoskeletal findings of viscerosomatic and somatovisceral reflexes are commonly found in patients with bladder infections.[2] These reflexes represent areas of spinal facilitation and altered tone of the autonomic nervous system.[3] Numerous studies done on animal models have demonstrated that somatic input can alter visceral function, including peristaltic and secretory activities.[2,4-9] Within the osteopathic concept these reflexes may be used diagnostically and therapeutically. Viscerosomatic reflexes are musculoskeletal changes driven by the irritation of the viscera. Somatovisceral reflexes can alter autonomic input to the viscera, potentially interfering with the organ's ability to respond to the irritation or disease. Viscerosomatic reflexes related to the lower urinary tract are typically found in the paraspinal muscles between the T10 and L1 vertebrae.[2,3] These can be treated with a variety of techniques best suited to the age, acuity, and disposition of the child.

Other areas of somatic dysfunction may influence visceral function via the autonomic nervous system. The parasympathetics to the bladder travel with the pelvic vasculature through the pelvic tissues. Fascial restrictions, tissue strains, or congestion in this area may affect the hemodynamics of the vasa nervorum supplying these nerves or may cause compression of the nerves themselves. Pelvic tissues may be treated using the principles of osteopathy in the cranial field, with indirect or direct techniques depending upon what is most appropriate for the child.

In addition to factors such as toileting habits, urological anomalies, and immune suppression, somatic dysfunction in the tissues of the pelvis needs to be considered in chronic or recurrent cystitis. When other etiologies have been ruled out, the inability of the child with recurrent bacterial cystitis to respond to antibiotics or resist reinfection may be due in part to impaired function of the respiratory/circulatory system in the pelvis. Venous and lymphatic congestion in the pelvis will impede the removal of inflammatory and cellular waste products and potentially impair delivery of nutrients and therapeutic agents to the involved area. The goal of osteopathic treatment in these cases is to improve venous and lymphatic function by correcting biomechanical strains that may interfere with function of the pelvic diaphragm. As previously discussed, viscerosomatic reflexes may also play a role in cystitis. The osteopathic approach to urinary problems typically focuses on the pelvis, sacrum, and lumbar areas.[1]

Burning dysuria, frequency, and itching are all sign of urethral irritation. Consequently, when urine analysis is negative and aseptic or chronic urethritis is suspected, one must consider mechanical irritation of the urethra. Urethral irritation may be caused by mechanical strains at the pubic symphysis. The urethra passes under the pubic symphysis, suspended in a connective tissue hammock. In females, the symphysis is cartilaginous throughout most of life with some degree of flexibility. According to the Mitchell model of sacral-pelvic mechanics,[2] dysfunctions of either innominate bone on the sacrum may produce a shear or strain at the symphysis pubis. This alteration in the relationship of the two pubic rami will produce tensions and stresses in the suspensory fascia of the urethra. If the strain is severe enough, the urethra may be compressed or torsioned, resulting in irritation and inflammation. A history of sport trauma or strain, such as those that might occur in track, gymnastics, or field games in which cleats are worn, is often associated with findings of pubic symphysis dysfunction. Various osteopathic techniques may be used to address the strain and remove the irritation from the urethra.

Somatic dysfunction of the pelvic floor may also play a role in producing symptoms of dysuria and frequency.[3] This may occur through direct irritation on the bladder and urethra or indirectly from venous and lymphatic congestion. Chapman reflexes and segmental somatic dysfunction in the thoracolumbar area have also been reported in patients with dysuria and frequency.[3] From an osteopathic perspective, techniques aimed at correcting mechanical strains in the pelvis and sacrum, improving function of the pelvic diaphragm, relieving tissue congestion, and facilitating involuntary motion of the sacrum are all indicated in the treatment of cystitis. Osteopathic manipulation would be done in conjunction with appropriate medical, herbal, or other therapeutic intervention as necessary. This is especially important in cases of recurrent or chronic cystitis, in which prolonged inflammation puts the child at risk for scarring, mucosal metaplasia, and renal disease.

Probiotics

There is reason to believe that probiotic therapy may provide therapeutic benefit for those with recurrent UTI, yeast vaginitis, and bacterial vaginosis,[1-3] but the data are not definitive. A study from 1973 first showed an association between freedom from UTI and the presence of vaginal lactobacilli.[4] In the past it was understood that *Lactobacillus acidophilus* constitutes the majority of the bacterial flora in a healthy vaginal environment, but this may not be true.[5,6] Lactobacilli found in yogurt may or may not colonize the vagina and thus might not offer a consistent clinical effect,[7,8] although studies that employed specific probiotic microbes do suggest colonization and therapeutic benefit.[9]

One double-blind trial was conducted with 585 infants in 12 Italian neonatal intensive care units. Newborns < 33 weeks gestational age or birth weight <1500 g were randomized to receive standard milk feed supplemented with 6 billion colony-forming units (CFU) of *Lactobacillus* GG once daily until discharge, starting with the first feed, or placebo. Both UTIs and necrotizing enterocolitis occurred less frequently in the group that received probiotic therapy, but the changes did not reach statistical significance. Bacterial sepsis was also more common in the probiotic group, but again not in a statistically significant manner.[10] A study using *Lactobacillus* vaginal suppositories to prevent UTI in adult women did show efficacy.[11] One case

report highlighted the successful daily use of 2 billion units of *Lactobacillus* DDS-1 prophylaxis against recurrent UTI in a 6 year old.[12] In a trial that focused on 13 women with recurrent candidal vaginitis, daily ingestion of 8 ounces of yogurt containing *L. acidophilus* decreased both candidal colonization and vaginal infection.[13] In contrast, a well-done adult study using either oral or vaginal lactobacilli to prevent post-antibiotic vulvovaginitis showed no benefit.[14]

A trial of probiotic therapy after antibiotic treatment for genitourinary tract infection makes sense, and yet supportive data are relatively sparse. The same may be said regarding a trial for vulvovaginal infections. Still, probiotic therapy is quite safe and may be needed only during the course of treatment and for 7 to 10 days beyond completion of therapy. Although some have recommended a delay between ingestion of antibiotic and probiotic, this author has found the precaution unnecessary.

Guidance with respect to choice of specific organisms and duration of therapy is sorely lacking. To further complicate matters, there seems little rationale behind the variety of dosages or combination of microbes employed in published studies. Similar dosages have been utilized often for distinct microbes, whereas widely disparate dosages have been employed by researchers studying the same probiotic. At this time, dosage recommendations are far from set in stone.

This author recommends using a 2- to 3-month trial of probiotic therapy employing well-studied organisms shown to be safe, such as *Lactobacillus* GG, *Lactobacillus plantarum*, *Lactobacillus paracasei*, *Lactobacillus reuteri*, or *L. acidophilus*. Dosing guidelines to consider are 10 billion CFU for children <12 kg and 20 billion CFU for children >12 kg. Treatment is extremely well tolerated, and palatability is not a common problem because the capsules can be opened and mixed into drinks or soft foods. Sometimes the agents are available as a powder as well. If effective, treatment can continue indefinitely. Use with extreme caution, if at all, for those children at risk for infectious complications (immunosuppression or use of immunosuppressive agents, presence of central venous catheter, prematurity).

References

Pediatric Diagnosis and Management

1. Lindert KA, Shortliffe LM: Evaluation and management of pediatric urinary tract infections, *Urol Clin North Am* 26:719-728, 1999.
2. Lettgen B: Urinary tract infections in childhood: old and new aspect [in German], *Klin Padiatr* 205:325-331, 1993 (abstract).
3. American Academy of Pediatrics. Committee on Quality Improvement. Subcommittee on Urinary Tract Infection: Practice parameter: the diagnosis, treatment, and evaluation of the initial urinary tract infection in febrile infants and young children, *Pediatrics* 103:843-852, 1999. Erratum in: *Pediatrics* 103:1052, 1999; 104:118, 1999; 105:141, 2000.
4. Behrman RE, Kliegman RM, Jenson HB, editors: *Nelson textbook of pediatrics*, ed 17, Philadelphia, 2004, Saunders.
5. Jadresic L, Cartwright K, Cowie N et al: Investigation of urinary tract infection in childhood, *Br Med J* 307:761-764, 1993.
6. Weir M, Brien J: Adolescent urinary tract infections, *Adolesc Med* 11:293-313, 2000.

7. Feld LG: Urinary tract infections in childhood: definition, pathogenesis, diagnosis, and management, *Pharmacotherapy* 11: 326-335, 1991.

8. Bourrillon A: Management of prolonged fever in infants [in French], *Arch Pediatr* 6:330-335, 1999 (abstract).

9. Watson AR: Urinary tract infection in early childhood, *J Antimicrob Chemother* 34(Suppl A):53-60, 1994.

10. Linshaw MA: Controversies in childhood urinary tract infections, *World J Urol* 17:383-395, 1999.

11. Roberts KB: The AAP practice parameter on urinary tract infections in febrile infants and young children. American Academy of Pediatrics, *Am Fam Physician* 62:1815-1822, 2000.

12. Feigin R, Cherry JD: *Textbook of pediatric infectious diseases*, ed 3, Philadelphia, 1992, Saunders.

13. Malhotra SM, Kennedy WA 2nd: Urinary tract infections in children: treatment, *Urol Clin North Am* 31:527-534, 2004.

14. Johansen TE: The role of imaging in urinary tract infections, *World J Urol* 22:392-398, 2004.

15. Rosenberg HK, Ilaslan H, Finkelstein MS: Work-up of urinary tract infection in infants and children, *Ultrasound Q* 17:87-102, 2001. Erratum in: *Ultrasound Q* 18:75, 2002.

16. Little L: Shorter antibiotic course for UTIs may be possible, *Infect Dis* 39:13, 2005.

17. Misselwitz J, Handrick W: Urinary tract infection in childhood— an overview: therapy [in German], *Kinderarztl Prax* 59:64-67, 1991 (abstract).

18. Smellie JM, Poulton A, Prescod NP: Retrospective study of children with renal scarring associated with reflux and urinary infection, *Br Med J* 308:1193-1196, 1994.

19. Nathanson S, Deschenes G: Urinary antimicrobial prophylaxis [in French], *Arch Pediatr* 9:511-518, 2002.

20. Raz R. Asymptomatic bacteriuria. Clinical significance and management, *Int J Antimicrob Agents* 22(Suppl 2):45-47, 2003.

Acupuncture

1. Loo M: *Pediatric acupuncture*, London, 2002, Elsevier.

2. Aune A, Alraek T, LiHua H et al: Acupuncture in the prophylaxis of recurrent lower urinary tract infection in adult women, *Scand J Prim Health Care* 16:37-39, 1998.

Chiropractic

1. Buerger MA: History and physical assessment. In Anrig CA, Plaugher G, editors: *Pediatric chiropractic*, Baltimore, 1998, Williams and Wilkins.

2. Vallone SA: Chiropractic management of a 7 year-old female with recurrent urinary tract infections, *Chiropractic Tech* 10:113-117, 1998.

3. Chaitow L: *Palpation skills: assessment and diagnosis through touch*, New York, 1997, Churchill Livingstone.

4. Hoffman D: *The holistic herbal*, Longmead, Shaftsbury, Dorset, United Kingdom, 1988, Element Books.

5. Zand J, Walton R, Rountree B: *Smart medicine for a healthier child*, Garden City Park, NY, 1994, Avery Publishing Group.

6. Gerard JW: Allergies and urinary tract infections: is there an association? *Pediatr* 48:994-995, 1971.

Herbs—Western

1. Haverkorn MJ, Mandigers J: Reduction of bacteriuria and pyuria using cranberry juice, *J Am Med Assoc* 272:590, 1994.

2. Avorn J, Manone M, Gurwitz JH et al: Reduction of bacteriuria and pyuria after ingestion of cranberry juice, *J Am Med Assoc* 271:751-754, 1994.

3. Kontiokari T, Sundqvist K, Nuutinen M et al: Randomised trial of cranberry-lingonberry juice and *Lactobacillus* GG drink for the prevention of urinary tract infections in women, Br Med J 2001;322:1571,2001.

4. Schlager TA, Anderson S, Trudell J et al: Effect of cranberry juice on bacteriuria in children with neurogenic bladder receiving intermittent catheterization, *J Pediatr* 135:698-702, 1999.

5. Foda MMR, Middlebrook PF, Gatfield CT et al: Efficacy of cranberry in prevention of urinary tract infection in a susceptible pediatric population, *Can J Urol* 2:98-102, 1995.

6. Waites KB, Canupp KC, Armstrong S et al: Effect of cranberry extract on bacteriuria and pyuria in persons with neurogenic bladder secondary to spinal cord injury, *J Spinal Cord Med* 27: 35-40, 2004.

7. Jackson B, Hicks LE: Effect of cranberry juice on urinary pH in older adults, *Home Healthcare Nurse* 15:199-202, 1997.

Homeopathy

1. *ReferenceWorks Pro 4.2,* San Rafael, Calif, 2008, Kent Homeopathic Associates.

Osteopathy

1. Kuchera ML, Kuchera WA: *Osteopathic considerations in systemic disease*, Columbus, Ohio, 1994, Greydon Press.

2. Beal MC: Viscerosomatic reflexes: a review, *J Am Osteopath Assoc* 85:786-801, 1985.

3. Willard FH: Autonomic nervous system. In Ward R, editor: *Foundations for osteopathic medicine,* ed 2, Philadelphia, 2003, Lippincott Williams and Wilkins.

4. Aihara Y, Nakamura H, Sato A et al: Neural control of gastric motility with special reference to cutaneo-gastric reflexes. In Brooks C, editor: *Integrative functions of the autonomic nervous system*, New York, 1979, Elsevier.

5. Pierau FK, Fellmer G, Taylor DCM: Somato-visceral convergence in cat dorsal root ganglion neurones demonstrated by double labelling with fluorescent tracers, *Brain Res* 321:63-70, 1984.

6. Sato A, Schmidt RF: Somatosympathetic reflexes: afferent fibers, central pathways, discharge characteristics, *Physiol Rev* 53: 916-947, 1973.

7. Sato A, Swenson S: Sympathetic nervous system response to mechanical stress of the spinal column in rats, *J Man Med* 7: 141-147, 1984.

8. Sato A: The reflex effects of spinal somatic nerve stimulation on visceral function, *J Man Physiol Ther* 15:57-61, 1992.

9. Sato A: Somatovisceral reflexes, *J Manipulative Physiol Ther* 18:597-602, 1995.

Probiotics

1. Reid G, Bruce AW: Urogenital infections in women: can probiotics help? *Postgrad Med J* 79:428-432, 2003.

2. Miller JL, Krieger JN: Urinary tract infections, cranberry juice, underwear, and probiotics in the 21st century, *Urol Clin North Am* 29:695-699, 2002.

3. Bruce AW, Reid G: Probiotics and the urologist, *Can J Urol* 10:1785-1789, 2003.

4. Bruce AW, Chadwick P, Hassan A et al: Recurrent urethritis in women, *Can Med Assoc J* 108:973-976, 1973.

5. Antonio MA, Hawes SE, Hillier SL: The identification of vaginal *Lactobacillus* species and the demographic and microbiologic characteristics of women colonized by these species, *J Infect Dis* 180:1950-1956, 1999.

6. Burton JP, Cadieux P, Reid G: Improved understanding of the bacterial vaginal microbiota of women before and after probiotic instillation, *Appl Environ Microbiol* 69:97-101, 2003.

7. Wood JR, Sweet RL, Catena A et al: In vitro adherence of *Lactobacillus* species to vaginal epithelial cells, *Am J Obstet Gynecol* 153:740-743, 1985.

8. Shalev E, Battino S, Weiner E et al: Ingestion of yogurt containing *Lactobacillus acidophilus* compared with pasteurized yogurt as prophylaxis for recurrent candidal vaginitis and bacterial vaginosis, *Arch Fam Med* 5:593-596, 1996.

9. Reid G, Bruce AW, Fraser N et al: Oral probiotics can resolve urogenital infections, *FEMS Immunol Med Microbiol* 30:49-52, 2001.

10. Dani C, Biadaioli R, Bertini G et al: Probiotics feeding in prevention of urinary tract infection, bacterial sepsis, and necrotizing enterocolitis in preterm infants. A prospective double-blind study, *Biol Neonate* 82:103-108, 2002.

11. Reid G, Bruce AW, Taylor M: Influence of three-day antimicrobial therapy and *Lactobacillus* vaginal suppositories on recurrence of urinary tract infections, *Clin Ther* 14:11-16, 1992.

12. Gerasimov SV: Probiotic prophylaxis in pediatric recurrent urinary tract infections, *Clin Pediatr* 43:95-98, 2004.

13. Hilton E, Isenberg HD, Alperstein P et al: Ingestion of yogurt containing *Lactobacillus acidophilus* as prophylaxis for candidal vaginitis, *Ann Intern Med* 116:353-357, 1992.

14. Pirotta M, Gunn J, Chondros P et al: Effect of *Lactobacillus* in preventing post-antibiotic vulvovaginal candidiasis: a randomised controlled trial, *Br Med J* 329:548, 2004.

Vomiting

Acupuncture May Loo

Herbs—Western Alan D. Woolf, Paula M. Gardiner, Lana Dvorkin-Camiel, Jack Maypole

Homeopathy Janet L. Levatin

Massage Therapy Agatha P. Colbert, Deborah Risotti

Naturopathy Matthew I. Baral

PEDIATRIC DIAGNOSIS AND MANAGEMENT

Vomiting is a nonspecific symptom that occurs frequently in children of all ages. The causes can range from food allergies, mild viral gastrointestinal (GI) infections to severe anatomical, metabolic, and chronic inflammatory conditions. The best differential approach to the child with vomiting is by age and by organ systems. Vomiting in newborns is usually due to congenital anatomical obstructions, inborn errors of metabolism, or sepsis. In infants, the causes can be acquired or milder congenital obstructive lesions such as pyloric stenosis, metabolic inborn errors of metabolism, food intolerance, gastroesophageal reflux, or psychosocial causes such as rumination after child abuse. Vomiting in older children has a long list of differentials that includes GI disorders such as gastroenteritis (most often due to viruses, but bacterial, protozoal, and helminthic gastroenteritis also occur, especially in developing countries), esophagitis, hepatitis, gastroesophageal reflux disease, intestinal obstructions, appendicitis, and inflammatory bowel disease; genitourinary disorders such as urinary tract infection, pyelonephritis, and renal obstructions; metabolic disorders; neurological conditions with increased intracranial pressure; various respiratory, cardiac, and gynecological disorders; drugs (especially chemotherapy); and postsurgery, all of which can have vomiting as part of the symptomatology. In addition, possible pregnancy, eating disorder, and drug abuse must be ruled out for vomiting in adolescents. Vomiting with motion sickness is obvious and benign but can be disruptive and inconvenient for the family.[1-11]

Conventional evaluation includes a comprehensive history, physical examination, and appropriate laboratory evaluations. Signs of dehydration should be quickly assessed, especially in infants and young children, to determine whether intravenous hydration needs to be instituted. Treatment is directed toward rehydration and management of specific disorders. Antiemetics are chosen according to the pathophysiology of vomiting: Antihistamines and anticholinergic agents are most effective in vomiting from vestibular and central nervous system causes. Dopamine and serotonin antagonists block the respective visceral chemoreceptor triggers.[12] Chemotherapy-induced acute emesis can be difficult to treat and may need a combination of a 5-hydroxytryptamine$_3$ (5-HT3) antagonist and dexamethasone.[13]

Fortunately, the majority of vomiting in children is mild, often due to acute viral gastroenteritis when the inflamed mucous membranes of the GI tract cause vomiting, frequently accompanied by watery diarrhea. Most infants and children can be rehydrated safely with oral rehydration solution. Antiemetics are not indicated in children with acute viral gastroenteritis (VGE).[14]

Complementary and alternative medicine (CAM) treatments can be incorporated in management of vomiting in children when the clinical presentation is compatible with acute VGE, in motion sickness, in mitigating the side effects of chemotherapy, in postoperative vomiting, or in diagnosed conditions when safe, nonchemical approaches can be incorporated as complementary modalities to alleviate discomfort without disrupting conventional treatment, such as in inflammatory bowel disease.

CAM THERAPY RECOMMENDATIONS

Acupuncture

Since the majority of pediatric vomiting is benign and short lived, children generally do not receive acupuncture treatment, and studies are difficult to conduct. The only situation in which controlled studies can be carried out is in prevention of postoperative nausea and vomiting (PONV). A frequent side effect of general anesthesia in children,[1] PONV can prolong recovery room stay and hospitalization and is one of the most common causes of hospital readmission after surgery. Currently available drugs still cannot completely control PONV and often present undesired adverse effects.[2]

Stimulation of acupuncture points has been shown to be effective in the prevention as well as treatment of PONV.[3] The most frequently used and studied acupoint is P6, pericardium 6, a well-known traditional Chinese medicine (TCM) point for controlling nausea and vomiting of any etiology. The classic texts state that P6 is a powerful point indicated for any "disharmony of the Stomach and Spleen" (i.e., the digestive system).[4] Current biochemical hypothesis presumes P6 acts on central emetic mechanisms to control nausea and vomiting.[5] Stimulation of P6 may produce an effect on neurotransmitters similar to that seen with other acupoints, such as Tai Chong (LR3), which has been found to increase indolamine metabolism, possibly leading to a decrease in various symptoms, including vomiting.[6]

Numerous randomized, controlled studies from all over the world evaluated the pediatric effect of P6 on PONV. A few studies will be included here. A randomized controlled trial (RCT) from the United States found bilateral P6 saline injections as effective as intravenous droperidol in controlling early PONV in children.[7] A prospective study in Turkey of 90 post-tonsillectomy children found that electrical stimulation at 20 Hz for 5 minutes via surface electrodes on P6 and Shangwan (CV13) was just as effective as a single dose of ondansetron, a 5-hydroxytryptamine type 3 antagonist. Side effects were often seen in the ondansetron group.[3] One U.S. study of 100 children, ages 2 to 12 years, compared acubands placed on P6 points and found no reduction in emesis in children following tonsillectomy.[8] However, another U.S. study of 4 to 18 year olds using low-frequency electrical stimulation for 20 minutes on the needled P6 acupoint (a stronger stimulation than the previous study) significantly reduced PONV, exerting similar effect as commonly used pharmacotherapies.[9] A randomized, prospective, controlled study in Croatia of 120 children undergoing hernia repair, circumcision, or orchidopexy found laser acupuncture on P6 acupoint was equally effective as metoclopramide in preventing PONV in these children.[1] A study from Israel of 90 children found acupuncture to be as effective as ondansetron in the prevention of post–dental surgery vomiting.[10]

Acupuncture in PONV with strabismus surgery in children has been studied extensively with varying results. A U.S. prospective, double-blind study of 66 children ages 3 to 12 years undergoing outpatient strabismus surgery found that P6 acupressure did not reduce the incidence of postoperative vomiting compared with placebo.[11] A Canadian randomized, double-blind, placebo-controlled study of 90 children older than 1 year found 5 minutes of P6 acupuncture and intravenous droperidol were equally ineffective in preventing vomiting within 48 hours of strabismus repair. Droperidol is associated with increased incidence of postoperative restlessness.[12]

A double-blind, randomized, placebo-controlled study from Austria involving children undergoing strabismus surgery used low-level laser stimulation on P6 for 15 minutes before induction of anaesthesia and 15 minutes after arriving in the recovery room. The incidence of vomiting was significantly lower in the laser stimulation group.[13] The same Austrian group applied an acupressure disc onto the Korean hand acupuncture point K-K9 (hand equivalent of P6). The incidence of vomiting was significantly reduced in children undergoing strabismus surgery.[14]

A group of researchers in Taiwan posit that stimulation of P6 can be ineffective in strabismus surgery because P6 may act only on hollow organs. They added three acupoints that were more relevant to the eyes: BL10 (Tianzhu), BL11 (Dazhu), and GB34 (Yanglinquan). Sixty-five children were randomized into placebo and acuplaster groups in which needleless acuplasters were applied to BL10, BL11, and GB34 on the night before surgery. The overall postoperative vomiting incidence was significantly decreased in the acuplaster patients. The authors concluded that the three acupoints might have diminished the parasympathetic stimulation resulting from surgical traction of eye muscles.[15]

Acupuncture is also used to treat vomiting associated with chemotherapy. In Canada, acupuncture is an option recommended for the prevention and management of acute chemotherapy-induced nausea and vomiting in children.[16] A multicenter, randomized crossover study from Germany found acupuncture reduced nausea and vomiting without the need for antiemetic medications in adolescent oncology patients. Acupuncture also enabled patients to experience higher levels of alertness during chemotherapy.[17]

Treatment Recommendations

Treatment of PONV: as noted in the previously mentioned studies.

For mild vomiting such as from gastroenteritis, food poisoning, or motion sickness:

P6; can also add ST 36, stimulate as follows:

Needling without electrical stimulation.

Apply south side of magnet facing downward on the acupoints.[18]

Massage the points in infants and young children.

Use laser stimulation.

Aromatherapy

See Chapter 46, Motion Sickness.

Herbs—Western

Some of the most common and long-used herbs for the treatment of motion sickness, nausea, and vomiting include ginger root, peppermint, chamomile, fennel and other calmative herbs. Ginger (*Zingiber officinale*) has been used as a remedy for dyspepsia and nausea for centuries. The authoritative German Commission E Monographs approves the use of ginger root as a treatment for dyspepsia and prophylactic against motion sickness.[1] Several RCTs and meta-analyses show mixed support for ginger's use as an antiemetic for nausea secondary to several conditions, including morning sickness, chemotherapy-associated nausea, postoperative nausea, and motion sickness.[2-7] In one clinical trial on motion sickness, 28 children aged 4 to 8 years received standardized preparation of ginger root (Zintona capsules) 30 minutes before the start of a 2-day trip and every 4 hours thereafter as necessary or 12.5 to 25 mg dimenhydrate 30 minutes before the start of the 2-day trip and every 4 hours thereafter as necessary. The physician rated the ginger as having good effectiveness in 100% of the children and rated dimenhydrate as having good effectiveness in 30.8% of the children. The dimenhydrate group reported more side effects (e.g., vertigo, increased salivation, stomachache, nausea, dry mouth, pallor, cold sweats), whereas the ginger-root group reported none.[6] Ginger is well tolerated, but in large doses it may cause abdominal discomfort, heartburn, or diarrhea.

Homeopathy

Before using this section, please see Appendix A, Homeopathy, for definitions of practitioner expertise categories and general information on prescribing homeopathic medicines.

Practitioner Expertise Category 1

There are no controlled clinical trials of homeopathic treatment for nausea and vomiting, although the homeopathic literature contains much evidence to support its use in the form of accumulated clinical experience.[1] Homeopathy can frequently treat early, acute vomiting very effectively, often preventing a trip for emergency care. For acute vomiting unassociated with other serious conditions, and before a child becomes significantly dehydrated because of fluid loss, it is safe to try homeopathic treatment prior to beginning conventional therapy. If the vomiting patient does not respond quickly to homeopathic treatment (prior to the onset of significant dehydration), then conventional care will be necessary for the patient.

The goal in treating vomiting homeopathically is to determine the single homeopathic medicine whose description in the materia medica most closely matches the symptom picture of the patient. Often mental and emotional states in addition to physical symptoms are considered. Once the medicine has been selected, it can be given orally or sublingually in the 30C potency after each episode of vomiting, up to six times per day. A few (4 to 6) granules of the medicine can also be diluted in 3 oz (90 mL) water, and a few drops can be placed in the patient's mouth whenever a dose is needed. The medicine does not need to be swallowed to be effective; the simillimum will work even if it remains in the mouth for only a brief period of time. If the medicine has not helped after six doses, then another homeopathic medicine should be tried or another form of therapy should be instituted as needed. Once symptoms have begun to resolve, the medicine can be given less frequently or stopped. It can be repeated again for a relapse of symptoms.

The following is a list of homeopathic medicines commonly used to treat patients with vomiting. It must be emphasized that this list is partial and represents some of the probable choices from the homeopathic materia medica. If the symptoms of a given patient are not represented here, further research in the homeopathic literature would be needed to find the simillimum.

Arsenicum album

Arsenicum album is particularly useful when the vomiting is secondary to food poisoning, but it may also be used for vomiting due to gastroenteritis. Burning stomach pains may be present, and the vomitus is acrid. The patient may be anxious and restless or exhausted and faint. There is marked chilliness. The symptoms are worse from 11 AM to 3 PM and/or from midnight to 3 AM.

Ipecacuanha

Ipecacuanha treats nausea and vomiting due to gastritis, as well as nausea and vomiting associated with cough or other respiratory conditions. The nausea is very severe and is often unrelieved by vomiting. There may be bloody vomiting (if the amount is significant, the child should be taken for emergency care). The child may be very irritable.

Nux vomica

Nux vomica treats nausea and vomiting with crampy pains, as well as retching. Constipation may occur with the nausea.

Symptoms are worse in the morning and worse after eating. The child is chilly, angry, and oversensitive.

Phosphorus

Phosphorus is a medicine to use when the patient craves cold or icy liquids but vomits them as soon as they become warm in the stomach.

Massage Therapy

Acupressure application to the acupuncture point P6 (Neiguan) to prevent and treat nausea and vomiting has been used in TCM. Several randomized, controlled studies have examined the use of acupressure wristbands for the treatment of postoperative or medication-induced nausea and vomiting.[1-6]

Two controlled studies on adults demonstrated that acupressure application to P6 significantly reduced the incidence of postoperative nausea and vomiting compared with controls.[1,2] One of these studies further compared the use of acupressure bands with traditional pharmaceutical antiemetic therapy. This study demonstrated that the use of the acupressure band in conjunction with ondansetron significantly reduced nausea, vomiting, and the need for rescue antiemetics and increased diet tolerance, quality of recovery, and patient satisfaction scores compared with patients who received either ondansetron or acupressure alone.[2] Children who received acupressure application preoperatively to the Korean acupuncture point K-K9 had reduced postoperative nausea and vomiting compared with controls.[3]

Prophylactic application of acupressure bands to P6 reduced emesis compared with controls in adult overdose patients after activated charcoal application.[4] Adult cancer patients treated with acupressure bands had decreased chemotherapy-induced nausea on the first day of chemotherapy administration compared with controls; however, there was no difference between the groups in the incidence of delayed-onset nausea and vomiting.[5] Adults who were treated with acupressure bands within the first 24 hours following a myocardial infarction experienced less nausea and vomiting in the 20 hours following the event compared to controls.[6]

Researchers report that the acupressure bands are well tolerated by the patients, with no complications.[1-6] Given the low risk and the potential efficacy of this therapy, use of acupressure bands for treatment of nausea and vomiting is worth investigating, especially when used as an adjunct to traditional antiemetic medications.

The research has demonstrated that acupressure bands and direct finger pressure application to P6 have both been effective. The P6 point is located approximately 2 finger widths (using the child's fingers to be in proportion with the child) above the wrist bone, on the dorsal aspect of the forearm, between the two tendons. Pressure may be applied in this location either with an acupressure band or finger. In the research cited, acupressure was applied from 30 minutes to 24 hours; it may be more practical to utilize the acupressure bands to maintain stimulation of this point.

Naturopathy

Several naturopathic therapies can be used to treat vomiting in children. They are generally safe and quite effective.

Ginger

Many of the studies on ginger have been done on the pregnant population. Ginger helped relieve nausea and vomiting in motion sickness and pregnancy.[1] In another study, 500 mg ginger orally or 10 mg vitamin B[6] three times per day for 3 days was shown to be helpful in nausea and vomiting of pregnancy.[2] Ginger may also be helpful in the treatment of chemotherapy-induced nausea and vomiting,[3] nausea from motion sickness,[4] and postoperative nausea and vomiting.[5]

A reasonable dose is 1 to 4 g/day or several cups of tea per day. Fresh ginger (equivalent of 1 teaspoon) is grated into a cup, hot water is poured over the herb, and the tea is steeped for 15 minutes. Honey or maple syrup may be added for taste.

Chamomile

Chamomile has been widely used as an herb to address many conditions of the GI tract because of its antiemetic and antispasmodic properties. It can be given to children with vomiting as an infusion of 1 to 2 teaspoons of the herb steeped in 1 cup of water; 1 to 3 cups several times per day may be consumed. The 1:5 alcohol tincture may be taken at 1 teaspoon three times per day.[6]

Vitamin B[6]

Extrapolating the use of vitamin B[6] for the treatment of nausea and vomiting in pregnancy,[7] its use may be beneficial in pediatric cases of vomiting, but more research is needed. A typical dose is 10 mg three times per day in children 1 year or older.

Black tea

Sipping black tea over the course of the day can also have an antiemetic effect. However, low levels of caffeine in black tea may keep a child awake, so dosing during the daytime may be best.

Slippery elm (Ulmus fulva)

Mary Bove, a naturopathic physician with extensive experience in the treatment of children, created an excellent recipe that has been effective. Add 1 teaspoon of ulmus powder, ¼ teaspoon cinnamon powder, and enough warm water to make a "gruel" or tea. Several cups per day may be consumed by children older than 1 year.

References

Pediatric Diagnosis and Management

1. Verma R: Vomiting. In Altschuler SM, Liacouras CA, editors: *Clinical pediatric gastroenterology*, Philadelphia, 1998, Churchill Livingstone.
2. Orenstein SR, Peters JM. Vomiting and regurgitation. In Kliegman RM, Greenbaum LA, Lye PS, editors: *Practical strategies in pediatric diagnosis and therapy*, ed 2, Philadelphia, 2004, Elsevier.
3. Behrman RE, Kliegman RM, Jenson HB, editors: *Nelson textbook of pediatrics*, ed 17, Philadelphia, 2004, Saunders.
4. Hiranrattana A, Mekmullica J, Chatsuwan T et al: Childhood shigellosis at King Chulalongkorn Memorial Hospital, Bangkok, Thailand: a 5-year review (1996-2000), *Southeast Asian J Trop Med Public Health* 36:683-685, 2005.
5. American Academy of Pediatrics Subcommittee on Chronic Abdominal Pain: North American Society for Pediatric Gastroenterology, Hepatology, and Nutrition: Chronic abdominal pain in children, *Pediatrics* 115:e370-e381, 2005.
6. Antonarakis ES, Hain RD: Nausea and vomiting associated with cancer chemotherapy: drug management theory and practice, *Arch Dis Child* 89:877-880, 2004.
7. Eberhart LH, Geldner G, Horle S et al: Prophylaxis and treatment of nausea and vomiting after outpatient ophthalmic surgery [in German], *Ophthalmologe* 101:925-930, 2004 (abstract).
8. Ida S: Evaluation and treatment of gastroesophageal reflux in infants and children [in Japanese], *Nippon Rinsho* 62:1553-1558, 2004 (abstract).
9. Kucik CJ, Martin GL, Sortor BV: Common intestinal parasites, *Am Fam Physician* 69:1161-1168, 2004.
10. Spinks AB, Wasiak J, Villanueva EV, et al: Scopolamine for preventing and treating motion sickness, *Cochrane Database Syst Rev* (3):CD002851, 2004.
11. Cezard JP: Managing gastro-oesophageal reflux disease in children, *Digestion* 69(Suppl 1):3-8, 2004.
12. Flake ZA, Scalley RD, Bailey AG: Practical selection of antiemetics, *Am Fam Physician* 69:1169-1174, 2004.
13. Roila F, Feyer P, Maranzano E et al: Antiemetics in children receiving chemotherapy, *Support Care Cancer* 13:129-131, 2005. Erratum in: *Support Care Cancer* 13:132, 2005.
14. Webb A, Starr M: Acute gastroenteritis in children, *Austr Fam Physician* 34:227-231, 2005.

Acupuncture

1. Butkovic D, Toljan S, Matolic M et al: Comparison of laser acupuncture and metoclopramide in PONV prevention in children, *Paediatr Anaesth* 15:37-40, 2005.
2. De Negri P, Ivani G: Management of postoperative nausea and vomiting in children, *Paediatr Drugs* 4:717-728, 2002.
3. Kabalak AA, Akcay M, Akcay F et al: Transcutaneous electrical acupoint stimulation versus ondansetron in the prevention of postoperative vomiting following pediatric tonsillectomy, *J Altern Complement Med* 11:407-413, 2005.
4. Deadman P, Al-Khafaji M: *A manual of acupuncture*, Ann Arbor, Mich, 1998, Journal of Chinese Medicine Publications.
5. Miller AD: Central mechanisms of vomiting, *Dig Dis Sci* 44 (8 Suppl):39S-43S, 1999.
6. Riederer P, Tenk H, Werner H et al: Manipulation of neurotransmitters by acupuncture (A preliminary communication), *J Neural Transm* 37:81-94, 1975.
7. Wang SM, Kain ZN: P6 acupoint injections are as effective as droperidol in controlling early postoperative nausea and vomiting in children, *Anesthesiology* 97:359-366, 2002.
8. Shenkman Z, Holzman RS, Kim C et al: Acupressure-acupuncture antiemetic prophylaxis in children undergoing tonsillectomy, *Anesthesiology* 90:1311-1316, 1999.
9. Rusy LM, Hoffman GM, Weisman SJ: Electroacupuncture prophylaxis of postoperative nausea and vomiting following pediatric tonsillectomy with or without adenoidectomy, *Anesthesiology* 96:300-305, 2002.
10. Somri M, Vaida SJ, Sabo E et al: Acupuncture versus ondansetron in the prevention of postoperative vomiting. A study of children undergoing dental surgery, *Anesthesia* 56:927-932, 2001.
11. Lewis IH, Pryn SJ, Reynolds PI et al: Effect of P6 acupressure on postoperative vomiting in children undergoing outpatient strabismus correction, *Br J Anaesth* 67:73-78, 1991.

12. Yentis SM, Bissonnette B: Ineffectiveness of acupuncture and droperidol in preventing vomiting following strabismus repair in children, *Can J Anaesth* 39:151-154, 1992.

13. Schlager A, Offer T, Baldissera I: Laser stimulation of acupuncture point P6 reduces postoperative vomiting in children undergoing strabismus surgery, *Br J Anaesth* 81:529-532, 1998.

14. Schlager A, Boehler M, Puhringer F: Korean hand acupressure reduces postoperative vomiting in children after strabismus surgery, *Br J Anaesth* 85:267-270, 2000.

15. Chu YC, Lin SM, Hsieh YC et al: Effect of BL-10 (tianzhu), BL-11 (dazhu) and GB-34 (yanglinquan) acuplaster for prevention of vomiting after strabismus surgery in children, *Acta Anaesthesiol Sin* 36:11-16, 1998.

16. Dupuis LL, Nathan PC: Options for the prevention and management of acute chemotherapy-induced nausea and vomiting in children, *Paediatr Drugs* 5:597-613, 2003.

17. Reindl TK, Geilen W, Hartmann R et al: Acupuncture against chemotherapy-induced nausea and vomiting in pediatric oncology. Interim results of a multicenter crossover study, *Support Care Cancer* 14:172-176, 2006.

18. Liu S, Chen Z, Hou J et al: Magnetic disk applied on Neiguan point for prevention and treatment of cisplatin-induced nausea and vomiting, *J Tradit Chin Med* 11:181-183, 1991.

Herbs—Western

1. Blumenthal M., editor: The complete German Commission E monographs: therapeutic guide to herbal medicines, Austin, Tex, 1998, American Botanical Council.

2. Arfeen Z, Owen H, Plummer JL et al: A double-blind randomized controlled trial of ginger for the prevention of postoperative nausea and vomiting, *Anaesth Intensive Care* 23:449-452, 1995.

3. Visalyaputra S, Petchpaisit N, Somcharoen K et al: The efficacy of ginger root in the prevention of postoperative nausea and vomiting after outpatient gynaecological laparoscopy, *Anaesthesia* 53:506-510, 1998.

4. Aikins Murphy P: Alternative therapies for nausea and vomiting of pregnancy, *Obstet Gynecol* 91:149-155, 1998.

5. Ernst E, Pittler MH: Efficacy of ginger for nausea and vomiting: a systematic review of randomized clinical trials, *Br J Anaesthesia* 84:367-371, 2000.

6. Careddu P: Motion sickness in children: results of a double-blind study with ginger (Zintona) and dimenhydrinate, *Eur Phytother* 6:102-107, 1999.

7. Jewell D, Young G: Interventions for nausea and vomiting in early pregnancy [see comment], *Cochrane Database Syst Rev* (1):CD000145, 2002. [Review; with 59 references.] [Update in *Cochrane Database Syst Rev* (4):CD000145, 2003; PMID: 14583914; update of *Cochrane Database Syst Rev* (2):CD000145, 2000; PMID: 10796155.]

Homeopathy

1. *ReferenceWorks Pro 4.2*, San Rafael, Calif, 2008, Kent Homeopathic Associates.

Massage Therapy

1. Ming JL, Kuo BI, Lin JG et al: The efficacy of acupressure to prevent nausea and vomiting in post-operative patients, *J Adv Nurs* 39:343-351, 2002.

2. White PF, Issioui T, Hu J et al: Comparative efficacy of acustimulation (ReliefBand) versus ondansetron (Zofran) in combination with droperidol for preventing nausea and vomiting, *Anesthesiology* 97:1075-1081, 2002.

3. Schlager A, Boeher M, Puhringer F: Korean hand acupressure reduces postoperative vomiting in children after strabismus surgery, *Br J Anaesth* 85:267-270, 2000.

4. Eizember FL, Tomaszewski CA, Kerns WP: Acupressure for prevention of emesis in patients receiving activated charcoal, *J Toxicol Clin Toxicol* 40:775-780, 2002.

5. Roscoe JA, Morrow GR, Hickok JT et al: The efficacy of acupressure and acustimulation wrist bands for the relief of chemotherapy-induced nausea and vomiting. A University of Rochester Cancer Center Community Clinical Oncology Program multicenter study, *J Pain Symptom Manage* 26:731-742, 2003.

6. Dent HE, Dewhurst NG, Mills SY et al: Continuous PC6 wristband acupressure for relief of nausea and vomiting associated with acute myocardial infarction: a partially randomized, placebo-controlled trial, *Complement Ther Med* 11:72-77, 2003.

Naturopathy

1. Koretz RL, Rotblatt M: Complementary and alternative medicine in gastroenterology: the good, the bad, and the ugly, *Clin Gastroenterol Hepatol* 2:957-967, 2004.

2. Sripramote M, Lekhyananda N: A randomized comparison of ginger and vitamin B6 in the treatment of nausea and vomiting of pregnancy, *J Med Assoc Thai* 86:846-853, 2003.

3. Dupuis LL, Nathan PC: Options for the prevention and management of acute chemotherapy-induced nausea and vomiting in children, *Paediatr Drugs* 5:597-613, 2003.

4. Grontved A, Brask T, Kambskard J et al: Ginger root against seasickness. A controlled trial on the open sea, *Acta Otolaryngol* 105:45-49, 1988.

5. Bone ME, Wilkinson DJ, Young JR et al: Ginger root—a new antiemetic. The effect of ginger root on postoperative nausea and vomiting after major gynaecological surgery, *Anaesthesia* 45:669-671, 1990.

6. Alschuler L. Seattle, 2000, Bastyr University.

7. Sahakian V, Rouse D, Sipes S et al: Vitamin B6 is effective therapy for nausea and vomiting of pregnancy: a randomized, double-blind placebo-controlled study, *Obstet Gynecol* 78:33-36, 1991.

Homeopathy: General Information on Prescribing and Administering Homeopathic Medicines

Janet Levatin

It is necessary for practitioners to understand the information in this appendix before recommending homeopathic treatment for any of the conditions included in this book. Therefore it is strongly suggested that this appendix and Chapter 5 in Section I of this book be read in their entirety (and subsequently referred to as needed) before practitioners utilize the homeopathic treatment recommendations in the chapters on individual medical conditions.

Who Can Be Treated Homeopathically?

One of the benefits of homeopathic treatment is that homeopathic medicines can be given to individuals at any age or stage of life, including infants, young children, and pregnant and nursing women. Homeopathic medicines can be given to people with medical conditions ranging from minor to serious. They can also be given to patients using other forms of treatment, both conventional and alternative, as there are essentially no interactions between homeopathic medicines and other substances or therapies.

Obtaining Homeopathic Medicines

Homeopathic medicines up to the 30C potency are usually available over the counter at health food stores or pharmacies and can also be obtained by mail order (see the list of homeopathic pharmacies and retail distributors at the end of this appendix).

Acute versus Chronic Prescribing

Homeopathy can be used to treat both chronic and acute conditions. For patients with chronic conditions, homeopathy can provide profound, long-lasting, curative changes; however, effective case taking, accurate case analysis and prescribing, and follow-up require a significant amount of training and expertise. It is appropriate for practitioners who have not had extensive training in the science and art of homeopathy to begin by prescribing for acute, self-limited conditions; therefore most of the treatment recommendations in this book are for acute conditions, although occasional treatment recommendations for chronic or recurrent conditions of low severity are included as well. With training and experience, interested practitioners can begin to treat more complex cases.

Gauging One's Level of Expertise

In order to help practitioners with varying levels of homeopathic training and experience determine which medical conditions may be appropriate for them to treat, the following practitioner expertise categories have been developed. Each medical condition in the book has been assigned to one or more categories.

Category 1

With the understanding that each case is unique and must be evaluated fully at the time of presentation, category 1 conditions usually can be treated homeopathically with a reasonable degree of safety and a reasonable chance of success by *clinicians who have only introductory training and limited experience in homeopathy*. Category 1 conditions include acute conditions of low severity and complexity and chronic or recurrent conditions of low severity and complexity.

Category 2

With the understanding that each case is unique and must be evaluated fully at the time of presentation, category 2 conditions usually can be treated homeopathically with a reasonable degree of safety and a reasonable chance of success by *clinicians who have a moderate amount of training and some clinical experience in homeopathy*. Category 2 conditions include acute conditions of low to moderate severity and complexity and chronic or recurrent conditions of low to moderate severity and complexity.

Category 3

With the understanding that each case is unique and must be evaluated fully at the time of presentation, safe and successful treatment of category 3 conditions usually requires extensive training in the art and science of homeopathy and should be undertaken only by *clinicians who have advanced training and extensive clinical experience in homeopathy*. Category 3 conditions include acute conditions of moderate to high severity and complexity and chronic or recurrent conditions of moderate to high severity and complexity, including psychiatric conditions and developmental disorders.

Homeopathic Methodology: Case Taking and Choosing a Homeopathic Medicine

Case taking for the purpose of prescribing a homeopathic medicine is described in detail in the Chapter 5 discussion of homeopathy and will be reviewed here in brief. During the interview, the patient's signs and symptoms of the patient are noted, as are any constitutional characteristics such as food cravings, thirst, and temperature sensitivity. Mental and emotional states should also be observed. After a patient's symptoms and general state are understood, the one homeopathic medicine whose symptom picture and general state are most similar to those of the patient, the simillimum, is chosen. The medicine will be found by studying homeopathic provings,[1] reading homeopathic materia medica,[1] and referring to homeopathic repertories[2] (see Chapter 5, discussion of homeopathy, for further information on the use of these reference books).

Prescribing One Medicine at a Time (The "Classical" Method)

It is best to use one homeopathic medicine at a time. Some systems of prescribing recommend that two or more homeopathically prepared (diluted and succussed) substances that involve combinations of two or more substances be given simultaneously. In addition, combination preparations containing two or more homeopathically prepared substances can be purchased over the counter by lay people for self-treatment; some practitioners recommend them as well. In this book, however, all treatment recommendations are for single medicine preparations (the "classical" method of homeopathic prescribing), unless explicitly stated otherwise in the text.

Potency, Dosage, and Administration of Homeopathic Medicines

Potency and Dosage Frequency

When choosing the potency of a homeopathic medicine, these general guidelines should be followed: usually lower potencies (up to 30C) are given for acute conditions of lower severity with few emotional and mental components in the presentation; higher potencies (200C and above) are given for acute conditions of higher severity, chronic conditions, and conditions with more emotional and mental components at presentation. (These are general guidelines to keep in mind as a homeopathic prescription is made. It must always be borne in mind that each case is unique and must be evaluated fully at the time of presentation.)

For most *acute conditions*, a homeopathic medicine in the 30C potency can be given and repeated one to three times per day, or even every few minutes for very acute conditions such as the onset of croup or the onset of an allergic reaction. In general, the more acute or extreme the patient's condition, the more frequently a medicine is repeated. When the patient begins to improve, the medicine can be given less frequently and then stopped. Usually a patient will continue to improve once the healing process has begun; should a relapse of symptoms occur, however, the medicine can be repeated. Sometimes increasing the potency to 200C or higher will be beneficial to

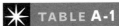

TABLE A-1

Guidelines for Choosing the Potency and Dosing Schedule for Homeopathic Medicines

ACUITY OF CONDITION	POTENCY	FREQUENCY OF ADMINISTRATION
Acute (mild)	30C or 200C	Two to four times daily or One to three times daily
Acute (severe)	30C or 200C	Every few minutes to four times daily
Chronic	200C or higher	One to two times daily

a patient with an acute illness. This strategy may be useful in the following situations: (1) for more acute medical problems such as the onset of croup or the onset of an allergic reaction or (2) if a patient is partially better after administration of a 30C medicine, but the progress of healing has stalled.

For *chronic conditions*, higher potencies (200C or higher) are usually given, and typically dosing is less frequent. These recommendations on potency and dosage frequency are summarized in Table A-1.

Medicines of any potency can be given to patients of any age when indicated for the patient's condition. In this book, usually the 30C potency is recommended, as this potency is often suitable for acute conditions of low to moderate severity, such as those included in this book.

Dosage Quantity and Administration Techniques

A dose of homeopathic medicine consists of two to five pellets or granules, which are administered sublingually or orally, from a spoon or medicine cup. (Unless otherwise noted in the sections for an individual condition, all treatments recommended are to be administered sublingually or orally. If a topical, ophthalmic, or intranasal preparation is recommended, it will be explicitly stated.)

For infants and small children, the medicine can be crushed and the crystals administered, or the medicine can be dissolved in purified or spring water and a small amount of the solution (2.5 to 10 mL) administered.*

Changing the Medicine

If no improvement in the patient's condition is seen after four to five doses of a homeopathic medicine, this means the medicine chosen probably is not correct and will not help. It should be stopped and another homeopathic medicine or another form of treatment begun, as needed.

---

*Physicians are accustomed to giving patients precise amounts of medicine, so recommendations that do not specify an amount of medicine based on age or weight seem unusual. According to homeopathic theory, however, the action of a homeopathic medicine is based on the "energetic" qualities of the medicine and is not dependent on a dose of medicine delivering a precise quantity of medicinal substance. The correct choice of medicine, not the amount given, is the most important determinant of the outcome of treatment. For this reason, the precise physical quantity of homeopathic medicine given is not critical.

Treating Patients Who Are Using Other Therapies

Homeopathic medicines can be given in the same time frame as herbs or conventional medicines, although the actual administration of the different medicines should be separated by at least 10 minutes (see later discussion). Homeopathic medicine can also be used in combination with manipulative and body-based methods. No deleterious interactions exist between homeopathic medicine and other modalities. For patients with chronic conditions who are beginning homeopathic treatment, initially it is best for them to continue taking any current conventional medicines. If more than one change is made at a time (starting a homeopathic medicine and withdrawing a conventional medicine), it may be difficult to interpret the patient's response to the homeopathic medicine. Additionally, the patient may experience an unnecessary increase in symptoms if a conventional medicine is withdrawn before the homeopathic medicine has begun to work.

Proper Handling of Homeopathic Medicines

Because homeopathic medicines contain dynamic energy, they can be inactivated or "antidoted" by various influences; therefore patients should be given the following guidelines for the correct use of the medicines:

- Patients should have nothing by mouth for at least 10 minutes before and after administration of a homeopathic medicine (water for a child or breastmilk for an infant may be given if the child or infant cannot wait).
- The medicines should not be exposed to bright sunlight, temperatures in excess of 120° F (49° C), excessive humidity, and strong odors such as camphor.
- Some patients taking homeopathic medicines may experience "antidoting" of their medicine by strong-tasting or strongly scented products such as coffee (including decaffeinated coffee), camphor-containing products, or strong mint. If a patient finds that a well-chosen homeopathic medicine is not helping his or her condition, he or she may need to refrain from these substances while undergoing homeopathic treatment.

Using Section II (Conditions) of This Book

The sections on homeopathic treatment of individual medical conditions contain short synopses of materia medica for some of the medicines commonly used to treat the conditions. The materia medica for a homeopathic medicine consists of a description of the symptoms and characteristics specific to the medicine that provide indications for prescribing the medicine. The goal in treating a patient homeopathically is to determine the single homeopathic medicine whose description in the materia medica most closely matches the symptom picture (physical, mental, and emotional) of the patient.

It may be necessary to refer to more than one condition section if the patient has a variety of symptoms. For example, if a child has otitis media and is also vomiting, the correct homeopathic medicine might be found in either the chapter on otitis media or the chapter on vomiting or may be represented in both sections. For a patient with a viral illness, one might consult the chapters on cough, fever, upper respiratory tract infection, vomiting, diarrhea, and/or others to find the simillimum.

It must be emphasized that the list of homeopathic medicines for each condition is partial and represents only some of the probable choices from the homeopathic materia medica. If the symptoms of a given patient are not represented in the relevant section(s), a search of the homeopathic literature would be needed to find the simillimum or another form of treatment would need to be rendered as needed.

In this book the summaries of materia medica in the chapters on individual conditions were adapted in part from Morrison's *Desktop Companion to Physical Pathology*,[3] Morrison's *Desktop Guide to Keynotes and Confirmatory Symptoms*,[4] Jonas and Jacobs' *Healing with Homeopathy*,[5] and other sources found in *ReferenceWorks*.[1]

Selected Homeopathic Resources

Sources of Homeopathic Medicines

Hahnemann Laboratories, Inc.
1940 Fourth Street, San Rafael, CA 94901

Helios Homeopathic Pharmacy
97 Camden Road, Tunbridge Wells, Kent TN1 2QR, United Kingdom

Ainsworths Pharmacy
36 New Cavendish Street, London W1G 8UF, United Kingdom

Homeopathy Overnight
929 Shelburne Avenue, Absecon NJ 08201

Homeopathic Books

Homeopathic Educational Services
2124B Kittredge Street, Berkeley, CA 94704

Minimum Price Books
PO Box 2187, Blaine, WA 98231

Whole Health Now
19552 Lemarsh Street, Northridge, CA 91324

Homeopathic Software

Kent Homeopathic Associates, Inc.
710 Mission Avenue, San Rafael, CA 94901

Homeopathic Organizations

American Institute of Homeopathy (AIH)
801 N. Fairfax Street, Suite 306, Alexandria, VA 22314

The AIH is a nonprofit trade association for medical and osteopathic physicians, dentists, advanced practice nurses, and physician assistants who practice homeopathy. The AIH works for its members to provide educational programs, promote legislative initiatives, and educate the public about homeopathy. Some AIH members teach courses for professionals.

National Center for Homeopathy (NCH)
801 North Fairfax Street, Suite 306, Alexandria, VA 22314

The mission of the NCH is to promote health through homeopathy. The NCH provides general education to the public through annual conferences and monthly newsletters. It also provides educational programs for professional homeopaths.

Selected Homeopathic Educational Opportunities

Luminos Homeopathic Courses, Ltd.
F-31, Bowen Island, BC V0N 1G0, Canada

Luminos Homeopathic Courses, Ltd., offers a distance learning course that provides a comprehensive introduction to homeopathy for beginners and less experienced practitioners. Live courses are for more experienced practitioners and are presented in a variety of locations.

Center for Education and Development of Clinical Homeopathy
P.O. Box 3, Edgemont, PA 19028

CEDH provides practical, clinical training in homeopathy to physicians in more than 20 countries and many U. S. cities. 136 hours of instruction are provided in a series of weekend seminars.

American Medical College of Homeopathy
2001 W. Camelback, Suite 150, Phoenix, AZ 85015

The American Medical College of Homeopathy offers a variety of onsite and distance learning programs. Beginning in 2001 they will offer a four-year, full-time program in classical homeopathy that will lead to a Doctor of Classical Homeopathy (DCH) degree.

References

1. *ReferenceWorks Pro 4.2,* San Rafael, Calif, 2008, Kent Homeopathic Associates.
2. *MacRepertory Pro 7.5,* San Rafael, Calif, 2008, Kent Homeopathic Associates.
3. Morrison R: *Desktop companion to physical pathology,* Nevada City, Calif, 1998, Hahnemann Clinic Publishing.
4. Morrison R: *Desktop guide to keynotes and confirmatory symptoms,* Albany, Calif, 1993, Hahnemann Clinic Publishing.
5. Jonas WB, Jacobs J: *Healing with homeopathy: the doctors' guide,* New York, 1996, Warner Books.

Acupuncture Meridians

✳ TABLE B-1

Standard International Nomenclature for the 14 Meridians

NAME OR MERIDIAN	ALPHABETIC CODE	
	AGREED	FORMER
Lung	LU	Lu, P
Large Intestine	LI	Co, Co, IC
Stomach	ST	S, St, E, M
Spleen	SP	Sp, LP
Heart	HT	H, C, Ht, He
Small Intestine	SI	Si, IT
Bladder	BL	B, Bi, UB
Kidney	KI	Ki, R, Rn
Pericardium	PC	P, Pe, HC
Triple Energizer	TE	T, TW, SJ, 3H, TB
Gallbladder	GB	G, VB, VF
Liver	LR	Liv, LV, H
Governor Vessel	GV	Du, Du Go, Gv, TM
Conception Vessel	CV	Co, Cv, J, REN, Ren

✳ TABLE B-2

Simple Tonification of Yin or Yang of an Organ/Meridian

ORGAN	YIN	YANG
Lung	LU-9—tonifies LU Yin	LU-9—tonifies LU QI LU-7 stimulates descent and dispersion of LU QI Circulates Wei Qi, releases exteriorly
Spleen	SP-6—tonifies Blood and Yin	SP-3—tonifies Spleen
Stomach	CV-12, SP-6—tonifies ST Yin	St=36—tonifies both St Qi and ST Yin
Heart	HT-7—tonifies Heart Blood	HT-5—tonifies Heart Qi
Kidney	KI-3—tonifies KI Yin, Essence KI-6 nourishes KI Yin	KI-3—tonifies KI Yang KI-7—tonifies KI Yang
Liver	LR-3—nourishes LR Blood and Yin	LR-3, LR 13 moves LR Qi

From Loo M: *Pediatric Acupuncture*, Edinburgh, 2002, Churchill Livingstone.

✳ TABLE B-3

Five-Element Points on All Meridians

MERIDIANS	WOOD	FIRE	EARTH	METAL	WATER
Yin Meridians					
LU	11	10	9	8	5
SP	1	2	3	5	9
HT	9	8	7	4	3
KI	1	2	3	7	10
PC	9	8	7	5	3
LR	1	2	3	4	8
Yang Meridians					
LI	3	5	11	1	2
ST	43	41	36	45	44
SI	3	5	8	1	2
BL	65	60	40	67	66
TE	3	6	10	1	2
GB	41	38	34	44	43

From Loo M: *Pediatric Acupuncture*, Edinburgh, 2002, Churchill Livingstone.

✳ TABLE B-4

Five-Element Horary Points

MERIDIANS	WOOD	FIRE	EARTH	METAL	WATER
LU				8	
SP			3		
HT		8			
KI					10
PC		8			
LR	1				
LI				1	
ST			36		
SI		5			
BL					66
TE		6			
GB	41				

From Loo M: *Pediatric Acupuncture*, Edinburgh, 2002, Churchill Livingstone.

TABLE B-5

Four-Point Tonification Protocol

Yin Organs

MERIDIANS	WOOD	FIRE	EARTH	METAL	WATER	LU	SP	HT	KI	PC	LR
LU*		−LU-10	**LU-9**				SP-3	HT-8			
SP	−SP-1	**SP-2**						**HT-8**			−LR-1
HT	**HT-9**				−HT-3				−KI-10		**LR-1**
KI			−KI-3	**KI-7**		LU-8	−SP-3				
PC	**PC-9**				PC-3				−KI-10		LR-1
LR			−LR-4		**LR-8**	−LU-8			**KI-10**		

Yang Organs

MERIDIANS	METAL	WATER	WOOD	FIRE	EARTH	LI	ST	SI	BL	TE	GB
LI				−LI-5	**LI-11**		ST-36	−SI-5			
ST			−ST-43	**ST-41**				SI-5			−GB-41
SI		−SI-2	**SI-3**						−BL-66		GB-41
BL	**BL-67**				−BL-40	**LI-1**	−ST-36				
TE		−TE-2	**TE-3**						−BL-66		GB-41
GB	−GB-44	**GB-43**				−LI-1			**BL-66**		

From Loo M: *Pediatric Acupuncture*, Edinburgh, 2002, Churchill Livingstone.

−, Sedation.

***Boldface** indicates tonification.

TABLE B-6

Four-Point Sedation Protocol

Yin Organs

MERIDIANS	WOOD	FIRE	EARTH	METAL	WATER	LU	SP	HT	KI	PC	LR
LU*		**LU-10**			−LU-5			**HT-8**	−KI-10		
SP		**SP-1**		−SP-5		−LU-8					**LR-1**
HT			−HT-7		**HT-3**		−SP-3		**KI-10**		
KI	−KI-1		**KI-3**				**SP-3**				−LR-1
PC			−PC-7		**PC-3**		−SP-3		**KI-10**		
LR		−LR-2	**LR-4**			**LU-8**		−HT-8			

Yang Organs

MERIDIANS	METAL	WATER	WOOD	FIRE	EARTH	LI	ST	SI	BL	TE	GB
LI		−LI-2		**LI-5**				SI-5	−BL-66		
ST		−ST-45	**ST-43**			−LI-1					GB-41
SI		**SI-2**			−SI-8		−ST-36		**BL-66**		
BL			−BL-65		**BL-40**		**ST-36**				−GB-41
TE		**TE-2**			−TE-10		−ST-36		**BL-66**		
GB	**GB-44**			−GB-38		**LI-1**		−SI-5			

From Loo M: *Pediatric Acupuncture*, Edinburgh, 2002, Churchill Livingstone.

−, Sedation.

***Boldface** indicates tonification.

TABLE **B-7**

Summary of Tonification Protocol

MERIDIANS	TONIFY		SEDATE	
LU	LU-9	SP3	LU-10	HT-8
SP	SP-2	HT-8	SP-1	LR-1
HT	HT-9	LR-1	HT-3	KI-10
KI	KI-7	LU-8	KI-3	SP-3
PC	PC-9	LR-1	PC-3	KI-10
LR	LR-8	KI-10	LR-4	LU-8
LI	LI-11	ST-36	LI-5	SI-5
ST	ST-41	SI-5	ST-43	GB-41
SI	SI-3	GB-41	SI-2	BL-66
BL	BL-67	LI-1	BL-40	ST-36
TE	TE-3	GB-41	TE-2	BL-66
GB	GB-43	BL-66	GB-44	LI-1

From Loo M: *Pediatric Acupuncture*, Edinburgh, 2002, Churchill Livingstone.

 TABLE **B-8**

Summary of Sedation Protocol

MERIDIANS	TONIFY		SEDATE	
LU	LU-10	HT-8	LU-5	KI-10
SP	SP-1	LR-1	SP-5	LU-8
HT	HT-3	KI-10	HT-7	SP-3
KI	KI-3	SP-3	KI-1	LR-1
PC	PC-3	KI-10	PC-7	SP-3
LR	LR-4	LU-8	LR-2	HT-8
LI	LI-5	SI-5	LI-2	BL-66
ST	ST-43	GB-41	ST-45	LI-1
SI	SI-2	BL-66	SI-8	ST-36
BL	BL-40	ST-36	BL-65	GB-41
TE	TE-2	BL-66	TE-10	ST-36
GB	GB-44	LI-1	GB-38	SI-5

From Loo M: *Pediatric Acupuncture*, Edinburgh, 2002, Churchill Livingstone.

 TABLE **B-9**

Summary of Dispersing Heat and Cold

ORGAN	TONIFY WATER POINT	SEDATE FIRE POINT	TONIFY HORARY WATER	SEDATE HORARY FIRE
Dispersing Heat				
Yin Organs				
LU*	**LU-5**	LU-10	**KI-10**	HT-8
SP	**SP-9**	SP-2	**KI-10**	HT-8
HT	**HT-3**	HT-8	**KI-10**	PC-8
KI	**KI-10**	KI-2	**KI-10**	HT-8
PC	**PC-3**	PC-8	**KI-10**	HT-8
LR	**LR-8**	LR-2	**KI-10**	HT-8
Yang Organs				
LI	**LI-2**	LI-5	**BL-66**	SI-5
ST	**ST-44**	ST-41	**BL-66**	SI-5
SI	**SI-2**	SI-5	**BL-66**	TE-6
BL	**BL-66**	BL-60	**BL-66**	SI-5
TE	**TE-2**	TE-6	**BL-66**	SI-5
GB	**GB-4E**	GB-38	**BL-66**	SI-5

ORGAN	SEDATE WATER POINT	TONIFY FIRE POINT	SEDATE HORARY WATER	TONIFY HORARY FIRE
Dispersing Cold				
Yin Organs				
LU	LU-5	**LU-10**	KI-10	**HT-8**
SP	SP-9	**SP-2**	KI-10	**HT-8**
HT	HT-3	**HT-8**	KI-10	**PC-8**
KI	KI-10	**KI-2**	KI-10	**HT-8**
PC	PC-3	**PC-8**	KI-10	**HT-8**
LR	LR-2	**LR-8**	KI-10	**HT-8**
Yang Organs				
LI	LI-2	**LI-5**	BL-66	**SI-5**
ST	ST-44	**ST-41**	LB-66	**SI-5**
SI	SI-2	**SI-5**	BL-66	**TE-6**
BL	BL-66	**BL-60**	BL-66	**SI-5**
TE	TE-2	**TE-6**	BL-66	**SI-5**
GB	GB-4E	**GB-38**	BL-66	**SI-5**

From Loo M: *Pediatric Acupuncture*, Edinburgh, 2002, Churchill Livingstone.

*Boldface indicates tonification.

✳ TABLE B-10

Five-Element Heat/Fire and Cold/Water Points

MERIDIANS	WOOD	FIRE	EARTH	METAL	WATER
LU	11	**10**	9	8	**5**
SP	1	**2**	3	5	**9**
HT	9	**8**	7	4	**3**
KI	1	**2**	3	7	**10**
PC	9	**8**	7	5	**3**
LR	1	**2**	3	4	**8**
LI	3	**5**	11	1	**2**
ST	43	**41**	36	45	**44**
SI	3	**5**	8	1	**2**
BL	65	**60**	40	67	**66**
TE	3	**6**	10	1	**2**
GB	41	**38**	34	44	**43**

From Loo M: *Pediatric Acupuncture,* Edinburgh, 2002, Churchill Livingstone.

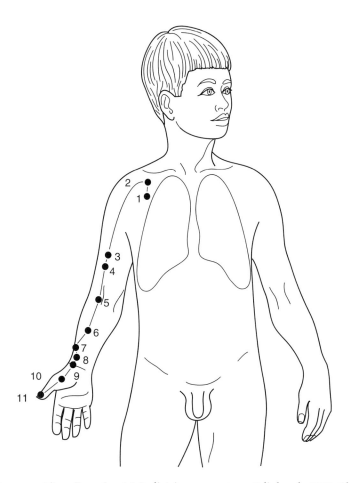

FIGURE B-1 The Lung meridian. *From Loo M:* Pediatric acupuncture, *Edinburgh, 2002, Churchill Livingstone.*

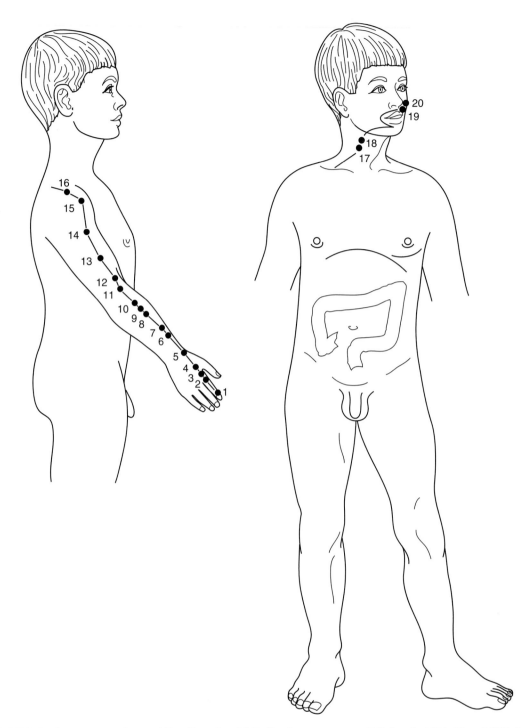

FIGURE B-2 The Large Intestine meridian. *From Loo M:* Pediatric acupuncture, *Edinburgh, 2002, Churchill Livingstone.*

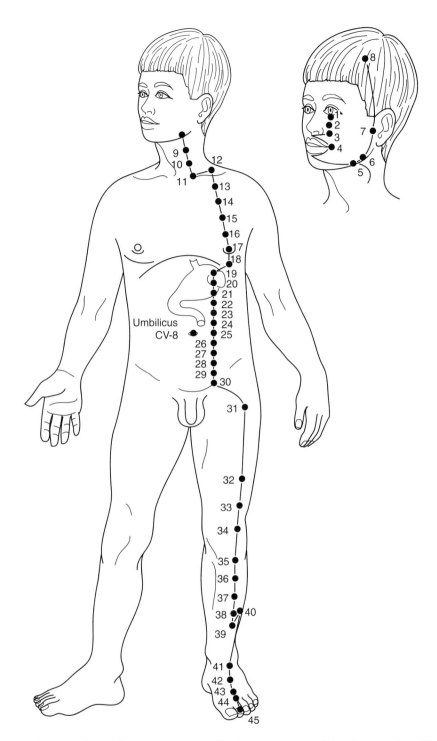

FIGURE B-3 The Stomach meridian. *From Loo M:* Pediatric acupuncture, *Edinburgh, 2002, Churchill Livingstone.*

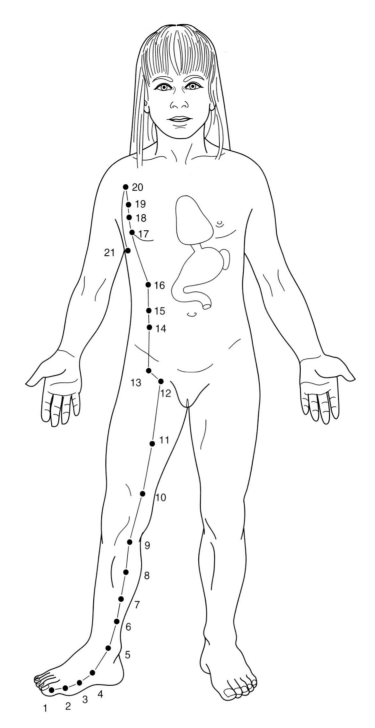

FIGURE B-4 The Spleen meridian. *From Loo M:* Pediatric acupuncture, *Edinburgh, 2002, Churchill Livingstone.*

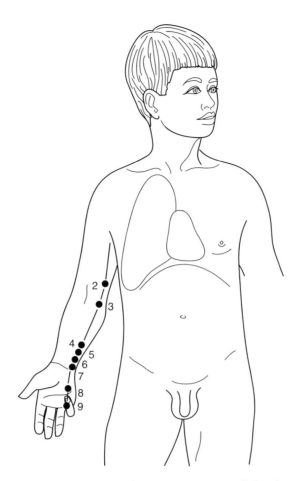

FIGURE B-5 The Heart meridian. *From Loo M:* Pediatric acupuncture, *Edinburgh, 2002, Churchill Livingstone.*

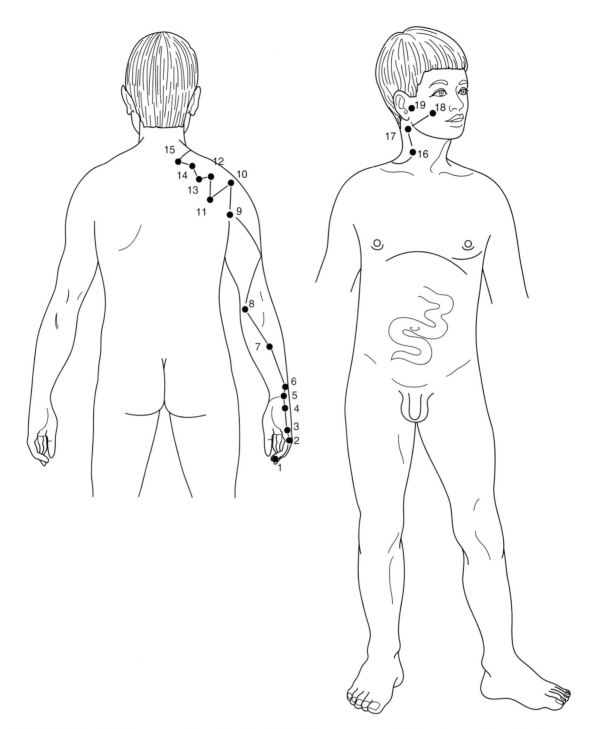

FIGURE B-6 The Small Intestine meridian. *From Loo M:* Pediatric acupuncture, *Edinburgh, 2002, Churchill Livingstone.*

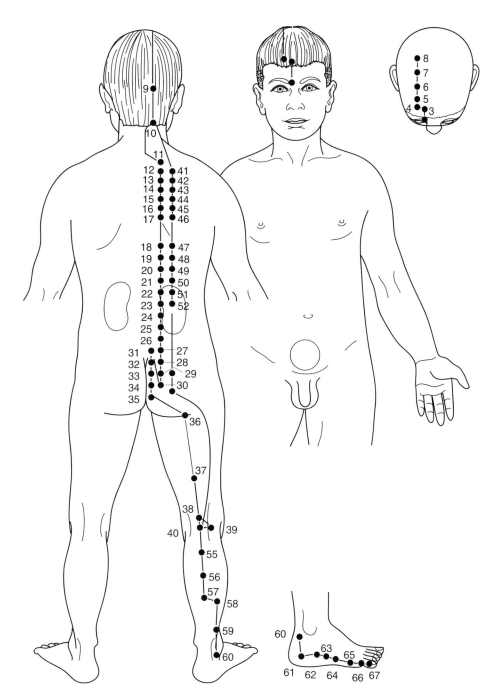

FIGURE B-7 The Bladder meridian. *From Loo M:* Pediatric acupuncture, *Edinburgh, 2002, Churchill Livingstone.*

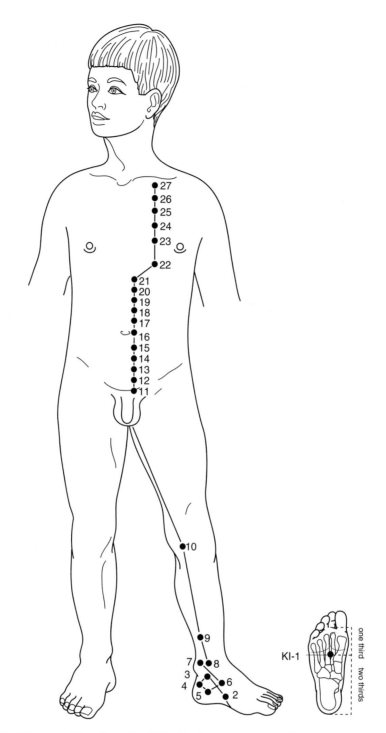

FIGURE B-8 The Kidney meridian. *From Loo M: Pediatric acupuncture, Edinburgh, 2002, Churchill Livingstone.*

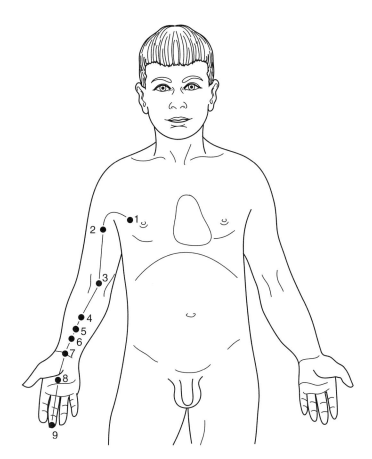

FIGURE B-9 The Pericardium meridian. *From Loo M:* Pediatric acupuncture, *Edinburgh, 2002, Churchill Livingstone.*

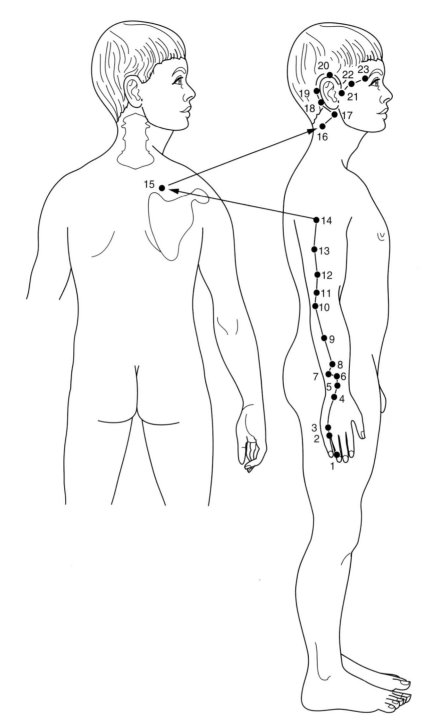

FIGURE B-10 The Triple Energizer meridian. *From Loo M:* Pediatric acupuncture, *Edinburgh, 2002, Churchill Livingstone.*

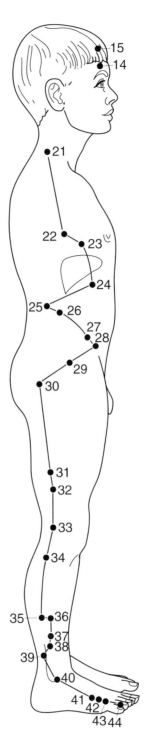

FIGURE B-11 The Gallbladder meridian. *From Loo M:* Pediatric acupuncture, *Edinburgh, 2002, Churchill Livingstone.*

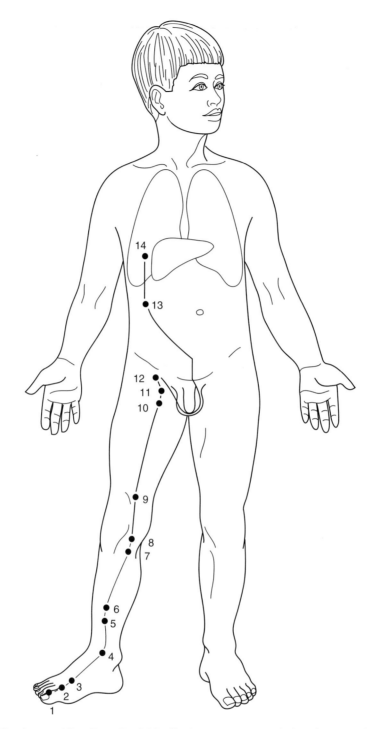

FIGURE B-12 The Liver meridian. *From Loo M:* Pediatric acupuncture, *Edinburgh, 2002, Churchill Livingstone.*

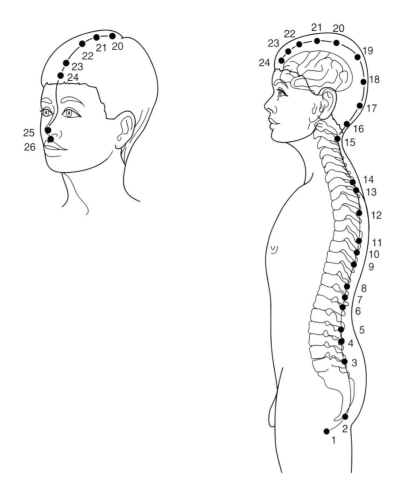

FIGURE B-13 The Governor Vessel meridian. *From Loo M:* Pediatric acupuncture, *Edinburgh, 2002, Churchill Livingstone.*

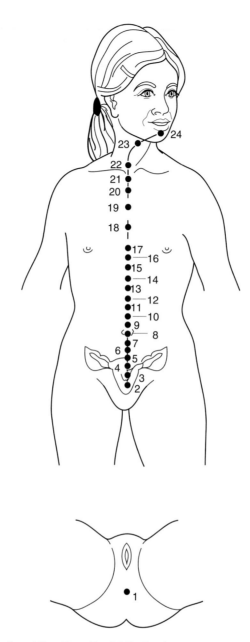

FIGURE B-14 The Conception Vessel meridian. *From Loo M:* Pediatric acupuncture, *Edinburgh, 2002, Churchill Livingstone.*

The major acupuncture points are shown in Figures B-15 to B-31.

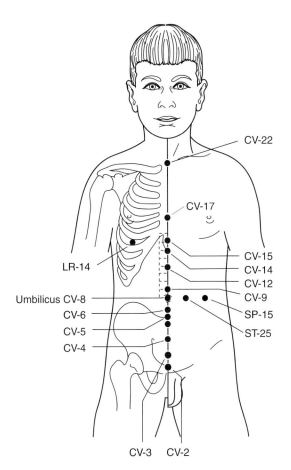

FIGURE B-15 Major points of the upper abdomen. *From Loo M:* Pediatric acupuncture, *Edinburgh, 2002, Churchill Livingstone.*

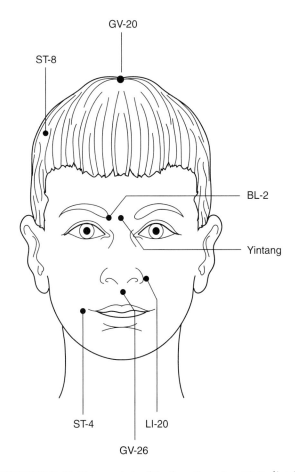

FIGURE B-16 Major points of the face. *From Loo M:* Pediatric acupuncture, *Edinburgh, 2002, Churchill Livingstone.*

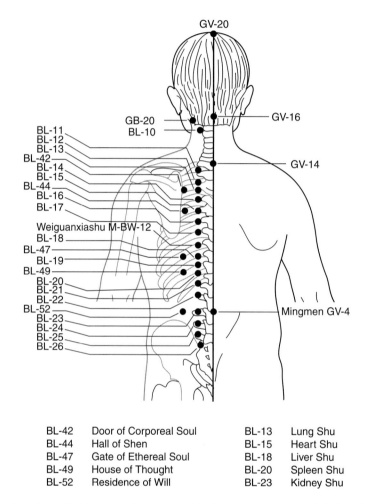

BL-42	Door of Corporeal Soul	BL-13	Lung Shu
BL-44	Hall of Shen	BL-15	Heart Shu
BL-47	Gate of Ethereal Soul	BL-18	Liver Shu
BL-49	House of Thought	BL-20	Spleen Shu
BL-52	Residence of Will	BL-23	Kidney Shu

FIGURE B-17 Major Governor Vessel and Bladder points. *From Loo M:* Pediatric acupuncture, *Edinburgh, 2002, Churchill Livingstone.*

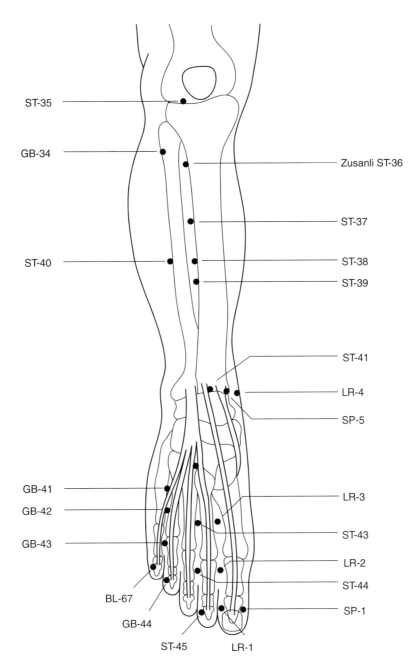

FIGURE B-18 Major points of the anterior lower leg. *From Loo M:* Pediatric acupuncture, *Edinburgh, 2002, Churchill Livingstone.*

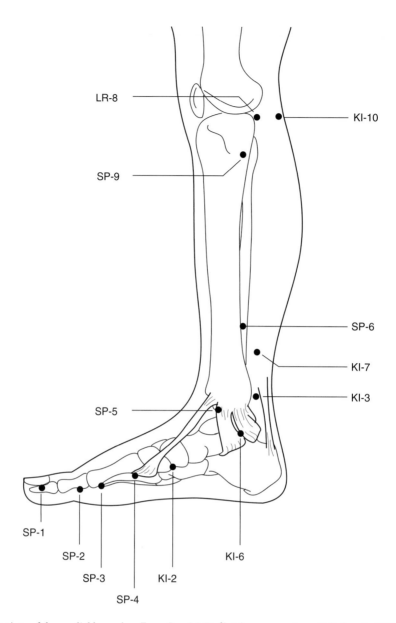

FIGURE B-19 Major points of the medial lower leg. *From Loo M:* Pediatric acupuncture, *Edinburgh, 2002, Churchill Livingstone.*

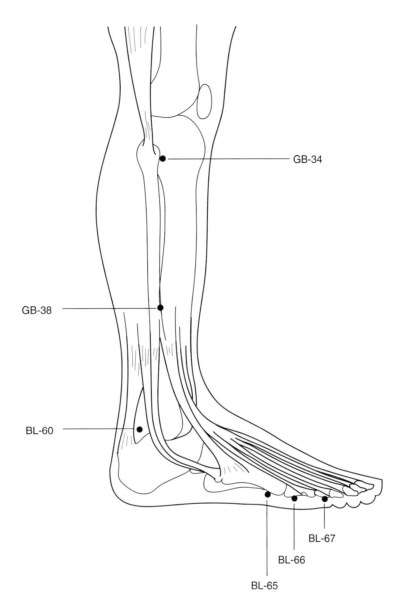

FIGURE B-20 Major points of the lateral lower leg. *From Loo M:* Pediatric acupuncture, *Edinburgh, 2002, Churchill Livingstone.*

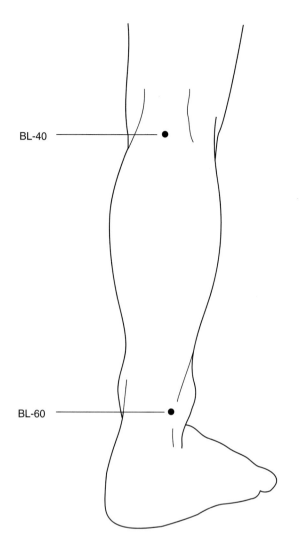

FIGURE B-21 Weizhong point BL40 on the leg. *From Loo M: Pediatric acupuncture, Edinburgh, 2002, Churchill Livingstone.*

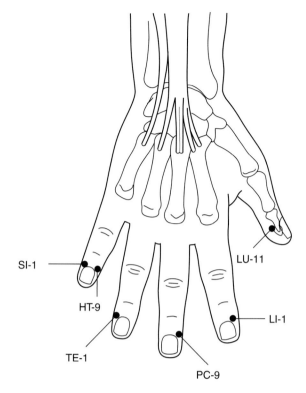

FIGURE B-22 Shaochong points on the hand for HT9. *From Loo M: Pediatric acupuncture, Edinburgh, 2002, Churchill Livingstone.*

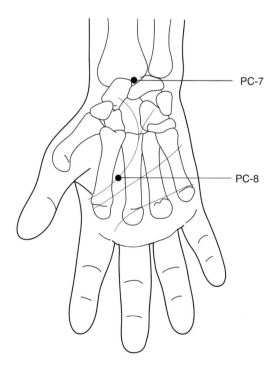

FIGURE B-23 Zhongchong points on the hand for the Pericardium channel. *From Loo M: Pediatric acupuncture, Edinburgh, 2002, Churchill Livingstone.*

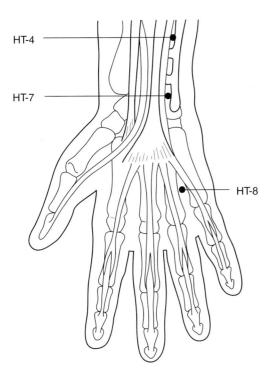

FIGURE B-24 Lingdao HT4 points on the hand. *From Loo M: Pediatric acupuncture, Edinburgh, 2002, Churchill Livingstone.*

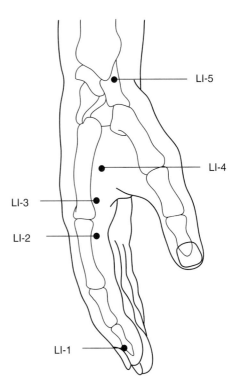

FIGURE B-25 Yangxi LI5 points on the hand. *From Loo M: Pediatric acupuncture, Edinburgh, 2002, Churchill Livingstone.*

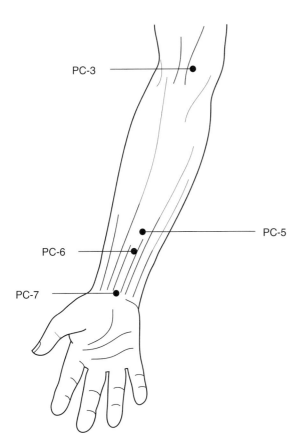

FIGURE B-26 Ximen PC4 points on the arm and hand. *From Loo M: Pediatric acupuncture, Edinburgh, 2002, Churchill Livingstone.*

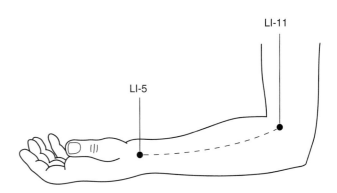

FIGURE B-27 Pianli LI6 points on the arm. *From Loo M: Pediatric acupuncture, Edinburgh, 2002, Churchill Livingstone.*

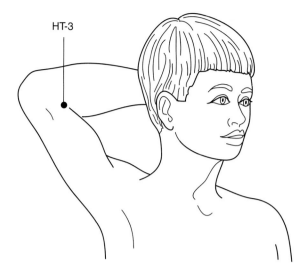

FIGURE B-28 Shaohai HT3 point. *From Loo M:* Pediatric acupuncture, *Edinburgh, 2002, Churchill Livingstone.*

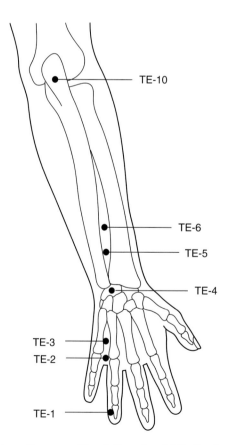

FIGURE B-29 Waiguan Triple Energizer points on the arm and hand. *From Loo M:* Pediatric acupuncture, *Edinburgh, 2002, Churchill Livingstone.*

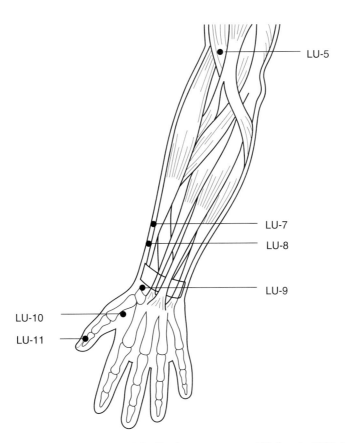

FIGURE B-30 Kongzui Lung points on the arm. *From Loo M:* Pediatric acupuncture, *Edinburgh, 2002, Churchill Livingstone.*

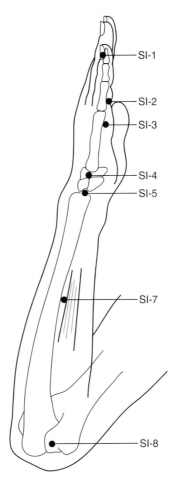

FIGURE B-31 Zhizheng Small Intestine points on the arm and hand. *From Loo M:* Pediatric acupuncture, *Edinburgh, 2002, Churchill Livingstone.*

Chinese Herbs

Randall Neustaedter, Jake Paul Fratkin

Dosage of Chinese Herbs for Children

Chinese herbal products can be valuable in the clinical practice for both acute and chronic pediatric disorders. They can be given to newborns and through all age groups.

Herbal products come available in a variety of forms, including pills, tablets, powder, liquids, and syrups. Pills are the most common form. For children who can swallow pills, those who are 7 to 10 years old should receive half the adult dosage; those older than 11 years should receive the full adult dosage. Children who cannot swallow pills can be given liquid or elixir according to the dosage prescribed by each commercial preparation.

Home Preparation

Pediatric elixir can also be prepared at home with any herbal tablets, powder, or granular extracts. The tablets can be ground into powder in a small household coffee grinder, and the powder is poured back into the original bottle, which should be clearly labeled. The powder form can be made into elixir and given as follows:

- Add a small amount of boiling water to ½ to 1 teaspoon of powder to form a gravy.
- Strain the liquid through a metal mesh strainer. This should make about 3 teaspoons of final liquid.
- Give the elixir in the following dosage with a pediatric syringe every 3 hours until symptoms are relieved:

  Infants younger 1 year: 2 mL

  1 to 4 years: increase by 1 mL for every year of life over age 1 (e.g., for age 1, give 2 mL; for age 3 years, give 4 mL, for age 1; up to a total of 4 mL)

  Age 5 and older: 6 mL, or 1 teaspoon

There have been concerns about heavy metals or pharmaceuticals in Chinese herbal medicines. Most of these reports are false, but it is always recommended that practitioners and patients use herbal products that are made using Good Manufacturing Practice (GMP) standards. These standards follow Australian standards for Chinese herbal products and are the most stringent in the world. They guarantee no heavy metals, pesticides, or prescription drugs. Most products imported into the United States are made in GMP factories.

Magnets

Agatha P. Colbert, Deborah Risotti

Caution: Do not allow children to play with magnets.

Application of Magnets to Acupuncture Points

Magnets are frequently applied to acupuncture points either as an alternative to needling or after the needles have been removed in order to prolong the effects of the acupuncture needling session. For children aged 1 to 5 years, 800-Gauss (G) ferrite magnets placed on acupuncture points are adequate as a 15-minute treatment. Many older children can be treated in the office setting with 6000-G or 9000-G area earth magnets for as long as to 15 to 20 minutes. These older children may be sent home with 800-G magnets taped to the same acupuncture points treated with the stronger magnets at the acupuncturist's office. The 800-G magnets with adhesives should remain in place no longer than 48 hours.

Application of Magnets to Larger Anatomical Areas

Magnetic devices that deliver static magnetic fields come in many sizes, shapes, and weights. Some are made of flexible materials that contour more readily to the body part, and some are ceramic blocks or discs. The surface field strength of each magnet and its depth of penetration vary according to its size, shape, polarity, and weight.

Types of Magnets Suggested for Treatments

800-G ferrite magnets (0.09 × 0.20 inch) have a tiny protrusion on the side of magnet that is designated as bionorth (−). These magnets may be obtained from OMS.

On 9000-G rare earth magnets (0.06 × 0.16 inch), the designated bionorth (−) side is marked with a small indentation. These magnets may be obtained from OMS.

3950-G ceramic block or disc magnets have a labeled bionorth side. These magnets may be obtained from Painfree Lifestyles or AHSM.

2450-Gauss Plastiform flexible magnets are ⅛-inch thick and available in 10 sizes. These magnets may be obtained from MagneCare or AHSM.

Neodymium nylon-coated Spot magnets of different Gauss strengths are available in thicknesses of 1 inch, ¾ inch, and ½ inch. These magnets may be obtained from Painfree Lifestyles.

Magnassager magnets are for use in massaging spastic muscles of children with cerebral palsy. These magnets may be obtained from Painfree Lifestyles.

Contact Information for Suppliers

Painfree Lifestyles: telephone, 800-480-8601
American Health Service Magnetics (AHMS): telephone, 800-635-7070
OMS Medical Supplies: telephone, 800-323-1839

✳ Index

Note: Page numbers followed by f indicate illustrations; t, tables; and b, boxed material.